Stroke
A practical guide to management

We can but apologise to our partners and children who we hope to see more of in the future. Unfortunately, there is never enough time for medical books to be written in the office, they are a family effort.

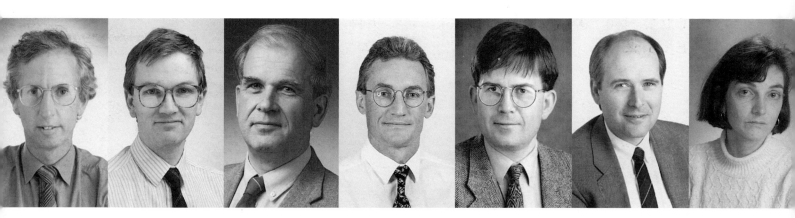

From left to right: C.P. Warlow   M.S. Dennis   J. van Gijn   G.J. Hankey   P.A.G. Sandercock   J.M. Bamford   J. Wardlaw

Stroke
A practical guide to management

C.P. Warlow   M.S. Dennis   J. van Gijn   G.J. Hankey
P.A.G. Sandercock   J.M. Bamford   J. Wardlaw

Foreword by H.J.M. Barnett

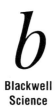

**Blackwell
Science**

© 1996 by
Blackwell Science Ltd
Editorial Offices:
Osney Mead, Oxford OX2 0EL
25 John Street, London WC1N 2BL
23 Ainslie Place, Edinburgh EH3 6AJ
350 Main Street, Malden
  MA 02148 5018, USA
54 University Street, Carlton
  Victoria 3053, Australia

Other Editorial Offices:
Blackwell Wissenschafts-Verlag GmbH
  Kurfürstendamm 57
  10707 Berlin, Germany

Blackwell Science KK
MG Kodenmacho Building
7-10 Kodenmacho Nihombashi
Chuo-ku, Tokyo 104, Japan

First published 1996
Reprinted 1997
Re-issued in paperback 1998

Set by Excel Typesetters Co., Hong Kong
Printed and bound in Great Britain
at the Bath Press, Bath

The Blackwell Science logo is a
trade mark of Blackwell Science Ltd,
registered at the United Kingdom
Trade Marks Registry

DISTRIBUTORS

Marston Book Services Ltd
PO Box 269
Abingdon Oxon OX14 4YN
(*Orders*: Tel: 01235 465500
          Fax: 01235 465555)

USA
Blackwell Science, Inc.
Commerce Place
350 Main Street
Malden, MA 02148 5018
(*Orders:* Tel: 800 759 6102
          617 388 8250
          Fax: 617 388 8255)

Canada
Copp Clark Professional
200 Adelaide St West, 3rd Floor
Toronto, Ontario M5H 1W7
(*Orders:* Tel: 416 597-1616
          800 815-9417
          Fax: 416 597-1617)

Australia
Blackwell Science Pty Ltd
54 University Street
Carlton, Victoria 3053
(*Orders:* Tel: 3 9347 0300
          Fax: 3 9347 5001)

A catalogue record for this title
is available from the British Library

ISBN 0-86542-874-3 (hbk)
ISBN 0-632-05005-5 (pbk)

Library of Congress Cataloging-in-Publication Data
Stroke: a practical guide to management/
  by Charles Warlow,
  with Martin Dennis . . . [*et al.*];
  foreword by Henry Barnett.
      p.   cm.
  Includes bibliographical references
  and index.
  ISBN 0-632-05005-5
    1. Cerebrovascular disease.
    I. Warlow, Charles, 1934–
    II. Dennis, Martin.
    [DNLM: 1. Cerebrovascular Disorders—therapy.
    WL 355 S9208   1996]
  RC 388.5.S847   1996
  616.8′1—dc20
  DNLM/DLC
  for Library of Congress   96-5661
                                               CIP

Contents

List of contributors

J.M. BAMFORD MD FRCP
Consultant Neurologist
St James' University Hospital
Beckett Street
Leeds, UK

M.S. DENNIS MD FRCP
Senior Lecturer in Stroke Medicine
Department of Clinical Neurosciences
Western General Hospital
Crewe Road
Edinburgh, UK

G.J. HANKEY MD MRCP FRACP
Consultant Neurologist
Department of Neurology
Royal Perth Hospital
Wellington Street
Perth
Western Australia
Australia

P.A.G. SANDERCOCK DM FRCP
Reader in Medical Neurology
Department of Clinical Neurosciences
University of Edinburgh
Western General Hospital
Crewe Road
Edinburgh, UK

J. VAN GIJN MD FRCPE
Professor and Chairman
University Department of Neurology
University Hospital of Utrecht
Utrecht
The Netherlands

J. WARDLAW MD MRCP FRCR
Senior Lecturer in Neuroradiology
Department of Clinical Neurosciences
University of Edinburgh
Western General Hospital
Crewe Road
Edinburgh, UK

C.P. WARLOW MD FRCP
Professor of Medical Neurology
Department of Clinical Neurosciences
University of Edinburgh
Western General Hospital
Crewe Road
Edinburgh, UK

Foreword

This book was enjoyable for its authors to create and promises to bring pleasure, interest and important guidance for all practitioners involved in the prevention and treatment of stroke.

Books about stroke are a new phenomenon. For decades, indeed for centuries, the occurrence of an insult to the brain from ischaemia or from haemorrhage was used to localise brain function or to describe syndromes. It was an academic pursuit and of little immediate value for the patients. Prevention and therapy remained elusive. Fortunately, revolutionary changes followed upon several sequential and contemporaneous developments: imaging of the blood vessels, the brain and the heart; explosive new knowledge about thrombosis and strategies to modify it; surgical techniques to remove the lesions of arterial degenerations and faults; and the maturation of the science of epidemiology, methodology and biostatistics which lead us on a path towards the practice of evidence-based medicine.

Stroke prevention can be realised effectively by attacking manageable and clearly identified risk factors, by altering thrombosis and by appropriately utilising surgical measures. Without question, these strategies will be refined further in the years ahead. Important new knowledge is appearing several times a year. This information is changing our abilities to treat stroke once it threatens. Even before that happens it is feasible to take measures which prevent the degenerative arterial processes, particularly artherosclerosis upon which so many strokes depend. As this volume goes to the printers, an air of optimism surrounds the possibility that we shall soon be able to reduce the amount of damage to a brain which has felt the early insults of ischaemia or haemorrhage. Specialised stroke units will be shifting into high gear to cope with the exciting prospects of providing genuine help for the ischaemic brain.

The commendable aim of the authors of this book has been to assist practitioners to make practical use of this rapidly expanding body of knowledge. Their aims are well satisfied. They have written their material in such a way as to assist us, at the bedside or in the clinic, in sorting out what is truly valuable, to point out what is likely to become valuable and to caution about therapeutic strategies which remain in the realm of speculation.

The authors have taken a novel approach to the production of a multi-author book. They have eschewed the common custom of pasting together a series of chapters and sections produced by individual authorities with a variety of styles, containing a lot of tiresome overlapping. Instead, as a group of colleagues and friends, they have engaged in a collaborative endeavour which makes use of all of their knowledge and ideas in the production of each chapter. Because they are all innovative leaders in the stroke field, the end product is both authoritative and readable. Because they are collectively a critical group they engage in a considerable but welcome amount of valid scientific criticism. They express due and expected cynicism about our professional tendency to cling to traditional unproved views. With an approach which is reader-friendly and even at times chatty, they have produced a remarkable distillation of what is currently useful to know and utilise in the field of cerebral vascular disease.

It is to be hoped that the pattern which they adopted in the writing of this book will be copied repeatedly by the authors of many other future medical scientific publications. Credibility is not lost by an engaging style. Readers will be grateful for it. The readers of this landmark publication will return regularly for help as the ever-changing tide of clinical material and clinical problems sweeps up to their out-patient clinics, wards and stroke units.

H.J.M. Barnett MD

Acknowledgements

We have had invaluable help and advice from many people in the preparation of this book. So thank you all, including:

Sheila Anderson
Chanpong Tangkanakul
Judi Clarke
Carl Counsell
Paut Greebe
Diane Fraser
Hazel Fraser
Mike McDowell
George MacIntyre

Lesley Moffatt
Lindsey Reynolds
Lesley Robertson
Gabriel Rinkel
Vicki Scoltock
Mark Smith
Trish Staniforth
Michael Watt
Graeme Wilson

Also, thank you to our teachers and colleagues from whom we have learned so many worthwhile things over the years:

Henry Barnett
Iain Chalmers
Rory Collins
Hans van Crevel
Richard Doll
Stuart Douglas
Barbara Farrell
C. Miller Fisher
Chris Foote
John Fry
Mike Gent

Michael Harrison
Bryan Matthews
Richard Peto
Geoffrey Rose
David Sackett
Jim Slattery
Rien Vermeulen
Ted Stewart-Wynne
Derick Wade
Eelco Wijdicks

Introduction

1.1   Aims and scope of the book

We, the authors of this book, regard ourselves as practising—and practical—doctors who look after stroke patients in very routine day-to-day practice. The book is for people like us: neurologists, geriatricians, stroke physicians, radiologists and general internal physicians. But, it is not just for doctors. It is also for nurses, therapists, managers and anyone else who wants practical guidance about all and any of the problems to do with stroke from aetiology to organisation of services, from prevention to occupational therapy and from any facet of cure to any facet of care. In other words, it is for anyone who has to deal with stroke in clinical practice. It is not a book for armchair theoreticians, who usually have no sense of proportion as well as difficulty in seeing the wood from the trees. Or, maybe, it is particularly for them so that they can be led back into the real world.

The book takes what is known as a problem-orientated approach. The problems posed by stroke patients are discussed in the sort of order that they are likely to present themselves. Is it a stroke? What sort of stroke is it? What caused it? What can be done about it? How can the patient and carer be supported in the short and in the long term? How can any recurrence be prevented? How can stroke services be better organised? Unlike traditional textbooks, which linger on dusty shelves, there are no 'ology' chapters. Aetiology, epidemiology, pathology and the rest represent just the tools to solve the problems so they are used when they are needed, and not discussed in isolation. For example,

to prevent strokes one needs to know how frequent they are (epidemiology), what types of stroke there are (pathology), what causes them (aetiology) and what evidence there is to support therapeutic intervention (randomised controlled trials). Clinicians mostly operate on a need-to-know basis and so when a problem arises they need the information to solve it at that moment, from inside their head, from a colleague, and we hope from a book like this.

1.2   General principles

To solve a problem one obviously needs relevant information. Clinicians, and others, should not be making decisions based on whim, dogma or the last case, although most do, at least some of the time, ourselves included. It is better to search out the reliable information based on some reasonable criteria of what is meant by reliable, get it into a sensible order, review it and make a summary which can be used at the bedside. If one does not have the time to do this—and who does for every problem?—then one has to search out someone else's systematic review. Or find the answer in this book. Good clinicians have always done all this intuitively, although recently the process has been blessed with the title of 'evidence-based medicine', and now even 'evidence-based patient-focused medicine'! In this book we have used the evidence-based approach, at least where it is possible to do so. Therefore, where a systematic review of a risk factor or a treatment is available we have cited it, and not just emphasised single studies done by us or our friends and with results to suit our prejudices. But, so often there is no good evidence or even any evidence at all available, and certainly no systematic reviews. What to do then? Certainly not what most doctors are trained to do: 'Never be wrong, and if you are, never admit it!' If we do not know something, we will say so. But, like other clinicians, we may have to make decisions even when we do not know what to do, and when nobody else does either. One can not always adopt the policy of 'if you don't know what to do, don't do it'. Throughout the book we will try to indicate where there is no evidence, or feeble evidence, and describe what *we* do and will continue to do until better evidence becomes available; after all, it is these murky areas of practice which need to be flagged up as needing to be researched. Moreover, in clinical practice, all of us ask respected colleagues for advice, not because they may know something that we do not, but because we want to know what they would do in a difficult situation.

1.3 Methods

We were all taught to look at the methods section of a scientific paper before anything else. If the methods are no good, then there is no point in wasting time and reading further. In passing, we do regard it as most peculiar that some medical journals still print the methods section in smaller letters than the rest of the paper. Therefore, before anyone reads further, perhaps we should describe the methods we have adopted.

It is now impossible for any single person to write a comprehensive book about stroke which has the feel of having been written by someone with hands-on experience of the whole subject. The range of problems is far too wide. Therefore, the sort of stroke book that we as practitioners want—and we hope others do too—has to be written by a group of people. Rather than putting together a hugely multi-author book, we thought it would be better and more informative, for ourselves as well as the readers, to write a book together which would take a particular approach (evidence based, if you will) and end up with a coherent message. After all, we have all worked together over many years, our views on stroke are more convergent than divergent, and so it should not be too terribly difficult to write a book together.

Like many things in medicine, and in life, this book started over a few drinks to provide the initial momentum to get going, on the occasion of a stroke conference in Geneva in 1993. At that time, we decided that the book was to be comprehensive but not to the extent of citing every known reference, that all areas of stroke must be covered, and who was

going to start writing which section. A few months later, the first drafts were then commented on in writing and in detail by all the authors before we got back together for a general discussion, again over a few drinks, but that time at the Stockholm stroke conference in 1994. Momentum restored, we went home to improve what we had written and the second draft was all sent round to everyone for comment in an attempt to improve the clarity, remove duplication, fill in gaps and expunge as much remaining neurodogma, neurofantasy and neuroastrology as possible. Our final discussion was held at the Bordeaux stroke meeting in 1995, and the drinks that time were more in relief and celebration that the end was in sight. Home we all went to update the manuscript and to make final improvements before handing over the whole lot to the publisher in January 1996.

This process may well have taken longer than a conventional multi-author book where all the sections are written in isolation. But, it was surely more fun and hopefully the result will provide a uniform and coherent view of the subject. It is, we hope, a 'How to do it' book, or at least a 'How we do it' book.

1.4 Using the book

This is not a stroke encyclopedia. Many very much more comprehensive books and monographs are available now, or soon will be. Nor is this really a book to be read cover to cover. Rather it is a book that we would like to be used on stroke units and in clinics to help illuminate stroke management at various different stages, both at the level of the individual patient and for patients in general. So we would like it to be kept handy and referred to when a problem crops up: how should swallowing difficulties be identified and managed? should an angiogram be done? is raised plasma fibrinogen a cause of stroke? how many beds should a stroke unit have? and so on. If a question is not addressed at all, then we would like to know about it so that it can be dealt with in the next edition, if there is to be one, which will clearly depend on sales, the publisher, and enough congenial European stroke conferences to keep us going.

It should be fairly easy to find one's way around the book from the chapter headings and the contents list at the beginning of each chapter. If that fails, then the index will do instead. We have used a lot of cross-referencing to guide the reader from any starting point and so to avoid constant reference to the index.

As mentioned earlier, we have tried to be as selective as possible with the referencing. On the one hand, we want to allow readers access to the relevant literature but, on the other hand, we do not want the text to be overwhelmed by references, particularly by references to unsound work. To be selective, we have tried to cite recent evidence-based systematic reviews and classic papers describing important work. Other references can probably mostly be found by those who want to dig deeper in the reference lists of the references we have cited.

Finally, we have liberally scattered what some would call practice points and others maxims throughout the book. These we are all prepared to sign up to, at least in early 1996. Of course, as more evidence becomes available, some of these practice points will become out of date.

1.5 Why a stroke book now?

Stroke has been somewhat of a Cinderella area of medicine, at least with respect to the other two of the three most common fatal disorders in the developed world, coronary heart disease and cancer. But, times are gradually changing, particularly in the last decade when stroke has been moving up the political agenda, when research has been expanding perhaps in the slipstream of coronary heart disease research, when treatments to prevent, if not treat, stroke have become available and when the pharmaceutical industry has taken more notice. It seems that there is now so much information about stroke that many of us practitioners are beginning to be overwhelmed. Therefore, now is a good time to try to capture all this information, digest it and then write down a practical approach to stroke management based on the best available evidence and research. This is our excuse for putting together what we know and what we do not know, what we do and why we do it.

Development of knowledge concerning cerebrovascular disease

2

'Our knowledge of disorders of the cerebral circulation and its manifestations is deficient in all aspects' was the opening sentence of the chapter on cerebrovascular diseases in a popular German textbook of neurology at the beginning of this century (Oppenheim, 1913). A good 80 years later, this avowal still holds true despite the considerable advances that have been made. In fact, the main reason for Oppenheim suggesting this, the limitations of pathological anatomy, is almost equally valid today. True, our methods of observation nowadays are no longer confined to the dead, as they were then, and they have been greatly expanded, first by angiography, then by brain imaging and measurement of cerebral blood flow and metabolism, and most recently by non-invasive methods of vascular imaging such as ultrasound and magnetic resonance angiography. Yet, our observations are still mostly anatomical, and after the event. We can identify patients at high risk, but only in rare instances are we able to reconstruct the dynamics of a stroke, even less for ischaemic than haemorrhagic stroke, where brain computerised tomography (CT) or magnetic resonance imaging (MRI) in the acute phase gives an indication of where a blood vessel has ruptured (although not why exactly there, and why at that time) and shows exactly how far the extravasated blood has invaded the brain parenchyma or the subarachnoid space. With ischaemic stroke, one may find a source of embolism in the heart or a large vessel, but the embolus itself usually escapes detection except by ultra-early angiography (Fieschi *et al.*, 1989) or transcranial ultrasound techniques (Zanette *et al.*, 1995). Only too often the physician is left with a dead piece of brain, without even the faintest clue about either the malefactor or the weapon. The few instances in which an ischaemic stroke is caught red-handed are made up by fatal events, e.g. massive infarction when an embolus is mechanically dislodged from the internal carotid artery (Beal *et al.*, 1981), or by haemorrhages occurring during a scanning procedure, such as rupture of an aneurysm during angiography (Hayakawa *et al.*, 1978; Saitoh *et al.*, 1995), or haemorrhagic transformation in several areas of an infarct at the same time in a patient on anticoagulant treatment (Franke *et al.*, 1990).

So it is with modesty, rather than in triumph, that we look back on the past. In each epoch the problems of stroke have been approached by the best minds, with the best tools available. But, many ideas in the past were wrong, as presumably are many of our own ideas. Even though we are firm believers in evidence-based medicine, some of our notions may well be based on paradigms that will not survive the test of time. Our knowledge may have vastly increased in the recent past but it is still a mere island in an ocean of ignorance.

2.1   Ideas change slowly

The history of medicine is usually described by a string of dates and names, linked to the discoveries that shaped our present knowledge. The interval between such identifiable advances is measured in centuries when we describe the art of medicine at the beginning of civilisation, but in mere years where our present times are chronicled. This leads to the impression that we are witnessing a dazzling explosion of knowledge. Some qualifications of this view are needed, however. First of all, any generation of mankind often takes a myopic view of history in that the importance of recent developments is overestimated. The Swedish Academy of Sciences therefore wisely waits for years, sometimes even decades, before awarding Nobel prizes, until scientific discoveries have withstood the test of time. When exceptions were made for the prize in medicine, the early accolades were often not borne out: Wagner-Jauregg's malaria treatment of neurosyphilis (1927) is no longer regarded as a landmark, and Moniz's prize (1949) for prefrontal leucotomy seems no longer justified, but at least he also introduced contrast angiography of the brain, although this procedure may again not survive beyond the end of this century. We can only hope that the introduction of X-ray CT by Hounsfield (Nobel prize for medicine in 1979) will be judged equally momentous by future generations as by ourselves.

Another important caveat in reviewing progress in medicine is that most discoveries gain ground only slowly. Even if new insights were quickly accepted by peer scientists, which was often not the case, it could still be decades before these had trickled down to the rank and file of medical practitioners. The mention of a certain date for a discovery may create the false impression that this change in medical thinking occurred overnight, like the exchange rate of the pound sterling. In most instances, this was far from the truth. An apt example is the extremely slow rate at which the concept of lacunar infarction became accepted by the medical community, despite its profound implications in terms of pathophysiology, treatment and prognosis. The first pathological descriptions date from around 1840 (Dechambre, 1838; Durand-Fardel, 1842) but it took the clinicopathological

correlations of C.M. Fisher in the 1960s before the neurological community and its textbooks started to take any notice (Fisher, 1965, 1969; Fisher & Curry, 1965). It was not until the instantaneous clinicoanatomical correlations provided by high-resolution techniques for brain imaging in the 1980s that no practising neurologist could avoid knowing about lacunar infarcts, some 150 years after the first description! It is best to become reconciled to the idea that a slow rate of diffusion of new knowledge is unavoidable. A contemporary survey amongst primary care physicians in the US, in which they were asked about their use of recent clinical advances (such as the determination of glycosylated haemoglobin as a measure for the control of diabetes) showed that between 20 and 50% of them were not aware of these advances, or were not using them (Williamson et al., 1989). The problem is one of all times. Biumi, one of the early pathologists, lamented in 1765: 'Sed difficile est adultis novas opiniones inserere, evellere insitas' (But it is difficult in adults to insert new opinions and to remove rooted ones). How slowly new ideas were accepted and acted upon, against the background of contemporary knowledge, can often be inferred from textbooks, particularly if written by full-time clinicians rather than by research-minded neurologists. An American textbook from 1923 even cites some observations of Morgagni, dating from 1761 (Jelliffe & White, 1923)! Therefore, we shall occasionally quote old textbooks to illustrate the development of thinking about stroke.

Conversely, a new discovery or even a new fashion may be interpreted beyond its proper limits and linger on as a distorted idea for decades. Take the discovery of vitamin B_1 deficiency as the cause of a tropical polyneuropathy almost a century ago; the notion that a neurological condition, considered untreatable almost by definition, could be cured by a simple nutritional supplement made such an impact on the medical community that in many Western countries vitamin B is still widely used as a panacea for almost any neurological symptom.

So there are at least two kinds of medical history, that of the front line and that of the medical profession as a whole. The landmarks are easy to identify only with the hindsight of present knowledge; in reality, new ideas often only gradually dawned on consecutive scientists, instead of the popular notion of a blinding flash of inspiration occurring in a single individual. For this reason, interpretations of the history of stroke are not always identical (Schiller, 1970; McHenry, 1981). A related problem, and one that we have only partly solved in this chapter, is that many important primary sources are not only scarce but also difficult to decipher, having been written in Latin.

2.2 The anatomy of the brain and its blood supply

From at least the time of Hippocrates (460–370 BC) the brain was identified with intelligence and thought and also with movements of the opposite side of the body, judging from the occurrence of unilateral convulsions after head wounds on the contralateral side (McHenry, 1969). Yet, stroke, or 'apoplexy' (being struck down), was defined as a sudden but mostly general, rather than focal, disorder of the brain. The pathogenesis was explained according to the humoral theory, based on the balance between the four humours: blood, phlegm, black bile and yellow bile. Anatomy played almost no part in these explanations. Apoplexy was often attributed to accumulation of black bile in the arteries of the brain, obstructing the passage of animated spirits from the ventricles (Clarke, 1963). Galen of Pergamon (131–201), a prolific writer and animal experimenter, further popularised the knowledge and tradition accumulated at the end of the Greek culture. Galen distinguished 'karos' from 'apoplexy', in that respiration was unaffected in the former condition (Galenus, edition of 1824). His texts (there are no known drawings of his observations) were to become the sole authority throughout the Dark and Middle Ages, when observations on the human body were precluded by its divine connotations. Any illustrations of the brain that are known from the 13th century (Albertus Magnus) or the next (Mundinus) are crude and schematic representations of Galenic theories, rather than attempts at copying the forms of nature.

Andries van Wesele (1514–64), the great Renaissance anatomist who Latinised his name to Andreas Vesalius, in 1543 produced the first accurate drawings of the brain in his famous book *De humani corporis fabrica libri septem*, with the help of the draughtsman Johan Stephaan van Calcar and the printer Oporinus in Basle. It was the same year in which Copernicus published *De revolutionibus*, proclaiming the sun and not the earth as the centre of the universe. Vesalius largely ignored the blood vessels of the brain, although he retracted an earlier drawing (Fig. 2.1) depicting a '*rete mirabile*', a network of blood vessels at the base of the brain that Galen had found in goats and that had been extrapolated to the human brain ever since (Clarke & Dewhurst, 1972). Before him, Berengario da Carpi had also denied the existence of the *rete* (Berengarius, 1523). Vesalius was vehemently attacked as an iconoclast of Galenic dogmas, but at first he did not go as far as outright opposition to the central Galenic tenet that the blood could pass through the septum between the right and left ventricle of the heart, allowing the mixture of blood and air and the elimination of 'soot'. Instead he praised the creator for hav-ing made the openings so small that nobody could detect them, another striking example of how the power of theories may mislead even the most inquisitive minds. Only later, in the 1555 edition of his *De humani corporis fabrica*, did he firmly state that the interventricular septum was tightly closed.

The decisive blow to the humoral theory came in 1628, through the description of the circulation by William Harvey (1578–1657), although it need no longer surprise us that it took many decades before these views were widely accepted. Harvey's work formed the foundation for the recognition of the role of blood vessels in the pathogenesis of stroke.

Thomas Willis (1641–75) is remembered not so much for having coined the term 'neurology', or for his iatrochemical theories, a modernised version of humoral medicine, but for his work on the anatomy of the brain, first published in 1664 (Meyer & Hierons, 1962), and especially for his description of the vascular interconnections at the base of the brain (Fig. 2.2). Before him, others had observed at least part of the circle (Fallopius, 1561; Casserio, 1627; Vesling, 1647; Wepfer, 1658), in the case of Casserio and Vesling even with an illustration. Undisputedly, it was Willis who most clearly grasped the functional implications of these anastomoses in a passage illustrating his proficiency in performing necropsies as well as postmortem experiments (from a posthumous translation; Willis, 1684):

> We have elsewhere shewed, that the *Cephalick* Arteries, viz. the *Carotides*, and the *Vertebrals*, do so communicate with one another, and all of them in different places, are so ingraffed one in another mutually, that if it happen, that many of them should be stopped or pressed together at once, yet the blood being admitted to the Head, by the passage of one Artery only, either the *Carotid* or the *Vertebral*, it would presently pass thorow all those parts exterior and interior: which indeed we have sufficiently proved by an experiment, for that Ink being squirted in the trunk of one Vessel, quickly filled all the sanguiferous passages, and every where stained the Brain it self. I once opened the dead Carcase of one wasted away, in which the right Arteries, both the *Carotid* and the *Vertebral*, within the Skull, were become bony and impervious, and did shut forth the blood from that side, notwithstanding the sick person was not troubled with the astonishing Disease.

It seems that the idea of infusing coloured liquids into blood vessels had been Christopher Wren's, and had been practised from 1659 onwards (Dewhurst, 1980).

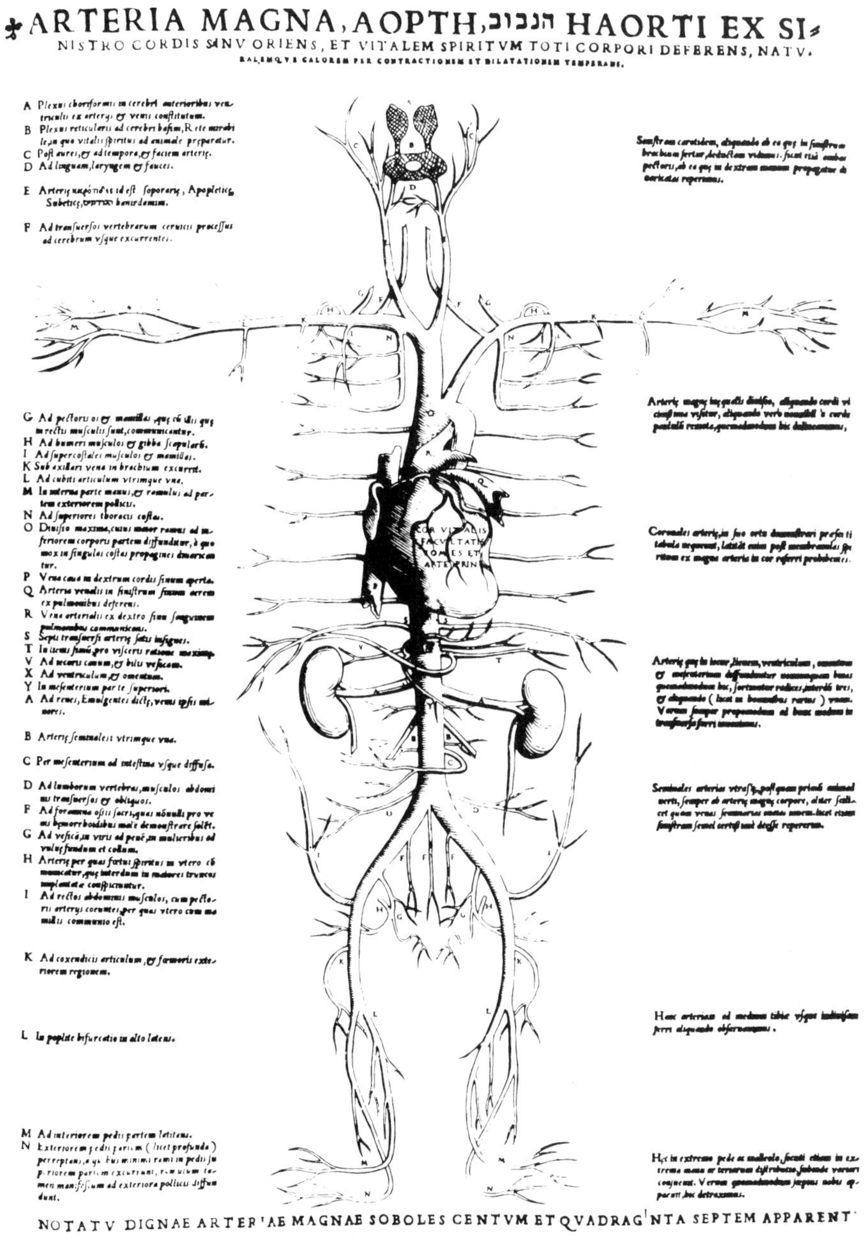

✤ ARTERIA MAGNA, AOPTH, הגדיב HAORTI EX SI✤

NISTRO CORDIS SINV ORIENS, ET VITALEM SPIRITVM TOTI CORPORI DEFERENS, NATV.

Figure 2.1 Plate depicting the blood vessels, from Vesalius' *Tabulae anatomicae sex*, of 1538. This shows the carotid arteries ending up in a network (B) at the base of the brain; the structures marked (A) represent the choroid plexus in the lateral ventricles. The network of blood vessels (*rete mirabile*) is found in oxen; Galen had assumed it was found also in the human brain, a belief perpetuated throughout the Dark and Middle Ages, up to the early Renaissance. Leonardo da Vinci has also drawn a (human?) brain with a *'rete mirabile'* at its base (Todd, 1991). Vesalius retracted the existence of a network in his atlas of 1543.

NOTATV DIGNAE ARTERIAE MAGNAE SOBOLES CENTVM ET QVADRAGINTA SEPTEM APPARENT

2.3 What happens in 'apoplexy'?

Willis's 'astonishing Disease', apoplexy, had of old intuitively been attributed to some ill-defined obstruction, whether from want of 'animal spirits' via the nerves in the tradition of Greek medicine, or, after Harvey's time, by deprivation of blood flow. Yet, it should be remembered that the notion of an intrinsic 'nervous energy' only slowly lost ground; even Boerhaave in the 18th century still echoed ancient notions in his explanation of apoplexy as a 'stoppage of the spirits' ('spiritus interceptio'; Boerhaave, 1959). In Table 2.1 we have provided a schematic representation of the development of ideas about apoplexy, and its relationship to arterial lesions, throughout the ages. That Willis had found 'bony' and 'impervious' arteries in patients who actually had not died from a stroke was probably the reason that he was not outspoken on the pathogenesis of apoplexy. His contemporaries, Wepfer, in Schaffhausen, and Bayle, in Toulouse, only

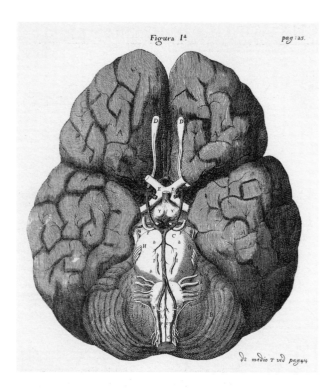

Figure 2.2 Illustration of the base of the brain from Willis's *Cerebri anatome* (1664), showing the interconnections between the right and left carotid systems, and also between these two and the posterior circulation. (From a drawing by Christopher Wren, the architect of St Paul's Cathedral in London.)

tentatively associated apoplexy with 'corpora fibrosa' (Wepfer, 1658) or with calcification of cerebral arteries (Bayle, 1677).

Wepfer not only recognised arterial lesions, but he also made one of the great advances in the knowledge about stroke by distinguishing between, on the one hand, arterial obstruction preventing the influx of blood and, on the other, extravasation of blood into the substance of the brain or the ventricular cavities, which were traditionally seen as an important source of mental energy. What still largely escaped him was the focal nature of apoplexia, which instead he mainly regarded as a process of global stunning. The four cases of haemorrhage Wepfer described were massive, at the base of the brain or deep in the parenchyma. In cases with obvious hemiplegia, incidentally a term dating back to Byzantine medicine in the 7th century (Paulus Aegineta, 625–90, edition of 1844), Wepfer suspected dysfunction of the ipsilateral rather than the contralateral side. He also observed patients who had recovered from apoplectic attacks, and he noted that those most liable to apoplexy were 'the obese, those whose face and hands are livid, and those whose pulse is constantly unequal'.

That the paralysis was on the opposite side of the apoplectic lesion was clearly predicted by Domencio Mistichelli from Pisa (Mistichelli, 1709) on the basis of his observation of the decussation of the pyramids (Fig. 2.3). A landmark in the recognition of the anatomical substrate of stroke was the work of Morgagni. In 1761 he published an impressive series of clinicopathological observations collected over a lifetime, in which he not only confirmed the notion of crossed paralysis but also firmly divided apoplexy into 'sanguineous apoplexy' and 'serous apoplexy' (and a third form which was neither serous nor sanguineous; Morgagni, 1761). A decade later, Portal rightly emphasised that it was impossible to distinguish between these two forms during life (Portal, 1781). It would be a grave anachronism, however, to assume that 'serous' (non-haemorrhagic) apoplexy was recognised as being the result of impaired blood flow, let alone of mechanical obstruction. Some even linked the arterial lesions with brain haemorrhages and not with the serous apoplexies (Baillie, 1793). Although we have seen that 17th-century scientists such as Bayle and Wepfer associated some non-haemorrhagic cases of apoplexy with obstruction of blood flow, in the 18th century medical opinion swayed towards 'vascular congestion', a kind of pre-haemorrhagic state. That explanation was propounded not only by Morgagni (Morgagni, 1761), but also by many of his con-

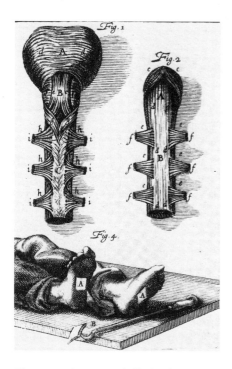

Figure 2.3 Illustration from Mistichelli's book on apoplexy (1709) in which he shows the decussation of the pyramids and also the outward rotation of the leg on the paralysed side.

Table 2.1 Development of ideas about 'apoplexy' and its relationship with arterial lesions.

Medical scientist	Ideas about 'apoplexy'		Medical scientist	Observations on arterial lesions	Historical events
	Haemorrhagic	Non-haemorrhagic			
Hippocrates (Kos) (460–370 BC)	Sudden loss of consciousness, as a result of brain disease				o Birth of Jesus Christ
Galenus (Pergamum and Rome) (131–201)	Sudden loss of consciousness, as a result of brain disease				
Wepfer (Schaffhausen) (1620–95)	Extravasation of blood in brain tissue (1658)		Wepfer	'Corpora fibrosa' (1658)	1642 Rembrandt paints *Night Watch*
			Bayle (Toulouse) (1622–1709)	Calcifications (1677)	1682 Peter I ascends Russian throne
Mistichelli (Pisa) (1675–1715)	Paralysis is unilateral, and crossed with respect to lesion (1709)		Willis (Oxford) (1621–75)	'Bony and impervious arteries' (1684)	1707 Union between England and Scotland
Boerhaave (Leiden) (1668–1738)	'Stoppage of the spirits'		Boerhaave	Narrowing due to cartilaginous change (1735)	1729 Bach writes *St Matthew's Passion*
Morgagni (Padua) (1682–1771)	'Sanguineous apoplexy' (1761)	'Serous apoplexy', extravasation of serum? (1761)	Baillie (London) (1761–1823)	Hardening of arteries associated with haemorrhage? (1795)	1776 Declaration of independence US
Rostan (Paris) (1790–1866)		'Ramollissement' (1820): —softening more frequent than haemorrhage —condition not inflammatory?	Rostan	Ossification of cerebral arteries (1820)	1815 Battle of Waterloo; Schubert writes *Erlkönig*
Lallemand (Montpellier) (1790–1853)		Cerebral softening is definitely inflammatory in nature (1824)	Lobstein (Strasburg) (1777–1835)	'Arteriosclerosis' (1829)	1829 Stephenson builds the railway engine called 'The Rocket'
Abercrombie (Edinburgh) (1780–1844)		Cerebral softening analogous to gangrene of limb? (1836)	Abercrombie	Due to ossification of arteries?	1837 Queen Victoria ascends to throne of British Empire
Carswell (London) (1793–1857)		Cerebral softening caused by obliteration of arteries? (one of possible causes; 1838)			1848 Year of revolutions; Louis Napoléon elected president of France
Rokitansky (Vienna) (1804–78)		'Encephalomalacia' (1844): —white, or serous (congestion) —red (inflammatory) —yellow (frequent; unexplained)			1859 Darwin publishes *The Origin of Species*
Cruveilhier (Paris) (1791–1874)		Cerebral softening caused by capillary congestion, secondary to 'irritation' (1862)			1863 Manet paints *Le Déjeuner sur l'herbe*
Virchow (Berlin) (1821–1902)		'Yellow softening' of the brain is secondary to arterial obliteration (Carswell); any inflammation is secondary (1856)	Virchow	Arteriosclerosis leads to thrombosis; thrombi may be torn off and lodge distally ('embolism') (1856)	1869 Opening of the Suez Canal 1871 Stanley meets Livingstone at Ujiji
Cohnheim (Berlin) (1839–84)		'Infarction' (stuffing) is haemorrhagic by definition, as opposed to ischaemic necrosis (1872)	Cohnheim	End-arteries most vulnerable; paradoxical embolism	1877 Bell invents telephone, Edison the phonograph
			Chiari (Prague) (1851–1916)	Thrombosis at the carotid bifurcation may cause secondary embolisation to brain (1905)	1895 Röntgen discovers X-rays in Würzburg 1907 Ehrlich introduces arsphenamine as treatment for syphilis

temporaries and followers (Portal, 1781; Hall, 1836; Burrows, 1846). Cheyne pointed out that, in patients who have survived a 'stroke of apoplexy' for a considerable time, autopsy may show a cavity filled with serum which is rusty yellow in colour and which may stain the substance of the adjacent brain tissue, but he may have been describing a residual lesion after cerebral haemorrhage rather than infarction (Cheyne, 1812).

The anatomical, organ-based approach exemplified by Morgagni reflected the Italian practice, in which the separation between physicians and surgeons was much less strict than in northern Europe with its more theoretical framework of medicine. The proponents of that school were Boerhaave (1668–1738) in Leiden and later Cullen (1710–90) in Edinburgh, both the most influential clinical teachers of their time. They established a nosological classification that was based much more on holistic theory, in terms of a disturbed system, than on actual observations at the level of the organ, at least with 20th-century hindsight (King, 1991). Probably our own time will be branded as the era of exaggerated reductionism! In the intellectual tradition of the Dutch–Scottish school, purely clinical classifications of apoplexy were proposed in the early 19th century by Serres (with and without paralysis), by Abercrombie (primary apoplexy, with deprivation of sense and motion, and sometimes with convulsions, a second type beginning with headache, and a third type with loss of power on one side of the body and of speech, often with recovery) and by Hope and Bennett (transient apoplexy, primary apoplexy with death or slow recovery, ingravescent apoplexy with partial recovery and relapse, and paraplexic apoplexy with paralysis) (Serres, 1819; Abercrombie, 1828; Hope *et al.*, 1840).

There are several reasons why the lesion in what we now call cerebral infarction was not actually identified until the middle of the 19th century. First, it was impossible to recognise ischaemic softening in patients who had usually died not long after their stroke. Fixation methods were not available until the end of the 18th century; Vicq d'Azyr, Marie Antoinette's physician, was the first to use alcohol as a tissue fixative (Vicq d'Azyr, 1786) and formaldehyde fixation was not employed until one-century later (Blum, 1893). Second, it is probable that many patients diagnosed as having died from apoplexy in fact had suffered from other conditions. If in our time the diagnosis can be wrong in as many as 13% of patients referred and subsequently admitted with a presumed stroke (Norris & Hachinski, 1982), the diagnostic accuracy was presumably no better in centuries past.

2.4 Cerebral infarction (ischaemic stroke)

It was Leon Rostan (1790–1866), a physician at the Salpêtrière in Paris, who clearly recognised softening of the brain as a separate lesion, distinct from haemorrhage, although the pathogenesis still escaped him. He published his findings in an unillustrated monograph, the first edition of which appeared in 1820 (Rostan, 1820). The lesions were most commonly found in the corpus striatum, thalamus or centrum ovale, but they also occurred in the cerebral cortex, brainstem and cerebellum. Old cases showed a yellowish-green discoloration, whereas if the patients had died soon after the event the colour of the lesion was chestnut or reddish. The softening might be so exteme as to lead to the formation of a cyst. In other patients it was difficult to detect any change in firmness or in colour.

Rostan distinguished softening of the brain from 'apoplexy', a term he no longer used for stroke in general, but which he regarded as being synonymous with haemorrhagic stroke. He supposed that softening of the brain was more frequent than brain haemorrhage, although some haemorrhages were secondary to softening. The clinical manifestations were thought to occur in two stages: first 'fugitive' disturbances in the use of a limb, in speech or in visual or auditory perception, sooner or later followed by hemiplegia and coma, in a slowly progressive fashion.

Although Rostan recognised 'ossification' of the cerebral arteries, he did not associate these lesions with cerebral softening via obstruction of the arterial system. That 'paradigm', in 20th-century terminology (Kuhn, 1962), had not yet entered medicine. But, at least he doubted the prevailing opinion that the lesion was some kind of inflammatory response; after all, there was redness and swelling (*rubor, tumor*), if not warmth and pain (*calor, dolor*), to complete the cardinal signs of inflammation delineated by Celsus in the first century AD. Rostan's contemporary Lallemand was much more outspoken and had little doubt that inflammation was at the root of cerebral softening (Lallemand, 1824). Twentieth-century doctors who find this difficult to understand should be aware that inflammation was one of the overriding medical paradigms from the middle of the 18th century until the middle of the next (King, 1991). Just as in our time some poorly understood disease conditions are explained in terms of slow virus infections or autoimmune disease, perhaps erroneously, inflammation seemed for a long time the most logical explanation for liquefaction of brain tissue.

The first hunch of a relationship between arterial disease and 'ramollissement', as many English writers continued to call brain softening in deference to Rostan, was voiced by Abercrombie, in a later edition of his textbook

(Abercrombie, 1836). He drew an analogy with gangrene, caused by 'failure of circulation', this in turn being secondary to 'ossification of arteries'. The role of arterial obstruction as a primary cause of softening of the brain was confirmed by others (Bright, 1831; Carswell, 1838), but the theory of inflammation continued to be defended by a few adherents (Cruveilhier, 1842; Durand-Fardel, 1843). Some were aware that apoplexy could be caused by 'cerebral anaemia' (as opposed to congestion), not only through loss of blood but also by a diminution of vascular pressure, particularly in the case of heart disease (Burrows, 1846).

Other missing links in the understanding of cerebral infarction were going to be provided by Rokitansky (1804–78) in Vienna and Virchow (1821–1902) in Berlin. Rokitansky divided cerebral softening (which he termed encephalomalacia) into three varieties: red (haemorrhagic) softening, inflammatory in nature; white softening (synonymous with 'serous apoplexy') caused by congestion and oedema; and, the most common variety, yellow softening, of which the pathogenesis was unknown. Virchow revolutionised medical thinking about vascular disease by firmly putting the emphasis on changes in the vessel wall rather than in the blood (Schiller called it the victory of 'solidism' over 'humoralism'; Schiller, 1970). He also firmly established that thrombosis of arteries was caused not by inflammation but by fatty metamorphosis of the vessel wall, even if he had to found his own journal before his papers were published (Virchow, 1847, 1856). For these changes in the arterial wall Virchow revived the term 'arteriosclerosis', first used by Lobstein (Lobstein, 1829). Virchow's disciple Julius Cohnheim introduced the word 'infarction' in a medical context, but strictly reserved it for haemorrhagic necrosis ('stuffing', by seeping of blood into ischaemic tissue, through damaged walls of capillaries) as opposed to ischaemic necrosis (Cohnheim, 1872).

2.5 Thrombosis and embolism

Virchow observed thrombosis secondary to atherosclerosis and also embolism (a term newly coined by him, at least in medical parlance) in patients with gangrene of the lower limbs caused by clots from the heart. He extrapolated these events to the cause of cerebral softening (Virchow, 1847):

> Here there is either no essential change in the vessel
> wall and its surroundings, or this is ostensibly
> secondary. I feel perfectly justified in claiming that
> these clots never originated in the local circulation but
> that they are torn off at a distance and carried along in
> the blood stream as far as they can go.

The relationship between vegetations on the heart valves and

stroke had in fact been suggested a century earlier by Boerhaave's pupil Gerard van Swieten, personal physician to the Austrian empress Maria Theresa and founder of the Viennese school of medicine (van Swieten, 1754):

> It has been established by many observations that these
> polyps occasionally attach themselves as excrescences
> to the columnae carneae of the heart, and perhaps then
> separate from it and are propelled, along with the
> blood, into the pulmonary artery or the aorta, and its
> branches . . . were they thrown into the carotid or
> vertebral arteries, could disturb—or if they completely
> blocked all approach of arterial blood to the brain—
> utterly abolish the functions of the brain.

For more than a century after Virchow's accurate pathological descriptions of arterial occlusions, the term 'cerebral embolism' was almost synonymous with embolism from the heart. Sources of embolism in the extracranial arteries were hardly considered until the 1960s, at least in teaching. By the same token, the term 'cerebral thrombosis' remained firmly entrenched in clinical thinking as being more or less synonymous with cerebral infarction without associated heart disease, the implication being that in these cases the site of the atheromatous lesion was in the intracranial vessels. For example, this is what the sixth edition of Brain's *Diseases of the Nervous System* says on the subject (Brain, 1968):

> Progressive occlusion of cerebral blood vessels impairs
> the circulation in the regions they supply. The effects of
> this depend upon the size and situation of the vessel,
> and the rate of onset of the occlusion particularly in
> relation to the collateral circulation. Actual obstruction
> of an artery by atheroma, with or without subsequent
> thrombosis, causes softening of the region of the brain
> supplied by the vessel.

That the notion of 'local atherosclerosis = local thrombosis' has persisted for such a long time must have been because of its appealing simplicity, not because there were no observations to the contrary. As long ago as 1905, Chiari had drawn attention to the frequency of atherosclerosis in the region of the carotid bifurcation and had suggested that embolisation of atheromatous material might be a cause of cerebral softening (Chiari, 1905), and not much later Hunt had described the relationship between carotid occlusion and stroke (Hunt, 1914).

The general acceptance of extracranial atherosclerosis as an important cause of cerebral ischaemia came only after two further developments. The first was the attention generated by Miller Fisher's studies, in which he re-emphasised the role of atherosclerosis at the carotid bifurcation, at least in patients of Caucasian descent (Fisher, 1951). He clinically correlated these lesions not only with contralateral hemiplegia but also with attacks of monocular blindness in the ipsilateral eye (Fisher, 1952). The second development was imaging. Cerebral angiography by direct puncture of the carotid artery had been introduced by Moniz in 1927 (Moniz, 1927, 1940), but imaging of the carotid bifurcation in patients with stroke became common only after the advent of catheter angiography (Seldinger, 1953), and later of ultrasound techniques for vascular imaging. These methods often showed abnormalities of the internal carotid artery near its origin, at least in patients with transient or permanent deficits from presumed ischaemia in the territory of the main trunk of the middle cerebral artery or one of its branches. If those patients are investigated early, within 6 hours of the attack, the site where the embolus has become impacted can be demonstrated even more often than its source, in about 75% of patients, by means of angiography (Fieschi *et al.*, 1989) or with transcranial Doppler monitoring (Zanette *et al.*, 1995). In some 40% of patients with temporary or permanent occlusion of large intracranial vessels no source of embolism can be found in the neck or in the heart. Pathological observations suggesting that the aorta may harbour atherosclerotic lesions (Soloway & Aronson, 1964) were recently confirmed in a large autopsy series (Amarenco *et al.*, 1992) and during life transoesophageal echocardiography may similarly detect sources of embolism in the aorta more often in these patients than in controls or in patients with known atheromatous lesions elsewhere in the cerebral circulation (Amarenco *et al.*, 1994).

Of course, there is more to ischaemic stroke than atherothrombotic occlusion of large vessels, but the history of small vessel disease and non-atheromatous causes of ischaemia is rather recent, and these subjects will be taken up in Chapters 6 and 7. Before concluding the sections on cerebral infarction, thrombosis and embolism, we should like briefly to draw attention to the term 'cerebrovascular accident', which enjoyed some undeserved popularity in the middle half of this century. The problem was that sometimes it was used as synonymous with cerebral infarction, at other times as denoting stroke in general. We can do no better than quote Schiller (1970):

> That rather blurry and pompous piece of nomenclature must have issued from the well-meant tendency to soften the blow to patients and their relatives, also from a desire to replace 'stroke', a pithy term that may sound unscientific and lacking gentility. 'Cerebrovascular accident (CVA)' can be traced to the early 1930s—between 1932, to be exact, when it was still absent from the 15th edition of *Dorland's Medical Dictionary*, and the following edition of 1936 where it first appeared.

This is the last time we shall mention cerebrovascular accident; there is, after all, nothing accidental about a stroke.

2.6 Transient ischaemic attacks (TIAs)

It is difficult to trace the first descriptions of what we now call TIAs of the brain or eye, because symptoms representing focal deficits were not clearly distinguished from non-specific symptoms of a more global nature such as fainting or headache (Hachinski, 1982).

Wepfer (1658) recorded that he had seen patients who recovered from hemiplegia in 1 day or less. An 18th-century account has been retrieved in the patient's own words, not muddled by medical interpretation (Kraaijeveld *et al.*, 1984), and therefore it is as lucid as it would have been today. The subject is Jean Paul Grandjean de Fouchy, writing in 1783, at the age of 76 years (Benton & Joynt, 1960):

> Toward the end of dinner, I felt a little increase of pain above the left eye and in that very instant I became unable to pronounce the words that I wanted. I heard what was said, and I thought of what I ought to reply, but I spoke other words than those which would express my thoughts, or if I began them I did not complete them, and I substituted other words for them. I had nevertheless all movements as freely as usual . . . I saw all objects clearly, I heard distinctly what was being said; and the organs of thought were, it seemed to me, in a natural state. This sort of paroxysm lasted almost a minute.

Once it had become established, in the middle of the 19th century, that cerebral softening was not caused by an inflammatory process but by occlusion of cerebral arteries, temporary episodes of ischaemia were recognised increasingly often (Wood, 1852; Jackson, 1875; Hammond, 1881; Gowers, 1893; Osler, 1911; Oppenheim, 1913). In the course of time, three main theories have been invoked to explain the pathophysiology of TIAs, at least in relation to atherosclerosis: the vasospasm theory, the haemodynamic theory and the thromboembolic theory (Hachinski, 1982).

2.6.1 The vasospasm theory

Arterial spasm as a cause of gangrene of the extremities was described by Raynaud in his doctoral thesis of 1862 (Raynaud, 1862). His theory of vasospasm was then extrapolated to the cerebral circulation (Peabody, 1891; Russel, 1909). The latter, writing about a 50-year-old farmer who had suffered three attacks of tingling and numbness in the right arm and the right side of the face, dismissed thrombosis ('Thrombus, once formed, does not break up and disappear in some mysterious way') and instead invoked a phenomenon of 'local syncope', analogous to Raynaud's disease or some cases of migraine: 'There must be some vessel constriction, local in site, varying in degree and in extent, coming and going, intermittent' (Russel, 1909). Even the great Osler mounted the bandwagon of the vasospastic theory to explain transient attacks of aphasia and paralysis: 'We have plenty of evidence that arteries may pass into a state of spasm with obliteration of the lumen and loss of function in the parts supplied' (Osler, 1911). Vasospasm remained the most popular theory to explain TIAs in the first half of the 20th century and provided the rationale for so-called cerebral vasodilators. Up to the 1980s this class of presumably useless drugs was still widely prescribed in some European countries, not only for TIAs but for 'senility' in general, and in France these drugs were the third most commonly prescribed category in 1982 (Payer, 1989).

In the front line of medicine, however, the vasospastic theory has gone into decline, first because the cerebral arteries are amongst the least reactive in the body (Pickering, 1948; Denny-Brown, 1951), and second because more plausible theories have emerged (see below). Only under strictly defined conditions can vasospasm be a causal factor in the pathogenesis of cerebral ischaemia, namely after subarachnoid haemorrhage or in association with migraine, and even in these conditions its role is disputable. Nevertheless, vasospasm has recently resurfaced as a possible cause of episodes of transient monocular blindness that are frequent and stereotyped and have no altitudinal distribution (Burger et al., 1991) or even of transient motor or sensory deficits not related to migraine (Call et al., 1988). Such events must be extremely rare.

2.6.2 The haemodynamic theory

The notion of 'low flow' as a cause of cerebral ischaemia should perhaps be attributed to Ramsay Hunt, who drew an analogy between the symptoms of carotid stenosis or occlusion and the symptoms of intermittent claudication in patients with severe peripheral arterial disease (Hunt, 1914). But, it was especially after 1951, when Denny-Brown suggested that TIAs might be caused by 'episodic insufficiency in the circle of Willis', that interest in the haemodynamic aspects of TIAs was fully aroused (Denny-Brown, 1951). Indeed, it was mainly the surgical community for which the concept of 'cerebral intermittent claudication' continued to have great appeal, despite the incongruity of the relatively constant blood flow to the brain and the large fluctuations in flow that occur in the legs, dependent on the level of activity, and despite the lack of support from clinical studies. When the blood pressure was artificially lowered, by means of hexamethonium and postural tilting, in 35 patients who had either experienced TIAs or who had known carotid artery disease, only one of the patients developed symptoms of focal cerebral ischaemia before a syncopal attack which sig-

nified global rather than focal ischaemia of the brain (Kendell & Marshall, 1963). Similarly, cerebral ischaemia with naturally occurring attacks of hypotension, such as cardiac arrhythmias, is almost always syncopal and not focal in nature (Reed et al., 1973), and cardiac arrhythmias do not occur more often in patients with TIAs than in controls (De Bono & Warlow, 1981). Once the first successful carotid reconstruction had been reported (Eastcott et al., 1954), the intuitive belief in the haemodynamic theory led to an ever-increasing number of carotid endarterectomies being performed (indeed, often called 'carotid disobstruction') in patients with and even without TIAs, despite the absence of any formal proof of efficacy. These developments caused understandable concern in the neurological community (Warlow, 1984; Barnett et al., 1984) and fortunately ended in well-designed clinical trials, which have served to define to a large extent the place of this operation (see Chapter 16).

That the haemodynamic theory does not apply to the majority of patients with TIAs is not to say that the exceptional patient can not suffer from 'misery perfusion'. In the presence of multiple occlusions or stenoses of the extracranial arteries, the haemodynamic reserve may be so poor that minor changes in systolic blood pressure can not be compensated for (see Section 6.5.5). Such triggering events include a change from a sitting to a standing position, turning the head, heating of the face or looking into bright light (Caplan & Sergay, 1976; Bogousslavsky & Regli, 1983; Ross Russell & Page, 1983). Perhaps for this small group of patients extracranial to intracranial bypass surgery has something to offer after all, despite the negative results of the controlled trial in a large but relatively unselected group of patients with occlusion of the internal carotid or middle cerebral artery (EC/IC Bypass Study Group, 1985).

2.6.3 The thromboembolic theory

In the 1950s C. Miller Fisher not only gave new impetus to some older observations about the relationship between stroke and atheromatous lesions of the carotid bifurcation, but he also provided evidence that the pathogenesis was more complex than could be explained by fixed arterial narrowing. First, he saw a patient in whom hemiplegia had been preceded by attacks of transient monocular blindness in the contralateral eye, 'the wrong eye' (Fisher, 1952). Second, through patient and extensive ophthalmoscopic observations, he saw that during an attack of transient monocular blindness white bodies passing slowly through the retinal arteries (Fig. 2.4), the whitish appearance and friability of the moving material suggesting that these were emboli, largely made up of platelets (Fisher, 1959). These findings

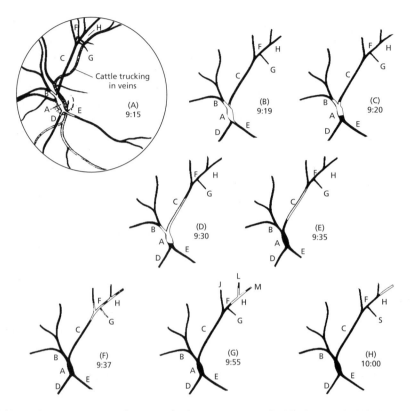

Figure 2.4 Diagrams of observations in a patient with an atttack of transient monocular blindness in the left eye (except the upper temporal quadrant); the attack had started at 8.55 AM, 20 minutes before the beginning of the observations. The column of blood in the retinal arteries was in some places interrupted by white segments, initially at the stems of the superior and inferior retinal arteries (A); also the column of blood in at least six venous branches of the superior half of the retina was broken into transverse bands. The white segments in the retinal arteries slowly passed through the superior temporal artery (B–H). At (C) the vision in the upper half of the visual field had returned. At (D) a fine trickle of erythrocytes moved slowly along one side of white segment AB to the superior nasal artery, and at (E) vision had also returned in the inferior temporal quadrant. After (H), when the column of blood had been completely restored, vision returned to normal. (From Fisher, 1959; by kind permission of the author and *Neurology*.)

were confirmed by Ross Russell (Ross Russell, 1961), whilst others saw atheromatous emboli in the retinal vessels, which did not move but had become impacted (Witmer & Schmid, 1958; Hollenhorst, 1961).

After these direct observations of the ocular fundus, additional—but more indirect—arguments corroborated the notion of artery-to-artery embolism as an important cause of TIAs.

1 In many patients with attacks involving the cortical territory of the middle cerebral artery there is an associated lesion of the internal carotid artery, but in only very few of them is the stenosis severe enough, with a residual lumen of 1–2 mm, for blood flow to be impaired below critical levels, even assuming there is no collateral circulation (Archie & Feldtman, 1981). In addition, the stenosis is constant but the

episodes of ischaemia transient, without evidence for cardiac arhythmias as an additional factor.

2 During carotid endarterectomy, fresh and friable thrombi have been seen to adhere to atheromatous plaques in the carotid bifurcation, especially in those patients who had experienced recent attacks (Gunning *et al*., 1964).

3 In patients with ocular as well as cerebral attacks, the two kinds of attacks occur after each other and almost never at the same time (Gunning *et al*., 1964).

4 Manual compression of the carotid artery may lead to dislodgement of atheromatous emboli to the cerebral circulation (Beal *et al*., 1981).

5 If patients continue to have TIAs after occlusion of the ipsilateral internal carotid artery, there is often an additional atheromatous lesion in the common carotid or external

carotid artery, these vessels at the same time being important collateral channels, supplying the hemisphere via retrograde flow in the ophthalmic artery (Bogousslavsky & Regli, 1983).

6 Asymptomatic emboli have been seen to flash up during angiography (Watts, 1982) and fibrin thrombi have been seen to pass through a cortical artery during craniotomy for a bypass procedure (Barnett, 1979). The recently developed technique of transcranial Doppler monitoring has uncovered an ongoing stream of high-intensity transient signals (HITS), probably small emboli, in patients with symptomatic carotid lesions (Markus, 1993). The HITS disappear after carotid endarterectomy (Siebler *et al.*, 1993), the rate depending on the interval since operation (van Zuilen *et al.*, 1995).

Whilst artery-to-artery thromboembolism from atheromatous plaques may seem the most important factor in explaining TIAs and ischaemic strokes, it is not necessarily the only one, not even in single patients. For example, it is probable that emboli have especially damaging effects in vascular beds that are chronically underperfused.

2.7 Intracerebral haemorrhage

As pointed out above, extravasation of blood into the brain parenchyma was first recognised by Wepfer (1658) and subsequently by Morgagni (1761). The cause remained obscure, and to a large extent still is (Adams & vander Eecken, 1953). In 1855, before blood pressure could be measured, Kirkes observed hypertrophy of the heart in 17 of 22 patients with fatal brain haemorrhage (Kirkes, 1855). Charcot and Bouchard in 1868 examined the brains of patients who had died from intracerebral haemorrhage and immersed these in running water; they found multiple, minute outpouchings of small blood vessels, so-called miliary aneurysms (Charcot & Bouchard, 1868). The irony of these two names being joined is that Bouchard, once Charcot's pupil, in later years generated much hostility between himself and his former chief, because he wanted to found a school of his own and to be considered the most influential man in the faculty of medicine (Satran, 1974; Iragui, 1986). It was in this adversarial atmosphere that in 1892 Bouchard, as president of the jury that had to decide about the competition for the rank of *professeur agrégé*, did not admit Charcot's pupil Babinski. Babinski subsequently left academic medicine by becoming chief of the Pitié hospital, where he devoted much time to the study of clinical signs, including the now famous 'toe sign'. The aneurysms described by Charcot and Bouchard were white or brownish-coloured nodules about 0.5–2.0 mm in diameter, attached to a small arteriole, most often in the basal ganglia (see Fig. 8.1). At the beginning of the present

century, Charcot and Bouchards's theory came under attack and some proposed that most of these dilatations were not aneurysms at all but occlusive thrombi at the site of rupture (Ellis, 1909); in Chapter 8 it is explained that some other 'miliary aneurysms' may in fact have been perivascular clots in perivascular (Virchow–Robin) spaces.

Alternative explanations for the pathogenesis of primary intracerebral haemorrhage included previous infarction of brain tissue and capillary vessels. The frequent co-existence of hypertension led Rosenblath to postulate that a renal toxin caused necrosis of vessel walls (Rosenblath, 1918) and Westphal to assume that arterial spasm was an intermediate factor (Westphal, 1932). Another theory was that arteries dilate and rupture only when a previous infarct has occurred, thus depriving the feeding vessel of its normal support (Hiller, 1935; Globus *et al.*, 1949; Schwartz, 1961). In the 1960s injection techniques revived the notion of microaneurysms (Ross Russell, 1963; Cole & Yates, 1967), although some still suspect that the injection pressures can artifactually distend or rupture vessel walls (Challa *et al.*, 1992).

It was at the beginning of the 20th century that amyloid angiopathy was recognised as a cause of primary intracerebral haemorrhage (Fischer, 1910; Scholz, 1938; Pantelakis, 1954). This type of haemorrhage occurs especially at the border of white and grey matter and not in the deep regions of the brain that are the most common sites of haemorrhages associated with microaneurysms. The first series of such patients appeared in the 1970s (Torack, 1975; Jellinger, 1977).

2.8 Subarachnoid haemorrhage

'Meningeal apoplexy' has intrigued not only practising physicians and anatomists but also medical historians (Ljunggren *et al.*, 1993). The disorder was not recognised until 3 years before the battle of Waterloo and in the next 125 years numerous accounts appeared that combined a few personal cases with attempts to review the entire world literature up to that time, the last being a heroic overview of 1125 patients (McDonald & Korb, 1939).

2.8.1 Diagnosis

The first unequivocal description of an aneurysm, although unruptured, was by Biumi in 1765, who saw it not on the circle of Willis but in the cavernous sinus (at the time called Vieussens' receptacle; Biumi, 1765). Morgagni (1761) had also mentioned dilatations of arteries that may have been aneurysms. In 1812 Cheyne provided the first illustration of lethal subarachnoid haemorrhage at the base of the brain (Fig. 2.5), but the aneurysm that must have been the source of the haemorrhage was not recognised at the time (Cheyne, 1812). One year later Blackall reported a postmortem observation in which the haemorrhage as well as the offending aneurysm (of the basilar artery) were identified (Blackall, 1813). Soon afterwards, Hodgson emphasised that the extravasated blood was contained under the arachnoid membrane (Hodgson, 1815). Serres, not aware of these publications, published two similar observations in a French periodical (Serres, 1826). In England, Bright added some further case reports in 1831, including an illustration of a pea-sized aneurysm on a branch of the middle cerebral artery (Bright, 1831). The erroneous notion that aneurysms are congenital malformations, caused by a defect in the muscular layer of the arterial wall (see Chapter 9), was first put forward in 1887 (Eppinger, 1887) and subsequently adopted by other writers (Wichern, 1912; Turnbull, 1914), to be perpetuated into contemporaneous textbooks and students' minds. Turnbull also pointed out, correctly, that syphilis was an extremely rare cause of aneurysms.

It took a long time before the clinical features were sorted out. Brinton (1852) pointed out that fatal rupture was not the only possible presentation of aneurysms, and that other manifestations were local pressure, convulsive attacks or inflammation (here he probably referred to cerebral infarction, which was barely recognised at the time; see Section 2.4); he also found that patients could harbour aneurysms without any symptoms at all. The sudden onset of the headache and the accompanying paralysis of the IIIrd cranial nerve in some patients with aneurysms at the origin of the posterior communicating artery from the internal carotid artery led Lebert (1866) to suppose that the diagnosis might be made during life, a feat that was to be achieved only rarely before the advent of vascular imaging (Bull, 1877; Cushing, 1923; Symonds, 1923).

Of the technical developments that would make it so much easier to establish the diagnosis of aneurysmal subarachnoid haemorrhage during life, the first was the lumbar puncture, introduced for therapeutic purposes in hydrocephalic patients (Quincke, 1891). Froin, in his thesis of 1904, analysed the cerebrospinal fluid for the presence of blood cells as well as of blood pigments, after haemolysis. The next advances were neuroradiological. The first angiographic visualisation of a cerebral aneurysm during life was reported in 1933 (Moniz, 1933), 6 years after the technique had been first applied (Moniz, 1927). In those days it remained a hazardous procedure (involving surgical dissection of the artery), to such an extent that someone like Cushing only rarely had his patients undergo it before neurosurgical exploration. Even today, in the era of selective catheterisation, the risks are far from negligible. Fortunately, the technique of magnetic resonance angiography is making rapid advances and may soon replace the invasive techniques, at least for diagnostic purposes (Atlas *et al.*, 1994; Korogi *et al.*, 1994). The greatest leap in our times was the advent of CT (Hounsfield, 1973); this technique made it possible to localise the extent of the haemorrhage in a precise fashion, to separate aneurysmal haemorrhage from non-aneurysmal haemorrhage and, by serial investigations, to detect and distinguish the most important complications: rebleeding, delayed ischaemia and hydrocephalus (see Chapter 13).

2.8.2 Surgical treatment

Carotid ligation was practised since the times of Ambroise Paré (1510–90) as a method to stop arterial bleeding in patients with neck wounds, and once aneurysms were recog-

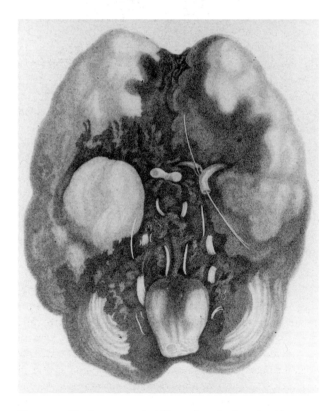

Figure 2.5 The first anatomical illustration of subarachnoid haemorrhage, from Cheyne (1812). A probe has been passed into the proximal end of the internal carotid artery and emerges at the presumed site of rupture; the offending aneurysm was not recognised at the time but presumably it was at the origin of the posterior communicating artery from the carotid artery, or at the anterior communicating artery complex.

nised as the cause of subarachnoid haemorrhage it was a logical step to consider this procedure as a method to decrease the risk of rebleeding (Bull, 1877). Hutchinson would actually have carried out the operation in 1875 had the patient not declined at the last moment, going on to survive for another 11 years (Hutchinson, 1875). Around 1886 it was Horsley who was one of the first who ligated the (common) carotid artery in the neck, for a tumorous aneurysm (Beadles, 1907). For decades this remained the only surgical intervention possible, but most patients were managed conservatively because the complications of surgery were considerable (Schorstein, 1940).

In 1931 the Edinburgh neurosurgeon Norman Dott, at that time only 33 years old, carried out the first intracranial operation for a ruptured aneurysm (Todd *et al.*, 1990). It was a more or less desperate attempt because the aneurysm had already rebled twice, leaving the patient comatose for some hours after the last episode and with some degree of right-sided hemiparesis and aphasia. To complicate matters further, the patient was a well-known Edinburgh solicitor, 53 years old and chairman of the board of governors of the Royal Hospital for Sick Children. But, both the patient and the young neurosurgeon were prepared to take the risk (Rush & Shaw, 1990). About the operation Dott (1932) wrote:

> A left frontal approach was employed and it was a difficult matter to elevate the tense and oedematous brain and identify the basal structures, which were bloodstained and largely embedded in clot. The left optic nerve was found and the internal carotid artery was defined at its outer side. This vessel was closely followed upwards, outwards and backwards to its bifurcation into the middle and anterior cerebral arteries. As this point was being cleared of tenacious clot a formidable arterial haemorrhage filled the wound. With the aid of suction apparatus, held closely to the bleeding point, we were able to see the aneurysm. It sprang from the upper aspect of the bifurcation junction; it was about 3 mm in diameter; blood spurted freely from its semidetached fundus. Meanwhile a colleague was obtaining fresh muscle from the patient's leg. A small fragment of muscle was accurately applied to the bleeding point and held firmly in place so that it checked the bleeding and compressed the thin walled aneurysmal sac. Thus it was steadily maintained for twelve minutes. As the retaining instrument was then cautiously withdrawn, no further bleeding occurred. The vessel was further cleared and thin strips of muscle were prepared and wound around it until a thick collar of muscle embedded the aneurysm and adjacent arterial trunks [Fig. 2.6].

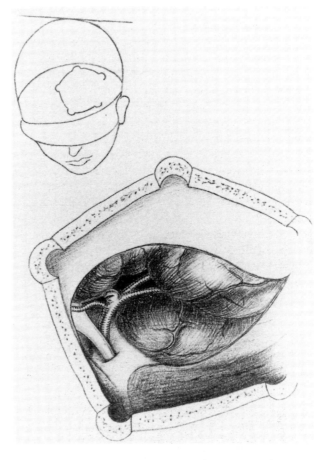

Figure 2.6 Norman Dott's drawing of the first intracranial operation for aneurysm. The proximal middle cerebral artery aneurysm was exposed and wrapped with muscle through a left frontal flap. (From Todd *et al.*, 1990; by kind permission of the authors and the *Journal of Neurology, Neurosurgery and Psychiatry*.)

The patient recovered well and a few weeks later Dott wrote, his sense of triumph carefully hidden: 'Mr. Colin Black's tibialis anticus seems to have stuck well to his internal carotid—he has gone for a holiday' (Rush & Shaw, 1990). In later years Dott and his patient went fishing together on a number of occasions and Mr Black's neurological condition remained good until he died from myocardial infarction 11 years after the momentous operation. Unfortunately, on later occasions the outcome with a direct approach to the aneurysm was often disappointing, if not fatal, and Dott reverted to ligating the internal carotid artery in the neck or the proximal anterior cerebral artery intracranially.

In 1937 Dandy was the first to use a clip to occlude the neck of the aneurysm that had bled (Dandy, 1938). Yet in some patients a clip could not be secured, and in those cases he often had to have recourse to so-called trapping, by clipping the parent vessel on either side of the aneurysm. Drake (1961) devised a technique for approaching basilar artery aneurysms, notoriously difficult until then, and managed to apply clips to them. In the 1960s, spring clips, which could be removed when placement was less than optimal, came into use and replaced the silver clips used by Dandy. Nevertheless, the direct operation of aneurysms remained dangerous and controlled trials of the efficacy of surgery were equivocal (see Chapter 13). Attempts to increase the safety of the operation included temporary cardiac arrest, hypotension and deep hypothermia, all without much success, although no formal trials were done.

In the 1980s, a consensus developed amongst neurosurgeons that direct operation of the aneurysm should best be delayed until 12–14 days after the initial haemorrhage. This regimen meant, of course, that a proportion of patients suffered rebleeding or other complications in the meantime. The gradual introduction of the operating microscope for aneurysm surgery in the 1970s made early operation (within 3 days) not only feasible but also fashionable, despite the dearth of evidence from controlled clinical trials (see Chapter 13). The medical management of patients with ruptured aneurysms has also improved in the last decade, especially with regard to the prevention of delayed ischaemia (see Chapter 13). This benefits patients regardless of the timing of operation, and from a strictly methodological point of view—there is no other view, to be honest—the question of the optimal time for operating on ruptured aneurysms should be regarded as unresolved.

2.9 Treatment and its pitfalls

Doctoring has always included treatment. In the past, medical management was almost invariably based on erroneous pathophysiological concepts, and the treatments were almost invariably ineffective, if not actually harmful, a situation often repeated in present times, and much more often than physicians and surgeons care to realise. Anyone who finds it amusing to read about 19th-century regimens, including measures such as bleeding, mustard poultices, castor oil and turpentine enemas as treatments for apoplexy, should read post-1950 treatises about the efficacy of vasodilator drugs or about transplantation of omentum to the intracranial cavity, as a chastening experience.

2.9.1 Clinical trials

The era of rational treatment dawned with the introduction of the randomised controlled clinical trial. These principles slowly gained acceptance after the landmark UK Medical Research Council trial of streptomycin in pulmonary tuberculosis with random assignment to treatment groups (Medical Research Council, 1948), but some forerunners had already used parallel control groups. Amongst these were James Lind in 1753 (lemons and oranges to prevent scurvy in sailors), Louis in 1835 (bleeding as a treatment for pneumonia, erysipelas or throat inflammation), Fibiger in 1898 (serum for diphtheria, with alternate assignment) and Ferguson *et al.* in 1927 (vaccines for the common cold, with concealment to patients).

Clinical trials in cerebrovascular disease were no exception to the rule that most methodological errors have to be committed before they are recognised, because the correct solutions are often counter-intuitive. The first trial of carotid endarterectomy excluded surgical mishaps from the analysis (Fields *et al.*, 1970); subsequently the operation boomed to worrying levels, until checked by methodologically sound trials (see Section 16.7.5). The first large trial of aspirin in stroke prevention evoked much controversy (Canadian Cooperative Study Group, 1978), for one thing because its initiators had chosen 'stroke or death' as the outcome event instead of stroke alone (Kurtzke, 1979); it took time for neurologists to realise that they treat whole patients rather than only their brains. Also, trials of anticoagulant drugs in brain ischaemia were too small, separately as well as collectively, to detect even large protective effects, apart from other shortcomings (Jonas, 1988).

2.9.2 Measuring outcome: the ghost of Gall

One of the greatest stumbling blocks in trials of acute stroke is the babel of tongues with regard to the measurement of outcome (van Gijn, 1992). Traditionally, so-called 'stroke scales' have been applied for this aim, analogous to scales for other neurological conditions, such as Parkinson's disease or multiple sclerosis. Although the stated purpose of 'stroke scales' is to measure outcome, these scales are nothing but codifications of the neurological examination, developed for no other purpose than that of localising lesions within the nervous system. With such a diagnostic approach, different functions of the nervous system are separately assessed: power of limbs, speech, visual fields, etc. This reductionist, mechanistic notion of brain function reflects the localisationists' position in the scientific battle that raged in the second half of the 19th century, the opposing party being that of equipotentiality.

The equipotentialists believed that the brain worked as a unitary system, brain tissue being omnipotent and flexible in its function. Consequently, brain damage would result in a decrease in the overall level of performance, but not in a loss of specific functions. The champion of the equipotentialists was the French physiologist Flourens, who supported his views with experiments on dogs and pigeons (Flourens, 1824). The opposing concept, that of localisation of specific functions, was propounded in a somewhat bizarre fashion by the anatomists Gall and Spurzheim (1819). They believed that every intellectual and moral property had its own position on the surface of the brain (Fig. 2.7) and that the degree of development of these dispositions could be identified by locating overlying protuberances on the skull (Fig. 2.8). However, the theory of localisation gained respectability after the stimulation experiments of Fritsch and Hitzig (1870) on anaesthetised dogs, in which they found that weak electrical currents applied through platinum electrodes to the anterior regions of the brain surface produced muscle contractions in the opposite half of the body. The clash between the adherents of the two theories culminated in 1881 at the Third International Congress of Medicine held in London (Thorwald, 1957). The equipotentialists were represented by the German physiologist Goltz, who showed the audience a dog in which a substantial portion of the

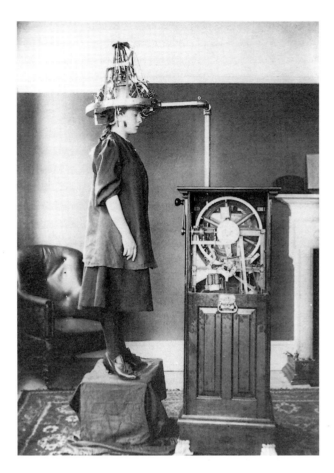

Figure 2.8 The pseudo-science of phrenology lived on well beyond the 19th century. The Lavery Electric Phrenometer of 1907 was intended to lend modern accuracy to the measurements of bumps on the skull. (Reproduced from Blakemore, 1977; by kind permission of the author and Cambridge University Press.)

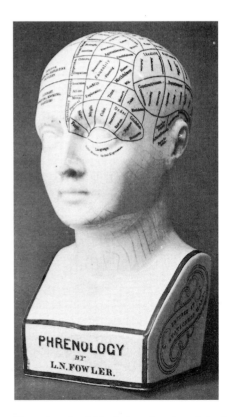

Figure 2.7 Phrenology head (Fowler); each region of the skull is supposed to represent a mental faculty, such as 'mirthfulness', 'perception of form' or 'ideality'.

brain had been removed by means of a hose, but who could still move all limbs, trunk and tail, and who had retained all his senses. Later, it would turn out that the lesions were less extensive than had been claimed, and on the same afternoon Ferrier showed two chimpanzees, one deaf after removal of the auditory cortex, the other limping with a hemiplegic gait after extirpation of the contralateral motor area (the sight of which led Charcot to exclaim: 'Mais c'est un patient!').

The localisationists had won the day, but they won too completely. The greater part of the brain has no 'primary' motor, sensory or cognitive tasks, and serves to connect and integrate the separate 'functions'. Similarly, everyday life consists of a multitude of tasks that are integrated and difficult to separate. Mood, initiative and speed of thinking are some of the essential features of human life that can be severely affected by stroke but are sadly ignored in 'stroke scales'. It is therefore naïve to try and rebuild an entire human being from separate 'functions', even apart from the insoluble problem of how to add up the different items to something meaningful. Patients are more than the sum of their signs (van Gijn & Warlow, 1992). A higher, more integrated level of measurement is needed; that is, scales should measure function not at the level of the organ but at the level of the person (disability scales), or even at the level of social interaction (handicap scales). What really counts for patients is what they can do in life, compared with what they want to do or were once able to do.

2.9.3 Meta-analysis and systematic reviews

Richard Peto and his collaborators have developed a method to overcome the problem that single studies may or may not show a significant difference in treated patients compared with controls, but that the magnitude of the difference can only be expressed as a confidence interval, which is usually wide. They developed a method of overviewing all related trials in a given field by which the differences between the treatment group and the control group in each trial are combined (Yusuf *et al.*, 1985). The key assumption is that, if a given treatment has any material effect on the incidence or outcome of disease, then the direction, although not necessarily the size, of this effect tends to be similar in different circumstances. If all available studies are combined, the confidence interval can be narrowed considerably and reviewer bias is avoided. There is a pressing need for up-to-date systematic reviews of all the available evidence regarding the various aspects of care of stroke patients — indeed, of all medical interventions. This need has led to the Cochrane Collaboration, which includes a stroke review group (Counsell *et al.*, 1995).

References

Abercrombie J (1828). *Pathological and Clinical Researches on Diseases of the Brain and Spinal Cord*. Edinburgh: Waugh & Innes.

Abercrombie J (1836). *Pathological and Practical Researches on Diseases of the Brain and Spinal Cord*, 2nd edn (from 3rd British edn). Philadelphia: Carey, Lea & Blanchard.

Adams RD, vander Eecken HM (1953). Vascular diseases of the brain. *Ann Rev Med* 4: 213–52.

Amarenco P, Duyckaerts C, Tzourio C, Henin D, Bousser MG, Hauw JJ (1992). The prevalence of ulcerated plaques in the aortic arch in patients with stroke. *N Engl J Med* 326: 221–5.

Amarenco P, Cohen A, Tzourio C *et al.* (1994). Atherosclerotic disease of the aortic arch and the risk of ischemic stroke. *N Engl J Med* 331: 1474–9.

Archie JP, Feldtman JP (1981). Critical stenosis of the internal carotid artery. *Surgery* 89: 67–70.

Atlas SW, Listerud J, Chung W, Flamm ES (1994). Intracranial aneurysms: depiction on MR angiograms with a multifeature-extraction, ray-tracing postprocessing algorithm. *Radiology* 192: 129–39.

Baillie M (1793). *The Morbid Anatomy of Some of the Most Important Parts of the Human Body*. London: J Johnson & G Nicol.

Barnett HJM (1979). The pathophysiology of transient cerebral ischemic attacks: therapy with antiplatelet antiaggregants. *Med Clin North Am* 63: 649–80.

Barnett HJM, Plum F, Walton JN (1984). Carotid endarterectomy —an expression of concern. *Stroke* 15: 941–3.

Bayle F (1677). *Tractatus de apoplexia*. Toulouse: B. Guillemette.

Beadles CF (1907). Aneurisms of the larger cerebral arteries. *Brain* 30: 285–336.

Beal MF, Park TS, Fisher CM (1981). Cerebral atheromatous embolism following carotid sinus pressure. *Arch Neurol* 38: 310–12.

Benton AL, Joynt RJ (1960). Early descriptions of aphasia. *Arch Neurol* 3: 205–22.

Berengarius J (1523). *Isagogae breves*. Bologna: Benedictum Hectoris.

Biumi F (1765). Observatio V: Carotis ad receptaculum Vieusenii aneurysmatica etc. In: Anonymous, ed. *Observationes anatomicae, scholiis illustratae*. Milan: S. & J. Lichtmans, 373–9.

Blackall J (1813). *Observations on the Nature and Cure of Dropsies*, 5th edn. London: Longman & Co.

Blakemore C (1977). *Mechanics of the Mind*. Cambridge: Cambridge University Press.

Blum F (1893). Der Formaldehyd als Härtungsmittel—vorläufige Mitteilung. *Z wiss Mikr mikr Technik* 10: 314–15.

Boerhaave H (1959). *Praelectiones de morbis nervorum (1730–1735)*. Leiden: Brill.

Bogousslavsky J, Regli F (1983). Delayed TIAs distal to bilateral occlusion of carotid arteries—evidence for embolic and hemodynamic mechanisms. *Stroke* 14: 58–61.

Brain R (1968). *Diseases of the Nervous System*, 6th edn. Oxford: Oxford University Press.

Bright R (1831). *Diseases of the Brain and Nervous System*. London: Longman, Rees, Orme, Brown & Green.

Brinton W (1852). Report on cases of cerebral aneurism. *Trans Pathol Soc Lond* 3: 47–9.

Bull E (1877). Akut hjerneaneurisma-okulomotoriusparalyse-meningealapoplexi. *Norsk Magasin for Laegevidenskapen* 7: 890–5.

Burger SK, Saul RF, Selhorst JB, Thurston SE (1991). Transient monocular blindness caused by vasospasm. *N Engl J Med* 325: 870–3.

Burrows G (1846). *On Disorders of Cerebral Circulation and on the Connection Between Affections of the Brain and Disease of the Heart*. London: Longman, Brown, Green & Longmans.

Call GK, Fleming MC, Sealfon S, Levine H, Kistler JP, Fisher CM (1988). Reversible cerebral segmental vasoconstriction. *Stroke* 19: 1159–70.

Canadian Cooperative Study Group (1978). A randomized trial of aspirin and sulfinpyrazone in threatened stroke. *N Engl J Med* 299: 53–9.

Caplan LR, Sergay S (1976). Positional cerebral ischaemia. *J Neurol Neurosurg Psychiatr* 39: 385–91.

Carswell R (1838). *Pathological Anatomy: Illustrations of the Elementary Forms of Disease*. London: Longman & Co.

Casserio G (1627). *Tabulae anatomicae (in Adrianus Spigelius' 'De humanis corporis fabrica', libri decem)*. Venice: Daniel Bucretius.

Challa VL, Moody DM, Bell MA (1992). The Charcot–Bouchard aneurysm controversy: impact of a new histologic technique. *J Neuropathol Exp Neurol* 51: 264–71.

Charcot JM, Bouchard C (1868). Nouvelles recherches sur la pathogénie de l'hémorrhagie cérébrale. *Arch Physiol Norm Pathol* 1: 110–27, 643–65, 725–34.

Cheyne J (1812). *Cases of Apoplexy and Lethargy with Observations on Comatose Patients*. London: Underwood.

Chiari H (1905). Über das Verhalten des Teilungswinkels des Carotis Communis bei der Endarteritis chronica deformans. *Verh Ddtsch Path Ges* 9: 326–30.

Clarke E (1963). Apoplexy in the Hippocratic writings. *Bull Hist Med* 37: 301–14.

Clarke E, Dewhurst K (1972). *An Illustrated History of Brain Function*. Oxford: Sandford Publications.

Cohnheim J (1872). *Untersuchungen uber die embolische processe*. Berlin: Hirschwald.

Cole FM, Yates PO (1967). The occurrence and significance of intracerebral micro-aneurysms. *J Pathol Bacteriol* 93: 393–411.

Counsell C, Warlow C, Sandercock P, Fraser H, Van Gijn J (1995). The Cochrane Collaboration Stroke Review Group: meeting the need for systematic reviews in stroke care. *Stroke* 26: 498–502.

Cruveilhier J (1842). *Anatomie pathologique du corps humain; descriptions avec figures lithographiés et coloriés; des diverses altérations morbides dont le corps humain est susceptible*. Paris: J.B. Baillière.

Cushing H (1923). Contributions to the clinical study of cerebral aneurysms. *Guy's Hosp Rep* 73: 159–63.

Dandy WE (1938). Intracranial aneurysm of internal carotid artery, cured by operation. *Ann Surg* 107: 654–7.

De Bono DP, Warlow CP (1981). Potential sources of emboli in patients with presumed transient cerebral or retinal ischaemia. *Lancet* i: 343–6.

Dechambre A (1838). Mémoire sur la curabilité du ramollissement cérébral. *Gaz Méd Paris* 6: 305–14.

Denny-Brown D (1951). The treatment of recurrent cerebrovascular symptoms and the question of 'vasospasm'. *Med Clin North Am* 35: 1457–74.

Dewhurst K (1980). *Thomas Willis's Oxford Lectures*. Oxford: Sandford Publications.

Dott N (1932). Intracranial aneurysms: cerebral arterio-radiography: surgical treatment. *Trans Med Chir Soc Edinb* 47: 219–40.

Drake CG (1961). Bleeding aneurysms of the basilar artery: direct surgical management in four cases. *J Neurosurg* 18: 230–8.

Durand-Fardel CLM (1842). Mémoire sur une altération particulière de la substance cérébrale. *Gaz Méd Paris* 10: 23–38.

Durand-Fardel CLM (1843). *Traité du ramollissement du cerveau*. Paris: J.-B. Baillière.

Eastcott HHG, Pickering GW, Robb CG (1954). Reconstruction of internal carotid artery in a patient with intermittent attacks of hemiplegia. *Lancet* ii: 994–6.

EC/IC Bypass Study Group (1985). Failure of extracranial–intracranial arterial bypass to reduce the risk of ischemic stroke: results of an international randomized trial. *N Engl J Med* 313: 1191–200.

Ellis AG (1909). The pathogenesis of spontaneous intracerebral hemorrhage. *Proc Pathol Soc Philadelphia* 12: 197–235.

Eppinger H (1887). Pathogenesis (Histogenesis und Aetiologie) der Aneurysmen einschliesslich des Aneurysma equi verminosum. *Arch Klin Chir* 35 (Suppl. 1): 1–563.

Fallopius G (1561). *Observationes anatomicae*. Venice: Marcus Antonius Ulmus.

Ferguson FR, Davey AFC, Topley WWC (1927). The value of mixed vaccines in the prevention of the common cold. *J Hyg* 26: 98–109.

Fibiger J (1898). Om serumbehandlung af difteri. *Hospitalstidende* 6: 309–25, 338–50.

Fields WS, Maslenikov V, Meyer JS, Hass WK, Remington RD, Macdonald M (1970). Joint study of extracranial arterial occlusion. V. Progress report of prognosis following surgery or nonsurgical treatment for transient ischemic attacks and cervical carotid artery lesions. *J Am Med Assoc* 211: 1993–2003.

Fieschi C, Argentino C, Lenzi GL, Sacchetti ML, Toni D, Bozzao L (1989). Clinical and instrumental evaluation of patients with ischemic stroke within the first six hours. *J Neurol Sci* 91: 311–21.

Fischer O (1910). Die presbyophrene Demenz, deren anatomische Grundlage und klinische Abgrenzung. *Z Gesamte Neurol Psychiatr* 3: 371–471.

Fisher CM (1951). Occlusion of the internal carotid artery. *Arch Neurol Psych* 65: 346–77.

Fisher CM (1952). Transient monocular blindness associated with hemiplegia. *Arch Ophthalmol* 47: 167–203.

Fisher CM (1959). Observations on the fundus oculi in transient monocular blindness. *Neurology* 9: 333–47.

Fisher CM (1965). Lacunes: small, deep cerebral infarcts. *Neurology* 15: 774–84.

Fisher CM (1969). The arterial lesions underlying lacunes. *Acta Neuropathol (Berl)* 12: 1–15.

Fisher CM, Curry HB (1965). Pure motor hemiplegia of vascular origin. *Arch Neurol* 13: 30–44.

Flourens MJP (1824). *Recherches expérimentales sur les propriétés et les fonctions du système nerveux, dans les animaux vertébrés*. Paris: Crevot.

Franke CL, Ramos LMP, Van Gijn J (1990). Development of multifocal haemorrhage in a cerebral infarct during computed tomography [letter]. *J Neurol Neurosurg Psychiatr* 53: 531–2.

Fritsch GT, Hitzig E (1870). Über die elektrische Erregbarkeit des Grosshirns. *Arch Anat Physiol Wiss Med* 37: 300–32.

Froin G (1904). *Les Hémorrhagies sous-arachnoidiennes et le méchanisme de l'hématolyse en général*. Paris: G. Steinheil.

Galenus (edition of 1824). *Opera omnia*. Leipzig: Cnobloch.

Gall FJ, Spurzheim JC (1819). *Anatomie et physiologie du système nerveux en général, et du cerveau en particulier, avec des observations sur la possibilité de reconnaÎtre plusieurs dispositions intellectuelles et morales de l'homme et des animaux, par la configurations de leurs têtes*. Paris: Schoell.

Globus JH, Epstein JA, Green MA, Marks M (1949). Focal cerebral hemorrhage experimentally induced. *J Neuropathol Exp Neurol* 8: 113–16.

Gowers WR (1893). *A Manual of Diseases of the Nervous System*, 2nd edn. London: J & A Churchill.

Gunning AJ, Pickering GW, Robb-Smith AHT, Ross Russell RW (1964). Mural thrombosis of the internal carotid artery and subsequent embolism. *Quart J Med* 33: 155–95.

Hachinski VM (1982). Transient cerebral ischemia: a historical sketch. In: Clifford Rose F, Bynum WF, eds. *Historical Aspects of the Neurosciences (Festschrift for M. Critchley)*. New York: Raven Press, 185–93.

Hall M (1836). *Lectures on the Nervous System and its Diseases*. London: Sherwood, Gilbert & Piper.

Hammond WA (1881). *Diseases of the Nervous System*. New York: D. Appleton.

Hayakawa I, Watanabe T, Tsuchida T, Sasaki A (1978). Perangiographic rupture of intracranial aneurysms. *Neuroradiology* 16: 293–5.

Hiller F (1935). Zirkulationsstörungen im Gehirn, eine klinische und pathologisch-anatomische Studie. *Arch Psychiatr Nervenkr* 103: 1–53.

Hodgson J (1815). *A Treatise on the Diseases of Arteries and Veins, Containing the Pathology and Treatment of Aneurisms and Wounded Arteries*. London: T Underwood.

Hollenhorst RW (1961). Significance of bright plaques in the retinal arterioles. *J Am Med Assoc* 178: 23–9.

Hope J, Bennett JH, Pritchard JC, Taylor RH, Thomson T (1840). Dissertations on nervous diseases. In: Tweedie A, ed. *Library of Practical Medicine*. Philadelphia: Lea & Blanchard.

Hounsfield GN (1973). Computerised transverse axial scanning (tomography): I. Description of system. *Br J Radiol* 46: 1016–22.

Hunt JR (1914). The role of the carotid arteries, in the causation of vascular lesions of the brain, with remarks on special features of the symptomatology. *Am J Med Sci* 147: 704–13.

Hutchinson J (1875). Aneurism of the internal carotid artery within the skull diagnosed eleven years before the patient's death: spontaneous cure. *Trans Clin Soc Lond* 8: 127–31.

Iragui VJ (1986). The Charcot–Bouchard controversy. *Arch Neurol* 43: 290–5.

Jackson JH (1875). A lecture on softening of the brain. *Lancet* ii: 335–8.

Jelliffe SE, White WA (1923). *Diseases of the Nervous System—a Text-book of Neurology and Psychiatry*. London: H & K Lewis.

Jellinger K (1977). Cerebrovascular amyloidosis with cerebral hemorrhage. *J Neurol* 214: 195–206.

Jonas S (1988). Anticoagulant therapy in cerebrovascular disease: a review and meta-analysis. *Stroke* 19: 1043–8.

Kendell RE, Marshall J (1963). Role of hypotension in the genesis of transient focal cerebral ischaemic attacks. *Br Med J* 2: 344–8.

King LS (1991). *Transformations in American Medicine—from Benjamin Rush to William Osler*. Baltimore: Johns Hopkins University Press.

Kirkes WS (1855). On apoplexy in relation to chronic renal disease. *Med Times Gaz* 11:515–16.

Korogi Y, Takahashi M, Mabuchi N *et al.* (1994). Intracranial aneurysms: diagnostic accuracy of three-dimensional, Fourier transform, time-of-flight MR angiography. *Radiology* 193: 181–6.

Kraaijeveld CL, Van Gijn J, Schouten HJ, Staal A (1984). Interobserver agreement for the diagnosis of transient ischemic attacks. *Stroke* 15: 723–5.

Kuhn TS (1962). *The Structure of Scientific Revolutions*. Chicago: Chicago University Press.

Kurtzke JF (1979). Controversy in neurology: the Canadian study on TIA and aspirin—a critique of the Canadian TIA study. *Ann Neurol* 5: 597–9.

Lallemand F (1824). *Recherches anatomo-pathologiques sur l'encéphale et ses dépendances*. Paris: Béchet.

Lebert H (1866). Über die Aneurysmen der Hirnarterien: eine Abhandlung in Briefen an Herrn Geheimrat Professor Dr. Frerichs. *Berl Klin Wochenschr* 3:209–405 (8 instalments).

Lind J (1753). *A Treatise of the Scurvy*. Edinburgh: Sands, Murray & Cochran.

Ljunggren B, Sharma S, Buchfelder M (1993). Intracranial aneurysms. *Neurosurg Quart* 3: 120–52.

Lobstein JFM (1829). *Traité d'anatomie pathologique*. Paris: Levrault.

Louis PCA (1835). *Recherches sur les effets de la saignée*. Paris: de Mignaret.

McDonald CA, Korb M (1939). Intracranial aneurysms. *Arch Neurol Psych* 42: 298–328.

McHenry LC (1969). *Garrison's History of Neurology*. Springfield: Charles C. Thomas.

McHenry LC (1981). A history of stroke. *Int J Neurol* 15: 314–26.

Markus H (1993). Transcranial Doppler detection of circulating cerebral emboli: a review. *Stroke* 24: 1246–50.

Medical Research Council (1948). Streptomycin treatment of pulmonary tuberculosis. *Br Med J* ii: 425–9.

Meyer A, Hierons R (1962). Observations on the history of the 'Circle of Willis'. *Med Hist* 6: 119–30.

Mistichelli D (1709). *Trattato dell' apoplessia*. Rome: A. de Rossi.

Moniz E (1927). L'encéphalographie artérielle, son importance dans la localisation des tumeurs cérébrales. *Rev Neurol Paris* 48: 72–90.

Moniz E (1933). Anévrysme intra-cranien de la carotide interne droite rendu visible par l'artériographie cérébrale. *Rev Oto-Neuro-Ophthalmol* 11: 198–203.

Moniz E (1940). *Die cerebrale Arteriographie und Phlebographie.* Berlin: Julius Springer.

Morgagni GB (1761). *De sedibus et causis morborum per anatomen indigatis libri quinque.* Vienna: ex typographica Remondiana.

Norris JW, Hachinski VC (1982). Misdiagnosis of stroke. *Lancet* i: 328–31.

Oppenheim H (1913). *Lehrbuch der Nervenkrankheiten für ärtzte und studierende.* Berlin: S Karger.

Osler W (1911). Transient attacks of aphasia and paralysis in states of high blood pressure and arteriosclerosis. *Can Med Assoc J* 1: 919–26.

Pantelakis S (1954). Un type particulier d'angiopathie sénile du système nerveux central: l'angiopathie congophile—topographie et fréquence. *Monatsschr Psychiatr Neurol* 128: 219–56.

Paulus Aegineta (edition of 1844). *The Seven Books (translated by Francis Adams).* London: The Sydenham Society.

Payer L (1989). *Medicine and Culture—Notions of Health and Sickness in Britain, the US, France and West Germany.* London: V Gollancz.

Peabody GL (1891). Relation between arterial disease and visceral changes. *Trans Assoc Am Physicians* 6: 154–78.

Pickering GW (1948). Transient cerebral paralysis in hypertension and in cerebral embolism with special reference to the pathogenesis of chronic hypertensive encephalopathy. *J Am Med Assoc* 137: 423–30.

Portal A (1781). Observations sur l'apoplexie. *Hist l'Acad Sci* 83: 623–30.

Quincke H (1891). Die Lumbalpunktion des Hydrocephalus. *Berl Klin Wochenschr* 28: 965–8.

Raynaud M (1862). *De l'asphyxie locale et de la gangrène symmétrique des extrémités.* Paris: L Leclerc.

Reed RL, Siekert RG, Merideth J (1973). Rarity of transient focal cerebral ischemia in cardiac dysrhythmia. *J Am Med Assoc* 223: 893–5.

Rosenblath L (1918). Über die Entstehung der Hirnblutung bei dem Schlaganfall. *Dtsch Z Nervenkr* 61: 10–143.

Ross Russell RW (1961). Observations on the retinal blood-vessels in monocular blindness. *Lancet* ii: 1422–8.

Ross Russell RW (1963). Observations on intracerebral aneurysms. *Brain* 86: 425–42.

Ross Russell RW, Page NGR (1983). Critical perfusion of the brain and retina. *Brain* 106: 434.

Rostan L (1820). *Recherches sur le ramollissement du cerveau. Ouvrage dans lequel on s'efforce de distinguer les diverses affections de ce viscère par des signes caractéristiques,* 1st edn. Paris: Béchet.

Rush C, Shaw JF (1990). *With Sharp Compassion: Norman Dott—Freeman Surgeon of Edinburgh.* Aberdeen: Aberdeen University Press.

Russel W (1909). A post-graduate lecture on intermittent closing of the cerebral arteries: its relation to temporary and permanent paralysis. *Br Med J* 2: 1109–10.

Saitoh H, Hayakawa K, Nishimura K et al. (1995). Rerupture of cerebral aneurysms during angiography. *Am J Neuroradiol* 16: 539–42.

Satran R (1974). Joseph Babinski in the competitive examination (agrégation) of 1892. *Bull NY Acad Med* 50: 626–35.

Schiller F (1970). Concepts of stroke before and after Virchow. *Med Hist* 14: 115–31.

Scholz W (1938). Studien zur Pathologieder Hirngefässe. II. Die drusige Entartung der Hirnarterien und -capillaren. *Z Gesamte Neurol Psychiatr* 162: 694–715.

Schorstein J (1940). Carotid ligation in saccular intracranial aneurysms. *Br J Surg* 28: 50–70.

Schwartz P (1961). *Cerebral Apoplexy—Types, Causes, and Pathogenesis.* Springfield, Ill.: Charles C Thomas.

Seldinger SI (1953). Catheter replacement of the needle in percutaneous arteriography. *Acta Radiol* 39: 368–78.

Serres ERA (1819). Nouvelle division des apoplexies. *Ann Méd Chir* 1: 246–363.

Serres ERA (1826). Observations sur la rupture des anévrysmes des artères du cerveau. *Arch Gén Méd* 10: 419–31.

Siebler M, Sitzer M, Rose G, Bendfeldt D, Steinmetz H (1993). Silent cerebral embolism caused by neurologically symptomatic high-grade carotid stenosis: event rates before and after carotid endarterectomy. *Brain* 116: 1005–15.

Soloway HB, Aronson SM (1964). Atheromatous emboli to central nervous system. *Arch Neurol* 11: 657–67.

Symonds CP (1923). Contributions to the clinical study of intracranial aneurysms. *Guy's Hosp Rep* 73: 139–58.

Thorwald J (1957). *Das Weltreich der Chirurgen.* Stutttgart: Steingrüben.

Todd EM (1991). *The Neuroanatomy of Leonardo da Vinci.* Park Ridge: American Association of Neurological Surgeons.

Todd NV, Howie JE, Miller JD (1990). Norman Dott's contribution to aneurysm surgery. *J Neurol Neurosurg Psychiatr* 53: 455–8.

Torack RM (1975). Congophilic angiopathy complicated by surgery and massive hemorrhage: a light and electron microscopic study. *Am J Pathol* 81: 349–65.

Turnbull HM (1914). Alterations in arterial structure, and their relation to syphilis. *Quart J Med* 8: 201–54.

van Gijn J (1992). Measurement of outcome in stroke prevention trails. *Cerebrovasc Dis* 2 (Suppl. 1): 23–34.

van Gijn J, Warlow CP (1992). Down with stroke scales! *Cerebrovasc Dis* 2: 244–6.

van Swieten G (1754). *Of the Apoplexy, Palsy and Epilepsy—Commentaries upon the Aphorisms of Dr. Herman Boerhaave.* London: J & P Knapton.

van Zuilen EV, Moll FL, Vermeulen FE, Mauser HW, Van Gijn J, Ackerstaff RG (1995). Detection of cerebral microemboli by means of transcranial Doppler monitoring before and after carotid endarterectomy. *Stroke* 26: 210–13.

Vesling J (1647). *Syntagma anatomicum, locis pluribus actum, emendatum, novisque iconibus diligenter exornatum.* Patavii:

Pauli Frombotti Bibliopolae.

Vicq d'Azyr F (1786). *Traité d'anatomie et de physiologie*. Paris: FA Didot.

Virchow RLK (1847). Ueber die akute Entzündung der Arterien. *Archiv Pathol Anat* 1: 272–378.

Virchow RLK (1856). Thrombose und Embolie: GefassentzÜndung und septische Infektion. In: Virchow RLK, ed. *Gesammelte abhandlungen zur wissenschaftlichen Medizin*. Frankfurt: Meidinger, 219–735.

Warlow C (1984). Carotid endarterectomy: does it work? *Stroke* 15: 1068–76.

Watts C (1982). External carotid artery embolus from the internal carotid artery 'stump' during angiography—case report. *Stroke* 13: 515–17.

Wepfer JJ (1658). *Observationes anatomicae, ex cadaveribus eorum, quos sustulit apoplexia, cum exercitatione de ejus loco affecto*. Schaffhausen: JC Suteri.

Westphal K (1932). Über die Entstehung und Behandlung der Apoplexia sanguinea. *Dtsch Med Wschr* 58: 685–90.

Wichern H (1912). Klinische Beiträge zur Kenntnis der Hirnaneurysmen. *Dtsch Zschr Nervenheilk* 44: 220–63.

Williamson JW, German PS, Weiss R, Skinner EA, Bowes F, IIIrd (1989). Health science information management and continuing education of physicians: a survey of US primary care practitioners and their opinion leaders. *Ann Intern Med* 110: 151–60.

Willis T (1684). *Dr. Willis's Practice of Physick*. London: Dring, Harper & Leigh.

Witmer R, Schmid A (1958). Cholesterinkristall als retinaler arterieller Embolus. *Ophthalmologica* 135: 432–3.

Wood GB (1852). *Treatise on the Practice of Medicine*. Philadelphia: Lippincott.

Yusuf S, Peto R, Lewis J, Collins R, Sleight P (1985). Beta blockade during and after myocardial infarction: an overview of the randomized trials. *Prog Cardiovasc Dis* 27: 335–71.

Zanette EM, Roberti C, Mancini G, Pozzilli C, Bragoni M, Toni D (1995). Spontaneous middle cerebral artery reperfusion in ischemic stroke: a follow-up study with transcranial Doppler. *Stroke* 26: 430–3.

Is it a vascular event?
Transient ischaemic attack or stroke

3

3.1   Definition of a vascular event

3.1.1   What is a transient ischaemic attack (TIA)?

A TIA is a clinical syndrome characterised by an acute loss of focal cerebral or monocular function with symptoms lasting less than 24 hours and which is thought to be due to inade-quate cerebral or ocular blood supply as a result of arterial thrombosis or embolism associated with arterial, cardiac or haematological disease (Hankey & Warlow, 1994). Abnormal but functionally unimportant focal neurological signs such as reflex asymmetry or an extensor plantar response may persist for longer (in about 5% of patients (Hankey *et al.*, 1991)) and cranial computerised tomography (CT) or magnetic resonance imaging (MRI) evidence of infarction may be present in an area of the brain relevant to the transient symptoms in at least 25% of patients (Awad *et al.*, 1986; Dennis *et al.*, 1990a; Hankey & Warlow, 1994). In patients with transient monocular symptoms, emboli may or may not be seen in the retina.

Because the diagnosis of TIA is clinical and can not be based on any specific diagnostic test, we have to rely on a certain constellation of clinical features that are thought to have a similar pathophysiological background (i.e. caused by focal cerebral or ocular ischaemia) and to be associated with similar outcomes (i.e. an increased risk of stroke and coronary events). Non-focal neurological symptoms such as faintness, non-specific dizzines, light-headedness, confusion, mental deterioration, incontinence, drop attacks or syncope do not suggest TIAs unless they are clearly accompanied by focal neurological symptoms (see Section 3.3.4). Neither do some focal neurological symptoms when they occur in isolation (such as rotational vertigo, diplopia or dysphagia) because these may all occur with diffuse cerebral ischaemia or in non-vascular conditions. Transient global amnesia (TGA) (see Section 3.3.2) and migraine attacks (see Section 3.3.2) are also not considered to be TIAs because their prognosis is much better than that of TIA patients (Hodges & Warlow, 1990a, b; Dennis & Warlow, 1992).

3.1.2 What is a stroke?

A stroke is a clinical syndrome characterised by rapidly developing clinical symptoms and/or signs of focal, and at times global (applied to patients in deep coma and those with subarachnoid haemorrhage), loss of cerebral function, with symptoms lasting more than 24 hours or leading to death, with no apparent cause other than that of vascular origin (Hatano, 1976). This definition embraces stroke due to cerebral infarction, primary intracerebral haemorrhage (PICH), intraventricular haemorrhage and most cases of subarachnoid haemorrhage (SAH); it does not include subdural haemorrhage, epidural haemorrhage, or intracerebral haemorrhage (ICH) or infarction caused by infection or tumour. The flaw in this definition is that it does not embrace the small subgroup of patients with SAH who are conscious and have no focal neurological signs apart from a stiff neck. A caveat therefore needs to be added to the standard definition of stroke: that the sudden onset of headache and isolated sign of meningism, without focal or global neurological dysfunction, can be a stroke due to SAH.

3.1.3 Do we need to distinguish between transient ischaemic attack (TIA) and stroke?

The duration of the symptoms of focal neurological dysfunction (i.e. less or more than 24 hours) is the only factor which distinguishes TIA from mild ischaemic stroke, even though most TIAs last minutes rather than hours (Fig. 3.1). Otherwise, patients with TIA and mild ischaemic stroke are qualitatively the same; they are of similar age and sex, have a similar prevalence of co-existent vascular risk factors (and probably therefore pathogenesis; see Section 6.1.1) and share the same long-term prognosis for serious vascular events (see Section 16.1.1). As the only distinction between TIA and mild ischaemic stroke is quantitative and purely arbitrary (being made by a World Health Organization (WHO) committee in 1978 (WHO, 1978), there is no press-

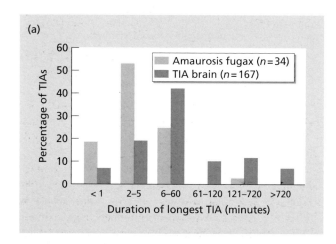

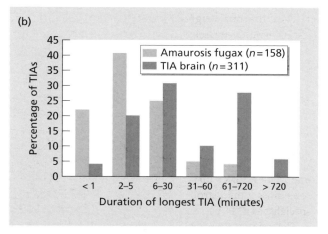

Figure 3.1 Histogram of the duration of the longest TIA before presentation amongst: (a) 184 TIA patients (of whom some had had amaurosis fugax and cerebral attacks) in the Oxfordshire Community Stroke Project; (b) 469 TIA patients in a hospital-referred series. (Adapted from Hankey & Warlow, 1994; reproduced with permission of WB Saunders Co. Ltd.)

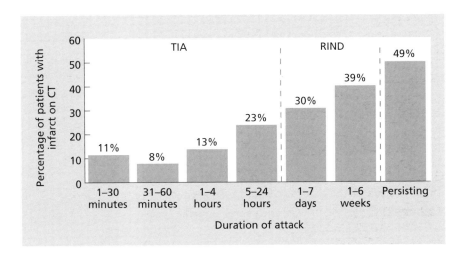

Figure 3.2 Duration of attack and percentage of patients with an appropriately sited low-density area on brain CT scan. RIND, a so-called reversible ischaemic neurological deficit. (Adapted from Koudstaal *et al.*, 1992; reproduced with permission of the *Journal of Neurology, Neurosurgery and Psychiatry*.)

ing need to distinguish them in clinical practice and clinical trials; it is probably more useful to distinguish patients with reversible ischaemic attacks (who recover in minutes, days or weeks) from those with major disabling ischaemic stroke and a permanent handicap.

Distinguishing between transient ischaemic attacks and mild ischaemic strokes is arbitrary and not particularly useful when considering prognosis and treatment. However, the distinction is important in differential diagnosis, case–control studies and in measuring stroke incidence.

It is useful, however, to distinguish between TIA and minor ischaemic stroke when formulating a differential diagnosis and when conducting incidence and case–control studies of cerebrovascular disease. This is because of the following.

1 The differential diagnosis of focal neurological symptoms lasting minutes (e.g. seizure, migraine) is quite different from that of attacks lasting several hours to days (e.g. intracranial tumour, intracranial haemorrhage).

2 Incidence studies of cerebrovascular disease are likely to achieve less complete case ascertainment for TIA than for stroke because patients who experience brief attacks (i.e. TIA) are more likely to ignore or forget them and less likely to report them to a doctor than patients who suffer more prolonged or disabling events (i.e. stroke). Nonetheless, it is important to check up on any TIAs that are reported because sometimes a mild stroke is incorrectly labelled by the non-specialist as a 'TIA'.

3 The reliability of the clinical diagnosis of stroke is much better than for TIA.

4 For case–control studies there is less change in haemostatic factors and no survival bias amongst TIA patients.

Are the findings on brain imaging relevant to the distinction?

Imaging of the brain of patients with TIA by CT or MRI has led some authors to suggest that patients with transient focal neurological symptoms lasting less than 24 hours but who have an anatomically appropriate area of presumed infarction on the scan should not be classified as TIAs but as 'cerebral infarction with transient signs' (CITS) (Waxman & Toole, 1983; Bogousslavsky & Regli, 1984; Murros *et al.*, 1989). The problems with this classification are as follow.

1 A CT, and now an MRI, scan becomes essential for the diagnosis of TIA and as technology advances the definition of a TIA would change.

2 The detection of ischaemic lesions by CT and MRI depends on the timing and resolution of the scan and the quality of the neuroradiologist (Awad *et al.*, 1986; Hommel *et al.*, 1990; Bryan *et al.*, 1991).

3 The relevant area on CT or MRI may not represent infarction occurring at the time of the TIA (it may be an old infarct or even an old haemorrhage).

4 A new diagnostic category would have to be made for patients with a clinically definite stroke who have a normal CT or MRI, which could hardly be called a 'TIA' (Hankey & Warlow, 1994).

Furthermore, there is a gradual increase in the percentage of patients with a relevant infarct on brain CT scan as the duration of symptoms increases, with no distinct change at 24 hours (Fig. 3.2). The most important clinical issue is whether the presence or absence of presumed brain infarction in TIA patients has any meaning as an independent predictor of subsequent important vascular events, such as stroke. At present, there appear to be no significant differences in the clinical features, prevalence of vascular risk factors and characteristics of the TIA in patients with and without a relevant infarct on CT (Dennis *et al.*, 1990a; Koudstaal *et al.*, 1991a; Eliasziw *et al.*, 1995), but it is uncertain whether the presence of such a 'TIA scar' is associated with an increased risk of future stroke (see Section 16.1) (Dennis *et al.*, 1990a; Dutch TIA Trial Study Group, 1993). Therefore, patients with clinically definite TIAs who have an appropriately sited and presumably ischaemic lesion on CT or MRI should have the fact noted but still be classified as having had a TIA and not a stroke, in the same way as patients who have some residual, but functionally insignificant, neurological signs are classified as a TIA if the *symptoms* really did resolve in 24 hours.

> *The brain CT and MRI scan appearances of presumed ischaemic lesions in the relevant part of the brain in patients presenting with transient ischaemic attack should not change the diagnosis of transient ischaemic attack to stroke.*

3.2 The clinical approach to the diagnosis of a vascular event

The first issue to address when evaluating a patient presenting with a suspected TIA or stroke is whether the symptoms (and signs) are those of a cerebrovascular event or not. As the cardinal features of a cerebrovascular event are the sudden onset of a loss of focal neurological function, the patient's *history* is obviously crucial for establishing the onset of the symptoms. If the symptoms have resolved at the time of assessment (as is usually the case in patients with suspected TIAs), the history is also the only avenue for determining the nature of the symptoms. However, if the patient still has a neurological deficit, it should be possible to establish the presence or absence of focal neurological signs (i.e. hemiparesis, dysphasia) by means of the neurological examination. The next issue is to determine whether any focal neurological signs are new (due to the TIA/stroke) or old (due to a previous neurological event or condition) and, if new, whether they have changed at all since the onset and, if so, in what way. This can frequently be resolved by asking the patient and family members whether they had noticed any of the deficits before the event, and whether any new features have developed subsequently, but this is only possible if they can actually recognise the deficit(s) being referred to (e.g. hemiparesis may be easily recognised but visual–spatial–perceptual dysfunction may not). Further clarification may be required through the use of special investigations such as CT or MRI scan, which might reveal evidence of recent or old cerebral infarction or haemorrhage, or other relevant brain pathology.

> *When a patient presents with a suspected transient ischaemic attack or stroke, the first question to answer is whether it really is a vascular event or not. This begins with and depends on a sound, carefully taken clinical history.*
>
> *The diagnosis of a cerebrovascular event is usually made at the bedside, not in the laboratory or in the X-ray department. It depends on the history of the sudden onset of focal neurological symptoms in the right milieu (usually an older patient with vascular risk factors) and the exclusion of other conditions which can present in a similar way.*

In this chapter we will work systematically through the diagnostic process required to determine whether the event was vascular in origin or not (Table 3.1). Eliciting and recognising the clinical features of a cerebrovascular event do not require a sophisticated knowledge of neurology but a careful history from the patient, observers, family members and friends, combined with a review of the patient's medical records (if available). The examination may not only confirm the presence of focal neurological signs in patients with a residual deficit but also uncover disorders not anticipated from the history (e.g. malignant hypertension with grade IV hypertensive retinopathy); provide information about the possible cause of the event (e.g. atrial fibrillation, elevated blood pressure, carotid bruits, cardiac murmurs, retinal emboli, etc.; see Section 6.5); and guide investigation and treatment (e.g. it is important to check that the femoral pulses are palpable before proceeding to contrast angiography or angioplasty). The art of diagnosis is to accord these features certain degrees of importance in isolation and in

Table 3.1 Model of the diagnostic process: is it a vascular event or not?

---

1 Are the neurological symptoms *focal* rather than *non-focal*?
2 Are the focal neurological symptoms *negative* rather than *positive*?
3 Was the *onset* of the focal neurological symptoms *sudden*?
4 Were the focal neurological symptoms *maximal at onset* rather than progressing over a period?

If the answer to all of these questions is yes, the symptoms are almost certainly caused by a vascular pathology (cerebral ischaemia or haemorrhage). The following question helps distinguish between TIA and stroke

5 How *long* did the focal neurological symptoms last for? or are they still present?

combination; combining the information often adds greatly to diagnostic accuracy.

Unavailable medical records may reflect laziness on the part of a physician who has not bothered to find them rather than the real lack of any records at all.

Initially, it is important to take the patient back to the event and to work through it in chronological order, recording the words used by the patient and not your interpretation of them. The critical information concerns the onset of the presenting neurological symptoms, their anatomical location (i.e. where in the body), nature (focal or non-focal, negative or positive quality) and temporal course, and the presence of any associated symptoms or relevant past history (Table 3.2) (Hankey, 1994).

3.2.1 The onset of the symptoms

Sudden onset

A patient with a TIA or stroke usually describes the abrupt onset of symptoms of focal neurological or monocular dysfunction, which are without warning and are more or less maximal at onset. If different parts of the body (e.g. face, upper limb and lower limb) are affected, the symptoms more often start at the same time in each of the affected body parts than intensify or spread ('march') from one part to another. It is the suddenness with which the neurological deficit develops that stamps the event as vascular. To check on this it is useful to ask the patient what they were doing at the time of onset of symptoms; if they do not remember, the onset was probably not that sudden. Sometimes, however, the focal neurological deficit develops over more than a few seconds or minutes; it may progress steadily over minutes or hours, it may develop in a saltatory (stuttering/stepwise) fashion over several hours, and occasionally it may develop over a few days. Figure 3.3 attempts to demonstrate this, and thus how it may not be possible to be certain whether the diagnosis is a TIA/stroke or not, but simply what the probabilities are. It is the level of uncertainty which determines the extent of the investigations to confirm the diagnosis.

Most ischaemic events start suddenly without any obvious precipitant. The symptoms may or may not worsen gradually or in a stepwise fashion, but nonetheless their onset is sudden.

Precipitants

More ischaemic and haemorrhagic strokes occur during the morning than later, especially between 8 and 10 AM, but

Table 3.2 Important clinical history to obtain from the patient, witness or family member in the consulting room or at the bedside.

1 The *onset* of the symptoms
   What day and at what time of the day did the symptoms start?
   What were you doing at the time?
      (i.e. were there any precipitating events such as certain activities or a change in posture?)
   Was the onset sudden?
      (if the time of onset can be specified and the patient or witness can describe what the patient was doing at the time, it almost certainly was sudden)
   Was the loss of function (neurological deficit) more or less maximal at onset; did it spread or progress in a stepwise, remitting or progressive fashion over minutes/hours/days; or were there fluctuations between normal and abnormal function?
2 The *anatomical location* of the symptoms
   Which parts of the body were affected?
      (e.g. was it all or part of the face, arm, leg; was it one or both eyes? Note: for some symptoms, such as 'dizziness', this is not applicable)
3 The *nature* of the neurological symptoms
   What exactly did you experience?
      Focal or non-focal symptoms
      Quality (i.e. 'negative', causing a loss of sensory, motor or visual function; or 'positive', causing limb jerking, tingling, hallucinations)
4 *Accompanying* symptoms
   Did you notice or feel anything else around the time of the attack or since?
      (e.g. headache, epileptic seizures, panic and anxiety, vomiting, hiccups, loss of consciousness, chest pain, palpitations, breathlessness, weight loss, skin rash, joint pains, pulsatile tinnitus)
5 The occurrence, date and nature of any *previous attacks* of TIA or stroke
6 The *past medical (particularly vascular) history*
   Hypertension, hypercholesterolaemia, diabetes mellitus, angina, myocardial infarction, intermittent claudication, arteritis
7 The *family history (particularly vascular)*
8 *Lifestyle habits/behaviours*
   Cigarette-smoking, alcohol consumption, diet, physical activity, medications

some also occur during sleep (Wroe *et al.*, 1992). It is not known whether there is also diurnal variation in onset of TIA. The cause of the circadian variation in stroke onset is unexplained. Indeed, the onset of symptoms of TIA and stroke is seldom associated with a precipitating event. Nevertheless, it is important to ask the patient exactly what he/she was doing at the onset of the event because a change in posture (Hankey & Gubbay, 1987), neck turning, exposure to bright or white light (Furlan *et al.*, 1979), exercise, a hot bath, a heavy meal (postprandial hypotension) (Kamata *et al.*, 1994) or sexual intercourse (Teman *et al.*, 1995) may

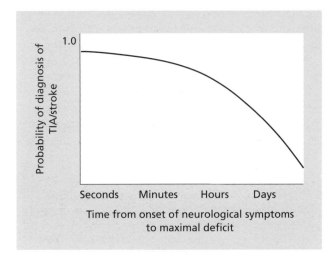

Figure 3.3 Graph illustrating that probability of an event being vascular depends on the time interval from onset of focal neurological symptoms to the maximal neurological deficit. If symptoms or signs increase over days or weeks, the diagnosis of stroke becomes less likely. This graph should *not* be interpreted as indicating that symptoms which last for seconds only are almost certainly vascular.

provoke cerebral and ocular ischaemic symptoms *in the right milieu* (i.e. in people with severe carotid and vertebrobasilar occlusive disease and a compromised collateral cerebral and ocular circulation; see Section 6.5.6). Of course, some of these stimuli may also provoke non-vascular symptoms, such as those due to hypoglycaemia (after a large carbohydrate meal) and seizures (after exposure to bright flashing lights). In addition, symptoms on waking from a general anaesthetic or cardiac arrest, or shortly after starting hypotensive drugs or vasodilators, or after undergoing cardioversion are compelling evidence for a haemodynamic cause (i.e. 'low-flow' TIA/stroke due to the combination of systemic hypotension, focal arterial stenosis/occlusion/compression and poor collateral circulation) (see Section 6.5.5). The last trimester of pregnancy and the puerperium are times when otherwise healthy young women may be predisposed to stroke as a result of paradoxical embolism from the venous system of the legs or pelvis, intracranial haemorrhage due to eclampsia, a ruptured arteriovenous malformation (AVM) and intracranial venous sinus thrombosis (see Section 7.11).

Occasionally, the aura of a previously experienced and otherwise unremarkable attack of migraine with aura persists for days or longer, the CT is normal or shows infarction, and the cause is attributed to arterial occlusion that may be due to vasospasm (see Section 7.5). The simultaneous occurrence of a TIA/stroke and a migraine attack may be coincidental and due to *chance* (both conditions are common; the prevalence of migraine in the general population is about 10% and ischaemic cerebrovascular disease is about 0.8%); *causal* (migraine may predispose to cerebral ischaemia by leading to platelet activation, arteriolar constriction and dehydration or cerebral ischaemia may trigger off a migraine attack) (Olesen *et al.*, 1993); or, a *misdiagnosis* (a stroke is misdiagnosed as migraine, e.g. carotid or vertebral artery dissection may cause headache and a neurological deficit due to thromboembolism that is misinterpreted as migraine); or a syndrome suggestive of stroke or migraine is a *manifestation of another disease* such as mitochondrial encephalomyopathy with lactic acidosis and stroke-like episodes (MELAS; see Section 7.15) or an AVM (see Section 8.2.2; Gubbay *et al.*, 1989; Easton, 1993; Welch, 1994).

Vigorous physical activity and coitus have been associated with haemorrhagic stroke, particularly SAH (see Section 5.3.1) However, apart from isolated case reports, there is no evidence that vigorous physical activity, coitus or stress precipitate TIAs and ischaemic stroke (Teman *et al.*, 1995). There is some evidence, however, that severely threatening life events in the preceding year may be one of the determinants of stroke onset (House *et al.*, 1990).

3.2.2 The anatomical location and nature of the neurological symptoms

The anatomical location (i.e. where in the body) and nature of the neurological symptoms of a TIA or stroke reflect the area of the brain that has been deprived of blood supply or compromised by haemorrhage and oedema. For example, if the corticospinal tract is deprived of blood supply at the level of the internal capsule the patient usually notices weakness in the contralateral face, arm and leg, whereas if the level of ischaemia is confined to the parasagittal motor cortex the weakness is usually confined to the contralateral leg (see Section 4.2.3).

Are the neurological symptoms focal or non-focal?

Focal neurological symptoms are those which arise from a disturbance in an identifiable focal area of the brain; for example, unilateral weakness or clumsiness, unilateral sensory loss, speech disorder and double vision (Table 3.3). On the other hand, non-focal symptoms are not anatomically localising; for example, light-headedness, faintness, 'dizziness', generalised weakness and drop attacks (Table 3.4). Non-focal symptoms alone, therefore, should not be interpreted as a TIA or stroke because they are seldom due to focal cerebral ischaemia. However, the neurological symp-

Table 3.3 Focal neurological and ocular symptoms.

Motor symptoms
Weakness or clumsiness of one side of the body, in whole or in part (hemiparesis)
Simultaneous bilateral weakness (paraparesis, quadriparesis)*
Difficulty swallowing (dysphagia)*
Imbalance (ataxia)*

Speech/language disturbances
Difficulty understanding or expressing spoken language (dysphasia)
Difficulty reading (dyslexia) or writing (dysgraphia)
Difficulty calculating (dyscalculia)
Slurred speech (dysarthria)*

Sensory symptoms
Somatosensory
    Altered feeling on one side of the body, in whole or in part (hemisensory disturbance)
Visual
    Loss of vision in one eye, in whole or in part (transient monocular blindness or amaurosis fugax)
    Loss of vision in the left or the right half or quarter of the visual field (hemianopia, quadrantanopia)
    Bilateral blindness
    Double vision (diplopia)*

Vestibular symptoms
A spinning sensation (vertigo)*

Behavioural/cognitive symptoms
Difficulty dressing, combing hair, cleaning teeth, etc.; geographical disorientation (visual–spatial–perceptual dysfunction)
Forgetfulness (amnesia)*

---

* As an *isolated* symptom, this does not necessarily indicate transient focal cerebral ischaemia.

Table 3.4 Non-focal neurological symptoms.

Generalised weakness and/or sensory disturbance
Light-headedness
Faintness
'Blackouts' with altered or loss of consciousness or fainting, with or without impaired vision in both eyes
Incontinence of urine or faeces
Confusion
Any of the following symptoms, if isolated*
    A spinning sensation (vertigo)
    Ringing in ears (tinnitus)
    Difficulty swallowing (dysphagia)
    Slurred speech (dysarthria)
    Double vision (diplopia)
    Loss of balance (ataxia)

---

* If these symptoms occur in combination, or with focal neurological symptoms, they may indicate focal cerebral ischaemia.

toms are not always easy to categorise; sensory and motor disturbances in a pseudo-radicular pattern (such as a wrist-drop or tingling in two or three fingers) may reflect focal neurological dysfunction (Kim, 1994); so may cognitive changes such as amnesia, but these can be difficult to characterise and quantify, particularly when transient. Vertigo, confusion and dysarthria may reflect either focal or non-focal pathology, dependng on whether other definitely focal neurological symptoms occur concurrently and wheter they occur in the right milieu.

> *Focal cerebral ischaemia causes focal neurological symptoms. Non-focal symptoms such as faintness, dizziness or generalised weakness are seldom, if ever, due to a transient ischaemic attack or stroke.*

What is the quality of the symptoms: negative or positive?

The symptoms of TIA and stroke are usually 'negative' in quality, representing a loss of function. Examples include loss of muscle power in a limb (rather than jerking of a limb), loss of sensation (rather than paraesthesia/tingling) and loss of vision (rather than seeing things such as flashing lights).

What functions are affected and how?

The physical functions that are affected by TIA and stroke reflect the areas of the brain that have been damaged (by ischaemia, haemorrhage or oedema), the extent of the damage and what the patient is doing at the time. The latter is particularly relevant for TIA patients because the neurological symptoms during a brief episode of ischaemia can only reflect the activities in which the patient was engaged during the attack. As many hours of wakefulness are spent in an alert state with eyes open, a keen sensorium, an upright posture and often speaking or reading, it is not surprising that most of the symptoms that TIA patients experience are of motor, somatosensory, visual or speech function (Table 3.5). Other, more transient activities, such as swallowing and calculation, are—not surprisingly—less frequently reported as being affected during a TIA.

Presumably TIAs, like strokes, can start during sleep, but the patient will be unaware of them if they have resolved before waking, there being no sequelae other than perhaps CT or MRI scan evidence of infarction if a scan is done (for some other reason) some time later. It is therefore crucial to ask the patient with suspected TIA what he/she was doing at the time of the event, not only to identify a possible precipitant (see Section 3.2.1) but to determine what functions could have been noticeably affected by the TIA. For example, if the patient was not engaged in conversation or

Table 3.5 Neurological symptoms during TIAs.

	Proportion (percentage of 184*)
Unilateral weakness, heaviness or clumsiness	50
Unilateral sensory symptoms	35
Slurred speech (dysarthria)	23
Transient monocular blindness	18
Difficulty speaking (dysphasia)	18
Unsteadiness (ataxia)	12
Dizziness (vertigo)	5
Homonymous hemianopia	5
Double vision (diplopia)	5
Bilateral limb weakness	4
Difficulty swallowing (dysphagia)	1
Crossed motor and sensory loss	1

* The proportion of TIA patients with various focal neurological symptoms from the Oxfordshire Community Stroke Project (Dennis, 1988); many patients had more than one symptom (e.g. weakness as well as sensory loss) and no patients had *isolated* dysarthria, ataxia, vertigo, diplopia or dysphagia.

did not try to speak or read during the event, it is impossible to know if dysphasia or dyslexia was present or not. Similarly, a weak leg may well not be noticed if the patient remained seated or supine.

Weakness

Motor symptoms, such as 'weakness', 'heaviness' and 'clumsiness', are the most common symptoms described by TIA and stroke patients (Table 3.5). Although usually accompanied by sensory symptoms of some sort, a minority do have pure motor symptoms. Even so, it is unnecessary to be dogmatic about the presence or absence of sensory symptoms in TIA patients because often a purely weak limb is described by the patient as 'numb' or 'dead', and this can be interpreted by the doctor as a combination of motor and sensory symptoms.

Weakness usually affects one side of the body: the face, arm or leg in isolation; each limb as a whole or in part (i.e. a pseudo-radicular distribution); or a combination of these. The occurrence of crossed weakness (i.e. weakness of one side of the face and the contralateral limbs) indicates a brainstem or multifocal disturbance. In many patients with suspected TIA, unilateral facial weakness is probably under-reported because they do not realise they have had facial weakness unless they have seen themselves in the mirror, or

the attack was witnessed by an observer. If there is a clear history of slurred speech, but no symptoms of cerebellar or bulbar dysfunction, it is reasonable to suspect facial weakness because this may cause dysarthria (if the patient attempts to speak). Having established that facial weakness was present, it can be even more difficult to determine which side of the face was weak. This is because the interpretation and recall of the patient and any witnesses may have been affected by anxiety and panic during the attack. Alternatively, the patient and witnesses may have suffered from left–right confusion or misinterpreted which side of the 'twisted' face was weak and which side was contracting. So, the side of the face which is reported to have been weak is very unreliable and can not be assumed to have been ipsilateral to the limb weakness, unless the patient was clearly dribbling from one side of the mouth or had clear sensory disturbance (as well as the weakness) on one side of the face.

Generalised weakness is a non-focal neurological symptom but is not always used by patients strictly to mean motor weakness; it is sometimes used as a word for fatigue, tiredness, lethargy and loss of balance. However, the sudden onset of clear-cut bilateral weakness (quadriparesis, paraparesis, bilateral facial weakness and face and contralateral hand weakness) together with symptoms of focal neurological (usually cranial nerve) dysfunction may be due to a TIA or stroke, in the brainstem. This is because the corticobulbar and corticospinal tracts from both cerebral hemispheres converge in the ventral brainstem, where they share a common blood supply (the basilar artery) and so may be concurrently affected by ischaemia or haemorrhage.

Unsteadiness is a fairly common symptom in TIA/stroke patients but, unless associated with clearly focal symptoms or residual neurological signs of weakness or ataxia, it can be difficult to decide whether the patient means weakness, incoordination, vertigo, presyncope or anxiety, or indeed a combination of these. Sometimes it is helpful to ask the patient whether he/she felt unsteady in the head or in the legs.

Movement disorders

Hemiballismus, unilateral asterixis, hemichorea and focal dystonia are uncommon but well-recognised manifestations of contralateral small deep vascular lesions of the subthalamic nucleus, striatum and thalamus (Kase *et al.*, 1981; Russo, 1983; Stell *et al.*, 1994), and involuntary tonic limb spasms may arise contralateral to ventral pontine brainstem infarction (Kaufman *et al.*, 1994). Episodes of 'limb-shaking', characterised by brief, repetitive, involuntary, coarse, irregular, wavering, trembling or jerking movements of the contralateral arm and/or leg, are one of the few symptoms of transient focal cerebral ischaemia that are 'positive' (Baquis *et al.*, 1985; Yanagihara *et al.*, 1985; Tatemichi *et al.*, 1990). In contrast to epileptic seizures, these attacks are usually due to severe carotid occlusive disease and are often provoked by postural change (from lying to sitting or standing up), by starting or increasing antihypertensive therapy, and by walking or by hyperextension of the neck, and they may be alleviated promptly by sitting or lying down, all of which suggest they are due to low flow rather than embolism (see Section 6.5.5). In some cases, such attacks have stopped after carotid endarterectomy (Stark, 1985; Baquis *et al.*, 1985). Transient cerebral ischaemia may also masquerade as paroxysmal dyskinesia; Hess *et al.* (1991) have described repetitive, stereotyped, involuntary, left arm movements (painless flexion and pronation of the wrist and elbow followed by abduction of the shoulder and hand behind the head) lasting 1–5 minutes in a patient with distal right internal carotid artery (ICA) occlusion and poor intracranial collateral circulation who, soon after, suffered a right-hemisphere ischaemic stroke.

Speech disturbances

Patients with TIA/stroke may complain of speech difficulty due to an articulatory and/or a language disturbance. If the patient describes slurred speech, as if drunk, and if the ability to understand and express spoken and written language is preserved, then the diagnosis is dysarthria, which is a disorder of articulation of sounds due to motor dysfunction as a result of cerebellar, pyramidal, extrapyramidal or facial nerve dysfunction. If the main difficulty is understanding or expressing spoken or written language, such as difficulty reading (can see the letters but can not make sense of them), difficulty writing even though the use of the hand is otherwise normal, difficulty producing sentences with words not being in their proper place or even non-words being used, then the diagnosis is dysphasia, and this is usually due to dominant frontotemporoparietal dysfunction (see Sections 4.2.5 and 15.30). If speech production is so severely affected that the patient is mute, it is important to ascertain whether it is a language deficit (dysphasia) or a motor deficit (dysarthria) which is present. This can be difficult in the acute stage but, as the patient recovers some speech, a more accurate assessment can be made. Also an anarthric patient will be able to follow written commands and write normally whereas an aphasic patient probably would not. Of course, dysphasia and dysarthria may co-exist.

Swallowing difficulties

Dysphagia is a common feature of acute stroke, as either a focal sign of the direct effects of the stroke on corticobulbar pathways or as a non-focal sign of the secondary effects of cerebral oedema, brain herniation or altered consciousness. However, it is not commonly recognised because it is not assessed particularly well and aspiration may be 'silent' (see Section 15.17) (Kidd *et al.*, 1993, 1995). Dysphagia is even less commonly reported by TIA patients, probably because any transient deficit is unlikely to coincide with eating or drinking and because dysphagia is not always a sign of focal neurological dysfunction (see Section 3.2.2).

Sensory symptoms

Somatosensory symptoms, when present, are usually described by the patient as numbness ('like the numbness I have after going to the dentist'), tingling or a dead sensation; occasionally as loss of temperature sensation when in the bath or shower; and very rarely as pain. In our experience, patients with a lot of pain in the body at the onset of the event often turn out to have a non-organic/functional disorder, and patients with severe localised limb pain tend to have other disorders, such as nerve-root compression in the neck or low back, or even myocardial infarction (MI) if the pain is down the arm or in the hand. Somatosensory symptoms are usually associated with motor symptoms but may occur in isolation. The anatomical distribution of somatosensory symptoms is usually unilateral, affecting the face, arm and/or leg, as it is for motor symptoms. However, it can be very difficult to interpret isolated transient sensory symptoms involving only a part of one extremity, or only one side of the face or around the mouth, during a single attack because they may be a manifestation of other disorders such as nerve or root entrapment (e.g. median neuropathy at the wrist, cervical radiculopathy in the neck), multiple sclerosis (MS), hyperventilation and even conversion hysteria (see Section 3.3.2). A recent review of 82 patients who were investigated for unilateral motor and/or sensory symptoms, without 'hard' neurological signs, found that a physical disorder was considerably more likely if the symptoms were on the right side of the body than on the left (Rothwell, 1994), supporting previous work suggesting that hyperventilation and conversion hysteria are associated with predominantly left-sided symptoms (Stern, 1977; Galin *et al.*, 1977; Blau *et al.*, 1983; Perkin & Joseph, 1986). The reason is uncertain, although it may be related to asymmetrical hemispheric function during altered mood; during anxiety states perception of left-sided visual and auditory stimuli is increased whereas in depression perception is greatest for right-sided stimuli (Liotti *et al.*, 1991).

'Neglect'

Visual–spatial–perceptual dysfunction, sometimes manifesting as 'neglect' of one side of the body or extrapersonal space, characteristically occurs in patients with dysfunction of the parietal lobe of the non-dominant cerebral hemisphere but can sometimes occur with dominant-hemisphere lesions. Relatives may report little more than 'confusion' or 'difficulty dressing' (Hier *et al.*, 1983; Devinsky *et al.*, 1988). Therefore, if suspected from the history, visuospatial problems should be carefully and systematically sought in the examination. If the deficit has persisted, neglect can be identified by tests that involve reading a menu, selecting named coins from an array on a card, indicating items of food on a plate, pointing to objects scattered around the room, cancelling or bisecting lines on a piece of paper, cancelling stars, clock-drawing and figure-copying (see Sections 4.2.5 and 15.29) (Stone *et al.*, 1992; Ishiai *et al.*, 1993).

Visual symptoms

Vision can be affected by both vascular and non-vascular diseases of the eye and brain. Visual symptoms associated with cerebral and retinal ischaemia are generally of three types: obscuration or loss of vision in one eye, in both eyes or double vision. Rarely, visual hallucinations occur.

Many patients have a great deal of difficulty describing visual symptoms. The first step in the assessment of a patient complaining of visual disturbance is to sort out whether the visual disturbance involved/involves one or both eyes. This can be particularly difficult in patients whose visual disturbance has resolved before the clinical assessment (i.e. TIA patients), and a frequent clinical problem is trying to differentiate a transient homonymous hemianopia from transient monocular blindness (TMB). Further clarification is required by asking the patient what they saw (was it only half of everything?) and whether they covered each eye in turn during the episode of visual disturbance. For patients without any residual visual disturbance it can be useful to cover one eye and ask the patient whether that reproduces the effect they experienced. It is important to interpret the patient's symptoms clearly because some patients use the term 'blackout' to mean bilateral blindness (and not syncope) and some patients who report 'blurred vision' in both eyes may actually be trying to describe double vision (see below). We find it useful to establish the severity of the visual disturbance; complete loss of vision, unable to find their way around, unable to recognise faces, unable to read.

> *When a patient complains of loss of vision in one eye, do not assume that the visual loss is or was monocular; it may have been a homonymous hemianopia.*

Isolated *homonymous hemianopia* is an uncommon symptom but a common sign in stroke patients and so it is essential to check the visual fields of all stroke patients for this important diagnostic and functional deficit, which may be unrecognised by the patient (and doctors). TIA patients may report that they 'saw half of everything' but more commonly they also have difficulty recognising and describing hemianopia, particularly if there are other symptoms (such as hemiparesis) which are more readily appreciated and described. They may simply describe 'blurred vision' or 'a shadow'. As stated above, patients often can not be certain whether or not 'visual loss in one eye' was really transient incomplete binocular visual loss (i.e. a homonymous hemianopia) or loss of vision in one eye only; to be sure, the patient has to have covered each eye in turn during the symptoms and noted the effect. Even so, it may not be possible to be really confident because a homonymous hemianopia does not necessarily split macular vision and may be interpreted by the patient as a loss of vision in one eye only. Similarly, if patients have only one functioning eye, it is almost impossible to distinguish a homonymous hemianopia from visual loss caused by ischaemia in the functioning eye, unless other symptoms of temporo-occipital dysfunction co-exist, such as dysphasia.

TMB or amaurosis fugax (AFx) (meaning literally 'fleeting blindness') are terms used interchangeably to describe the abrupt onset, over seconds, of loss of vision (greyish haze or black) in one eye. There are several causes; one is transient ischaemia in the territory of supply of the ophthalmic, posterior ciliary or central retinal artery. Typically, the symptoms arise spontaneously, without provocation, but they may be precipitated by bright or white light, a change in posture, exercise, a hot bath or a heavy meal, particularly in patients with severe ipsilateral carotid occlusive disease (see Section 6.5.5). The visual loss is generally painless (although some patients do complain of a dull ache or numbness in or above the eye) and usually complete immediately. It is often described by the patient as if a blind or shutter had come down from above or — less often — up from below. Occasionally, however, the visual loss is restricted to either the upper or lower half of the visual field and, even less frequently, to the peripheral nasal and/or temporal field (in which case, be suspicious that the visual loss is or was binocular). Patchy and sectorial loss may also occur but presumably is less likely to be noticed by the patient (Bogousslavsky *et al.*, 1986). Flashing lights, shooting stars, scintillations or other positive phenomena in the area of impaired vision occasionally arise during retinal or optic nerve ischaemia (Goodwin *et al.*, 1987), but are far more commonly encountered during migraine or glaucoma, in which case the onset is not sudden and the symptoms are not maximal at onset. Vision commonly recovers rapidly after several seconds to a few (usually less than 5) minutes, but sometimes not for several hours. If the visual loss is persistent (i.e. beyond several hours), the patient may have infarcted the optic nerve or retina. If ophthalmoscopy reveals pallor of all or a section of the retina (due to cloudy swelling of the retinal ganglion cells), then the diagnosis is retinal infarction (Fig. 3.4). Additional findings of retinal infarction may include an afferent pupillary defect, embolic material in the retinal arteries or arterioles (which can also be seen after AFx or in asymptomatic individuals) and a cherry-red spot over the fovea (due to accentuation of the normal fovea, which is devoid of ganglion cells, by the opalescent halo) in cases of central retinal artery occlusion (Fig. 3.5). If there is a visual field defect, such as an absolute or relative inferior altitudinal hemianopia, inferior nasal segmental loss or central scotoma, and if opthalmoscopy reveals swelling of a segment or all of the optic disc (which may be indistinguishable from that seen with raised intracranial pressure), pallor of the disc, flame-shaped haemorrhages near the disc and distended veins (Fig. 3.6), then the diagnosis is likely to be anterior ischaemic optic neuropathy (AION) (see Section 3.4.3). Monocular blindness may not be the only symptom; other symptoms may occur at the same or different times, such as contralateral hemiparesis and hemisensory deficit due to

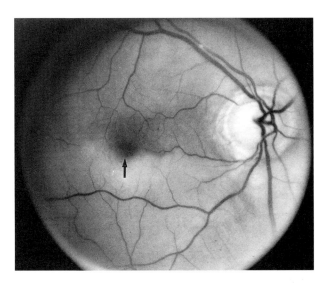

Figure 3.5 Ocular fundus photograph showing a cherry-red spot over the fovea (arrow), due to accentuation of the normal fovea, which is devoid of ganglion cells, by the opalescent halo, in a patient with retinal artery occlusion.

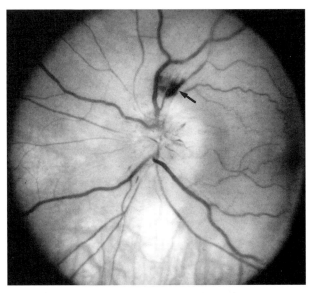

Figure 3.6 Fundus photograph of the eye of a patient with anterior ischaemic optic neuropathy due to occlusion of the posterior ciliary arteries as a result of giant cell arteritis. Note the oedema of the optic disc and flame-shaped haemorrhages (arrow).

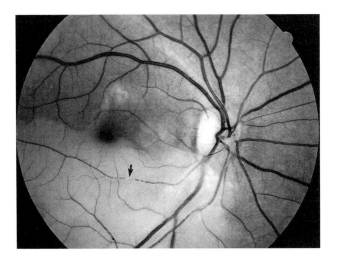

Figure 3.4 Ocular fundus photograph of a patient with inferior temporal branch retinal artery occlusion showing pallor of the inferior half of the retina due to cloudy swelling of the retinal ganglion cells caused by retinal infarction. The inferior temporal branch arteriole is attenuated and contains embolic material (arrow).

emboli (or low flow) to the ipsilateral cerebral hemisphere as a result of severe ipsilateral carotid disease (Pessin *et al.*, 1977). TMB may recur, usually in a stereotyped fashion, but the area of visual impairment may vary from one episode to the next, depending on which part of the retina is ischaemic.

Upon exposure to bright sunlight or white light, some patients with severe stenosis or occlusion of one or both ICAs may experience a *visual disturbance in one or both eyes* consisting of subacute (developing over minutes rather than seconds) blurring, dimming or constriction of the visual field from the periphery to the centre of vision of the involved eye, objects appearing bleached like a photographic negative, scotomata or complete visual loss; a shade or blind effect is most unusual (see Section 6.5.5) (Furlan *et al.*, 1979; Wiebers *et al.*, 1989; Sempere *et al.*, 1992). Such transient episodes of monocular or binocular blindness are presumed to be due to low flow and are typically less rapid in onset than the brief transient attacks of embolic origin, and sight returns more gradually. The symptoms are considered to result from choroidal (choriocapillaris) ischaemia causing a delay in the regeneration of visual pigments in the retinal pigment epithelial layer. Sunglasses may be an effective symptomatic treatment.

Sudden, spontaneous and simultaneous dimming or loss of vision in all of the visual field of both eyes is presumed to be due to bilateral occipital lobe (visual cortices and optic radiations) ischaemia/infarction caused by an embolus to the top of the basilar artery, or to both posterior cerebral arteries. If the visual symptoms occur in isolation (without associated symptoms of focal cerebral ischaemia, seizures or reduction in consciousness) in an elderly patient and if they resolve within 24 hours, they are probably due to a TIA of the occipital lobes, because the prognosis for subsequent stroke and other serious vascular events is similar to the prognosis of other elderly TIA patients (Dennis *et al.*, 1989a). However, when this occurs in adolescents and young adults, investigations are unlikely to reveal a cause and the long-term prognosis appears benign (Bower *et al.*, 1994).

Sometimes, bilateral blindness is denied by the patient (Anton's syndrome). The denial of blindness signifies involvement of the association areas adjacent to the primary visual cortex, but otherwise the pathogenesis is as unclear as that of the denial of left hemiplegia or for anosognosia in general. Perhaps the right-hemisphere component is crucial.

Transient *double vision* in isolation may or may not be an indication of a brainstem ischaemic event (e.g. it could be due to myasthenia gravis). However, transient diplopia in association with other symptoms of brainstem or cerebellar dysfunction, such as unilateral or bilateral motor or sensory disturbances, vertigo, ataxia or dysarthria, usually signifies a vertebrobasilar circulation TIA. Persistent diplopia can be confirmed at the time of examination by observing dysconjugate eye movements. If the patient complains of diplopia and the eye movements appear normal, the following questions may help.

1 Is the double vision present when one eye is closed (monocular diplopia) or only when both eyes are open (binocular diplopia)? Monocular diplopia is due to intraocular pathology causing light rays to be dispersed on to the retina (e.g. corneal disease, cataract, vitreous haemorrhage) or to functional (non-neurological) disturbance; it is not due to paralysis of extraocular muscles. Binocular diplopia is usually due to extraocular muscle weakness or imbalance.

2 Are the images separated side by side (horizontal), one above the other (vertical) or at an angle to one another (oblique)? Horizontal diplopia is seen with lateral or medial rectus weakness or underaction associated with abducens nerve or oculomotor nerve palsy and internuclear ophthalmoplegia. Vertical and oblique diplopia occur with oculomotor and trochlear nerve palsies and skew deviation.

3 In which direction of gaze are the images separated maximally? The distance between the true image ('good' eye) and the false image (eye with paretic muscle) increases in the direction of action of the paretic muscle so that maximum separation of images occurs in the direction of action of the affected muscle. For example, if the patient looks to the left and there is maximum separation of images, then either the left lateral rectus or the right medial rectus muscle is affected.

4 To detect which extraocular muscle is weak, one can ask 'In which eye is the image fainter?' The fainter image is seen by the eye with the paralysed muscle. Alternatively, as the more peripherally seen image is the false image (seen by the eye having the paretic muscle), the paretic extraocular muscle can be detected by asking the patient to look at an object (i.e. on the left) and to state whether the outside image (the far left) or inside image disappears when the examiner's hand is placed over one (the right) eye. If the patient notes that the inside image (true image) disappears, then it can be deduced that the peripheral/outside image (false image) is seen by the eye that was not covered (the left eye) and that the left lateral rectus is the defective muscle. This can be confirmed by asking the patient to look left and, upon experiencing horizontal diplopia, covering the left eye and noting that the outside/peripheral image disappears.

Visual hallucinations can occur in patients with stroke involving the occipital, temporal and parietal cortices as well as the eye, optic pathways and cerebral peduncle (see Section 15.27.3). Visual hallucinations secondary to occipital lesions most commonly consist of elementary (unformed) visual perceptions, sensations of light and colours, simple geometric figures and movements. Posterior temporal lesions, involving the association cortex, result in more complex (formed) visual hallucinations, consisting of faces and scenes that may include objects, pictures and people (Kolmel, 1985; Cohen *et al.*, 1992; Martin *et al.*, 1992). Lesion in the high mesencephalon, particularly the pars reticulata of the substantia nigra, may give rise to the so-called 'peduncular hallucinosis' of Lhermitte, in which the hallucinations are purely visual, appear natural in form and colour, move about as in an animated cartoon, and are usually considered to be unreal, abnormal phenomena (i.e. insight is preserved) (McKee *et al.*, 1990). More commonly, however, visual hallucinations are due to other disorders, such as migraine and partial seizures (in which case, the hallucinations are usually unformed), psychosis or an adverse effect of a drug.

Vertigo

Vertigo, or a sensation of rotational movement or spinning, may be symptom of dysfunction of the labyrinth in the inner ear, the vestibular nerve, the vestibular nucleus in the lateral medulla or the pathways from the vestibular nucleus to the vestibular cortex, which is probably at the posterior end of the insula (Grad & Baloh, 1989; Baloh, 1992; Oas & Baloh, 1992; Brandt *et al.*, 1995). When it occurs together with other clear-cut brainstem symptoms, such as diplopia or bilateral sensorimotor disturbance, it can be considered a focal symptom of brainstem dysfunction, and if it came on suddenly then it is likely to be vascular in origin. However, when it occurs in isolation (as a solitary symptom), it may represent dysfunction of the vestibular nucleus in the lateral medulla, the vestibular nerve or the superior vestibular labyrinth in the inner ear and, therefore, can not be considered a definite focal neurological symptom (and so should not be classified as a TIA or stroke). Although vertigo in isolation *can* theoretically be due to a TIA or stroke (i.e. due to ischaemia of the vestibular labyrinth), it is far more commonly caused by disorders of the peripheral vestibular apparatus (e.g. benign paroxysmal positional vertigo, vestibular neuronitis (see Section 3.3.2)) or episodes of non-rotatory dizziness, such as orthostatic hypotension or hyperventilation. So, unless vertigo is associated with other concurrent brainstem symptoms, it should not be classified as a definite TIA or stroke (and, of course, neither should non-rotatory dizziness or light-headedness).

> *Vertigo is a sensation of rotation or spinning. By itself it can not be regarded as a definite symptom of brainstem ischaemia because exactly the same sensation can occur in labyrinthine disorders, such as benign positional vertigo.*

Hearing loss

Sudden unilateral hearing impairment, with or without ipsilateral tinnitus, is a symptom of dysfunction of the cochlea, vestibulocochlear nerve or cochlear nucleus. Recognised causes include trauma, tympanic membrane rupture, viral and other infections, acoustic neuroma and toxic and metabolic disorders. Whether sudden unilateral hearing loss without vertigo or other brainstem dysfunction is ever due to vascular disease is unknown, because histopathological examination of the temporal bone and labyrinth at autopsy is not performed routinely and, if it is, it is usually carried out some time after the onset of hearing loss, which may have resolved or been forgotten by the clinicians looking after the patient during the final illness. Nevertheless, there is some histopathological evidence of labyrinthine infarction due to vascular disease (Kimura & Perlman, 1958; Gussen, 1976; Belal, 1980). Several cases of sudden-onset permanent hearing loss of presumed vascular origin have been described (see Section 4.4.7; Hankey & Dunne, 1987; Matsushita *et al.*, 1993). Greater uncertainty prevails as to whether transient deafness in isolation is ever due to a TIA in the internal auditory artery territory; it probably does occur in patients with advanced vertebrobasilar atheroma, but other causes of sudden hearing loss need to be excluded.

Amnesia

Although transient forgetfulness can not be regarded as a focal neurological symptom, there are cases in which transient or persistent amnesia may be the sole or primary symptom of TIA or stroke. Historically, the term 'amnesic stroke' was used only in patients with bilateral ischaemic or haemorrhagic lesions of the limbic system (i.e. amygdala, hippocampus, thalamus) due to occlusion of the top of the basilar artery or both posterior cerebral arteries, but it is being increasingly recognised that amnesia may also arise and persist as a result of ischaemia or haemorrhage of the amygdala, hippocampus or thalamus on only one side of the brain, usually the left (Hankey & Stewart-Wynne, 1988; Ott & Saver, 1993). Most patients with unilateral amnesic stroke have evidence of ischaemia/infarction in the territory of supply of the left posterior cerebral, anterior choroidal or thalamic penetrating arteries (Ott & Saver, 1993). Most episodes of transient amnesia in isolation (TGA), however, are not due to ischaemia (see Section 3.3.2); amnesia due to vascular disease is usually associated with other focal neurological symptoms or signs of posterior circulation dysfunction, whilst transient amnesia due to a partial epileptic seizure is usually brief, associated with an aura and automatisms and likely to recur (see Section 3.3.2).

Confusion

Confusion is not a focal neurological symptom *per se* (it

tends to be a symptom of systemic upset causing a metabolic/toxic encephalopathy), but a patient may *appear* confused because of an underlying focal neurological disturbance such as dysphasia, visual–spatial–perceptual disturbance, hemianopia or amnesia. These functions therefore need to be carefully assessed in anyone who is said to be confused (see Section 3.3.4).

3.2.3 Associated symptoms

The presence of associated symptoms are more useful in discerning whether the pathogenesis is vascular or not than whether the symptoms are focal or non-focal.

Headache

Headache occurs in about one-sixth of patients at the onset of a TIA of the brain and eye (Koudstaal *et al.*, 1991b), about 25% of patients with acute ischaemic stroke, about 50% of patients with ICH and nearly all patients with SAH (Vestergaard *et al.*, 1993; Arboix *et al.*, 1994; Jorgensen *et al.*, 1994; Kumral *et al.*, 1995) (see Sections 6.5.6 and 15.9). The site of any headache is, if lateralised, usually ipsilateral to the lesion and is often above the affected eye in patients with AFx who experience headache. The headache is usually continuous and not throbbing and rather mild in intensity. Of course, the headache may not only be determined by the site of the vascular insult but also by the underlying pathology. The presence of headache in anyone presenting with ischaemia of the brain or eye demands immediate exclusion of giant cell arteritis (see Section 7.2). Similarly, the presence of severe pain on one side of the head, face, eye or neck or at the back of the head and neck at around the time of onset is highly suggestive of carotid or vertebral arterial dissection (see Section 7.1) or of ICH or SAH. Ischaemia and infarction of the cerebral cortex or structures supplied by the posterior circulation cause headache more often than small, deep, lacunar infarcts (Koudstaal *et al.*, 1991b; Vestergaard *et al.*, 1993; Jorgensen *et al.*, 1994; Kumral *et al.*, 1995) (see Section 15.9).

The cause of the headache associated with TIA is unknown. As cerebral ischaemia activates platelets (Lane *et al.*, 1983; Shah *et al.*, 1985), Edmeads (1979, 1983) has suggested that the headache is due to the release of vasoactive substances, such as serotonin and prostaglandins, from platelets activated by cortical cerebral ischaemia. Other possibilities include distortion or dilatation of collateral blood vessels, arterial dissection and mechanical (stretch or haemorrhage) stimulation of intracranial nociceptive afferents (Kumral *et al.*, 1995). Of course, some of the headaches are probably due to anxiety and muscle tension.

Other causes of headache with focal neurological signs include migrainous stroke, meningitis and intracranial venous sinus thrombosis, but usually there are other clues to these diagnoses.

Epileptic seizures (see also Sections 6.5.6 and 15.8)

About 3% of patients with acute stroke have a past history of epileptic seizures, one-third of these occurring for the first time in the previous year (Burn *et al.*, 1996). About 2% of patients have an epileptic seizure at the onset of the stroke; about 50% are generalised and 50% partial seizures (Burn *et al.*, 1994). Seizures at stroke onset are more common in patients presenting with a total anterior circulation syndrome and in those with haemorrhagic stroke (PICH or SAH) rather than ischaemic stroke, and are associated with an increased risk of further seizures. More importantly, seizures may mimic stroke and lead to difficulties in making the diagnosis of stroke and in judging the severity.

Symptoms of panic and anxiety

The sudden loss of limb, speech or eye function is a frightening experience, which often evokes considerable anxiety and panic in patients and carers, particularly in the first if not in later attacks. Patients may consequently hyperventilate and in turn develop presyncopal symptoms or unilateral or peripheral sensory symptoms; these include perioral and distal limb paraesthesia bilaterally, and even unilateral sensory symptoms (usually left- more than right-sided (Rothwell, 1994)). Under these circumstances it is important to try and meticulously distinguish between the primary (TIA/stroke) and secondary (panic/anxiety) symptoms. The timing of the symptoms is one clue; palpitations occurring immediately before or concurrently with TIA/stroke, rather than following the attack, are more suggestive of the underlying cause (i.e. hypotension due to cardiac arrhythmia) than any psychological consequences.

Vomiting

Vomiting is very rare during TIA and is even uncommon in patients with stroke. When it does occur, it suggests either a posterior fossa stroke (because of vertigo in some cases and presumably because of direct involvement of the 'vomiting centre' in the area postrema in the floor of the fourth ventricle in other cases) or a large supratentorial stroke (usually a haemorrhage) causing raised intracranial pressure (Mohr *et al.*, 1978). Vomiting within 2 hours of stroke onset is highly predictive of ICH (Allen, 1983).

Hiccups

Hiccups consist of brief bursts of intense inspiratory activity, involving the diaphragm and inspiratory intercostal muscles, with reciprocal inhibition of the expiratory intercostal muscles. Glottic closure occurs almost immediately after the onset of diaphragmatic contraction, generating the characteristic sound and sense of discomfort. Hiccups usually resolve spontaneously after a few minutes but if they persist for days they may indicate underlying structural or functional disturbances of the medulla (affecting the region of the vagal nuclei and the nucleus tractus solitarius) or of afferent or efferent nerves to the respiratory muscles (Howard, 1992). Hiccups are a well-recognised phenomenon in patients with lateral medullary infarction but may occur with any lesion of the medullary region that is associated with respiratory control. Neurogenic hiccup rarely occurs in isolation, however; associated brainstem or long tract signs are usually evident (see Section 15.10). We are not aware of any reports of hiccups occurring as part of a TIA but suspect that they do occur.

Transient loss of consciousness

Transient loss of consciousness usually does not indicate a TIA unless accompanied, before or after, by clear-cut focal neurological symptoms. However, beware of Todd's paresis following an epileptic seizure; this can also present as transient loss of consciousness followed by a hemiparesis. When loss of consciousness does occur during a TIA, it seems to be associated with brainstem or bihemispheric ischaemia, or ischaemia of the deep diencephalic and mesencephalic structures superimposed on widespread bihemispheric ischaemia, as a result of either bilateral carotid or vertebrobasilar occlusive disease (Yanagihara *et al.*, 1989).

> *Loss of consciousness during a transient ischaemic attack is extremely unusual.*

Loss of consciousness is also uncommon in stroke patients, particularly soon after the onset. When it does occur, it is suggestive of a posterior fossa stroke, a large supratentorial ICH, or an SAH if there are no focal neurological symptoms or signs to suggest a focal brain lesion. Large cerebral infarcts do not usually cause coma until 2–3 days after stroke onset (see Sections 4.2.2 and 15.3).

3.2.4 Severity of symptoms

Only the most severe strokes cause the patient to become suddenly quadriplegic or comatose, an event that is so dramatic that it is easy to understand how the terms 'apoplexy'

and 'stroke' have been used to describe it. Most strokes are less severe and can consist of only trivial focal neurological symptoms or signs that may not even be noticed by the patient, let alone arouse any concern or apparent need for medical attention. Between these two extremes there are all grades of severity. The severity depends on the neuroanatomical site, extent and duration of the vascular insult. Indeed, TIAs can also cause very severe neurological deficits, but transiently, as well as mild deficits that may not be recognised or may not prompt a visit to the doctor.

3.2.5 Past history

Although prior cerebrovascular events are not particularly common (about 10–15% of stroke patients give a history of prior TIAs (Dennis *et al.*, 1989b; Sandercock *et al.*, 1989)), their presence favours a vascular basis for the present symptoms, particularly if they are the same symptoms and possibly caused by ischaemia in the same arterial territory (e.g. loss of vision in the left eye on one occasion followed by dysphasia and right arm and leg weakness on a later occasion could all be due to left carotid artery territory ischaemia). The clinical history should therefore include an enquiry into any previous symptoms suggestive of cerebrovascular disease (Table 3.6).

As most patients are naturally quite naïve about the functions of the nervous system, it is safest not to assume any knowledge and to ask specific questions such as 'have you

Table 3.6 Check-list of previous symptoms of cerebrovascular disease.

Have you ever been told that you have had a stroke, mini-stroke, TIA or brain attack?

If so, when did this occur and can you describe what happened?

Have you ever suddenly
    Lost vision or gone blind in one eye?
    Had double vision for more than a few seconds?
    Had jumbled speech, slurred speech or difficulty talking?
    Had weakness or loss of feeling in the face, arm or leg?
    Had clumsiness of the arm or leg?
    Had unsteadiness walking?
    Had a spinning (dizzy) sensation?
    Lost consciousness?

How long did the symptoms last?

Do you still have these symptoms?

Did you see a doctor about the episode and, if so, who was it and what were you told, and were you admitted to hospital?

What medications/drugs are you taking (particularly aspirin, warfarin)?

---

ever had weakness on one or both sides of your face, arms or legs?' This is because many TIA and stroke patients attribute focal neurological symptoms (i.e. blindness, weakness, sensory loss) to a disturbance of the organ involved (i.e. the eyes or the limbs) rather than a disturbance of the brain. Consequently, they may fail to recognise that a previous TIA or stroke (e.g. causing right face and arm weakness) may have been related to their present symptoms (e.g. dysphasia) and so may not volunteer information about it. Also, temporary symptoms are frequently attributed to environmental causes, such as the heat, a draught or lying on a nerve.

It is also important to ask more than once about previous neurological symptoms; many patients have told us several days after their TIA or stroke about prior TIAs, having not recalled them when asked at their first consultation. Sometimes this is because anxiety and panic at the time of the recent attack or, perhaps more likely, at the time of the consultation impairs recall. Of course, a few patients are affected by altered consciousness or amnesia during the event and can not recall it exactly and others may not wish to disclose such information for fear of potential repercussions for their employment or driving status. It is the doctor's responsibility to explore these possibilities with insight, sensitivity and confidentiality, and this frequently involves talking to family members, friends and the patient's general practitioner and reviewing the patient's medical records. Sometimes a detailed history of previous episodes helps confirm an alternative diagnosis, such as migraine or epilepsy. Similarly, it is important to know what drugs the patient is taking because sometimes they are a marker of a forgotten event (e.g. aspirin, warfarin, antiepileptic, antihypertensive, antimigraine drugs) or increase the likelihood that the present event is vascular (e.g. when on warfarin).

Vascular risk factors

Knowledge of the presence of vascular risk factors (see Section 6.2.3) or markers of arterial disease, such as advanced age (Fig. 3.7), high blood pressure, cigarette-smoking, high plasma cholesterol, atrial fibrillation, ischaemic and valvular heart disease, diabetes mellitus and intermittent claudication, is useful for deciding whether or not an event was likely to have been vascular and the possible mechanism. In other words, 'is this the right milieu for a vascular event to occur or not?' For example, an episode of focal limb weakness in a person aged 30 years without vascular risk factors is more likely to be due to a non-vascular lesion (e.g. MS) than a vascular lesion, whereas a similar event in a 70 year old with hypertension, intermittent claudication and carotid bruits is extremely likely to be vascular (and probably ischaemic rather than haemorrhagic).

> *Transient ischaemic attack and stroke most commonly occur in late middle and old age, usually in a patient with vascular risk factors or diseases such as hypertension or intermittent claudication. Transient focal neurological symptoms in young patients without vascular risk factors are unlikely to be due to vascular disease.*

3.2.6 Physical signs (see also Section 6.5.7)

If relevant focal neurological signs are still present at the time of the clinical examination, it may be possible to more confidently confirm a diagnosis of stroke and more accurately localise the responsible brain lesion (it is exceptionally rare to examine someone during a TIA). These signs will be dis-

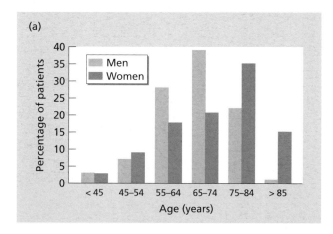
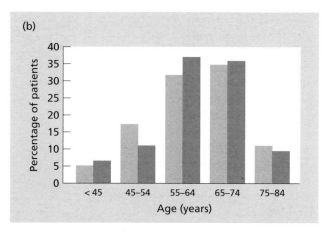

Figure 3.7 Age and sex composition of: (a) 184 TIA patients in the Oxfordshire Community Stroke Project; (b) 469 TIA patients in a hospital-referred series of TIA patients. (Adapted from Hankey & Warlow, 1994; reproduced with permission of WB Saunders Co. Ltd.)

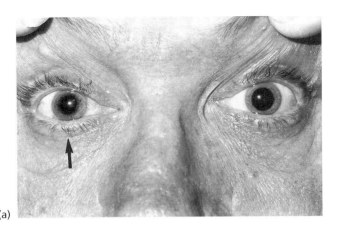 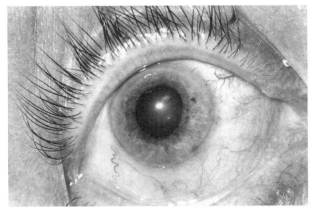

(a)   (b)

Figure 3.8 (a) Photograph of a patient's eyes. The right eye (arrow) is affected by ischaemic oculopathy. (b) Note the episcleral vascular congestion, cloudy cornea, neovascularisation of the iris (rubeosis of the iris) and mid-dilated pupil on external examination of the eye, which indicate chronic anterior segment ocular ischaemia due to carotid occlusive disease. (Reproduced from Hankey & Warlow, 1994; reproduced with permission of WB Saunders Co. Ltd.)

cussed in Chapter 4. This section will deal only briefly with some physical signs which, if present, may help resolve whether or not the lesion is vascular.

Eye

If the eye is red and painful with a fixed, semidilated, oval pupil and cloudy/steamy cornea, then acute glaucoma is the likely cause of any visual disturbance (see Section 3.4.1). Finding episcleral vascular congestion, a cloudy cornea, neovascularisation of the iris (rubeosis iridis) and a sluggishly reactive mid-dilated pupil on external examination of the eye indicate chronic anterior segment ocular ischaemia due to carotid occlusive disease (Fig. 3.8; see Section 6.5.7), or small vessel disease in a diabetic. Arrest of blood flow in retinal vessels can be seen during ophthalmoscopy by exerting light finger pressure on the globe.

Ophthalmoscopy may reveal emboli of varying composition. The most common type are the bright orange or yellow crystals of cholesterol that originate from ulcerated atheroma in proximal arteries and usually appear in showers. Although cholesterol crystals are white, they appear orange or golden because their thin fish-scale contour permits blood to pass above and below them and thus produce their characteristic refractile appearance (Fig. 3.9). Most of the crystals, because of their small size, thin flat structure and lack of adhesiveness and cohesiveness, flush through the retinal arterioles rapidly and leave behind only the larger crystals or stacks of crystals at some of the forks in the arterioles. They rarely occlude the larger vessels, although it is probable that large clumps of crystals briefly occlude the central artery of the retina, producing TMB, and then break up and flush through the retina. Commonly accompanying the choles-

terol crystals are less numerous white plugs of fibrin, platelets or fatty material from the same ulcerating atheromatous plaque. They occur in all sizes and nearly always occlude the arteriole in which they lodge. Other less common types of emboli include calcium, micro-organisms (septic), fat and tumour cells. Calcium emboli are chalky white angular crystals that tend to arise in patients with calcific aortic stenosis and completely and permanently occlude the central retinal artery (behind the cribriform plate) or one of the branch retinal arterioles near the optic disc, causing reti-

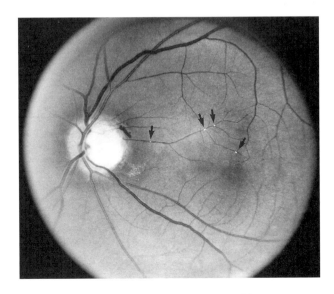

Figure 3.9 Ocular fundus photograph showing golden orange cholesterol crystals (Hollenhorst plaques) in the cilioretinal artery (arrows). The cilioretinal artery is present in only about one-third of people. It originates from a branch of the short posterior ciliary artery and supplies the macula.

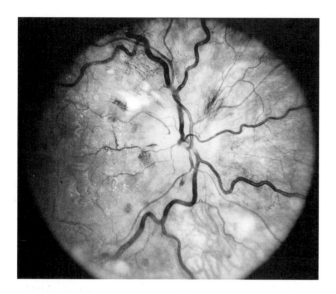

Figure 3.10 Ocular fundus photograph showing narrowing and tortuosity of retinal arterioles, arteriovenous nipping, retinal haemorrhages and papilloedema. These are the features of hypertensive retinopathy seen in malignant hypertension.

nal infarction. Septic emboli are white and may be very small, producing small white infarcts, sometimes encircled by haemorrhage (Roth spots), or larger fluffy emboli that can occlude the central retinal artery or one of its branches. Tumour emboli rarely enter the retinal circulation because they tend to be too large; they usually metastasise through the larger vessels that supply the choroidal circulation. The presence of narrowing, focal irregularity/constriction and tortuosity of retinal arterioles, arteriovenous nipping and fluffy white patches of transudate ('cotton-wool patches'), which are thought to be small focal infarcts in the inner layers of the retina, indicate long-standing hypertension and, if papilloedema and retinal haemorrhages are also present, this indicates malignant hypertension, which is very rare these days (Fig. 3.10). Of course, although finding hypertensive retinopathy supports a vascular aetiology, it does not necessarily mean that the patient's presenting complaint was vascular.

The presence of retinal haemorrhages in a patient with an acute neurological event is strong evidence of a haemorrhagic stroke, provided they are not just a reflection of hypertensive or diabetic retinopathy. They are usually caused by a very sudden increase in intracranial pressure, which is transmitted to the distal optic nerve sheath, where it causes a temporary obstruction of retinal venous outflow. The subsequent rise in retinal venous pressure leads to secondary bleeding from retinal veins and capillaries (Fahmy, 1973). The appearance of the haemorrhage depends on its site.

Small dot and blot haemorrhages lie in the deep retinal layers; linear haemorrhages in the superficial (nerve fibre) layer; 'thumbprint' haemorrhages with frayed borders are preretinal or superfical retinal; and large fluid subhyaloid haemorrhages lie between the retina and the internal limiting membrane. Subhyaloid haemorrhages (large round haemorrhages with a fluid level) and other types of retinal haemorrhage can be seen in some patients with SAH (Keane, 1979). Other possible causes of subhyaloid haemorrhage in a patient with suspected stroke include conditions that cause a rapid increase in intracranial pressure (such as acute hydrocephalus and sudden expansion of a massive cerebral haemorrhage), bleeding diatheses, intravenous drug abuse, haemorrhagic retinal infarction due to embolism from infective endocarditis, carbon monoxide poisoning and highaltitude stress (Keane, 1979).

Cardiovascular

Eliciting evidence of recent (within the last 3–6 months) myocardial infarction, or signs of splinter haemorrhages, atrial fibrillation, a cardiac murmur or cardiac failure are suggestive (but not diagnostic) of embolism from the heart, whereas absent peripheral pulses, elevated blood pressure and carotid and femoral bruits are more suggestive, but not diagnostic, of atherothromboembolic disease (Table 3.7).

3.2.7 Recurrence of symptoms

TIAs often occur only once but they may recur, and recur frequently, up to several times a day (Fig. 3.11) (Dennis, 1988; Hankey *et al.*, 1991, 1992). Consequently, by the time the patient presents to the doctor, he/she may have suffered several TIAs. Recurrent TIAs may sometimes be remarkably stereotyped or they may be quite different in terms of the 'type' of attack (i.e. the nature of the symptoms). It is important to remember that very frequent (i.e. more than daily) recurrent episodes of suspected TIA, particularly those that do not respond to antithrombotic treatment, may be partial seizures or in some way psychogenic (see Section 3.3.2).

3.3 Differential diagnosis of transient cerebral ischaemic attacks

As the symptoms of TIA usually resolve within about 15–60 minutes (and within 24 hours by definition), the diagnosis of a TIA is almost always based entirely on the clinical history. However, the history may not be very clear for a number of reasons: the patient may have forgotten the symptoms, because of either poor memory or delay in presenting to

Table 3.7 Clinical features (i.e. the milieu) influencing the probability that the event was vascular.

Very likely to be vascular, almost definite

History and physical signs suggestive of infective endocarditis (i.e. fever, splinter haemorrhages, cardiac murmur)

Frequent carotid-distribution TIAs and focal, long, loud bruit over the carotid artery on the symptomatic side

Recent myocardial infarction (in last 3–4 weeks)

Atrial fibrillation and rheumatic heart disease

Likely to be vascular but less definite

Atrial fibrillation and non-rheumatic valvular heart disease (but 10% of fibrillating stroke patients have PICH as the cause of the stroke)

Arterial bruits anywhere (e.g. carotid, orbital, cardiac, aortic, femoral)

Prosthetic heart valve, taking anticoagulants (but some strokes are haemorrhagic, and some TIAs are related to co-existent carotid artery disease)

Unlikely to be vascular (particularly if neurological symptoms are transient)

Less than 40 years of age, no symptomatic vascular disease, no vascular risk factors

medical attention; the symptoms may have been remembered but are difficult to describe (e.g. transient homonymous hemianopia); or the patient may have been so frightened by the attack that he/she was more preoccupied

with the immediate outcome than the exact nature of the deficit. All of these problems are more common in the elderly. Even if one can obtain an accurate history, it is sometimes difficult to know whether the symptoms are those of a TIA. This is because we are still uncertain about certain aspects of the definition of TIA. For example, how short can a TIA be (i.e. is a sudden focal neurological deficit, particularly a sensory deficit, of less than 5-seconds' duration a TIA?) and how often, if ever, is vertigo in isolation really a TIA? In view of the difficulties that may be encountered with history-taking and defining the limits of a TIA, it is not surprising that the diagnosis of TIA is subject to considerable inter- and intraobserver variation.

> *Amongst the conditions that may present like a transient ischaemic attack, the most important to exclude are those which are serious and yet treatable, such as hypoglycaemia, Stokes–Adams attacks due to heart block, subdural haematoma, benign structural intracranial lesions (such as meningioma) and partial epileptic seizures.*

3.3.1 Interobserver variation in the diagnosis of transient ischaemic attack (TIA)

For every patient who presents to his/her general practitioner with a definite TIA, there are many more who present with transient neurological symptoms due to other disorders. For example, in the Oxfordshire Community Stroke Project (OCSP), 512 patients were referred by their general practitioner or attending hospital doctor with a diagnosis of 'possible TIA', of whom 317 (62%) were considered by the OCSP neurologists *not* to have had a TIA (Table 3.8). In

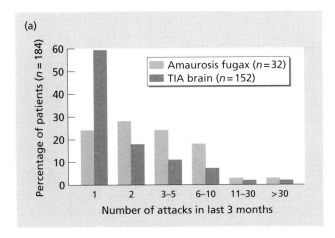
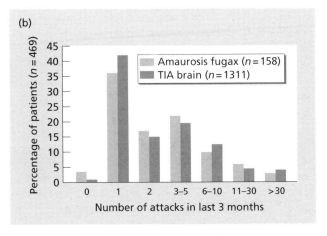

Figure 3.11 Histogram of the number of TIAs in the 3 months before presentation amongst: (a) 184 TIA patients in the Oxfordshire Community Stroke Project; (b) 469 TIA patients in a hospital-referred series. (Adapted from Hankey & Warlow, 1994; reproduced with permission of WB Saunders Co. Ltd.)

Table 3.8 Breakdown by diagnosis of all 512 patients with transient neurological symptoms notified to the OCSP with suspected TIAs. (Modified from Dennis *et al.*, 1989b.)

Not TIAs		TIAs	
Migraine	52	Incident TIAs	184
Syncope	48	Prevalent TIAs	11
Possible TIA*	46		
'Funny turn'†	45		
Isolated vertigo	33		
Epilepsy	29		
TGA	17		
Lone bilateral blindness‡	14		
Isolated diplopia	4		
Drop attack	3		
Intracranial meningioma	2		
Miscellaneous	24		
Total	317		195

* Possible TIA was diagnosed in patients with transient focal neurological symptoms in whom the clinical features were not sufficiently clear to make a diagnosis of definite TIA or of anything else.
† 'Funny turn' was used to describe transient episodes of only non-focal symptoms not due to any identifiable condition (e.g. isolated and transient confusion).
‡ Lone bilateral blindness was later considered to be a TIA, after following up these patients and noting their similar prognosis to patients with definite TIA (see Section 3.2.2).

another study, 30% of the patients originally classified by their doctors as having TIAs were reclassified as not having TIAs when their records were reviewed by a stroke specialist (Calanchini *et al.*, 1977). This problem is not unique to general practitioners and hospital doctors; Kraaijeveld *et al.* (1984) investigated the interobserver agreement for the diagnosis of TIA of the brain amongst eight senior and interested neurologists from the same department who interviewed 56 patients in alternating pairs. Both neurologists agreed that 36 patients had a TIA and 12 had not, but they disagreed about eight (kappa = 0.65; for perfect agreement kappa would be 1.0).

Even experienced neurologists show considerable interobserver variability in the diagnosis of transient ischaemic attack.

Possible explanations for disagreement

There are several factors which can increase the chance of clinical disagreement (Sackett *et al.*, 1991). The main one is difficulty eliciting and interpreting the history of the event accurately in the absence of any confirmatory physical signs.

Previous studies have shown that clinicians differ in the interpretation of even isolated elements of the history, such a 'blurred or foggy vision' (Sisk *et al.*, 1970; Calanchini *et al.*, 1977; Shinar *et al.*, 1985; Koudstaal *et al.*, 1986, 1989). Another problem, as outlined above, is that the definition of TIA lacks specific detail about which symptoms are focal neurological symptoms (e.g. vertigo alone?) and what is the lower time limit for the duration of symptoms (e.g. <5 seconds?), mainly because these issues are unresolved (Hankey & Warlow, 1994).

Strategies to reduce interobserver variation in the diagnosis of transient ischaemic attack

Sackett *et al.* (1991) highlight the clinical skills required to obtain an accurate and useful history (Table 3.9), and six strategies for preventing or minimising clinical disagreement (Table 3.10). If these principles are applied with a knowledge of the diagnostic criteria for TIA (Table 3.11), then diagnostic inconsistency should be minimised. If there is still uncertainty about the diagnosis at the end of the history, then the findings of the examination and special investigations aimed at detecting vascular diseases and risk factors may be useful; the odds of a TIA are reduced considerably if the patient is young and has no vascular risk factors, and are enhanced considerably if the patient is elderly, has several

Table 3.9 Clinical skills required to obtain an accurate and useful history. (Modified from Sackett *et al.*, 1991.)

The ability to
1 establish understanding
2 establish information
3 interview logically
4 listen
5 interrupt
6 observe non-verbal cues
7 establish a good relationship
8 interpret the interview
9 tell the story in plain language
10 tell the story in chronological order
11 make the story 'human'

i.e. like this
This 85-year-old widow was standing up at the kitchen bench peeling potatoes at 7 PM on the 26th November 1994, with her daughter, when she suddenly stopped talking, dropped the potato peeler she was holding and fell to the floor. She was unable to get up and has not been able to speak or move her right arm or leg since . . .

Not like this
This lady developed sudden dysphasia and right hemiparesis . . .

Table 3.10 Strategies for preventing or minimising clinical disagreement. (Adapted from Sackett *et al.*, 1991.)

1 Assess the patient in a suitable consulting environment (i.e. quiet room, minimal interruptions, necessary equipment available: ophthalmoscope, sphygmomanometer, etc., telephone on desk to call witnesses (to clarify history) or colleagues (to obtain advice))
2 Clarify and confirm key points
  (a) Repeat key elements of the history or examination
  (b) Corroborate important findings with witnesses, documents and, if necessary, appropriate tests
  (c) Ask 'blinded' colleagues to see the patient also (i.e. at ward teaching sessions)
3 Report evidence as well as inference, making a clear distinction between the two, reporting exactly what the patient said and then your interpretation (e.g. 'the patient complained of heaviness of the right arm and leg' and *not* 'the patient complained of right-sided weakness' or 'the patient complained of right hemiparesis')
4 Apply the art and social sciences of medicine, as well as the biological sciences of medicine

---

vascular risk factors, has evidence of vascular disease (e.g. carotid or femoral bruits, absent peripheral pulses) or has symptomatic vascular disease elsewhere (e.g. angina, intermittent claudication).

Diagnostic conformity can only be achieved if precise diagnostic criteria are available which are valid, reliable and generally accepted (Kessler *et al.*, 1991). In the case of TIA, however, it is difficult to determine the validity of any diagnostic criteria for TIA because there is no gold standard for the diagnosis. Kraaijeveld *et al.* (1984) used more explicit criteria for the diagnosis of TIA, which also allow for differentiation between carotid and vertebrobasilar TIA, and these have been modified (Table 3.11) (Sandercock, 1991). More widespread and consistent consideration, discussion and application of these criteria should enhance diagnostic accuracy and interobserver agreement and thereby improve patient management and care (Shinar *et al.*, 1985). However, as the diagnostic criteria become more specific, sensitivity is sacrificed and so an increasing number of genuine TIAs may be discarded and left untreated. If, on the other hand, diagnostic criteria become less specific, there may be a tendency to overdiagnose TIA and this can also have adverse consequences, such as the loss of a job, driver's or pilot's licence, money and self-esteem and inappropriate treatment.

If the history is elicited by a second physician, a subsequent comparison of the symptoms as well as their interpretation may lead to a greatly increased reliability of the diagnosis (Koudstaal *et al.*, 1986). Teaching hospitals in particular are in a privileged position to apply this powerful but expensive diagnostic 'instrument' but, even so, it is still unrealistic except for the occasional very difficult case.

The use of check-lists, written in simple language, has been shown to be effective in clinical studies (Koudstaal *et*

Table 3.11 Diagnostic criteria for TIA.

Nature of symptoms
Focal neurological or monocular symptoms (see Table 3.3)

Quality of symptoms
'Negative' symptoms, representing a loss of focal neurological or monocular function (e.g. weakness, numbness, dysphasia, loss of vision)

Rarely, 'positive' symptoms occur (e.g. pins and needles, limb shaking, scintillating visual field abnormality)

Time course of symptoms
Onset: abupt, starting in different parts of the body (e.g. face, arm, leg) at more or less the same time, without intensification or spread ('march'); deficit maximal usually within a few seconds

Offset: symptoms resolve more gradually but completely, usually within 1 hour and, by definition, always within 24 hours. Very brief attacks, lasting only seconds, are unusual except for AFx
(Note: we do not know how brief an attack of AFx can be and still be classified as AFx due to transient ischaemia; perhaps 10 seconds or so?)

Associated symptoms
TIAs usually occur without warning

Antecedent symptoms are rare but may reflect the cause (e.g. neck and face pain due to carotid dissection, headache due to giant cell arteritis). Otherwise, antecedent symptoms (e.g. headache, nausea or epigastric discomfort) usually suggest migraine or epilepsy

Headache may occur during and after a TIA; it is to be distinguished from migraine headache

Loss of consciousness is almost never due to a TIA; it usually suggests syncope or epilepsy

Neurological signs
Following symptomatic recovery, a few physical signs, such as reflex asymmetry or an extensor plantar response, which are not significant functionally, may be elicited

Brain CT or MRI scan
Small areas of low density, consistent with brain infarction, in a relevant part of the brain may be present

Frequency of attacks
TIAs often recur, but very frequent stereotyped attacks raise the possibility of partial seizures (sometimes due to an underlying structural abnormality such as an AVM, chronic subdural haematoma or cerebral tumour) or hypoglycaemia

al., 1986) and is likely to be useful for computer-aided diagnosis and further research studies but, although check-lists may encourage more thorough history-taking, the symptoms still have to be interpreted correctly.

The difficulties of establishing a uniform consensus between clinicians about the diagnosis of TIA has led some investigators to develop and evaluate computer-based systems to improve the intra- and interobserver variation in the diagnosis (Reggia *et al.*, 1984). If validated, these systems could have a role beyond research studies if they were practical enough to be programmed into a computerised hospital or practice network.

We would recommend that in patients who present with transient symptoms that might suggest a TIA, but who have additional symptoms that are too vague or uncharacteristic or which occurred in unusual circumstances, the diagnosis of 'possible TIA' should be made and further evidence sought by talking to witnesses of the event and by reassessing the patients after any further attack (which is hopefully not a stroke!) (Whisnant *et al.*, 1990).

3.3.2 Differential diagnosis of transient focal neurological symptoms of sudden onset (Table 3.12)

The most common conditions confused with cerebral TIAs are migraine, syncope, labyrinthine vertigo, partial epileptic seizures and TGA. The most important conditions to exclude are hypoglycaemia and Stokes–Adams attacks due to complete heart block (less so, partial seizures and structural intracranial lesions) because these conditions are treatable and, if not treated, are potentially dangerous (Fig. 3.12).

> *There are many conditions which can cause transient focal neurological symptoms that clinically mimic transient ischaemic attack and stroke. Some are both serious and treatable.*

Migraine

Migraine with aura (classical migraine) differs from TIA in that it usually starts in younger patients who may have a family history of migraine. It begins with an aura that commonly consists of positive symptoms of focal cerebral or retinal dysfunction that develop gradually over 5–20 minutes and lasts less than 60 minutes (Olesen, 1988; Welch & Levine, 1990; Blau, 1991). The most common aura consists of homonymous, unilateral or central visual symptoms, such as flashes of light, zigzag lines, scintillations or fortification spectra, which gradually 'build up', expand and migrate across the visual field. Somatosensory or motor distur-

Table 3.12 Causes of transient focal neurological attacks (see Section 3.3.2).

Focal cerebral ischaemia (i.e. TIA)
Migraine aura (with or without headache)
Partial (focal) epileptic seizures
TGA
Intracranial structural lesion
    Tumour
    Giant aneurysm
    AVM
    Chronic subdural haematoma
MS
Labyrinthine disorders
    Ménière's disease
    Benign paroxysmal positional vertigo
    Benign recurrent vertigo
    Labyrinthitis
Metabolic disturbances
    Hypoglycaemia
    Hyperglycaemia
    Hypercalcaemia
    (Hyponatraemia)
Peripheral nerve lesions
    Mononeuropathy/radiculopathy
Myasthenia gravis
Psychological
    Hyperventilation attacks
    Panic attacks
    Somatisation

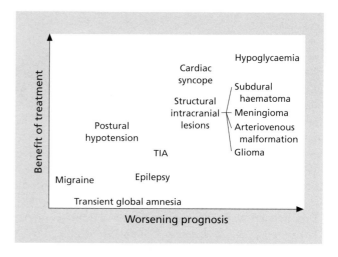

Figure 3.12 Figure showing some of the differential diagnoses of TIA in terms of how treatable they are and how dangerous they may be if not treated. It is important to consider the conditions which have the worst prognosis untreated but for which we have effective treatments (e.g. hypoglycaemia and cardiac syncope due to complete heart block) before diagnosing less serious or less treatable conditions (e.g. migraine or TGA).

bances, such as paraesthesias or heaviness in one or more limbs, may also occur and evolve and spread over a period of minutes in a 'marching' fashion (e.g. spread of tingling from hand to arm to face to tongue over several minutes). The serial progression from one accompaniment to another without delay, such as from visual symptoms to paraesthesias to dysphasia, is quite characteristic. Sometimes, however, the symptoms are negative and consist of 'blind patches' (often a homonymous hemianopia) and, rarely, even loss of colour vision (Lawden & Cleland, 1993). Headache, nausea and/or photophobia follow the neurological aura symptoms immediately or after an interval of less than 1 hour, and often there is associated photophobia and phonophobia, which clearly help to distinguish migraine attacks from TIA. The headache usually lasts 4–72 hours.

Patients who regularly experience migraine aura and a typical headache not infrequently suffer identical auras at other times, but without headache, and this should not cause confusion with TIAs. However, diagnostic difficulty may arise when a patient *without* known classical migraine presents following their first-ever episode of transient positive symptoms of focal neurological dysfunction, with the typical features of a migraine aura, but without any associated headache (Peatfield, 1987), particularly if the patient is older and has one or more vascular diseases and risk factors. Of course, if the patient is young (i.e. less than about 40 years of age), and particularly a young woman with a normal heart, it is most unlikely that the symptoms are those of a TIA caused by arterial thromboembolism (perhaps explaining why young female patients with suspected TIA, with or without a family history of migraine, do not seem to have any higher risk of stroke than other women of the same age (Holt Larsen *et al.*, 1990)). In any case, a careful history eliciting the slow onset and spread of neurological symptoms, particularly if positive and visual, should clinch the diagnosis of migraine.

Several series of older patients with presumed 'migraine aura without headache', as defined by Dennis and Warlow (1992), have been described (Whitty, 1967; Fisher, 1971, 1980, 1986). In our study, 50 patients diagnosed as migraine aura without headache and 50 age- and sex-matched patients from the same neurology clinic diagnosed as definite TIAs were prospectively followed for up to 10 years (Dennis & Warlow, 1992). Only one migraine patient suffered a subsequent serious vascular event (an MI), compared with three TIA patients who suffered a stroke and two others who died from vascular disease. The relative odds of a stroke occurring in a TIA patient compared with a 'migraine aura without headache' patient was 7.6 (95% confidence interval (CI): 0.8–74), and the relative odds of any serious vascular event (stroke, MI or vascular death) was 3.8 (95% CI: 0.8–19),

suggesting that patients with the clinical characteristics of 'migraine aura without headache' have a lower risk of vascular events than patients with TIA. These patients need reassurance that they have not 'had a stroke' and therefore do not require any aggressive and potentially hazardous investigations or treatments, apart from sensible control of any vascular risk factors, like anyone else. Some patients with a history of migraine with aura (classical migraine) do have an increased risk of ischaemic stroke, even after controlling for a number of known vascular risk factors. However, it has not been established whether migraine *per se* is a causal risk factor for stroke, whether vascular factors associated with migraine (i.e. altered blood flow and platelet aggregability) play a causal role in stroke or whether migraine is a marker of an increased risk of stroke that is unrelated to the migraine attack (see Section 7.5).

> A 55-year-old man, who had previously been well, described an episode when he had noted a heaviness and slight pins and needles in his right arm whilst driving home from a business meeting. By the time he arrived home, his arm was returning to normal but when he tried to speak to his wife he could only garble a few inappropriate words and when he tried to read the evening newspaper it did not make sense. He also noted a 'jazzy' effect in his right visual field, which fluctuated over the next few hours. He went to bed and his wife called the doctor, who arrived about 1-hour later. The doctor found his speech to be normal apart from a slight hesitancy, and by this time he was able to read again, although his vision was still not normal. He awoke the next morning entirely well. The physician who saw him about 3-weeks later elicited a family history of migraine, although the patient had never previously suffered from migraine himself. A diagnosis of migraine aura without headache was made and the patient was reassured. No investigations were carried out. He remained well over the next 4 years, although he had occasional recurrences of the visual symptoms.

Epilepsy

Partial (focal) seizures can be distinguished from TIAs because they usually cause sudden positive sensory or motor phenomena which spread *quickly* to adjacent body parts over 1 minute or so. Although positive sensory phenomena, such as tingling, can occur in TIAs, they tend to arise in all affected body parts at the same time (i.e. in the face, arm and leg together), whereas the symptoms of seizures spread from one body part to another over 1 minute of so (cf. migraine aura, where any spread is over several minutes; see above).

Negative motor symptomatology, such as postictal or Todd's paresis, is a well-recognised phenomenon that may follow a partial motor seizure or a generalised seizure with focal onset (Todd, 1856), but this should be obvious from the history unless the patient was asleep or is aphasic and there is no witness. The difficulty arises in the very rare patient in whom epileptic seizures actually cause transient 'negative' symptoms during the electrical discharge (Globus *et al.*, 1982; Lee & Lerner, 1990). One then has to rely on other factors, such as the patient's age, any past history of seizures and the nature of the symptoms. For example, transient speech arrest (as opposed to aphasia with muddled language output) which is characterised by the sudden onset of a cessation of speech, often accompanied by aimless staring and subsequent amnesia for the details of the episode, is usually epileptic in origin rather than ischaemic (Cascino *et al.*, 1991). Transient aphasia (Suzuki *et al.*, 1992) and, rarely, bilateral blindness (Bauer *et al.*, 1991) or amnesia (Hodges & Warlow, 1990a; Kopelman *et al.*, 1994) can also be epileptic.

Distinguishing between seizures and TIAs can occasionally be very difficult. Sometimes it requires prolonged and careful observation of, and interaction with, the patient (and witness) over several visits. The diagnosis should not be rushed as patients may have several types of attacks with different causes. Initially, it is important to explain the diagnostic uncertainty to the patient and the reasons why it is necessary to establish the precise diagnosis; to exclude a structural intracranial lesion (with CT scan); to advise the patient not to drive or put themselves in a position in which they would be a danger to themselves or others if they were to have another attack; and not to proceed with carotid surgery (if this had already been planned). The interictal electroencephalogram (EEG) can be misleading (except that a patient having several episodes a day is unlikely to have a normal EEG if the attacks really are seizures). Ambulatory or telemetered EEG examination is subject to artefact and requires skilled and careful analysis because of the potential for false-positive diagnoses of epilepsy. Nevertheless, it is helpful if the attack is recorded with an accompanying accurate record of what the patient did at the time. Concomitant videorecording is therefore very useful. Prolactin estimation after a suspected seizure can be helpful, because a raised serum prolactin level occurs characteristically, but not always, after generalised tonic–clonic seizures (peaking at 15–20 minutes after the seizure and declining to baseline levels by 60 minutes). However, a less convincing rise occurs after partial seizures, which unfortunately is exactly where the confusion with TIA usually arises (Rao *et al.*, 1989). Also, the predictive value of prolactin levels in the diagnosis

of epilepsy depends on the population under study, the interval since the last seizure and the criteria chosen for abnormality of prolactin levels. Some authors propose a level above 18 ng/ml, others say above 23 ng/ml, others suggest twice the upper limit of normal and yet others propose a level that is two to three times the baseline prolactin level (Yerby *et al.*, 1987; Fisher *et al.*, 1991). If the last criteria are required, a baseline prolactin level is necessary for comparison. If more than one suspected seizure has occurred, the time interval since the last seizure needs to be considered because serum prolactin levels decline after repetitive seizures which have a seizure-free interval of less than 24 hours (Malkowicz *et al.*, 1995).

If partial seizures are suspected an MRI examination of the brain should perhaps be performed to seek a focal structural lesion too small to be seen on CT, such as mesial temporal sclerosis, a hamartoma or a tumour, usually in a frontal or temporal lobe.

> *A 64-year-old woman described about 20 attacks of pins and needles in her right arm and leg over a period of 6 weeks. Each attack lasted for about 5 minutes and there were no associated symptoms. On closer examination, she said that the sensation started in the right foot and then over a period of about 1 minute spread 'like water running up my leg' to involve the whole leg and arm. Each attack was identical. A cranial CT scan showed a glioma in the left parietal lobe. A diagnosis of partial sensory seizures secondary to the glioma was made.*

Transient global amnesia

TGA is a very characteristic clinical syndrome which typically occurs in a middle-aged or elderly person. There is a sudden disorder of memory, which is often mistaken as confusion (Fisher & Adams, 1964; Hodges, 1991). For some hours, the patient can not memorise any current information (anterograde amnesia) and often can not recall more distant events as well over the past weeks or years (retrograde amnesia) (Hodges & Ward, 1989; Evans *et al.*, 1993). There is no loss of personal identity (patients know who they are), personality, problem-solving, language and visuospatial function and the patient can perform complex activities, such as driving a motor car. The patient seems healthy but repetitively asks the same questions and has to be reminded continually of what he/she has just done. There are no other symptoms, apart from headache perhaps. The retrograde amnesia tends to diminish with recovery but probably leaves a short retrograde gap in all cases. Recovery is complete but, after the event, the patient can not remember anything which happened during the amnesic period. Recurrences are not very common—about 3%/year (Hodges & Warlow, 1990a,b; Melo *et al.*, 1992; Easton, 1995).

Although no cause is found in most patients, it is possible that a small proportion are due to transient brain ischaemia, a small proportion to epilepsy and a greater proportion to migraine; the vast majority are of unknown aetiology. The reason for suspecting that a cerebrovascular aetiology may underlie the occasional patient with TGA is that sometimes a stroke may give rise to a pure amnesic syndrome if it is confined to the anterior thalamus (mammillothalamic tract), hippocampus and even hypothalamus (Hankey & Stewart-Wynne, 1988; Sorensen *et al.*, 1995). More commonly, however, amnesia following a stroke is accompanied by other signs of midbrain, thalamic or temporal lobe dysfunction, such as somnolence, vertical gaze palsies and corticospinal and spinothalamic tract signs. Other reasons why a cerebrovascular aetiology is unlikely to be the cause of most cases of isolated TGA are that there is no significant difference in the prevalence of vascular diseases and risk factors between patients with TGA and age- and sex-matched normal controls; there is a lower prevalence of vascular risk factors in TGA patients than in matched TIA controls; and the prognosis of TGA patients for serious vascular events is strikingly better than that of TIAs (Hodges & Warlow, 1990a). As yet, we can not distinguish the small subgroup of patients with TGA due to possible transient cerebral ischaemia from the much larger proportion of TGA patients due to another mechanism (possibly migraine/vasospasm), who have a better prognosis than TIA patients. There is no difference in the prevalence of epilepsy between TGA patients and control groups, but an important minority (7%) of TGA cases go on to develop epilepsy, usually within 1 year of presentation (Hodges & Warlow, 1990a). These patients tend to have had shorter attacks of TGA, lasting less than 1 hour, and have already experienced more than one attack at the time of presentation. It must be presumed that in this minority of cases with 'TGA' the cause was temporal lobe epileptic seizures from the beginning. Epilepsy may therefore initially masquerade as TGA, but only in a small minority of patients. Consequently, the occurrence of TGA should generally not restrict holders of an ordinary driving licence from continuing to drive (Cartlidge, 1991).

Migraine is more common in TGA patients than in control groups (Hodges & Warlow, 1990a; Melo *et al.*, 1992). It seems that the association between migraine and TGA is also biologically plausible, as there are some theoretical reasons to implicate migraine in the pathogenesis of TGA (Hodges & Warlow, 1990a,b). Three studies of single-photon emission CT (SPECT) imaging have revealed marked bilateral hypo-perfusion of the medial temporal lobes during the TGA attack, which resolved several weeks afterwards (Evans *et al.*, 1993). However, it is not known whether the perfusion defect is primary or secondary to a fall in metabolism due to other factors. Hodges (1991) has hypothesised that diverse stressful precipitants may trigger a release of an excitotoxic neurotransmitter (such as glutamate), which then temporarily shuts down normal memory function in the medial temporal regions via the mechanism of spreading depression, and this in turn leads to a fall in cerebral perfusion.

Intracranial structural lesions

Although *intracranial tumours* often cause focal brain dysfunction, the onset of symptoms and signs is usually gradual over several days or weeks and not abrupt like TIAs. Occasionally, however, perhaps if there is bleeding into a tumour, there can be a sudden focal neurological deficit, although this usually lasts longer than 24 hours. Greater diagnostic difficulty arises when a tumour causes a partial and non-convulsive seizure, with or without postictal (Todd's) paresis, or intermittent focal neurological symptoms (so-called 'tumour attacks') that do not seem to be epileptic in origin (Daly *et al.*, 1961; Fowler, 1970; Weisberg & Nice, 1977; Ross, 1983; Fritz *et al.*, 1983; Davidovitch & Gadoth, 1988). Amongst 2449 patients suspected strongly enough by their neurologist of having had a TIA or mild stroke to be randomised in the UK-TIA aspirin trial, 11 (0.4%) were found later to have an intracranial neoplasm (glioma or meningioma) and one had a vascular malformation (UK-TIA Study Group, 1993). The clinical features associated with these 'tumour attacks' were focal jerking or shaking, pure sensory phenomena, loss of consciousness and isolated aphasia or speech arrest. With time, a more obvious epileptic syndrome often declares itself.

Possible explanations for transient neurological symptoms in patients with cerebral tumour include the following.
1 Partial seizures.
2 Spreading depression of Leao (as some suppose occurs in migraine).
3 Vascular 'steal', leading to focal brain ischaemia adjacent to the tumour.
4 A sudden change in intracranial pressure, as may occur following haemorrhage into a tumour.
5 Vessel encasement or direct compression by the tumour mass.
6 Indirect compression of vessels by herniating tissue or coning (usually a preterminal event).
7 An inaccurate clinical history; for example, the patient may have actually experienced the gradual onset of headache

and neurological symptoms, on reflection the symptoms may have been clearly epileptic, and the relatives may not have communicated that the patient had not been him/herself for some time.

> *A 78-year-old woman complained of many attacks of weakness and clumsiness of the left arm over a period of 4 months. The weakness came on suddenly, lasted for between 10 and 45 minutes, and was not associated with any other symptoms. In between attacks, she had no symptoms. A diagnosis of transient ischaemic attack was made by both her general practitioner and the neurologist, and she was started on aspirin. A cranial CT scan was performed later because the attacks continued, and this showed a meningioma involving the right frontal lobe (Fig. 3.13). A final diagnosis of 'tumour attacks' was made but, in view of the patient's age, the neurosurgeon thought an operation was not advisable.*

Intracranial aneurysms and *cerebral AVMs* can cause transient focal neurological deficits mimicking a TIA, and even AFx (Fisher *et al.*, 1980; Ross, 1983; Bogousslavsky *et al.*, 1985). Possible explanations are embolisation of thrombus from within an aneurysm, vascular steal around an

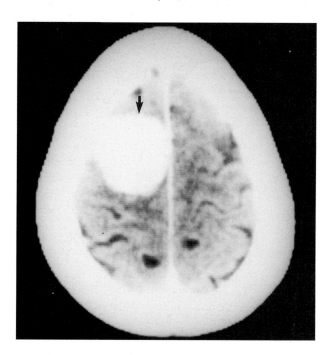

Figure 3.13 Brain CT scan after injection of contrast showing a meningioma involving the posterior part of the frontal lobe (arrow) of a patient presenting with a history suggestive of a TIA. Over 3 months this elderly lady had had eight attacks of a sudden onset of weakness affecting the contralateral arm, each lasting a few minutes. Between attacks the neurological examination was entirely normal.

AVM, a partial seizure or a small intraparenchymal haemorrhage (see Section 7.4; Bogousslavsky *et al.*, 1985).

Intracranial haemorrhage

ICH usually causes prolonged or permanent focal neurological dysfunction, but there are isolated reports of neurological deficits that have resolved within a few days (Scott & Miller, 1985; Dennis *et al.*, 1987), and it is possible that a very small haemorrhage, in the internal capsule or thalamus for example, may cause a transient hemiparesis resolving within 24 hours. However, it can be very difficult to be sure from the history. For example, 'I got better in 24 hours' does not necessarily mean 'I got completely back to normal', and it is the latter which we are referring to here when defining a TIA. To our knowledge, ICH has not been reported to cause focal neurological symptoms that have definitely resolved within 24 hours.

> *A 77-year-old man, whilst standing in his garden, suddenly developed weakness of the right arm and unsteadiness on walking. He had no headache or vomiting. He sat down and within 3 hours was 'better', although on closer questioning his arm did not return to normal for about 3 days. A cranial CT scan performed 8-days later showed a small intracerebral haemorrhage in the left putamen.*

Transient focal neurological symptoms, such as aphasia and speech arrest, may occur as a consequence of a *chronic subdural haematoma* (Melamed *et al.*, 1975; Williams, 1979; Noda *et al.*, 1981; Moster *et al.*, 1983). Although subdural haematomas occur in all age groups, they are more frequent amongst the elderly, in chronic alcoholics and in patients receiving anticoagulant drugs or who have another bleeding diatheiss. About 50% of patients recall sustaining a head injury, which may have been mild. Additional clues to the diagnosis are headache (present in about 80% of cases), clouding of consciousness and focal neurological signs, particularly if they change or fluctuate. Such rather imprecise symptoms may remotely suggest a subacute delirious reaction or even dementia. The diagnosis is usually confirmed by cranial CT or MRI scan but sometimes the haematoma is of the same density (isodense) as normal brain tissue and may be difficult to detect, unless there is mass effect causing unilateral compression of sulci and ventricles or midline shift (Fig. 3.14) (Davenport *et al.*, 1994). The EEG may show focal delta-activity, but this is non-specific (Nicoli *et al.*, 1990). In a few cases, a subdural haematoma may prove to be an incidental finding and the TIA can be attributed to more commonly recognised factors, such as carotid artery disease (Moster *et al.*, 1983). The pathogenesis of the tran-

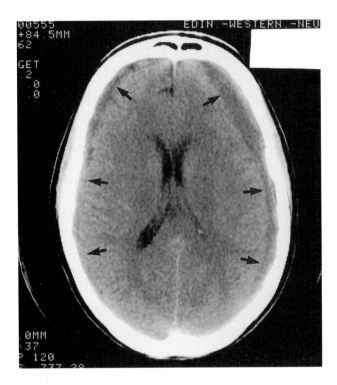

Figure 3.14 Brain CT scan showing bilateral subdural haematomata (arrows) in a patient in atrial fibrillation who was taking warfarin and who presented with a week-long history of intermittent headache on waking and three episodes of weakness, each lasting about 5 minutes. The first attack affected her left hand, the others her right leg. No drainage procedure was carried out but the warfarin was stopped and her symptoms and the subdurals resolved.

sient neurological dysfunction is unknown but may be epileptic (Nicoli *et al.*, 1990).

Multiple sclerosis

Patients with MS usually develop focal neurological symptoms in their third or fourth decade (as opposed to the seventh and eighth decades for TIA). The onset is usually subacute, coming on over days or even weeks. However, sometimes symptoms start abruptly and so can mimic a TIA, particularly if the initial presentation is one of optic neuritis, unilateral myelitis or a dystonic limb attack (Twomey & Espir, 1980; Drulovic *et al.*, 1993). Nevertheless, the diagnosis is seldom difficult because these patients are usually young women without any vascular diseases or risk factors, the symptoms are as often positive as negative, there are usually more neurological signs than symptoms (compared with TIA and stroke, in which there are often more symptoms than signs), and some may have subclinical evidence of dis-

ease in other parts of the central nervous system that can be readily detected clinically or by MRI.

Labyrinthine disorders

When patients complain of an illusionary sense of movement, the first steps are to establish that the symptom is true vertigo (see Section 3.2.2) and to localise the disturbance to the brainstem (central) or to the vestibulocochlear nerve or labyrinth (peripheral). It is not so much the character of the vertigo that helps to localise the disorder but the associated features and the character of the attacks. For example, vertigo accompanied by features of intrinsic brainstem dysfunction, such as diplopia and face and limb sensory disturbance, and normal hearing points to a central cause, whereas vertigo associated with auditory or ear symptoms is usually due to a peripheral cause. Vertical nystagmus occurs only with brainstem lesions, whereas horizontal or rotatory nystagmus may occur in either (although it tends to outlast the symptoms with brainstem lesions).

Ménière's disease is characterised by repeated, more or less regular, crises of quite severe rotatory or whirling vertigo, which can be acute in onset and last from several minutes up to a few days. Varying degrees of nausea and vomiting, unilateral (initially) low-pitched tinnitus, sensorineural deafness and a feeling of fullness or pressure in the ear are almost always present as well (Ludman, 1990). It usually begins in middle age.

Benign paroxysmal positional vertigo is characterised by recurrent episodes of vertigo and nystagmus that occur only after suddenly changing the position of the head, such as looking up, rolling over in bed and turning the head toward the affected ear, lying down, bending over and straightening up (Baloh, 1987; Baloh *et al.*, 1993; Lempert *et al.*, 1995). The vertigo is usually severe but very brief in duration, lasting less than 1 minute, and usually less than 15 seconds. Hearing is normal. There may be a history of recent head trauma, viral illness, stapes surgery or chronic middle ear disease. The diagnosis is established from the history and the Dix–Hallpike manoeuvre (Dix & Hallpike, 1952; Baloh, 1987; Denholm, 1993). The patient is moved quickly from a sitting to a supine position and the head tilted over the end of the examination couch until it has been lowered about 30° below the level of the couch, and it is simultaneously turned 30–40° to one side. If the test is positive, there is a latent interval of a few seconds after which the patient experiences a paroxysm of vertigo and rotatory/torsional nystagmus, with the upper pole of the eye beating toward the floor and the undermost ear, usually lasting less than 15 seconds and no more than 30–40 seconds. The vertigo and nystagmus then stop, a phenomenon known as adaptation. If the patient sits up again, the direction of vertigo and nystagmus often reverse direction. If the manoeuvre is repeated, the vertigo and nystagmus become less apparent and 'fatigue' but can be reproduced after a period of rest. Any nystagmus induced by this test which does not fit with this description may be central in origin and warrants further neurological investigation.

Benign recurrent vertigo can occur at any age and is characterised by sudden attacks of vertigo and nystagmus that last from 20 to 30 minutes to 1 to 2 hours, and are sometimes followed by positional vertigo and a feeling of imbalance for days to weeks (Slater, 1979). Sometimes there are associated features that suggest that this is a migraine variant (i.e. the timing of the attack in conjunction with sudden relaxation of tension (Matthews, 1975)), but the pathophysiology remains uncertain. Audiometry and caloric tests are normal and the patient recovers without any cause being found.

'Viral' labyrinthitis (or so-called vestibular neuronitis) is characterised by the acute or subacute onset of a single attack of severe vertigo with consequential nausea, nystagmus, vomiting and ataxia but without deafness or tinnitus, which lasts for several days and is followed by a feeling of imbalance and some positional vertigo for a few weeks (Buchele & Brandt, 1988). It tends to occur in young to middle-aged adults, usually following an antecedent upper respiratory tract infection. Examination discloses vestibular paresis (absent or diminished response to caloric stimulation of the horizontal semicircular canal). Hearing is normal. It is thought that the superior part of the vestibular nerve trunk is affected, possibly by a viral infection.

Vertigo due to intracranial structural lesions is usually associated with other focal neurological symptoms and signs that allow for neuroanatomical localisation to the brainstem, thalamus, temporal lobe or parietal association cortex (Schneider *et al.*, 1968). Rarely, vertigo may occur as part of a seizure disorder. Vestibular epilepsy is a cortical vertigo syndrome secondary to focal discharges from either the temporal lobe or the parietal association cortex, both of which receive bilateral vestibular projections from the ipsilateral thalamus (Kogeorgos *et al.*, 1981; Brandt, 1991).

Metabolic disturbances

Metabolic disturbances, such as hypoglycaemia (Ravid, 1928; Montgomery & Pinner, 1964; Rother *et al.*, 1992), hypercalcaemia (Longo & Witherspoon, 1980) and, less convincingly, hyponatraemia (Faris & Poser, 1964; Ruby & Burton, 1977), are well recognised but very rare causes of TIA-like focal neurological symptoms.

Hypoglycaemia generally causes hunger, generalised weakness, dizziness, rapid palpitations, profuse sweating and an altered mental state (confusion and reduced consciousness). However, in some patients, hypoglycaemia causes isolated and transient focal neurological symptoms, most often a right hemiparesis (see Section 6.5.6). Consciousness is preserved and there is a striking absence or unawareness of the usual systemic manifestations of hypoglycaemia (Wallis *et al.*, 1985; Foster & Hart, 1987; Amiel, 1993; Mitrakou *et al.*, 1993). In the elderly, and in diabetic patients with autonomic neuropathy, the explanation may be a blunted end-organ response to counter-regulatory hormones (i.e. catecholamines) secreted in response to hypoglycaemia (Hoeldtke *et al.*, 1982; Brierley *et al.*, 1995). By the time a doctor arrives, the patient has often recovered and the blood glucose may well have returned to normal. Persisting focal deficits are unusual (Malouf & Brust, 1985). Attacks of nocturnal hypoglycaemia may be unrecognised as such because they are followed by 'rebound hyperglycaemia' (Silas *et al.*, 1981).

The most common times that hypoglycaemic attacks occur are at night, on waking in the morning and after exercise.

The cause of the hypoglycaemia is almost always hypoglycaemic drugs, and very rarely hyperinsulinism, due to an insulinoma for example. Therefore, if diabetic patients receiving insulin or oral hypoglycaemic agents present with focal or generalised neurological symptoms (particularly if at night, on waking or after exercise), a plasma glucose level should be estimated at a similar time of day or at the time of any further attack. If the blood glucose is normal at the time of the attack, then it is unlikely that it was due to hypoglycaemia. However, if the blood glucose is normal shortly after the event, a true hypoglycaemic attack can not be excluded. Sometimes, the hypoglycaemia can only be demonstrated by frequent blood samples during the day and particularly the night.

If the patient has a history compatible with hypoglycaemia but does not have symptoms at the time of examination, hospitalisation for a 72-hour fast has traditionally been required to try and answer two questions. First, does the patient have fasting hypoglycaemia? Second, if so, is the hypoglycaemia associated with hyperinsulinism? Neither question is easy to answer. Plasma glucose, insulin, C peptide and cortisol should be measured every 6 hours. There is no definitive lower limit of plasma glucose that unequivocally defines pathological hypoglycaemia during a 72-hour fast; values as low as 1.2 mmol/L (22 mg/dl) may occur in normal women without symptoms. On balance, a presumptive diagnosis of hypoglycaemia is probably justified if the plasma glucose falls below 2.5 mmol/L (45 mg/dl) in venous blood at any time during the fast, provided typical symptoms are induced. The diagnosis of hypoglycaemia is strengthened if the symptoms are rapidly relieved by administration of carbohydrate. If symptoms are not produced, the diagnosis of hypoglycaemia should be made with caution, or not at all. On the other hand, the importance of mistaking hypoglycaemia for a TIA or some other 'funny turn' can not be overemphasised; excessive oral hypoglycaemic or insulin therapy in a diabetic patient that provokes recurrent hypoglycaemia sufficient to cause neurological symptoms is likely to result in permanent neurological damage, or even death if unrecognised, whereas prompt rocognition and modification of diabetic treatment should prevent further attacks and serious sequelae. Failure to diagnose hyper- and hypoglycaemia may also lead to inappropriate tests (e.g. CT scan, duplex ultrasound, carotid angiogram, etc.).

Peripheral nerve lesions

It is surprising how often TIAs have to be distinguished from a median neuropathy at the wrist (carpal tunnel syndrome), an ulnar neuropathy at the elbow or cervical radiculopathy in the neck as the cause of intermittent focal neurological symptoms in the hand or arm (Dawson *et al.*, 1990). The distinction can be quite difficult when patients report a brief episode of numbness or tingling in the hand or arm without any other associated symptoms. In these situations, an entrapment neuropathy is more likely if the symptoms have been, or can be, precipitated by any posture or movement, if they occur at night whilst in bed or upon awakening from sleep, and if sensory symptoms have a painful or unpleasant tingling ('positive') quality. We have also seen patients who present with symptoms of transient (days to weeks) focal neurological dysfunction in the leg of apparently sudden onset as a result of other peripheral mononeuropathies (e.g. sciatic) or radiculopathies (e.g. lumbosacral root compression due to disc herniation).

Myasthenia gravis

Although the symptoms of myasthenia gravis usually come on gradually, there are instances of fairly rapid development, sometimes precipitated by an infection (usually respiratory), drugs or emotional upset. The muscles of the eyes (levator palpebrae and extraocular muscles) and, less often, the face, jaw, throat and neck are the first to be affected (causing ptosis, diplopia, dysarthria or dysphagia), but in rare cases the initial complaint may be of limb weakness. The subsequent clinical course of a fluctuating oculofaciobulbar palsy can then be mistaken for a (brainstem) TIA but the weakness tends to persist (if left untreated) and to increase as the day wears on. Fatiguability can be demonstrated objectively by asking the patient to sustain the activity of the symptomatically involved muscles (i.e. ask the patient to look at the ceiling for 2–3 minutes without blinking (increasing ptosis) or to fixate in lateral or vertical gaze (increasing diplopia)). Conversely, muscle power improves after a brief rest, or in response to intravenous edrophonium (Tensilon).

Psychological

Many patients have recurrent attacks of transient focal (or non-focal) neurological dysfunction which do not have an organic basis. Some have a somatisation disorder, which has been defined as 'the tendency to experience and communicate psychological distress in the form of physical symptoms and to seek medical help for them' (Samuels, 1995). The diagnostic criteria for somatisation disorder are listed in Table 3.13. Attacks that are emotionally based take several forms, such as hyperventilation attacks, panic attacks, anxiety attacks, swoons, tantrums and deliberate simulation (Betts, 1990). Functional overbreathing (hyperventilation) usually causes bilateral limb and perioral sensory symptoms, but occasionally the symptoms are confusingly unilateral (Blau *et al.*, 1983) and usually it is the left limbs which are affected (see Section 3.2.2). Features distinguishing these attacks from TIAs include the patient's age (usually young) and sex (usually female), the circumstances of the attack, the lack of underlying vascular risk factors, the presence of other inexplicable symptoms, the lack of any objective neurological signs other than those which are clearly hysterical, and often the emotional context (anxiety, indifference or ambivalence).

Table 3.13 Diagnostic criteria for somatisation disorder. (Adapted from the American Psychiatric Association, 1994.)

History of many physical complaints starting before the age of 30 years

During the course of the current disturbance, each of the following
  Four pain symptoms
  Two gastrointestinal symptoms
  One sexual symptom
  One pseudoneurological symptom

Each symptom, after appropriate investigation, can not be fully explained by known general medical conditions or the direct effects of a substance, or when there is a related general medical condition, complaints or impairments are more than expected from history, physical examination or laboratory findings

Symptoms are not intentionally produced or feigned

3.3.3 Clinical approach to the differential diagnosis of transient focal neurological symptoms of sudden onset

A careful history needs to be taken about the timing of the attacks, the nature of the symptoms and any associated symptoms and what medications the patient has taken. A plasma glucose and electrocardiogram (ECG) should also be done in most, if not all, patients with suspected TIA, but a random plasma glucose level may not be helpful in trying to establish or exclude the diagnosis of hypoglycaemic attacks (see Section 3.3.2); it is more useful for the diagnosis of diabetes (see Section 6.6.1). A structural intracranial lesion (such as a meningioma, glioma, subdural haematoma, vascular malformation or giant aneurysm) is rarely the cause of an apparent 'TIA'; limited data indicate that the yield of CT for detecting structural lesions is about 1% in patients with suspected TIA (Hankey & Warlow, 1992, 1994) (see below).

Role of cranial CT and MRI

The main purpose of cranial CT (or MRI) in suspected TIA patients is to detect an underlying structural intracranial lesion which may present like a TIA; it is not to detect low-density lesions (presumed infarcts) or to exclude PICH, as it is in patients with stroke, because definite ICH has not been reported to cause focal neurological symptoms lasting less than 24 hours (see Section 3.3.2). However, if a patient is seen during a TIA (when it is not known how long the symptoms are going to last) and if the patient has been taking anticoagulants or is being considered for antithrombotic therapy, then CT is indicated to exclude PICH.

As the yield from routine screening of TIA patients with CT is very low for detecting structural lesions, and as the cost of CT probably exceeds that of both the neurological consultation and the initial investigations combined, the routine examination of every TIA patient with CT must be very carefully considered (see Section 6.6.3). The small minority of 'TIA' patients with structural intracranial lesions who will be missed by not performing a CT scan are likely to continue to have symptoms (and so return to the doctor) and their outcome is unlikely to be altered by a short delay in diagnosis. It is our impression that the small yield of structural brain lesions from CT is almost always in patients with carotid territory 'TIAs' and there is some evidence to suggest that performing CT in patients with vertebrobasilar territory TIAs and TMB is a waste of resources (Kingsley et al., 1980). We believe that CT should be reserved for patients with more than one TIA of the brain (and not at all if the attacks affect the eye only), particularly if they are in the carotid territory, and for those being considered for carotid endarterec-

tomy (to avoid operating on someone with a symptomatic meningioma, for example), but acknowledge that this is controversial (Martin et al., 1991). The CT scan should initially be a non-contrast study. Contrast should be used subsequently if a meningioma, giant aneurysm or AVM is suspected, or alternatively MRI and MR angiography should be undertaken. For patients who continue to have vertebrobasilar TIAs despite optimal medical therapy, and in whom a cranial CT scan is unhelpful and an abnormality in the posterior fossa is still suspected, an MRI study should be done because, although more expensive, MRI images of the posterior fossa (and also the cerebral hemispheres) are superior to CT for detecting infarcts and, of more relevance for management, structural lesions such as vascular malformations (Davis et al., 1989; Hommel et al., 1990; Edelman & Warach, 1993). However, even MRI is not 100% sensitive in detecting brainstem infarcts (Besson et al., 1992).

The data on the cost-effectiveness of CT and MRI in TIA patients are very poor and there is a need for a methodologically sound, prospective, multicentre study of this question, particularly in view of the considerable cost implications of a policy of 'CT or MRI for all suspected TIA patients'.

Role of EEG

The indication for an EEG is when the clinical diagnosis of TIA is in doubt and partial (focal or localisation-related) seizures are a possibility (Faught, 1993). About 35% of all patients with epilepsy consistently have epileptiform discharges on the waking interictal EEG, 50% do so on some occasion with repeated recording and about 15% never do (Chadwick, 1990). These figures vary according to the type of epilepsy; amongst patients who present with a first seizure, epileptiform abnormalities on the EEG are present in a higher proportion with idiopathic generalised seizures than with partial seizures.

3.3.4 Differential diagnosis of non-focal neurological symptoms of sudden onset

Non-focal neurological symptoms (see Table 3.4) should not be accepted as evidence of a TIA if they occur in isolation, without any associated definite focal neurological symptoms (Landi, 1992).

Syncope/transient loss of consciousness

Syncope is defined by loss of consciousness and postural tone due to a sudden fall in blood flow to the brain (Kapoor, 1991). Sometimes loss of consciousness may occur abruptly without any warning (e.g. syncope due to aortic stenosis, complete heart block), but more commonly there is history of a preceding (and sometimes *only*) feeling of light-headedness, faintness or 'dizziness' (not rotational vertigo), bilateral dimming or loss of vision (not to be confused with lone bilateral blindness), sounds seeming to be distant, generalised weakness, and symptoms of adrenergic activity such as nausea, hot and cold feelings and sweating. Additional clinical features during unconsciousness include multifocal, arrhythmic, myoclonic jerks (in up to 90% of cases), head turns, oral automatisms, righting movements (sustained head-raising or sitting up), eye movements (upward or lateral deviation of the eyes) and visual and auditory hallucinations, all of which may lead to an erroneous diagnosis of epilepsy (Lempert *et al.*, 1994). There are usually no *focal* neurological symptoms, unless the drop in blood pressure occurs in the presence of severe occlusive arterial disease in the neck or impaired cerebral autoregulation due to a previous stroke. During the attack, the patient is pale, sweaty/clammy and floppy, rather than cyanosed and rigid. The pulse may be absent or difficult to feel (but this can not be relied on) and the patient may be incontinent of urine. If the patient is lying flat and is not held upright (by someone or an obstacle), then consciousness is regained within seconds and there is very little mental confusion or difficulty in recalling the warning symptoms (unless there has been head trauma).

The key to the diagnosis of syncope is a sound clinical history (Hoefnagels *et al.*, 1991). Making a correct diagnosis is important because some causes are quite serious (e.g. Stokes–Adams attacks) and if misdiagnosed as a TIA may lead to the patient being denied an effective and possibly life-saving treatment (e.g. pacemaker implantation).

The conscious state depends on the integrity of the brainstem reticular activating system interacting (through its ascending pathways) with both cerebral hemispheres (Plum & Posner, 1985). Therefore, to disturb consciousness, the function of the brainstem or both cerebral hemispheres needs to be disturbed. Although brief episodes of loss of consciousness, sometimes during paroxysms of coughing (Linzer *et al.*, 1992), are well recognised in some patients with vertebrobasilar occlusive disease and, rarely, in patients with bilateral carotid occlusive disease due to presumed bihemispheric ischaemia (Yanagihara *et al.*, 1989), they are far more frequently due to hypotension (or systemic disorders and generalised epileptic seizures) (Kapoor, 1991).

> *If a patient presents with syncope, exclude epilepsy and heart disease. Transient ischaemic attacks very rarely lead to loss of consciousness.*

Transient unresponsiveness in the elderly

Sometimes elderly patients are found, usually early in the morning or in the afternoon, profoundly unresponsive without other neurological signs and they recover completely within 12 hours (Haimovic & Beresford, 1992). These episodes may recur and all diagnostic tests are unremarkable; the EEG usually shows only diffuse slowing of the background rhythm. Whether this is a sleep disorder or not is unknown (Rao *et al.*, 1994).

Drop attacks

Sudden loss of postural tone causing the patient to fall suddenly to the ground without any obvious reason has been ascribed to epilepsy, tumours in the region of the foramen magnum or third ventricle, vertebrobasilar 'insufficiency' associated with atheromatous vascular disease or cervical spondylosis, vestibular disease, myxoedema, old age and even subconscious guilt. In the vast majority of cases, however, no cause is found and the episode is called a 'cryptogenic drop attack' (Stevens & Matthews, 1973).

Drop attacks are defined as falling without warning, not apparently due to any malfunction of the lower limbs, not induced by change of posture or movement of the head and not accompanied by vertigo or other sensation (Stevens & Matthews, 1973). The definition does include patients in whom it is not possible to exclude, with absolute certainty, momentary loss of consciousness for the duration of the fall. However, attacks from which recovery is delayed by any factor other than the effects of any injury sustained in the fall are not drop attacks.

Amongst 40 patients evaluated by Stevens and Matthews (1973), all were women and the average age at onset was 44 years. The fall occurred whilst walking in all but one patient and could not be attributed to wearing high-heeled shoes. During follow-up, drop attacks continued to occur as an isolated symptom for many years and, although distressing, were not associated with any serious prognostic implications. The sex ratio, circumstances of the falls and favourable prognosis suggest that the cause reflects differences between the two sexes in the mechanism of walking rather than in any central neurological disturbance.

The most common differential diagnosis is vertebrobasilar ischaemia, but here there is usually some warning that the patient is going to fall—additional brainstem symptoms, such as vertigo or diplopia; the patient may be unable to rise immediately after the fall despite not injuring him/herself, and the symptoms are sometimes precipitated by a change in head or body posture (see Section 6.5.6).

Narcolepsy

Narcolepsy is part of a distinct neurological syndrome of excessive daytime sleepiness and abnormalities of rapid eye movement (REM) sleep, which, when associated with cataplexy, is often called 'classic narcolepsy'. Cataplexy is loss of muscle tone, usually precipitated by excitement or emotion, and is virtually unique to the narcolepsy syndrome (Aldrich, 1990). Laughter is the most common precipitant, but other forms of emotion and athletic activities can induce cataplexy. Severe attacks cause complete paralysis except for the respiratory muscles, whereas the more common partial episodes cause patients to drop objects or to sit down or stop walking. Momentary attacks are common and generally last less than 1 minute. Prolonged episodes may be associated with hallucinations. Rarely, cataplexy that is almost continuous ('status cataplecticus') may occur. Although sleepiness usually begins several months before the onset of episodes of cataplexy, up to 10% of patients have cataplexy initially and 10–15% develop cataplexy 10 or more years after the onset of sleepiness. The multiple sleep latency test is the most useful diagnostic technique; more than 80% of patients with the narcolepsy syndrome have a mean sleep latency of less than 5 minutes and at least two REM periods at the onset of sleep during the procedure (Amira *et al.*, 1985).

Giddiness/dizziness

'Giddiness' or 'dizziness' is a symptom that commonly prompts referral as a suspected TIA. More often than not, however, the diagnosis is something else. The first step is to distinguish rotatory vertigo from non-specific giddiness. A determined attempt must be made to define as closely as possible the patient's actual sensations, and direct and pointed questions must be asked; for example, 'is it a spinning feeling or just a light-headedness?' (Matthews, 1975). Descriptions that include a subjective or objective illusion of motion, such as spinning or whirling, which is usually so unpleasant that it makes the patient feel nauseated and also unable to stand, denote what is meant by vertigo (see Section 3.3.2). Feelings of light-headedness, swaying, a swimming feeling, walking on air, queer head or faintness (often with accompanying feelings of panic, palpitations or breathlessness) without a feeling of motion are non-specific symptoms, which may be caused by a wide variety of systemic disturbances (usually systemic hypotension or overbreathing). Precipitating factors and premonitory symptoms may be of diagnostic value, as also may be the mode of onset (whether sudden or gradual), the duration and the presence of any associated symptoms such as deafness, tinnitus and ear pain or fullness (Ahmad *et al.*, 1992) (see Section 3.3.2). Not infrequently,

the 'dizziness' does not even come from the head, but from the eyes (i.e. poor vision) or legs (i.e. weakness, proprioceptive sensory loss or incoordination).

Confusion

The term 'confusion' is imprecise. In general, it means an inability to think with customary clarity, coherence and speed. However, the definition of 'thinking' is also imprecise because this is a term that refers variably to problem solving or to coherence of ideas about a subject. Nevertheless, the key to sorting out the cause of apparent 'confusion' or 'difficulty thinking' is to appreciate the common clinical features of confusion (disorientation, impaired attention and concentration, an inability to properly register immediate events and to recall them later, and a diminution of all mental activity), and that there are several different causes that need to be considered and sought such as inattentiveness; disorders of language; disorders of memory (verbal and visual) and cognition; and apathy. All too frequently, alert stroke patients with dysphasia or visual–spatial–perceptual dysfunction (and subsequent frustration) are misdiagnosed as confused (and agitated), and are consequently exposed to unnecessary investigations (to exclude infections, tumours, metabolic disturbances and non-convulsive status epilepticus) and are mistreated (with the cessation of some necessary drugs and the prescription of unnecessary sedative/hypnotic drugs).

3.4 Differential diagnosis of transient monocular blindness (TMB) (amaurosis fugax (AFx))

TMB is a symptom and is often referred to as AFx. It is commonly caused by ischaemia of the retina (usually as a result of atherothromboembolism from the origin of the ipsilateral ICA or embolism from the heart) or ischaemia of the anterior optic nerve (usually due to thrombosis of the posterior ciliary artery). However, there are other causes of TMB which are important to differentiate because the prognosis and treatments differ (Table 3.14). Many are uncommon and frequently go unrecognised if the patient is not examined during the acute episode.

> *Transient monocular blindness and amaurosis fugax are two different terms for describing the same symptom: blurring or loss of vision in the whole or part of the visual field of one eye.*

Table 3.14 Causes and mechanisms of TMB (AFx).

RETINA

Vascular
Low retinal artery perfusion
    ICA atherothromboembolism or other arterial disorders (e.g.
      dissection, etc., see Table 6.3)
    Embolism from the heart (see Section 6.4)
    Retinal migraine (see Section 3.3.2)
High resistance to retinal perfusion
    Intracranial AVM (see Section 3.4.1)
    Central or branch retinal vein thrombosis (see Section 3.4.1)
    Raised intraocular pressure (glaucoma) (see Section 3.4.1)
    Raised intracranial pressure (blowing the nose)
    Increased blood viscosity (see Section 7.6)
    Malignant arterial hypertension (see Sections 3.4.3 and 3.5.6)
Retinal haemorrhage (see Section 3.4.1)

Non-vascular
Paraneoplastic retinopathy (see Section 3.4.2)
Phosphenes (see Section 3.4.2)
Lightning streaks of Moore (see Section 3.4.2)
Chorioretinitis (see Section 3.4.2)

OPTIC NERVE

Vascular (anterior ischaemic optic neuropathy) (see Section 3.4.3)
Systemic hypotension
Arteritis (e.g. giant cell) (see Section 7.2)
Malignant arterial hypertension

Non-vascular
Papilloedema (see Section 3.4.4)
Optic neuritis and Uhthoff's phenomenon (see Section 3.4.4)
Dysplastic coloboma

EYE/ORBIT
Vitreous haemorrhage (see Section 3.4.5)
Reversible diabetic cataract (see Section 3.4.5)
Lens subluxation (see Section 3.4.5)
Orbital tumour (e.g. optic nerve-sheath meningioma): gaze-evoked
    loss of vision (see Section 3.4.5)

3.4.1 Retinal vascular

Retinal vasculitis

Retinal vasculitis, inflammation of or around the arteries and/or veins of the eye, may lead to monocular or binocular visual loss of acute or subacute onset, which may be transient or permanent. There may be a history of recent viral infection or evidence of systemic disease, such as sarcoidosis, Behçet's disease and systemic lupus erythematosus. Indirect ophthalmoscopy of the fundus through a dilated pupil may reveal sheathing around retinal arterioles and veins (which may be focal or extensive), arteriolar occlusion, causing retinal infarction or haemorrhage and even neovascularisation in the affected area, macular oedema or retinal detachment

(Sanders, 1987). Viruses such as varicella-zoster and cytomegalovirus can cause severe necrotising retinal vasculitis, which results in areas of white dead retina and, when these areas are extensive, there may be retinal detachment. Slit-lamp examination and fluorescein angiography show that sheathed areas leak dye into the retina (due to breakdown of the normal blood–retinal barrier) and often there is retinal and macular oedema. There may also be evidence of an associated inflammatory process within the eye, such as vitritis or anterior uveitis, or features of systemic diseases, such as sarcoidosis, Behçet's disease or toxoplasmosis. Sometimes, however, there may be no underlying disease detectable (Sanders, 1987).

Retinal migraine

Migraine with aura (classical migraine) is usually ushered in by 'positive' binocular visual symptoms (see Section 3.3.2). Transient monocular visual symptoms followed by unilateral pulsatile headache have been described in patients with known migraine and this is classified as 'retinal migraine' (Hedges & Lackman, 1976). Retinal migraine is much more difficult to diagnose if there is no headache associated with the attacks. TMB as a result of thromboembolism and retinal migraine are distinguished on the basis of the patient's symptoms; the former is characterised by the abrupt onset of 'negative' monocular visual phenomena (blindness), which is painless and usually lasts only a few minutes, whilst the latter is characterised by the gradual build-up of transient monocular visual impairment (i.e. scotoma or blindness), which is usually incomplete and may be associated with 'positive' visual symptoms (e.g. scintillations) lasting for up to 1 hour and a pulsatile headache or orbital pain (Blau, 1992; Blau & MacGregor, 1993). Sometimes it can be difficult to distinguish between retinal ischaemia and retinal migraine, particularly in older patients. Attacks of positive visual phenomena lasting longer than expected for retinal ischaemia (5 minutes or so) not infrequently turn out to be associated with angiographic evidence of ipsilateral ICA stenosis (Goodwin et al., 1987). It has therefore been suggested that the results of non-invasive investigations, such as carotid ultrasound, may help distinguish the two — i.e. the presence of tight stenosis of the ICA on the symptomatic side is suggestive of retinal ischaemia (due to artery-to-artery embolism) and the absence of carotid disease favours retinal migraine (Sandercock & Smart, 1990). However, this is only circumstantial evidence.

Patients have been described with frequent (one to 30 episodes per day), stereotyped episodes of brief (lasting < 3 minutes) unilateral visual loss caused by presumed vasospasm (Burger et al., 1991). Fundus examination during the episodes of blindness showed constriction of the retinal arteries and segmentation in a thin and slowly moving column of blood. The calibre of the retinal vessels was restored with the return of vision. Another patient has been reported in whom multiple daily episodes of brief unilateral visual loss stopped when the patient was treated with a calcium channel blocker, suggesting that vasospasm may have been the underlying mechanism (Winterkorn & Teman, 1991). The same authors have also reported another patient with recurrent episodes of TMB associated with sexual intercourse, which stopped after he began to take 20 mg of nifedipine by mouth 0.5 hours before expected intercourse (Teman *et al.*, 1995). However, as there is really no proof of vasospasm, we have to be very cautious in the interpretation of these observations.

The results of prognostic studies showing that patients with retinal ischaemia have a better prognosis than patients with TIA of the brain (Dennis *et al.*, 1990b; Hankey *et al.*, 1991, 1992; Dutch TIA Trial Study Group, 1993) suggest that a considerable proportion of these patients may have been cases of retinal migraine or something else benign; those who proceeded to subsequent vascular events, such as stroke or retinal infarction, were presumably true cases of retinal ischaemia due to carotid stenosis, heart disease or other less common conditions, such as arteritis and procoagulant states (Tippin *et al.*, 1989; Gutrecht *et al.*, 1991; O'Sullivan *et al.*, 1992).

The question therefore arises, how do we define retinal migraine: is it a diagnosis based on the clinical symptoms and signs, the results of investigations, the response to treatment or the prognosis? It has been traditionally diagnosed on the basis of the clinical history but this may be non-specific and it is seldom possible to examine the patient during the episode to see if 'vasospasm' is present. It has therefore been suggested that the presence or absence of carotid disease (whether coincidental or not), the response to treatment and the prognosis may help determine the diagnosis. For practical purposes, if it is not possible to confidently distinguish retinal ischaemia and migraine from the history, the patient should be assessed, investigated and treated as a case of retinal ischaemia, but carotid angiography should only be undertaken if duplex carotid ultrasound shows tight carotid stenosis on the symptomatic side. Using the prognosis as a definition is of course unhelpful in clinical practice.

Dural arteriovenous malformation

Anterior and middle fossa dural AVMs may very rarely cause TMB, probably because of transient lowering of retinal arterial pressure associated with shunting of blood away from the ophthalmic artery to the malformation (Bogousslavsky *et al.*, 1985).

Central or branch retinal vein thrombosis

Thrombosis of the central retinal vein or branch retinal vein sometimes presents with attacks of TMB; the visual loss tends to be patchy rather than complete. The fundoscopic appearance is characteristic and consists of engorged retinal veins and multiple retinal haemorrhages (Fig. 3.15) (Hayreh, 1976).

Glaucoma

In narrow-angle (closed-angle, angle-closure) glaucoma, the apposition of the peripheral iris to the trabecular meshwork blocks filtration at the angle. The extent of angle closure determines the decrease in outflow and in turn the increase in intraocular pressure. Elevated intraocular pressure reduces perfusion pressure of the eye and may reduce blood flow to the choroid, retina and disc (Best *et al.*, 1969). Transient monocular visual disturbance may occur, particularly in poor light when the pupil is dilated (Fisher, 1967; Ravits & Seybold, 1984). The onset is usually subacute; vision may be decreased, blurred, foggy or smoke-like; and the patient may see haloes around lights. Some patients complain of light sensitivity during the attack and most, but not all, have eye pain. The symptoms may last from a few minutes to hours. The presence of eye pain and the stereotyped recurrence of attacks under certain lighting conditions can be useful clues to the diagnosis, particularly if the eye is red, the cornea

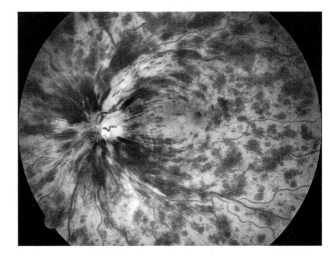

Figure 3.15 Ocular fundus photograph showing engorged retinal veins and multiple retinal haemorrhages due to central retinal vein thrombosis.

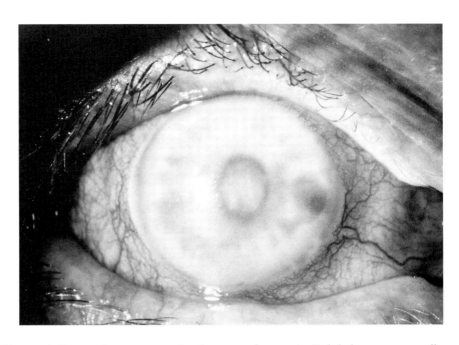

Figure 3.16 Photograph of the eye of a patient with acute glaucoma. Note the congested sclera, cloudy cornea and oval pupil.

cloudy and the pupil oval in shape (Fig. 3.16). Intraocular pressure should be checked but it is not always raised between attacks.

Retinal and other intraocular haemorrhage

Retinal haemorrhage, if small or located in the periphery of the retina, may cause sudden reduced vision in one eye which resolves within hours. The diagnosis should be evident on ophthalmoscopy, particularly if the pupil is dilated. Similarly, vitreous and anterior chamber haemorrhage may cause TMB (Amaurosis Fugax Study Group, 1990). The cause may be evident from the history; for example, sudden visual loss caused by preretinal haemorrhages within the macula may occur during physical exertion, sexual activity or Valsalva manoeuvre (Friberg *et al.*, 1995).

3.4.2 Retinal non-vascular

Paraneoplastic retinopathy

Transient episodes lasting seconds to minutes of painless monocular dimming of the central field of vision and overwhelming visual glare and photosensitivity when exposed to bright light are suggestive of not only photoreceptor dysfunction due to transient retinal ischaemia but also paraneoplastic retinopathy (Jacobsen *et al.*, 1990). Patients may also experience transient bizarre entoptic symptoms (alterations in normal light perception resulting from intraoptic phenomena, akin to the subjective perception of light resulting from mechanical compression of the eyeball) (Keltner *et al.*,

1983; Jacobsen *et al.*, 1990). Ophthalmoscopy usually reveals attenuated retinal arterioles, electroretinography demonstrates abnormal cone and rod-mediated responses, and antiretinal antibodies may be identified in the serum (Grunwald *et al.*, 1985). Over the subsequent months, progressive visual loss occurs, during which time a small cell carcinoma of the lung often declares itself.

Phosphenes

Phosphenes are flashes of light and coloured spots which are induced by eye movement in a dark environment and occur in the absence of luminous stimuli. They may occur with disease of the visual system at many different sites, such as optic neuritis in the recovery phase, perhaps as a result of the mechanical effects of movement of the optic nerve. However, mechanical pressure on the normal eyeball may also induce a phosphene, as every child discovers, by stimulating the retina. Phosphenes may also occur in a healthy dark-adapted closed eye after a saccade (flick phosphene).

Lightning streaks of Moore

In a dark environment elderly people frequently experience recurrent, brief, stereotypic, vertical flashes of light in the temporal visual field of one eye, which are elicited by eye movement. These are known as Moore's lightning streaks and are benign. It is believed that, with advanced age, the posterior vitreous may collapse and detach from the retina, leading to persistent vitreoretinal adhesions. The mechanical forces associated with eye movement exert traction on the

59

macula and retina, and induce the photopsias (subjective sensations of sparks or flashes of light) (Zaret, 1985).

Chorioretinitis

Macular disease due to chorioretinitis or retinal pigmentary degeneration can sometimes lead to loss of vision in bright light (Severin *et al.*, 1967; Glaser *et al.*, 1977).

3.4.3 Optic nerve vascular

Anterior ischaemic optic neuropathy (AION)

AION is due to ischaemia in the territory of supply of the posterior ciliary arteries, which are branches of the ophthalmic artery and supply the anterior part of the optic nerve, the choroid and outer retina (Hayreh, 1975). Because the optic disc is close to an arterial border zone between the territories of the two major posterior ciliary arteries and, because the border zone is situated at the furthest periphery of the arterial tree, it is liable to selective ischaemia when the systemic blood pressure falls, when the intraocular pressure rises or when there is occlusive disease of local small arteries (Anonymous, 1984). The most common cause of AION is therefore reduced perfusion pressure caused by a marked fall in systemic blood pressure or a rise in intraocular pressure, or a combination of the two. Less often, AION is caused by thrombotic or embolic occlusion of the posterior ciliary arteries or of the arterioles feeding the anterior part of the optic nerve (Hayreh, 1975). Thrombotic occlusion of the posterior ciliary arteries can be caused by giant cell arteritis (Fig. 3.17) and other types of vasculitis, such as polyarteritis nodosa. Atherosclerosis is another presumed cause (Boghen & Glaser, 1975; Goodwin, 1985), given that patients with AION have an increased prevalence of hypertension and diabetes and an increased risk of subsequent cerebrovascular and cardiovascular events (Guyer *et al.*, 1985), but we are not aware of any histological proof of atheromatous occlusion of these arteries. Embolic occlusion seems to occur much less frequently than thrombotic occlusion, but this impression may be based partly on our inability to see the emboli in these vessels on ophthalmoscopy, as compared with the easily seen emboli in the retinal arteries. Nevertheless, multiple emboli in the vessels of the anterior part of the optic nerve have been demonstrated histologically in AION (Lieberman *et al.*, 1978). The usual source of embolism is presumably the proximal carotid circulation, but this remains uncertain (Reich *et al.*, 1990).

Ischaemia of the optic disc is characterised clinically by the abrupt onset of painless visual loss in one eye. This may involve the whole field but tends to be more severe in the

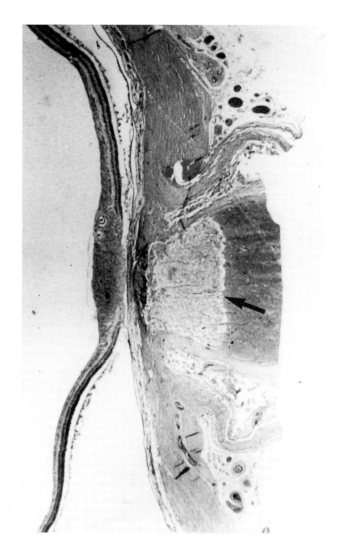

Figure 3.17 Photomicrograph of anterior ischaemic optic neuropathy caused by giant cell arteritis. Arrow indicates the infarcted optic nerve head. (Courtesy of Dr J. F. Cullen, Western General Hospital, Edinburgh.)

lower quadrants because the upper segment of the optic disc is more vulnerable to ischaemia (Hayreh, 1981). In the early stages, the circulation may be so precariously balanced that minor postural change may have profound effects on the degree of visual loss. The visual loss is often severe, non-progressive and prolonged, but it can be brief (and present as TMB) and it can be progressive over several hours or days. In AION due to giant cell arteritis, the visual loss may develop in both eyes within a few days and, rarely, almost simultaneously. On examination, the visual acuity varies from 6/6 to no light perception, so that normal visual acuity does not exclude AION. Almost any part of the visual field can be affected but usually the visual field defects are nerve fibre bundle defects characteristic of an optic disc disorder. An altitudinal hemifield defect (loss of either the upper or, more frequently, the lower half of the field in one eye) is particularly common, as is inferior nasal segmental loss and central scotoma. The disc may appear normal at first, but within a few days it becomes pale and swollen, often with small flame-shaped haemorrhages radiating from the disc margin (ischaemic papillopathy), distended veins and, occasionally, cotton-wool spots due to ischaemic change in the surrounding retina (see Fig. 3.6). The swelling may involve only one segment of the disc or be more marked in one segment than in another. The disc swelling is attributed partly to leakage of plasma from damaged blood vessels and partly to arrest of axoplasmic transport along damaged nerve fibres. The disc swelling may be indistinguishable from that seen with raised intracranial pressure, and sometimes the disc has a pale appearance and, in about 50% of the eyes with AION due to giant cell arteritis, the disc swelling has a chalky white appearance (Hayreh, 1981). Later, the swelling subsides to be succeeded by optic atrophy with attenuation of the small blood vessels on the disc surface. The prognosis for recovery of vision is variable. Many patients recover good central vision but are left with arcuate and sectorial visual field defects corresponding to loss of bundles of nerve fibres. In other patients visual loss may be complete and permanent.

Malignant arterial hypertension

Some patients with malignant hypertension experience TMB due to ischaemia of the optic nerve head (Hayreh et al., 1986). Associated headache, seizures, encephalopathy, renal impairment, high blood pressure and characteristic ophthalmoscopic features of hypertension, such as arterial narrowing and tortuosity, arteriovenous nipping, optic disc oedema and retinal haemorrhages point to the diagnosis (see Fig. 3.10).

3.4.4 Optic nerve non-vascular

Papilloedema

Patients with papilloedema (Fig. 3.18) from any cause may experience transient visual blurring or obscurations, with or without photopsias (Hayreh, 1977). The visual loss in chronic papilloedema is often postural, occurring as patients get up from a chair (or bend over), and may involve either eye alone or both eyes together. The explanation may be transient optic nerve ischaemia secondary to a relative decrease in orbital blood flow as a result of raised cerebrospinal fluid (CSF) pressure in the subarachnoid space around the optic nerve and increased pressure in the veins

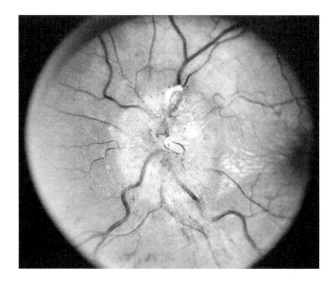

Figure 3.18 Ocular fundus photograph showing papilloedema. Note the congested swollen disc, loss of the physiological cup, blurred disc margins and congested retinal veins.

draining the optic nerve head. A history of episodes of visual blurring or blindness in someone with papilloedema should lead to urgent investigation and appropriate action, because permanent visual loss will eventually follow, gradually or suddenly.

Optic neuritis

Patients with optic nerve demyelination due to MS may experience transiently decreased vision in one or both eyes during exercise (Uhthoff's symptom) or in association with other causes of increased temperature, emotional stress, increased illumination, eating, drinking, smoking and menstruation. The pathophysiology of Uhthoff's symptom is unknown, although a reversible conduction block in demyelinated nerve fibres secondary to an increase in body temperature or to changes in blood electrolyte levels or pH is believed to play a role (Scholl et al., 1991). Ophthalmoscopy may be normal but if the optic nerve head is inflamed the optic disc may be swollen and look similar to papilloedema.

Optic disc anomalies

Transient monocular visual obscurations are occasionally associated with an elevated optic disc without increased intracranial pressure. Examples include congenital anomalies of the optic disc, such as drüsen or posterior staphyloma (Seybold & Rosen, 1977).

3.4.5 Eye/orbit

Transient changes in the ocular media or intraocular pressure, such as vitreous floaters, vitreous haemorrhage, anterior chamber haemorrhage, lens subluxation, reversible cataract (in a diabetic) and glaucoma may cause transient monocular visual disturbance (Ravits & Seybold, 1984; Paylor *et al.*, 1985). Most of these conditions can be excluded by a competent ophthalmological examination. Intraorbital masses, such as an optic nerve sheath meningioma, may produce gaze-evoked TMB; the blindness is limited to the duration of gaze in the affected direction and the visual acuity usually returns to normal about 30 seconds after the eye moves back to the primary position; the loss of vision is possibly caused by a reduction in flow to the blood vessels surrounding the optic nerve itself (Wilkes *et al.*, 1979; Brown & Sheilds, 1981; Bradbury *et al.*, 1987).

> *Patients with transient monocular blindness must have a competent ophthalmological examination to exclude primary disorders of the retina, optic disc and media before jumping to the conclusion that the explanation is vascular disease.*

3.5 Differential diagnosis of stroke

The clinical differentiation of 'stroke' from 'not a stroke' is accurate more than 95% of the time if there is a clear history (from the patient or carer) of focal brain dysfunction of sudden onset (or first noticed on waking), and if there is a residual relevant focal neurological deficit present at the time of the clinical examination (Allen, 1983; Sandercock *et al.*, 1985). This is particularly true if the patient is elderly or has other vascular diseases or risk factors, because the prevalence, i.e. the prior (or pretest) probability, of stroke is greater in elderly people with vascular disease than in younger people who have no evidence of vascular disease. Of course, the accuracy of the diagnosis of stroke also depends on the timing of the assessment; it can occasionally be difficult to distinguish stroke from non-stroke within the first few hours of presentation but, as time evolves, other history or physical signs frequently declare themselves and improve diagnostic accuracy. On the other hand, it can also be difficult if patients are seen a long time after the onset of their stroke, when they may not be clear about the onset and nature of their symptoms.

Sometimes, it is not possible to obtain a history of the onset, or even the nature, of the symptoms because the patient is unconscious, confused, demented or dysphasic and there is nobody who can provide information about how quickly the symptoms were likely to have developed. In these patients in particular, the presence of a persistent focal neurological deficit may not be due to stroke but to head trauma, encephalitis, brain abscess, brain tumour or a chronic subdural haematoma. The presence of symptoms or signs that are unusual in uncomplicated stroke, such as papilloedema and unexplained fever, should call into question the clinical diagnosis. Also, a persistent focal neurological deficit may be due to a previous stroke and the clinical presentation is caused by a non-vascular problem such as pneumonia. Without information about the rate of onset and progression of symptoms, it is crucial to search for indirect clues to the pathogenesis in the past history and physical examination and to continue to assess the patient over time for the development of new signs such as fever, and for the natural recovery that characterises non-fatal stroke (as opposed to tumour).

The absence of a persistent focal neurological deficit by no means excludes a stroke in patients who have suffered a sudden decline in neurological function. It may simply represent a delay in presentation, so the signs have resolved, or it may be that the signs are subtle (but nevertheless functionally important to the patient) and have been missed. For example, patients may have a visual–spatial–perceptual disorder (e.g. dressing apraxia) but no weakness in the limbs, due to a non-dominant parietal lesion, subtle cognitive dysfunction, due to a vascular lesion in the frontal lobe(s) or thalamus, or truncal and gait ataxia, due to a cerebellar stroke, which may not be apparent (or elicitable) if the patient is not sat up or got ut of bed (Dunne *et al.*, 1986; Mori & Yamadori, 1987). These are the sort of deficits that may be missed (but should not be) on busy ward rounds after carotid endarterectomy or coronary artery bypass surgery, or indeed any time.

> *In patients without obvious focal neurological signs, look specifically for: visual–spatial–perceptual dysfunction, such as constructional apraxia, sensory inattention/extinction, loss of discriminative sensations, proprioception or graphaesthesia, impaired two-point discrimination, neglect and anosognosia, etc.; a visual field deficit; dysphasia; cognitive dysfunction; and gait or trunk ataxia.*

The conditions that may be mistaken clinically and radiologically for a stroke are listed in Table 3.15.

3.5.1 Epileptic seizures

Epileptic seizures are one of the most common causes of misdiagnosis of stroke. In a series of 821 consecutive patients admitted to an acute stroke unit, the initial diagnosis of 'stroke' proved to be epileptic seizures in 4% (Norris &

Table 3.15 Differential diagnosis of stroke.

Diagnosis	Key features
Epileptic seizure + postictal neurological deficit (see Section 3.5.1)	History from witness, positive symptoms (e.g. focal limb jerking), EEG
Structural intracranial lesions (see Section 3.5.2) Subdural haematoma (acute, chronic) Tumour (primary, secondary) AVM	Gradual onset, headache, confusion, drowsiness, seizures, papilloedema fluctutation, tendency to worsen rather than improve
Metabolic/toxic encephalopathy (see Section 3.5.3) Hyponatraemia Hypocalcaemia Hepatic encephalopathy Wernicke–Korsakoff syndrome	Confusion, seizures, altered consciousness Global brain dysfunction Global brain dysfunction Global brain dysfunction Alcoholic, confusion, ataxia, nystagmus, neuropathy, reduced blood transketolase, response to thiamine
Hypoglycaemia	Timing and recurrence of attacks, usually diabetic on hypoglycaemic treatment
Non-ketotic hyperglycaemia	Global brain dysfunction (delirium, coma), seizures, involuntary movements
Alcohol and drug intoxication	Seizures, global brain dysfunction
Head injury (see Section 3.5.4)	History, signs of head trauma
Encephalitis/cerebral abscess (see Section 3.5.5)	Gradual onset, fever, seizures, systemic infection
Hypertensive encephalopathy (see Section 3.5.6)	Subacute onset, headache, confusion, seizures, altered consciousness, high blood pressure, hypertensive retinopathy
MS (see Section 3.5.7)	Young, subacute onset, previous attacks, MRI, CSF
Creutzfeldt–Jakob disease (see Section 3.5.8)	Subacute onset, dementia, myoclonus, EEG
Peripheral nerve lesion (see Section 3.5.9)	Lower motor neurone or dermatomal signs
Functional (hysteria/malingering) (see Section 3.5.10)	Inconsistencies, concurrent emotional conflict, past history of previous episodes of hysteria or psychiatric problems, hard objective neurological signs lacking, 'give-way weakness'

Hachinski, 1982). The usual scenario is a patient with postictal confusion, stupor, coma or hemiparesis in whom the preceding seizure was unwitnessed or unrecognised. Clues to the diagnosis of seizures instead of stroke can be obtained by taking a careful history from the family or patient of previous seizures before admission or of similar episodes (i.e. of confusion and hemiparesis) shown to be due to epilepsy, by continuing to observe the patient in hospital for evidence of further seizures and by performing an EEG to see if any epileptic features are present (Norris & Hachinski, 1982).

Recurrent partial epileptic seizures that are secondary to a previous stroke can sometimes cause a prolonged exacerbation of the initial neurological deficit rather than a temporary exacerbation (e.g. Todd's paresis of aphasia) and so be mistaken for a recurrent stroke (Bogousslavsky *et al.*, 1992; Hankey, 1993). The diagnosis depends on an accurate history of events before the onset of the neurological deficit (e.g. epigastric discomfort and olfactory or gustatory hallucinations due to an initial partial sensory seizure) and serial CT or MRI scans showing no extension of the previous lesion or a new lesion.

3.5.2 Structural intracranial lesions

In less than 5% of patients who are diagnosed clinically as having an acute stroke, the brain CT or MRI scan reveals a structural intracranial lesion such as a subdural haematoma, tumour (e.g. meningioma) or AVM. In such cases, there has usually been some doubt about the rate of onset of the focal neurological deficit.

Subdural haematoma

Subdural haematoma may rarely present with the abrupt onset of focal neurological signs and so mimic a stroke (Luxon & Harrison, 1979). In one series, three of the 821 patients admitted with a diagnosis of stroke were eventually shown to have a subdural haematoma (Norris & Hachinski, 1982). Each patient had a confusional state and minimal neurological signs starting 3 days to 3 weeks previously. Therefore, suspect subdural haematoma if there is evidence of: focal neurological symptoms and signs (i.e. hemiparesis, aphasia) of subacute onset; persistent headache; more confusion and drowsiness than expected from the neurological deficit; a progressive or fluctuating clinical course; a bleeding diathesis; anticoagulant use; alcohol abuse; head injury in the preceding few weeks (which only about 50% of patients recall); or ventricular decompression for hydrocephalus.

In the acute phase, brain CT scan usually shows a unilateral area of hyperdensity in the subdural space, ipsilateral effacement of sulci and mass effect causing shift of the mid-

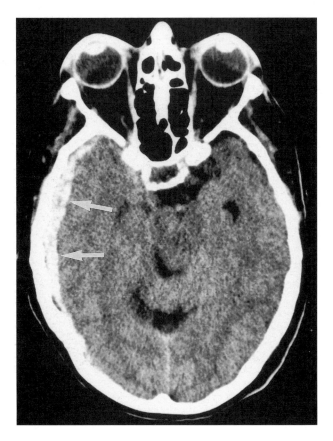

Figure 3.19 Plain (non-contrast) brain CT scan showing a unilateral area of hyperdensity in the subdural space (arrows) due to an acute subdural haematoma, with ipsilateral effacement of sulci and mass effect causing shift of the midline and distortion of the ventricular system.

line and distortion of the ventricular system (Fig. 3.19). There is a transitional stage, however, between 7 and 21 days, during which clotted blood evolves on CT scan from a region of hyperintensity to one of isointensity and this can easily be missed, particularly if the subdural haematomas are bilateral and so there is little if any evidence of midline shift or asymmetrical ventricular compression (see Fig. 3.14; Davenport *et al.*, 1994). Thereafter, the haematoma becomes hypodense and thus more easily visible. MRI is more sensitive than CT for detecting subdural haematomas.

Tumour

Although stroke is a common cause of progressing neurological deficit over hours or even days, it is also important to consider intracranial tumours in the differential diagnosis of a patient with progressing neurological deficit, particularly if the rate of progression is slower (over several days/weeks/months) and there is a history of recent headache or

epileptic seizures, signs of papilloedema or any evidence of a primary extracranial source of malignancy. All nine (1%) of the 821 patients with suspected stroke studied by Norris and Hachinski (1982) who turned out to have a cerebral tumour had a hemiparesis gradually evolving over several weeks to several months. Three of these patients presented with seizures and five had papilloedema on admission, a finding which is most uncommon in acute stroke.

Papilloedema is very uncommon in acute stroke.

Occasionally, tumours can give rise to focal neurological deficits that arise suddenly and may even be followed by recovery, so mimicking a TIA or stroke (Daly *et al.*, 1961; Weisberg & Nice, 1977). The usual cause is a Todd's paresis following a partial seizure associated with a tumour or haemorrhage into a tumour. The brain tumours that tend to bleed are glioblastoma, choroid plexus papilloma, meningioma, neuroblastoma, melanoma, hypernephroma, lymphoma, endometrial carcinoma and choriocarcinoma (see Section 5.3.4). The CT scan may disclose ICH in an unusual location or associated with a lot of oedema, or multiple haemorrhages, or it may show other metastatic deposits

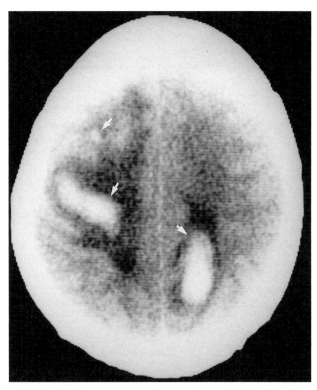

Figure 3.20 Plain CT scan showing multiple areas of high density (arrows) due to spontaneous ICH into what turned out at postmortem to be metastases from choriocarcinoma.

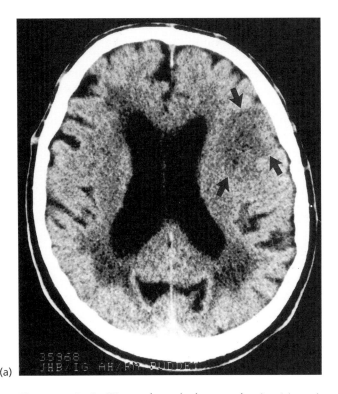
(a)

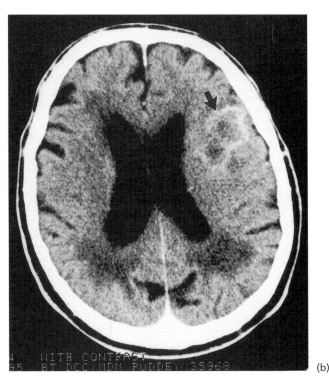
(b)

Figure 3.21 Brain CT scan of a cerebral tumour showing: (a) a region of low attenuation (due to cerebral oedema) with imprecise boundaries (arrows) and some mass effect, causing effacement of sulci; (b) after intravenous injection, iodinated contrast material leaks into the tumour and is seen on CT as an area of diffuse or peripheral enhancement (arrow).

(Fig. 3.20). If there has been no haemorrhage into the tumour, CT scan usually shows a region of low attenuation (due to cerebral oedema) with imprecise boundaries and some mass effect, causing effacement of sulci or ventricular compression. If there is a breakdown of the blood–brain barrier, as commonly occurs in patients with cerebral tumours, then intravenous injection of iodinated contrast material leaks into the tumour and is seen on CT as an area of diffuse or peripheral enhancement (Fig. 3.21). A similar, but nevertheless distinctive, appearance of enhancement of the gyri, which may be seen within 1–2 weeks of a recent cerebral infarct, is also due to breakdown of the blood–brain barrier (Fig. 3.22). Although this has been referred to as 'luxury perfusion', we believe this is an inappropriate term because the appearance has nothing to do with extra perfusion; it is a result of contrast leaking from damaged capillaries.

If the clinical examination and CT are ambiguous, patients should be followed up clinically (because with a tumour they usually deteriorate, with new or more severe symptoms and signs) and a follow-up CT or MRI should be performed within a few weeks to a few months (depending of the patient's progress) to see if the lesion has resolved or, if it is a tumour, continued to grow.

Arteriovenous malformation (see Section 8.2.2)

When AVMs become symptomatic, they generally do so by causing seizures or haemorrhage into the brain and occasionally haemorrhage into the subarachnoid space. Sometimes they cause intermittent or fluctuating focal neurological symptoms, which are probably due to vascular steal or microhaemorrhage, in brainstem AVMs in particular (Abe *et al.*, 1989; Anonymous, 1989). Brain CT scan, with and without contrast, MRI or cerebral angiography may be required to make the diagnosis, but AVMs can be suspected clinically if there is cutaneous evidence of the Sturge–Weber syndrome, a cranial bruit (which is uncommon), the clinical features of hereditary haemorrhagic telangiectasia or a past history of SAH or seizures.

3.5.3 Metabolic/toxic encephalopathy

Encephalopathies due to metabolic or toxic distrubances generally cause subacute evolution of an altered conscious state, with or without systemic disturbance, and few if any focal neurological signs (perhaps only generalised hyperreflexia, with or without extensor plantar responses). However, sometimes metabolic disturbances present with

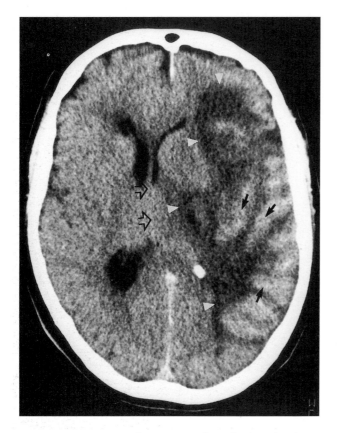

Figure 3.22 Brain CT (with contrast) performed 8 days after the stroke onset showing a region of low attenuation consistent with infarction (arrowheads) in the vascular territory of the middle cerebral artery, and a serpiginous gyral pattern of high attenuation due to breakdown of the blood–brain barrier (arrows). There is considerable mass effect with displacement of midline structures (open arrows), effacement of the ventricle and obliteration of sulci.

focal neurological symptoms and signs, which may be acute in onset and mimic a stroke (Norris & Hachinski, 1982; Berkovic *et al.*, 1984). These include hyponatraemia (cf. central pontine myelinolysis), hypocalcaemia, hepatic failure, Wernicke–Korsakoff syndrome, hypoglycaemia and non-ketotic hyperglycaemia; the hyperosmolarity of hyperglycaemia can itself cause regional reduction of cerebral blood flow, focal neurological deficits, stroke-like syndromes and cerebral infarction (Maccario, 1968; Duckrow *et al.*, 1985; Lin & Chang, 1994).

Amongst 1460 consecutive patients admitted to an acute stroke unit, Berkovic *et al.* (1984) found that in 10 (0.7%) the cause was a metabolic encephalopathy, such as hypoglycaemia (three cases), hyperglycaemia (three), hyponatraemia (three) and hypoxia (one). The conventional symptoms and signs of the metabolic disorders were frequently minimal or absent, but common clinical clues to the diagnosis were a

confusional state and focal seizures (both of which are unusual in stroke). In a similar study by Norris and Hachinski (1982), there were 23 patients (2.8%) who were misdiagnosed as an acute stroke and who presented in a state of confusion or impaired consciousness that was not due to epilepsy; seven patients were intoxicated with drugs or alcohol, seven had psychogenic disorders, three had senile confusional states, three subdural haematoma and three metabolic encephalopathy, including hepatic encephalopathy.

Hypoglycaemia

Although hypoglycaemia usually causes symptoms of adrenergic activity, such as sweating and tachycardia, sometimes there are only focal neurological features without the adrenergic symptoms and so the attack may mimic a stroke. The patient is almost always being treated for diabetes with hypoglycaemic agents but may have factitious hypoglycaemia; an insulinoma; clinical evidence of Addison's disease; hypopituitarism; hypothyroidism; sepsis; terminal malignancy or liver failure; have been starving; or be on drugs whose adverse effects include hypoglycaemia (Rother *et al.*, 1992). The symptoms tend to be stereotyped in an individual and usually occur before meals (i.e. before breakfast or during the night, after fasting for some time), after exercise or 2–3 hours after ingestion of sugars and starch, and are relieved by glucose administration. The blood glucose is usually less than 2.5 mmol/L at the onset of the attack but may have normalised spontaneously or with glucose supplementation later.

> If a diabetic patient presents with a suspected stroke early in the morning, it is imperative that hypoglycaemia be considered, and treated if the diagnosis is confirmed and the patient has not recovered spontaneously.

Wernicke's disease

Wernicke's disease (thiamine-deficient encephalopathy) can sometimes be mistaken for a stroke because of an unusually sudden onset of diplopia (due to abducens and conjugate gaze palsies and nystagmus), ataxia and mental confusion, either singly or, more often, in various combinations (Harper *et al.*, 1986; Victor *et al.*, 1989). It is due to thiamine deficiency and is seen mainly, although not exclusively, in alcoholics (Vortmeyer *et al.*, 1992). The diagnosis can be difficult because the history of symptom onset may be unclear due to recent alcohol intoxication or the presence of Korsakoff psychosis. *Korsakoff psychosis* (amnesic or amnestic confabulatory state) is a unique mental disorder, in which retentive memory is impaired out of all proportion to other cognitive functions in an otherwise alert and responsive patient. It is often associated with alcoholism and malnutrition, but it may be a symptom of other disorders that cause lesions in the temporal lobes or diencephalon (e.g. infarction, surgical resection, herpes simplex virus infection, hypoxic encephalopathy, Alzheimer's disease, tumours of the third ventricle). In the alcoholic, nutritionally deficient patient, the Korsakoff amnesic state is usually associated with Wernicke's disease and is termed the Wernicke–Korsakoff syndrome.

Clues to the diagnosis are the nature of the clinical features, signs of peripheral neuropathy in more than 80% of patients, postural hypotension (autonomic neuropathy), disordered cardiovascular function (tachycardia, exertional dyspnoea, minor ECG abnormalities) and impaired capacity to discriminate between odours (in the chronic stage of the disease due to a lesion of the medial dorsal nucleus of the thalamus). The diagnosis can be confirmed by showing a marked reduction in blood transketolase activity (transketolase is one of the enzymes of the hexose monophosphate shunt and requires thiamine pyrophosphate as a cofactor) and a striking restoration toward normal of the transketolase and the clinical features even within hours of the administration of thiamine; completely normal values of transketolase are usually attained within 24 hours. Failure of the ocular palsies to respond to thiamine within a few days should raise doubts about the diagnosis of Wernicke's disease. The medial thalamic and periaqueductal lesions are also usually well demonstrated on MRI of the brain (Fig. 3.23).

If Wernicke's disease or hypoglycaemia is a diagnostic possibility, take blood (for red cell transketolase, thiamine and glucose levels) and then treat immediately with thiamine and glucose; do not waste time waiting for the results to come back.

3.5.4 Head injury

Head injury and stroke can co-exist or predispose to each other. For example, head injury may cause intracranial haemorrhage, which can be mistaken for a primary stroke if the patient is amnesic for the injury and has no external scalp evidence of injury. Head injury can also lead to ischaemic stroke as a result of arterial dissection in the neck or head (see Section 7.1). On the other hand, stroke can precipitate a fall, causing head injury and, if the CT scan shows intracranial haemorrhage, the primary stroke event may be missed (Berlit *et al.*, 1991; Sakas *et al.*, 1995). An accurate history from relevant people (the patient, witnesses, family members, ambulance officers and family doctor) is essential to try

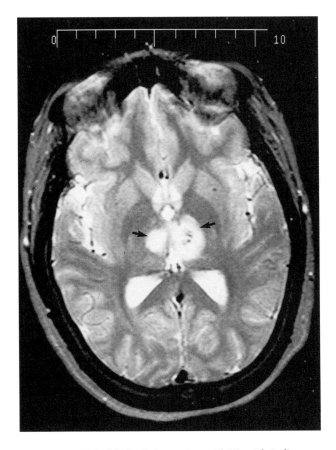

Figure 3.23 MRI of the brain in a patient with Wernicke's disease. She presented with an abrupt onset of double vision followed within a few minutes by a depressed level of consciousness (Glasgow Coma Scale E1 V1 M5) and was initially diagnosed as an acute stroke. She had a complete vertical and horizontal ophthalmoplegia with no response to oculocephalic manoeuvres or caloric testing. She responded rapidly to 100 mg of thiamine given intravenously. The MRI shows bilateral lesions in the medial periventricular thalamic regions (arrows), which extended into the midbrain, the floor of the third ventricle and the upper part of the oculomotor nucleus.

and sort this out. The radiological findings can also shed some light on the cause; intracranial haemorrhages from head injury tend to be more common in the frontal and anterior temporal regions, superficial and multiple and there may be accompanying extension into the subarachnoid space and associated skull fractures (Fig. 3.24).

3.5.5 Encephalitis/cerebral abscess/ subdural empyema

If a patient with a focal neurological deficit has an altered conscious state and a fever, then localised infection (meningoencephalitis, brain abscess or subdural empyema) needs

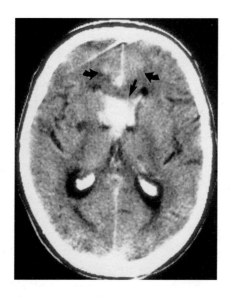

Figure 3.24 Brain CT scan showing SAH in a patient who presented with confusion following a head injury. There is blood in the anterior interhemispheric fissure (arrow) in a pattern suggestive of SAH, but the presentation apparently following a head injury and the suggestion of frontal haemorrhagic contusions (curved arrows) clouded the interpretation of the CT scan and delayed recognition of the true pathology (aneurysmal haemorrhage).

to be considered (and perhaps even treated empirically), particularly if there is no other cause for the fever (such as pneumonia, urinary tract infection or deep venous thrombosis). There may also be a history of subacute evolution of systemic upset (fever, malaise, lethargy) and focal neurological symptoms as well as evidence of seizures, meningism or a predisposing condition such as sinusitis, mastoiditis, otitis, thrombophlebitis, pneumonia or congenital heart disease.

The EEG, brain CT, MRI scan and CSF are usually characteristically abnormal and suggestive (Mauser *et al.*, 1986; Saul *et al.*, 1986; Khan *et al.*, 1995). For example, the parasitic infection cysticercosis may present like a stroke, but the patient will have lived in an endemic area and the CT scan often shows an area of calcification within a cyst as well as scattered foci of parenchymal calcification (McCormick *et al.*, 1982). In unilateral subdural empyema, the EEG shows extensive unilateral depression of cortical activity and focal delta waves lasting up to 2 seconds (Mauser *et al.*, 1986) and the CT shows a non-homogeneous lenticular or semilunar extracerebral lesion with mass effect. However, the CT can be normal early in subdural empyema. Likewise, brain CT or MRI of a cerebral abscess usually shows a low-density lesion which is not in a specific vascular territory and which has peripheral ring enhancement following intravenous contrast, but sometimes the presentation can be acute and the

typical CT findings of an abscess can be delayed for several weeks after the onset of the focal neurological deficit (Kong *et al.*, 1993; Hogan, 1994). It can also be difficult do distinguish radiologically herpes simplex encephalitis (HSE) of the frontotemporal lobes from a middle cerebral artery territory infarct (Fig. 3.25). So, if the patient has focal neurological signs and is systemically unwell with fever and has what looks like a normal CT scan, then an abscess, subdural empyema or meningoencephalitis needs to be excluded by MRI scan, EEG and CSF examination (Mauser *et al.*, 1986; Saul *et al.*, 1986).

3.5.6 Hypertensive encephalopathy

Although malignant hypertension with hypertensive encephalopathy is now rare, it is still seen, most commonly in patients with a history of hypertension, but also in

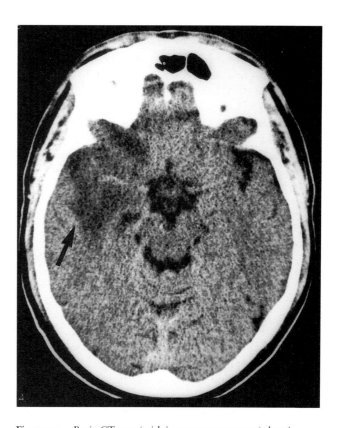

Figure 3.25 Brain CT scan (with intravenous contrast) showing a region of low intensity in the right temporal lobe (arrow) due to HSE. Note how it can sometimes be difficult to distinguish HSE of the frontotemporal lobes from a middle cerebral artery territory infarct radiologically, but usually the site of the encephalitis does not conform to a specific vascular territory and the radiological characteristics of the lesion are different: low density with patchy high density (due to haemorrhagic necrosis) and oedema.

patients with acute hypertension whose autoregulation is normal and easily exceeded by a rapid rise in blood pressure (i.e. associated with conditions such as pre-eclampsia, acute nephritis, phaeochromocytoma, renin-secreting tumour, ingestion of sympathomimetic drugs and tricyclic antidepressants, ingestion of tyramine in conjunction with a monoamine oxidase inhibitor, head injury, autonomic hyperactivity in patients with Guillain–Barré syndrome or spinal cord disorders, and with baroreceptor reflex failure after bilateral carotid endarterectomy) (Calhoun & Oparil, 1990; Ille *et al.*, 1995). Encephalopathy rarely develops in patients with long-standing hypertension until the diastolic blood pressure exceeds 150 mmHg, because their upper limit of anticoagulation is 'set' higher. On the other hand, a previously normotensive young woman with eclampsia or acute glomerulonephritis, for example, may have encephalopathy with a diastolic blood presure of 100 mmHg or less.

The clinical picture is usually dominated by the subacute onset of headache, nausea, vomiting, confusion, declining conscious state, blurred vision, seizures and focal or generalised weakness (Healton *et al.*, 1982). Physical signs include disorientation, obtundation, focal neurological signs, generalised or focal seizures and hypertensive retinopathy (including papilloedema). The cause is thought to be widespread cerebral oedema resulting from a failure of cerebral blood flow autoregulation. Hypertensive encephalopathy can sometimes be mistaken for a stroke, particularly if there is doubt about the onset of symptoms (i.e. if the patient is confused or obtunded) and if the blood pressure is only moderately elevated; even a severely elevated blood pressure can be a consequence of stroke as well as a cause of stroke (see Section 15.7).

3.5.7 Multiple sclerosis (MS)

MS can sometimes present abruptly with a focal neurological deficit and so mimic a stroke (Harper *et al.*, 1981; Galer *et al.*, 1990; Drulovic *et al.*, 1993). However, the patients are usually quite young (< 40 years of age); the onset is often more subacute over days to weeks; the location and shape of the lesions on brain CT or MRI are usually fairly characteristic (i.e. discrete round or oval lesions in the white matter of the cerebral or cerebellar hemispheres and brainstem, in the corpus callosum and adjacent to the temporal horns of the lateral ventricles, not corresponding to territories supplied by specific cerebral arteries); the CSF usually shows a raised lymphocyte count, raised immunoglobulin G (IgG) and oligoclonal bands, which are not present in the serum (Drulovic *et al.*, 1993); and there may be a history of previous episodes of focal neurological dysfunction which were more typical of MS, such as optic neuritis or transverse

myelitis. However, none of these features is specific; for example, oligoclonal bands may also be found in patients with acute stroke, particularly if due to vasculopathies associated with Behçet's disease, systemic lupus erythematosus and sarcoidosis (see Section 7.2; Markowitz & Kokmen, 1983; McLean *et al.*, 1995).

3.5.8 Creutzfeldt–Jakob disease (CJD)

CJD typically presents with a combination of rapidly progressive dementia and myoclonus, which may be accompanied by symptoms and signs of visual, pyramidal and cerebellar dysfunction. However, CJD may occasionally present acutely with a stroke-like syndrome. Amongst a series of 532 patients with 'definite' or 'probable' CJD, the onset was sufficiently abrupt to be diagnosed as a stroke in 30 cases (5.6%); the diagnosis was made by a consultant physician or neurologist in 28 cases and even fulfilled the standard WHO criteria for stroke in two (McNaughton & Will, 1994). Of 29 patients who had a CT scan, five (17%) were reported to have a low-density lesion like an 'infarct' that was appropriate to the clinical signs, and a further five showed 'other' infarct-like areas.

It is difficult to understand how the pathology of CJD could lead to a sudden onset of focal neurological dysfunction and, indeed, that is rarely the case, even in the above series. More commonly, the symptoms evolve over hours to days to weeks and continued observation and follow-up of the patient reveals progressive cognitive impairment, multifocal neurological deficits and, in particular, myoclonus. The EEG usually progressively changes and becomes more specific for CJD.

> *If a 'stroke' patient deteriorates and develops myoclonus or dementia, think of Creutzfeldt–Jakob disease and do an EEG.*

3.5.9 Peripheral nerve lesions

Peripheral nerve (e.g. radial nerve palsy (Norris & Hachinski, 1982)) or nerve-root lesions may occasionally give rise to the sudden onset (or sudden awareness, on waking up from sleep) of focal sensory or motor symptoms. These symptoms can be confused with a 'pseudoradicular' stroke, which may be seen with small lesions confined to the contralateral pre- or postcentral gyrus, corona radiata or thalamus (Omae *et al.*, 1992; Kim, 1994). However, the physical signs of a peripheral nerve lesion (i.e. lower motor neurone signs and/or sensory loss to pain in a dermatomal distribution) are different from those of an intracranial cortical/subcortical lesion, which tend to be associated with upper motor neurone signs and/or loss of discriminative/ 'cortical' sensations, such as joint position sense and two-point discrimination ability.

3.5.10 Functional symptoms and signs

Hysterical conversion (unconscious) and malingering (conscious) can be diagnostic problems in older as well as younger patients, but are uncommon in older patients who do not have a past psychiatric history of some sort. The history tends to be vague and inconsistent and may disclose evidence of social disruption or personality disturbance or a past history of other functional disorders or unexplained somatic symptoms (see Table 3.13). There may or may not be some evidence of potential for gain and, if so, the gain is almost always 'primary' (solution of emotional conflict) rather than 'secondary' (financial compensation). Sometimes there is a 'model' with a real illness (e.g. a friend or family member with a stroke).

The examination findings are helpful. For those with apparent weakness, there are no hard signs of upper or lower motor neurone dysfunction (such as abnormal reflexes, extensor plantar response) and no pressure sores. Voluntary effort is inappropriate and intermittent; there is simultaneous contraction of agonist and antagonist muscles; excessive effort in irrelevant muscle groups; prominent verbal grunts; and with encouragement it is possible to elicit full muscle power even though it is often only momentary and interspersed with episodes of apparent lack of muscle power ('give-way weakness'). There is also inconsistency in what the patient can and can not do during the examination and in between times; for example, the patient may be unable to lift either leg off the bed but can sit up from the supine position and walk (Norris & Hachinski, 1982).

Apparent sensory loss tends to be inconsistent in location and when it is consistent it more frequently involves the left side of the body (Rothwell, 1994) and is non-reproducible, inconsistent with function (e.g. absent joint position sense but normal gait with eyes closed), incompatible with normal sensory anatomy and intermittent (e.g. with eyes shut, the patient responds normally to the examiner touching the tip of the index finger and asking the patient to touch the tip of his/her nose with it, but later the patient appears to have loss of sensation to formal light touch testing in the same finger). Other clues to functional sensory loss include nonsense behaviour (e.g. patient responds 'no' to being touched in the numb area), vibration sense being lost on just one side of the sternum, numbness with circular borders in the limbs or sensory loss on the trunk which changes side when the patient is turned over. Visual function in patients complaining of bilateral blindness who have a normal neuro-ophthalmological examination and who are suspected of malingering can be inferred by testing for optokinetic nystagmus and noting the presence of the optokinetic response, which can not be voluntarily suppressed. Peripheral sensory nerve action potentials, nerve conduction studies and somatosensory, motor and visual evoked potentials are normal, but it is often not necessary to resort to these.

It is important, however, to be very careful when diagnosing focal neurological symptoms and signs as functional, and to do so only after repeated observation, because sometimes conditions such as carotid and vertebral artery dissection and myasthenia gravis in young people can produce variable neurological signs and have a normal series of baseline investigations (McCormick & Halbach, 1993).

> It is not uncommon for patients with an organic problem to have functional overlay as well, as if to try and draw attention to their real underlying problem.

3.5.11 The role of brain CT and MRI scan in the differential diagnosis of stroke

The diagnosis of stroke is largely clinical, and the role of imaging studies such as CT and MRI is to assist in establishing the clinical diagnosis, underlying pathology (see Chapter 5) and cause (see Chapters 6 and 8). The main indications are when there is doubt about the clinical diagnosis of stroke versus non-stroke intracranial pathology; for distinguishing PICH from infarction (see Section 5.3); and for identifying specific pathophysiological subtypes of cerebral infarction and haemorrhage (see Section 5.3.5) (Wardlaw, 1994). There may be doubt about the clinical diagnosis of stroke in up to 20% of patients with suspected stroke (Sandercock et al., 1985; Wardlaw, 1994), particularly when the history is unclear about the onset (? sudden) of focal neurological symptoms (e.g. because of coma, dysphasia, confusion, no witness); when the clinical features are atypical for stroke (e.g. gradual onset, seizures, no clear focal neurolgical signs); when the clinical course is atypical (e.g. progression/worsening of the neurological deficit after onset); when the patient is young (age < 50 years) with no vascular risk factors (i.e. low pretest probability of stroke); and when SAH is suspected (Table 3.16).

The choice of CT or MRI will depend on local availability, cost and effectiveness. If CT is available, it should be performed as soon as possible in all patients because it is the best technique for diagnosing or excluding early ICH (see Section 5.3.4) and it is essential to image suspected SAH (see Section 5.5.3); MRI is no substitute and will miss SAH.

Table 3.16 Indications for brain CT (or MRI) in suspected stroke (see also Section 6.6.3).

---

1 To help distinguish 'stroke' from 'non-stroke'
  Doubt about clinical diagnosis of stroke
  Unclear history of sudden onset of focal neurological symptoms
    (i.e. because of coma, dysphasia, confusion, no witness)
  Atypical clinical features
    (i.e. gradual onset, seizures, no clear focal neurological signs)
  Atypical progression/worsening of 'stroke' after onset
  Young patient (age <50 years) with no vascular risk factors
2 To distinguish ICH from cerebral infarction (CT must be done as soon as possible, certainly within 10 days of stroke)
3 SAH suspected (CT prior to lumbar puncture where possible; not MRI, see Section 5.3.3)

Note: the sudden onset of a focal neurological deficit is, by definition, a stroke syndrome (or a TIA if the deficit resolves within 24 hours), even if the CT scan is normal, provided other possibilities have been excluded, such as MS and psychogenic behaviour (see Table 3.15)

Table 3.17 Circumstances in which brain MRI is preferable to CT (see also Section 5.3.6).

---

1 More than 10 days has elapsed since stroke onset, CT scan shows a low-density area that could have been infarction or resolving haemorrhage and it is essential to know whether the stroke was ischaemic or haemorrhagic
2 When CT scan is negative and it is crucial to be able to localise the infarct (this is only very occasionally); MRI is more likely to image the lesion
3 Arterial dissection is a suspected cause of cerebral infarction (see Section 7.1)

> *Brain CT scan is required, and is the investigation of choice, to identify intracranial haemorrhage, but it needs to be performed within a few days of stroke onset.*

In the acute stage (within 5 hours of symptom onset) of clinically definite ischaemic stroke, CT will show abnormalities consistent with the diagnosis in about 50% of cases (Horowitz *et al.*, 1991). CT will not show an infarct in a variable proportion of ischaemic strokes, particularly small deep infarcts and posterior fossa infarcts, and, if the CT is performed early, within 24 hours of onset. MRI will more often confirm the site of cerebral infarction suspected clinically but this, as yet, is rarely necessary; the immediate priority is to exclude ICH. So MRI is not necessarily better than CT (Mohr *et al.*, 1995). Furthermore, CT is an excellent technique for ill, confused patients—as many stroke patients

are—and MRI is a more difficult technique to apply. MRI should be reserved for difficult cases (Table 3.17).

3.5.12 The role of EEG in the differential diagnosis of stroke

The role of the EEG in patients with suspected stroke is to help determine whether there is a seizure focus in patients in whom the clinical diagnosis is in doubt (e.g. in patients with suspected postictal paresis or suspected non-convulsive status epilepticus who may present with the sudden onset of a confusional state) and the CT scan is normal or shows a lesion that is not typical of an infarct or PICH; and if there is any suspicion of CJD or HSE (e.g. clinical deterioration with new neurological signs, particularly myoclonus and cognitive decline, or hemiparesis, dysphasia and fever). The EEG is not useful for *diagnosing* stroke; in other words, stroke is a clinical diagnosis and there are no EEG features that are specific for stroke. The usual EEG findings in acute stroke are a localised reduction of normal cortical rhythms and a major surrounding slow-wave abnormality with individual waves of less than 1 Hz (Binnie & Prior, 1994). Focal EEG slowing, however, is not specific; it only indicates the presence and side of lesion (Faught, 1993).

Although the EEG may help distinguish between small deep (lacunar) and cortical infarction (MacDonnell *et al.*, 1988; Kappelle *et al.*, 1990), the clinical features and brain CT or MRI scan are more effective tools for doing this.

References

Abe M, Kjellberg RN, Adams RD (1989). Clinical presentations of vascular malformations of the brainstem: comparison of angiographically positive and negative types. *J Neurol Neurosurg Psychiatr* 52: 167–75.

Ahmad N, Wilson JA, Barr-Hamilton RM, Kean DM, MacLennan WJ (1992). The evaluation of dizziness in elderly patients. *Postgrad Med J* 68: 558–61.

Aldrich MS (1990). Narcolepsy. *N Engl J Med* 323: 389–94.

Allen CMC (1983). Clinical diagnosis of the acute stroke syndrome. *Quart J Med* 208: 515–23.

Amaurosis Fugax Study Group (1990). Current management of amaurosis fugax. *Stroke* 21: 201–8.

Amiel S (1993). Reversal of unawareness of hypoglycaemia. *N Engl J Med* 329: 876–7.

American Psychiatric Association (1994). *Diagnostic and Statistical Manual of Mental Disorders*, 4th edn. Washington: American Psychiatric Association.

Amira SA, Johnson TS, Logowitz NB (1985). Diagnosis of narcolepsy using multiple sleep latency test: analysis of current laboratory criteria. *Sleep* 8: 325–31.

Anonymous (1984). Ischaemia of the optic disc. *Lancet* ii: 1391–2.

Anonymous (1989). Vascular malformations in the brainstem. *Lancet* ii: 720–1.

Arboix A, Massons J, Oliveres M, Arribas MP, Titus F (1994). Headache in acute cerebrovascular disease: a prospective clinical study in 240 patients. *Cephalgia* 14: 37–40.

Awad I, Modic M, Little JR, Furlan AV, Weinstein M (1986). Focal parenchymal lesions in transient ischaemic attacks: correlation of computed tomography and magnetic resonance imaging. *Stroke* 17: 399–402.

Baloh RW (1987). Benign positional vertigo: clinical and oculographic features in 240 cases. *Neurology* 37: 371–8.

Baloh RW (1992). Stroke and vertigo. *Cerebrovasc Dis* 2: 3–10.

Baloh RW, Jacobsen K, Honrubia V (1993). Horizontal semicircular canal variant of benign positional vertigo. *Neurology* 43: 2542–9.

Baquis GD, Pessin MS, Scott RM (1985). Limb shaking—a carotid TIA. *Stroke* 16: 444–8.

Bauer J, Schuler P, Feistel H, Hilz MJ, Stefan H (1991). Blindness as an ictal phenomenon: investigations with EEG and SPECT in two patients suffering from epilepsy. *J Neurol* 238: 44–6.

Belal A Jr (1980). Pathology of vascular sensorineural hearing impairment. *Laryngoscope* 90: 1831–9.

Berkovic SF, Bladin PF, Darby DG (1984). Metabolic disorders presenting as stroke. *Med J Aust* 140: 421–4.

Berlit P, Rakicky J, Tornow K (1991). Differential diagnosis of spontaneous and traumatic intracranial haemorrhage. *J Neurol Neurosurg Psychiatr* 54: 1118.

Besson G, Hommel M, Clavier I, Perret J (1992). Failure of magnetic resonance imaging in the detection of pontine lacune. *Stroke* 23: 1535.

Best M, Blumenthal M, Futterman HA *et al.* (1969). Critical closure of intraocular blood vessels. *Arch Ophthalmol* 82: 385–92.

Betts T (1990). Pseudoseizures: seizures that are not epilepsy. *Lancet* ii: 163–4.

Binnie CD, Prior PF (1994). Electroencephalography. *J Neurol Neurosurg Psychiatr* 57: 1308–19.

Blau JN (1991). The clinical diagnosis of migraine: the beginning of therapy. *J Neurol* 238: S6–S11.

Blau JN (1992). Classical migraine: symptoms between visual aura and headache onset. *Lancet* 340: 355–6.

Blau JN, MacGregor EA (1993). Retinal migraine. *Lancet* 342: 1185.

Blau JN, Wiles CM, Solomon FS (1983). Unilateral somatic symptoms due to hyperventilation. *Br Med J* 286: 1108.

Boghen DR, Glaser JS (1975). Ischaemic optic neuropathy: the clinical profile and natural history. *Brain* 98: 689–708.

Bogousslavsky J, Regli F (1984). Cerebral infarction with transient signs (CITS): do TIAs correspond to small deep infarcts in internal carotid artery occlusion? *Stroke* 15: 536–9.

Bogousslavsky J, Vinuela F, Barnett HJM, Drake CG (1985). Amaurosis fugax as the presenting manifestation of dural arteriovenous malformation. *Stroke* 16: 891–3.

Bogousslavsky J, Martin R, Regli F, Despland P-A, Bolyn S (1992). Persistent worsening of stroke sequelae after delayed seizures. *Arch Neurol* 49: 385–8.

Bogousslavsky J, Hachinski VC, Boughner DR, Fox AJ, Vinuela F, Barnett HJM (1986). Clinical predictors of cardiac and arterial lesions in carotid transient ischaemic attacks. *Arch Neurol* 43: 229–33.

Bower S, Dennis M, Warlow C, Jordan N, Sagar H (1994). Long term prognosis of transient lone bilateral blindness in adolescents and young adults. *J Neurol Neurosurg Psychiatr* 57: 734–6.

Bradbury PG, Levy IS, McDonald WI (1987). Transient uniocular visual loss on deviation of the eye is association with intraorbital tumours. *J Neurol Neurosurg Psychiatr* 50: 615–19.

Brandt T (1991). Vestibular epilepsy. In: *Vertigo: Its Multisensory Syndromes*. London: Springer-Verlag, 91–7.

Brandt Th, Botzel K, Yousry T, Dieterich M, Schulze S (1995). Rotational vertigo in embolic stroke of the vestibular and auditory cortices. *Neurology* 45: 42–4.

Brierley EJ, Broughton DL, James OFW, Alberti KGMM (1995). Reduced awareness of hypoglycaemia in the elderly despite an intact counter-regulatory response. *Quart J Med* 88: 439–45.

Brown GC, Sheilds JA (1981). Amaurosis fugax secondary to presumed cavernous haemangioma of the orbit. *Ann Ophthalmol* 13: 1205–9.

Bryan RN, Levy LM, Whitlow WD, Killian JM, Preziosi TJ, Rosario JA (1991). Diagnosis of acute cerebral infarction: comparison of CT and MR imaging. *Am J Roentgenol* 157: 585–94.

Buchele W, Brandt Th (1988). Vestibular neuritis—a horizontal semicircular canal paresis? *Adv Oto-Rhino-Laryngol* 42: 157–61.

Burger SK, Saul RF, Selhorst JB, Thurston SE (1991). Transient monocular blindness caused by vasospasm. *N Engl J Med* 325: 870–3.

Burn J, Dennis M, Bamford J, Sandercock P, Wade D, Warlow C (1995). Epileptic seizures after a first ever in a lifetime stroke: the Oxfordshire Community Stroke Project. *Br Med J* (in press).

Calanchini PR, Swanson PD, Gotshall RA *et al.* (1977). Cooperative study of hospital frequency and character of transient ischaemic attacks: IV. The reliability of diagnosis. *J Am Med Assoc* 238: 2029–33.

Calhoun DA, Oparil S (1990). Treatment of hypertensive crisis. *N Engl J Med* 323: 1177–83.

Cartlidge NEF (1991). Transient global amnesia: recurrences are rare and patients may drive. *Br Med J* 302: 62–3.

Cascino GD, Westmoreland BF, Swanson TH, Sharbrough FW (1991). Seizure-associated speech arrest in elderly patients. *Mayo Clin Proc* 66: 254–8.

Chadwick D (1990). Diagnosis of epilepsy. *Lancet* 336: 291–5.

Cohen L, Verstichel P, Pierrot-Deseilligny C (1992). Hallucinatory vision of a familiar face following right temporal haemorrhage. *Neurology* 42: 2052.

Daly DD, Svien HJ, Yoss RE (1961). Intermittent cerebral symptoms with meningiomas. *Arch Neurol* 5: 287–93.

Davenport RJ, Statham PFX, Warlow CP (1994). Detection of bilateral isodense subdural haematomas. *Br Med J* 309: 792–4.

Davidovitch S, Gadoth N (1988). Neurological deficit simulating transient ischaemic attacks due to intracranial meningioma. *Eur Neurol* 28: 24–6.

Davis SM, Donnan GA, Tress BM *et al.* (1989). Magnetic resonance imaging in posterior circulation infarction: impact on diagnosis and management. *Aust N Z J Med* 19: 219–25.

Dawson DM, Hallett M, Millender LH (1990). *Entrapment Neuropathies*, 2nd edn. Boston: Little, Brown & Co., 38.

Denholm SW (1993). Benign paroxysmal positional vertigo. *Br Med J* 307: 1507–8.

Dennis MS (1988). *Transient ischaemic attacks in the community.* Doctor of Medicine thesis, University of London.

Dennis MS, Warlow CP (1992). Migraine aura without headache: transient ischaemic attack or not? *J Neurol Neurosurg Psychiatr* 55: 437–40.

Dennis MS, Bamford JM, Molyneux AJ, Warlow CP (1987). Rapid resolution of signs of primary intracerebral haemorrhage in computed tomograms of the brain. *Br Med J* 295: 379–81.

Dennis MS, Bamford JM, Sandercock PAG, Warlow CP (1989a). Lone bilateral blindness: a transient ischaemic attack. *Lancet* i: 185–8.

Dennis MS, Bamford JM, Sandercock PAG, Warlow CP (1989b). Incidence of transient ischaemic attacks in Oxfordshire, England. *Stroke* 20: 333–9.

Dennis MS, Bamford JM, Sandercock PAG, Warlow CP (1989c). A comparison of risk factors and prognosis for transient ischaemic attacks and minor ischaemic strokes: the Oxfordshire Community Stroke Project. *Stroke* 20: 1494–9.

Dennis MS, Bamford JM, Sandercock PAG, Molyneux A, Warlow CP (1990a). Computerised tomography in patients with transient ischaemic attacks: when is a transient ischaemic attack not a transient ischaemic attack but a stroke? *J Neurol* 237: 257–61.

Dennis M, Bamford J, Sandercock P, Warlow C (1990b). Prognosis of transient ischaemic attacks in the Oxfordshire Community Stroke Project. *Stroke* 21: 848–53.

Dennis MS, Burn JPS, Sandercock PAG, Bamford JM, Wade DT, Warlow CP (1993). Long-term survival after first-ever stroke: the Oxfordshire Community Stroke Project. *Stroke* 24: 796–800.

Devinsky O, Bear D, Volpe BT (1988). Confusional states following posterior cerebral artery infarction. *Arch Neurol* 45: 160–3.

Dix M, Hallpike C (1952). The pathology, symptomatology and diagnosis of certain common disorders of the vestibular system. *Ann Otol Rhinol Laryngol* 32: 364.

Drulovic B, Ribaric-Jankes K, Kostic VS, Sternic N (1993). Sudden hearing loss as the initial monosymptom of multiple sclerosis.

Neurology 43: 2703–5.

Duckrow RB, Beard DC, Brennan RW (1985). Regional cerebral blood flow decreases during hyperglycaemia. *Ann Neurol* 17: 267–72.

Dunne JW, Leedman PJ, Edis RH (1986). Inobvious stroke: a cause of delirium and dementia. *Aust N Z J Med* 16: 771–8.

Dutch TIA Trial Study Group (1993). Predictors of major vascular events in patients with a transient ischaemic attack or nondisabling stroke. *Stroke* 24: 527–31.

Easton JD (1993). Treatment for preventing migraine-related stroke. *Cerebrovasc Dis* 3: 244–7.

Easton JD (1995). The diagnostic evaluation of transient global amnesia. *Cerebrovasc Dis* 5: 212–16.

Edelman R, Warach S (1993). Magnetic resonance imaging. *N Engl J Med* 328: 708–16.

Edmeads J (1979). The headaches of ischaemic cerebrovascular disease. *Headache* 19: 345–9.

Edmeads J (1983). Complicated migraine and headache in cerebrovascular disease. *Neurol Clin* 1: 385–97.

Eliasziw M, Streifler JY, Spence JD, Fox AJ, Hachinski VC, Barnett HJM, for the North American Symptomatic Carotid Endarterectomy Trial (NASCET) Group (1995). Prognosis for patients following a transient ischaemic attack with and without a cerebral infarction on brain CT. *Neurology* 45: 428–31.

Evans J, Wilson B, Wraight P, Hodges JR (1993). Neuropsychological and SPECT scan findings during and after transient global amnesia: evidence for the differential impairment of remote episodic memory. *J Neurol Neurosurg Psychiatr* 56: 1227–30.

Fahmy JA (1973). Fundal haemorrhages in ruptured intracranial aneurysms. 1. Material, frequency, and morphology. *Acta Ophthalmol* 51: 189–98.

Faris AA, Poser CM (1964). Experimental production of focal neurological deficit by systemic hyponatraemia. *Neurology* 14: 206–11.

Faught E (1993). Current role of electroencephalography in cerebral ischaemia. *Stroke* 24: 609–13.

Fisher CM (1967). Some neuro-ophthalmological observations. *J Neurol Neurosurg Psychiatr* 30: 383–92.

Fisher CM (1971). Cerebral ischaemia, less familiar types. *Clin Neurosurg* 18: 267–336.

Fisher CM (1980). Late-life migraine accompaniments as a cause of unexplained transient ischaemic attacks. *Can J Neurol Sci* 7: 9–17.

Fisher CM (1986). Late-life migraine accompaniments—further experience. *Stroke* 17: 1033–42.

Fisher CM, Adams RD (1964). Transient global amnesia. *Acta Neurol Scand* 40 (Suppl. 9): 1–83.

Fisher M, Davidson RI, Marcus EM (1980). Transient focal cerebral ischaemia as a presenting manifestation of unruptured cerebral aneurysms. *Ann Neurol* 8: 367–72.

Fisher RS, Chan DW, Bare M, Lesser RP (1991). Capillary prolactin measurement for diagnosis of seizures. *Ann Neurol* 29:

187–90.

Foster JW, Hart RG (1987). Hypoglycaemic hemiplegia: two cases and a clinical review. *Stroke* 18: 944–6.

Fowler GW (1970). Meningioma and intermittent aphasia of 44 years duration. *J Neurosurg* 3: 100–2.

Friberg TR, Braunstein RA, Bressler NM (1995). Sudden visual loss associated with sexual activity. *Arch Opthalmol* 113: 738–42.

Fritz VU, Levien LJ, Hagen DJ (1983). Cerebral tumours mimicking transient cerebral events. *South Afr J Surg* 21: 243–50.

Furlan AJ, Whisnant JP, Kerns TP (1979). Unilateral visual loss in bright light: an unusual symptom of carotid artery occlusive disease. *Arch Neurol* 36: 675–6.

Galer BS, Lipton RB, Weinstein S, Bello L, Solomon S (1990). Apoplectic headache and oculomotor palsy: an unusual presentation of multiple sclerosis. *Neurology* 40: 1465–6.

Galin D, Diamond R, Braff D (1977). Lateralisation of conversion symptoms: more frequent on the left. *Am J Psychiatr* 134: 578–80.

Glaser JS, Savino PJ, Sumers KD, McDonald SA, Knighton RW (1977). The photostress recovery test in the clinical assessment of visual function. *Am J Ophthalmol* 83: 255–60.

Globus M, Lavi E, Alexander F, Oded A (1982). Ictal hemiparesis. *Eur Neurol* 21: 165–8.

Goodwin JA (1985). Acute ischaemic optic neuropathy. *J Am Med Assoc* 254: 951–2.

Goodwin JA, Gorelick PB, Helgason CM (1987). Symptoms of amaurosis fugax in atherosclerotic carotid artery disease. *Neurology* 37: 829–32.

Grad A, Baloh RW (1989). Vertigo of vascular origin: clinical and electronystagmographic features in 84 cases. *Arch Neurol* 46: 281–4.

Grunwald GB, Klein R, Simmonds MA, Kornguth SE (1985). Autoimmune basis for visual paraneoplastic syndrome in patients with small cell lung carcinoma. *Lancet* i: 658–61.

Gubbay SS, Hankey GJ, Tan NTS, Fry JM (1989). Mitochondrial encephalomyopathy with steroid dependence. *Med J Aust* 151: 100–7.

Gussen R (1976). Sudden deafness of vascular origin: a human temporal bone study. *Ann Otol Rhinol Laryngol* 85: 94–100.

Gutrecht JA, Kattwinkel N, Stillman MJ (1991). Retinal migraine, chorea, and retinal artery thrombosis in a patient with primary antiphospholipid antibody syndrome. *J Neurol* 238: 55–6.

Guyer DR, Miller NR, Auer CL *et al.* (1985). The risk of cerebrovascular and cardiovascular disease in patients with anterior ischaemic optic neuropathy. *Arch Ophthalmol* 103: 1136–42.

Haimovic IC, Beresford HR (1992). Transient unresponsiveness in the elderly: report of five cases. *Arch Neurol* 49: 35–7.

Hankey GJ (1993). Prolonged exacerbation of the neurological sequelae of stroke by post-stroke partial epileptic seizures. *Aust N Z J Med* 23: 306.

Hankey GJ (1994). Cerebrovascular disease: a clinical approach. *Rev Clin Gerontol* 4: 289–310.

Hankey GJ, Dunne JW (1987). Five cases of sudden hearing loss of presumed vascular origin. *Med J Aust* 147: 188–90.

Hankey GJ, Gubbay SS (1987). Focal cerebral ischaemia and infarction due to antihypertensive therapy. *Med J Aust* 46: 412–14.

Hankey GJ, Stewart-Wynne EG (1988). Amnesia following thalamic haemorrhage: another stroke syndrome. *Stroke* 19: 776–8.

Hankey GJ, Warlow CP (1992). Cost-effective investigation of patients with suspected transient ischaemic attacks. *J Neurol Neurosurg Psychiatr* 55: 171–6.

Hankey GJ, Warlow CP (1994). *Transient Ischaemic Attacks of the Brain and Eye.* London: WB Saunders.

Hankey GJ, Slattery JM, Warlow CP (1991). The prognosis of hospital-referred transient ischaemic attacks. *J Neurol Neurosurg Psychiatr* 54: 793–802.

Hankey GJ, Slattery JM, Warlow CP (1992). Transient ischaemic attacks: which patients are at high (and low) risk of serious vascular events? *J Neurol Nerosurg Psychiatr* 55: 640–52.

Harper CG, Bajada S, Chakera T, Cook R (1981). Acute central nervous system disorder mimicking stroke. *Med J Aust* 1: 136–8.

Harper CG, Giles M, Finlay-Jones R (1986). Clinical signs in the Wernicke–Korsakoff complex: a retrospective analysis of 131 cases diagnosed at necropsy. *J Neurol Neurosurg Psychiatr* 49: 341–5.

Hatano S (1976). Experience from a multicentre stroke register: a preliminary report. *Bull WHO* 54: 541–53.

Hayreh SS (1975). *Anterior Ischaemic Optic Neuropathy.* New York: Springer-Verlag.

Hayreh SS (1976). So-called 'central retinal vein occlusion': I. Pathogenesis, terminology, clinical features. *Ophthalmologica* 172: 1–13.

Hayreh SS (1977). Optic disc oedema in raised intracranial pressure: IV. Associated visual disturbances and their pathogenesis. *Arch Ophthalmol* 95: 1566–79.

Hayreh SS (1981). Anterior ischaemic optic neuropathy. *Arch Neurol* 38: 675–8.

Hayreh SS, Servais GE, Virdi PS (1986). Fundus lesions in malignant hypertension, V. hypertensive optic neuropathy. *Ophthalmology* 93: 74–87.

Healton EB, Brust JC, Feinfeld DA, Thomson GE (1982). Hypertensive encephalopathy and the neurologic manifestations of malignant hypertension. *Neurology* 32: 127–32.

Hedges TR, Lackman RD (1976). Isolated ophthalmic migraine in the differential diagnosis of cerebro-ocular ischaemia. *Stroke* 7: 379–81.

Hess DC, Nichols FT, Sethi KD, Adams RJ (1991). Transient cerebral ischaemia masquerading as paroxysmal dyskinesia. *Cerebrovasc Dis* 1: 54–7.

Hier DB, Mondlock J, Caplan LR (1983). Behavioural

abnormalities after right hemisphere stroke. *Neurology* 33: 337–44.

Hodges JR (1991). *Transient Global Amnesia: Clinical and Neuropsychological Aspects.* London: WB Saunders.

Hodges JR, Ward CD (1989). Observations during transient global amnesia. *Brain* 112: 595–620.

Hodges JR, Warlow CP (1990a). The aetiology of transient global amnesia: a case–control study of 114 cases with prospective follow-up. *Brain* 113: 639–57.

Hodges JR, Warlow CP (1990b). Syndromes of transient amnesia: towards a classification. A study of 153 cases. *J Neurol Neurosurg Psychiatr* 53: 834–43.

Hoefnagels WAJ, Padberg GW, Overweg J, van der Velde EA, Roos RAC (1991). Transient loss of consciousness: the value of the history for distinguishing seizure from syncope. *J Neurol* 238: 39–43.

Hoeldtke RD, Boden G, Shuman CR, Owen OE (1982). Reduced epinephrine secretion and hypoglycaemia in diabetic autonomic neuropathy. *Ann Intern Med* 96: 459–63.

Hogan RE (1994). Sudden 'stroke-like' onset of hemiparesis due to bacterial brain abscess. *Neurology* 44: 569–70.

Holt Larsen B, Soelberg Sorensen P, Marquardsen J (1990). Transient ischaemic attacks in young patients: a thromboembolic or migrainous manifestation? A 10 year follow up study of 46 patients. *J Neurol Neurosurg Psychiatr* 53: 1029–33.

Hommel M, Besson G, Le Bas JF et al. (1990). Prospective study of lacunar infarction using magnetic resonance imaging. *Stroke* 21: 546–54.

Horowitz SH, Zito JL, Donnarumma R, Patel M, Alvir J (1991). Computed tomographic–angiographic findings within the first five hours of cerebral infarction. *Stroke* 22: 1245–53.

House A, Dennis M, Mogridge L, Hawton K, Warlow C (1990). Life events and difficulties preceding stroke. *J Neurol Neurosurg Psychiatr* 53: 1024–8.

Howard RS (1992). Persistent hiccups. *Br Med J* 305: 1237–8.

Ille O, Woimant F, Pruna A, Corabianu O, Idatte JM, Haguenau M (1995). Hypertensive encephalopathy after bilateral carotid endarterectomy. *Stroke* 26: 488–91.

Ishiai S, Sugishita M, Ichikawa T, Gono S, Watabiki S (1993). Clock-drawing test and unilateral spatial neglect. *Neurology* 43: 106–10.

Jacobsen DM, Thirkill CE, Tipping SJ (1990). A clinical triad to diagnose paraneoplastic retinopathy. *Ann Neurol* 28: 162–7.

Jorgensen HS, Jespersen HF, Nakayama H, Raaschou HO, Olsen TS (1994). Headache in stroke: the Copenhagen Stroke Study. *Neurology* 44: 1793–7.

Kamata T, Yokota T, Furukawa T, Tsukagoshi H (1994). Cerebral ischaemic attack caused by postprandial hypotension. *Stroke* 25: 511–13.

Kapoor WN (1991). Diagnostic evaluation of syncope. *Am J Med* 90: 91–106.

Kappelle LJ, van Huffelen AC, van Gijn J (1990). Is the EEG really normal in lacunar stroke? *J Neurol Neurosurg Psychiatr* 53:

63–6.

Kase CS, Maulsby GO, deJuan E, Mohr JP (1981). Hemichorea–hemiballism and lacunar infarction in the basal ganglia. *Neurology* 31: 452–5.

Kaufman DK, Brown RD, Karnes WE (1994). Involuntary tonic spasms of a limb due to a brainstem lacunar infarction. *Stroke* 25: 217–19.

Keane JR (1979). Retinal haemorrhages: its significance in 100 patients with acute encephalopathy of unknown cause. *Arch Neurol* 36: 691–4.

Keltner JL, Roth AM, Chang RS (1983). Photoreceptor degeneration: possible autoimmune disorder. *Arch Ophthalmol* 101: 564–9.

Kessler C, Freyberger HJ, Dittmann V, Ringelstein EB (1991). Interrater reliability in the assessment of neurovascular diseases. *Cerebrovasc Dis* 1: 43–8.

Khan S, Yaqub BA, Poser CM, Al Deeb SM, Bohlega S (1995). Multiphasic disseminated encephalomyelitis presenting as alternating hemiplegia. *J Neurol Neurosurg Psychiatr* 58: 467–70.

Kidd D, Lawson J, Nesbitt R, MacMahon J (1993). Aspiration in acute stroke: a clinical study with videofluoroscopy. *Quart J Med* 86: 825–9.

Kidd D, Lawson J, Nesbitt R, MacMahon J (1995). The natural history and clinical consequences of aspiration in acute stroke. *Quart J Med* 88: 409–13.

Kim JS (1994). Restricted acral sensory syndrome following minor stroke: further observation with special reference to differential severity of symptoms among individual digits. *Stroke* 25: 2497–502.

Kimura R, Perlman HB (1958). Arterial obstruction of the labyrinth: cochlear changes. *Ann Otol Rhinol Laryngol* 67: 5–24.

Kingsley DPE, Radue EW, Du Boulay EPGH (1980). Evaluation of computed tomography in vascular lesions of the vertebrobasilar territory. *J Neurol Neurosurg Psychiatr* 43: 193–7.

Kogeorgos J, Scott DF, Swash M (1981). Epileptic dizziness. *Br Med J* 282: 687–9.

Kolmel H (1985). Complex visual hallucinations in the hemianopic field. *J Neurol Neurosurg Psychiatr* 48: 29–38.

Kong HL, Ong BKC, Lee TKY, Cheah JS (1993). Melioidosis of the brain presenting with a stroke syndrome. *Aust N Z J Med* 23: 413–14.

Kopelman MD, Panaayiotopoulos CP, Lewis P (1994). Transient epileptic amnesia differentiated from psychogenic 'fugue': neuropsychological, EEG, and PET findings. *J Neurol Neurosurg Psychiatr* 57: 1002–4.

Koudstaal PJ, Gerritsma JGM, van Gijn J (1989). Clinical disagreement on the diagnosis of transient ischaemic attack: is the patient or the doctor to blame? *Stroke* 20: 300–1.

Koudstaal PJ, van Gijn J, Staal A, Duivenvoorden HJ, Gerritsma JGM, Kraaijeveld CL (1986). Diagnosis of transient ischaemic attacks: improvement of interobserver agreement by a check-list in ordinary language. *Stroke* 17: 723–8.

Koudstaal PJ, van Gijn J, Lodder J *et al.* for the Dutch Transient Ischaemic Attack Group (1991a). Transient ischaemic attacks with and without a relevant infarct on computed tomographic scans cannot be distinguished clinically. *Arch Neurol* 48: 916–20.

Koudstaal PJ, van Gijn J, Kappelle LJ for the Dutch TIA Study Group (1991b). Headache in transient or permanent cerebral ischaemia. *Stroke* 22: 754–9.

Koudstaal PJ, van Gijn J, Frenken CWGM *et al.* for the Dutch Transient Ischaemic Attack Group (1992). TIA, RIND, minor stroke: a continuum, or different subgroups? *J Neurol Neurosurg Psychiatr* 55: 95–7.

Kraaijeveld CL, van Gijn J, Schouten HJA, Staal A (1984). Interobserver agreement for the diagnosis of transient ischaemic attacks. *Stroke* 15: 723–5.

Kumral E, Bogousslavsky J, Van Melle G, Regli F, Pierre P (1995). Headache at stroke onset: the Lausanne Stroke Registry. *J Neurol Neurosurg Psychiatr* 58: 490–2.

Landi G (1992). Clinical diagnosis of transient ischaemic attacks. *Lancet* 339: 402–5.

Lane DA, Wolff S, Ireland H, Gawel M, Foadi M (1983). Activation of coagulation and fibrinolytic systems following stroke. *Br J Haematol* 53: 655–8.

Lawden MC, Cleland PG (1993). Achromatopsia in the aura of migraine. *J Neurol Neurosurg Psychiatr* 56: 708–9.

Lee H, Lerner A (1990). Transient inhibitory seizures mimicking crescendo TIAs. *Neurology* 40: 165–6.

Lempert T, Bauer M, Schmidt D (1994). Syncope: a videometric analysis of 56 episodes of transient cerebral hypoxia. *Ann Neurol* 36: 233–7.

Lempert T, Gresty MA, Bronstein AM (1995). Benign positional vertigo: recognition and treatment. *Br Med J* 311: 489–91.

Lieberman MF, Shahi A, Green WR (1978). Embolic ischaemic optic neuropathy. *Am J Opthalmol* 86: 206–10.

Lin J-J, Chang M-K (1994). Hemiballism–hemichorea and non-ketotic hyperglycaemia. *J Neurol Neurosurg Psychiatr* 57: 748–50.

Linzer M, McFarland TA, Belkin M, Caplan L (1992). Critical carotid and vertebral arterial occlusive disease and cough syncope. *Stroke* 23: 1017–20.

Liotti M, Sava D, Rizzolatti G, Carrarra PI (1991). Differential hemispheric asymmetries in depression and anxiety: a reaction time study. *Biol Psychiatr* 29: 887–99.

Longo DL, Witherspoon JM (1980). Focal neurological symptoms in hypercalcaemia. *Neurology* 30: 200–1.

Ludman H (1990). Menière's disease. *Br Med J* 301: 1232–3.

Luxon LM, Harrison MJ (1979). Chronic subdural haematoma. *Quart J Med* 48: 43–53.

Maccario M (1968). Neurological dysfunction associated with nonketotic hyperglycaemia. *Arch Neurol* 19: 535–6.

McCormick GF, Halbach VV (1993). Recurrent ischaemic events in two patients with painless vertebral artery dissection. *Stroke* 24: 598–602.

McCormick GF, Zee C, Heiden J (1982). Cysticercosis cerebri: review of 127 cases. *Arch Neurol* 39: 534.

MacDonnell RAL, Donnan GA, Bladin PF, Berkovic SF, Wriedt CHR (1988). The electroencephalogram and acute ischaemic stroke: distinguishing cortical from lacunar infarction. *Arch Neurol* 45: 520–4.

McKee AC, Levine D, Kowall NW, Richardson EP Jr (1990). Peduncular hallucinosis associated with isolated infarction of the substantia nigra pars reticulata. *Ann Neurol* 27: 500.

McLean BN, Miller D, Thompson EJ (1995). Oligoclonal banding of IgG in CSF, blood–brain barrier function, and MRI findings in patients with sarcoidosis, systemic lupus erythematosus, and Behcet's disease involving the nervous system. *J Neurol Neurosurg Psychiatr* 58: 548–54.

McNaughton HK, Will RG (1994). Creutzfeldt–Jakob disease presenting acutely as stroke: an analysis of 30 cases. *Ann Neurol* 36: 313.

Malkowicz DE, Legido A, Jackel RA, Sussman NM, Eskin BA, Harner RN (1995). Prolactin secretion following repetitive seizures. *Neurology* 45: 448–52.

Malouf R, Brust JCM (1985). Hypoglycaemia: causes, neurological manifestations and outcome. *Ann Neurol* 17: 421–30.

Markowitz H, Kokmen E (1983). Neurologic diseases and the cerebrospinal fluid immunoglobulin profile. *Mayo Clin Proc* 58: 273–4.

Martin JD, Valentine J, Myers SI *et al.* (1991). Is routine CT scanning necessary in the preoperative evaluation of patients undergoing carotid endarterectomy? *J Vasc Surg* 14: 267–70.

Martin R, Bogousslavsky J, Regli F (1992). Striatocapsular infarction and 'release' visual hallucinations. *Cerebrovasc Dis* 2: 111–13.

Matsushita K, Naritomi H, Kazui S *et al.* (1993). Infarction in the anterior inferior cerebellar artery: magnetic resonance imaging and auditory brainstem responses. *Cerebrovasc Dis* 3: 206–12.

Matthews WB (1975). *Practical Neurology*, 3rd edn. London: Blackwell Scientific Publications, 76.

Mauser HW, van Huffelen AC, Tulleken CAF (1986). The EEG in the diagnosis of subdural empyema. *Electoencephalogr Clin Neurophysiol* 64: 511–16.

Melamed E, Lavy S, Reches A (1975). Chronic subdural haematoma simulating transient cerebral ischaemic attacks: case report. *J Neurosurg* 42: 101–3.

Melo TP, Ferro JM, Ferro H (1992). Transient global amnesia: a case control study. *Brain* 115: 261–70.

Mitrakou A, Fanelli C, Veneman T *et al.* (1993). Reversibility of unawareness of hypoglycaemia in patients with insulinomas. *N Engl J Med* 329: 834–9.

Mohr JP, Caplan LR, Melski J *et al.* (1978). The Harvard Cooperative Stroke Registry: a prospective registry. *Neurology* 28: 754–62.

Mohr JP, Biller J, Hilal SK *et al.* (1995). Magnetic resonance versus computed tomographic imaging in acute stroke. *Stroke* 26: 807–12.

Montgomery BM, Pinner CA (1964). Transient hypoglycaemic hemiplegia. *Arch Intern Med* 114: 680–4.

Mori E, Yamadori A (1987). Acute confusional state and acute agitated delirium: occurrence after infarction in the right middle cerebral artery territory. *Arch Neurol* 44: 1139–43.

Moster ML, Johnston DE, Reinmuth OM (1983). Chronic subdural haematoma with transient neurological deficits: a review of 15 cases. *Ann Neurol* 14: 539–42.

Murros KE, Evans GW, Toole JF, Howard G, Rose LA (1989). Cerebral infarction in patients with transient ischaemic attacks. *J Neurol* 236: 182–4.

Nicoli F, Milandre L, Lemarquis P, Bazan M, Jau P (1990). Hématomes sous-duraux chroniques et déficits neurologiques transitoires. *Rev Neurol* 146: 256–63.

Noda S, Kawada M, Umezaki H (1981). A case of chronic subdural haematoma simulating transient cerebral ischaemic attacks. *Clin Neurol* 21: 271–3.

Norris JW, Hachinski VC (1982). Misdiagnosis of stroke. *Lancet* i: 328.

Oas JG, Baloh RW (1992). Vertigo and the anterior inferior cerebellar artery syndrome. *Neurology* 42: 2274–9.

Olesen J (1988). Classification and diagnostic criteria for headache disorders, cranial neuralgias and facial pain. *Cephalgia* 8 (Suppl. 7): 19–28.

Olesen J, Friberg L, Olsen TK et al. (1993). Ischaemia-induced (symptomatic) migraine attacks may be more frequent than migraine-induced ischaemic insults. *Brain* 116: 187–202.

Omae T, Tsuchiya T, Yamaguchi T (1992). Cheiro-oral syndrome due to lesions in the corona radiata. *Stroke* 23: 599–601.

O'Sullivan F, Rossor M, Elston JS (1992). Amaurosis fugax in young people. *Br J Ophthalmol* 76: 660–2.

Ott BR, Saver JL (1993). Unilateral amnesic stroke. *Stroke* 24: 1033–42.

Paylor RR, Selhorst JB, Weinberg RS (1985). Reversible monocular cataract simulating amaurosis fugax. *Ann Opththalmol* 17: 423–5.

Peatfield RC (1987). Can transient ischaemic attacks and classical migraine always be distinguished? *Headache* 27: 240–3.

Perkin GD, Joseph R (1986). Neurological manifestations of the hyperventilation syndrome. *J Roy Soc Med* 79: 448–50.

Pessin MS, Duncan GW, Mohr JP, Poskanzer DC (1977). Clinical and angiographic features of carotid transient ischaemic attacks. *N Engl J Med* 296: 358–62.

Plum F, Posner JB (1985). *Diagnosis of Stupor and Coma*, 3rd edn. Philadephia: FA Davis.

Rao ML, Stefan H, Bauer J (1989). Epileptic but not psychogenic seizures are accompanied by simultaneous elevation of serum pituitary hormones and cortisol levels. *Neuroendocrinology* 49: 33–9.

Rao TH, Schneider LB, Lupyan Y (1994). Transient unresponsiveness in the elderly. *Arch Neurol* 51: 644.

Ravid JM (1928). Transient insulin hypoglycaemic hemiplegias. *Am J Med Sci* 175: 756–9.

Ravits J, Seybold ME (1984). Transient monocular visual loss from narrow angle glaucoma. *Arch Neurol* 41: 991–3.

Reggia JA, Tabb R, Price TR, Banko M, Hebel R (1984). Computer-aided assessment of transient ischaemic attacks: a clinical evaluation. *Arch Neurol* 41: 1248–54.

Reich KA, Giansiracusa DF, Strongwater SL (1990). Neurologic manifestations of giant cell arteritis. *Am J Med* 89: 67–72.

Ross TR (1983). Transient tumour attacks. *Arch Neurol* 40: 633–6.

Rother J, Schreiner A, Wentz K-U, Hennerici M (1992). Hypoglycaemia presenting as basilar artery thrombosis. *Stroke* 23: 112–13.

Rothwell PM (1994). Investigation of unilateral sensory or motor symptoms: frequency of neurological pathology depends on side of symptoms. *J Neurol Neurosurg Psychiatr* 57: 1401–2.

Ruby RJ, Burton JR (1977). Acute reversible hemiparesis and hyponatraemia. *Lancet* i: 1212.

Russo LS (1983). Focal dystonia and lacunar infarction of the basal ganglia: a case report. *Arch Neurol* 40: 61–2.

Sackett DL, Haynes RB, Guyatt GH, Tugwell P (1991). *Clinical Epidemiology: A Basic Science for Clinical Medicine*, 2nd edn. Boston: Little, Brown and Co., 19–49.

Sakas DE, Dias LS, Beale D (1995). Subarachnoid haemorrhage presenting as head injury. *Br Med J* 310: 1186–7.

Samuels AH (1995). Somatisation disorder: a major public health issue. *Med J Aust* 163: 147–9.

Sandercock PAG (1991). Recent developments in the diagnosis and management of patients with transient ischaemic attacks and minor ischaemic stroke. *Quart J Med* 286 (78): 101–12.

Sandercock PAG, Smart SE (1990). Migraine or amaurosis fugax? The value of ultrasound. *Scot Med J* 35: 147.

Sandercock P, Molyneux A, Warlow C (1985). Value of computed tomography in patients with stroke: Oxfordshire Community Stroke Project. *Br Med J* 290: 193–7.

Sandercock PAG, Warlow CP, Jones LN, Starkey IR (1989). Predisposing factors for cerebral infarction: the Oxfordshire Community Stroke Project. *Br Med J* 298: 75–80.

Sanders M (1987). Retinal arteritis, retinal vasculitis, and autoimmune retinal vasculitis. *Eye* 1: 441–6.

Saul RF, Gallagher JG, Mateer JE (1986). Sudden hemiparesis as the presenting sign in cryptococcal meningitis. *Stroke* 17: 753–4.

Schneider RC, Calhoun HD, Crosby EC (1968). Vertigo and rotational movement in cortical and subcortical lesions. *J Neurol Sci* 6: 493–516.

Scholl GB, Song H-S, Wray SH (1991). Uhthoff's symptom in optic neuritis: relationship to magnetic resonance imaging and development of multiple sclerosis. *Ann Neurol* 30: 180–4.

Scott WR, Miller BR (1985). Intracerebral haemorrhage with rapid recovery. *Arch Neurol* 42: 133–6.

Sempere AP, Duarte J, Coria F, Claveria LE (1992). Loss of vision by the colour white: a sig]n of carotid occlusive disease. *Stroke* 23: 1179.

Severin SL, Tour RL, Kershaw RH (1967). Macular function and the photostress test 2. *Arch Ophthalmol* 77: 163–7.

Seybold ME, Rosen PN (1977). Peripapillary staphyloma and amaurosis fugax. *Ann Opthalmol* 9: 1139–41.

Shah AB, Beamer N, Coull BM (1985). Enhanced *in vivo* platelet activation in subtypes of ischaemic stroke. *Stroke* 16: 643–7.

Shinar D, Gross CR, Mohr JP *et al.* (1985). Interobserver variability in the assessment of neurologic history and examination in the Stroke Data Bank. *Arch Neurol* 42: 557–65.

Silas JH, Grant DS, Maddocks JL (1981). Transient hemiparetic attacks due to unrecognised nocturnal hypoglycaemia. *Br Med J* 282: 132–3.

Sisk C, Ziegler DK, Zileli T (1970). Discrepancies in recorded results from duplicate neurological history and examination in patients studied for prognosis in cerebrovascular disease. *Stroke* 1: 14–18.

Slater R (1979). Benign recurrent vertigo. *J Neurol Neurosurg Psychiatr* 42: 363–7.

Sorenson EJ, Silbert PL, Jack CR, Parisi JE (1995). Transient amnestic syndrome after spontaneous haemorrhage into a hypothalamic pilocystic astrocytoma. *J Neurol Neurosurg Psychiatr* 58: 761–3.

Stark SR (1985). Transient dyskinesia and cerebral ischaemia [letter]. *Neurology* 35: 445.

Stell R, Davis S, Carroll WM (1994). Unilateral asterixis due to a lesion of the ventrolateral thalamus. *J Neurol Neurosurg Psychiatr* 57: 878–80.

Stern DB (1977). Lateral distribution of conversion reactions. *J Nerv Mental Dis* 164: 122–8.

Stevens DL, Matthews WB (1973). Cryptogenic drop attacks: an affliction of women. *Br Med J* 1: 439–42.

Stone SP, Patel P, Greenwood RJ, Halligan PW (1992). Measuring visual neglect in acute stroke and predicting its recovery: the visual neglect recovery index. *J Neurol Neurosurg Psychiatr* 55: 431–6.

Suzuki I, Shimizu H, Ishijima B *et al.* (1992). Aphasic seizure caused by focal epilepsy in the left fusiform gyrus. *Neurology* 42: 2207–10.

Tatemichi TK, Young WL, Prohovnik I, Gitelman DR, Correll JW, Mohr JP (1990). Perfusion insufficiency in limb-shaking transient ischaemic attacks. *Stroke* 21: 341–7.

Teman AJ, Winterkorn JMS, Weiner D (1995). Transient monocular blindness associated with sexual intercourse. *N Engl J Med* 333: 393.

Tippin J, Corbett JJ, Kerber RE, Schroeder E, Thompson HS (1989). Amaurosis fugax and ocular infarction in adolescents and young adults. *Ann Neurol* 26: 69–77.

Todd RB (1856). *Clinical Lectures on Paralysis*. London: Churchill.

Twomey JA, Espir MLE (1980). Paroxysmal symptoms as the first manifestations of multiple sclerosis. *J Neurol Neurosurg Psychiatr* 43: 296–304.

UK-TIA Study Group (1993). Intracranial tumours that mimic transient cerebral ischaemia: lessons from a large multicentre trial. *J Neurol Neurosurg Psychiatr* 56: 563–6.

Vestergaard K, Andersen G, Nielsen MI, Jensen TS (1993). Headache in stroke. *Stroke* 24: 1621–4.

Victor M, Adams RD, Collins GH (1989). *The Wernicke–Korsakoff Syndrome and Related Neurologic Disorders Due to Alcoholism and Malnutrition*, 2nd edn. Philadelphia: Davis.

Vortmeyer AO, Hagel C, Laas R (1992). Haemorrhagic thiamine deficient encephalopathy following prolonged parenteral nutrition. *J Neurol Neurosurg Psychiatr* 55: 826–9.

Wallis WE, Donaldson I, Scott RS, Wilson J (1985). Hypoglycaemia masquerading as cerebrovascular disease (hypoglycaemic hemiplegia). *Ann Neurol* 18: 510–12.

Wardlaw JM (1994). Is routine computed tomography in strokes unnecessary? *Br Med J* 309: 1498–500.

Waxman SG, Toole JF (1983). Temporal profile resembling TIA in the setting of cerebral infarction. *Stroke* 14: 433–7.

Weisberg LA, Nice CN (1977). Intracranial tumour simulating the presentation of cerebrovascular syndromes: early detection with cerebral computed tomography. *Am J Med* 63: 517–24.

Welch KMA (1994). Relationship of stroke and migraine. *Neurology* 44 (Suppl. 7): S33–S36.

Welch KMA, Levine SR (1990). Migraine-related stroke in the context of the International Headache Society Classification of Head Pain. *Arch Neurol* 47: 458–62.

Whisnant JP and colleagues for the National Institute of Neurological Disorders and Stroke (1990). Classification of cerebrovascular diseases III. *Stroke* 21: 637–76.

Whitty CWM (1967). Migraine without headache. *Lancet* ii: 283–5.

WHO (World Health Organization) (1978). Cerebrovascular Disorders: a Clinical and Research Classification. Geneva: World Health Organization, Offset Publication No. 43.

Wiebers DO, Swanson JW, Cascino TL, Whisnant JP (1989). Bilateral loss of vision in bright light. *Stroke* 20: 554–8.

Wilkes SR, Troutmann JC, DeSanto LW, Campbell RJ (1979). Osteoma: an unusual cause of amaurosis fugax. *Mayo Clin Proc* 54: 258–60.

Williams RS (1979). Chronic subdural haematoma simulating transient cerebral ischaemic attacks. *Ann Neurol* 5: 597.

Winterkorn JMS, Teman AJ (1991). Recurrent attacks of amaurosis fugax treated with calcium channel blocker. *Ann Neurol* 30: 423–5.

Wroe SJ, Sandercock P, Bamford J, Dennis M, Slattery J, Warlow C (1992). Diurnal variation in incidence of stroke: Oxfordshire community stroke project. *Br Med J* 304: 155–7.

Yanagihara T, Klass DW, Piepgras DG, Houser OW (1989). Brief loss of consciousness in bilateral carotid occlusive disease. *Arch Neurol* 46: 858–61.

Yanagihara T, Sundt TM, Piepgras DG (1988). Weakness of the lower extremity in carotid occlusive disease. *Arch Neurol* 45: 297–301.

Yerby MS, van Belle G, Friel PN, Wilensky AJ (1987). Serum prolactins in the diagnosis of epilepsy: sensitivity, specificity, and predictive value. *Neurology* 37: 1224–6.

Zaret BS (1985). Lightning streaks of Moore: a cause of recurrent stereotypic visual disturbance. *Neurology* 35: 1078–81.

Where is the lesion? 4

4.1 General introduction

Once the clinical diagnosis of stroke (versus not-stroke) has been made, one should then consider how extending the diagnostic process might help in the subsequent investigation and management of the patient. Table 4.1 lists some other reasons for subclassifying patients with stroke, which, whilst not all of immediate value to the individual patient, may be helpful when considering the general management of stroke and overall burden to the community. It is stating the obvious to say that, at present, there is no uniformity of subclassification either within or between countries, or often amongst different patients of an individual physician. The reasons are undoubtedly complex, but in this chapter we have attempted to describe a framework which might go some way towards improving the situation.

Making 'the diagnosis' in a patient with stroke is a multilevel process, which is set out in Table 4.2. To begin with, one is faced by a patient with symptoms and signs resulting in impairments and disabilities. In general, these will be related to the site and size of the damaged brain parenchyma. Thus, one should be trying to determine where the lesion is and how extensive it is. Then, possibly with the results of suitable investigations, one needs to try and determine the pathological type of the stroke and the aetiological mechanism, i.e. what the vascular lesion is. Finally, during the phase of rehabilitation, the disability and handicap experienced by the patient and his/her carers needs to be assessed, i.e. what the functional consequences of the stroke are. Thus, the diagnostic process should consist of a hierarchy of complementary stages.

The complete diagnostic formulation in a patient presenting with a stroke consists of a series of complementary stages which occur over a variable length of time.

Table 4.1 Potential benefits of subclassifying stroke.

Aid cost-effective search for causal factors (see Sections 6.5 and 6.7)
Improve prognostication for functional outcome, survival and
  recurrence (see Sections 10.2.7 and 16.1.3)
Stratify entry to clinical trials (see Chapter 11)
Aid assessment of case mix in individual units (see Section 17.6.3)
Aid audit of management (see Section 17.6.2)

Table 4.2 The diagnostic process.

1 Is it a stroke? (see Chapter 3)
2 Which part of the brain has the stroke affected? (see Chapter 4)
3 What pathological type of stroke is it? (see Chapter 5)
4 What disease process caused the stroke? (see Chapters 6–8)
5 What are the functional consequences of the stroke? (see
Chapter 15)

There are numerous schemes of subclassification which focus on the vascular lesion itself (e.g. Foulkes *et al.*, 1988; Adams *et al.*, 1993). Many were developed for specific research projects in specialist institutions. Inherent in most of them is an entirely understandable desire to establish the pathophysiological factors underlying every individual stroke, since it is with this knowledge that rational treatments aimed both at limiting the acute damage and at secondary prevention will be developed and deployed. However, even with the most intensive investigation protocols, such diagnostic certainty remains elusive in up to 40% of patients (Sacco *et al.*, 1989). There is also evidence of only moderate inter-rater reliability for such classifications (Gordon *et al.*, 1993).

We just do not have the knowledge or the technology to determine the exact mechanism of stroke in every patient.

Although there are many instruments for assessing impairment, disability and handicap, there is no generally agreed method of classification in these areas, which probably reflects the continuing problems of measuring many of the deficits objectively and accurately. One would include here many of the clinical stroke scales, prognostic scores, activity of daily living scales, quality of life measures, etc. (see Section 17.6.3).

In view of all this, it is perhaps surprising that relatively little attention has been paid to developing classifications based on the site and size of the parenchymal brain lesion. To some extent, this may be because it was anticipated that the advances in neuroimaging would make any clinically based classification redundant. But, although imaging has

certainly aided our understanding of the anatomical substrate underlying some of the deficits and is of undoubted benefit in the subclassification of primary intracerebral haemorrhage (PICH) and subarachnoid haemorrhage (SAH) (see Sections 4.4.4 and 5.5.3), it has so far failed to provide a useful framework for classification of ischaemic stroke and transient ischaemic attack (TIA). Furthermore, any classification which places an undue reliance on the results of investigations will be difficult to use in routine clinical practice for every patient because of factors such as the following.
1 The variable availability of such investigations.
2 The perceived appropriateness of using a particular investigation for an individual patient (e.g. because of the degree of pre- or post-stroke disability).
3 The variability of the results arising from both observer- and technology-dependent factors (see Chapter 5).
4 The speed with which any classification needs to be made (e.g. particularly for acute treatments; see Chapter 11).

It is also important to recognise the limitations of both clinical and instrumental data; neither will be 100% sensitive and specific, although there is a tendency for the results of investigations to be perceived, almost automatically, as the gold standard. This may partially explain the tendency for the literature to overemphasise exceptions to general clinical rules. In reality, however, even the most sophisticated images have to be interpreted (just like physical symptoms and signs) and one should not ignore the potential for considerable inter- and intrarater variability or for there to be a learning curve (see Section 5.3.5).

One should not presume that the results of investigations will be any more sensitive and specific than the clinical findings.

The traditional teaching of cerebrovascular neurology is based on the general assumption that particular symptoms and signs arise from restricted areas of damaged brain parenchyma, which, in turn, receive their vascular supply in a predictable manner. There is a large classical literature describing patterns of neurological deficit which are linked to a particular pattern of vascular lesions, including a myriad of eponymous clinical syndromes. Although these are of value to those interested in exploring the subtleties of cerebral localisation, and are the stock in trade of many neurologists' clinical demonstrations, the original descriptions were often of only a handful of cases. Consequently, the sensitivity, specificity and generalisability of many of the clinicoanatomical correlations have rarely been tested on large, unselected groups of patients with stroke. What is clear is that many of the 'classical' vascular syndromes occur infrequently (at least in their pure forms), and even when they do they rarely have particularly distinctive causes. Thus, they are of limited practical value to jobbing clinicians. Additionally, the descriptions nearly always relate to ischaemic rather than haemorrhagic strokes and, although one might argue that this is perfectly acceptable in the context of a high proportion of patients having brain computerised tomography (CT) or magnetic resonance imaging (MRI) scans, there will remain a large number of clinicians worldwide who do not have ready access to such technology.

> *Despite being well known, many of the 'classical' vascular syndromes occur rather infrequently in routine clinical practice.*

To be of use, any system of classification should have a clear purpose and be applicable to all (or almost all) patients with stroke; it needs to provide a skeleton on which fragments of information about an individual patient can be hung in an orderly manner. Ideally, a 'core' skeleton which could be used in everyday practice could also be built on both by scientists and clinicians according to their access to, or the applicability of, various investigations. Used in this way, a system of classification should also facilitate the integration of research findings from the university centres into everyday practice. Wherever one practises cerebrovascular medicine, the unifying starting point is going to be the patient presenting with symptoms and signs. What is needed is a system that synthesises this information in a manner that allows reference to the vascular anatomy and directs one towards the most efficient way of determining the most likely aetiological mechanism. In this chapter we will discuss features of the clinical examination of patients with stroke which assist parenchymal localisation and identification of clinically relevant neurological deficits (see Section 4.2); review the relevant vascular anatomy (see Section 4.3); and suggest a system which brings together these seemingly disparate types of classification (see Section 4.4).

4.2 Symptoms and signs of the brain lesion

4.2.1 Introduction

It should go without saying that physicians must continually make efforts to refine their clinical abilities if the deficits resulting from stroke are to be recognised and documented accurately. It is surprising how rarely one sees this mentioned in textbooks; yet, if, for example, they were radiologists beginning to use a new imaging modality, it would be accepted that there would need to be training and even after that there would be a continuous learning process. A failure to recognise or, conversely, a tendency to overinterpret a clinical sign is no different from failing to report an infarct on CT or reporting a Virchow–Robin space as an infarct on MRI. It has been shown that the accuracy of the clinical diagnosis of lacunar stroke (see Section 4.4.6), albeit when judged against neuroimaging, is significantly better when the clinician had a specific interest in cerebrovascular disease (Lodder *et al.*, 1994). There are many texts devoted to the honing of clinical skills and the recognition of the many subtle (and interesting) facets of disturbed function of the nervous system. This section is not intended, therefore, to give a comprehensive account of the subject. However, there are some aspects which seem particularly relevant to the diagnosis and management of patients with cerebrovascular disease.

> *Clinical skills need to be developed, maintained and updated as necessary.*

4.2.2 Disturbance of conscious level
(see also Section 15.3)

Consciousness may be defined as 'the state of awareness of the self and the environment', whilst coma is the total absence of such awareness (Plum & Posner, 1980). Vascular diseases are probably the second most common cause of non-traumatic coma after metabolic/toxic disorders, and up to 20% of patients with stroke may have some impairment of consciousness (Bogousslavsky *et al.*, 1988; Melo *et al.*, 1992). Furthermore, conscious level is a very important predictor of survival and functional outcome (see Section 10.2.7).

Although consciousness is usually considered to have two components, alertness (or arousal) and content (or the sum of cognitive and affective mental functions), when dealing with a predominantly focal disorder such as stroke, where there are frequently cognitive deficits, one tends to consider the 'conscious level' in the more restricted sense of level of alertness. Terms such as 'drowsy', 'obtunded' and 'stuporous' are imprecise, and therefore liable to variable interpretation, and fail to reflect the continuum of alertness between coma and normality. The Glasgow Coma Scale (GCS) (Table 4.3) (Teasdale & Jennett, 1974) provides a more structured way of describing conscious level and is often part of the standard nursing observation form. It was developed for patients with head injury, and some care is needed when applying it to patients with stroke. It should be stressed to nursing staff that the motor deficit should be assessed in the 'normal' arm and leg and not on the side with the motor deficit. One should take more note of each subscore than of the total, since specific focal deficits, and particularly global aphasia, depress the overall score disproportionately to the level of alertness. Nevertheless, any deterioration should prompt the clinician to consider whether

Table 4.3 The GCS.

	Score
Eye opening	
None	E1
To painful stimuli	E2
To command/voices	E3
Spontaneously with blinking	E4
Motor response (best response in unaffected limbs)	
None	M1
Arm extension to painful stimulus	M2
Arm flexion to painful stimulus	M3
Arm withdraws from painful stimulus	M4
Hand localises painful stimulus	M5
Obeys commands	M6
Verbal response	
None	V1
Sounds but no recognisable words	V2
Inappropriate words/expletives	V3
Confused speech	V4
Normal	V5

Note: the scale was developed for use with patients with head injury. When using it for patients with stroke, it is important that staff are trained to record the best response in the 'good' limbs and not the paretic limbs. One must also be aware of the possible confounding effects of aphasia.

it is because of the progression of the neurological deficit or because of non-vascular factors, such as infection, metabolic disturbance or the effect of drugs (see Section 15.5).

The Glasgow Coma Scale provides a structured way of describing conscious level which avoids the ambiguities of terms such as drowsy, obtunded and stuporous.

Consciousness is dependent on the proper functioning of the ascending reticular activating system (ARAS). This is a complex functional rather than anatomical grouping of neural structures in the upper brainstem, the subthalamic region and the thalamus (mainly the intralaminar nuclei) (Brodal, 1981b). Focal lesions which impair consciousness tend to either disrupt the ARAS directly (i.e. mainly infratentorial lesions) or are large supratentorial lesions, which cause secondary brainstem compression (Fig. 4.1). Almost instantaneous loss of consciousness suggests either an SAH or an intrinsic brainstem haemorrhage. However, some episodes of loss of consciousness in patients with vascular disease remain unexplained. A few of these may be due to ischaemia in the territory of small, perforating arteries which supply the reticular activating system in the brainstem (Sherrington & Bamford, 1996).

Depression of the conscious level is most likely to occur in patients with displacement of midline structures, although transtentorial herniation is not invariable (Ropper, 1986). A large intracerebral haematoma, and particularly a cerebellar haematoma, may result in loss of consciousness over a few hours due to secondary brainstem compression. Early impairment of consciousness from a supratentorial *infarct* is most unusual. This is probably because the associated cerebral oedema responsible for the mass effect, and so the midline shift, usually takes 1–2 days to develop, although evidence of transtentorial herniation may be present within 24 hours (Shaw *et al.*, 1959; Silver *et al.*, 1984). Torvik and Jorgensen (1964) and Greenhall (1977) showed that infarction of the complete middle cerebral artery (MCA) territory is needed before significant lateral and caudal displacement of midline structures occurs.

Very early impairment of conscious level is most commonly associated with haemorrhagic strokes.

Although they occur relatively infrequently, there are a number of clinical syndromes where patients have impaired responsiveness but do not seem to be in coma. The neuroanatomical and management implications of these states are important. Probably the most important to recognise is the *locked-in syndrome*. This is a state of motor de-

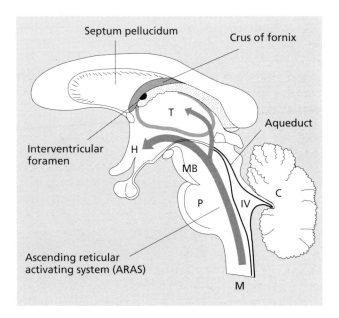

Figure 4.1 Diagrammatic representation in the sagittal plane of the subcortical areas involved in consciousness (especially the ARAS). C, cerebellum; H, hypothalamus; M, medulla; MB, midbrain; P, pons; T, thalamus; IV, fourth ventricle.

efferentation, where there is usually severe paralysis not only of the limbs but also of the neck, jaw and face. Indeed, the only muscles remaining under voluntary control may be those concerned with vertical eye movements and the ability to blink. All this occurs with clear, and often extremely distressing, retention of awareness. The patient is unable to communicate by word or movement other than blinking or moving the eyes up and down, but is fully aware of the surroundings and attempts to respond to them. There is usually an extensive, bilateral lesion in the ventral pons, which interrupts the descending motor tracts, but the medial longitudinal fasciculus (MLF) in the rostral pontine tegmentum is spared—hence the preservation of vertical eye movements (Fig. 4.2)—as is the ARAS. Horizontal eye movements are usually absent because of damage to the paramedian pontine reticular formation (PPRF) or to the VIth cranial nerves themselves. In this situation, cognitive functions must be considered normal and the patient given a full explanation of his/her predicament. One often needs to reiterate this to other staff and take appropriate account of the normal cognition when planning long-term care, since prolonged survival in this state is possible (Katz *et al.*, 1992).

> *The relatives and staff caring for patients with the locked-in syndrome need reminding regularly that cognitive functions and awareness are normal.*

Akinetic mutism is another state where there is limited responsiveness to the environment, although the patients appear alert (or at least wakeful) in that their eyes are open and there is active gaze. However, in contrast to the locked-

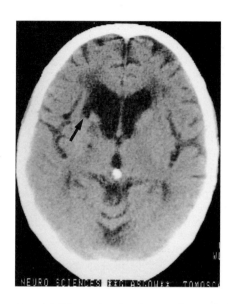

Figure 4.3 An axial CT scan showing the typical area of infarction (arrow) resulting from occlusion of the RAH.

in syndrome, the physical examination does not reveal evidence of a major lesion of the sensorimotor pathways. At its most extreme, patients may lie with open eyes, follow objects and become agitated or even say the occasional appropriate word following noxious stimuli (thus distinguishing the state from that of coma or persistent vegetative state), but otherwise do not respond to their environment, although catatonic posturing may occur (Cairns *et al.*, 1941; Plum & Posner, 1980). *Abulia* is a term used to describe a less severe presentation of reduced spontaneous movement and speech (Fisher, 1995). Such patients often appear to have a marked flatness of affect but, with adequate stimulation, can be shown to have relatively preserved cognition.

Both akinetic mutism and abulia occur with bilateral damage to the cingulum, caudate nuclei and anterior limb of the internal capsule. Although they are most commonly seen after head injury or in multi-infarct states, they may occur with unilateral infarction of the caudate or occlusion of the recurrent artery of Heubner (RAH) (Fig. 4.3). It has been suggested that the clinical features may arise because of an alteration of dopaminergic extrapyramidal modulatory signals from the caudate to the frontal lobe. Treatment with dopamine agonists has been reported to be of benefit (Ross & Stewart, 1981; Barrett, 1991). A similar clinical picture may occur with strokes affecting the thalamus and upper midbrain, but then there is usually an associated disorder of vertical eye movements.

The persistent vegetative state is mentioned for completeness, although it rarely occurs because of a focal vascular

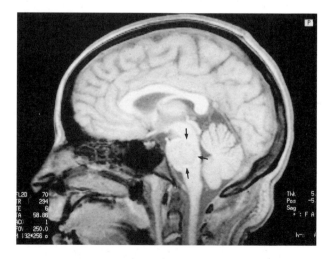

Figure 4.2 A T1-weighted, sagittal MRI scan showing a ventral pontine infarct (arrows) in a patient with the locked-in syndrome. When the site of the lesion is compared with that of the ARAS in Fig. 4.1, one can see why consciousness was preserved.

Table 4.4 Disorders of consciousness.

Causes of impaired consciousness after stroke
Primary damage to subcortical structures (e.g. thalamus) or to the
reticular activating system in the brainstem (e.g. brainstem
haemorrhage)
Secondary damage to reticular activating system in the brainstem
(e.g. large supratentorial stroke with transtentorial herniation
due to oedema)
Co-existing metabolic derangement (e.g. hypoglycaemia, renal or
hepatic failure)
Drugs

Decreased responsiveness without impaired consciousness
Locked-in syndrome
Akinetic mutism
Abulia
Severe extrapyramidal bradykinesia
Severe depression
Catatonia
Hysterical conversion

event. Here there appears to be wakefulness and preserved
autonomic function but total lack of cognition. It is usually
the result of a diffuse insult to the cerebral cortex (e.g. trauma, hypoxia) but with relative sparing of the brainstem
(Jennett & Plum, 1972; Spudis, 1991; Howard & Miller,
1995).

All these states of altered responsiveness should be distinguished from other physical disorders, such as extreme
extrapyramidal bradykinesia/bradyphrenia, and also from
psychiatric conditions, such as catatonia, depression or hysteria (Table 4.4).

4.2.3 Disturbance of the motor system

The corticospinal tract descends from the primary and supplementary motor cortex, the fibres converging in the corona
radiata. There is evidence from primates, however, that the
corticospinal tracts contain a significant number of fibres
from cortical areas other than the primary and supplementary motor areas, particularly the parietal lobe (Russell &
DeMeyer, 1961). The fibres then pass through the internal
capsule, predominantly in the posterior limb, and enter the
brainstem. Here, the fibres lie in the cerebral peduncles of the
midbrain and the base of the pons before entering the
medullary pyramids. The majority of fibres decussate in the
lower medulla and come to lie in an anterolateral position in
the spinal cord, although a variable proportion remain
uncrossed and this may be of some clinical relevance (Fig.
4.4) (Chollet *et al.*, 1991).

For the clinician, the diagnostic problem lies not with the

hemiplegic patient with increased tone, deep tendon reflexes
and an extensor plantar response but rather with the patient
with a deficit at the other end of the spectrum of severity.
When taking the history, descriptions such as 'heaviness'
and 'numbness' should not simply be accepted as evidence of
motor and sensory disturbance, respectively. In our experience the terms are used interchangeably (and are often cul-
turally determined) and a little more interrogation is often
rewarding. Similarly, care should be taken before accepting a
patient's or relative's description of the lateralisation of a
facial weakness. They should be asked, 'Which side
"dropped" and did saliva trickle from one side of the
mouth?' (see Section 3.3.2).

> *Patients use terms such as 'heaviness' and 'numbness'
> interchangeably; further questioning is needed to
> distinguish motor and sensory deficits.*

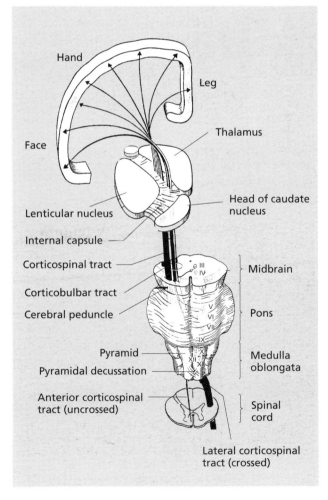

Figure 4.4 Diagrammatic representation of the corticospinal and
corticobulbar tracts.

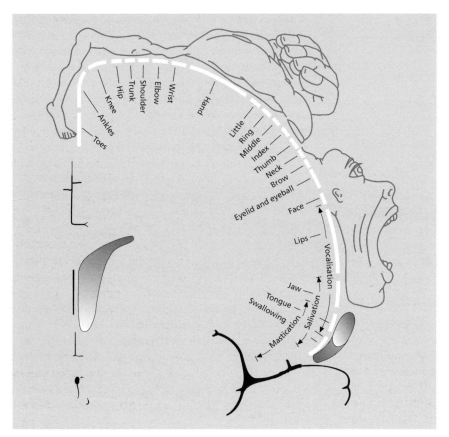

Figure 4.5 Topographical organisation of the motor cortex in the cerebral hemisphere (the motor homunculus). (After Penfield & Rasmussen, 1950.)

The relative size of areas of the motor cortex which, when stimulated, will result in movement of a particular body part is traditionally portrayed by the homunculus (or manikin) (Penfield & Boldrey, 1937). Although the absolute neuroanatomical relationships may be incorrect (Schott, 1993), in cerebrovascular practice it remains useful as an *aide-mémoire*. The very large cortical representation of the hand (Fig. 4.5) has two important effects. First, it is possible for a stroke just to affect this area of the cortex without involving other neural pathways. The resulting deficit, the so-called 'cortical hand', is often not recognised as being due to a stroke because of the restricted pure motor deficit, the lack of any change in muscle tone or in deep tendon reflexes, and the flexor plantar response. Often the probem is thought to be due to a peripheral nerve lesion but closer analysis reveals that this would require simultaneous involvement of the median, ulnar and radial nerves. Of course, small infarcts causing such a deficit are often not visualised on CT scanning!

> *The 'cortical hand syndrome' is often attributed to a peripheral nerve lesion, but closer analysis reveals that this would require simultaneous involvement of the median, ulnar and radial nerves, a most unlikely occurrence.*

The second effect is that subtle abnormalities of motor function may be detectable in the hand at a time when there is no objective weakness. It has been shown that impairment of fine finger movements (or rapid hand movements) is the most sensitive clinical test of corticospinal function (Louis *et al.*, 1995). This equates with functional problems reported by patients who, in the face of normal power, often have difficulty controlling pens, etc., and may describe the problem as 'clumsiness', although they are much more likely to notice this in their normally dominant hand. This is probably due to a subtle increase in co-contraction of antagonist muscles secondary to the reduced input to the spinal motor neurones. Ipsilateral descending motor pathways have been postulated to be involved in the recovery of certain voluntary motor activities after stroke (Chollet *et al.*, 1991), although as yet there is no neurophysiological support for this hypothesis (Palmer *et al.*, 1992).

> *The impairment of fine finger or rapid hand movements is probably the most sensitive clinical test of corticospinal function.*

Drift from the horizontal of the outstretched arm with the eyes closed is often suggested as a good screening test of motor function (Fig. 4.6). However, it must be remembered

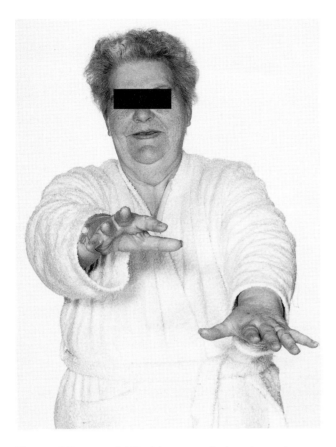

Figure 4.6 Downward drift of the outstretched arm in a patient with a mild corticospinal motor deficit.

Although there is moderate inter-rater agreement about the presence or absence of weakness (Table 4.5), it is clear from the above discussion that the standard methods of grading power (e.g. the Medical Research Council (MRC) system) are of limited value in patients with stroke (see Section 15.21). The anatomical extent rather than the severity of the motor deficit is of more importance for clinicoanatomical correlation, and, from a functional point of view, a description of some action the patient can not perform is often of more value (e.g. hold a cup of water, comb hair).

More attention should be focused on the anatomical extent of the weakness and the functional consequences rather than trying to grade the severity.

One sometimes encounters patients who at one moment seem to have a dense hemiplegia (usually left-sided) and yet, very soon afterwards, are observed to move the 'paralysed' limbs. The pattern is so odd that a somatisation disorder might be suspected. Other patients may appear to have a complete hemiplegia, without movement in either the arm or the leg when tested on the bed, but then can actually walk. This pattern can be seen with the so-called capsular warning syndrome or crescendo small vessel TIAs (Donnan *et al.*, 1995), but in such cases the episodes seem much more dis-

that there are several potential causes for this, although the patterns of drift may be subtly different. These include loss of proprioception, when the fingers tend to move independently—so-called 'piano-playing' or 'pseudoathetosis'; neglect (see Section 4.2.5), when there tend to be much larger-amplitude movements, including upwards; or cerebellar dysfunction (see Section 4.2.7), when there tend to be larger-amplitude oscillations, particularly if sharp downward pressure is applied to the arm. Thus, as a screening test for motor dysfunction, it is quite sensitive but not very specific and should be used in conjunction with the examination of fine finger movements. Minor motor deficits affecting the leg are best detected by rapid tapping of the foot against the examiner's hand, when striking asymmetry of the rate or rhythm may be present. Additionally, the patient's gait should be observed carefully.

Drift from the horizontal of the outstretched arm with the eyes closed is a good screening test of motor function but is not very specific.

Table 4.5 Interobserver agreement for neurological signs in stroke patients.

Signs examined	Kappa value	
	Lindley *et al.* (1993)	Shinar *et al.* (1985)
Conscious level	0.60	0.38
Confusion	0.21	NS
Dementia	NS	0.34
Weakness of arm	0.77	NS
Weakness of hand	0.68	0.58 (R) 0.49 (L)
Weakness of leg	0.64	NS
Weakness of face	0.63	0.51 (R) 0.66 (L)
Sensory loss on hand	0.19	0.50 (R) 0.32 (L)
Sensory loss on arm	0.15	NS
Dysphasia/language	0.70	0.54
Dysarthria	0.51	0.53
Visuospatial dysfunction	0.44	NS
Hemianopia	0.39	0.40
Cerebellar signs/ataxia	0.46	0.45
Cranial nerve palsy	0.34	NS
Extraocular movement disorder	0.30	0.77

L, left; NS, not stated; R, right.

crete. It can also occur in patients with a haemodynamically significant internal carotid artery (ICA) stenosis, presumably due to subtle changes in distal perfusion pressure. However, the majority are patients where this seems to be a manifestation of an inattention/neglect syndrome or even apraxia (see Section 4.2.5). In patients who are recovering from what appears to be an extensive non-dominant hemisphere stroke, as the inattention/neglect begins to resolve, what seems to be a dense hemiplegia may improve very rapidly, a fact that needs to be borne in mind when predicting the eventual functional outcome. It has been suggested that these phenomena may be responsible for the excess of left over right hemiplegias that has been reported in some large series of stroke (Sterzi *et al.*, 1993).

It is always important to see if a patient can walk, provided there is no risk to the patient or physician, whatever the motor deficit when tested on the bed; a severe deficit may be due to neglect and not weakness, whilst no deficit at all may be associated with profound ataxia of gait.

Another situation in which a patient may move an apparently paralysed limb is as part of certain reflex movements, e.g. yawning, coughing or crying. These associated reactions or synkinesias are not voluntary, but anxious relatives may see them and become overly optimistic about the patient's recovery. Additionally, movements of the normal limb may evoke mirror movements in the paralysed limb. Occasionally, one encounters patients who describe jerking movements of the limbs prior to the onset of a fixed deficit (although this itself may only last a few minutes) (Baquis *et al.*, 1985). The distinction from focal motor epilepsy may be difficult (see Sections 3.2.2 and 3.3.2). This pattern has been reported with internal boundary-zone infarcts (Chambers & Bladin, 1995) and can also occur with cortical infarcts. It may be associated with critical ischaemia and thus may be associated with high-grade ICA stenosis or occlusion (Fig. 4.7). However, such a syndrome should always be an indication for brain imaging, even if a patient has had other episodes which have been considered to be due to cerebrovascular disease, since tumours may present in this manner, i.e. with focal epileptic seizures (Coleman *et al.*, 1993).

Anxious relatives should be counselled concerning involuntary movements or associated reactions that they may witness and to which they might attach too much prognostic significance.

Although spasticity (see Section 15.20) may be ascribed to lesions of the corticospinal tract, it is almost certainly dependent on the influence of extrapyramidal motor pathways. Indeed, lesions of the medullary pyramid, which is the section of the corticospinal tract most clearly separated from the other motor systems, result in a flaccid weakness. Strokes which cause extensive destruction of the cortex may also be associated with flaccidity, whilst early, severe spasticity may be seen with small lesions in the basal ganglia.

An extensor plantar response is but one part of a nociceptive spinal flexion reflex, which, in its complete form (the

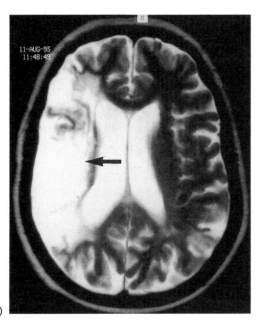

(a)

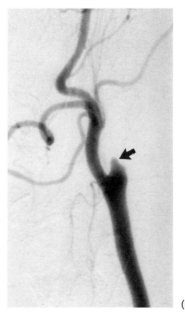

(b)

Figure 4.7 A patient presented with several episodes of jerking of the left arm, which were initially thought to be epileptic. A cranial CT scan was normal. Three-days later he awoke with a left hemiparesis. A T2-weighted axial MRI scan (a) showed an extensive area of infarction in an area usually supplied by the MCA (arrow) and an intra-arterial angiogram (b) showed occlusion of the ipsilateral ICA (arrow).

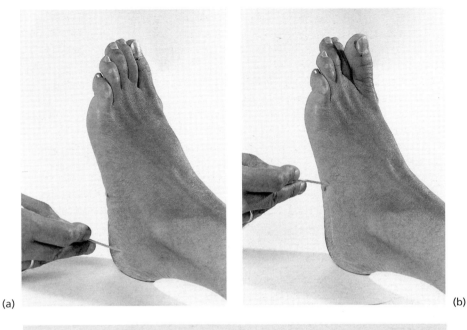

(a)

(b)

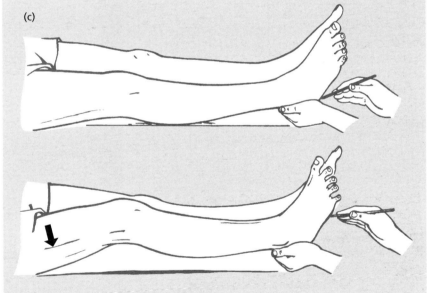

(c)

Figure 4.8 (a,b) The Babinski sign, evoked in this case by stroking the lateral part of the dorsum rather than the sole of the foot in order to avoid voluntary withdrawal. The tendon of extensor hallucis longus can be seen on the dorsum of the hallux and the foot. (c) The Babinski sign involves contraction of the extensor hallucis longus simultaneously with other muscles which shorten the leg: tibialis anterior, the hamstrings (arrow) and tensor fasciae latae. (From van Gijn, 1995; reproduced with permission of the author and the *Postgraduate Medical Journal*.)

sign of Babinski), involves flexion at the hip, knee and ankle as well as extension of the great toe (Fig. 4.8) (van Gijn, 1995). Failure to appreciate this perhaps explains, in part, the rather poor reliability of the sign (Louis *et al.*, 1995). Although its presence signifies a lesion of the corticospinal tract, it is not an invariable accompaniment of such lesions.

Whilst the presence of a Babinski response signifies a lesion of the corticospinal tract, it is not an invariable accompaniment of such lesions.

4.2.4 Disturbance of the sensory system

The main sensory pathways are shown in Fig. 4.9. There are broadly two types of sensory message passing from the periphery to the brain. Somatic sensation (also known as cutaneous or exteroceptive) includes light touch, pain and temperature modalities. These impulses are conveyed in the spinothalamic tracts, which cross the midline at spinal level and then ascend through the spinal cord and brainstem. Fibres carrying similar sensory impulses from the face enter

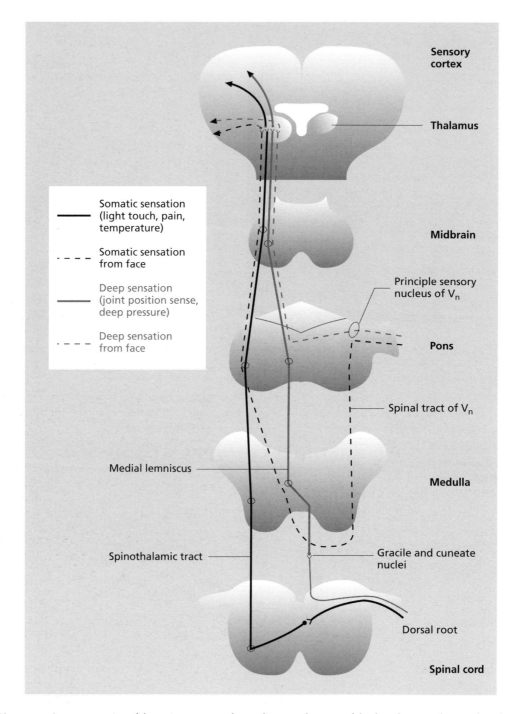

Figure 4.9 Diagrammatic representation of the main sensory pathways between the entry of the dorsal root to the spinal cord and the sensory cortex.

the ipsilateral, descending (or spinal) trigeminal nucleus and cross the midline in the upper cervical spinal cord. They then ascend through the medulla, close to the medial lemniscus, and separate to join the spinothalamic tract in the pons.

Deep (or proprioceptive) sensation refers to joint position sense and deep pressure. The relevant fibres are primarily in the ipsilateral posterior columns, synapsing in the gracile and cuneate nuclei. Decussation occurs in the medulla, after which the fibres ascend through the brainstem in the medial lemniscus. Fibres carrying similar sensory impulses from the face enter the primary trigeminal nucleus in the pons and cross the midline at this level to form the trigeminal lemniscus, which lies adjacent to the medial lemniscus. All these ascending fibres converge towards the midbrain and project, in the main, to the posterior group of thalamic nuclei and in particular to the ventroposterior–lateral (VPL) nuclei. Lesions of the thalamus often involve all sensory modalities, although deep sensation may be more affected than somatic sensation (Brodal, 1981a; Sacco *et al.*, 1987).

From the thalamus there are two main projections. The first is to the postcentral or primary somatic cortex. Here there is somatotopic representation, with the leg uppermost and the face lowermost. The afferent projection is mainly from the dorsal column/medial lemniscus and is concerned with sensory discrimination. A second projection is to the area adjacent to the upper part of the Sylvian fissure and insula. Here there is less discrete localisation but, in general, the face is rostral and the leg caudal. Interestingly, stimulation of this area may result in bilateral symptoms. Also, localised lesions in this area may give a sensory deficit without symptoms. Lesions confined to the parietal lobe are generally regarded as affecting higher-level 'discriminatory' functions (i.e. proprioception, two-point discrimination, stereognosis) rather than primary modalities, although there are cases in the literature (referred to as 'pseudothalamic') where the opposite pattern has occurred.

It is widely recognised that the formal testing of the sensory system is one of the most unreliable parts of the neurological examination (see Table 4.5). Additionally, patients often lack the ability to describe unusual sensations in a manner that allows accurate classification. The descriptions that are used seem to vary between cultures. Furthermore, one gets the impression that certain symptoms (e.g. those experienced in central post-stroke pain (see Section 15.23))are outside the realm of common experience. In general, therefore, one should take due note of sensory symptoms even in the absence of a deficit on examination. Paraesthesia, for example, is presumed to occur because of partial damage to the sensory tracts, which become hyperexcitable (perhaps akin to brisk reflexes), such that ectopic impulses are generated either spontaneously or after a normal stimulus-evoked volley of impulses. There will quite frequently be no detectable sensory loss. Indeed, assuming the patients are able to communicate and do not have neglect, the only situation when they will have sensory loss without sensory symptoms is when there is a restrictive problem of discriminatory rather than primary sensory function (due to a parietal lesion), something that is uncommon in clinical practice. Conversely, care needs to be taken over the interpretation of very transient sensory symptoms which can be within the range of normal experience, although the clinician should not accept uncritically the patients' common interpretation of sensory symptoms that they had 'trapped a nerve' or been 'lying in a draught'.

Formal testing of the sensory system is the most unreliable part of the neurological examination, and the physician should always take due note of sensory symptoms, even in the absence of a deficit on examination.

As with other aspects of examination, the physician dealing with patients with stroke needs to have a repertoire of tests allowing adjustment to particular circumstances, since it will be impossible to conduct the 'standard' examination of sensation in the presence of drowsiness, dysphasia or dementia. However, in most cases there will at least be a 'normal' side to permit comparison of response. The physician should always remember that patient (and doctor) fatigue will impair the reliability of results and tired patients become increasingly suggestible. In such cases one may have to rely on identifying a difference in response between the patient's right and left side to either predominantly somatic sensory stimuli, such as pinprick, or deep pressure, e.g. squeezing the Achilles tendon. The presence of severe visuospatial disturbance may make meaningful sensory testing impossible.

The physician should always remember that patient, and doctor, fatigue will impair the reliability of the results of sensory testing and tired patients become increasingly suggestible.

Somatic sensation should be tested in the standard manner, using a wisp of cotton wool and an appropriate pin (i.e. not a hypodermic needle!). Proprioception may be assessed with the patient's arms outstretched, the fingers spread and the eyes closed. The examiner should look for drift of the patient's arm in a pseudoathetoid or 'piano-playing' manner. This can be amplified by asking the patient to touch the tip of his/her nose with the forefinger whilst the eyes remain closed, when those with disturbed proprioception will repeatedly miss the target. This screening test will assess proprioception around proximal as well as distal joints, but, as mentioned above (see Section 4.2.3), drift can also be due to a motor deficit or neglect/inattention. Therefore, if possible, one should always attempt the traditional method of testing joint position sense of the distal interphalangeal joints. If there is dysphasia, it is sometimes worth asking the patient to indicate with gesture the direction of movement. Romberg's test is rarely of value unless lower-limb motor function is entirely normal.

Testing higher cortical sensory function is really only of value when the primary modalities are intact. For example, asterognosis (which is an inability to identify an object by palpation, e.g. a coin placed in the palm of the hand and the patient being able to move and feel it with the ipsilateral fingers) may be associated with lesions of the contralateral parietal cortex. However, it must be distinguished from the much more common stereo-anaesthesia, where the inability to identify the object occurs because of disruption of the lower sensory tracts, i.e. it is not purely a question of discrimination. Additionally, and to reinforce the point that one should always compare the two sides, it needs to be distinguished from tactile agnosia, where the inability to recognise the object is present in *both* hands. This usually occurs with a posterior dominant-hemisphere lesion. Other tests worth considering are letter-writing in the palm of the hand and formal testing of two-point discrimination, but one has to say that the number of patients with stroke where such tests are both relevant and practicable is very small.

Sensory extinction is the situation where the patient fails to register a tactile stimulus on one side of the body when both sides are stimulated simultaneously, but will register the same stimulus when given independently to each side separately. This is a form of visuospatial disturbance (see Section 4.2.5) and was previously known as perceptual rivalry.

Some patients have restricted sensory syndromes which affect unusual combinations of bodily parts. The most frequently encountered is the cheiro-oral syndrome, where there is a sensory abnormality over the perioral area and ipsilateral palm. In some patients, the foot may be involved and, in both the hand and foot, certain digits may be affected whilst others are spared (a pseudoradicular distribution). Although lesions at most levels of the sensory pathways can give these patterns, lesions in the ventroposterior nucleus (VPN) of the thalamus are the most likely (Kim, 1994; Kim & Lee, 1994). It is thought that sensory projections from the face (with a particularly large representation for the lips), hand and foot are somatotopically arranged in the ventral portion of the nucleus, and the fingertips have particularly large representation areas, with that for the thumb more medial and the little finger more laterally. The projection areas for the trunk and proximal limbs are relatively small and sited more dorsally and therefore may be selectively spared. However, a similar proximity of projection areas through the corona radiata and in the sensory cortex may also occur and, consequently, lesions in these areas may also result in the cheiro-oral syndrome. An isolated deficit in a pseudoradicular distribution (most often involving the thumb and forefinger) is probably more often caused by a cortical lesion, because a stroke of any given size would affect fibres from a more restricted anatomical area in the cortex than in the thalamus. Bilateral symptoms may occur from midpontine lesions, because the sensory fibres from the mouth, arm and leg are once again arranged somatotopically in the medial lemnisci. Other theories which may account for these syndromes have been discussed by Kim (1994).

4.2.5 Disturbance of higher cerebral function

Because of its sheer complexity, higher cerebral function, whilst being one of the most fascinating aspects of neurological practice, is often perceived as one of the most difficult areas for the average clinician. This need not be so if one remembers that the roles (and information needs) of clinicians, neuropsychologists and remedial therapists are very different. It is perfectly respectable for the clinician dealing with stroke patients to be able to identify cognitive disorders in general terms to facilitate diagnosis, lesion localisation and basic management. This does not require detailed assessment batteries, which may help the neuropsychologist to investigate specific neural mechanisms or the therapist to monitor the rehabilitation process. Therefore, in this section we will concentrate on the bedside or clinical assessment of disturbances of higher cerebral function.

> *The clinician dealing with stroke patients should be able to identify cognitive disorders in general terms, without resorting to detailed assessment batteries, in order to facilitate diagnosis, lesion localisation and basic management.*

There is continuing debate amongst neuropsychologists about how localised (or not) certain cerebral functions are, but, in general, it is useful to distinguish those functions which are 'distributed', i.e. involve several areas of the cortex, such as attention, concentration, memory and higher-order social behaviour (see Section 15.28), from more 'localised' functions, such as speech and language (see Section 15.30), visuospatial function and praxis (see Section 15.20; Hodges, 1994). However, it must be remembered that few tests are absolutely specific for a single area of cognition. Clearly, it is important for the physician to determine the handedness of an individual patient, but the descriptions below assume left-hemisphere dominance.

> *Few tests are absolutely specific for a single area of cognition.*

Attention and concentration

Attention is not synonymous with wakefulness. Failure of attention results in patients being unable to sustain concentration and they appear distractable. It depends on the integrated activity of the neocortex (predominantly the prefrontal, posterior parietal and ventral temporal lobes), the thalamus and brainstem. Disorientation may be a consequence of a more severe disorder of attention and it also has an impact on memory function. From a practical point of view, if there is a significant disorder of attention, then extreme care is required when interpreting the results of

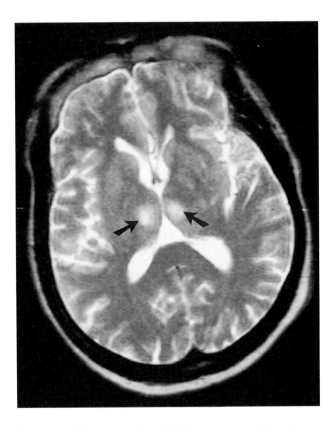

Figure 4.10 A T2-weighted, axial MRI scan showing bilateral thalamic infarction (arrows) in a patient with a major cardiac source of embolism (atrial fibrillation plus left atrial thrombus). The patient also sustained infarction in both cerebellar hemispheres at the same time as the thalamic infarction.

Table 4.6 Bedside testing of attention.

Orientation (in person, time and place)
Digit span forwards and backwards
Recite months of year or days of week backwards
Serial subtraction of 7s

testing higher-order functions. Attention and concentration can be assessed at the bedside using the tests shown in Table 4.6.

It is difficult to test higher-order cerebral functions if there is a significant disorder of attention.

Memory

Many patients with stroke are of an age when there is a natural decline in memory. Furthermore, attentional problems after stroke can result in failure to register new information. Therefore, although many patients complain of memory problems, it may be difficult to identify those that are the direct result of the vascular disease. The important structures for memory are the medial temporal lobes and the thalamus (particularly the dorsomedial nuclei), i.e. structures usually supplied by the posterior circulation, although disorders of the frontal lobes may also influence memory.

The nomenclature of memory and theories about memory processing are changing (Hodges, 1994). One method of dividing the memory function is into 'explicit' (that which is available to conscious access) and 'implicit' (that which relates to learned responses and conditioned reflexes). Explicit memory may be 'episodic' (dealing with specific events and episodes that have been personally experienced) or 'semantic' (which deals with knowledge of facts, concepts and the meaning of words). The terms short- and long-term memory are used loosely by clinicians and often rather differently by neuropsychologists. The current prevailing opinion is that there is a 'working memory' for very short-term or immediate recall of verbal and spatial material and a number of systems which work in parallel dealing with long-term memory for different types of material. However, for the clinician, who will know more or less precisely the time of the stroke, distinguishing anterograde amnesia (failure to acquire new memories) from retrograde amnesia (failure to recall previously learnt material) is probably more useful. With most memory disorders caused by the vascular lesion, new information may be registered but will not be retained for more than a few minutes. Additionally, there will usually be a degree of retrograde amnesia. This is important because impaired concentration or attention, which is common after stroke, can significantly impair the retention of new information, but recall of past events is usually intact. Severe amnesia is usually the result of bilateral lesions (particularly of the thalamus; Fig. 4.10). Verbal memory is affected predominantly by left-hemisphere lesions and non-verbal memory by right-hemisphere lesions, although the latter often has much less impact on functional abilities. Suggested methods for assessing memory are set out in Table 4.7.

Table 4.7 Bedside testing of memory.

Check that patient is attentive (see Table 4.6) and that language function is adequate (see Table 4.8)

Working memory
Give patient a name, address and name of a flower
Ensure that they have registered the information
Test the patient 3-, 5- and possibly 10-minutes later

Long-term memory
Ask patient to describe recent events on the ward
Ask about significant historical events and major events in the
patient's life, e.g. date of marriage

The terms short- and long-term memory are used loosely by clinicians and often rather differently by neuropsychologists. In patients with stroke, the terms anterograde and retrograde amnesia may be of more value.

Speech and language

Disorders of speech and language are commonly encountered in patients with stroke (see Section 15.30). At the outset, it is important to stress that the two are not synonymous, in that reading and writing are also important language functions. Furthermore, the production (or expression) and comprehension (or reception) of speech should be considered separately. The analysis of such disorders can be of value in localising the lesion, although this is probably overrated in everyday cerebrovascular practice. However, the recognition of specific problems is important for the management and advice given to both patients and their carers. The primary distinction to be made is between aphasia/dysphasia (which is defined as an acquired disorder of the production and/or comprehension of spoken and/or written language) and anarthria/dysarthria (which is defined as a disorder of articulation).

Disorders of speech and language are not synonymous; reading and writing are also important language functions which should be assessed.

In the acute phase of stroke, many patients are mute, i.e. there is a total loss of expressive speech. The majority will have severe aphasia, but a few will be anarthric. Anarthria may occur as part of a pseudobulbar palsy or with a single lesion involving both sides of the brainstem. With both aphasia and anarthria, other neurological symptoms and signs (and, in particular, dysphagia with anarthria) will usually be present as well. Cortical dysarthria and aphemia are

terms used when the patient is mute but comprehension, reading and writing are intact and there are no signs to suggest a bulbar palsy. Despite this, it is probably best regarded as a form of expressive aphasia. It has been reported with lesions in the anterior frontal lobe.

Many types of aphasia have been described. Although in general non-fluent (expressive) aphasias are more likely to be due to lesions of the dominant frontal lobe (although not necessarily confined to Broca's area (Mohr *et al.*, 1978)) and fluent (receptive) aphasias to more posterior lesions (but not necessarily confined to Wernicke's area), most patients with stroke have a combination referred to as mixed (or, if severe, global) aphasia. Typically, this occurs with extensive lesions within the MCA territory (see Section 4.3.2) and is usually associated with a right hemiparesis and hemianopia. There is a general tendency in everyday clinical practice to underestimate the receptive component, particularly if the clinician does not go beyond questions requiring a yes/no answer or simple social conversation. Occasionally, one encounters patients with non-fluent aphasia in whom repetition is intact. This is termed transcortical motor aphasia and is usually caused by lesions restricted to the anterior cerebral artery (ACA) territory (see Section 4.3.2). The equivalent fluent aphasia with normal repetition (termed transcortical sensory aphasia) occurs with strokes in the left temporo-occipital region and therefore may result from lesions in the usual territory of the posterior cerebral artery (PCA) (see Section 4.3.3). Lesions of the thalamus may also result in predominantly non-fluent aphasia, in which case they may be associated with fluctuating alertness (see Section 4.3.3).

Another type of language disorder that may result from PCA territory strokes which involve the medial aspect of the left occipital lobe and the splenium of the corpus callosum is alexia, with or without agraphia. There is usually a right visual field defect but no hemiparesis, and it is thought that the lesion in the splenium interrupts the transfer of visual information from the normal left visual field (right occipital lobe) to the damaged left-hemisphere language areas.

Dysarthria should only be diagnosed with confidence if all the aspects of language function described above are intact. Care must be taken if the patient is being assessed after the acute phase, since during the recovery from milder forms of aphasia articulation may be impaired and the evidence of language dysfunction difficult to detect.

It is important not to assume that dysarthria is always due to a brainstem or cerebral lesion. It can occur with facial weakness in a hemispheric stroke and it can be very severe indeed with bilateral hemispheric lesions.

As with other aspects of the examination, the physician

has to judge how relevant detailed testing actually is, since in the majority of patients with stroke the language disorders are anything but subtle. Table 4.8 sets out a scheme of bedside testing which will detect most speech and language problems. The moderate inter-rater reliability for the detection of dysphasia (see Table 4.5) reflects the difficulties of performing detailed testing in many patients with stroke, especially where there may be associated deafness, confusion, etc.

The assessment of language function may be difficult or impossible in those with severe deafness and/or confusion.

Table 4.8 Bedside testing of speech and language function.

First ensure any hearing-aid is switched on and working and that appropriate, clean spectacles are worn! Also check that you are using the patient's native language

Spontaneous speech
Consider output (whether fluent or non-fluent), articulation and
content:
during history-taking
for a structured task (e.g. 'describe your surroundings')

Auditory comprehension
Simple yes/no questions (e.g. is Russia the capital of Moscow? Can
dogs fly? Do you put your shoes on before your socks?)
Give commands (being careful not to use non-verbal cues) of one,
two and three steps using common objects, such as the
manipulation of three different-coloured pens (care needed
that complex motor tasks do not involve the use of limbs with
significant weakness or apraxia)

Naming
Ask the patient to name objects, parts of objects, colours, body
parts, famous faces (certain groups, particularly the naming of
people, may be more severely affected. If visual agnosia is present,
use auditory/tactile presentation, e.g. bunch of keys)

Repetition
'West Register Street' (difficult if dysarthric)
'No ifs, ands or buts' (difficult if aphasic)

Reading
Aloud, e.g. from a book or newspaper
Comprehension of the same piece

Writing
Spontaneous ('why have you come into hospital?')
Dictation ('the quick brown fox jumped over the lazy dog')
Copying

Articulation
p/p/p/p (tests particularly orbicularis oris)
t/t/t/t (tests particularly anterior tongue)
k/k/k/k (tests particularly posterior tongue and palate)

Visuospatial dysfunction

Many patients with stroke fail to respond to stimulation of, or to report information from, the side contralateral to the cerebral lesion. The underlying mechanisms of such 'neglect' are much debated, but currently most authorities consider it to be a modality-specific disorder of attention rather than a primary defect of sensory processing. A number of different types and/or degrees of severity of neglect occur in patients with stroke and, in many, a combination of somatic sensory deficits and disturbed visual perception, as well as conceptual negation of deficits, contribute to the clinically apparent 'neglect': hence, the use of the broader term 'visuospatial dysfunction'. Such phenomena are almost certainly more severe in posterior parietal lesions of the non-dominant hemisphere, particularly those that extend to the visual association areas. Although they can occur with left-hemisphere lesions, their detection is often hindered by co-existent language disturbances and inability to use the dominant hand (see Table 15.39). Visuospatial problems are major causes of disability and handicap and impede the functional recovery of the patient (see Section 15.29).

There are two broad categories of neglect.
1 *Intrapersonal neglect*, i.e. with respect to the patient's own body. The clinically apparent problem may range from, at its most severe, denial either of the limb itself (*non-belonging*) or of the deficit, e.g. a paralysed limb (*anosognosia*), through showing no concern for the deficit (*anosodiaphoria*) and a tendency to ignore the limb (*inattention*), to sensory (or visual) *extinction*, when the deficit is only elicited when there is simultaneous stimulation of both sides. *Dressing apraxia*, which is occasionally seen in a pure form, is when a patient is unable to dress despite having no apparent weakness, sensory or visual loss, or neglect. It probably occurs because of a combination of disordered body image, sensory and visual inattention rather than being a true apraxia.
2 *Extrapersonal (topographical) neglect* refers to the patient's abnormal response to the environment and may be recognised by abnormalities either of spontaneous actions or of response to various tasks, such as drawing, copying, constructional tasks, cancellation and line-bisection tests. Unfortunately, many such tests rely on there being reasonable motor function of the dominant hand, and are impossible to perform if there are significant communication or visual problems.

By simply observing how patients respond to their environment and carry out tasks one can often deduce the presence of visuospatial problems (Fig. 4.11). An obvious example would be if a patient (without a hemianopia) does not register the doctor's presence when approached from one side, even when spoken to. Alternatively, they might be unable to find their way back to their hospital bed having been taken to the toilet, suggesting geographical disorientation. The nurses and therapists are often better placed than the doctor to witness such behaviour, so it is important that these staff are trained to recognise and report these problems to other members of the team.

One can often deduce the presence of visuospatial problems by simply observing how the patient responds to the environment and carries out tasks around the ward.

Although many tests to identify and quantify visuospatial dysfunction have been described, the gold standard against which the tests are evaluated is often regarded as the opinion of an occupational therapist (Stone *et al.*, 1991). Therefore, although test batteries may be more objective and repeatable, they may not be any more valid than a bedside assessment. Also, one could reasonably argue that these test batteries are not particularly relevant, because they do not test functionally important tasks such as washing, dressing and feeding. Despite their limitations in routine clinical practice, test batteries are undoubtedly useful in further characterising deficits in selected patients with difficult or persistent problems, in helping to explain patient's functional problems and in research (see Section 15.29). Table 4.9 sets out a bedside examination which should detect significant visuospatial dysfunction and Table 4.10 a glossary of terms used. Figure 4.12 shows the type of abnormal drawing of a flower that may occur when there has been a non-dominant parietal stroke. Drawing a clock face is a commonly used test (Fig. 4.13), although recent studies have reported that it may not be specific for visual neglect (Ishiai *et al.*, 1993) but rather reflect other cognitive problems (Watson *et al.*, 1993). Of the many cancellation tasks available, the star cancellation test is probably the most sensitive and is easy to use (Fig. 4.14) (Halligan *et al.*, 1989), although it is only one component of the Behavioural Inattention Test. Many aspects of these assessments of visuospatial function require subjective judgements to be made by the physician, which probably accounts for the relatively poor inter-rater reliability (see Table 4.5).

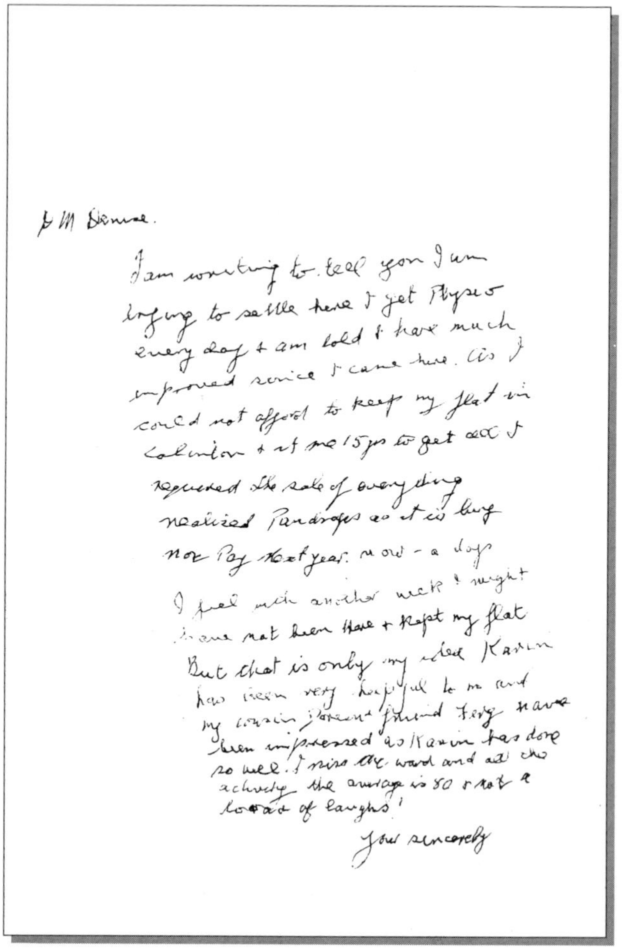
Dr M Dennis.
I am writing to tell you I am
trying to settle here I get Physio
every day + am told I have much
improved since I came here. as I
could not afford to keep my flat in
London + it me 15 yrs to get out I
required the sale of everything
realized Pandropes as it is long
now Pay next year. now - a days
I feel with another week I might
have not been there + kept my flat
But that is only my idea Karin
has been very helpful to me and
my cousin Doreen friend Terry have
been impressed as Karin has done
so well. I miss the ward and all the
activity the average is 80 + not a
lot of laughs!
Yours sincerely

Figure 4.11 A letter from a patient with left visual neglect.

Apraxia is defined as a loss of ability to perform learned movements which can not be explained by weakness, sensory loss, incoordination, inattention and other perceptual disorders, or by failure to understand the command. Patients have difficulty with or are incapable of miming actions, imitating how an object is used or even making symbolic gestures, even though at other times they may be observed making the individual movements that would be needed to perform the action. In general, they will have most difficulty miming the action, less difficulty imitating the examiner and least difficulty when actually given the object to use. The

Table 4.9 Bedside test of visuospatial function.

Is the patient aware of, and reacting appropriately to his/her deficit?
Observe the patient's response to the environment
Observe the patient's ability to carry out a specific task
Check for sensory and visual extinction (see Sections 4.2.4 and 4.2.5)
Copy a simple picture, e.g. a flower (see Fig. 4.11)
Perform the star cancellation test (see Fig. 4.13)

Table 4.10 Glossary of terms describing disorders of visuospatial function.

Hemi-inattention Where the patient's behaviour during examination suggests an inability to respond appropriately to environmental stimuli on one side, e.g. people approaching, noises or activity in the ward

Sensory or tactile extinction Where the patient fails to register a tactile stimulus (light touch) on one side of his/her body when both sides are stimulated simultaneously (i.e. double simultaneous stimulation) but where the patient has registered the stimulus when each side was stimulated independently

Visual inattention or extinction Where the patient fails to register a visual stimulus (e.g. finger movement) in one homonymous visual field when the same stimulus is presented to both fields simultaneously but where the patient had no field defect on normal testing

Allaesthesia Where the patient consistently attributes sensory stimulation on one side to stimulation of the other. This is related to right/left confusion, where the patient consistently moves the limbs on one side when requested to move the limbs on the other

Anosognosia Where the patient denies the presence of a neurological impairment on one side, most often weakness

Non-belonging Where the patient denies ownership of the limbs on one side of their body or even attributes the limb to another person

RELATED PHENOMENA SEEN IN PARIETAL LOBE DYSFUNCTION

Anosodiaphoria Refers to an indifference to a perceived weakness or other impairment

Astereognosia Where the patient is unable to recognise objects placed in the affected hand

Graphaesthesia Where the patient is unable to identify a number drawn on the palm of the affected hand

Geographical disorientation Where the patient becomes lost in familiar surroundings despite being able to see

Dressing apraxia (dyspraxia) Where the patient is unable to dress despite having no apparent weakness, sensory loss or visual or neglect problems. We have seen occasional patients with apparently isolated dressing dyspraxia

more sequences there are to the action, the more difficult it is and so the more sensitive the test. These relatively common problems are sometimes referred to as ideomotor apraxias and may be distinguished from ideational apraxias, when the patient has difficulty performing a sequence of movements even though the individual movements can be performed normally. However, the latter probably occurs very rarely in a pure form and the distinction of ideomotor and ideational apraxias is of little value to clinicians.

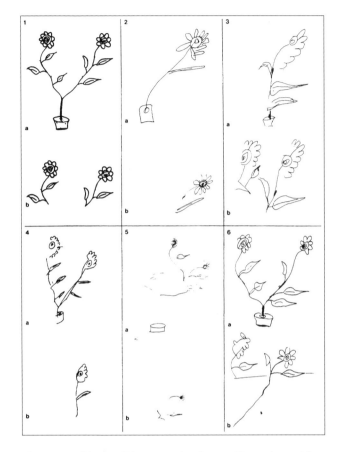

Figure 4.12 Abnormalities on copying flowers. Five patients with damage to the right hemisphere were asked to copy the pictures (a) and (b) in panel 1. These figures illustrate the variations seen in copying tasks. 1, normal test. 2, this patient has mainly neglected the information on the left side of the page. 3, this patient has omitted the left-hand components of the objects but has shifted attention to the right-hand side of another object placed to the left of the neglected space. 4, this patient has drawn the right side of both flowers in the pot but has completely neglected the left of the two separate flowers. 5, this patient has transposed objects in the left field to the right field, i.e. both flowers are drawn on a single stem. This phenomenon has been likened to allaesthesia, which has been reported for tactile and visual modalities. 6, this patient has produced a 'hallucinatory' rabbit in the left field when copying the separate flowers. This has been termed a 'metamorphopsia' and when restricted to one visual field has been likened to lateralised confabulations, which may occasionally be seen in patients with neglect. (Reproduced with permission of Marshall & Halligan (1993) and the *Journal of Neurology*.)

It is thought that the programmes of learned movements (engrams) reside predominantly in the subcortex of the left hemisphere; clearly the left superior temporal region (Wernicke's area) will be required for interpretation of the command. Messages then pass to the left premotor frontal

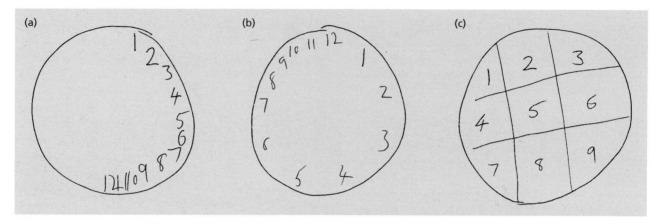

Figure 4.13 (a) Drawing of a clock face by a patient with left visuospatial disturbance after a stroke. This shows crowding of digits on the right and neglect of the left side of the clock face. (b) Drawing of a clock face by a confused, elderly patient who had not had a stroke. The crowding of digits on the left occurs because of a failure of planning. Many normal people insert 12, 3, 6 and 9 before the other numbers. (c) A rather bizarre drawing of a clock face by a patient with strokes affecting both cerebral hemispheres.

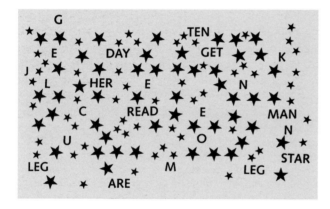

Figure 4.14 Star cancellation test. The chart is placed in front of the patient, who is asked to cross out all the small stars whilst ignoring the large stars and letters. (Reproduced with permission of Thames Valley Test Company, 7–9 The Green, Flempton, Bury St Edmunds, Suffolk IP28 6EL, UK.)

cortex and finally, via the anterior corpus callosum, to the right premotor frontal cortex (Fig. 4.15). Lesions in the posterior left hemisphere may result in bilateral apraxia (because the message is not transmitted), those in the premotor areas are usually associated with a hemiparesis and therefore apraxia may only be apparent in the non-paralysed limbs, and finally a lesion of the corpus callosum may cause isolated apraxia of the left limbs, with normal function of the right limbs. In patients with stroke, the main problem is being sure that they have understood the command, because lesions of the relevant areas will often result in aphasia. Nevertheless, DeRenzi *et al.* (1980) reported that with an imitation test (i.e. no verbal command) 80% of patients with aphasia also had evidence of apraxia. In some patients orofacial apraxia may contribute to post-stroke dysphagia and dysarthria.

The clinician should always consider this type of problem in patients where there seems to be a disparity between the degree of deficit as tested on the bed (when one often gives the patient relatively simple commands) and their functional abilities. It is also important to be aware that such patients may perform the same acts reflexly and they should not be misinterpreted as having a somatisation disorder. Table 4.11 suggests ways of screening for apraxia. Dressing and constructional apraxias, which usually occur when there is a right-hemisphere lesion, are best considered as disorders of visuospatial function rather than true apraxias (see above). Although the term verbal or speech apraxia may be used by speech and language therapists when there are repeated phonemic substitutions, in practice such patients usually also have evidence of dysphasia and/or dysarthria. We are not aware of any data to indicate the inter-rater reliability for detecting apraxias but suspect it might not be very high.

Apraxia should always be considered as a potential explanation where there seems to be a disparity between the degree of deficit as tested on the bed (when one often gives the patient relatively simple commands) and their functional abilities.

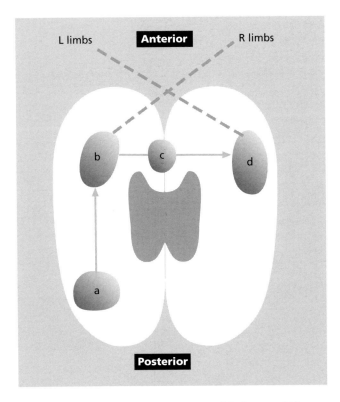

Figure 4.15 Diagrammatic representation of the lesions which can result in apraxia. (a) The dominant temporoparietal cortex is the probable site of the programmes of learned movements (engrams). Lesions here result in bilateral apraxias due to failure to transmit the motor information to the frontal lobes, although they may be difficult to identify because the interpretation of the command may also be affected by a receptive aphasia. (b) Although lesions of the dominant frontal lobe will often be associated with an expressive aphasia, comprehension is usually relatively spared. The apraxia may only be apparent in the left limbs, since there will usually be a right hemiparesis. (c) Lesions in the anterior corpus callosum may result in isolated apraxia of the left limbs, because of failure of transmission of the motor information to the right frontal lobe, whilst the right arm and leg move normally. (d) Lesions of the non-dominant frontal lobe are not usually associated with clinically apparent apraxias, because there will usually be a left hemiparesis.

4.2.6 Disturbance of the visual system

When trying to assess the visual disturbances that occur in patients with cerebrovascular disease, one should consider the problem under three broad headings: the reception of visual stimuli by the eyes; the transmission of the visual information from the eyes to the occipital cortex; and the interpretation of the visual information in the visual cortex.

It may be difficult to test visual acuity formally (e.g. with a Snellen chart) in patients with acute stroke because of drowsiness, aphasia or the fact that they are bed-bound, but at least testing with a hand-held acuity chart or simply using everyday written material should be attempted. Many stroke patients are elderly and therefore concomitant diseases, such as glaucoma, senile macular degeneration, cataracts and diabetic retinopathy, are common. It is important to identify them at an early stage, because they may make rehabilitation significantly more difficult. Indeed, the improved visual acuity that follows a cataract extraction may make the difference between a patient with residual disability from a stroke being able to live independently (and safely) or not. Because of the very large representation of the macula area in the occipital cortex even patients with complete homonymous hemianopias (see below) do not have significantly reduced visual acuity *per se*. The various patterns of visual loss related to specific anatomical lesions are shown in Fig. 4.16.

One should be surprised if elderly patients attempt, never mind accomplish, tests of visual acuity without clean spectacles.

Reduction of visual acuity in one eye suggests that the problem lies anterior to the optic chiasma. In patients with vascular disease, the most common symptom is amaurosis fugax, i.e. transient monocular blindness (see Section 3.2.2). In this condition (or retinal artery occlusion), the patient describes either total visual obscuration (in which case it is particularly important to ask if they covered each eye during

Table 4.11 Bedside testing of praxis.

Extremities
Ask the patient to
Mime the use of a pen, comb and toothbrush
Imitate examiner's use of the same objects
Use the actual objects
Orofacial
Ask the patient to
Whistle
Put tongue out
Blow out cheeks
Cough
*Serial actions**
Ask the patient to
Mime putting the address on a letter
Then seal it
Then put a stamp on it

* Traditionally the test was to mime taking out, lighting and smoking a pipe or cigarette. This would almost constitute a reflex action in many stroke patients and should not be encouraged!

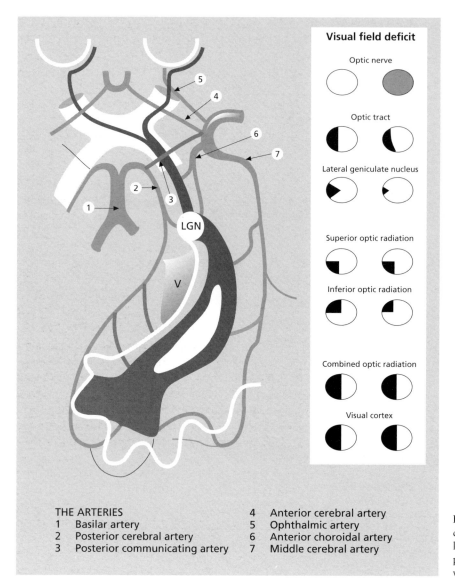

Visual field deficit

Optic nerve

Optic tract

Lateral geniculate nucleus

Superior optic radiation

Inferior optic radiation

Combined optic radiation

Visual cortex

LGN

V

THE ARTERIES
1 Basilar artery
2 Posterior cerebral artery
3 Posterior communicating artery
4 Anterior cerebral artery
5 Ophthalmic artery
6 Anterior choroidal artery
7 Middle cerebral artery

Figure 4.16 Diagram of the visual field deficits which may result from vascular lesions at various sites on the visual pathway and the relationship to the vascular supply.

the attack since many people describe loss of a homonymous hemifield as loss of vision in one eye) or a partial defect. This partial defect is almost always an inferior or superior altitudinal defect, since it reflects the arterial supply of the retina. Homonymous altitudinal defects (i.e. present in the same part of both visual fields) may occur from infarction of the occipital calcarine cortex restricted to either the superior or inferior border of the sulcus, but in practice such cases are very rare.

Sudden, complete visual loss is an uncommon but extremely distressing condition. The first question (which is rarely relevant in the vascular age group) is whether it is functional and not due to any physical disorder at all. This is best detected with an optokinetic drum or a long piece of

material with vertical stripes (e.g. a scarf or tape measure) since it is impossible to voluntarily suppress nystagmus if there is visual function. The second question is where is the lesion. Lesions anterior to the lateral geniculate nucleus will result in loss of the pupillary light reflex (the relevant fibres entering the pretectal nuclei in the brainstem before passing to the Edinger–Westphal nuclei). Anterior ischaemic optic neuropathy (see Section 3.4.3) may result in a small central scotoma (which, nonetheless, can cause severe reduction in visual acuity), an altitudinal defect or, more typically, sudden complete loss of vision. The optic nerve head may be swollen or pale. With bilateral occipital lobe infarction, which may occur with occlusion of both PCAs, the occipital pole may be preserved by MCA collaterals (see Section 4.3.2;

Miller, 1982), but the visual deficit still occurs, because of involvement of the optic radiations. Denial of the visual deficit may sometimes occur, with subsequent confabulation (Anton's syndrome). The involvement of more anterior (association area) occipital lobe structures in such cases is also suggested by the pattern of recovery, which, when it does occur, tends to be through a phase of visual agnosia. In middle-aged and elderly people, one presumes that transient bilateral visual loss or dimming, which should be considered a vascular syndrome, is due to short-lived ischaemia in both PCA territories (Dennis *et al.*, 1989).

Vascular lesions affecting the optic chiasm symmetrically (when one might detect a bitemporal hemianopia) are rare. Indeed, the only vascular lesion of note would be a large aneurysm from the circle of Willis.

Homonymous visual field deficits (i.e. loss of vision in the corresponding part of the visual fields in both eyes) signify a retrochiasmal lesion. In theory, if the deficit in the two eyes is entirely congruous, the lesion is likely to be in the calcarine cortex of the occipital lobe (otherwise known as the striate cortex because of its 'striped' appearance at autopsy). On the other hand, incongruous deficits are more likely to be due to lesions of the optic tracts. Distinguishing the two types in bedside cerebrovascular practice is probably of little practical relevance. Lesions of the lateral geniculate nucleus (LGN) of the thalamus may result in homonymous horizontal sectoranopia (i.e. a segmental defect which respects the vertical but not the horizontal meridian) (Frisen, 1979), but these rarely occur in isolation.

The optic radiations pass from the LGN as the most posterior structures of the internal capsule. Involvement at this level is probably one of the causes of hemianopia in extensive MCA territory infarction, but the radiations do not seem to be affected by occlusion of a single perforating artery. Restricted lesions of the inferior optic radiation between the LGN and the calcarine cortex, where the fibres swing over the temporal horn of the lateral ventricle and deep into the temporal lobe (Meyer's loop), result in a homonymous superior quadrantanopia. Lesions of the equivalent fibres passing superiorly through the parietal lobe should result in a homonymous inferior quadrantanopia, but this is rarely identified in practice, presumably because those occurring in the dominant hemisphere are likely to be associated with aphasia and those in the non-dominant hemisphere with neglect or inattention. If the entire calcarine cortex or optic tract on one side is damaged, there will be a complete homonymous hemianopia, including macular vision. Sparing of macular vision with an otherwise complete hemianopia does occur in PCA territory infarction. The conventional explanation of this phenomenon is that the infarction is confined to the cortical surface (thereby sparing the optic radiations) but that the macular cortex is spared because it receives sufficient collateral supply from the terminal branches of the MCA (see Section 4.3.2; Miller, 1982).

Ultimately, most patients with a stroke who have a visual field defect are reported as having an homonymous hemianopia. When the hemianopia is an isolated feature, it is most likely to be due to a lesion in the occipital lobe. When this is due to infarction, it will most often be due to occlusion of the PCA (Trobe *et al.*, 1973). Embolism is probably the most frequent cause, but giant cell arteritis and migraine are other aetiologies which need to be considered (Kaul *et al.*, 1974). A homonymous hemianopia rather than an inferior quadrantanopia is frequently present in patients with MCA lesions, despite the fact that the MCA is traditionally considered to supply the area through which the superior but not the inferior radiation passes. However, in some patients, the territory supplied by the MCA extends much more posteriorly than is apparent on standard 'maps' (see Section 4.3.2) and, thus, an MCA lesion could produce a homonymous hemianopia by interrupting the converging optic radiations. In other patients, the MCA territory ischaemia will be secondary to a lesion in the ICA. The hemianopia might then occur because, in a proportion of people, the PCA derives its blood supply from the anterior circulation. Also, there might be ischaemia of the optic tracts or LGN when the relevant perforating arteries arise from the carotid system (see Section 4.3.2). Perhaps the most likely explanation, however, is that in many patients there is a mixture of a true visual field loss and visual inattention.

Visual agnosia is the state when primary visual perception is intact but the patient is unable to comprehend the meaning of the object without resorting to the use of other sensory modalities such as touch. *Prosopagnosia* is a syndrome where patients can not recognise familiar faces, even though they can describe them. In its pure form it is very rare but can result in enormous distress if a patient denies recognising his/her close family. Most lesions causing visual agnosia are in the anterior part of the dominant occipital lobe (the so-called visual association areas) and the angular gyrus, although the majority of cases of prosopagnosia have occurred with bilateral lesions (Hodges, 1994).

Assessment of the visual fields

Assessment of the visual fields must be tailored to the patient's overall condition and it is important that the physician has a repertoire of methods and does not give up simply because 'formal' testing by confrontation is impossible because the patient is drowsy, dysphasic, cognitively impaired or just can not sit up. It is important to remember that kinetic testing (i.e. using moving objects, waggling fingers, etc.) is a less sensitive way of detecting deficits than static methods such as counting fingers or comparing colours in each hemifield (i.e. there is a dissociation between the visual perception of form and movement). Furthermore, although standard texts suggest that it should be easy to distinguish a true hemianopia from visual inattention, the reality with many patients with stroke is that one is left saying that there is probably 'an abnormality' of the visual field. If the patients can understand and communicate, one should first ask them to describe what they see in front of them, perhaps using the same text as for testing visual acuity, and ideally testing each eye individually. After that, hold up fingers sequentially in each quadrant of vision and ask the patient to count them. Following this, try and perform simultaneous finger-counting to detect evidence of visual extinction. Testing of the visual fields with automated perimetry is extemely tiring and of little value in the acute situation. Indeed, it may produce bizarre deficits which are normally associated with non-organic disorders. However, it may be necessary when there is doubt about driving eligibility (see Section 15.32.2).

> *Although testing of the visual fields using conventional confrontation methods is often impossible because the patient is drowsy, dysphasic, cognitively impaired or just can not sit up, one can usually use other methods to determine whether or not there is an abnormality of the visual field.*

If, for whatever reason, the patient can not follow commands, one will need to use quite gross stimuli to be sure of eliciting and identifying a response if the visual fields are intact. Examples include seeing if there is any response to moving a brightly coloured object in one hemifield, getting a colleague to approach the patient from one side, or seeing whether the patient blinks when a threatening stimulus (e.g. a quickly moving finger) is brought towards the eye (although one needs to be careful that the associated air current is not simply stimulating a corneal reflex). A hemianopia is almost always associated with an ipsilateral loss of this blink reflex, although the reverse is not always true. An asymmetrical response to any of these tests suggests that a field defect, inattention, neglect or a combination of these is present. It is not surprising, given these difficulties, that the inter-rater reliability of the assessment of visual fields is relatively poor (see Table 4.5).

4.2.7 Disturbance of the brainstem and cerebellum

Vascular disease affecting the brainstem and cerebellum can, on the one hand, result in combinations of physical signs which allow the clinician to pinpoint the site of the lesion with great accuracy, whilst, on the other hand, it may produce extremely subtle symptoms that are easily overlooked or dismissed. Having said that, the classical descriptions of localised lesions in the brainstem are infrequently encountered, probably because many patients have lesions at several sites. The manifestations of brainstem lesions are best considered under the headings of: conscious level; pupillary reactions; external ocular movements; other cranial nerve palsies; the descending motor and ascending sensory tracts; the descending sympathetic pathway; and cerebellar and vestibular function. Diagrammatic cross-sections at various levels through the brainstem are shown in Fig. 4.17.

Conscious level

The assessment of conscious level has been dealt with in Section 4.2.2.

Pupillary reactions

Brainstem involvement in the control of the pupils is in two parts; there are sympathetic pupillodilator fibres, which descend ipsilaterally from the hypothalamus through the brainstem (see below), and parasympathetic pupilloconstrictor fibres, which enter the Edinger–Westphal nucleus (a distinct part of the IIIrd nerve nuclear complex) and exit alongside the IIIrd nerve itself (Fig. 4.18). The response of the pupils to light, both direct and consensual, and accommodation should be tested. Because of the functional separation of fibres within the IIIrd nerve nuclear complex, IIIrd nerve palsies from midbrain vascular lesions may or may not involve dilatation of the pupil. On the other hand, in an unconscious patient with extensive damage to the midbrain (either due to intrinsic pathology or secondary to pressure from above), the pupils will both be fixed and either dilated or in a midposition (4–5 mm), depending on whether the sympathetic as well as the parasympathetic fibres are involved. Bilateral 'pinpoint' pupils in an unconscious patient suggest a massive lesion in the pons, always assuming there is no evidence of drug overdose. This is thought to be due to a combination of damage to the sympathetic fibres and irritation of the parasympathetic fibres (lesions solely of sympathetic fibres do not usually result in such intense pupilloconstriction). Despite this, the pupils will react to a bright light, but this may be difficult to observe (Plum & Posner, 1980).

> *In elderly patients with stroke, always remember that they may be using pupilloconstrictor drops for glaucoma.*

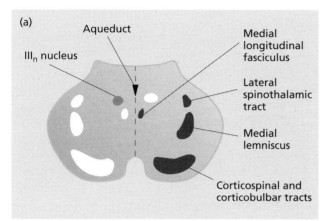

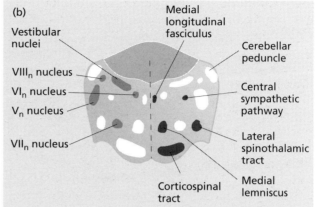

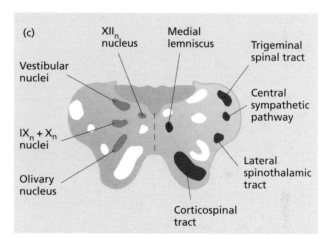

Figure 4.17 Diagrammatic representation of the main anatomical structures within the brainstem: (a) midbrain; (b) pons; (c) medulla.

External ocular movements

If the patient is conscious, communicative and cooperative the eye movements can be tested in the normal way. However, it is difficult to do this if patients can not follow commands. In such cases, observe spontaneous movements in each direction to confirm the absence of a gaze palsy. One can also stimulate the patient to look in each direction by doing something 'interesting' in different fields of vision, e.g. following the examiner's face rather than a finger or a pen. This also has the advantage that the examiner can continually reinforce the command 'watch my nose'.

The patient may be stimulated to look in each direction by doing something 'interesting' in different fields of vision, e.g. following the examiner's face rather than a finger or a pen.

Even though it is sometimes claimed to be a pathognomonic sign of multiple sclerosis, vascular disease can cause an internuclear ophthalmoplegia (failure of adduction in the adducting eye, with nystagmus in the abducting eye), due to involvement of the MLF on the side of the adducting eye,

although it tends to be unilateral rather than bilateral, as is the case in multiple sclerosis (Fig. 4.19) (Chadwick, 1993). A failure of conjugate horizontal gaze to one side can occur with ischaemia of the ipsilateral paramedian pontine reticular formation. Additional involvement of the ipsilateral MLF (with failure of adduction of the ipsilateral eye on attempted gaze to the other side) may result in the so-called 'one and a half syndrome', where the only remaining horizontal eye movement is abduction of the contralateral eye.

Nystagmus of brainstem or cerebellar origin is probably best appreciated by asking the patient to fixate on, and then follow, a moving target. Remember that a few irregular 'jerks' of the eyes are often seen in normal people when they move their eyes, particularly at the extremes of lateral gaze. In patients with vascular disease, it is the pattern of associated signs that is of more use in localising the lesions than attempts to analyse the nystagmus itself. Nystagmus may arise from vascular lesions of the vestibulolabyrinthine system, but these may be either ischaemia of the end-organs or due to involvement of the vestibular nuclei in the brainstem (see Section 4.3.3). In the latter, there are likely to be other signs of brainstem disturbance. Vertical nystagmus is

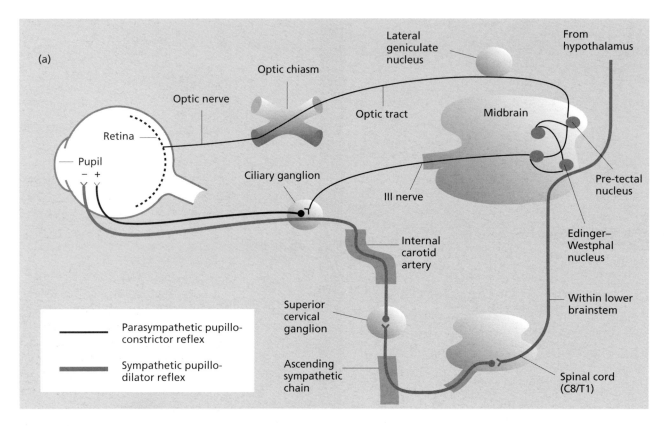

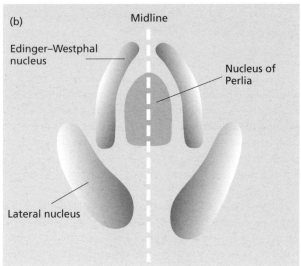

Figure 4.18 The neurogenic control of pupil size. (a) An outline of the parasympathetic and sympathetic pathways involved in pupilloconstriction and pupillodilatation, respectively. (b) The IIIrd nerve nuclear complex consists of: (i) the Edinger–Westphal nuclei concerned with parasympathetic innervation of the pupils; (ii) the midline nucleus of Perlia concerned with convergence and accommodation; (iii) the lateral nuclei, which innervate the levator palpebrae, superior recti, inferior obliques, medial recti and inferior recti. It is possible for vascular lesions to result in ischaemia of the lateral nuclei (resulting in an extraocular palsy) but spare the pupilloconstrictor fibres from the Edinger–Westphal nuclei.

more likely to result from a lesion of the tegmentum of the brainstem or cerebellum. Convergence and retraction nystagmus are considered indicative of midbrain disease (Plum & Posner, 1980).

> *In patients with stroke who have nystagmus, it is the pattern of the associated signs that is of more use in localising the lesion than detailed analysis of the nystagmus itself.*

Ocular bobbing is a sign which is usually only present with impaired conscious level and extensive pontine disease. The spontaneous rapid downward movement of the eyes is followed by a slow drift back to the original position (Fisher, 1964). It is thought to occur because of the tendency of such patients to have roving eye movements but, without any horizontal gaze, the only observable movements are in the vertical plane. A number of related disorders which are

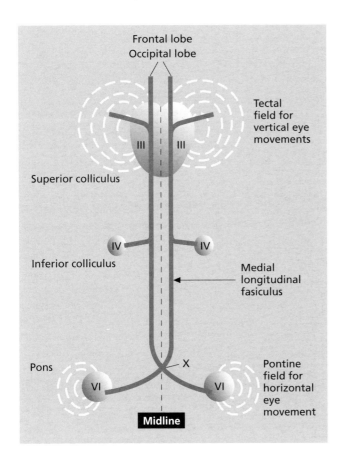

Figure 4.19 The role of the MLF in the control of conjugate gaze. Conjugate gaze requires coordinated action of the IIIrd, IVth and VIth nerve nuclei in the brainstem. The MLF links these nuclei and also provides the pathway for inputs from the frontal eye field (for voluntary movements) and the occipital lobe (for reflex movements), as well as the tectal field for vertical eye movements and the pontine field for horizontal eye movements. X indicates the site of the lesion which results in the classical bilateral internuclear ophthalmoplegia often associated with multiple sclerosis. Vascular lesions more often result in a unilateral internuclear ophthalmoplegia, presumably because they are more likely to respect the midline than a plaque of demyelination. Following a cortical lesion, there may be reduced ipsilateral input to the MLF/pontine field for lateral gaze, resulting in conjugate deviation of the eyes towards the lesion. Conversely, a lesion of the pons may prevent ipsilateral lateral gaze and there may be conjugate deviation of the eyes away from the side of the lesion.

probably due to a disturbance of saccadic eye movements are associated with cerebellar disease. These include ocular dysmetria (where there is overshoot of the eyes on attempted fixation), ocular flutter (where there are occasional bursts of rapid horizontal oscillations) and so-called square wave jerks (Kennard *et al.*, 1994).

The patient may complain that static objects are oscillating either from side to side or up and down. This is termed oscillopsia. It can occur with nystagmus or any of the other tonic abnormalities of movement, but these can sometimes be difficult to demonstrate. The symptom, although uncommon, can be extremely distressing and disabling. Loss of optokinetic nystagmus may occur with unilateral parietal lesions, but there will usually be many additional signs to suggest such a lesion.

Other cranial nerve palsies

The likely combinations of cranial nerve palsies that may occur in patients with vascular disease can be deduced from Fig. 4.17. Nuclear lesions of the VIIth nerve will involve both the upper and lower parts of the face. If the examiner is uncertain whether a weakness is present or whether it is simply the normal side-to-side asymmetry, it may be useful to ask the patient to attempt to whistle, an action which requires fine control of the facial muscles. The gag reflex alone does not constitute an adequate examination of the IXth and Xth cranial nerves, nor is it a good indicator of swallowing ability (see Section 15.17). Sensation on the two sides of the soft palate should be tested individually using an orange-stick, elevation of the palate should be observed and the patient asked to cough. Failure to oppose the vocal cords adequately will result in some air escaping, and such a finding should alert the physician that the patient may have swallowing difficulties.

Descending motor and ascending sensory tracts

From the point of view of localising the lesion, the important point about the descending motor and ascending sensory tracts is the level of decussation (see Figs. 4.4 and 4.9) and the separation of the various sensory modalities, as described earlier (see Section 4.2.4).

Descending sympathetic pathway

Interruption of the descending sympathetic pathway in the brainstem results in a complete ipsilateral Horner's syndrome, i.e. miosis, ptosis and loss of sweating on the side of the face. On its own, it is of little localising value; for example, it can also occur with carotid dissection (see Section 7.1).

Cerebellar and vestibular function

The most common manifestation of cerebrovascular disease involving the cerebellum or its connections is truncal ataxia. Frequently, there are no cerebellar signs when the limbs are examined on the bed, and therefore the problem may be overlooked if the patient's gait is not examined. If the disorder is mild, sudden changes in position may be the most sensitive way of detecting an abnormality. It is also worth asking about the impact of loss of visual fixation, e.g. in the dark, in a shower. Most ataxic syndromes are worse when visual fixation is lost, although that would also be true for patients with disordered proprioception.

> *Cerebellar disorders may not be identified if the patient's gait is not examined.*

Signs in the limbs are traditionally considered to need involvement of the cerebellar hemispheres rather than the midline structures. Care must be taken when faced with a resolving hemiparesis, since at this time cerebellar-like signs can be elicited which are probably just a manifestation of the impaired corticospinal control. This is most relevant when trying to distinguish the lacunar syndromes of pure motor hemiparesis and ataxic hemiparesis (AH) (see Section 4.4.6).

Many patients complain of 'dizziness', either around the onset of a stroke or at other times, but this term is too imprecise to be of localising value, even between carotid and vertebrobasilar (VB) territories, although it is probably more frequent in the latter. It is, however, worth distinguishing between vertigo, dysequilibrium and other sensory experiences.

1 Vertigo may be defined as any subjective or objective illusion of motion (usually rotation) or position. This is caused by an imbalance of tonic signals from the otolith and semicircular canals to the vestibular nuclei. When an isolated phenomenon, and particularly when induced by postural changes, it has long been viewed as a symptom of peripheral rather than central dysfunction. It is clear, however, that not only labyrinthine ischaemia but also some cerebellar strokes and even lesions of more central pathways may mimic these symptoms (Huang & Yu, 1985). In general, peripheral lesions are more often associated with hearing loss or tinnitus than central lesions, there are no other neurological symptoms and signs, and the resolution of the symptoms tends to be quite rapid. The distinction from benign paroxysmal positional vertigo (BPPV) may be difficult, but the duration of vertigo in BPPV is usually only a matter of seconds and there will be the characteristic fatiguable nystagmus during Hallpike's manoeuvre. Although most cases are probably due to debris in the posterior semicircular canal, it must be remembered that BPPV may occur as a sequel of labyrinthine ischaemia, although the attacks of vertigo should not then be interpreted as being due to recurrent ischaemia (Lempert *et al.*, 1995).

2 Dysequilibrium is a sensation of imbalance when standing or walking. This may be due to impairment of vestibular, sensory, cerebellar or motor function and consequently may be due to lesions in many parts of the nervous system.

3 Other sensory experiences, such as light-headedness, swimminess or a feeling of passing out are of no localising value. They may be associated with more diffuse cerebral ischaemia but may also occur with anxiety states, panic attacks and hyperventilation.

The tendency to label any episode of 'dizziness', especially in the elderly, as 'VB ischaemia' (VBI) or, even worse, VB insufficiency should be strongly resisted. One sees all too frequently patients who have complained of 'dizziness' when turning their neck (very common in general practice), have then had a cervical spine X-ray which shows some degenerative changes (extemely common in the elderly population) and are then told that they are 'trapping the blood supply to the brain'. What little work there is to support this theory is mainly based on postmortem studies (Toole & Tucker, 1960; Koskas *et al.*, 1992) or dyamic arteriography in highly selected patient (Ruotolo *et al.*, 1992). Furthermore, many of the patients initially described under this banner had clear focal disturbances of brainstem and occipital lobe function (see Section 6.5.6; Williams & Wilson, 1962). For the vast majority of patients with non-focal symptoms, the terms simply engender undue anxiety about impending strokes and divert attention from more likely explanations, such as labyrinthine dysfunction.

> *The tendency to label any episode of 'dizziness', especially in the elderly, as 'vertebrobasilar ischaemia' or vertebrobasilar insufficiency should be strongly resisted.*

Sudden, unilateral deafness is probably an underrecognised symptom of vascular occlusion (see Section 3.2.2). Pontine and midbrain lesions may be associated with both auditory and visual illusions/hallucinations. Auditory hallucinations tend to be more complex than tinnitus and less formed than those in temporal lobe epilepsy. Visual hallucinations may be colourful and include bizarre, complex, formed images. The patients have insight that the visual and auditory phenomena are not real (see Section 3.2.2).

Finally, vascular diseases are a relatively common cause of brainstem death. The detailed issues surrounding this issue are beyond the scope of this text but have recently been reviewed (Conference of Medical Royal Colleges and their Faculties in the United Kingdom, 1976, 1979, 1995).

4.3 The cerebral arterial supply

4.3.1 Introduction

In order for the information from the clinical history and examination to be formulated in a manner which will have as much relevance as possible to the underlying vascular lesion, the clinician needs to have a working knowledge of the cerebral blood supply. This will also be required for planning investigations and possible treatment. However, the general assumption that the vascular supply of the brain parenchyma follows a predictable pattern (as depicted in many textbooks) certainly should not be accepted without closer scrutiny. Many classifications refer to 'standard' maps of the areas of distribution of individual arteries, especially those that have been produced as cross-sectional templates to correspond with CT/MRI sections (e.g. Damasio, 1983). From knowing the site and size of the lesion, these maps are then used to 'identify' the occluded artery. Certain sites are identified as arterial boundary zones and further assumptions are then often made about the underlying pathophysiological process (i.e. low flow rather than thrombo-embolism (see Section 6.5.5)). However, it is clear from recent work that the cerebral circulation is a dynamic system with large inter- and intra-individual variability (i.e. between hemispheres and even varying with time) (van der Zwan et al., 1992) and that atheroma or other arterial disease in one part of the system may have complex and relatively unpredictable effects elsewhere. The description below attempts to relate each section of the vascular anatomy to the symptoms and signs commonly encountered in clinical practice. Most of the discussion refers to ischaemic stroke syndromes, but the overall parenchymal localisation is as applicable to cases of PICH (see Table 8.5).

The cerebral vascular anatomy can be described in two main parts, the anterior (carotid) and posterior (VB) systems. For each system there are three components: the extracranial arteries, the major intracranial arteries and the small (in terms of diameter) superficial and deep perforating arteries (Table 4.12). These groups of arteries have different structural and functional characteristics. The extracranial vessels (e.g. the common carotid artery (CCA)) have a trilaminar structure (intima, media and adventitia) and act as capacitance vessels (Fig. 4.20a). A limited number of anastomotic channels exist between these arteries. The larger intracranial arteries (e.g. the MCA) have potentially important anastamotic connections over the pial surface (vander Eecken & Adams, 1953) and at the base of the brain, via the circle of Willis and choroidal circulation (see below). The adventitia of these arteries is thinner than that of the extracranial vessels, with little elastic tissue (Fig. 4.20b). The media is also thinner, although the internal elastic lamina is thicker (such changes occurring gradually as the arterial diameter decreases). Thus, these vessels are more rigid than extracranial vessels of similar size. The small, deep perforating (e.g. the lenticulostriate arteries (LSAs)) and superficial perforating arteries from the pial surface are pre-

Table 4.12 Which arterial territory are the neurological problems in?

	Likely arterial territory		
	Carotid	Either	VB
Dysphasia	+		
Monocular visual loss	+		
Unilateral weakness*		+	
Unilateral sensory disturbance*		+	
Dysarthria†		+	
Ataxia†		+	
Dysphagia†		+	
Diplopia†			+
Vertigo†			+
Bilateral simultaneous visual loss			+
Bilateral simultaneous weakness			+
Bilateral simultaneous sensory disturbance			+
Crossed sensory/motor loss			+

* Usually assumed to be 'carotid'.
† In isolation these symptoms are not normally regarded as indicating a TIA.
Note: whether the neurological symptoms are transient or persistent and irrespective of whether there are abnormal neurological signs, it can be all but impossible to be sure of which arterial territory is involved, because so often it can be either carotid or VB. This is because of individual variation in arterial anatomy and the pattern of any arterial disease affecting the collateral circulation, and because one function can be distributed through both arterial territories (e.g. the corticospinal tract is supplied in the cerebral hemispheres by the carotid system and then, in the brainstem, by the VB system). Sometimes brain imaging can help if one lesion is found in a relevant place (e.g. if a patient with a hemiplegia has just one infarct in the contralateral pons on MRI, then it is more likely to have been due to VB than carotid ischaemia). Arterial imaging is unhelpful, because so often a symptomatic lesion in one artery is associated with asymptomatic lesions in other arteries.

dominantly end-arteries, with very limited anastomotic potential, and are primarily resistance vessels (Fig. 4.20c). The overall resistance in any section of the arterial tree is inversely proportional to the vascular density, which, on average, is approximately four times greater in grey matter (cortical and subcortical) than in white matter (van der Zwan, 1991).

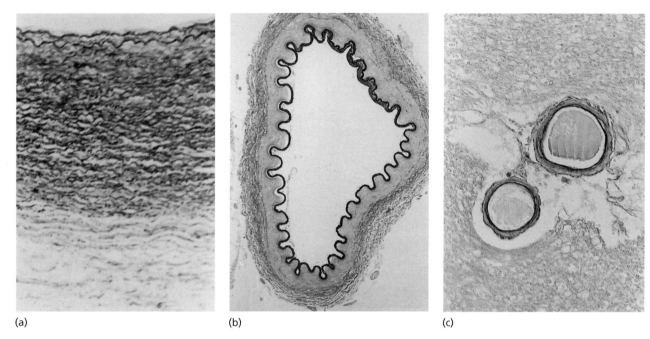

(a)   (b)   (c)

Figure 4.20 (a) ICA just above the common carotid bifurcation (Elastic van Gieson (EVG) ×120). The intima is barely visible, lying inside an ill-defined internal elastic lamina. The relatively thick media is rich in elastic tissue. The adventitia is thin and poorly defined. (b) Cross-section of MCA (EVG ×50). The intima is barely visible, and lies internal to the internal elastic lamina, which shows mild focal reduplication. Both media and adventitia are thinner than in extracranial arteries of comparable size. The media is virtually devoid, and the adventitia, in elastic tissue. There is no definite external elastic lamina. (c) A pair of basal ganglionic perforating vessels (EVG ×250). Each of these vessels has an indistinct internal elastic lamina, and a media composed of two to three layers of smooth muscle cells; arterioles are devoid of an internal elastic lamina. (Photographs courtesy of Dr G. Alistair Lammie, Department of Neuropathology, University of Edinburgh.)

4.3.2 The anterior (carotid) system

Common carotid artery

The left CCA usually arises directly from the left side of the aortic arch, whereas the right CCA arises from the innominate (brachiocephalic) artery (Fig. 4.21). The CCAs ascend through the anterior triangle of the neck and, at the level of the thyroid cartilage, they divide into the ICA and the external carotid artery (ECA). Throughout, the CCA is intimately associated with the ascending sympathetic fibres. Thus, lesions of the CCA (trauma, dissection or sometimes thrombotic occlusion) may cause an ipsilateral oculosympathetic palsy (Horner's syndrome), with involvement of sudomotor fibres to the face. Damage to the CCA, or thrombus within it, may also result in carotidynia, a syndrome characterised by tenderness over the artery and pain referred to the ipsilateral frontotemporal region. It may be the site of radiotherapy-induced damage (see Section 7.9).

> *Lesions of the common carotid artery may cause an ipsilateral oculosympathetic palsy (Horner's syndrome), with involvement of sudomotor fibres to the face.*

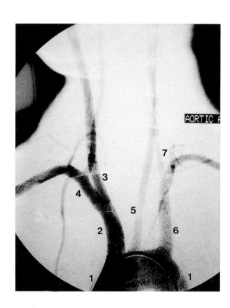

Figure 4.21 Arch aortogram showing the origins of the major vessels: 1, aortic arch; 2, innominate artery; 3, right CCA; 4, right subclavian artery; 5, left CCA; 6, left subclavian artery; 7, left vertebral artery.

Carotid bifurcation

The carotid bifurcation is usually at the level of the thyroid cartilage, but the exact site may vary by several centimetres. It contains the carotid body. The ICA is usually posterior to the ECA. The carotid body and carotid sinus nerve receive their blood supply from the ECA (Fig. 4.22). The bifurcation is one of the most common sites for atheroma to develop, and it is over this area that bruits should be listened for (see Section 6.5.7). However, there is no way of telling on auscultation whether a bruit arises from the ICA, ECA or both. One practical point relates to carotid duplex scanning. In general, the bifurcation and ICA/ECA for a few centimetres distal to the bifurcation are visualised. However, in patients with a high bifurcation significant difficulties may be encountered.

The carotid body responds to increases in the arterial partial pressure of oxygen (PaO_2), blood flow or arterial pH and decreases in $PaCO_2$ or blood temperature. It has a modulatory role on pulse rate, blood pressure and hypoxic ventilatory drive. Increased discharges in the carotid sinus nerve can be caused by stretching of the wall of the carotid sinus and will increase the depth and rate of respiration and increase peripheral vascular resistance. Carotid sinus hypersensitivity is probably an under-recognised cause of collapse in the elderly but is not necessarily associated with structural disease of the bifurcation.

External carotid artery

In patients with cerebrovascular disease, the branches of the ECA (ascending pharyngeal, superior thyroid, lingual, occipital, facial, posterior auricular, internal maxillary and superficial temporal) are mainly of interest because of the potential for anastamoses with branches of the intracranial ICA.

In the presence of an extracranial ICA occlusion or severe stenosis, blood flow may be maintained to the ipsilateral intracranial circulation by ECA–ICA collaterals (see below). It has been suggested that amaurosis fugax can occur due to intermittent failure of perfusion through ECA–ICA collaterals because of stenosis of the ECA origin, particularly when there is ipsilateral ICA occlusion or severe stenosis. The branches of the ECA may be affected by giant cell arteritis (see Section 7.2). Palpable pulsation of the temporal artery may be reduced or absent with ipsilateral CCA or ECA occlusion and, conversely, may be increased when there is ipsilateral ICA occlusion. The presence of extracranial branches distinguishes the ECA from the ICA on arterial studies (Fig. 4.22).

Internal carotid artery

The ICA on both sides ascends through the foramen lacerum in the skull base. Along the petrosal section there are small branches to the tympanic cavity and the artery of the pterygoid canal, which may anastamose with the internal maxillary artery, a branch of the ECA.

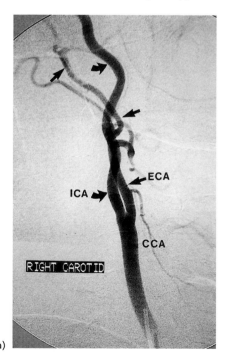

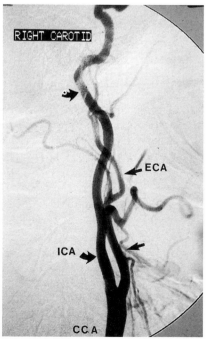

Figure 4.22 (a) Selective carotid angiogram (anteroposterior projection). (b) Selective carotid angiogram (lateral projection). ECA and its branches, straight arrows; ICA, curved arrows.

(a)

(b)

Torvik and Jorgensen (1966) demonstrated in an autopsy series that in 78% of cases with an ICA occlusion there was evidence of infarction ipsilateral to the occlusion, although many had not caused any symptoms. When neurological symptoms do occur, they may be due to artery-to-artery embolism, low distal flow or local arterial thrombosis. The clinical picture may range from a transient disturbance of cortical function to the 'full house' of hemiplegia, hemi-anaesthesia, hemianopia and profound disturbance of higher cortical function. Around the origin of the ICA are the superior laryngeal and hypoglossal nerves, which may be affected by operative procedures (see Section 16.7.4). The ICA may be affected at this level by atheroma, trauma causing arterial dissection (when the neck is hyperextended and/or rotated and the artery stretched over the transverse process of C1/2) or pseudoaneurysms which may be a source of emboli (see Section 7.1); spontaneous arterial dissection with little or no such trauma (see Section 7.1); or a local arteritis secondary to paratonsillar infections (see Section 7.8).

Carotid siphon

The S-shaped carotid siphon lies within the venous plexus of the cavernous sinus adjacent to cranial nerves III, IV, V1, V2 and VI, which run in the lateral wall of the sinus. There are several small branches (the most important of which is the meningohypophyseal trunk), which may anastamose with branches of the ECA. One congenital variant worth noting is the persistence of the trigeminal artery, which may arise from the ICA as it enters the cavernous sinus and links with the basilar artery (BA), usually between the superior cerebellar artery (SCA) and the anterior inferior cerebellar artery (AICA).

Atheroma may affect the ICA in the siphon. Although it may be a cause of embolism, flow restriction and, in a few cases, complete occlusion, the resulting symptoms will be similar to those originating from more proximal ICA sources. The degree of atheroma is not necessarily related to that at the carotid bifurcation. On the other hand, *cavernous sinus thrombosis* classically presents with varying degrees of ophthalmoplegia, chemosis and proptosis (sometimes bilateral, because the venous plexus communicates across the midline) in a patient with evidence of facial or sinus sepsis (Fig. 4.23). Aneurysms at the level of the cavernous sinus are relatively common and may present with IIIrd nerve dysfunction (see Section 9.1.1). If there is rupture of the artery which is confined by the sinus, then a *carotico-cavernous fistula* may develop. The typical picture is of pulsatile proptosis, with ophthalmoplegia and reduced visual acuity.

Supraclinoid internal carotid artery

The short supraclinoid portion of the ICA lies in the subarachnoid space and is related to the IIIrd cranial nerve. The most important branch is the ophthalmic artery, which enters the orbit through the optic foramen. This and the other branches of the ophthalmic artery (lacrimal, supraorbital, ethmoidal, palpebral) are probably the most important potential anastamotic links with the ECA (Fig. 4.24).

Amaurosis fugax or transient monocular blindness may be due to emboli passing from the ICA to the ophthalmic artery (Fisher, 1959). However, a large proportion of such patients have no evidence of ICA disease, and local atheroma within the ophthalmic arterial system remains a possibility. Fixed deficits come from retinal artery occlusion (usually considered embolic (see Section 3.2.2) and ischaemic optic neuropathy (see Section 3.4.3), although the latter is surprisingly infrequent with ICA occlusion, presumably because of collateral flow. The combination of ocular and cerebral hemi-

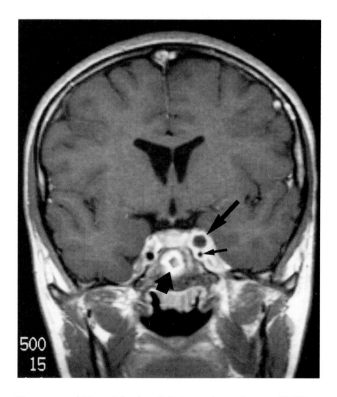

Figure 4.23 A T1-weighted, gadolinium-enhanced, coronal MRI scan showing thrombosis within the cavernous sinus. The thrombus (long arrow) is seen separate from the flow void in the left carotid artery (short arrow). Enhancement is seen in the sphenoid sinus (broad arrow), which is due to infection. The patient had a fever, chemosis and a partial IIIrd nerve palsy.

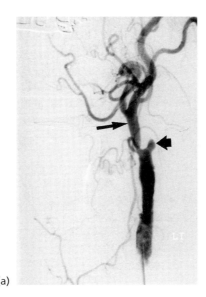
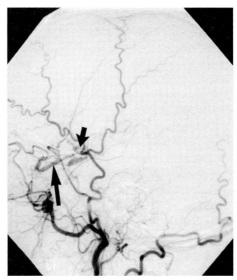

Figure 4.24 (a) Selective intra-arterial angiogram showing occlusion of the left ICA (short arrow) and filling of the ECA (long arrow). (b) Intracranial views of the same angiogram (lateral projection, left common carotid injection) showing retrograde filling of the ophthalmic artery (long arrow) from the ECA, which provides a collateral supply to the distal ICA (short arrow).

(a)

(b)

sphere ischaemic attacks on the same side is a strong pointer towards a severe ICA stenosis or occlusion, although the symptoms rarely occur simultaneously. When ICA occlusion occurs, the distal extent of the thrombus may end at the level of the ophthalmic artery. The supraclinoid ICA may be involved by inflammatory/infective processes, such as tuberculous meningitis, in the basal subarachnoid space.

> *The combination of ocular and cerebral hemisphere ischaemic attacks on the same side is a strong pointer towards a severe internal carotid artery stenosis or occlusion.*

Posterior communicating artery (PCoA)

The next branch of the ICA is usually the PCoA. Arising from the dorsal aspect of the ICA, it tracks caudally to join the PCA (Fig. 4.25). The PCoA may give off small branches, which contribute to the blood supply of the basal ganglia.

Aneurysms at the origin of the PCoA may present with a painful IIIrd nerve palsy with pupillary involvement, or SAH (see Section 9.3.2). In a few patients, both PCoAs are absent. This may result in much more marked symptomatology from lesions of the VB system than in patients with a functionally intact circle of Willis (see below).

Anterior choroidal artery (AChA)

Just before its terminal bifurcation into the ACA and MCA, the ICA gives rise to the AChA (Fig. 4.26). Although a rela-

tively small branch which gains it name because of supplying the choroid plexus, it may also supply important structures such as the globus pallidus, anterior hippocampus, uncus, lower part of the posterior limb of the internal capsule and rostral portions of the midbrain, including the cerebral peduncle. It accompanies the optic tract and supplies the

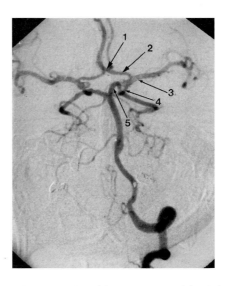

Figure 4.25 Demonstration of the components of the circle of Willis by intra-arterial angiography (anteroposterior projection). The whole of the circle is filled from a selective left vertebral artery injection in a patient who had bilateral ICA occlusions. The components are: 1, anterior communicating artery; 2, ACA; 3, MCA; 4, PCoA; 5, PCA.

LGN and the rostral part of the optic radiation. It may anastamose with the posterior choroidal artery (PChA) (a branch of the PCA).

Isolated occlusion of the AChA may be more often due to intrinsic disease of the artery rather than thrombosis or embolism from more proximal sources (see Section 6.5.2). AChA territory infarcts typically produce a contralateral hemiparesis and hemisensory deficit, the latter often sparing proprioception. There may also be dysfunction of higher cortical modalities, such as language and visuospatial function, which has been attributed to extension of the ischaemia to the lateral thalamus. Large AChA territory infarcts have an additional visual field defect. This can be a hemianopia (due to ischaemia of the optic tract), but the pathognomonic pattern is considered to be a homonymous horizontal sectoranopia due to involvement of the LGN (Frisen, 1979; Helgason, 1995).

Distal internal carotid artery

At the bifurcation of the ICA, the main continuing branch is usually the MCA, whilst the smaller ACA and the PCoA form the anterior portion of the circle of Willis (see Fig. 4.25). This is not a common site for atheroma but can be the superior extent of a carotid dissection (see Section 7.1). It is also a site of aneurysm formation (see Section 9.1.1).

Circle of Willis

In the embryo, a large branch from the ICA provides most of the blood supply to the occipital lobes. From this branch the future PCoA and post-communicating (P2) segment of the PCA will develop and, in general, will link with the pre-communicating (P1) segment of the PCA, which develops from the VB system. According to Padget (1948), the arterial components of the circle of Willis and the origins of its branches (i.e. the ACAs, the PCAs, the anterior communicating artery (ACoA) and the PCoAs) are formed by 6–7 weeks of gestation (see Fig. 4.25). At this stage, the PCoA and the P1 segment of the PCA are usually of approximately similar diameter and contribute equally to the supply of the P2 segment of the PCA. Van Overbeeke *et al.* (1991) showed that this 'transitional' configuration is present in nearly 80% of fetuses under 20 weeks' gestation, but over the next 40 weeks (and particularly between the 21st and 29th weeks of gestation, which coincides with the period of most rapid growth of the occipital lobes) there is a change in the configuration. In the majority, the P1 segment of the PCA will become larger than the PCoA, resulting in the 'adult' configuration, where the occipital lobes are supplied primarily by the VB system. However, in a minority, the PCoA will become larger and the occipital lobes will obtain most of their blood supply from the carotid circulation, a situation which is referred to as a 'fetal' configuration. The 'transition-

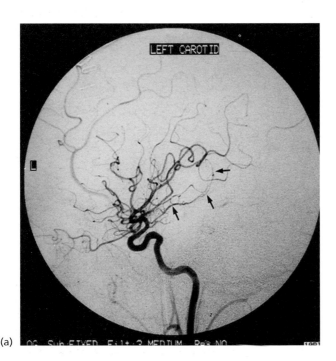

(a)

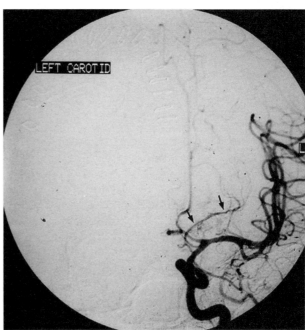

(b)

Figure 4.26 Angiogram of AChA (arrows). (a) Lateral and (b) anteroposterior views of a left carotid angiogram.

al configuration' may persist in less than 10% of adults (Riggs & Rupp, 1963). The exact proportions of the different configurations are difficult to estimate from the literature because of the very variable selection criteria that have been used (van Overbeeke *et al.*, 1991).

Anomalies of the circle of Willis are reported in between 48% (Alpers & Berry, 1963) and 81% (Riggs & Rupp, 1963) of cases, depending on selection criteria, and certainly seem to be more prevalent in cases where there has been cerebrovascular pathology (Alpers & Berry, 1963). The distribution of the abnormalities found in Riggs and Rupp's (1963) study of 994 cases is shown in Fig. 4.27. In this study, hypoplasia of part of the anterior part of the circle of Willis was found in 13%, of the posterior part in 32% and of both parts in 36%. They noted that, when there was maldevelopment of either the P1 segment of the PCA or the precommunicating (A1) segment of the ACA, there was usually an ectopic origin of the distal branches. Taken alongside the haemodynamic consequences of the hypoplastic segments of the circle of Willis (Hillen, 1986), these anatomical factors are likely to result in considerable variation in the area of

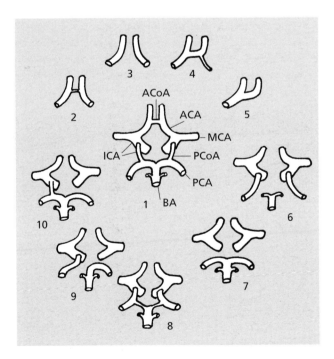

Figure 4.27 Anomalies of the circle of Willis. In the centre is a complete circle of Willis (1). There are 21 possible variants. Those involving the ACA and ACoA are shown at the top (2–5) and some of those involving the PCoA below (6–10). The anterior part of the circle provides poor collateral supply in 24% of people and no collateral supply in 7%. The most common anomaly of the PCoA is its direct origin from the ICA (6 and 9 above) which occurs in 30% of subjects. BA, basilar artery.

supply of the major intracerebral arteries and the ability of the cerebral circulation to respond to changes in perfusion when more proximal arteries are diseased (see below). Not surprisingly, one can not identify any particular clinical symptomatology related to the anomalies of the circle of Willis.

Anterior cerebral artery

The ACA arises as the medial branch of the bifurcation of the ICA, at the level of the anterior clinoid process. The proximal A1 segments of the ACAs pass medially and forward over the optic nerve or chiasm and corpus callosum to enter the interhemispheric fissure, where they are linked by the ACoA (Fig. 4.28). The distal 'post-communicating' segments run together in the interhemispheric fissure and then continue backwards as the pericallosal and callosomarginal arteries. Other branches include the orbitofrontal, frontopolar, anterior, middle and posterior internal frontal, paracentral and superior and inferior parietal arteries. The potential minimum and maximum areas of supply are shown in Fig. 4.29 (van der Zwan *et al.*, 1992).

Isolated infarction of the ACA territory is comparatively rare, other than when due to 'vasospasm' complicating SAH (see Section 13.6). This may be due in part to the fact that if the proximal ACA is occluded, the distal ACA may obtain a blood supply from the other ACA via the ACoA. Bilateral ACA territory infarction should always prompt a search for an aneurysm which may have bled recently, although it may also occur when both ACAs receive their supply from the same carotid artery via the ACoA, or due to crossover of distal branches in the interhemispheric fissure. The majority of cases of ACA territory infarction are probably due to either cardiogenic embolism or artery-to-artery embolism from an occluded or stenosed ICA (Bogousslavsky & Regli, 1990).

> *Bilateral anterior cerebral artery territory infarction should always prompt a search for an aneurysm which may have bled recently.*

The motor deficit in the leg usually predominates over that in the arm and is often most marked distally, in contrast to that from cortical MCA infarcts (Critchley, 1930). When the arm is affected, it is usually thought to be due to extension of the ischaemic area to the internal capsule (Bogousslavsky & Regli, 1990), although in some cases it may also be a form of motor 'neglect' due to involvement of the supplementary motor area. There is often no sensory deficit, but when present it is usually mild. When the motor deficit is bilateral, ACA territory infarction needs to be distinguished from a lesion in the spinal cord or brainstem. The same applies to

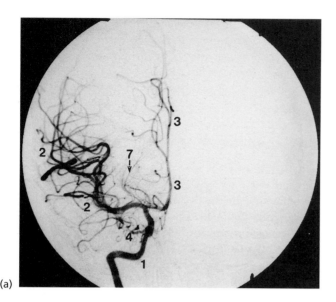
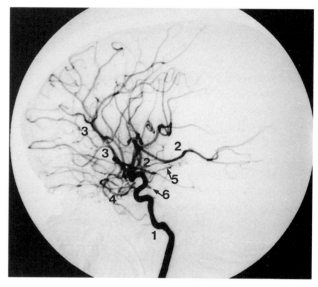

Figure 4.28 Angiogram of the anterior intracranial circulation: (a) anteroposterior projection; (b) lateral projection. 1, ICA; 2, MCA and its branches; 3, ACA and its branches; 4, ophthalmic artery; 5, anterior choroidal artery; 6, vestigial stump of PCoA (normal variant); 7, lenticulostriate arteries.

sensory deficits, but these are usually mild. Other frontal lobe features may be present, including urinary incontinence, lack of motivation or, paradoxically, agitation and social disinhibition. Abulia and akinetic mutism (see Section 4.2.2) may occur, usually with bilateral lesions. A grasp reflex may be elicited if the motor deficit in the hand is not too great. Various aphasic syndromes have been described, and these are usually attributed to involvement of the supplementary motor area (rather than Broca's area). Typically, there will be reduced spontaneous output but preserved repetition. These patients may be mute immediately after the onset of the stroke (see Section 4.2.5). Occlusion of the ACA can result in apraxias (see Section 4.2.5; Kazui & Sawada, 1993) and other disconnection syndromes. Interruption of frontocerebellar tracts can result in incoordination of limbs, which may mimic cerebellar dysfunction and, when there is an ipsilateral corticospinal deficit, may mimic the lacunar syndrome of homolateral ataxia and crural paresis (HACP) (see below; Bogousslavsky *et al.*, 1992). Amnesic disorders are also encountered, particularly after rupture of an ACoA aneurysm. The 'alien-hand sign' refers to a variety of dissociative movements between right and left hands due to a lesion of the mesial frontal lobe and/or corpus callosum (McNabb *et al.*, 1988).

Recurrent artery of Heubner

The RAH is an inconstant branch of the ACA, which, if present, usually arises around the level of the ACoA. It may supply the head of the caudate, the inferior portion of the

anterior limb of the internal capsule and the hypothalamus (Fig. 4.3). The deficit from unilateral occlusion of the RAH depends on the extent of the capsular supply. Weakness of the face and arm, often with dysarthria, is said to be characteristic (Critchley, 1930). The syndromes of akinetic mutism or abulia (see Section 4.2.2) may occur but are usually associated with bilateral lesions.

Deep perforating arteries (medial striate)

A variable number of small branches of the ACA and ACoA enter the anterior perforated substance and may supply the anterior striatum, the ventral anterior limb of the internal capsule and the anterior commissure. They may also supply the optic chiasm and tract (see Fig. 4.16) (Perlmutter & Rhoton, 1976). As with the RAH, if the medial striate arteries contribute to the vascular supply of the internal capsule, weakness of the face and arm may occur.

Middle cerebral artery main stem

The first segment of the MCA tracks laterally between the upper surface of the temporal lobe and the inferior surface of the frontal lobe until it reaches the Sylvian fissure (see Fig. 4.28). The lenticulostriate arteries (LSAs) arise from the proximal part of the MCA stem (see below).

Atheroma may develop *in situ*, but this is uncommon in Caucasians and more frequent in Orientals. Therefore, in Caucasians the mechanism of occlusion tends to be either

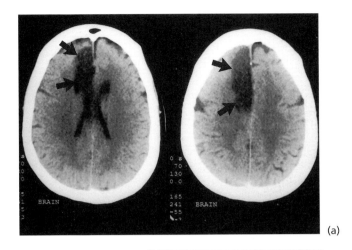

(a)

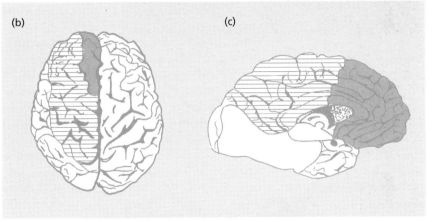

(b)   (c)

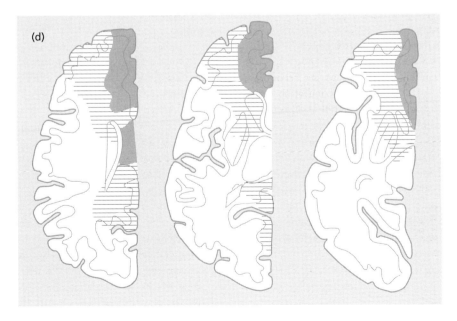

(d)

Figure 4.29 Ischaemia in the territory of the ACA. (a) The typical appearance on axial CT scan of ACA territory infarction (arrows). (b, c) However, there is great inter-individual and interhemispheric variability in the area supplied by the ACA. The hatched areas show the only part of the cortex on the superolateral surface (b) and the medial surface (c) of the hemisphere, which was always supplied by the ACA in a large pathological study (van der Zwan, 1991). The horizontal lines represent the maximum extent of the area which may be supplied by the ACA in some patients. (d) A similar degree of variability exists for the intracerebral territory supplied by the ACA. The figure shows the minimum (hatched) and maximum (horizontal lines) areas of supply at three levels in the same pathological study. (Redrawn with permission of Dr A. van der Zwan.)

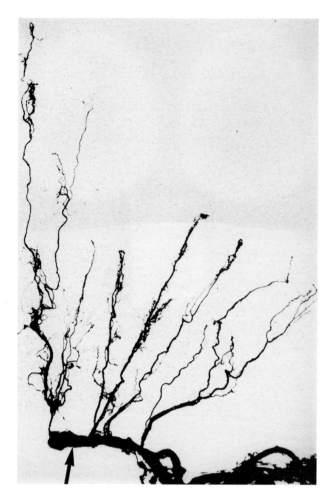

Figure 4.30 Autopsy demonstration of the deep perforating arteries arising from the main stem of the MCA (arrow).

impaction of an embolus or extension of a more proximal thrombus (e.g. from the ICA) (Olsen *et al.*, 1985; Fieschi *et al.*, 1989). Occlusion of the MCA stem is nearly always symptomatic. In most cases, the occlusion occurs in the proximal stem, thereby involving the LSAs, and consequently there is ischaemia of both the deep and superficial territory of the MCA. Typically, this presents as a contralateral hemimotor and sensory deficit, hemianopia and disturbance of the relevant higher cortical functions (e.g. dysphasia if in the dominant hemisphere). If the cortical collateral supply from the ACA and PCA is good, the brunt of the ischaemia may fall on the subcortical structures, resulting in a striatocapsular infarct, because thrombus occludes the origins of the deep perforating arteries, which are functional end-arteries. Nevertheless, there is often cortical ischaemia without infarction and consequently the clinical symptoms can be very similar (see below). If the occlusion is more distal in the

stem and there is no ischaemia in the LSA territory, the leg may be relatively spared, because most fibres will originate in cortical areas usually supplied by the ACA (Ueda *et al.*, 1992).

Middle cerebral artery deep perforating arteries (lenticulostriate)

From the main MCA stem a variable (usually 6–12) number of LSAs branch at right angles to the parent artery and enter the anterior perforated substance. They may supply the lentiform nucleus, lateral head of the caudate nucleus, anterior limb of the internal capsule, part of the globus pallidus and dorsal parts of the internal capsule (Fig. 4.30).

When a thrombus in the MCA stem lies over the origins of all of the LSAs, a 'comma'-shaped infarct may develop, a so-called striatocapsular infarct (Fig. 4.31) (see Section 6.5.2). About one-third of cases will a have a potential cardiac source of embolism, one-third will have stenotic or occlusive disease of the ICA and one-third will have stenosis or occlusion confined to the MCA stem (Weiller, 1995). Angiographic studies have shown that MCA stem occlusion of this type may often be relatively short-lived, presumably due to fragmentation of the embolus (Olsen *et al.*, 1985; Fieschi *et al.*, 1989). The deficit in the limbs tends to be motor rather than sensory and is often similar in the arm and leg. In about 70% there are symptoms of cortical dysfunction, although these may be mild and resolve rapidly. The pathogenesis of the cortical symptoms is much debated but seems most likely to be due to actual cortical ischaemia, which is not imaged by CT or MRI, although it may be detected by functional imaging, such as positron emission tomography (PET) and single-photon emission CT (SPECT) (Weiller, 1995). The alternative explanations include de-afferentation of the cortex, direct interruption of subcortical–cortical pathways or involvement of subcortical structures which subserve language functions. Hemianopia is an unusual feature.

Occlusion of a *single* LSA results in a 'lacunar infarct' (Fig. 4.32), there being no functional anastamoses between adjacent perforating arteries. It should be stressed that this is a pathological term, and for clarity the radiological equivalent should probably be referred to as a 'small, deep infarct' (Donnan *et al.*, 1993). Most occlusions of single, deep perforating arteries from the MCA stem are probably caused by local vasculopathies rather than embolism, although the number of pathologically verified cases is very small (see Section 6.3). There is considerable interindividual variation in the number of LSAs, but in general the largest area is supplied by the most lateral branch. Additionally, the vol-

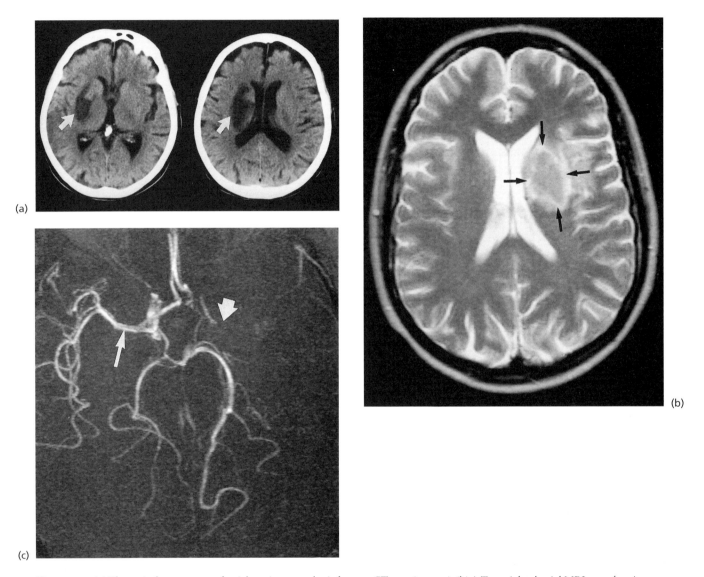

Figure 4.31 (a) The typical appearance of a right striatocapsular infarct on CT scan (arrows). (b) A T2-weighted axial MRI scan showing a left striatocapsular infarct (arrows) and (c) MR angiogram from the same patient showing lack of flow in the proximal segment of the left MCA (broad arrow). Normal flow is seen in the right MCA (narrow arrow). The patient had had a recent anterior myocardial infarction and it was presumed that an embolus had lodged in the proximal left MCA (see also Fig. 6.14e).

ume of an individual infarct will depend on the actual site of occlusion, i.e. the more proximal the occlusion in the LSA the larger the lacune. The tendency for studies not to consider imaged lesions greater than 1.5 cm diameter as the radiological equivalent of lacunes is probably flawed, the figure emanating originally from pathological studies (Fisher, 1965b). When the results of acute imaging and subsequent autopsy have been reported, the lesion at autopsy was significantly smaller (Donnan *et al.*, 1982). Single lacunes *may*

present with one of the classical 'lacunar syndromes' (see Section 4.4.6) or with isolated movement disorders, such as hemiballismus. However, the majority of lâcunes (80%) are clinically silent (or at least clinically unrecognised), occurring most frequently in the lentiform nucleus (Fisher, 1965b).

Multiple supratentorial lacunes, also referred to as *état lacunaire*, may present as a pseudobulbar palsy, with or without *marche à petits pas*. This abnormality of gait super-

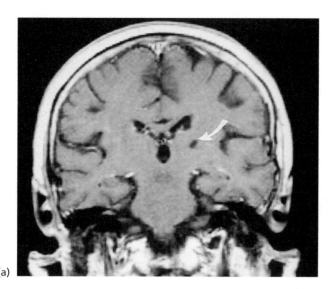

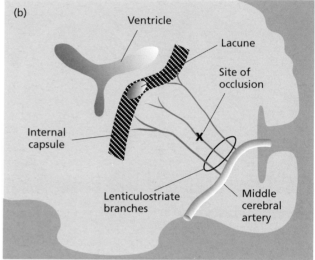

Figure 4.32 (a) The typical appearance of a small, deep infarct confined to the territory of a single, deep perforating artery on a T1-weighted, coronal MRI scan (arrow). (b) Diagrammatic representation of the case demonstrating the likely underlying vascular process.

ficially resembles that of Parkinson's disease, but debate continues as to whether a true Parkinsonian syndrome can occur from small, deep infarcts in the basal ganglia (Critchley, 1929; Eadie & Sutherland, 1964; Parkes *et al.*, 1974; Friedman *et al.*, 1986). It is important to distinguish *état lacunaire* from the dilatations of perivascular spaces which are often present in the basal ganglia of hypertensive individuals and may be difficult to differentiate on MRI scans (Hauw, 1995). These are not due to infarction and have not been convincingly associated with any particular clinical presentation.

Middle cerebral artery cortical branches

In the Sylvian fissure, the MCA usually bifurcates to give superior and inferior divisions. The superior division usually gives rise to the orbitofrontal, prefrontal, pre-Rolandic, Rolandic, anterior parietal and posterior parietal branches, whilst the inferior division usually gives rise to the angular, tempero-occipital, posterior temporal, middle temporal, anterior temporal and temperopolar branches. However, there are many variations in this pattern. The potential minimum amd maximum area of supply of these branches is shown in Fig. 4.33 (van der Zwan *et al.*, 1992). At their origins, the luminal diameter of these vessels is usually about 1 mm, but by the time they anastomose with the branches of the ACA and PCA (vander Eecken and Adams, 1953) they are usually less than 0.2 mm in diameter. There is no signifi-

cant collateral supply between individual branches of the MCA.

Local disease of the branches is unlikely except in the context of cerebral vasculitis, and the main occlusive mechanisms are probably embolism or low flow secondary to more proximal vascular lesions (Olsen *et al.*, 1985; Bogousslavsky *et al.*, 1990). The usual clinical syndrome resulting from occlusion of the superior division is much the same as for the MCA stem, but in general the motor and sensory deficits are greater in the face and arm than in the leg. Occlusion of the inferior division usually causes a hemianopia or superior quadrantanopia and fluent aphasia but relatively mild problems in the limbs, although higher level discriminatory sensory functions may be affected. A similar pattern can, however, occur with occlusion of the PCA (see Section 4.3.3). The area of infarcted cortex can be very small; indeed, the distinction on CT from cortical atrophy can be very difficult (see Section 5.3.5). As a result, some very restricted clinical deficits may occur. For example, it has been shown that isolated arm weakness is much more likely to occur from a cortical than a subcortical lesion (Boiten & Lodder, 1991a). Although there is a large volume of classical neurological literature correlating various restricted 'MCA' syndromes (most of which include some disturbance of higher cortical function) with ischaemia or haemorrhage in specific areas of brain parenchyma (Foix & Levy, 1927; Waddington & Ring, 1968), the interindividual variability of the vascular anatomy means that it is virtually impossible

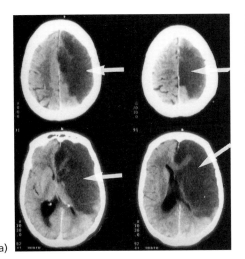

(a)

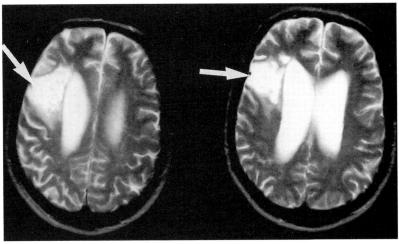

(b)

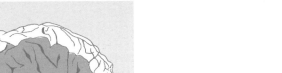

(c)

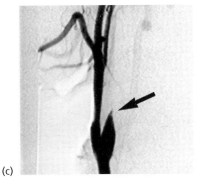

(d)

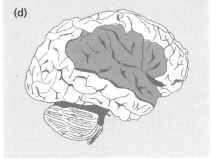

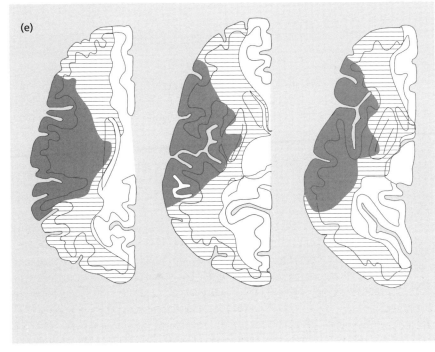

(e)

Figure 4.33 Ischaemia in the territory of the MCA. (a) The typical appearance on axial CT scan of extensive MCA territory infarction (arrows) in a patient who had an occluded main stem of the MCA. (b) The typical appearance on T2-weighted axial MRI scan of MCA branch occlusion (arrows). (c) The patient whose scan is shown in (b) was a young man who had dissected his proximal ICA (arrow) in a road accident. The intra-arterial digital subtraction angiogram shows a smooth, tapering, complete occlusion of the proximal ICA, typical of dissection. (d) However, there is great interindividual and interhemispheric variability in the area supplied by the MCA. The hatched area shows the only part of the cortex on the lateral surface of the hemisphere, which was always supplied by the MCA in a large pathological study (van der Zwan, 1991). (e) A similar degree of variability exists for the intracerebral territory supplied by the MCA. The figure shows the minimum (hatched) and maximum (horizontal lines) areas of supply at three levels in the same pathological study. (Redrawn with permission of Dr A. van der Zwan.)

to link them reliably with occlusions of particular MCA branches. Furthermore, many of the reports do not deal with deficits in the acute phase of stroke.

Middle cerebral artery medullary perforating arteries

MCA medullary perforating arteries arise from the cortical arteries of the surface of the hemispheres. They are usually 20–50 mm in length and descend to supply the subcortical white matter (i.e. the centrum ovale or centrum semi-ovale, which are interchangeable terms, it seems), converging centripetally towards the lateral ventricle (Fig. 4.34). These are functional end-arteries and their distal fields are part of the internal border zone (see Section 4.3.4).

Isolated infarcts of the centrum ovale are rare (Uldry & Bogousslavsky, 1995). The majority are small (< 1.5 cm diameter) and probably arise from the occlusion of a single medullary perforating artery, although this has never been verified pathologically. The spectrum of clinical presentation is similar to that of single deep perforating artery occlusions, with the classical lacunar syndromes of pure motor hemiparesis, sensorimotor stroke and ataxic hemiparesis predominating. In such cases there is rarely evidence of large vessel disease or cardioembolism. Larger infarcts in this area present with a syndrome similar to more extensive MCA cortical infarction, with weakness/sensory loss which is more marked in the face and arm than leg, dysphasia or visuospatial disturbance and, if the optic radiation is involved, a visual field defect. These are more often associated with large vessel disease (ICA/MCA occlusion or stenosis). The potential explanations for deficits of 'cortical' modalities are similar to those for striatocapsular infarction, i.e. ischaemia without necrosis, deafferentation of the cortex or involvement of subcortical structures subserving 'cortical' functions, but there is less evidence to support any individual mechanism.

4.3.3 The posterior vertebrobasilar (VB) system

The VB system develops quite separately from the carotid system and is subject to many more changes during fetal development. It is this that probably accounts for the much greater individual variation.

Precerebral vertebral artery (VA)

The right VA arises as the first branch of the right subclavian artery (which arises from the innominate artery), whilst the left VA arises as the first branch of the left subclavian artery (which arises directly from the aortic arch) (see Fig. 4.21). The course of the VA is traditionally divided into segments.

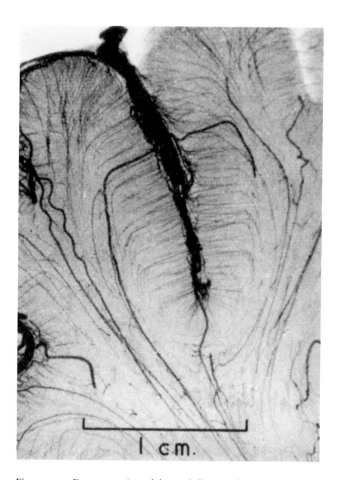

Figure 4.34 Demonstration of the medullary perforating arteries arising from the cortical surface. (Courtesy of Dr Nigel Hyman, Radcliffe Infirmary, Oxford, UK.)

The first segment is from the origin to the transverse foramen at either C5 or C6. The next segment is within the transverse foramina from this level to C2. The third segment circles the arch of C1 and passes between the atlas and occiput. The major branch outside the skull is the single, midline anterior spinal artery, formed by a contribution from both VAs.

The origin of the VA can be affected by atheroma, either within the VA itself or by overlying plaque in the larger parent vessel, and may be the site of occlusion or source of emboli (Caplan & Tettenborn, 1992b). It may also be involved in inflammatory disorders, such as that in Takayasu's arteritis (see Section 7.2). The extracranial VA may also be the site of arterial dissection (see Section 7.1; Caplan & Tettenborn, 1992a). Trapping of the VA by cervical spondylosis is frequently cited as a cause of symptoms attributed to 'VBI', but, in reality, both the symptoms and the X-ray changes of cervical spondylosis are common in the vascular age group and rarely is there a convincing cause-and-effect relationship (see Section 6.5.6). However, thrombus may form in the VA after prolonged or unusual neck posturing (Caplan & Tettenborn, 1992a).

Intracranial vertebral artery

The fourth segment of the VA is intracranial, until the two arteries unite to form the BA at the pontomedullary junction (Fig. 4.35). As the VAs pierce the dura, there is a decrease in the adventitia and media, with marked reduction in both medial and external elastic laminae. There may be branches which supply the medulla.

As with the ICA, occlusion of the VA may be asymptomatic. At the other extreme, there may be extensive infarction of the lateral medulla and inferior cerebellar hemisphere. Dissection of the VA may present with SAH (Caplan & Tettenborn, 1992a). The subclavian steal syndrome occurs when there is haemodynamically significant stenosis of the subclavian artery proximal to the origin of the VA. In this situation, the direction of blood flow is normal in the contralateral VA but reversed in the ipsilateral VA, with blood passing into the axillary artery from the VA. The pulse and blood pressure will be lower in the affected arm. Exercise of the ipsilateral arm

increases the flow away from the hindbrain, which may cause symptoms of brainstem dysfunction. However, it is noteworthy that reversed flow in VA is a common finding on ultrasound and angiographic studies in patients with no neurological symptoms (see Section 16.10; Hennerici et al., 1988).

> *Reversed flow in one vertebral artery is a common finding in patients with no neurological symptoms.*

Posterior inferior cerebellar artery (PICA)

The PICAs usually arise from the intracranial VA, although one may be absent in up to 25% of patients (Fig. 4.35). Also, the VA may terminate in the PICA. Small branches from the PICA may supply the lateral medulla, but more frequently there are direct branches from the VA between the ostium of PICA and the origin of the BA (Duncan et al., 1975). There are medial and lateral branches of the PICA, the medial branch usually supplying the cerebellar vermis and adjacent hemisphere and the lateral branch the cortical surface of the cerebellar tonsil and suboccipital cerebellar hemisphere.

Historically, occlusion of the PICA has been linked to lateral medullary infarcts, causing Wallenberg's syndrome. This consists of an ipsilateral Horner's syndrome (descend-

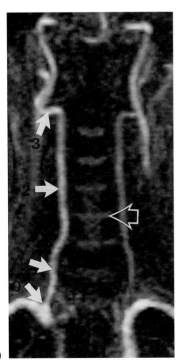

(a)

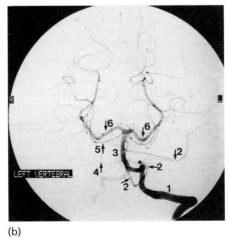

(b)

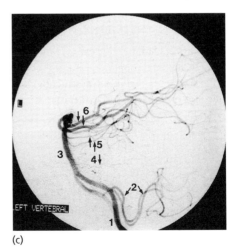

(c)

Figure 4.35 Angiographic demonstration of the VB system. (a) Anteroposterior projection of an MR angiogram showing the extracranial VAs. The numbers refer to the segments of the artery; o, the origin and the open arrow shows an intravertebral disc. (b) Anteroposterior projection of an intra-arterial angiogram showing: (1) distal VA, (2) posterior inferior cerebellar artery, (3) BA, (4) anterior inferior cerebellar artery, (5) superior cerebellar artery, (6) PCA. (c) Lateral projection of an intra-arterial angiogram showing the arteries as numbered above.

ing sympathetic fibres), loss of spinothalamic function over the contralateral limbs (spinothalamic tract) and ipsilateral face (descending trigeminal tract), vertigo, nausea, vomiting and nystagmus (vestibular nuclei), ipsilateral ataxia of limbs (inferior cerebellar peduncle) and ipsilateral paralysis of palate, larynx and pharynx (nucleus ambiguus), resulting in dysarthria, dysphonia and dysphagia (see Fig. 4.17). As with other 'classical' eponymous brainstem syndromes, the complete form of Wallenberg's syndrome is relatively infrequent in clinical practice. However, syndromes which do not involve the lateral medulla are now recognised as being more frequent. They usually present with vertigo, headache, ataxia (of gait and limbs) and nystagmus. Another striking symptom is ipsilateral axial lateropulsion (Amarenco *et al.*, 1991), which seems to the patient like a lateral displacement of the centre of gravity. Isolated vertigo is recognised increasingly in cases of PICA infarction (Duncan *et al.*, 1975; Huang & Yu, 1985). Infarcts restricted to either the medial or lateral branches of PICA usually have a benign outcome (Kase *et al.*, 1993).

Basilar artery

The general pattern of branches from the BA is of short paramedian (perforating) branches, which supply the base of the pons to either side of the midline and also the paramedian aspects of the pontine tegmentum. As with the anterior circulation, the frequency of infarction from occlusion of such perforating arteries has probably been underestimated, although infarcts arising from the BA disease are less well documented, partly because of the difficulty of imaging such infarcts with CT and the fact that angiography of the VB system so seldom has any clinical utility. The lateral aspects of the base of the pons and the tegmentum are supplied by pairs of short and long circumferential arteries, which also supply the cerebellar hemispheres.

Occlusion of a single paramedian artery, resulting in a restricted infarct in the brainstem, can present with any of the classical lacunar syndromes (see Section 4.4.6). Disturbances of eye movement (either nuclear or internuclear) may also occur from such lesions, either in isolation or in addition to pure motor deficits (e.g. Weber's syndrome) (Hommel *et al.*, 1990b; Fisher, 1991). Unlike the anterior circulation, where intrinsic disease of the ACA or MCA stem is uncommon, occlusion of the mouth of a single perforating artery by a plaque of atheroma in the parent artery (BA) needs to be considered alongside intrinsic small vessel disease as the underlying mechanism (Caplan, 1989). The 'locked-in syndrome' occurs with bilateral infarction, or haemorrhage, of the base of the pons (see Section 4.2.2 and Fig. 4.2).

The 'top of the basilar syndrome' is a constellation of symptoms and signs which may occur when an embolus impacts in the rostral BA, resulting in bilateral ischaemia of rostral brainstem structures and of the PCA territories (Caplan, 1980). The syndrome consists of variable pupillary responses, supranuclear paresis of vertical gaze, ptosis or lid retraction, sleep disorders, hallucinations, involuntary movements, such as hemiballismus (from involvement of rostral brainstem structures), visual abnormalities, such as cortical blindness (from involvement of the occipital lobes) or an amnesic state (from involvement of the temporal lobes or thalamus).

Sometimes the BA becomes elongated (and therefore tortuous) and dilated. This is known as dolichoectasia, and the importance of this may have been underestimated (see Section 6.2.2; Schwartz *et al.*, 1993). There are four potential consequences.

1 The dilated artery may directly compress the brainstem, resulting in a mixture of cranial nerve and long-tract signs.
2 The disruption of laminar flow predisposes to *in situ* thrombosis which may occlude the origins of the paramedian or long circumferential branches.
3 There may be distal embolisation from the areas of *in situ* thrombosis.
4 The changes in contour of the BA may result in distortion around the origins of the perforating arteries (Fig. 4.36).

Anterior inferior cerebellar artery

The AICAs originate from the caudal BA (see Fig. 4.35) and give off branches to the rostral medulla and base of the pons before supplying the rostral cerebellar structures. In most cases, they also give rise to the labyrinthine and internal auditory arteries, but these may come directly from the BA or, occasionally, the SCA or PICA. They are effectively end-arteries. The labyrinthine artery supplies the VIIth and VIIIth cranial nerves within the auditory canal and, on entering the inner ear, divides into the common cochlear and anterior vestibular arteries. The common cochlear artery then divides into the main cochlear artery, which supplies the spiral ganglion, the basilar membrane structures and the stria vascularis, whilst the posterior vestibular artery supplies the inferior part of the saccule and the ampulla of the semicircular canal. The anterior vestibular artery supplies the utricle and ampulla of the anterior and horizontal semicircular canals (Baloh, 1992).

Isolated occlusion of the AICA is probably relatively uncommon, but when it does occur there is almost always infarction in both the cerebellum and the pons (Amarenco &

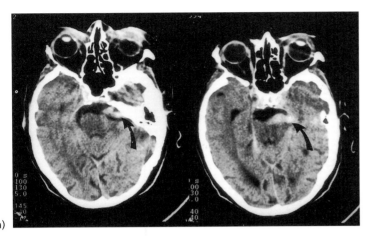

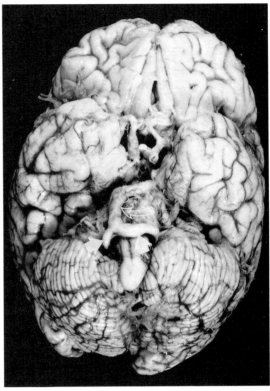

(a)

(b)

Figure 4.36 (a) Axial CT scan showing dolichoectasia of the BA extending into the cerebellopontine angle (arrow). At this stage the patient presented with trigeminal neuralgia. (b) Autopsy demonstration of the VA (closed arrows) and BA (open arrow) of same patient 2-years later, following massive infarction of the brainstem and cerebellum.

Hauw, 1990b). Symptoms tend to be tinnitus, vertigo and nausea, with an ipsilateral Horner's syndrome, an ipsilateral nuclear facial palsy, dysarthria, nystagmus, ipsilateral trigeminal sensory loss, cerebellar ataxia (in the ipsilateral limbs) and sometimes a hemiparesis (i.e. similar to the lateral medullary syndrome with the VIIth and VIIIth nerve lesions replacing those of the IXth and Xth nerves and a hemiparesis). Occlusion of the internal auditory artery is probably an under-recognised cause of sudden unilateral deafness, which may occur in isolation, as may vertigo (Amarenco et al., 1993). Occlusion of the AICA is probably most often secondary to atherosclerosis in the BA or anomalies such as dolichoectasia.

Superior cerebellar artery

The SCA arises from the BA, immediately before its terminal bifurcation (see Fig. 4.35). It usually supplies the dorsolateral midbrain and has branches to the superior cerebellar peduncle and superior surface of the cerebellar hemispheres. The 'classical' syndrome of occlusion of the whole territory of the SCA includes an ipsilateral Horner's syndrome, limb ataxia and tremor, with contralateral spinothalamic sensory loss, upper motor neurone type facial palsy and sometimes a contralateral IVth nerve palsy. In its pure from, it is rare; however, it is often associated with other infarcts in the distal territory of the BA and may have a poor prognosis (Amarenco & Hauw, 1990a). Infarcts which only involve the cerebellar territory of the SCA, on the other hand, have a benign prognosis (Amarenco et al., 1991; Struck et al., 1991). In these cases, headache, limb and gait ataxia, dysarthria, dizziness and vomiting are most prominent, but cases with some of these deficits in isolation have been reported, due to occlusion of the distal branches (Amarenco et al., 1994). Vertigo is much less common in SCA than PICA or AICA territory infarction (Kase et al., 1993). Embolism (either cardiac or artery-to-artery) is considered the most frequent cause of both complete and partial SCA territory infarcts.

The arterial supply of the cerebellum

The cerebellum is supplied by the three long circumferential arteries (PICA, AICA, SCA) described above. The PICA usually supplies the inferior surface, the AICA the rostral surface and the SCA the tentorial surface. Territorial infarction is considered most likely to be due to thromboembolism, particularly from the heart or the BA. However, these arterial systems also have perforating arteries. Cortical infarction in the cerebellum is of two types: (i) infarction perpendicular to the cortical rim at the boundary zone between perforating arteries (which lack anastamoses); and (ii) infarction that parallels the cortical rim and is the boundary zone between the SCA and PICA. Small, deep infarcts occur within the deep white matter of the cerebellar hemispheres, usually around the deep boundary zones. Unlike other small, deep infarcts, the predominant mechanism may be hypoperfusion secondary to large vessel atherosclerosis (Fig. 4.37) (Amarenco, 1995).

> *Cerebellar infarction may be misdiagnosed as 'labyrinthitis' or even upper gastrointestinal pathology if nausea and vomiting are prominent.*

Posterior cerebral artery

The two PCAs are usually the terminal branches of the BA (see Fig. 4.35). The P1 segments of the PCAs pass around the cerebral peduncles and come to lie between the medial surface of the temporal lobe and the upper brainstem. From this portion of the PCA small paramedian mesencephalic arteries and the thalamic–subthalamic arteries arise to supply the medial midbrain, the thalamus and part of the lateral geniculate body. In about 30% of patients, these vessels arise from a single pedicle and therefore bilateral midbrain infarction can result from a single PCA occlusion. After the PCoA (from which the polar arteries to the thalamus usually arise), there are the thalamogeniculate arteries and the PChA, which supply the thalamus. Once the PCA has passed around the free medial edge of the tentorium, it usually divides into two divisions, with a total of four main branches. The anterior division gives rise to the anterior and posterior temporal arteries, whilst from the posterior division the calcarine and parieto-occipital arteries arise. The potential minimum and maximum areas of supply of these branches are shown in Fig. 4.38 (van der Zwan *et al.*, 1992). During early fetal development, the ICA supplies most of the posterior aspect of the cerebral hemispheres and brainstem through the PCoA. In some adults this pattern persists, with only a vestigial BA–PCA connection (Riggs & Rupp, 1963; van Overbeeke *et al.*, 1991).

Occlusions of the PCA origin are probably most often embolic and may occur subsequent to the arrest of an embolus at the basilar bifurcation (Caplan, 1980). As with occlusion of the main stem of the MCA, ischaemia can occur in both the deep and superficial territory of the PCA. Occlusion

of the deep perforating branches of the PCA results in ischaemia of the thalamus and upper brainstem, as described below. Such patients may have a hemiparesis in addition to their visual defects and so mimic extensive MCA territory infarction (Hommel *et al.*, 1990a, 1991). Visual field defects are the most commonly encountered syndrome from PCA infarction. A macular-sparing homonymous hemianopia may occur because collateral flow from the MCA spares the occipital pole and the optic radiation is not involved. More restricted infarcts can result in small homonymous sectoranopias. Bilateral occipital infarction may result in cortical blindness (see Section 4.2.6). When visual function is less severely affected, disorders of colour vision (discrimination, naming) may be apparent. Transient ischaemia in the PCA territory may give 'positive' visual phenomena which are very similar to those of classical migraine (Fisher, 1986). Visual perseverations, such as seeing an object several times despite continued fixation, and continuing to see an object as an after-image (palinopsia) (Critchley, 1951) may also occur. Disorders of language function may occur from PCA territory infarction, probably due to involvement of the thalamus (see below) or its projection fibres. There is dispute about whether the patterns of dysphasia that are seen are in any way characteristic. Sometimes there is a fluent dysphasia, whilst at other times there seems to be a specific naming problem. Alexia, with or without agraphia, may result from left PCA occlusion (see Section 4.2.5). Amnesic disorders may occur because of direct involvement of the temporal lobes, the thalamus or the mamillothalamic tract (Clarke *et al.*, 1994). Typically, there is marked amnesia for recent events. Non-dominant-hemisphere PCA territory infarcts may result in disorders of visuospatial function.

The arterial supply of the thalamus

The thalamus is involved in about 25% of all VB strokes (Bogousslavsky, 1995), but usually in combination with other structures. The blood supply to the thalamus comes from four groups of arteries, which over the years have, confusingly, been called several different names (Fig. 4.39). Unlike other small deep infarcts, those in the thalamus produce a wide range of clinical syndromes, which can make clinical localisation difficult.

1 The thalamic–subthalamic (also known as the paramedian, thalamoperforating, posterior internal optic) arteries arise from the proximal PCA. They are usually 200–400 μm in luminal diameter. In addition to supplying the thalamus, branches also go to the rostral midbrain. In 30% of people the branches to the two thalamic hemispheres have a common pedicle from just one PCA. They supply the posteromedial thalamus, including the nucleus of the MLF,

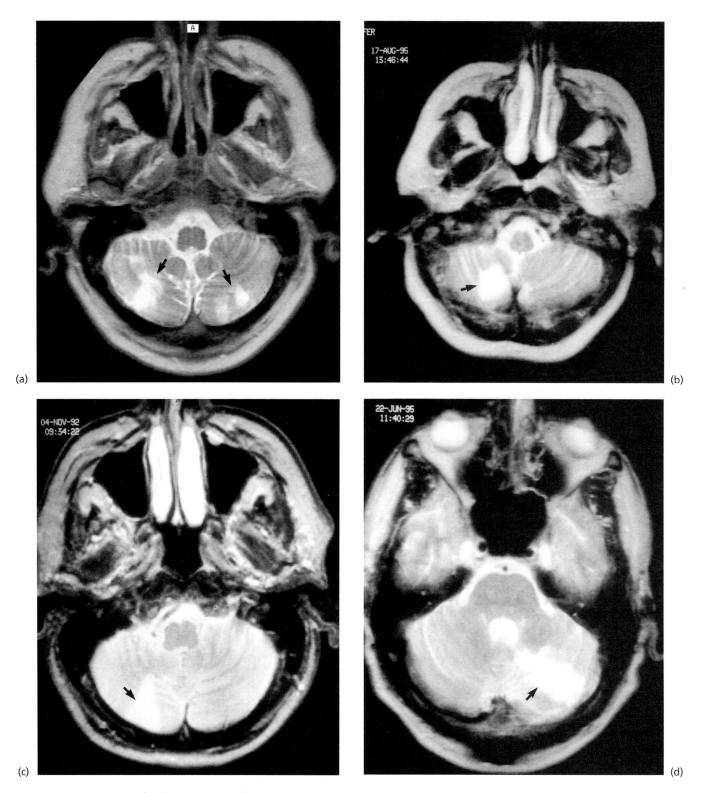

Figure 4.37 Montage of MRI scans (and one CT scan) showing various cerebellar infarcts. (a) Bilateral small cerebellar cortical infarcts in the PICA territories. (b) Unilateral small right cerebellar cortical infarct (medial branch of PICA). (c) Cortical infarct in the right PICA territory. (d) Left cerebellar cortical infarct (lateral branch of superior cerebellar artery).

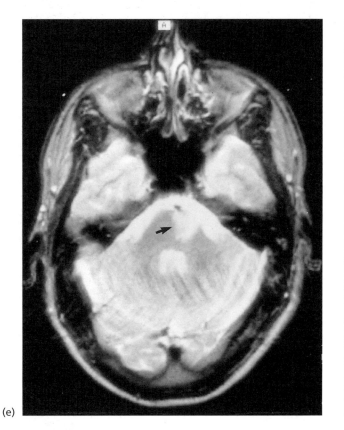

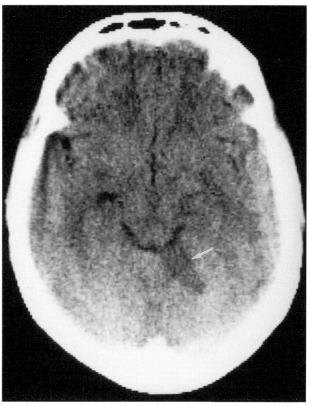

(e)

(f)

Figure 4.37 *Continued*. (e) Infarct in the left brainstem just inferior to the pons (perforating branch of BA). (f) CT scan showing left superior cerebellar infarct (medial branch of superior cerebellar artery).

the posterior dorsomedial nucleus and the intralaminar nuclei.

The typical syndrome of unilateral infarction is of acute depression of conscious level, neuropsychological disturbances and impaired upgaze, with little or no motor or sensory disturbance. The neuropsychological abnormalities are difficult to distinguish from cortical syndromes. The symptoms resulting from bilateral infarcts due to occlusion of the common vascular pedicle are similar to those from unilateral infarction but are usually much more severe. Additionally, the syndrome of akinetic mutism can occur (see Section 4.2.2). Amnesic syndromes are most likely to occur when there is involvement of the dorsomedial nucleus, and mood disturbances may mimic frontal lobe syndromes. Thalamic dementia consists of impaired attention, slowed responses, apathy, poor motivation and amnesia.

2 The polar (also known as the tuberothalamic, anterior internal optic) arteries usually arise from the PCoA, although in about 30% the artery is absent and the vascular supply comes from the thalamic–subthalamic arteries. They supply the anteromedial and anterolateral areas, including

the dorsomedial nucleus, the reticular nucleus, the mamillothalamic tract and part of the ventrolateral nucleus.

The deficits from polar infarcts are mainly neuropsychological. Typically, left-sided infarcts will result in a dysphasia which is non-fluent, with normal comprehension and repetition. Right-sided infarcts may result in hemineglect syndromes and impaired visuospatial processing. Bilateral polar infarcts may result in acute amnesia.

3 The thalamogeniculate arteries are five or six small branches arising from the more distal PCA. These are the equivalent of the LSAs of the MCA and are usually 400–800 μm in luminal diameter. They supply the ventrolateral thalamus, including the VPL and medial nuclei.

Pure sensory stroke (PSS) is a typical lateral thalamic deficit due to occlusion of the thalamogeniculate arteries. There may be a full hemianaesthesia or there may be partial syndromes such as cheiro-oral, cheiro-podo-oral and pseudoradicular sensory loss (see Section 4.2.4). The deficit may involve all modalities or spare pain and temperature sensation (Sacco *et al.*, 1987). If there is extension to the internal capsule, a sensorimotor stroke (SMS) may occur

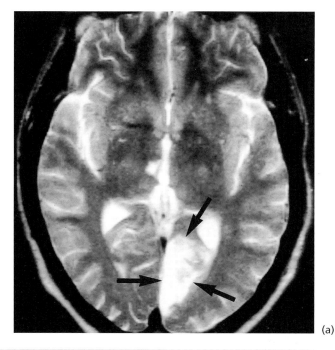

(a)

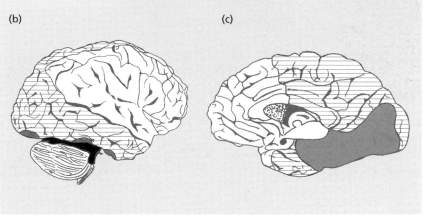

(b)   (c)

Figure 4.38 Ischaemia in the territory of
the PCA. (a) The typical appearance on
T2-weighted axial MRI scan of PCA
territory infarction (arrows). (b, c)
However, there is great interindividual
and interhemispheric variability in the
area supplied by the PCA. The hatched
areas show the only part of the cortex on
the lateral surface (b) and the medial
surface (c) of the hemisphere, which was
always supplied by the PCA in a large
pathological study (van der Zwan, 1991).
The horizontal lines represent the
maximum extent of the area which may
be supplied by the PCA in some patients.
(d) A similar degree of variability exists
for the intracerebral territory supplied by
the PCA. The figure shows the minimum
(hatched) and maximum (horizontal lines)
areas of supply at three levels in the same
pathological study. (Redrawn with
permission of Dr A. van der Zwan.)

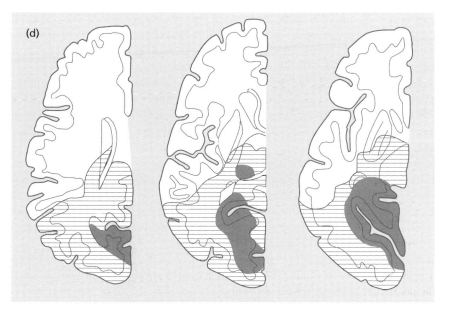

(d)

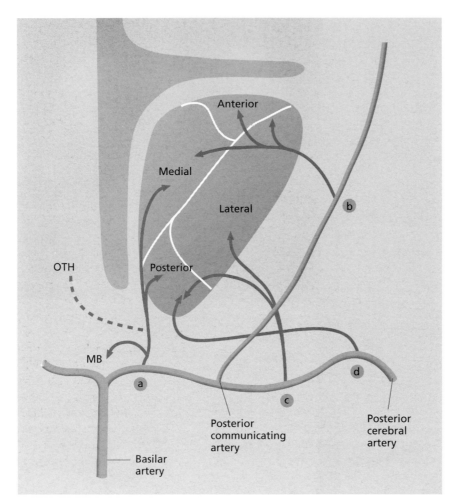

Figure 4.39 Diagrammatic representation of the arterial supply of the thalamus. The branches are: (a) thalamic–subthalamic (paramedian, thalamoperforating, posterior internal optic) arteries. In addition to the thalamus, branches supply the midbrain (MB) and in about 30% the branches to the other thalamic hemisphere (OTH) arise from a common pedicle; (b) polar (tuberothalamic, anterior internal optic) arteries; (c) thalamogeniculate arteries; (d) posterior choroidal arteries.

(Mohr *et al.*, 1977). Hemiataxia is also a typical feature of involvement of the contralateral ventrolateral nucleus because of interruption of fibres in the dentatorubrothalamic pathway. The clinical features are suggestive of cerebellar dysfunction and are not explained by proprioceptive loss.

The Dejerine–Roussy syndrome (Dejerine & Roussy, 1906; Caplan *et al.*, 1988) is caused by more extensive lateral thalamic infarction and consists of a mild contralateral hemiparesis, marked hemianaesthesia, hemiataxia, astereognosis and frequently paroxysmal pain/hyperaesthesia and choreoathetotic movements. The original cases had extension of the infarcts into the internal capsule and towards the putamen, although most of the features of this syndrome result from involvement of the VPN and ventrolateral nucleus of the thalamus.

4 Finally, there is the supply from the medial and lateral PChAs, which also arise from the PCA. These supply the pul-

vinar and posterior thalamus, the geniculate bodies and the anterior nucleus.

Involvement of the PChA presents typically with visual field deficits (upper or lower homonymous quadrantonopia, homonymous horizontal sectoranopia), although some will have associated neuropsychological deficits.

The thalamic arteries were traditionally considered to be end-arteries, but recent work suggests that functional anastamoses do occur (Bogousslavsky, 1995). It is perhaps for this reason that the aetiology of thalamic infarcts is much more variable than that of other small, deep infarcts.

4.3.4 Arterial boundary zones

Arterial boundary zones may be defined as those areas of brain parenchyma where the distal fields of two or more adjacent arteries meet (see Section 6.5.5). The potential clinical relevance is that one might predict that these areas would be particularly vulnerable to haemodynamic stresses, such as hypotension. There are two types of boundary zone.

1 Those where functional anastamoses between the two arterial systems exist (e.g. on the pial surface between the major cerebral arteries (vander Eecken & Adams, 1953) and to a lesser extent at the base of the brain between the choroidal circulations).

2 Those at the junction of the distal fields of two non-anastamosing arterial systems (e.g. deep perforating and pial medullary perforating arteries).

With the former, the boundary zone will occur at points of equal pressure between the two arterial systems. Consequently, changes in arterial pressure in one of the systems may result in a shift of the boundary zone towards the compromised artery (see Figs 4.29, 4.33 & 4.38). With the latter, the boundary zone is likely to be more or less fixed in the individual hemisphere (Fig. 4.40). Both types of boundary zone are present in the cerebellum (see above).

The impression that might be gained from the clinicoradiological literature is that the major boundary zones occur at symmetrical, predictable sites in the hemispheres (Damasio, 1983). Consequently, in some classifications of stroke, imaged infarcts in these areas are considered most likely to be haemodynamic rather than embolic in origin. As has been shown in Figs 4.29, 4.33, 4.38 and 4.40, recent work has suggested that, for both types of boundary zone, there is considerable inter- and intra-individual variation (van der Zwan *et al.*, 1992). We do not believe it is possible to identify 'typical' CT or MRI patterns associated with boundary-zone infarction, given the very real difficulty of identifying them *in vivo* (see Section 6.5.5).

4.4 Subclassification in clinical practice

4.4.1 Introduction

There is a tendency to consider subclassification simply from the point of view of the acute-phase clinician (particularly those engaged in research), whereas, in reality, it has the potential to refine the practice of many other medical and paramedical professionals, as well as health care purchasers and planners (see Table 4.1). It has been noted that the first group tend to produce classifications relating to the vascular mechanism of stroke, but it is striking how few long-term natural history studies there are of strokes subdivided in this way and how little there is in the literature about the reliability of such classifications. Other health professionals are more interested in the clinical deficits and functional consequences resulting from the parenchymal lesion for which longer-term outcome data are available, although no single method of classification predominates. Whilst it is unrealistic to expect any single method to cater for all the disparate

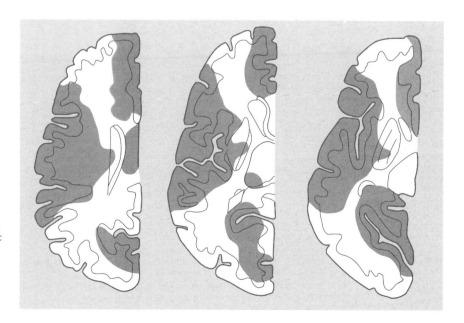

Figure 4.40 Variability of the internal boundary zones. The shaded areas represent the minimum areas of intracerebral supply at three levels of the ACA, MCA and PCA in a large pathological study (van der Zwan, 1991), as shown individually in Figs 4.29d, 4.33c and 4.38d. The adjacent unshaded area represents the area of variation within which the boundaries between these territories was found. (Redrawn with permission of Dr A. van der Zwan.)

requirements, it would seem logical to attempt to bring together the core features of both the parenchymal anatomy and the vascular anatomy and pathophysiology in a manner which permits a hierarchical development to suit individual requirements, i.e. one should be looking to identify groups of parenchymal lesions likely to be caused by broadly similar vascular mechanisms which would also have a distinctive prognosis. In many ways, this is simply an extension of the traditional neurological teaching of first determining the site of the lesion, since this nearly always narrows the range of possible pathological mechanisms. Furthermore, a *primary* method of subclassification should, if possible, be applicable to *all* patients during life, irrespective of age, disability and geographical location, and in practical terms this means a clinical rather than an investigation-based classification. Finally, it is worth stating that anyone using any classification must be blessed with a healthy dose of realism. No classification is ever going to be 100% sensitive and specific. Clinical medicine is not like that and cerebrovascular disease is no exception. These are always going to be exceptions to the rules and one definition of clinical acumen might be the ability to sense when such exceptions are likely to occur.

4.4.2 Classification by duration of symptoms

We have seen already that the distinction between stroke and TIA (i.e. whether symptoms persist for more or less than 24 hours) is arbitrary and does not have any rational pathophysiological basis (see Section 3.1.3). Similarly, there is no evidence to suggest that a distinction between 'major stroke' and 'minor stroke' or reversible ischaemic neurological deficit (RIND), the latter being variously defined as cases where symptoms resolve in less than 1 or 3 weeks, conveys any useful pathophysiological information. Apart from the fact that any stroke may be caused by cerebral haemorrhage or infarction, an identical vascular lesion (of which ICA occlusion would be a good example) might give any of these temporal patterns or even be asymptomatic. To the physician seeing patients with stroke acutely, the fact that the complete classification may not be made accurately in all cases until at least 1 week has elapsed means that the system is only of value retrospectively. Furthermore, contrary to what one might think, it does not impart any useful information about residual disability, since the persistence of tingling in one hand for more than 1 week would be classified as a 'major stroke' in just the same way as a patient who had a dense hemiplegia. The tendency for some physicians to use the terms 'minor' and 'major' as a type of shorthand to describe the level of residual disability simply leads to confusion.

4.4.3 The role of neuroimaging: ischaemic stroke

Superficially, a method of subclassification based on the imaged site of parenchymal infarction or ischaemia and then describing this in terms of the likely vascular territory involved would be attractive and, indeed, is quite often referred to in the literature. However, the arguments against this include the following.

1 The enormous inter- and intra-individual variability of the vascular supply to the brain (see Section 4.3).
2 The current limitations of even the most sophisticated imaging technology to produce reliable results in *all* patients with stroke, particularly within hours of onset of ischaemic stroke (see Section 5.3.5).
3 The problems with generalisability of such a system even if images were available (as they may well be in the future), given current problems with funding health care worldwide.
4 The lack of data correlating cross-sectional imaging with outcome.
5 The illogicality of basing a system on imaging 'holes in the brain' when the current thrust of acute treatments is to prevent such holes appearing.

This reinforces the argument for the primary method of subclassification to be clinically based. Further support comes from the many recent community-based studies of stroke, which have provided data on prognosis and have used some form of clinical examination (which can be applied almost universally), *supplemented* in some studies by ancillary investigations (which may be applied to a subset of patients, selected according to individual circumstances). The conclusions of such studies are much more likely to equate with everyday clinical practice worldwide than those from hospital-based data banks in academic hospitals.

4.4.4 The role of neuroimaging: primary intracerebral haemorrhage (PICH)

An issue that is rarely addressed by most systems of classification is that there are obvious differences between haemorrhages and infarcts, not least because haemorrhages do not respect vascular–anatomical boundaries. As we will see in Chapter 5, the accurate differentiation of infarcts and haemorrhages requires CT or MRI scanning. Furthermore, unlike infarcts, PICHs are almost always visualised immediately on CT scan, and therefore it seems reasonable to describe PICH as deep (ganglionic), cortical (lobar), massive (ganglionic plus lobar), brainstem and cerebellar (see Chapter 8). However, not all physicians will have ready access to CT scanning, and so there is an advantage to having a primary method of classification which is able to classify strokes irrespective of their pathological type, at least until that is known as a result of later CT scanning. Although the discussion below relates primarily to infarcts, the syndromes described may equally be caused by PICH.

4.4.5 The clinical subclassification of stroke

Having taken the history and performed a physical examination, the physician should have established which brain functions have been affected by the stroke. These clinical findings then need to be used to identify groups of patients in a manner which will bring together both the clinical sequelae (i.e. the site and size of the parenchymal lesion) and the pathology/aetiology (i.e. the pattern and nature of the vascular lesion).

Traditional clinically based classifications have distinguished anterior (carotid) circulation strokes and posterior (VB) circulation strokes (see Table 4.12). It seems reasonable to retain this division, since such strokes tend to have characteristic clinical features, the distribution of underlying vascular mechanisms (e.g. embolism versus *in situ* thrombosis) may be different (although this may have been overstated in the past (Caplan & Tettenborn, 1992b)) and certain investigations (e.g. carotid duplex) and treatments (e.g. carotid endarterectomy) are only appropriate to one of the vascular territories. In terms of the intracranial circulation (both anterior and posterior), there are striking differences between the structure, anastamotic potential, vascular pathology and functional areas of the brain perfused by: small, deep perforating arteries; cortical branch arteries; and the main stems of the parent arteries (Table 4.13). There is also good evidence that the prognosis of these groups differs (see Section 10.2.7). A case can therefore be made for further subdividing anterior and posterior circulation strokes into those that are restricted to deep, subcortical areas (supplied by small perforating arteries), those that are restricted to superficial cortical areas (supplied by small pial branch arteries) and finally those which involve both deep and cortical structures (implicating the whole area of supply).

Next, one needs to consider whether these subgroups can be identified clinically with reasonable reliability. Perhaps rather surprisingly, given their relative obscurity until recent years, the greatest amount of information is available for the group of strokes due to occlusion of a single, deep perforating artery and these will be considered first.

4.4.6 Lacunar syndromes (LACS)

The occlusion of a single, deep perforating artery results in a restricted area of infarction known as a 'lacune' (Fig. 4.41; see Section 6.3). The term 'lacune' is a pathological one and unfortunately there are very few cases in the literature with precise clinicoradiological–pathological correlation. If only cross-sectional imaging is available, the term 'small, deep infarct' is preferred (Donnan *et al.*, 1993), with the presumption that the imaged area of infarction is within the territory of a single perforating artery. The majority of lacunes occur in areas such as the lentiform nucleus and are thought to be clinically 'silent' (or at least unrecognised). Although these may be important in some patients with cognitive decline, they do not need to be considered further when considering patients presenting with a 'stroke'. Other lacunes, however, occur at strategic sites such as in the internal capsule and pons, where clinically eloquent ascending and descending neural tracts are concentrated, with the result that an exten-

Table 4.13 Functional characteristics of arteries.

Deep perforating arteries
Limited anastamotic potential
Very restricted areas of infarction
Small vessel disease most likely cause

Cortical branch arteries
Anastamotic potential via pial collaterals
Thus, variable area of ischaemia
Embolism or distal hypoperfusion most likely cause

Main parent arteries
Anastamotic potential via circle of Willis, extracranial connections and pial collaterals
Thus, variable area of ischaemia
Embolism or *in situ* thrombosis most likely cause

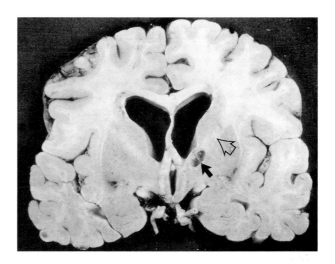

Figure 4.41 Autopsy demonstration of a lacune (closed arrow) in the internal capsule (open arrow).

sive clinical deficit can occur from an anatomically small lesion (see Figs 4.4 & 4.9). If one considers the basic neurovascular pattern described earlier, lesions at such sites are inherently less likely to have a major impact on higher cognitive or visual function than those affecting the cortex.

Initially, a small number of clinical syndromes were correlated with relevant lacunes at subsequent autopsy (Fisher, 1965a; Fisher & Cole, 1965; Fisher & Curry, 1965; Fisher, 1967). These came to be regarded as the 'classical' LACS, although before the advent of CT/MRI the sensitivity and specificity of these relationships were impossible to test. The widespread use of CT/MRI has also resulted in many more syndromes being associated with small, deep infarcts (Fisher, 1991). It could be argued that these should all be included as LACS, but rare associations, perhaps due to idiosyncratic variations in the vascular anatomy, whilst of immense interest to researchers, are of little practical use to clinicians (Bamford, 1995). Consequently, a recently proposed classification of subcortical infarction suggested that the term LACS should be restricted to a clinical situation where the likely mechanism of infarction 'involves transient or permanent occlusion of a single perforating artery with a high degree of probability', i.e. that this mechanism is the *usual* cause of a particular syndrome (Donnan *et al.*, 1993; see Section 6.5.3).

Pure motor stroke (PMS)

PMS is probably the most 'classical' as well as the most frequently encountered of all LACS and will be described in detail, since it exemplifies many of the core features of LACS. The association of pure motor deficits and lacunes was noted early in the 20th century (Hauw, 1995), but the clinical 'rules' for diagnosing PMS were not set out until much later, by Fisher and Curry (1965). They defined the syndrome as 'a paralysis complete or incomplete of the face, arm and leg on one side unaccompanied by sensory signs, visual field defect, dysphasia, or apractagnosia. In the case of brainstem lesions the hemiplegia will be free of vertigo, deafness, tinnitus, diplopia, cerebellar ataxia, and gross nystagmus.' The definition allowed sensory symptoms but not signs to be present. It was stressed that 'this definition applies to the acute phase of the vascular insult and does not include less recent strokes in which other signs were present to begin with, but faded with the passage of time', e.g. aphasia. This puts into clinical terminology the fundamental neuroanatomical concepts of LACS (Table 4.14). For a patient to present with symptoms and signs which fulfil the above criteria, it is most likely that the stroke has been caused by a lesion in an area where the motor tracts are closely packed together, since a lesion of the motor cortex sufficiently extensive to involve the face, arm

Table 4.14 Lacunar syndromes (LACS).

Definition
Maximum deficit from a single vascular event
No visual field deficit
No new disturbance of higher cortical function
No signs of brainstem disturbance*

Categories of LACS
PMS
PSS
Ataxic hemiparesis (including dysarthria clumsy-hand syndrome and homolateral ataxia and crural paresis)
SMS

To be acceptable as a PMS, PSS or SMS, the relevant deficit must involve at least two out of three areas of the face, arm and leg, and, with particular reference to the arm, should involve the whole limb and not just the hand

* In the future some brainstem syndromes may be reclassified as LACS (see Sections 4.4.6 and 4.4.7).

and leg areas of the homunculus would almost certainly involve neural pathways subserving higher cognitive or visual functions. It so happens that most of the relevant anatomical areas (e.g. internal capsule, pons) obtain their vascular supply from deep perforating arteries.

> *Patients presenting with lacunar syndromes have no aphasia, no visuospatial disturbance, no visual field defect, no clear disturbance of brainstem function and no drowsiness at* any *time after their stroke.*

In the original report of nine autopsied cases, six of the lacunes were in the internal capsule and three in the basis pontis, which emphasises the point that the same clinical syndrome may occur with occlusion of a perforating artery from the MCA or the BA. Since then, cases of PMS have been reported with lacunes in other sites along the pyramidal tract, including the corona radiata, the cerebral peduncle and the medullary pyramid (Bamford & Warlow, 1988). However, in general, the anatomical distribution in large series seems to be broadly in keeping with the original pathological observations.

In the early 1980s, the clinicoanatomical correlation of cases with more restricted pure motor deficits associated with small, deep infarcts was reported (Donnan *et al.*, 1982; Rascol *et al.*, 1982). Although in theory one might include any case with a pure motor deficit, the more restricted a deficit is, the more likely it is to arise from a cortical infarct, which spares other modalities. By common usage (which tends to reflect clinical utility), a LACS is usually considered to include only deficits involving the whole of the face and arm, or the whole of the arm and leg. Such cases are probably best regarded as 'partial' rather than 'classical' LACS (Bamford, 1995), but many large studies that have reported on clinicoanatomical correlations have combined the two groups and it is not possible to comment on the sensitivity and specificity of classical and partial LACS separately in predicting the site of the lesion. However, it seems likely that the partial LACS are still most likely to be associated with small, deep infarcts, although it should be stressed that the definitions used stated that the *whole* of the arm or leg should be affected, something one suspects is often overlooked. The small, deep infarcts associated with these partial LACS tend to occur in the corona radiata or the junctional zone between it and the capsule, where fibres are relatively more dispersed (Donnan *et al.*, 1982).

> *Only deficits involving the whole of the face and arm or the whole of the arm and leg should be accepted as partial lacunar syndrome and not more restricted deficits which are more likely to be of cortical origin.*

Pure sensory stroke

The sensory counterpart of PMS is encountered much less frequently. Although the definition in the original paper (Fisher, 1965a) suggested that there should be objective sensory loss, in a later paper Fisher (1982) noted that there could be cases with persistent sensory symptoms in the absence of objective signs. A case of a partial PSS has been verified pathologically (Fisher, 1978a). Most small, deep infarcts causing PSS are in the thalamus, in keeping with the original pathological studies. The lesions causing PSS are the smallest of the symptomatic small, deep infarcts.

Homolateral ataxia and crural paresis (HACP), dysarthria clumsy-hand syndrome (DCHS) and ataxic hemiparesis (AH)

Unlike the general acceptance of PMS and PSS as 'classical' LACS, this group of syndromes is less accepted as 'lacunar', although they were initially described at about the same time. This may be because of the difficulty of interpreting some physical signs and the fact that they are less common. Cases of HACP were described as having weakness of the lower limb, especially the ankle and toes, a Babinski sign and 'striking dysmetria of the arm and leg on the same side' (Fisher & Cole, 1965). In the DCHS, although the deficit was described as being 'chiefly of dysarthria and clumsiness of one hand', two of the three original cases had signs suggestive of pyramidal dysfunction in the ipsilateral leg and

both had an ataxic gait (Fisher, 1967). Indeed, in his later paper, Fisher (1978b) draws the cases together under the new term AH. The relevant lacunes were all in the basis pontis and he attributed the variable distribution of the weakness in different cases to the involvement of motor fibres where they are relatively dispersed by the pontine nuclei. It has been reported that, if 'rigid' clinical criteria are used, the syndrome predicts a lesion in the contralateral pontine base (Glass *et al.*, 1990). On the other hand, Bogousslavsky *et al.* (1992) suggest that true HACP may be most frequently seen from partial ACA infarcts. They make the point that many other cases reported with CT evidence of corona radiata 'lacunes' have had much more extensive deficits. Sensory variants of AH have been reported, but there is no evidence that the anatomical and clinical issues raised are significantly different from those between PMS and SMS (see below).

> *Limb ataxia does not necessarily imply a cerebellar stroke in the presence of ipsilateral pyramidal signs.*

Sensorimotor stroke

The inclusion of SMS as a classical LACS is based on a single case with autopsy, which appeared almost a decade after the reports of the other classical LACS (Mohr *et al.*, 1977). This case was due to a lacune in the VPN of the thalamus, but there was also pallor of the adjacent internal capsule. Although there were marked sensory and motor signs which persisted, the sensory symptoms preceded the motor ones. There is also autopsy support for an infarct primarily within the internal capsule being able to cause SMS (Tuszynski *et al.*, 1989). Groothuis *et al.* (1977) reported a similar syndrome occurring after a small haemorrhage in the same place. The authors made the point that a sensory deficit can occur from lesions of the posterior limb of the internal capsule, presumably by interruption of the thalamocortical pathways. Allen *et al.* (1984) reported 12 cases of SMS examined soon after onset, 11 of whom had low-attenuation areas on brain CT. When superimposed they were slightly larger and extended more medially than cases with PMS, abutting the posterolateral aspect of the thalamus, but were still within the usual territory of a single perforating artery. In an MRI study (Hommel *et al.*, 1990b), the infarcts in cases of SMS were larger than for other LACS, although still thought to equate with lacunes. In the Stroke Data Bank, where SMS was the most frequent LACS after PMS, 31% had a lesion in the posterior limb of the internal capsule, 22% had a lesion in the corona radiata, 7% in the genu of the capsule, 6% in the anterior limb of the capsule and only 9% in the thalamus (Chamorro *et al.*, 1991). The lesions in the corona radiata were on average almost twice as large as those in the capsule, but both were larger than the corresponding values for the PMS group. MRI scanning has disclosed that in some hitherto unrecognised cases the lesion is in the medial part of the medulla (Kim *et al.*, 1995).

The parenchymal lesion

Table 4.15 summarises the clinicoradiological correlations for the various LACS and imaged small, deep infarcts in large studies. Overall, about 10% of patients presenting with a LACS will have a lesion other than a small, deep infarct on a scan which *might* explain the neurological symptoms. The proportion of such 'atypical' patients does seem to be higher for SMS than for the other syndromes and therefore particular care should be taken with this group.

The vascular lesion

Any of the 'classical' LACS may be caused by a small haemorrhage, and this accounts for about 5% of cases in community studies (Bamford & Warlow, 1988). In the pre-CT era, this fact may have been of some clinical utility, and it may still be in countries with limited access to CT, where theraputic decisions may have to be made on the basis of probability rather than absolute evidence. There is no direct

information about the cause of the occlusion of single perforating arteries, except in a handful of cases. Asymptomatic (smaller) lacunes are probably most often the consequence of occlusion by lipohyalinosis, when the usual diameter of the vessel is less than $100\,\mu m$ (Fisher, 1969). Symptomatic lacunes are probably most often the result of occlusion by microatheroma, when the vessel diameter is around $400\,\mu m$ (Fisher, 1979). Some cases, particularly those with basilar perforating artery occlusion, may be caused by obstruction of the mouth of the perforating artery by an atheromatous plaque within the parent artery (Fisher & Caplan, 1971). Although an embolic mechanism is possible (Millikan, 1995), epidemiological evidence suggests that there is a low frequency of significant carotid stenosis (Tables 4.16 & 4.17) or cardiac source of embolism (Boiten & Lodder, 1995) (see Section 6.3).

From the above it can be seen that a classical LACS does not reliably distinguish whether the occluded perforating artery arises from the anterior or posterior systems, although in older series (e.g. Rochester, Minnesota: Turney *et al.*, 1984) it seems likely that they would always have been considered as anterior circulation strokes. More recently, it has been recognised that small deep infarcts are the usual cause of certain brainstem syndromes (usually a PMS plus a cranial nerve palsy or eye movement disorder) (Hommel *et al.*, 1990b). Before simply accepting these alongside the classical LACS, the even greater paucity of pathological studies

Syndrome	study	Setting	Imaging	n	Non-lacunar (%)
PMS	Bamford *et al.* (1987)	Community	CT	49	1 (2)
	Hommel *et al.* (1990b)	Hospital	MR	35	0 (0)
	Arboix & Marti-Vilalta (1992)	Hospital	CT/MR	137	12 (9)
PSS	Bamford *et al.* (1987b)	Community	CT	7	0 (0)
	Hommel *et al.* (1990b)	Hospital	MR	12	1 (8)
	Arboix & Marti-Vilalta (1992)	Hospital	CT/MR	45	3 (7)
AH	Bamford *et al.* (1987)	Community	CT	9	0 (0)
	Hommel *et al.* (1990b)	Hospital	MR	28	2 (7)
SMS	Bamford *et al.* (1987)	Community	CT	43	2 (5)
	Hommel *et al.* (1990b)	Hospital	MR	8	1 (12)
	Landi *et al.* (1991)	Hospital	CT	34	3 (11)
	Lodder *et al.* (1991)	Hospital	CT	47	5 (11)
	Huang *et al.* (1987)	Hospital	CT	37	8 (21)
	Arboix & Marti-Vilalta (1992)	Hospital	CT/MR	42	8 (19)
All	Wardlaw *et al.* (1996)	Hospital	CT	19	2 (11)
	Boiten and Lodder (1991b)	Hospital	CT	109	11 (10)
	Ricci *et al.* (1991)	Community	CT	56	2 (4)

Table 4.15 Clinicoradiological correlations of LACS.

Table 4.16 Carotid duplex findings by clinical subtype: degree of stenosis ipsilateral to the site of infarction. (From Mead *et al.*, in press.)

	Stenosis of ipsilateral ICA				
	0–30%	31–69%	70–99%	Occlusion	Total
Total anterior circulation syndrome	51 (65%)	3 (4%)	5 (6%)	19 (24%)	78
Partial anterior circulation syndrome	50 (60%)	7 (8%)	13 (15%)	14 (17%)	84
LACS	64 (88%)	6 (8%)	1 (1%)	2 (3%)	73
Posterior circulation syndrome	15 (88%)	1 (6%)	1 (6%)	0 (0%)	17

Table 4.17 Angiographic findings according to infarct size on brain CT. (From Olsen *et al.*, 1985.)

Infarct size on brain CT	MCA occlusion	Significant ICA disease	Neither	Total
Large	14	6	0	20
Medium	14	6	5	25
Small	0	1	14	15
None	1	1	11	13

should be recognised. As noted above, the vascular pathology may be different, with atheroma overlying the mouth of the penetrating artery being more frequent than in the anterior circulation (Fisher & Caplan, 1971). Consequently, these types of deficit are not generally included in studies reporting the prognosis of patients with LACS, but this position may need to be reviewed in the light of new MRI studies.

4.4.7 Posterior circulation syndromes (POCS)

Although there are some clinical syndromes due to well-localised lesions within the VB system which, along with their eponymous names, are an integral part of 'classical neurology' (e.g. Weber's, Millard–Gubler, Wallenberg's syndrome), in practice such syndromes are rarely seen in their pure form. Indeed, in many ways, the clinical consequences of a given vascular lesion are probably less predictable than for other arteries, because of the greater prevalence of developmental anomalies and the fact that, instead of a paired system of arteries in which the luminal diameter decreases as one moves distally, this is the only example in the body of two large arteries joining to form a single larger artery. Additionally, until the advent of MRI, clinicoradiological correlation was difficult because of the poorer performance of CT in the posterior fossa compared with the supratentorial compartment. Angiography was also performed much less

frequently than for anterior circulation strokes, because it did not lead to any change in the management, such as vascular surgery. A further problem is that, in Caucasians at least, intrinsic disease of the intracranial portion of the posterior circulation is more common than in the anterior circulation. The possible impact on small vessel ischaemia has already been commented on. Consequently, at the present time one must recognise that this grouping is relatively crude and POCS encompasses a heterogeneous group of stroke (see Section 6.5.4).

The clinical syndromes

The clinical deficits which point to the lesion being in the distribution of the VB system are shown in Table 4.18. Other symptoms and signs which may be present in patients with POCS but are not of useful localising value include Horner's syndrome, nystagmus, dysarthria and hearing disturbance. Occasionally, an otherwise typical POCS may be associated with disturbance of higher cerebral function, e.g. aphasia, agnosias. This should not come as a surprise, given the variable supratentorial territory supplied by the PCAs (see Section 4.3.3; Hommel *et al.*, 1990a, 1991), and these cases should still be considered as POCS.

Table 4.18 Posterior circulation syndromes (POCS).

Any of
Ipsilateral cranial nerve palsy (single or multiple) with contralateral motor and/or sensory deficit
Bilateral motor and/or sensory deficit
Disorder of conjugate eye movement (horizontal or vertical)
Cerebellar dysfunction without ipsilateral long-tract deficit (as seen in ataxic hemiparesis)
Isolated hemianopia or cortical blindness

Cases where there is disturbance of higher cortical function alongside any of the above should be considered as POCS

The parenchymal lesion

In the Oxfordshire Community Stroke Project (OCSP), of 109 patients presenting with POCS, of whom 90 had a CT scan within 28 days of stroke onset or autopsy, nine (10%) were due to PICH (Bamford, 1986). In the study from Lund, seven of 39 (18%) patients with POCS had a PICH (Lindgren *et al.*, 1994). In the OCSP, of the remaining 81 patients with CT or autopsy, 19 showed an infarct within the usual distribution of the VB system, 60 showed no relevant lesion and two showed an 'inappropriate' infarct (an MCA branch occlusion and multiple small, deep infarcts) (Bamford, 1986). Of 24 cases of POCS not due to haemorrhage in the Studio Epidemiologico sulla Incidenza delle Vasculopatie Acute Cerebrali (SEPIVAC) study, none had inappropriate lesions on CT (Ricci *et al.*, 1991). In a more recent hospital-based study, Wardlaw *et al.* (1996) reported that, of 13 patients diagnosed as POCS and not due to haemorrhage, eight (62%) had a cerebellar, PCA or brainstem infarct visible on CT, whilst the other five had 'negative' CT.

As mentioned above, with the increasing use of MRI, it has been realised that certain syndromes are usually due to small, deep infarcts, compatible with occlusion of a single perforating artery. The two groups which fall into this category are those that generally have a pure motor deficit with, additionally, disorders of eye movement or a single cranial nerve (e.g. Weber's syndrome, PMS plus IIIrd nerve palsy), and those where there is an isolated internuclear ophthalmoplegia. They have been referred to as extended LACS (Bamford, 1995). The only detailed study of this issue was reported by Hommel *et al.* (1990b), where all 21 cases presenting with these so-called extended LACS had evidence of a small, deep infarct on MRI. What is not known at present is the spectrum of clinical syndromes that may be caused by such lesions in the brainstem.

The vascular lesion

Traditionally, pathological series have suggested that within the carotid circulation the ratio of embolism to *in situ* thrombosis is about 3 : 1, whilst in the VB circulation this ratio is reversed (Escourelle, 1978). Recent workers have questioned this (Caplan & Tettenborn, 1992b; Caplan *et al.*, 1992) and it seems likely that at least some of the difference is the result of the inevitable selection bias that occurs in pathological series. In their recent study, Caplan and Tettenborn (1992b) reported that 43% of VB infarcts were due to large artery occlusive disease, 20% were due to artery-to-artery emboli, 19% were due to cardiogenic embolism and 18% were due to small vessel disease. It seems likely that, because of the shape of the BA, emboli would be more likely to arrest in the upper portion of the artery. Amongst 93 cases of isolated homonymous hemianopia due to a vascular lesion, 80 (96%) were due to PCA occlusion (Trobe *et al.*, 1973).

The POCS are probably the most heterogeneous group in terms of both the parenchymal and the vascular lesion, and in the future there is likely to be increasing distinction between those due to small and large vessel disease. There is a tendency for POCS to be underdiagnosed in non-specialist centres. In our view this is due most often to a failure to appreciate that truncal or gait ataxia is present because no one bothers to sit or stand the patient up.

4.4.8 Total anterior circulation syndromes (TACS)

At the other end of the spectrum of clinical severity from most patients with LACS, hospital clinicians in particular are familiar with the patient who has a complete hemiplegia, hemianopia and evidence of higher cortical dysfunction (especially language or visuospatial function). Additionally, some impairment of consciousness is often present, which can make formal testing difficult. Such patients are likely to be admitted to hospital more frequently than those with LACS (Bamford *et al.*, 1986).

The clinical syndrome

The clinical features of TACS (Table 4.19) are a hemiplegia (usually with an ipsilateral hemisensory loss), a visual field deficit on the same side and a new disturbance of higher cerebral function referable to the same hemisphere.

The parenchymal lesion

In the OCSP, of 107 patients presenting with TACS, of whom 73 had a CT scan within 28 days of onset or autopsy, 18 (25%) were due to PICH (Bamford, 1986). In the study from Lund, 13 of 67 patients with TACS (19%) had PICH (Lindgren *et al.*, 1994). Amongst the non-haemorrhagic cases in the OCSP, 52 (95%) showed evidence of extensive infarction within the usual distribution of at least the MCA. There were only three patients with 'inappropriate', but possibly clinically relevant, lesions (two with multiple small, deep infarcts, one with a single internal capsule infarct). In the SEPIVAC study, of 42 cases with TACS not due to haemorrhage, one had a restricted area of cortical infarction within the MCA territory, but otherwise there were no 'inappropriate' lesions on CT (Ricci *et al.*, 1991). Allen (1984), who used the term 'full house' for this clinical pattern, reported that the volume of infarction as judged

Table 4.19 Total anterior circulation syndrome (TACS).

All of
Hemiplegia contralateral to the cerebral lesion*
Hemianopia contralateral to the cerebral lesion
New disturbance of higher cerebral function (e.g. dysphasia,
  visuospatial disturbance)

---

* Although it has never been tested formally, one gains the
impression that the more severe the motor deficit the less likely are
there to be mistakes made with respect to clinicoradiological
correlation.

by CT was significantly greater than for patients with lesser
deficits. A similar result was reported by Lindgren *et al.*
(1994) (Table 4.20). Finally, Wardlaw *et al.* (1996) reported
that 30 of 33 (91%) patients classified as TACS and due to
infarction had large or medium-sized MCA territory infarcts
on CT, or large subcortical infarcts. One had a small cortical
infarct but there had been a rapid resolution of the patient's
clinical deficit. Two had an infarct involving the whole of the
usual left PCA territory (Hommel *et al.*, 1990a, 1991).

> Up to 25% of all patients presenting with a total anterior
> circulation syndrome have an underlying primary
> intracerebral haemorrhage.

The vascular lesion

Foix and Levy (1927) recognised that this pattern of deficit
was associated with occlusion of the proximal main trunk of
the MCA and that infarction occurred in both the deep and
superficial territories. They also recognised that, on occasion, the extent of infarction in the superficial territory was
not as extensive and they presumed this reflected functionally effective leptomeningeal collaterals. This is a similar argument to that relating to striatocapsular infarction (see
Section 4.3.2). Olsen *et al.* (1985) reported that, in 20 cases

of extensive hemispheric infarction as judged by CT, 14 had
evidence of MCA occlusion and the other six had either
occlusion or more than 75% stenosis of the ipsilateral ICA.
Mead *et al.* (in press) reported that, amongst patients with
non-haemorrhagic TACS who had an early carotid duplex
examination, 30% had either occlusion or more than 70%
ICA stenosis ipsilateral to the cerebral lesion (see Table
4.16).

Perhaps the biggest 'catch', as exemplified by the study
of Wardlaw *et al.* (1996), is the ability of PCA territory
ischaemia to produce a TACS. This has been described in
detail by Hommel *et al.* (1990a, 1991) and Chambers *et al.*
(1991). In general, such cases have a relatively mild hemiparesis but marked aphasia (not always fluent) and a visual
field deficit. The motor deficit occurs because of involvement
of the small, perforating arteries arising from the proximal
PCA, which supply the upper midbrain. The other situation
worth noting is that occasionally one sees a patient very early
on who appears to have a PMS. However, 24-hours later
they have a TACS. This probably occurs when there is
thrombus in the proximal MCA trunk. Because the basal
ganglia have a high metabolic rate, the symptoms (and in
some cases the changes on CT) will first be apparent in this
area.

> Occasionally, a total anterior circulation syndrome
> results from occlusion of the posterior cerebral artery. In
> such cases, there is often a relatively mild hemiparesis but
> a marked aphasia and visual field loss.

4.4.9 Partial anterior circulation syndromes (PACS)

The final group of syndromes have less extensive deficits
than TACS and yet do not fulfil the specific criteria for
LACS, either because of the presence of higher cortical
deficits or because the motor/sensory deficit is too restricted
in anatomical terms.

Table 4.20 Volume of infarction on brain CT according to clinical subtype.

	TACS (ml) $n = 41$	PACS (ml) $n = 41$	LACS (ml) $n = 38$	POCS (ml) $n = 18$
Lindgren *et al.* (1994)	91.8	18.8	4.2	8.5
Allen (1984)	134.3	(a) 60.2	3.0	(e) 7.0
		(b) 44.5		(f) 31.8
		(c) 40.6		
		(d) 14.0		

(a) Hemiplegia + hemianopia; (b) hemiplegia + higher cerebral dysfunction; (c) hemianopia +
higher cerebral dysfunction; (d) lone higher cerebral dysfunction; (e) brainstem; (f) lone
hemianopia.
PACS, partial anterior circulation syndrome.

The clinical syndromes

The clinical features of PACS are set out in Table 4.21. In general, these are patients with definite disturbance of higher cortical function whose deficit is not as extensive as those with TACS or who have restricted motor and/or sensory deficits which do not fulfil the criteria for a LACS.

The parenchymal lesion

In the OCSP, of 135 patients presenting with PACS, of whom 113 had a CT scan within 28 days of stroke onset or autopsy, seven (6%) were due to PICH (Bamford, 1986). In the study from Lund, eight of 69 patients with PACS (12%) had a PICH (Lindgren *et al.*, 1994). Amongst the non-haemorrhagic cases in the OCSP, 103 showed evidence of infarction within the usual distribution of the MCA or ACA or had a 'normal' scan. There were 'inappropriate' but potentially clinically relevant lesions in three cases (one with multiple small, deep infarcts, one with a thalamic infarct and one with an infarct of the anterior internal capsule) (Bamford, 1986). In the SEPIVAC study, of 160 patients with PACS not due to haemorrhage, three had infarcts on CT in the posterior circulation, six had small, deep infarcts and three had extensive areas of MCA territory infarction (Ricci *et al.*, 1991). Allen (1984) showed that patients with the clinical features of PACS had lesions on CT generally extending into the cortex but significantly smaller than patients with a 'full house' or TACS. This was confirmed by Lindgren *et al.* (1994) (see Table 4.20). Wardlaw *et al.* (1996) reported that 27 of 43 (63%) patients classified as PACS and due to infarction had small or medium-sized MCA territory infarcts on CT or large subcortical infarcts. Three other cases had CT lesions which might be deemed appropriate to the syndrome; two had 'boundary-zone' infarcts and one had a large cortical infarct in the MCA territory. Five cases had small deep

Table 4.21 Partial anterior circulation syndromes (PACS).

Any of
Motor/sensory deficit + hemianopia
Motor/sensory deficit + new higher cerebral dysfunction
New higher cerebral dysfunction + hemianopia
Pure motor/sensory deficit less extensive than for LACS (e.g. monoparesis)
New higher cerebral dysfunction alone

When more than one type of deficit is present, they must all reflect damage in the same cerebral hemisphere

---

infarcts (all left-sided), one had an infarct involving the whole of the usual right PCA territory and seven had 'negative' scans.

The vascular lesion

In an angiographic study of 25 cases with medium (1.5–3.0 cm) areas of infarction on CT, 14 had early angiographic evidence of MCA occlusion, six had ICA occlusion and five had no significant angiographic lesion (Olsen *et al.*, 1985). Mead *et al.* (in press) reported that 32% of patients with non-haemorrhagic PACS had either occlusion or more than 70% stenosis of the ICA ipsilateral to the cerebral lesion (see Table 4.16).

There are certainly patients, who are often very elderly, where it can be difficult to decide whether they should be classified as a PACS or a TACS, usually because of uncertainty about the presence of higher cerebral dysfunction or a visual field deficit. If one is not certain about a deficit, it is usually best to consider it absent and therefore the majority should be considered as PACS. The exception is if the patient is drowsy, which, if due to the cerebral lesion, would be indicative of an extensive lesion and the patient should be classified as a TACS. At the other end of the spectrum, one should be quite rigid about applying the rules describing the extent of a motor or sensory deficit, which ought to be present before diagnosing a LACS (i.e. only when there is involvement of the face, arm and leg or the whole of the face and arm, or the whole of the arm and leg).

4.4.10 Syndromes of uncertain origin

The physician will, for a variety of reasons, occasionally have difficulty allocating cases with confidence on clinical grounds to one of the four groups; for example, the patient may have had a previous stoke, be demented or have had a limb amputated for peripheral vascular disease. In such cases, it may be unclear what *new* neurological deficits have arisen from the current stroke. In research studies, such as the OCSP, cases who died before clinical assessment was possible were also included in this group. This is a situation where the results of any brain imaging *may* assist the primary classification, i.e. point towards the most likely clinical syndrome. This can be of value both in clinical practice (for reasons discussed in Section 4.4.11) and in research studies, where it will help minimise the risk of bias being introduced, particularly when considering the outcome of the groups.

It is worth stressing that it is the pattern of clinical symptoms and signs at the time of maximum deficit that were

Table 4.22 Formulating the clinical findings.

1	Unilateral weakness (and/or sensory deficit) affecting face
2	Unilateral weakness (and/or sensory deficit) affecting arm
3	Unilateral weakness (and/or sensory deficit) affecting hand
4	Unilateral weakness (and/or sensory deficit) affecting leg
5	Unilateral weakness (and/or sensory deficit) affecting foot
6	Dysphasia, dyslexia, dysgraphia (i.e. dominant hemisphere cortical)
7	Visuospatial disorder/inattention/neglect (i.e. non-dominant hemisphere)
8	Homonymous hemianopia or quadrantanopia
9	Brainstem/cerebellar signs other than ataxic hemiparesis
10	Other deficit

TACS:	1 + 2 + 3 + 4 + 5 + 6 + 7
LACS:	1 + 2 + 3 + 4 + 5 or 1 + 2 + 3 or 2 + 3 + 4 + 5
POCS:	8 or 9 or 8 + 9
PACS:	other combinations excluding 9 and 10

used in the original clinicoradiological correlation study (Bamford *et al.*, 1991). Thus, one will encounter patients who, very soon after the onset of their stroke seem to have a PMS that would fit the description of a LACS, but who, 24-hours later, have a deficit in the pattern of a TACS. This will occur because with an ICA or MCA occlusion the territory of the deep, perforating arteries may become ischaemic more quickly (and deeply) than the overlying cortex. At the present time, it is uncertain how often such changes in syndrome allocation would occur if patients were seen within 6 hours of onset, but it is clearly an important question for those involved with hyperacute stroke treatment trials.

4.4.11 Using the clinical classification

Any system of classification will not become widely accepted unless it is easy to use and conveys useful information to the clinician. How do the clinical syndromes described above measure up to this challenge? The necessary information is, by and large, easy (and inexpensive) to collect from virtually all patients with stroke. The check-list in Table 4.22 can be incorporated into stroke clerking or admission forms as an *aide-mémoire*. Lindgren *et al.* (1994) reported that the inter-observer agreement for the allocation of clinical subtypes between the initial 'routine' clinical clerking (albeit using a protocol) and another performed within 1 week by one of the authors was 92% (kappa 0.89). Table 4.23 shows the sensitivity, specificity, positive and negative predictive value of the clinical syndromes when judged against subsequent CT scanning. Each syndrome occurs frequently in patients with stroke (Fig. 4.42), which should promote pattern recognition, particularly by junior medical staff.

The syndromes provide the clinician with some indication of the likelihood of a stroke being due to cerebral haemorrhage (unlikely with LACS but more likely with TACS), because in the OCSP 25% of the TACS, 10% of the

Table 4.23 The clinical classification of cerebral infarcts versus brain CT as the gold standard showing the site and size of the lesion.

Clinical subtype		Sensitivity	Specificity	Positive predictive value	Negative predictive value
TACI:	a	0.95	1.00	1.00	0.99
	b	0.98	0.99	0.93	0.99
	c	0.97	0.96	0.94	0.99
PACI:	a	0.97	0.98	0.96	0.99
	b	0.92	0.91	0.98	0.91
	c (b)	0.95	0.90	0.84	0.97
	(w)	0.94	0.82	0.67	0.97
LACI:	a	0.97	0.96	0.91	0.99
	b	0.96	0.97	0.90	0.99
	c (b)	0.77	0.98	0.89	0.94
	(w)	0.71	0.92	0.63	0.94
POCI:	a	0.97	1.00	1.00	0.99
	b	1.00	1.00	1.00	1.00
	c (b)	0.81	1.00	1.00	0.97
	(w)	0.73	0.95	0.61	0.97

a, OCSP (Bamford, 1986); b, SEPIVAC (Ricci *et al.*, 1991); c, Wardlaw *et al.* (1996) (b) best- and (w) worst-case scenario. LACI, lacunar infarct; PACI, partial anterior circulation infarct; POCI, posterior circulation infarct; TACI, total anterior circulation infarct. Note: Table 4.23 shows that, in two large community-based studies, there was very good sensitivity, specificity and positive and negative predictive value for the diagnosis of the clinical syndromes in patients with infarction, when judged against lesions on CT which were considered to be 'appropriate' for the syndrome (e.g. small deep infarct for patients with LACI). However, in both studies, a 'normal' CT scan was considered appropriate for both LACI and PACI and, therefore, in the hospital-based study of Wardlaw *et al.* (1996), a 'best'- and 'worst'-case scenario (i.e. assuming that all normal scores were appropriate or inappropriate, respectively) was presented. Even with the worst-case scenario, the clinical syndromes still performed at a level which is useful in clinical practice.

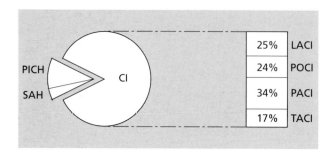

Figure 4.42 The distribution of clinical subtypes of cerebral infarction in the OCSP. CI, cerebral infarction; LACI, lacunar infarction; PACI, partial anterior circulation infarction; POCI, posterior circulation infarction; TACI, total anterior circulation infarction.

POCS, 6% of the PACS and 5% of the LACS were caused by intracerebral haemorrhage. This in no way obviates the need for CT scanning to make a definitive distinction between infarct and haemorrhage, but, unfortunately, many clinicians continue to have restricted access to such facilities (see Chapter 5). The syndromes predict the volume of cerebral infarction in patients with ischaemic stroke (see Table 4.20). Thus, very rapidly, clinical staff can predict which patients are at greatest risk of developing impairment of conscious level and, for example, be at risk of aspiration (TACS and POCS) (see Section 15.17). The nursing staff and the relatives can then be alerted to the possibility. Impairment of consciousness developing in a patient with LACS should prompt a search for an alternative explanation, since such patients will not develop significant cerebral oedema.

Since the syndromes predict the volume of cerebral infarction, not surprisingly they predict outcome (see Section 10.2.7). Not only does this allow more accurate information to be given to the patients and their relatives, it also allows early, realistic discharge planning to begin. More research is required into whether given deficits occurring as part of different syndromes have different patterns of recovery. Since the syndromes can be determined immediately by junior medical staff, they can be used to stratify patients in large clinical trials of treatments for acute stroke (International Stroke Trial Pilot Study Collaborative Group, 1996).

The syndromes provide the clinician with an indication of the most likely underlying vascular pathology (see Section 6.7). TACS/PACS are likely to be caused by large vessel disease and therefore the clinician should be thinking about car-

diac sources of embolism or carotid atherosclerosis. If access to, for example, carotid duplex is restricted, one could argue that cases of PACS, where there is a significant chance of finding a more than 70% ICA stenosis in a patient who has a good chance of making an excellent physical recovery and where the risk of early recurrence may be greatest (Bamford *et al.*, 1991), should take precedence over patients with LACS. Furthermore, in trials of thrombolysis, it may be logical to distinguish TACS/PACS from LACS. If a patient presents with a LACS, the clinician should not be surprised if there is no lesion on the CT scan, carotid duplex or cardiac echo and should not 'chase' excessively rare causes of stroke without some good reason.

References

Adams HP Jr, Bendixen BH, Kappelle LJ *et al.* and the TOAST investigators (1993). Classification of subtype of acute ischemic stroke: definitions for use in a multicenter clinical trial. *Stroke* 24: 35–41.

Allen CMC (1984). *The accurate diagnosis and prognosis of acute stroke.* MD thesis, University of Cambridge.

Allen CMC, Hoare RD, Fowler CJ, Harrison MJG (1984). Clinico-anatomical correlations of uncomplicated stroke. *J Neurol Neurosurg Psychiatr* 47: 1251–4.

Alpers BJ, Berry RG (1963). Circle of Willis in cerebral vascular disorders. *Arch Neurol* 8: 398–402.

Amarenco P (1990). The spectrum of cerebellar disorders. *Neurology* 41: 973–9.

Amarenco P (1995). Small, deep cerebellar infarcts. In: Donnan GA, Norrving B, Bamford JM, Bogousslavsky J, eds. *Lacunar and Other Subcortical Infarctions.* Oxford: Oxford University Press, 208–13.

Amarenco P, Hauw J-J (1990a). Cerebellar infarction in the territory of the superior cerebellar artery: a clinicopathologic study of 33 cases. *Neurology* 40: 1383–90.

Amarenco P, Hauw J-J (1990b). Cerebellar infarction in the territory of the anterior and inferior cerebellar artery. *Brain* 113: 139–55.

Amarenco P, Rosengart A, DeWitt LD, Pessin MS, Caplan LR (1993). Anterior inferior cerebellar artery territory infarcts: mechanisms and clinical features. *Arch Neurol* 50: 154–61.

Amarenco P, Levy C, Cohen A, Touboul P-J, Roullet E, Bousser M-G (1994). Causes and mechanisms of territorial and nonterritorial cerebellar infarcts in 115 consecutive cases. *Stroke* 25: 105–12.

Amarenco P, Roullet E, Goujon C, Cheron F, Hauw J-J, Bousser M-G (1991). Infarction of the anterior part of the rostral cerebellum. *Neurology* 41: 253–8.

Arboix A, Marti-Vilalta JL (1992). Lacunar syndromes not due to lacunar infarcts. *Cerebrovasc Dis* 2: 287–92.

Baloh RW (1992). Stroke and vertigo. *Cerebrovasc Dis* 2: 3–10.

Bamford J, Sandercock P, Jones L, Warlow C (1987). The natural history of lacunar infarction: the Oxfordshire Community Stroke Project. *Stroke* 18: 545–51.

Bamford J, Sandercock P, Dennis M, Burn J, Warlow C (1991). Classification and natural history of clinically identifiable subtypes of cerebral infarction. *Lancet* 337: 1521–6.

Bamford JM (1986). *The classification and natural history of acute cerebrovascular disease.* MD thesis, University of Manchester.

Bamford JM (1995). Lacunar syndromes—are they still worth diagnosing? In: Donnan GA, Norrving B, Bamford JM, Bogousslavsky J, eds. *Lacunar and Other Subcortical Infarctions.* Oxford: Oxford University Press, 32–43.

Bamford JM, Warlow CP (1988). Evolution and testing of the lacunar hypothesis. *Stroke* 19: 1074–82.

Bamford JM, Sandercock PAG, Warlow CP, Gray JM (1986). Why are acute stroke patients admitted to hospital? The Oxfordshire Community Stroke Project. *Br Med J* 292: 1369–72.

Baquis GD, Pessin MS, Scott RM (1985). Limb shaking: a carotid TIA. *Stroke* 16: 444–8.

Barrett K (1991). Treating organic abulia with bromocriptine and lisuride: four case studies. *J Neurol Neurosurg Psychiatr* 54: 718–21.

Bogousslavsky J (1995). Thalamic infarcts. In: Donnan GA, Norrving B, Bamford JM, Bogousslavsky J, eds. *Lacunar and Other Subcortical Infarctions.* Oxford: Oxford University Press, 149–70.

Bogousslavsky J, Regli F (1990). Anterior cerebral artery territory infarction in the Lausanne Stroke Registry: clinical and etiologic patterns. *Arch Neurol* 47: 144–50.

Bogousslavsky J, Martin R, Moulin T (1992). Homolateral ataxia and crural paresis: a syndrome of anterior cerebral artery territory infarction. *J Neurol Neurosurg Psychiatr* 55: 1146–9.

Bogousslavsky J, van Melle G, Regli F (1988). The Lausanne Stroke Registry: analysis of 1000 consecutive patients with first stroke. *Stroke* 19: 1083–92.

Bogousslavsky J, van Melle G, Regli F (1990). Middle cerebral artery pial territory infarcts: a study of the Lausanne Stroke Registry. *Ann Neurol* 25: 555–60.

Boiten J, Lodder J (1991a). Isolated monoparesis is usually caused by superficial infarction. *Cerebrovasc Dis* 1: 337–40.

Boiten J, Lodder J (1991b). Lacunar infarcts: pathogenesis and validity of the clinical syndromes. *Stroke* 22: 1374–8.

Boiten J, Lodder J (1995). Risk factors for lacunar infarction. In: Donnan GA, Norrving B, Bamford JM, Bogousslavsky J, eds. *Lacunar and Other Subcortical Infarctions.* Oxford: Oxford University Press, 56–69.

Brodal A (1981a). The somatic afferent pathways. In: *Neurological Anatomy in Relation to Clinical Medicine,* 3rd edn. Oxford: Oxford University Press, 46–147.

Brodal A (1981b). The reticular formation. In: *Neurological Anatomy in Relation to Clinical Medicine,* 3rd edn. Oxford: Oxford University Press, 394–447.

Cairns H, Oldfield RC, Pennybacker JB, Whitteridge D (1941). Akinetic mutism with an epidermoid cyst of the 3rd ventricle. *Brain* 64: 273–90.

Caplan LR (1980). 'Top of the basilar syndrome'. *Neurology* 30:

72–9.

Caplan LR (1989). Intracranial branch atheromatous disease: a neglected, understudied, and underused concept. *Neurology* 39: 1246–50.

Caplan LR, Tettenborn B (1992a). Vertebrobasilar occlusive disease: review of selected aspects. 1. Spontaneous dissection of extracranial and intracranial posterior circulation arteries. *Cerebrovasc Dis* 2: 256–65.

Caplan LR, Tettenborn B (1992b). Vertebrobasilar occlusive disease: review of selected aspects. 2. Posterior circulation embolism. *Cerebrovasc Dis* 2: 320–6.

Caplan LR, Dewitt LD, Pessin MS, Gorelick PB, Adelman LS (1988). Lateral thalamic infarcts. *Arch Neurol* 45: 959–64.

Caplan LR, Amarenco P, Rosengart A *et al.* (1992). Embolism from vertebral artery origin occlusive disease. *Neurology* 42: 1505–12.

Chadwick D (1993). The cranial nerves and special senses. In: *Brain's Diseases of the Nervous System,* 10th edn. Oxford: Oxford University Press, 77–126.

Chambers BR, Bladin CF (1995). Internal watershed infarction. In: Donnan GA, Norrving B, Bamford JM, Bogousslavsky J, eds. *Lacunar and Other Subcortical Infarctions.* Oxford: Oxford University Press, 139–48.

Chambers BR, Brooder RJ, Donnan GA (1991). Proximal posterior cerebral artery occlusion simulating middle cerebral artery occlusion. *Neurology* 41: 385–90.

Chamorro A, Sacco RL, Mohr JP *et al.* (1991). Clinical–computed tomographic correlations of lacunar infarction in the Stroke Data Bank. *Stroke* 22: 175–81.

Chollet F, DiPiero V, Wise RJS, Brooks DJ, Dolan RJ, Frackowiak RSJ (1991). The functional anatomy of motor recovery after stroke in humans: a study with positron emission tomography. *Ann Neurol* 29: 63–71.

Clarke S, Assal G, Bogousslavsky J *et al.* (1994). Pure amnesia after unilateral left polar thalamic infarct: topographic and sequential neuropsychological and metabolic (PET) correlations. *J Neurol Neurosurg Psychiatr* 57: 27–34.

Coleman RJ, Bamford JM, Warlow CP (for the UK TIA Study Group) (1993). Cerebral tumours that mimic transient cerebral ischaemia—lessons from a large multi-centre trial. *J Neurol Neurosurg Psychiatr* 56: 563–6.

Conference of Medical Royal Colleges and their Faculties in the United Kingdom (1976). Diagnosis of brain death. *Br Med J* ii: 1187–8.

Conference of Medical Royal Colleges and their Faculties in the United Kingdom (1979). Diagnosis of brain death. *Br Med J* i: 332.

Conference of Medical Royal Colleges and their Faculties in the United Kingdom (1995). Criteria for the diagnosis of brain stem death. *J Roy Coll Phys* 29: 381–2.

Critchley M (1929). Arteriosclerotic Parkinsonism. *Brain* 52: 23–83.

Critchley M (1930). The anterior cerebral artery and its syndromes. *Brain* 53: 120–65.

Critchley M (1951). Types of visual perseveration: palinopsia and illusory visual spread. *Brain* 74: 267–99.

Damasio H (1983). A computed tomographic guide to the identification of cerebral vascular territories. *Arch Neurol* 40: 138–42.

Dejerine J, Roussy G (1906). Le syndrome thalamique. *Rev Neurol* 14: 521–32.

Dennis MS, Bamford JM, Sandercock PAG, Warlow CP (1989). Lone bilateral blindness: a transient ischaemic attack? *Lancet* i: 185–8.

DeRenzi E, Motti F, Nichelli P (1980). Imitating gestures: a quantitative approach to ideomotor apraxia. *Arch Neurol* 37: 6–10.

Donnan GA, Tress BM, Bladin PF (1982). A prospective study of lacunar infarction using computerized tomography. *Neurology* 32: 49–56.

Donnan GA, Norrving B, Bamford JM, Bogousslavsky J (1993). Subcortical infarction: classification and terminology. *Cerebrovasc Dis* 3: 248–51.

Donnan GA, O'Malley HM, Quang L, Hurley S, Bladin PF (1995). The capsular warning syndrome and lacunar transient ischaemic attacks. In: Donnan GA, Norrving B, Bamford JM, Bogousslavsky J, eds. *Lacunar and Other Subcortical Infarctions.* Oxford: Oxford University Press, 47–55.

Duncan GW, Parker SW, Fisher CM (1975). Acute cerebellar infarction in the PICA territory. *Arch Neurol* 32: 364–8.

Eadie MS, Sutherland JM (1964). Arteriosclerosis and Parkinsonism. *J Neurol Neurosurg Psychiatr* 27: 237–40.

Escourelle R (1978). *Manual of Basic Neuropathology.* Philadelphia: Saunders.

Fieschi C, Argentino C, Lenzi GL, Sacchetti ML, Toni D, Bozzao L (1989). Clinical and instrumental evaluation of patients with ischemic stroke in the first six hours. *J Neurol Sci* 91: 311–22.

Fisher CM (1959). Observations of the fundus occuli in transient monocular blindness. *Neurology* 9: 333–47.

Fisher CM (1964). Ocular bobbing. *Arch Neurol* 11: 543–6.

Fisher CM (1965a). Pure sensory stroke involving face, arm and leg. *Neurology* 15: 76–80.

Fisher CM (1965b). Lacunes—small, deep cerebral infarcts. *Neurology* 15: 774–84.

Fisher CM (1967). A lacunar stroke: the dysarthria–clumsy hand syndrome. *Neurology* 17: 614–17.

Fisher CM (1969). The arterial lesion underlying lacunes. *Acta Neuropathol (Berl)* 12: 1–15.

Fisher CM (1978a). Thalamic pure sensory stroke: a pathologic study. *Neurology* 28: 1141–4.

Fisher CM (1978b). Ataxic hemiparesis: a pathologic study. *Arch Neurol* 35: 126–8.

Fisher CM (1979). Capsular infarcts: the underlying vascular lesions. *Arch Neurol* 36: 65–73.

Fisher CM (1982). Lacunar strokes and infarcts: a review. *Neurology* 32: 871–6.

Fisher CM (1986). The posterior cerebral artery syndrome. *Can J Neurol Sci* 13: 232–9.

Fisher CM (1991). Lacunar infarcts—a review. *Cerebrovasc Dis* 1: 311–20.

Fisher CM (1995). Abulia. In: Bogousslavsky J, Caplan LR, eds. *Stroke Syndromes.* Cambridge: Cambridge University Press, 182–7.

Fisher CM, Caplan LR (1971). Basilar artery branch occlusion: a cause of pontine infarction. *Neurology* 21: 900–5.

Fisher CM, Cole M (1965). Homolateral ataxia and crural paresis: a vascular syndrome. *J Neurol Neurosurg Psychiatr* 28: 48–55.

Fisher CM, Curry HB (1965). Pure motor hemiplegia from vascular origin. *Arch Neurol* 13: 30–44.

Foix C, Levy M (1927). Les ramollissements sylviens: syndromes des lésions en foyer du territoire de l'artère sylvienne et de ses branches. *Rev Neurol (Paris)* 11: 1–51.

Foulkes MA, Wolf PA, Price TR *et al.* (1988). The Stroke Data Bank: design, methods, and baseline characteristics. *Stroke* 19: 547–54.

Friedman A, Kang UJ, Tatemichi TK, Burke RE (1986). A case of parkinsonism following striatal lacunar infarction. *J Neurol Neurosurg Psychiatr* 49: 1087–8.

Frisen L (1979). Quadruple sectoranopia and sectorial optic atrophy: a syndrome of the distal anterior choroidal artery. *J Neural Neurosurg Psychiatr* 42: 590–4.

Glass JD, Levey AI, Rothstein JD (1990). The dysarthria–clumsy hand syndrome: a distinct clinical entity related to pontine infarction. *Ann Neurol* 27: 487–94.

Gordon DL, Bendixen BH, Adams HP Jr, Clarke W, Kappelle LJ, Woolson RF and the TOAST investigators (1993). Interphysician agreement in the diagnosis of subtypes of acute ischemic stroke: implications for clinical trials. *Neurology* 43: 1021–7.

Greenhall RCD (1977). *Pathological findings in acute cerebrovascular disease and their clinical implications.* DM thesis, University of Oxford.

Groothuis DR, Duncan GW, Fisher CM (1977). The human thalamocortical sensory path in the internal capsule: evidence from a small capsular haemorrhage causing a pure sensory stroke. *Ann Neurol* 2: 328–31.

Halligan PW, Marshall JC, Wade DT (1989). Visuospatial neglect: underlying factors and test sensitivity. *Lancet* ii: 908–11.

Hauw J-J (1995). The history of lacunes. In: Donnan GA, Norrving B, Bamford JM, Bogousslavsky J, eds. *Lacunar and Other Subcortical Infarctions.* Oxford: Oxford University Press, 3–15.

Helgason CM (1995). Anterior choroidal artery territory infarction. In: Donnan GA, Norrving B, Bamford JM, Bogousslavsky J, eds. *Lacunar and Other Subcortical Infarctions.* Oxford: Oxford University Press, 131–8.

Hennerici M, Klemm C, Rautenberg W (1988). The subclavian steal phenomenon: a common vascular disorder with rare neurologic deficits. *Neurology* 38: 669–73.

Hillen LH (1986). A mathematical model of the flow in the circle of Willis. *J Biomech* 19: 187–94.

Hodges J (1994). *Cognitive Assessment for Clinicians.* Oxford: Oxford University Press.

Hommel M, Moreau DO, Besson G, Perret J (1991). Site of arterial occlusion in the hemiplegic posterior cerebral artery syndrome. *Neurology* 41: 604–5.

Hommel M, Besson G, Pollak P, Kahane P, Lebas JF, Perret J (1990a). Hemiplegia in posterior cerebral artery occlusion. *Neurology* 40: 1496–9.

Hommel M, Besson G, Le Bas JF *et al.* (1990b). Prospective study of lacunar infarction using magnetic resonance imaging. *Stroke* 21: 546–54.

Howard RS, Miller DH (1995). The persistent vegetative state. *Br Med J* 310: 341–2.

Huang CY, Yu YL (1985). Small cerebellar strokes may mimic labyrinthine lesions. *J Neurol Neurosurg Psychiatr* 48: 263–5.

Huang CY, Woo E, Yu YL, Chan FL (1987). When is sensorimotor stroke a lacunar syndrome? *J Neurol Neurosurg Psychiatr* 50: 720–6.

International Stroke Trial Pilot Study Collaborative Group (1996). Study design of the International Stroke Trial (IST), baseline data and outcome of 984 randomised patients in the pilot study. *J Neurol Neurosurg Psychiatr* 60: 371–6.

Ishiai S, Sugishita M, Ichikawa T, Gono S, Watabiki S (1993). Clock drawing test and unilateral spatial neglect. *Neurology* 43: 106–10.

Jennett B, Plum F (1972). Persistent vegetative state after brain damage: a syndrome in search of a name. *Lancet* i: 734–7.

Kase CS, Norrving B, Levine SR *et al.* (1993). Cerebellar infarction: clinical and anatomical observations in 66 cases. *Stroke* 24: 76–83.

Katz RT, Haig AJ, Clark BB, DiPaola RJ (1992). Longterm survival, prognosis and life-care planning for 29 patients with chronic locked-in syndrome. *Arch Phy Med Rehab* 73: 403–8.

Kaul SN, DuBoulay GH, Kendall BE, Ross Russell RW (1974). Relationship between visual field defect and arterial occlusion in posterior circulation. *J Neurol Neurosurg Psychiatr* 37: 1022–30.

Kazui S, Sawada T (1993). Callosal apraxia without agraphia. *Ann Neurol* 33: 401–3.

Kennard C, Crawford TJ, Henderson C (1994). A pathophysiological approach to saccadic eye movements in neurological and psychiatric disease. *J Neurol Neurosurg Psychiatr* 57: 881–5.

Kim JS (1994). Restricted acral sensory syndrome following minor stroke: further observation with special reference to differential severity of symptoms among individual digits. *Stroke* 25: 2497–502.

Kim JS, Lee MC (1994). Stroke and restricted sensory syndromes. *Neuroradiology* 36: 258–63.

Kim JS, Kim HG, Chung CS (1995). Medial medullary syndrome: report of 18 new patients and a review of the literature. *Stroke* 29 (9): 1548–52.

Koskas F, Comizzoli I, Gobin YP *et al.* (1992). Effects of spinal mechanics on the vertebral artery. In: Berguer R, Caplan LR, eds. *Vertebrobasilar Arterial Disease*. St Louis, QMP, 15–28.

Landi G, Anzalone N, Cella E, Boccardi E, Musicco M (1991). Are sensorimotor strokes lacunar strokes? A case–control study of lacunar and non-lacunar strokes. *J Neurol Neurosurg Psychiatr* 54: 1063–8.

Lempert T, Gresty MA, Bronstein AM (1995). Benign positional

vertigo: recognition and treatment. *Br Med J* 311: 489–91.

Lindgren A, Norrving B, Rudling O, Johansson BB (1994). Comparison of clinical and neuroradiological findings in first-ever stroke: a population-based study. *Stroke* 25: 1371–7.

Lindley RI, Warlow CP, Wardlaw JM, Dennis MS, Slattery J, Sandercock PAG (1993). Interobserver reliability of a clinical classification of acute cerebral infarction. *Stroke* 24: 1801–4.

Lodder J, Boiten J, Raak L, Heuts van Raak L (1991). Sensorimotor syndrome relates to lacunar rather than to non-lacunar cerebral infarction. *J Neurol Neurosurg Psychiatr* 54: 1097.

Lodder J, Bamford J, Kappelle J, Boiten J (1994). What causes false clinical prediction of small, deep infarcts. *Stroke* 25: 86–91.

Louis ED, King D, Sacco R, Mohr JP (1995). Upper motor neuron signs in acute stroke: prevalence, interobserver reliability, and timing of initial examination. *J Stroke Cerebrovasc Dis* 5: 49–55.

McNabb AW, Carol WM, Mastaglia FL (1988). 'Alien-hand' and loss of bimanual co-ordination after dominant anterior cerebral artery territory infarction. *J Neurol Neurosurg Psychiatr* 51: 218–22.

Marshall JC, Halligan PW (1993). Visuo-spatial neglect: a new copying test to assess perceptual parsing. *J Neurol* 240: 37–40.

Mead GE, Murray H, Farrell A, Picton AJ, O'Neill PA (in press).

Melo P, de Mendonca A, Crespo M, Carvalho M, Ferro JM (1992). An emergency room based study of stroke coma. *Cerebrovasc Dis* 2: 93–101.

Miller NR (ed.) (1982). Vascular supply of the visual pathways. In: *Walsh and Hoyt's Clinical Neuro-ophthalmology*, 4th edn. Baltimore: Williams and Wilkins, 104–7.

Millikan CH (1995). About lacunes. In: Donnan GA, Norrving B, Bamford JM, Bogousslavsky J, eds. *Lacunar and Other Subcortical Infarctions*. Oxford: Oxford University Press, 23–8.

Mohr JP, Kase CS, Meckler RJ, Fisher CM (1977). Sensorimotor stroke due to thalamocapsular ischemia. *Arch Neurol* 34: 734–41.

Mohr JP, Pessin MS, Finkelstein S, Funkenstein HH, Duncan GW, Davis KR (1978). Broca aphasia: pathologic and clinical. *Neurology* 28: 311–24.

Olsen TS, Skriver EB, Herning M (1985). Cause of cerebral infarction in the carotid territory: its relations to the size and the location of the infarct and to the underlying vascular lesion. *Stroke* 16: 459–66.

Padget H (1948). The development of the cranial arteries in the human embryo. *Contrib Embryol* 32: 205–61.

Palmer E, Ashly P, Hajek VE (1992). Ipsilateral fast corticospinal pathways do not account for recovery in stroke. *Ann Neurol* 32: 519–25.

Parkes JD, Marsden CD, Rees JE *et al.* (1974). Parkinson's disease, cerebral arteriosclerosis, and senile dementia. *Quart J Med* 43: 49–61.

Penfield W, Boldrey E (1937). Somatic motor and sensory representation in the cerebral cortex of man as studied by electrical stimulation. *Brain* 60: 389–443.

Penfield W, Rasmussen T (1950). *The Cerebral Cortex of Man*. New York: Macmillan.

Perlmutter D, Rhoton AL Jr (1976). Microsurgical anatomy of the anterior cerebral–anterior communicating–recurrent artery complex. *J Neurosurg* 45: 259–72.

Plum F, Posner JB (1980). The pathologic physiology of signs and symptoms of coma. In: Plum F, Posner JB, eds. *The Diagnosis of Stupor and Coma*. Philadelphia: FA Davis.

Rascol A, Clanet M, Manelfe C, Guiraud B, Bonafe A (1982). Pure motor hemiplegia: CT study of 30 cases. *Stroke* 13: 11–17.

Ricci S, Celani MG, Caputo N (1991). SEPIVAC: a community-based study of stroke incidence in Umbria, Italy. *J Neurol Neurosurg Psychiatr* 54: 695–8.

Riggs HE, Rupp C (1963). Variation in form of circle of Willis. *Arch Neurol* 8: 8–14.

Ropper A (1986). Lateral displacement of the brain and level of consciousness in patients with acute hemispheral mass. *N Engl J Med* 314: 953–8.

Ross ED, Stewart RM (1981). Akinetic mutism from hypothalamic damage: successful treatment with dopamine agonists. *Neurology* 31: 1435–9.

Ruotolo C, Hazan H, Rancurel G, Kieffer E (1992). Dynamic arteriography. In: Berguer R, Caplan LR, eds. *Vertebrobasilar Arterial Disease*. St Louis: QMP, 116–23.

Russell JR, DeMeyer W (1961). The quantitative cortical origin of pyramidal axons of *Macaca rhesus*, with some remarks on the slow rate of axolysis. *Neurology* 11: 96–108.

Sacco RL, Bello JA, Traub R, Brust JCM (1987). Selective proprioceptive loss from a thalamic lacunar stroke. *Stroke* 18: 1160–3.

Sacco RL, Ellenberg JH, Mohr JP *et al.* (1989). Infarcts of undetermined cause: the NINCDS Stroke Data Bank. *Ann Neurol* 25: 382–90.

Schwartz A, Rautenberg W, Hennerici M (1993). Dolichoectatic intracranial arteries: review of selected aspects. *Cerebrovasc Dis* 3: 273–9.

Schott GD (1993). Penfield's homunculus: a note on cerebral cartography. *J Neurol Neurosurg Psychiatr* 56: 329–33.

Shaw CM, Alvord EC, Berry RG (1959). Swelling of the brain following ischaemic infarction with arterial occlusion. *Arch Neurol* 1: 161–77.

Sherrington CS, Bamford JM (1996). Coma due to brainstem ischaemia—is it always an indicator of grave prognosis? *J Neurol Neurosurg Psychiatr* (in press).

Shinar D, Gross CR, Mohr JP (1985). Interobserver variability in the assessment of neurologic history and examination in the Stroke Data Bank. *Arch Neurol* 42: 557–65.

Silver FL, Norris JW, Lewis AJ, Hachinski VC (1984). Early mortality following stroke: a prospective view. *Stroke* 3: 492–6.

Spudis EV (1991). The persistent vegetative state—1990. *J Neurol Sci* 102: 128–36.

Sterzi R, Bottini G, Celani MG (1993). Hemianopia, hemianaesthesia, and hemiplegia after right and left hemisphere damage: a hemispheric difference. *J Neurol Neurosurg Psychiatr* 56: 308–10.

Stone SP, Wilson B, Wroot A *et al.* (1991). The assessment of visuo-spatial neglect after acute stroke. *J Neurol Neurosurg Psychiatr* 54: 345–50.

Struck LK, Biller J, Bruno A *et al.* (1991). Superior cerebellar artery territory infarction. *Cerebrovasc Dis* 1: 71–5.

Teasdale G, Jennett B (1974). Assessment of coma and impaired consciousness: a practical scale. *Lancet* ii: 81–4.

Toole JF, Tucker SH (1960). Influence of head position upon cerebral circulation. *Arch Neurol* 2: 616–23.

Torvik A, Jorgensen L (1964). Thrombotic and embolic occlusions of the carotid arteries in an autopsy series. 1. Prevalence, location and associated disease. *J Neurol Sci* 1: 24–39.

Torvik A, Jorgensen L (1966). Thrombotic and embolic occlusions of the carotid arteries in an autopsy series. 2. Cerebral lesions and clinical course. *J Neurol Sci* 3: 410–32.

Trobe JD, Lorber ML, Schlezinger NS (1973). Isolated homonymous hemianopia. *Arch Ophthalmol* 89: 377–81.

Turney TM, Garraway WM, Whisnant JP (1984). The natural history of hemispheric and brainstem infarction in Rochester, Minnesota. *Stroke* 15: 790–4.

Tuszynski MH, Petito CK, Levy DE (1989). Risk factors and clinical manifestations of pathologically verified lacunar infarctions. *Stroke* 20: 990–9.

Ueda S, Fugitsu K, Inomori S, Kuwabara T (1992). Thrombotic occlusion of the middle cerebral artery. *Stroke* 23: 1761–6.

Uldry P-A, Bogousslavsky J (1995). Acute infarcts in the centrum ovale. In: Donnan GA, Norrving B, Bamford JM, Bogousslavsky J, eds. *Lacunar and Other Subcortical Infarctions*. Oxford: Oxford University Press, 171–80.

Vander Eecken HM, Adams RD (1953). The anatomy and functional significance of the meningeal arterial anastamoses of the human brain. *J Neuropathol Exp Neurol* 12: 132–57.

van der Zwan A (1991). *The variability of the major vascular territories of the human brain*. Doctoral thesis, University of Utrecht.

van der Zwan A, Hillen B, Tulleken CAF, Dujovny M, Dragovic L (1992). Variability of the territories of the major cerebral arteries. *J Neurosurg* 77: 927–40.

van Gijn J (1995). The Babinski reflex. *Postgrad Med J* 71: 645–8.

van Overbeeke JJ, Hillen B, Tulleken CAF (1991). A comparitive study of the circle of Willis in fetal and adult life: the configuration of the posterior bifurcation of the posterior communicating artery. *J Anat* 176: 45–54.

Waddington MM, Ring BA (1968). Syndromes of occlusions of middle cerebral artery branches: angiographic and clinical correlations. *Brain* 91: 685–96.

Wardlaw JM, Dennis MS, Lindley RI, Sellar RJ, Warlow CP (1996). The validity of a simple clinical classification of acute ischaemic stroke. *J Neurol* 243: 274–9.

Watson YI, Arfken CL, Birge SJ (1993). Clock completion: an objective screening test for dementia. *J Am Geriatr Soc* 41: 1235–40.

Weiller C (1995). Striatocapsular infarcts. In: Donnan GA, Norrving B, Bamford JM, Bogousslavsky J, eds. *Lacunar and*

Other Subcortical Infarctions. Oxford: Oxford University Press, 104–16.

Williams D, Wilson TG (1962). The diagnosis of the major and minor syndromes of basilar insufficiency. *Brain* 85: 741–74.

What pathological type of stroke is it?

5

5.1   Introduction

Diagnosis of the pathological type of stroke is important, because treatment, prognosis and secondary prevention are different for ischaemic and haemorrhagic stroke. In practical day-to-day terms, most patients will have one of the common causes of stroke, i.e. ischaemic stroke due to the complications of atherothrombosis (see Section 6.2), intracranial small vessel disease (see Section 6.3) or embolism from the heart (see Section 6.4); primary intracerebral haemorrhage (PICH), due to hypertension, for example (see Section 8.3); or subarachnoid haemorrhage (SAH), due to a ruptured saccular aneurysm (see Section 9.1). A small minority will have an unusual underlying cause of their PICH, an odd presentation of SAH, a tumour presenting as a stroke or an odd cause of ischaemic stroke, such as venous infarction. Thus, whilst most strokes seen clinically and on imaging are due to some-

thing which is common, it is important not to assume that all strokes are. Some strokes will be due to unusual causes. If there is something odd about either the clinical presentation or the imaging, then it is important to look for an explanation. This point will be illustrated with examples where appropriate.

5.2   Frequency of different pathological types of stroke

It is important to consider the frequency of a condition when evaluating a diagnostic method. The community-based studies of stroke incidence are described in Section 17.2.1, and are mentioned here as background to the clinical and imaging diagnosis of stroke type. In the Oxfordshire Community Stroke Project (OCSP), the Studio Epidemiologics

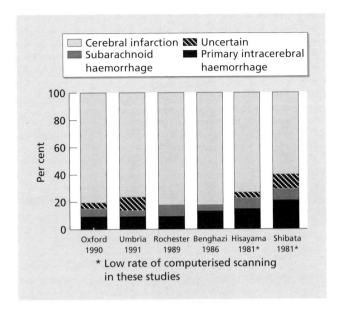

Figure 5.1 Histogram of cause of first-ever stroke by pathological type in the community-based studies. Oxford 1990, the OCSP (Bamford *et al.*, 1990); Umbria, the SEPIVAC study (Ricci *et al.*, 1991); Rochester, Rochester, Minnesota, US (Broderick *et al.*, 1989); Benghazi (Ashok *et al.*, 1986); Hisayama, Japan (Ueda *et al.*, 1981); Shibata, Japan (Tanaka *et al.*, 1981). Note that the Japanese studies had lower computerised tomography scan and autopsy rates than the later studies which may in part explain the larger proportion of strokes attributed to PICH. (The figure was prepared by Dr Richard Lindley, The Royal Victoria and Western General Hospitals, Edinburgh, UK.)

sulla Incidenza della Vasculopatie Acute Cerebrali (SEPI-VAC) from Umbria in Italy and the studies from Rochester in Minnesota, Benghazi in Libya, Hisayama and Shibata in Japan and Perth in Australia, the majority of strokes (about 80%) were due to cerebral infarction (Fig. 5.1) (Tanaka *et al.*, 1981; Ueda *et al.*, 1981; Ashok *et al.*, 1986; Ward *et al.*, 1988; Broderick *et al.*, 1989; Bamford *et al.*, 1990; Ricci *et al.*, 1991). About 10% were due to PICH, 5% to SAH and, except in Rochester and Benghazi, in 5% the cause was uncertain or due to non-vascular pathology (the Rochester and Benghazi studies did not have an 'uncertain' classification). There was, in general, reasonable consistency between these studies, although older studies from Japan had higher PICH rates, consistent with much anecdotal information that cerebral haemorrhage is considerably more common in Oriental than in Caucasian populations.

However, in hospital there is a bias towards admitting the more 'severe' strokes, and so a greater proportion of haemorrhages (perhaps as much as 20%, depending on the speciality) and a greater proportion of large cortical and extensive brainstem/cerebellar infarcts. Thus, in hospitals

one will generally see fewer patients with minor cortical or brainstem strokes. Furthermore, in both community- and hospital-based studies, a small proportion of 'strokes' turn out to be due to tumours or infections or some other non-vascular pathology presenting as a 'stroke' (see Section 3.5; Tanaka *et al.*, 1981; Ueda *et al.*, 1981; Ward *et al.*, 1988; Bamford *et al.*, 1990; Sotaniemi *et al.*, 1990; Ricci *et al.*, 1991). There may be clues to a non-vascular cause for a 'stroke' in that the history or examination is atypical; for example, a recent epileptic seizure, increasing headaches, stuttering onset or previous malignant disease should all alert one to a possible non-vascular pathology. Fortunately, cross-sectional brain imaging can usually sort out most non-vascular causes (Fig. 5.2).

5.3 Differentiating ischaemic stroke from primary intracerebral haemorrhage (PICH)

From a practical point of view, the first important step in classification is the distinction of cases of ischaemic stroke from those due to PICH. This distinguishes groups of stroke with differing causes, prospects for survival and recurrence, and will also influence decisions about medical and surgical treatments. Whilst clinical paradigms can be of some assistance (see Section 5.3.1), the gold standard for making the

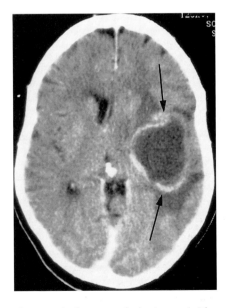

Figure 5.2 Computerised tomography brain scan (with contrast) from a patient who presented with a stroke (sudden-onset right hemiparesis), but whose scan shows a large primary brain tumour with considerable mass effect (probably a glioblastoma—arrows) to be the cause of symptoms. (Note the scan was done first without contrast, which was then given to clarify the picture.)

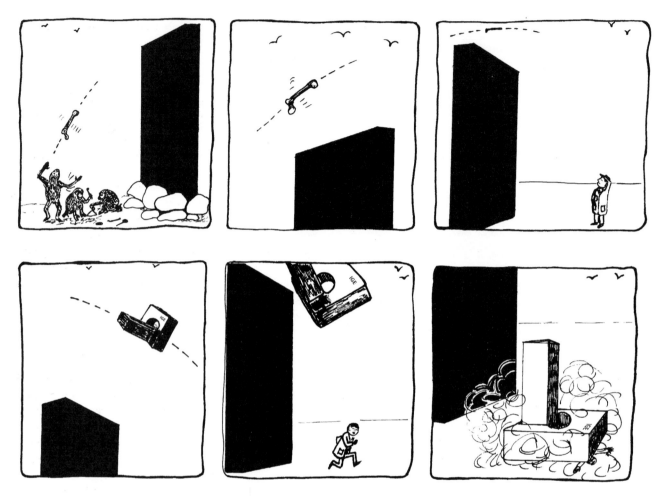

Figure 5.3 'Beware the double-edged sword of technology.' The cartoon depicts the evolution of the use of 'tools' from the dawn of man to the present day, but tools must be used with intelligence, otherwise our good intentions may backfire! (Adapted from *2001 Space Odyssey*, with apologies to Stanley Kubrick.)

distinction is either computerised tomography (CT) or magnetic resonance imaging (MRI) brain scanning (see Sections 5.3.3 and 5.3.6).

There are three issues to be considered in assessing the reliability of the clinical diagnosis of stroke: (i) there is the question of the diagnosis of stroke itself (i.e. is it a stroke or not?); (ii) whether the stroke is due to an infarct or a haemorrhage; and (iii) particularly in ischaemic stroke, the site and size of the lesion (i.e. anterior versus posterior circulation, lacunar versus cortical, etc.). The first and third of these have been discussed in Chapters 3 and 4 and will not be mentioned further here. The second is the basis for this chapter and requires the use of CT or MRI scanning. However, before proceeding further, there is one key point worth emphasising which underpins the use of imaging tests generally: it is essential for the correct conduct of the radiological examination that the radiologist has all the relevant information, including time from symptom onset, relevant past history

and current background information; otherwise the investigation may not be conducted in the correct way to get the information required and misleading reports may be issued (Fig. 5.3).

> *For the correct conduct and interpretation of diagnostic imaging, give the radiologist all the relevant information, especially: how long ago the stroke occurred; any previous strokes; the clinical features of this stroke; history of malignant disease; and any concurrent illnesses (e.g. renal failure, infection).*

With respect to stroke, it is occasionally difficult to differentiate a tumour from an infarct or partially resolved haematoma on the initial scan: haematomas may mimic tumours radiologically at certain phases in their evolution (see Section 5.3.4), and tumours may mimic infarcts (see Fig. 5.2) (Cameron, 1994). Therefore, it may be necessary to re-scan the patient after several weeks, when vascular lesions and tumours can usually be distinguished by the different pattern of their evolution with time.

5.3.1 Clinical scoring methods

Having made the clinical diagnosis of stroke, the next step is to decide which of the two main pathologies is responsible, infarct or intracerebral haemorrhage. How good is the clinical distinction between the two? In the past, the clinical features considered typical of PICH were caused by very large intraparenchymal and intraventricular haemorrhages and SAHs—for example, drowsiness and severe headache. When CT scanning became available, it was soon clear that many smaller PICHs were not associated with these 'typical' features. Therefore, a number of clinical scoring systems were devised specifically to differentiate PICH from infarction, for use when CT scanning was less available than it is now: the Allen (1983) and the Siriraj (Pounguarin et al., 1991) scores and a recent method suggested by Besson et al. (1995). Although these systems do increase clinical diagnostic accuracy, prospective studies have shown that, even in patients with a low probability (<10%) of cerebral haemorrhage on the basis of these scores, at least 7% (with the Allen) and 5% (with the Siriraj) of patients actually had an intracerebral haemorrhage on brain CT (Celani et al., 1992, 1994; Lindley et al., 1993; Weir et al., 1994; Hawkins et al., 1995). Thus, even with a complex and fairly time-consuming clinical scoring method used by physicians experienced in stroke, and even in patients with the lowest probability of haemorrhage, the clinical differentiation of ischaemic stroke from haemorrhage will still be wrong, importantly wrong, in up to 10% of patients. It is likely that less experienced clinicians would

be wrong even more often. For example, Fig. 5.4 shows a patient who had less than a 5% chance of haemorrhage using the Siriraj score, but brain CT showed a thalamic haematoma as the cause of the stroke.

No clinical scoring method can absolutely reliably differentiate ischaemic stroke from primary intracerebral haemorrhage. To do this, brain CT or MRI is required.

Therefore, the problem with these scoring systems is that they miss small PICHs, and these are often in the very patients in whom the distinction of PICH from infarct is most important. Although it may be acceptable to rely on the scores in some circumstances, for example in some aspects of epidemiological work—although this was debated by Hawkins et al. (1995)—and to speed randomisation in some acute stroke treatment trials, it may not be in others (e.g. prior to anticoagulant treatment). CT and MRI are the only methods of reliably distinguishing infarct from haemorrhage (see Sections 5.3.3 and 5.3.6).

5.3.2 Cerebrospinal fluid (CSF) examination

Examination of the CSF is clearly important in suspected SAH (see Section 5.5.3), but to differentiate ischaemic stroke from PICH it is both a complete waste of time and even occasionally dangerous when there is a possibility of raised intracranial pressure. In the pre-CT era, CSF examination was more widely used in the diagnosis of all kinds of neurological diseases for which there are now much better diagnostic tests. Abnormalities of the CSF cell and protein contents do occur following ischaemic stroke and PICH, but they are so unreliable and non-specific as to be probably worse than relying on clinical features to make the distinction (Fishman, 1992).

Examination of the cerebrospinal fluid is useless to differentiate ischaemic stroke from primary intracerebral haemorrhage.

5.3.3 CT scanning

The earliest reports of brain CT scanning in cerebrovascular disease quickly showed how valuable it was for differentiating between cerebral haemorrhage and infarction (and other pathologies, such as tumours) as the cause of acute focal neurological symptoms. Ambrose (1973) stated that 'in the overall investigation of cerebrovascular disease, computerised tomography will, without doubt, come to be an invaluable means of distinguishing between haemorrhage and infarction.' In 1974 Paxton and Ambrose reported positive CT findings in all 66 patients with intracranial haemorrhage and in 27 of 55 patients with cerebral infarction, and

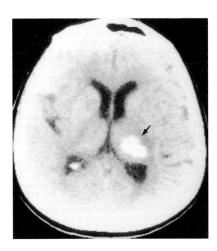

Figure 5.4 CT brain scan of a patient presenting within 24 hours of a stroke, who had less than a 5% chance of having a PICH (by the Siriraj score). The CT brain scan shows a primary thalamic haemorrhage (arrow) to be the cause of the stroke.

observed density changes in the evolution of the infarcted brain tissue (Paxton & Ambrose, 1974). Kistler *et al.* (1975) and Kinkel and Jacobs (1976) reported CT scans of 111 patients with stroke. The quality of scans was poor by today's standards: pixels were large, scan times slow and processing algorithms less sophisticated, all of which limited the visualisation of small infarcts and of subtle changes in the early stages of larger infarcts. However, they found that virtually all patients with a permanent neurological deficit had a defect in the appropriate area on brain CT, whereas patients with transient ischaemic attacks (TIAs) did not. They also noted mass effect in the early stages of large cerebral infarcts, which, as a result, could be confused with cerebral tumours. In 43% of patients whose scan showed PICH, the clinical diagnosis had been acute ischaemic stroke and the haemorrhage would not have been diagnosed without CT. This was one of the first indications of how unreliable clinical criteria are in differentiating infarct from haemorrhage.

CT brain scan technique for stroke

A standard brain CT consists of axial images through the whole brain, starting at the skull base and ending at the vertex, at 1.0-cm intervals. This usually produces about 10 sequential images. The slices may be contiguous or overlapping or leave gaps of a few millimetres in between, depending on the age of the scanner. A state-of-the-art mid-1980s scanner performed 10 slices through the whole brain and produced the images in about 10 minutes. A modern mid-1990s spiral CT scanner will produce the same set of images in about 20 seconds. Images can be done at narrower intervals to show fine detail, or in different planes of section to avoid bone artefacts, and at very fast scan speeds to reduce motion artefact. With modern scanners being so fast, there is a great temptation to 'do a few extra slices' or to do brain scans more readily, but it should be noted that an average brain CT scan exposes the patient to the equivalent of 1 year of average background radiation (Royal College of Radiologists, 1995). Pregnancy is a relative contraindication to brain CT; it can be done when necessary with careful shielding of the abdomen. Intravenous contrast may be given to help clarify lesions, but generally it is not required in the investigation of stroke and may cause diagnostic confusion. It is much better to do a non-enhanced scan first; contrast may be used afterwards if necessary.

> *A simple routine brain scan, i.e. about 10 slices through the whole brain at 1-cm intervals without intravenous contrast, is usually all that is required for acute stroke. This will exclude primary intracerebral haemorrhage, although it may not show the site of any infarction.*

The availability of CT scanning varies, depending on local numbers of scanners and practice. In areas where scanners are scarce, and so where the radiology department is very busy, a few simple manoeuvres may help smooth the path of the stroke patient to the CT scanner. Always inform the radiology department of the request for a scan as early as possible in the day; there is nothing more infuriating than being asked to do a scan at 4 PM when the patient has been languishing in the hospital since 8 AM. If the patient is immobile and can not transfer, send him/her on a trolley; if dependent and the radiology department has few nurses, which applies to most, then send a nurse escort to look after the patient whilst in the scanning department. Good communication between clinician and radiologist helps their interdependent relationship enormously. Feedback to the radiologist on what has happened to patients is always appreciated.

5.3.4 The appearance of primary intracerebral haemorrhage (PICH) on brain CT

Recent haemorrhage

Acute parenchymatous haemorrhage is of higher density than normal brain parenchyma, typically about 80 Hounsfield units (HU) compared with 35 HU (Figs 5.4 & 5.5). The density increase occurs, as far as we know, virtually immediately and is thought to be due to both the haemoglobin content and the matrix of the static blood (or clot). There have been a few reports of cerebral haemorrhages observed whilst the patient was in the CT scanner which confirm the immediacy of the change (Masson *et al.*, 1984; Francke *et al.*, 1990). As soon as blood stops moving, its density increases to appear 'whiter' on CT. This is true whether the blood is in the subarachnoid space, in the brain parenchyma or in an embolus or thrombus blocking a large intracranial artery (see Section 5.3.5).

The area of high attenuation is usually rather circumscribed (most often rounded or oval) and tends to be of homogeneous density (an exception being the appearance of a blood/fluid level in some large haematomas; see below). It is surrounded by a variable amount of low attenuation, caused by a combination of oedema and ischaemic necrosis of compressed brain. In addition to the increased density, intracerebral haematomas exert mass effect, depending on their size and site, compressing and damaging adjacent structures. If large, supratentorial haematomas cause herniation of the temporal lobe through the tentorial hiatus, with compression of vital brainstem structures, or of the ipsilateral parasagittal cortex under the falx, with compression of the ipsilateral and dilatation of the contralateral lateral ventricles (Fig. 5.5, and see Section 11.1.5).

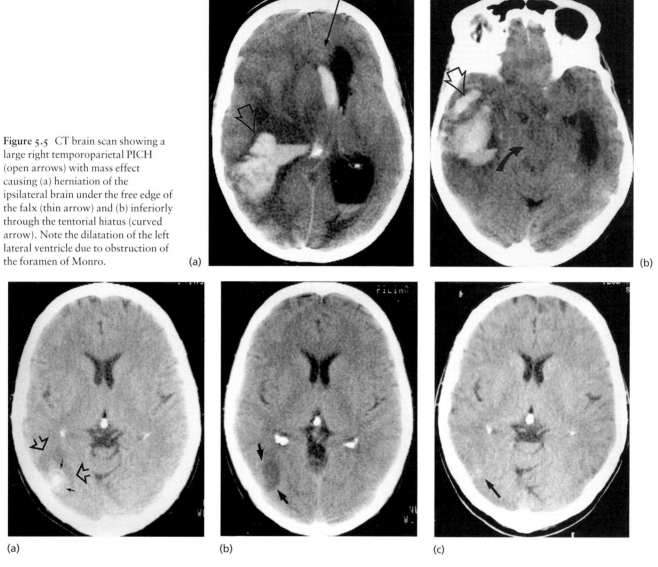

Figure 5.5 CT brain scan showing a large right temporoparietal PICH (open arrows) with mass effect causing (a) herniation of the ipsilateral brain under the free edge of the falx (thin arrow) and (b) inferiorly through the tentorial hiatus (curved arrow). Note the dilatation of the left lateral ventricle due to obstruction of the foramen of Monro.

(a)

(b)

(a)

(b)

(c)

Figure 5.6 Sequence showing the change in the appearance of haemorrhage on CT brain scan with time. (a) About 4 days after the stroke, there is a hyperdense lesion (fresh blood) in the right occipital cortex (small arrows) with surrounding hypodensity (open arrows) due to oedema. Scanning sooner after the stroke would have shown slightly more solid hyperdensity (but of similar size) but less hypodense rim (as it takes 1 day or so for the oedema to develop). Very fresh haemorrhage is seen in Figs 5.4 and 5.5. (b) About 3 weeks after the stroke, the hyperdensity has completely disappeared leaving a hypodense lesion (arrows) which could easily be mistaken for an infarct without the prior scan. (c) About 10 weeks after the stroke, the lesion has virtually vanished (arrow). The final diagnosis was PICH—cerebral angiography and follow-up scans failed to reveal any underlying structural cause. A larger haemorrhagic lesion would probably have left a residual 'hole' in the brain parenchyma of CSF density.

Haemorrhage in the brain is visible on CT immediately. It does not take a few hours to develop its distinct appearance.

Evolution in appearance of the haematoma with time

The density of the haematoma decreases with time due to the breakdown of haemoglobin, becoming isodense with brain within a few days to a few weeks, depending on its size, although it might still have mass effect (Fig. 5.6). Later it becomes hypodense, so that, on CT performed weeks to a few months after the stroke, the haematoma appears as a defect of CSF (i.e. water) density. At this late stage—in fact, at any stage beyond the time when the haematoma becomes isodense—a haematoma may look identical to an old infarct (Dennis *et al.*, 1987). The additional problem of distinguishing PICH and haemorrhagic transformation of an infarct (HTI) will be discussed below (see Section 5.4). Although large haematomas may remain visible for many weeks, small haematomas become hypodense more quickly, so to be sure of differentiating a haematoma from an infarct the CT scan should be performed as soon as possible, preferably within a few days of onset (Dennis *et al.*, 1987). This may not be practical in patients who are not admitted to hospital, but in any case scanning should be done as soon as it is practical.

Late appearance of the haematoma

After many months the process of haematoma resorption is complete and all that may be left is a small, slit-like cavity containing fluid of CSF density, or no abnormality at all (Sung & Chu, 1992; Bradley, 1994). Frequently there is also an *ex vacuo* effect, such as enlargement of the lateral ventricle or sulci adjacent to the site of the former haemorrhage. 'Pseudocalcification'—dotted or linear high density on brain CT—around the wall of the cavity has been described after large basal ganglia haematomas. This is thought to be due to visible deposition of haemosiderin and haematoidin (Sung & Chu, 1992). In a small proportion of patients, 'pseudocalcification' is the only visible evidence on late CT of previous haemorrhage. In some patients, one may simply see an *ex vacuo* effect without any cavity.

> *Brain CT must be done within a few days of the stroke, preferably within 24 hours, to exclude a parenchymal haemorrhage.*

Does intravenous contrast help?

The use of intravenous contrast in the acute phase can complicate rather than clarify matters, although it may be necessary if an arteriovenous malformation (AVM) or a haemorrhagic metastasis is suspected. In the first few days, contrast has very little effect on the appearance of the haematoma, even if an AVM is present, because the haematoma and its mass effect obliterate all visible signs of enhancement. Contrast can be useful if haemorrhage into a metastasis is suspected, because it might show up deposits elsewhere in the brain, not visible on the unenhanced scan, thus establishing the diagnosis. After about 1 week, ring

enhancement around the haematoma can be seen, very similar to the enhancement around tumours and abscesses (Fig. 5.7). Follow-up CT with contrast, preferably after any mass effect has settled, may be of value in showing tumours or cryptic vascular malformations, but MRI is more sensitive and specific (see Section 5.3.6).

Do all haemorrhages show up on CT?

Given a relatively artefact-free scan, all haemorrhages of sufficient volume to cause a clinically apparent stroke will be visualised, assuming that the CT scan was done within the correct time frame, as discussed above. A recent paper describing a small series of anaemic patients has suggested that, despite the concern that haematomas might not look 'white' on CT because of their reduced haemoglobin content, in practice it is likely that they are all readily visible (Pierce *et al.*, 1994). The most difficult area of the brain in which to see haemorrhage is in the posterior fossa, because of frequent bone artefacts. Additional thin sections at 0.5-cm slice intervals, instead of the standard 1.0 cm, may be helpful.

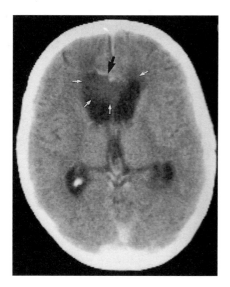

Figure 5.7 CT brain scan of a patient who presented with a 2-week history of confusion, and some headache. The CT scan shows a hypodense mass in the right frontal lobe and corpus callosum (white arrows), which showed some enhancement with intravenous contrast (black arrow) and was interpreted as being a tumour. However, a biopsy showed only features of resolving haemorrhage, and a subsequent angiogram demonstrated the underlying anterior communicating artery aneurysm. The right frontal mass was simply a 2-week old haematoma, showing how rapidly even quite sizeable haematomas can lose their 'whiteness' on CT.

Is there any underlying cause of the haematoma?

The underlying cause may sometimes be inferred (traumatic, aneurysmal, AVM, or into a tumour, or an arterial or venous HTI) from the extent, site and distribution of blood and any associated features (see Section 8.9.2). A recent study suggested that a fluid-blood level in an acute intracerebral haematoma on CT occurs more frequently in patients with a coagulopathy, but the study was retrospective; furthermore, the interpretation of a fluid-blood level must partly depend on the age of the haematoma, because in our and others' experience many large haematomas go through a phase where there is a fluid level (Pfleger *et al.*, 1994).

Intraparenchymal haematomas secondary to aneurysm rupture are discussed in greater detail in Section 9.4.1. They occur in parts of the brain adjacent to the common sites of aneurysms, sometimes not in association with visible subarachnoid blood. Absence of subarachnoid blood might be because the patient was scanned late and the blood has cleared from the subarachnoid space, or because there was little leakage of blood into the subarachnoid space at the time of rupture. Typical sites include the inferomedial parts of the frontal lobes (anterior communicating artery aneurysm), the temporal or inferolateral parietal lobe (middle cerebral artery (MCA) aneurysm) and the cerebellar hemisphere (posterior inferior cerebellar artery aneurysm). In patients with an underlying AVM, abnormal arteries or areas of calcification close to or in the haematoma may be visible, although in the acute stage a large haematoma can obliterate all signs of the underlying AVM on CT, MRI and even catheter angiography. Follow-up imaging, once the haematoma and its mass effect have resolved, is required to demonstrate small AVMs (see Section 8.9.4).

Haemorrhage into a tumour is unusual but may be the presenting feature. Primary brain tumours associated (occasionally) with haemorrhage include glioblastoma, lymphoma, neuroblastoma, choroid plexus papilloma and meningioma. Secondary brain tumours presenting with haemorrhage are more frequent, although still relatively rare, and include melanoma, choriocarcinoma and thyroid, renal, lung and breast carcinoma. Multiple, mainly peripheral, haemorrhages in a patient with an appropriate past history, and with contrast enhancement, should suggest the diagnosis. *Multiple haematomas* can also occur in amyloid angiopathy and intracranial venous thrombosis (see Sections 5.3.5 and 8.2.5). It should be said that 'unusual' causes of PICH are being increasingly recognised and, with more experience, we should be able to identify more of these on imaging.

Amyloid angiopathy. Haemorrhage due to amyloid angiopathy tends to be large, rather patchy and diffuse, have a fluid level and occur in multiple sites, either simultaneously or sequentially (Fig. 5.8). The haematoma is typically peripheral, i.e. involves the cortex, and may break through on to the surface of the brain. The patients tend to be elderly, but we have seen pathologically proved amyloid angiopathy in patients in their 50s (see Section 8.2.3).

Cerebral venous occlusive disease will be discussed in more detail below (see Sections 5.3.5 and 8.2.5) and can present as lesions which are mainly haemorrhagic. Deep bilateral haematomas occur in deep cerebral vein occlusion. Cortical haematomas with finger-like structures and surrounding low density with excessive mass effect occur in cortical vein thrombosis. Both may occur with or without signs of sinus thrombosis, such as the 'empty delta sign' (Figs 5.9 & 5.10).

5.3.5 The appearance of ischaemic stroke on brain CT

Early CT signs of infarction

In the first decade of CT, infarct visibility was limited by the technology. Campbell *et al.* (1978) examined 141 patients admitted to hospital with acute ischaemic stroke as soon after the onset as possible, and again 7-days later, and com-

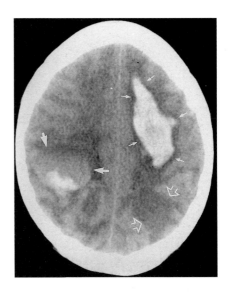

Figure 5.8 CT brain scan showing typical features of cerebral amyloid angiopathy. There are at least three different haematomas in different parts of the brain (left frontoparietal, right parietal and left occipital lobes) all of different ages (small arrows, thick arrows and open arrows, respectively) (see also Fig. 8.6).

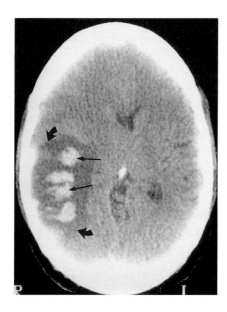

Figure 5.9 CT brain scan of a right parietal cortical venous infarct taken within 6 hours of the onset of symptoms. There is a well-defined hypodense lesion (curved arrows) affecting grey and white matter with some mass effect in the right parietal region. There are finger-like areas of haemorrhage in the centre of the lesion (thin arrows). Note also the rest of the right hemisphere appears slightly swollen, although is of normal density (note the midline shift) (see also Figs 5.10 & 5.16).

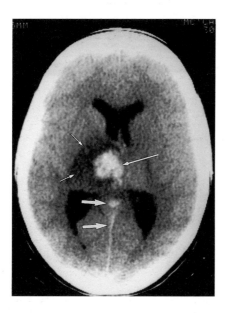

Figure 5.10 CT brain scan (unenhanced) showing a right thalamic haematoma (thin arrow) due to infarction secondary to a thrombosis of the deep cerebral veins. Note the increased density in the straight sinus (thick arrows) due to the thrombus in the sinus, and the general brain swelling, and low density around the haemorrhage (small arrows) indicating the venous infarct (see also Figs 5.9 & 5.16).

pared the results with radionuclide scanning. They found that more than 50% of the ischaemic lesions were detected on the first CT scan and 66% on the second scan, compared with 58% on radionuclide scanning (the only alternative non-invasive diagnostic tool available at the time). It was considered unusual to see changes of infarction on brain CT prior to 24–48 hours of onset, although occasional ischaemic lesions were seen as early as 3–6 hours (Inoue *et al.*, 1980; Wall *et al.*, 1982). More recently, with improved CT technology, subtle early signs of cerebral infarction have been recognised. Loss of visualisation of the insular ribbon and loss of outline of the lentiform nucleus have been reported within 3 hours of onset in ischaemic strokes of the basal ganglia, probably reflecting the increased sensitivity of modern scanners (Fig. 5.11; Tomura *et al.*, 1988; Truwit *et al.*, 1990). Loss of the normal grey–white-matter differentiation and effacement of the overlying cortical sulci are early signs of cortical infarction. Small infarcts probably appear later than large ones, because there is less tissue altering its density, so lacunar infarcts (LACIs) are less likely to show up in the first 24 hours and sometimes do not do so at all (see below) (Fig. 5.12) (Donnan *et al.*, 1982; Bamford *et al.*, 1987; Bonke *et al.*, 1989; Lindgren *et al.*, 1994). Small infarcts in the brainstem and cerebellum are particularly difficult to visualise with CT because of artefacts arising from the petrous bones; this is probably less problematic with modern scanning technology and thinner scan sections (Savoiardo, 1986).

Hyperdense artery sign is another early, indirect, sign of ischaemic stroke (Fig. 5.13). It represents the visualisation of acute large cerebral artery occlusion as an increased density in the artery (see Section 6.6.3; Gacs *et al.*, 1982; Yang *et al.*, 1990, Bastianello *et al.*, 1991; Leys *et al.*, 1992). However, the reliability of this sign is uncertain. It may be valid in young patients, in whom the arteries tend to be less calcified, but elderly patients frequently have calcified artery walls, particularly around the carotid siphon, which may produce a similar appearance; evidence of calcification persists on rescanning, but not the hyperdense artery sign, which disappears in a few days. In one series of 36 acute ischaemic stroke patients presenting within 4 hours of the onset of MCA territory stroke, the hyperdense artery sign was present in 50% of the occlusions proved on angiography done within 6 hours of onset (Bastianello *et al.*, 1991). In a larger series of 272 consecutive patients with first-ever stroke CT-scanned within 12 hours of symptom onset, Leys *et al.* (1992) found a hyperdense MCA in 73 (27%) patients, which was 41% of those with an MCA territory infarct. The sign was not dependent on cerebrovascular risk factors and was more likely to occur in cortical and large, deep MCA infarcts. It

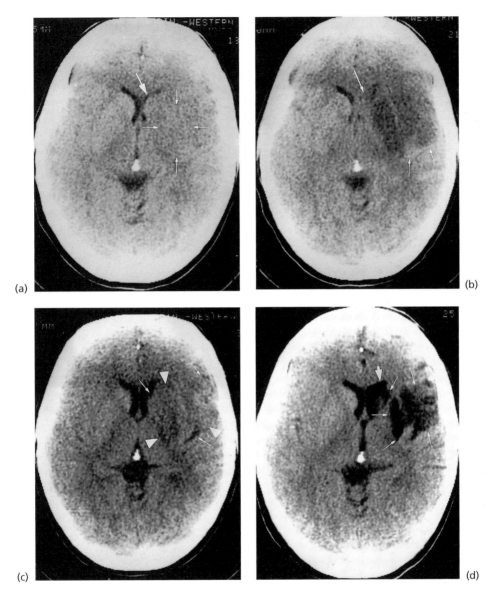

Figure 5.11 Sequence of CT brain scans to demonstrate the evolution of the appearance of a left MCA infarct with time. (a) At 3 hours after the stroke, there is loss of visibility of the normal basal ganglia and insular cortex (thin arrows indicate where the outline should be—compare with the right basal ganglia which are clearly seen), slight swelling seen as slight compression of the frontal horn of the left lateral ventricle (thick arrow). (b) At 3 days the infarct is more hypodense and clearly demarcated and swollen. There is complete effacement of the left lateral ventricle (thin arrow) and small areas of increased density at the infarct margins suggest petechial haemorrhage (small arrows). The latter may not be seen—the infarct may simply appear uniformly hypodense with very distinct sharp margins at this stage. Note that the infarct is wedge-shaped and involves cortex and adjacent white matter. (c) At 2 weeks the swelling has subsided (the frontal horn of the lateral ventricle and the cortical sulci are clearly seen—arrows), the hypodensity has nearly gone and the lesion has similar density to normal brain due to the 'fogging' effect (see Fig. 5.14). At this stage the lesion can be almost impossible to see despite being a sizeable infarct. Arrowheads indicate the margins of the infarct. (d) At 3 months the lesion is a shrunken, CSF-containing hole (arrows). The surrounding normal structures show an *ex vacuo* effect—the frontal horn of the left lateral ventricle has expanded to take up space vacated by the damaged brain (arrowhead).

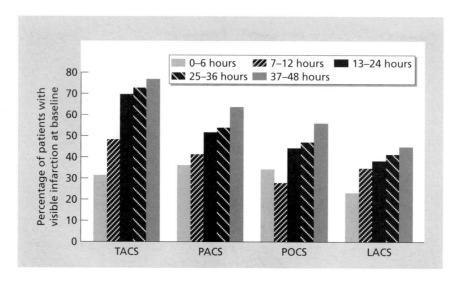

Figure 5.12 Data from the First International Stroke Trial showing the effect of time and stroke clinical syndrome on the visibility of infarcts on CT scanning. The visibility of infarcts increases with time over the first 2 days from the onset of the stroke, and the larger the infarct the more often it is visible (i.e. total anterior circulation syndrome (TACS) infarcts show up more than lacunar syndrome (LACS), etc.). PACS, partial anterior circulation syndrome; POCS, posterior circulation syndrome. (The figure was prepared by Dr Paul Dorman, Western General Hospital, Edinburgh.)

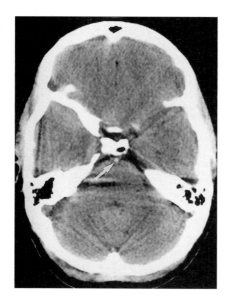

Figure 5.13 An unenhanced CT brain scan from a 28-year-old woman presenting with features of a large brainstem stroke, obtained within 6 hours of onset. The basilar artery is hyperdense indicating that it is thrombosed (arrow). There is a suggestion of some low density in the pons with effacement of the fourth ventricle indicating a pontine infarct, but the appearance is subtle. MRI confirmed a large pontine infarct.

was not an independent predictor for poor outcome; 20% of the patients with the sign recovered within 2 weeks. It disappeared within a few days and was always related to an

occlusion of the MCA in patients who had angiography, giving a specificity of 100% but a sensitivity of only 30%. It has also been associated with larger infarcts (Tomsick *et al.*, 1990). However, others have found the hyperdense artery sign in only 5% of patients with acute cerebral infarction (Yang *et al.*, 1990). Hankey *et al.* (1988) described a hyperdense basilar artery in four patients with posterior circulation strokes.

All of these studies were in hospital-admitted patients, who were therefore more likely to have had a 'severe' stroke. In community-based studies, it is likely that the hyperdense artery sign is much less frequent. Therefore, the hyperdense artery sign is probably a reasonably reliable indicator of an occluded cerebral artery when the hyperdensity is visible at a distance from the carotid siphon, e.g. in the proximal MCA or its branches, and particularly in younger patients. An absent sign is certainly not a reliable indicator of a patent artery.

Evolution of the CT appearance of infarction

Evolution of the CT appearance of infarction is illustrated in Fig. 5.11. Initially, the lesion has ill-defined margins and slight swelling and is somewhat hypodense compared with normal brain. The infarct becomes more clearly demarcated and hypodense during the first few days (Hakim *et al.*, 1983; Skriver *et al.*, 1990). The swelling is usually maximal around the third to fifth days and this gradually subsides during the second and third week (Clasen *et al.*, 1980; Terent *et al.*,

1981; Hakim *et al.*, 1983; Skriver *et al.*, 1990; Wardlaw *et al.*, 1993). However, occasionally infarct swelling can occur very rapidly, within the first 24 hours, to cause brain herniation, generally with very extensive infarcts. The amount of infarct swelling and the rate at which it appears vary between patients, for reasons which are not understood. On balance, swelling is most apparent in large infarcts but presumably also occurs in small ones, although it is difficult to see and is probably clinically less important. Extensive infarct swelling may compress adjacent normal brain and cause herniation (see Section 11.1.5). The presence of recent haemorrhage in the infarct produces areas of increased density relative to both normal brain and the infarcted tissue, and presumably contributes to any swelling (see Section 5.4).

Fogging. During the second week the infarct gradually increases in density, sometimes becoming isodense, so that it is indistinguishable from normal brain. This is the so-called 'fogging effect' and without close inspection even quite sizeable infarcts may be overlooked (see Figs 5.11 & 5.14). The 'fogging effect' may make the infarct impossible to see on CT scans done at this time. It is less pronounced in large infarcts, but may lead to underestimation of infarct size. It does not occur in all infarcts and the rate of occurrence varies between reports. Skriver and Olsen (1981) observed it in 54% of cases scanned 10 days after onset, whereas Becker *et al.* (1979) found it at some time in all

cases examined with six consecutive CT scans within 42 days of stroke. The 'fogging effect' may last for up to 2 weeks and then the infarct becomes progressively more hypodense.

Eventually a sharply demarcated, atrophic, hypodense (similar to CSF) defect remains (see Fig. 5.11). Although old infarcts usually have sharply demarcated borders, it is not possible to tell with certainty how old an infarct is, something that is often overlooked when ascribing particular clinical symptoms to lesions seen on CT.

Effect of intravenous contrast

In the first 4–6 days, intravenous X-ray contrast has very little effect on the appearance of an infarct (Wing *et al.*, 1976; Davis *et al.*, 1977); but, in the second and third weeks contrast enhancement occurs, frequently corresponding with the time of maximal blood–brain barrier breakdown and positivity of radioisotope scans (Inoue *et al.*, 1980; Pullicino & Kendall, 1980). The mechanism is probably a combination of blood–brain barrier breakdown, neovascularisation and impaired autoregulation (Sage, 1982). The enhancement can be very marked in children and young adults (Fig. 5.15). Hayman *et al.* (1981) suggested that early prominent contrast enhancement in large infarcts correlated strongly with massive haemorrhagic transformation later in the course of the infarct. They suggested that this was due to severe early vasogenic oedema; however, most of their patients had large

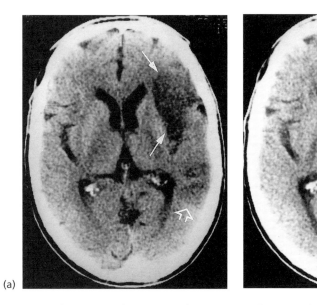

(a)

(b)

Figure 5.14 CT brain scans to demonstrate 'fogging'. (a) Obtained 3 days after onset of a right hemiparesis showing an obvious infarct (hypodense area) in the left parietal cortex and adjacent white matter (arrow). The patient had also had a stroke 2-years previously, seen as the small hypodense area in the posterior left temporal region (open arrow). (b) Obtained at 14 days after onset. The recent infarct in the anterior left parietal region is almost invisible—it is now mainly isodense with normal brain and there is no mass effect—due to 'fogging'.

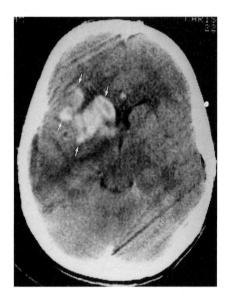

Figure 5.15 CT brain scan (with intravenous contrast) obtained at 10 days after a right basal ganglia infarct in a 10-year-old girl. There is marked serpiginous enhancement of the infarct (arrows) attributed to breakdown of the blood–brain barrier and 'luxury perfusion'.

infarcts with a poor prognosis and were therefore probably more likely to develop haemorrhagic transformation anyway (Lodder, 1984; see Section 5.4). The tendency to enhance with contrast gradually resolves over the following few weeks. It has been suggested that stroke patients deteriorate as a result of intravenous contrast, although the relationship was not statistically significant (Kendall & Pullicino, 1980). It is certainly possible that extravasation of neurotoxic contrast agents could be harmful, but the majority of patients described in the paper had large infarcts with a poor prognosis in any case. Fortunately, in practice, it is rarely necessary to give intravenous contrast as a diagnostic aid.

Is early infarct visibility on CT important?

The significance of visualisation of decreased density in the ischaemic tissue in the very early phase within a few hours of stroke onset is uncertain. It has been suggested that early visualisation may indicate more profound ischaemia. For example, Higano *et al.* (1990), using positron emission tomography (PET) scanning in nine stroke patients with MCA occlusion, found that the hypodensity on CT corresponded with the areas of brain with the lowest cerebral blood flow. Also, there is accumulating evidence that early visualisation of an infarct may carry a worse prognosis than if the patient had the same neurological deficit with no

infarct visible. In the American Nimodipine Study, a *post hoc* analysis showed that a subgroup with no infarct visible on their pre-treatment CT scan had a better outcome than those with a visible infarct, although the 'blindness' of the CT review is not clear (American Nimodipine Study Group, 1992). In the European Cooperative Acute Stroke Study (ECASS), there was a suggestion that patients with an infarct visible on their pre-randomisation CT scan done within 6 hours of the stroke onset had a worse prognosis than those with a normal CT scan, but, as the review of the scans was not blind to subsequent scans, it is difficult to exclude bias (Hacke *et al.*, 1995). von Kummer *et al.* (1994) found that early infarct visibility in patients with angiographically proved MCA occlusion was associated with a much worse clinical outcome than patients without early hypodensity. In the International Stroke Trial (IST), patients with an infarct visible on their CT scan done within 48 hours of the stroke onset had a worse prognosis than those with a normal scan and the same clinical stroke syndrome (see Fig. 5.12) (IST Collaborative Group, 1995). On multiple regression analysis, early infarct visibility was an independent adverse prognostic variable, despite quite a lot of 'noise' in the data collection (partly due to the scans not being reviewed centrally). Therefore, it seems likely that early infarct visibility indicates a profound depth of ischaemia, which in turn indicates a marked drop in blood flow to a largish area of brain, which in turn suggests that the outcome will be poor.

Appearances of established infarction: can we infer anything about the cause of the infarct?

A typical established large artery infarct is wedge-shaped, of decreased density compared with normal brain and sharply demarcated and occupies a recognisable vascular territory (Damasio, 1983; Savoiardo, 1986). LACIs, thought to arise from occlusion of a single perforating artery (see Section 6.3), are less than 1.5 cm in diameter, usually rounded in shape and sited in the deep white matter, basal ganglia and pons (Donnan *et al.*, 1982; Bamford *et al.*, 1987; Bamford & Warlow, 1988; Bonke *et al.*, 1989). Boundary-zone infarcts lie in areas of the brain at the edges of the large artery vascular territories, i.e. in the parieto-occipital region for the MCA/posterior cerebral artery and over the vertex for the anterior cerebral artery/MCA boundary zone, or in the internal boundary zone at the junction of the deep and superficial arterial supply areas (Damasio, 1983; Torvik, 1984; Graeber *et al.*, 1992). However, the boundary-zone areas have recently been shown to be potentially more extensive than previously thought, and very variable between and within individuals (see Sections 4.3.4 and 6.5.5; van der Zwan & Hillen, 1991). Therefore, in any individual patient, it is very difficult to decide from brain imaging whether an infarct has arisen from occlusion of a cortical branch of the MCA, which might be embolic, or from poor perfusion due to an internal carotid artery occlusion (Graeber *et al.*, 1992; Lang *et al.*, 1995).

Striatocapsular infarcts are larger than lacunes and occur in the deep white matter and basal ganglia, with preservation of the overlying cortex (see Sections 4.3.2 and 6.6.3). They are thought to arise from transient occlusion of the MCA main stem, prolonged occlusion of the MCA main stem with good cortical collaterals or occlusion of multiple lenticulostriate artery origins from atheroma of the MCA (Weiller *et al.*, 1990; Angeloni *et al.*, 1991; Donnan *et al.*, 1991). These patterns are illustrated in Fig. 6.14.

How often is an appropriate infarct visible on CT?

In the study by Lindgren *et al.* (1994), an appropriate infarct was seen in 43% of patients with a LACI scanned within 2 days of onset, rising to 75% when scanned more than 16 days after the stroke. The corresponding figures for total anterior circulation infarct (TACI), partial anterior circulation infarct (PACI) and posterior circulation infarct (POCI) patients scanned within 2 days were 44%, 41% and 43%, and more than 16 days were 55%, 64% and 56%, respectively. The proportion of TACI patients with a visible infarct was perhaps rather low in their study compared with others, including our own (Wardlaw *et al.*, 1996), but the principle of increasing infarct visibility with interval from stroke onset is well demonstrated. In the IST, infarct visibility increased with time from onset in the first 48 hours (see Fig. 5.12) and the highest proportion of patients with visible infarction was in the TACI group. In general, the greater the volume of infarcted tissue, the more often the infarct is visible on CT scanning. It is uncertain just how many patients with a clinically definite stroke *never* have an appropriate infarct visible on brain CT, but the proportion is probably quite high (up to 50%) and depends on the timing of the scan, the age of the scanner, the thickness of the slices, the cooperation of the patient, the size and age of the infarct, the vigilance and interest of the radiologist and possibly some pathophysiological characteristic of the lesion itself. However, the main reason for doing the scan is to exclude a haemorrhage (or a tumour or infection) as the cause of the symptoms, and if the scan is normal the presumptive diagnosis is of ischaemic stroke.

> *Brain CT only shows the relevant infarct in 50–60% of patients with an ischaemic stroke. Absence of a visible infarct does not mean that the patient has not had a stroke.*

How well do the clinical and CT diagnoses of lesion site correspond?

The site of the lesion on brain CT correlates relatively well with the clinical syndrome (Manelfe *et al.*, 1981; Damasio, 1983; Saito *et al.*, 1987; Zeumer & Ringelstein, 1987; Anderson *et al.*, 1994; Lindgren *et al.*, 1994; Wardlaw *et al.*, 1995). The MCA territory is the most frequently involved on CT (60%), followed by the posterior cerebral artery (14%), the anterior cerebral artery (5%), the posterior fossa (5%) and the multiple territories or boundary zones (14%) (Savoiardo *et al.*, 1996). There are now at least three published studies comparing stroke syndrome defined clinically, using the OCSP classification, with the site of the infarct as demonstrated by cross-sectional imaging (see Section 4.4.11; Anderson *et al.*, 1994; Lindgren *et al.*, 1994; Wardlaw *et al.*, 1996). In each study, there was reasonable agreement between the clinical and CT diagnosis of lesion site. In the Perth study, the allocation of the stroke clinical syndrome was made retrospectively from the patients' notes and then compared with the lesion site shown by CT or at postmortem (Anderson *et al.*, 1994). This may have introduced errors in the clinical diagnosis. In the other two studies, the stroke clinical syndrome was allocated prospectively and therefore the results may be more reliable. In each study, a proportion of the patients had, of course, 'normal' imaging— that is, the imaging did not show an appropriate recent infarct — and these cases were analysed differently. In the Perth study, about one-third of the PACI, LACI and POCI patients did not show a relevant lesion on CT, and these scans were not included in the assessment of the accuracy of the clinical diagnosis of lesion site (Anderson *et al.*, 1994). Lindgren *et al.* (1994) used multiple CT and MRI scans at different times after the stroke and so had fewer patients whose scan did not show a relevant lesion, but it is not clear how they were accounted for in the analysis. It is unlikely that any imaging technique, no matter how sophisticated, will ever be able to demonstrate *all* infarcts, even though, for example, T2-weighted MRI can demonstrate areas of altered signal in the appropriate area of the brain after as brief an insult as a TIA (Hommel *et al.*, 1994). The problem for comparative studies of imaging (and pathology) with the clinical diagnosis of lesion site is what to do with the 'normal' or 'inappropriate' scans. Should they be discounted from the study and only scans which show a recent lesion included? In that case, a false estimate of the accuracy of the clinical diagnosis might arise, either falsely high or falsely low, because the 'normal' scans, had they shown a lesion, might have displayed it in a different part of the brain from that predicted clinically (e.g. a small deep white-matter infarct instead of a predicted cortical infarct in a PACI patient). Therefore, including the 'normal' scans in the analysis is important, and the result can be expressed as the 'best' and 'worst' possible agreement; in the former, one assumes that all the patients with normal scans had a lesion in the area predicted clinically and, in the latter, one assumes that the lesion is elsewhere.

In studies of stroke lesion site, diagnosed clinically versus radiologically and which have used other classifications, the level of agreement between clinician with pin and tendon hammer and radiologist with scanner has been no better (Bamford, 1992). For example, in the Stroke Data Bank, a classification was used based on the likely pathophysiological cause of the stroke, i.e. large artery atherosclerosis, lacunar, cardiac embolism, tandem arterial pathology, infarct of unknown origin, or other. This classification was heavily dependent on the use of imaging, despite which it proved impossible to allocate a likely mechanism for the stroke in 40% of patients (Sacco *et al.*, 1989). In the National Institute of Neurological Diseases and Stroke (NINDS) classification, with subdivisions according to the pathological mechanism, the clinical category and the arterial distribution, numerous assumptions must be made for which there is no good evidence; for example, that cardioembolic strokes are of exceptionally rapid onset and not preceded by TIAs (Kittner *et al.*, 1990). The Trial of ORG 10172 in Acute Stroke Therapy (TOAST) Trial classification, which divides strokes into atherothromboembolic, cardioembolic, small vessel thrombotic, other and unknown, found that the initial clinical classification agreed with the final diagnosis after diagnostic tests in only 65%, and 15% of patients remained without a clear stroke subtype identification (Madden *et al.*, 1994). Finding a potential source of embolism does not mean that it was the cause of the stroke, and in a significant proportion of patients there is more than one potential cause (see Section 6.7). Thus, the problem is compounded rather than simplified by using a complex classification, and the problem of 'normal' scans has not been surmounted by using multiple imaging modalities.

Distinction of arterial infarcts from other pathologies on CT

Whilst many infarcts arising from arterial occlusion are easy to diagnose from their site, shape, density and appropriate clinical features, other pathologies can occasionally produce very similar appearances, which may be confusing.

Venous infarcts (see Section 8.2.5) are uncommon and frequently misdiagnosed as arterial infarcts, intracerebral haemorrhages or tumours on CT. However, in our experience there are often clues which should point to the correct diagnosis. Many are overlooked simply because the pos-

sibility of venous infarction is not even considered (Table 5.1). Cerebral venous disease consists of a spectrum, varying from the effects of sinus thrombosis, without any parenchymal change, at one extreme to purely parenchymal lesions, due to cortical vein thrombosis (infarction with or without haemorrhage) without sinus thrombosis, at the other end. The clinical presentation and radiological appearance in any individual patient depend on the balance of these components. Venous infarcts can usefully be thought of in two parts: the primary features of the parenchymal lesion, and the secondary features of sinus thrombosis, which may or may not be present. Venous infarcts are typically of low density and may be wedge-shaped, like arterial infarcts, but the key differentiating features are that: they often do not quite fit the usual site of an arterial infarct; they are much more swollen for their size than an equivalent-sized arterial infarct; there may be swelling in the hemisphere beyond the low-density area; and they often contain haemorrhage (Fig. 5.16) (Virapongse *et al.*, 1987; Perkin, 1995). The haemorrhage is typically in the centre of the low-density area and may be patchy and finger-like in distribution (see Fig. 5.10), whereas in arterial infarcts the haemorrhage is usually around the edges. The high density of a thrombosed cortical vein or sinus may also be visible. After intravenous contrast, there may be an 'empty delta' sign in the venous sinus and serpiginous enhancement at the edges of the infarct (Fig. 5.17).

Table 5.1 Differentiation of arterial from venous infarcts.

	Arterial	Venous
Shape	Wedge or rounded	Usually wedge if cortical, rounded if deep
Number occurring simultaneously	Usually single	May be multiple
Density	Early: slightly hypodense Later: hypodense	Early obvious hypodensity
Margins	Indistinct early, distinct after several days	Distinct early
Swelling	Develops over days usually	Marked, appears very early
Haemorrhage	Infrequent, peripheral	Frequent, central finger-like
Additional signs	Hyperdense artery sign	Of venous *sinus* thrombosis

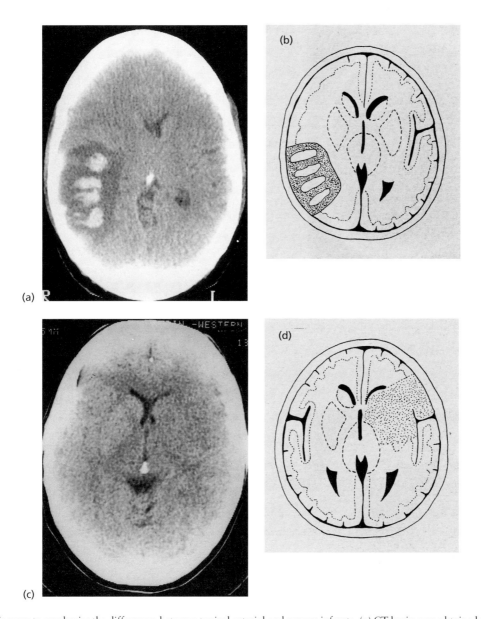

Figure 5.16 Diagram to emphasise the differences between typical arterial and venous infarcts. (a) CT brain scan obtained within 6 hours of symptom onset showing a right parietal venous infarct. (b) Drawing of (a) to emphasise the key features: the margins are clearly seen and the lesion is very hypodense even at such a short time after onset; there is marked swelling both within the infarct and within the rest of the hemisphere beyond the infarct; and there are central areas of haemorrhage. (c) CT brain scan obtained within 6 hours of symptom onset showing a left parietal arterial infarct. (d) Drawing of (c) to emphasise the key features: the margins are ill defined and the lesion is only slightly hypodense compared with normal brain; there is only slight swelling within the infarct and none beyond it; and there is no haemorrhage (see also Figs 5.9, 5.10 & 5.17).

Encephalitis, if relatively focal in distribution, can look exactly like an infarct, although this is rare. The typical appearance of encephalitis with involvement of the medial temporal lobes should not cause confusion, but we have seen patients with low-density areas in the temporoparietal region associated with rising herpes simplex titres, which resolved following treatment with acyclovir (Fig. 5.18). The

important message is that the radiology should be reviewed with all the clinical information and, if in doubt, other diagnostic tests must be done, such as an electroencophalogram (EEG) or MRI scan.

Cerebritis can look like an infarct, although the lesion is usually not wedge-shaped and involves more white matter than

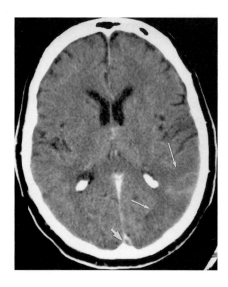

Figure 5.17 CT brain scan (enhanced) showing a left occipital venous infarct (thin arrows) with a thrombosis of the superior sagittal sinus as shown by the 'empty delta' sign (thick arrow) (see also Figs 5.9, 5.10 & 5.16).

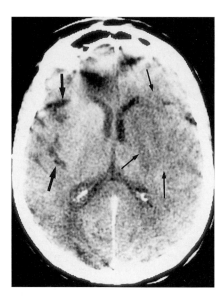

Figure 5.18 CT brain scan in a 70-year-old woman with a right hemiparesis, confusion and drowsiness, showing an extensive area of low density in the left temporoparietal region including the basal ganglia. The appearance is subtle, but there is loss of the outline of the normal basal ganglia (thin arrow) and loss of the overlying cortical sulci indicating slight swelling (compare with the easily seen right parietal sulci—short arrows). The initial clinical diagnosis was of a stroke (infarct), but 1-week later the patient deteriorated and the CT scan showed extensive haemorrhage in the left temporoparietal region. Subsequent autopsy confirmed the diagnosis of herpes simplex encephalitis.

cortex, and the clinical information should allow the distinction to be made.

Tumours. Occasionally, a peripheral metastasis with a lot of white-matter oedema can mimic an infarct on CT, although usually the density is lower than one would expect in an infarct, and administration of contrast may show up a cortical nodule (Fig. 5.19). If there is still doubt, a repeat CT a few weeks later will usually sort out the pathology, because infarcts and tumours evolve differently.

> *Time is a useful diagnostic tool. If in doubt whether a lesion is a tumour or infarct on CT, repeat the scan in a few weeks' time. Infarcts get smaller (usually), whereas tumours stay the same or get bigger.*

Interobserver variability in the analysis of CT scans of stroke patients

Interobserver reliability in reporting CT scans in patients with cerebrovascular disease has not been studied extensively. High levels of agreement (substantial to perfect) were demonstrated in a study of the interpretation of scans in patients with dementia and in another study of patients with stroke (Lee *et al.*, 1987; Shinar *et al.*, 1987). However, in the study by Shinar *et al.* (1987), all observers had free access to relevant clinical details, so their interpretation of the scan may have been biased. A study by Bonke *et al.* (1989), in which a group of neurologists and radiologists reviewed the same two CT brain scans from patients with a lacunar stroke (camouflaged by an assortment of other scans), accompanied by misleading clinical information, showed that the diagnosis of lacunar infarction did not appear to be biased by informing the observer that the patient was thought clinically to have had a stroke. The lack of bias with knowledge of clinical details may have been because the study was small and may not be a true reflection of the difficulties encountered in routine practice when faced with a CT scan showing multiple 'holes in the brain' and generalised atrophy. The first makes the diagnosis of recent lacunar infarction difficult, because it is impossible to decide which 'hole' is the relevant one unless serial scans show a new 'hole' developing, and the last makes the diagnosis of a small cortical infarct difficult (when is a large sulcus actually an infarct?). Interobserver reliability in the interpretation of site of infarction, amount of swelling in the acute stage and haemorrhagic transformation of medium to large infarcts was evaluated in a study by two experienced neuro-radiologists and six trainee radiologists, using a simple method of classifying stroke CT scans (Wardlaw & Sellar, 1994). The agreement was excellent between the two

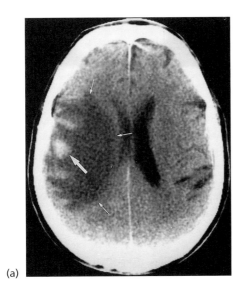
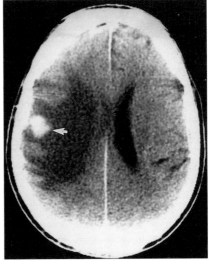

(a)
(b)

Figure 5.19 CT brain scan of a 60-year-old man who presented with a stroke obtained 2-days later showing a tumour which looks like an infarct. (a) Unenhanced scan shows an extensive right parietal low-density area (thin arrows) with a high-density area in the cortex (thick arrow). This could be misinterpreted as an area of haemorrhage, however. (b) Following intravenous contrast the cortical high-density area enhances (arrow) consistent with a tumour nodule. The low density is therefore all due to oedema. It was in fact a solitary secondary brain tumour, as a subsequent chest X-ray showed a previously undiagnosed primary bronchial carcinoma.

experienced neuroradiologists and good between the trainees and one of the experts. A further study of the effect of interobserver variability in the diagnosis of haemorrhagic transformation on CT showed good agreement for the diagnosis of infarct site and haematomas, but was less good for minor amounts of petechial haemorrhage (Rimdusid *et al.*, 1995). In this study, most of the scans showed small infarcts or were normal.

5.3.6 MRI

Historical note and practical points regarding use of MRI

MRI became a clinical tool in the early 1980s. The equipment is expensive, both to purchase and to run, and MRI was initially little used in acute stroke. It is not a practical technique for acutely ill patients; the patient must be placed inside a tube-like structure, which makes access for monitoring and administering anaesthetics difficult; the patient must lie still, usually for at least 5 minutes at a time, although recent fast scanning techniques now mean that diagnostic images may be acquired in seconds; and many acute stroke patients are confused, restless and frightened by the noise and vibration of the scanner, which is rather like being in the engine-room of a very large ship or like loud machine-gunfire. Despite faster image acquisition with modern scanners, the first-line investigation for stroke patients will prob-

ably continue to be CT in the immediate future, reserving MRI for 'difficult cases' and research. However, as MRI scanners become less expensive and more 'open-access', and therefore more user-friendly, their use will expand. The great advantages of MRI are not only its superior pathoanatomical cross-sectional imaging properties, but the same machine's ability to perform angiography and measure cerebral blood flow non-invasively; to provide diffusion and perfusion imaging and spectroscopy to elucidate mechanisms of brain damage in ischaemia and how experimental treatments might modify these; and, by functional imaging, to elucidate mechanisms of brain recovery.

Routine brain imaging with MRI

A routine MRI brain image consists of a midline sagittal localising view of the brain, usually T1-weighted, followed by axial T2 and either proton density or T1-weighted images covering the whole brain. It is well beyond the scope or intention of this chapter to describe the differences between these sequences, or indeed what they mean, but in simple terms it is useful to think of T2-weighted images as showing brain water content (so CSF and areas of oedema will show up as high-signal areas, i.e. white) and proton density and T1-weighted images as showing brain structure. Other MRI techniques are described briefly below.

Contraindications to MRI

All patients should be screened for MRI compatibility at MRI scanning departments before they enter the magnetic field, but the key contraindications will be mentioned here to help avoid inappropriate referrals: pacemakers, intracranial aneurysm clips and definite metallic intraocular foreign bodies. Metallic prostheses, foreign bodies other than in the eyes, some ventriculoperitoneal shunts, some artificial heart valves and first trimester of pregnancy are all relative contraindications which are useful for the MRI department to know about well in advance, so that the individual patient's circumstances can be checked (to see whether MRI scanning will be possible without undue risk) and to tailor the scan to the patient.

Appearance of haemorrhage on MRI

Appearance of haemorrhage on MRI is governed by the paramagnetic properties of haemoglobin breakdown products and so it changes with time (Bradley, 1994). Freshly extravasated red blood cells contain oxyhaemoglobin, which does not have any paramagnetic properties, so there may be little immediate signal change and, although a lesion may be visible, the differentiation from infarction is difficult within the first few hours. In practice currently, this is not a problem because so few patients are scanned very early and, even when they are, in our experience there has been enough signal change to make the distinction. Once enough deoxyhaemoglobin has formed (which takes about 24 hours), clear changes will be seen and the typical appearance is of a hypointense (dark) T1 image and a markedly hypointense (dark) T2 image. Within the first week, methaemoglobin is formed in the red cells and gradually the T1 image becomes hyperintense (bright), whilst the T2 image remains dark. Following this, as the methaemoglobin becomes extracellular and the haematoma liquefies, the T2 image becomes hyperintense (bright) as well as the T1 image. After several weeks, T2 images become bright in the centre with a very dark rim, and T1 images are bright centrally and moderately dark around the rim, and these changes presumably persist for life (Fig. 5.20). The exact timing and degree of these signal changes vary with the strength of the magnet, which compartment of the brain the haemorrhage lies in, abnormal haemostatic mechanisms, haematocrit and the exact scan sequence used (Bradley, 1994). There are sequences which are very sensitive to the presence of haemoglobin breakdown products, e.g. 'Flash2D' T2 (gradient

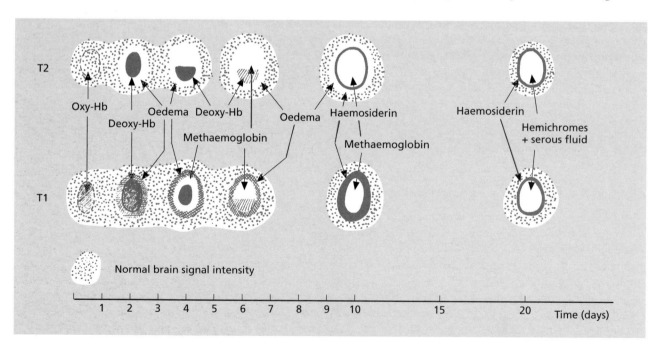

Figure 5.20 Diagram of the change in the appearance of parenchymal brain haemorrhage on MRI. The top row shows the typical appearance on T2-, and the lower row on T1-weighted imaging. The normal brain is represented by the stippled background. To a certain extent, the exact appearance and timing of the changes depends on the field strength of the magnet. The most important things to remember are that intracellular deoxyhaemoglobin (Deoxy-Hb) is dark on T1 and T2, methaemoglobin is bright on T1 and T2, and haemosiderin is dark on T1 and T2. Haemosiderin persists in the margins of a haematoma for years after the original haemorrhage. Oxy-Hb, oxyhaemoglobin.

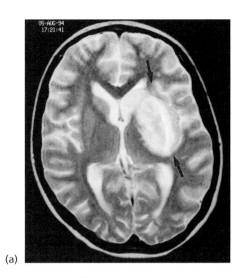
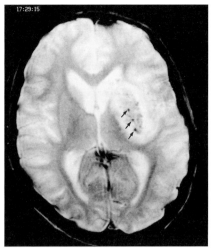

(a) (b)

Figure 5.21 MR scan of a 5-day-old left striatocapsular infarct to show the extreme sensitivity of appropriate MR sequences to tiny areas of petechial haemorrhage. (a) T2-weighted spin-echo sequence shows the infarct (arrows), but no haemorrhage. (b) T2-weighted gradient-echo 'haem' sequence shows tiny low-signal areas within the infarct due to tiny amounts of petechial haemorrhage (arrows) such as would normally only be visible to the pathologist. The clinical relevance of this is uncertain.

echo T2), which shows petechial haemorrhage in infarcts, previously visible only to the pathologist (Fig. 5.21). The clinical relevance of being able to see such tiny amounts of haemorrhage is uncertain and may just be more upsetting to clinicians than useful.

> *For all practical purposes, the characteristic signal changes of parenchymal haemorrhage on MRI persist for life; therefore, haematomas can be identified even years after they have occurred.*

Is there an underlying cause of the haemorrhage?

MRI is probably better than CT at sorting out the underlying cause of an intracerebral haemorrhage (see Section 8.9.3). For example, it demonstrates venous sinus disease, multiple pinpoint metastases, features of vasculitis, primary tumours and AVMs, which are all generally less visible on CT. MRI venography can confirm sinus occlusion (Dormont *et al.*, 1994; Vogl *et al.*, 1994; Yuh *et al.*, 1994). MRI may also have a useful role in sorting out whether a lesion *was* an infarct or a haematoma in patients who present late after their stroke, too late for CT to make the distinction reliably. MRI shows the characteristic signal changes for many years, probably for life, which indicate that the lesion was predominantly haemorrhagic at its inception. However, the usefulness of this has not been formally assessed, and, in any case, it is probably better to encourage patients to present as early as possible, through public health and general practitioner education, rather than relying on 'salvage' by MRI.

Early MRI signs of infarction

The earliest ischaemic changes detectable with routine MRI (i.e. not with spectroscopy or diffusion imaging) are loss of the normal flow void in the symptomatic artery (within minutes of onset), which is the MRI equivalent of the hyperdense artery sign on CT; swelling on T1-weighted images without signal change on T2-weighted images (3 hours); signal changes on T2-weighted images (8 hours); and signal change on T1-weighted images (16 hours) (Kertesz *et al.*, 1987; Baker *et al.*, 1991; Yuh *et al.*, 1991; Ida *et al.*, 1994).

It has been said that it is difficult to differentiate between acute cerebral haemorrhage and acute cerebral infarction in the first 24 hours (Brant-Zawadski *et al.*, 1987; Hayman *et al.*, 1991). In our experience, this has not been a problem, possibly because it is rare to get a stroke patient into the MRI scanner within 12 hours of onset. After the first few hours, MRI is much more sensitive to haemorrhage than CT, because of the paramagnetic effects of deoxyhaemoglobin (see above). Tiny areas of haemorrhagic transformation not visible on CT can be identified, which might influence the use of anticoagulants in the future, although at the moment there is insufficient knowledge of their risks and benefits with such minor areas of (petechial) haemorrhage for this information to be much use (Bryan *et al.*, 1991).

MRI can sometimes detect signal changes in appropriate areas of the brain lasting up to several days after TIAs (Yuh *et al.*, 1991; Hommel *et al.*, 1994). Pronounced brain parenchymal cortical enhancement following intravenous gadolinium injection has been described within the first 24 hours after onset in patients with a TIA, partial arterial occlusion and isolated boundary-zone infarcts (Sato *et al.*, 1991; Yuh *et al.*, 1991; Ida *et al.*, 1994).

Evolution of the appearance of infarction on MRI

The general principles of recognition of infarcts from their shape and site in the brain, and any relationship to the underlying mechanism, are the same as were described for CT scanning above. Thus, the infarct swells and many of the other features change according to the same time frame. In the second week after infarct onset, diffuse increase in signal (brightness on T2-weighted images) of gyri overlying the infarct is often visible. This is thought to be due to neovascular capillary proliferation, or loss of autoregulation in leptomeningeal collaterals, and is visible for up to 8 weeks after onset (Brant-Zawadski *et al.*, 1987; DeWitt *et al.*, 1987). It is mirrored by a similar appearance on CT scanning, attributed to areas of breakdown of the blood–brain barrier corresponding with the gyriform petechial haemorrhages seen at postmortem (Inoue *et al.*, 1980). In the second to third week after onset, some infarcts become isodense with normal brain on CT (fogging effect) and, as they may have lost most of their mass effect by that stage, are difficult to identify. Recent MRI studies have shown changes in T1 (increased signal) and in T2 (decreased signal) suggestive of diffuse haemorrhage in the second to third week. This is probably due to diffuse petechial haemorrhage from leaky capillaries, with diapedesis of red blood cells (Torigoe *et al.*, 1990; Bryan *et al.*, 1991), and would fit with the 'fogging effect' on CT, as the thinly spread red blood cells would cause a diffuse increase in Hounsfield numbers, raising the low density of the lesion to that of normal brain parenchyma.

Late appearance of infarction on MRI

After several weeks, the infarcted brain appears as an area with similar signal characteristics to CSF, i.e. bright on T2 and dark on T1, with an *ex vacuo* effect on the surrounding brain. Other long-term effects of ischaemic stroke seen on MRI include Wallerian degeneration, visible as atrophy and low density in the white matter of the brainstem, and the late effects of any haemorrhagic transformation (DeWitt *et al.*, 1987).

How rapidly and how often do infarcts become visible on MRI?

On routine T1- and T2-weighted imaging, large infarcts are often visible within 6 hours (Hasso *et al.*, 1994; Ida *et al.*, 1994). Diffusion-weighted imaging can show abnormalities

within minutes of the stroke in animals and presumably also in humans (although this is more difficult to test), but currently is a less widely available and more cumbersome technique (Chien *et al.*, 1992; Warach *et al.*, 1995). It certainly shows appropriate lesions when patients have been scanned within 30 minutes of the stroke. As mentioned above, MRI abnormalities may be visible in the brain after as brief an insult as a TIA, but, on the other hand, not all patients with a clinically definite stroke have a corresponding MRI abnormality (Alberts *et al.*, 1992). Of patients who subsequently develop MRI changes, about 15% will show abnormalities within 8 hours and 90% within 24 hours (Kertesz *et al.*, 1987). Of note is that 30% of patients showing changes within 24 hours show an increase in size of the abnormal signal area on follow-up scan. However, at present it is unclear whether this imaged abnormality represents irretrievably damaged brain or whether the ischaemic penumbra is also being imaged. More widespread use of MRI in ischaemic stroke will make the relevance of early infarct visibility with different MRI scanning methods clearer. MRI is able to detect small infarcts well, especially lacunes (Bryan *et al.*, 1991). Furthermore, in patients with numerous 'holes in the brain', gadolinium-enhanced MRI demonstrates which is the recent lacune, because it will enhance whereas older lesions will not (Elster, 1992; Samuelsson *et al.*, 1994). MRI is more sensitive to small lesions in the brainstem and posterior fossa than CT, because there is no interference from bone artefacts (Simmons *et al.*, 1986).

5.3.7 Comparative studies of CT and MRI in acute stroke

There have been a few studies comparing the visibility of lesions on brain CT and MRI in acute stroke. Simmons *et al.* (1986), in a retrospective study, found that infarcts in the posterior fossa were visible in 14 of 14 patients using MRI, compared with only seven of 14 on CT. Bryan *et al.* (1991) found a visible relevant infarct in 82% (of 31 patients) on MRI but in only 58% on CT within 24 hours, and in 88% on both techniques on repeat scan at 1 week. MRI showed more areas of haemorrhage on the follow-up scans than CT. Neither study stated the actual timing of the scans, both studies were very small and both technologies have advanced since then. More recently, Mohr *et al.* (1995), in a prospective blinded study, identified patients within 3 hours of stroke onset and compared the infarct visibility on CT and MRI obtained 'concurrently'. In 80 patients, there were 75 infarcts (35 major and 11 minor hemispheric, 17 brainstem and 15 LACIs) and five haemorrhages. CT (non-contrast) and MRI (T2-weighted and proton-density-weighted) were equal in their ability to demonstrate early infarction or haematoma. Some patients with an initially positive CT or MRI scan had returned to normal, neurologically, by 24 hours, and CT was better than MRI at predicting whether or not this neurological improvement occurred. There was a marginally significant correlation between early positive brain imaging by either modality and the severity of the stroke. Thus, although MRI is more sensitive for posterior fossa infarcts and LACIs, CT is probably equally good at demonstrating early infarct changes in cortical strokes.

> *At present, 'routine' CT and MRI are probably equally good at demonstrating early cortical infarcts and primary intracerebral haemorrhage, but MRI is superior for lacunar and posterior fossa infarcts.*

5.3.8 Advanced MRI techniques

MRI permits other useful methods of examining the brain, including MR angiography to demonstrate the arteries and veins; regional cerebral blood flow measurement; diffusion- and perfusion-weighted imaging to demonstrate very early ischaemic changes; MRI spectroscopy to show the effect of ischaemia on brain metabolites; and functional MRI to identify areas of the brain which control body function. The details of these techniques are beyond the scope of this chapter, but there are excellent reviews describing each technique, as detailed below.

MR angiography

MR angiography allows the acquisition of images of blood vessels, without injection of contrast, by using the signal characteristics of flowing blood (Baker *et al.*, 1991; Fisher *et al.*, 1992; Warach *et al.*, 1992). This technique is not yet practical for acute ischaemic stroke, because the patient must keep very still for the longish scanning time, but it is promising for the assessment of carotid stenosis in patients being considered for carotid endarterectomy (see Section 6.6.4) and is also being evaluated for the detection of intracranial aneurysms (see Section 9.4.3; Fisher *et al.*, 1992; Huston *et al.*, 1993). It may become more practical for ischaemic stroke with the very fast scan times which are now available.

Diffusion-weighted MRI

Diffusion-weighted MRI exploits the Brownian motion of water molecules in the brain and has demonstrated abnormalities in ischaemic tissue within 14 minutes of onset in animal models (Fisher & Sotak, 1992). In stroke patients, initial studies have shown alteration of water diffusibility in the infarcted tissue, which varied both within the lesion and with time (Chien *et al.*, 1992; Warach *et al.*, 1995). The significance of these changes in relation to clinical outcome, the extent of the ischaemic penumbra, the influence of experimental treatments for ischaemic stroke and the effect of reperfusion have yet to be evaluated.

Perfusion-weighted MRI

Perfusion-weighted MRI to examine the cerebral microcirculation can also be performed, but, again, information from stroke patients so far is limited (Baker *et al.*, 1991; Zigun *et al.*, 1993; Rother *et al.*, 1994). Perfusion imaging relies on the paramagnetic properties of injected agents, such as gadolinium, to identify parts of the brain with reduced blood flow through the capillary microcirculation. Like the other techniques mentioned above, it is relatively difficult to apply in confused ischaemic stroke patients, but this problem will lessen with fast scan techniques. Perfusion imaging has demonstrated lesions in patients in appropriate areas of the brain within 6 hours of the stroke when the T1 and T2 images were normal (Rother *et al.*, 1994). Thus, along with diffusion-weighted imaging, it may in future turn out to be a useful way of identifying the degree of reduction in blood flow and the extent of any ischaemic penumbra in ischaemic stroke.

MRI spectroscopy

MRI spectroscopy can demonstrate metabolic changes in ischaemic tissue *in vivo*, particularly hydrogen, phosphate, carbon, fluorine and sodium metabolism (Bottomley, 1989; Baker *et al.*, 1991; Howe *et al.*, 1993; Ross & Michaelis, 1994). N-Acetylaspartate (considered to be a marker of 'normal neurones'), creatine and phosphocreatine, choline-containing compounds, lactate and pH have all been measured in preliminary studies in stroke patients, but it is still too early yet to be certain of the significance of the changes (Howe *et al.*, 1993; Saunders *et al.*, 1995). It may be possible to study the evolution of metabolite changes in ischaemic stroke and the response to drug treatment *in vivo* using these techniques.

Functional MRI

When a part of the cerebral cortex becomes metabolically active, its blood flow increases, thereby changing the MRI signal obtained from this volume of brain (Ellis, 1993; Kwong, 1995). For example, if the subject is asked to undertake a task, such as wriggling a finger, whilst in the MRI scanner, and the MRI prior to the movement is compared with the image during the task, the difference between the two demonstrates the area of cortex activated by the function. Therefore, areas of the brain which are taking over the function of damaged areas can be identified and the pattern of brain compensation to injury studied during recovery from ischaemic stroke or head injury or in patients with brain tumours. However, the technique is difficult and great care is required to obtain meaningful results. The subject must keep his/her head very still and only perform the requested task, as inadvertent movement of other parts of the body will show up on MRI and be misleading. Nonetheless, the technique shows promise for the future by allowing insights into normal brain function as well as recovery from injury.

5.3.9 Other 'sophisticated' methods of imaging cerebral ischaemia

Single-photon emission CT (SPECT)

SPECT is an isotope technique in which cross-sectional images of the brain are obtained using either a rotating gamma-camera or a dedicated SPECT scanner and computerised reconstruction of the data from the emitted radiation. Various isotopes are available for SPECT scanning, such as hexamethyl propylene amine oxime (HMPAO) (Ceretec), which images regional perfusion differences and therefore can identify infarcts early, or xenon-133, which can measure regional cerebral blood flow quantitatively (Witt *et al.*, 1991). However, the equipment to perform SPECT is not all that widely available, the scanning times are long (20 or more minutes) and so problems due to movement artefacts can arise from restless stroke patients, and the isotopes are expensive. A potential source of error, which is particularly relevant to ischaemic stroke, is that blood–brain barrier breakdown alters the behaviour of the isotope and hence the accuracy and interpretation of the images (Merrick, 1990).

SPECT can demonstrate appropriate lesions within a few hours of stroke onset. In patients with a TIA, up to 60% will have an appropriate abnormality if examined within 24 hours of onset (deBruine *et al.*, 1990). In acute ischaemic stroke, SPECT demonstrates an area of relative hypoperfusion corresponding with the ischaemic tissue in most patients studied (Hayman *et al.*, 1989; deBruine *et al.*, 1990; Limburg *et al.*, 1990). In the first week after the stroke, the relative blood flow in the infarct may be increased or decreased, corresponding with luxury perfusion or persistent hypoperfusion, respectively (Moretti *et al.*, 1990). It has also been shown that abnormalities are visible not only in the infarct itself, but also in remote parts of the brain, such as the opposite cerebral hemisphere or the contralateral cerebellum in cerebral cortical infarcts (Raynaud *et al.*, 1989; Bowler *et*

al., 1995; Infeld *et al.*, 1995). This has given rise to the concept of 'diaschisis' or 'shut-down' of areas of the brain not directly involved in the infarct itself but whose function is in some way influenced, possibly through association fibres. There is some evidence of clinical correlates of 'shut-down' of these areas in terms of symptoms and signs not fully explained by loss of the area of brain directly involved in the infarct (Andrews, 1991; Bowler *et al.*, 1995).

Positron emission tomography (PET)

PET has the capability to depict a variety of physiological processes, from glucose metabolism to neuroreceptor density, thus allowing study of the normal workings of the brain as well as the consequences of pathology. The data, which arise by collection and analysis of complicated signals from positron-emitting isotopes, can be displayed as colour-coded tomographic pictures (Frackowiak, 1985). PET has been available since the 1970s, but the imaging equipment and isotopes are extremely expensive, the scan times are prolonged and the patient must keep very still. Therefore, PET is likely to remain a research tool with limited clinical applications for the foreseeable future (Dobkin & Mintun, 1993). PET studies in ischaemic stroke have provided evidence that the ischaemic penumbra really does exist in humans and that neural tissue in the penumbra may survive for up to 48 hours (Heiss, 1992; Heiss *et al.*, 1992).

5.4 Differentiating haemorrhagic transformation of an infarct (HTI) from primary intracerebral haemorrhage (PICH)

HTI is an aspect of stroke pathophysiology which is particularly difficult to assess and is fraught with what may turn out to be misconceptions as to clinical relevance. The exact frequency of HTI is almost impossible to assess because postmortem studies are biased towards severe strokes and only give a 'snapshot' of the brain at the point of death, leaving one to speculate on events earlier in the course of the stroke. Imaging studies offer some improvement, although they have all been small and there has never been one published where every patient had either a follow-up CT scan or a postmortem, so they inevitably give a biased estimate of the frequency of HTI and its clinical associations (see below). More information on risk factors, the influence of antithrombotic treatment and the role of reperfusion will become available from the present randomised trials of antithrombotic and thrombolytic treatments (see Chapter 11).

HTI can usefully be thought of as being asymptomatic (picked up on imaging but not associated with worsening of symptoms) or symptomatic (definite deterioration in symptoms associated with the appearance of new haemorrhage into an infarct on imaging). HTI is also described as 'petechial' (little areas of patchy haemorrhage without frank haematoma) or as a haematoma, although definitions vary, which accounts for some of the variability of HTI rates in published studies.

Appearance of haemorrhagic transformation of an infarct on CT or MRI

Typically HTI is distinguished from PICH by the lack of homogeneity of the haemorrhagic area which lies within, or on the edge of, an area of low density confined to a single arterial territory, i.e. within a presumed infarct. However, it is clear that some cases which appear radiologically to be parenchymal haematomas are due to HTI occurring within hours of stroke onset (Fig. 5.22), the so-called intra-infarct haematomas (Bogousslavsky *et al.*, 1991). The HTI can look so like a PICH that, without a prior scan showing no haemorrhage, the patient would have been labelled as PICH. The size of this problem will become clearer with more experience of early scanning. Currently, however, there are no absolute rules for distinguishing early HTI obliterating the infarct from a true PICH.

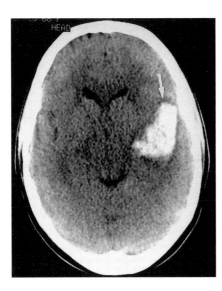

Figure 5.22 CT brain scan showing very early haemorrhagic transformation of a left temporal arterial infarct. The CT scan was obtained within 3 hours of onset of a right hemiparesis and shows a fairly dense haematoma in the left temporal region (arrow). Angiography immediately after the scan showed the proximal left MCA main stem to be occluded by an embolus with dilated lenticulostriate arteries (collateral supply). The source of the embolus was never found. A repeat angiogram at 2 months showed that the left MCA had recanalised.

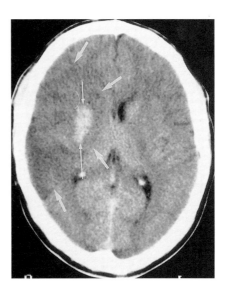

Figure 5.23 CT brain scan showing petechial haemorrhage (thin arrows) into a right temporoparietal infarct (thick arrows) obtained at 36 hours after the stroke. The haemorrhage was not particularly dense, unlike a haematoma.

Haemorrhagic transformation of an infarct can occur very early after stroke onset and make the infarct look just like a primary intracerebral haemorrhage.

The more commonly seen forms of HTI consist of serpiginous areas of increased density (whiteness) on CT (or of appropriate signal characteristics on MRI) at the margins of the infarct (Fig. 5.23); more obvious patchy areas of increased density throughout the infarct; or frank haematomas exerting mass effect (see Fig. 5.22). In large infarcts involving the cortex, curvilinear bands of increased density may be seen at the cortical edge, at the junction of the lesion with white matter and within the lesion in the second and third weeks after the stroke. These areas also enhance markedly when X-ray contrast is given (Davis *et al.*, 1977) and are thought to correspond with areas where the capillaries are leaky, where there is blood–brain barrier breakdown and where there is frank petechial haemorrhage at postmortem (Inoue *et al.*, 1980).

The influence of observer variability and visual perception

Some of the wide range of reported rates of petechial haemorrhage must be due to interobserver variation in reporting, but this is less likely to affect focal haematomas (Wardlaw & Sellar, 1993; Rimdusid *et al.*, 1995). The visual perception of the density of normal brain is influenced by the density of adjacent tissue, such that normal brain next to the low density of an infarct looks to be of higher density than it really is and so can be mistaken for areas of haemorrhage (Fig. 5.24).

To avoid this mistake, the density of the brain can be measured on the CT console to distinguish petechial haemorrhage from normal brain.

Frequency of haemorrhagic transformation of an infarct

Studies using CT and MRI scanning have suggested that haemorrhagic transformation of some degree occurs in 15–45% of patients for petechial haemorrhage (Hornig *et al.*, 1986; Okada *et al.*, 1989) and in about 5% for symptomatic parenchymatous haematoma formation (Lodder, 1984). This may be an under- or overestimate for the following reasons: the studies were all small and few were of consecutive patients or prospective; not all patients were followed up, only survivors or those who remained in hospital for the study period; the definition of HTI was not stated in all the publications; the influence of interobserver variability was not taken into account; the generation of scanner used varied and hence the sensitivity of the diagnosis of HTI; and the number of patients given antithrombotic drugs was often not stated. Thus, it is very difficult to tease

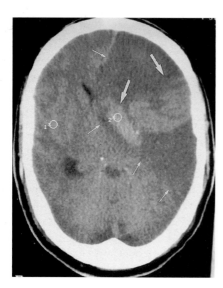

Figure 5.24 CT brain scan to illustrate the effect of altered brain density on visual perception. The scan was obtained from a 40-year-old man at 24 hours after a left MCA occlusion causing an extensive left hemispheric infarct (thin arrows). The areas of hyperdensity (thick arrows) within the low density of the infarct were interpreted as being due to haemorrhage by the clinician due to their apparent brightness. However, the actual density when measured on the CT scanning console was the same as normal grey matter, indicating that the areas of hyperdensity were in fact islands of surviving, i.e. non-infarcted, brain and not haemorrhage at all. Area 1 (normal right insular cortex) was 51 HU and area 2 (apparent increased density within the left infarct) was 46 HU. Blood generally registers at around 70–80 HU.

out from the published studies of HTI what its true rate really is.

More information is becoming available from the control groups of the recent randomised trials of thrombolytic and antithrombotic drugs, such as Multicentre Acute Stroke Trial—Italy (MAST-I) and the IST, but even so not all patients had a follow-up scan (or postmortem). In MAST-I, 69 of the 622 patients randomised died and did not have a second CT scan or postmortem (Multicentre Acute Stroke Trial—Italy (MAST-I) Group, 1995). In 10% of the control patients the infarct became haemorrhagic but without symptoms and in 1% the HTI was symptomatic. In the pilot phase of the IST, 7% of patients who had a pre-randomisation and a follow-up CT scan developed any HTI (3% had a focal haematoma), but 75% of the patients were taking antithrombotic drugs (the treatment code will not be broken until the end of the trial in 1996) (Rimdusid *et al.*, 1995).

Factors associated with haemorrhagic transformation of an infarct and its clinical relevance

This is also somewhat difficult to tease out from published studies, which have so far tended to be small and possibly biased. However, the available evidence suggests that HTI is more frequent in large infarcts (and therefore possibly after cardioembolic stroke) and that its occurrence is associated with a worse clinical outcome (Lodder, 1984; Hart & Easton, 1986; Hornig *et al.*, 1986; Beghi *et al.*, 1989; Okada *et al.*, 1989; Bozzao *et al.*, 1992; Lindley *et al.*, 1992; Pessin *et al.*, 1992; Rimdusid *et al.*, 1995). However, the associations and clinical relevance may become clearer from the results of the recent large thrombolysis and antithrombotic drug trials.

Influence of antithrombotic drugs

Haemorrhagic transformation can occur spontaneously in patients treated without anticoagulants (Bogousslavsky & Regli, 1985; Ott *et al.*, 1986). Patients with HTI have even continued on anticoagulants without worsening of the haemorrhage or symptomatic deterioration (Ott *et al.*, 1986; Dickmann *et al.*, 1988; Pessin *et al.*, 1992). Some non-randomised series have found little apparent effect on the rate of haemorrhage with antithrombotic treatment (Vemmos *et al.*, 1994; Chamorro *et al.*, 1995) as have the randomised studies so far available, although they are too small to give a reliable answer (Crepin-Leblond *et al.*, 1994; Kay *et al.*, 1994). The true effect of antithrombotic treatment on HTI will hopefully be resolved by the large randomised controlled trials which are under way at the moment, although it now seems fairly clear that thrombolytic drugs do cause HTI (see Section 11.5).

Possible mechanisms of haemorrhagic transformation of an infarct

Traditionally HTI was considered to occur when an arterial occlusion, usually cardioembolic in origin, resulted in ischaemia of the distal capillary bed and then, when fragmentation of the embolus occurred, this ischaemic area was subjected to arterial pressure, resulting in rupture of the necrotic arterioles and capillaries (Fisher & Adams, 1951). This concept arose from work in postmortem brains, but this is biased towards patients who die in the early stages of their stroke and who are therefore more likely to have had a large cerebral infarct. The signs of haemorrhage resolve with time, so that, in patients dying weeks or months after their stroke, it may no longer be possible to distinguish the relative contribution of infarct and haemorrhage in the residual lesion. The postmortem studies of Fisher and Adams (1951) suggested that in most cases of HTI the cause of infarction was an embolus (origin unspecified) which had broken up and moved distally, exposing the ischaemic tissue to arterial blood pressure, leading to haemorrhage. Of 373 brains with vascular occlusion (123 with presumed embolism, 89 with presumed thrombosis and 161 of uncertain cause), 66 had haemorrhagic infarction and in 63 there was evidence of embolism as the cause of stroke. They did not discuss the possibility that some of their infarcts with open arteries might have been due to venous thrombosis (see Section 5.3.5), nor did they say how the evidence of embolism was obtained.

The idea that embolism is the cause of HTI has become rather entrenched, to the point of HTI being used in some studies as diagnostic of embolic (usually implied cardiac origin) stroke (Lodder et al., 1986). Closer examination of the literature on HTI shows that the situation is more complicated than the reperfusion–haemorrhagic transformation hypothesis would suggest (Pessin et al., 1992). Shortly before Fisher and Adam's (1951) work became so widely publicised and accepted, Globus and Epstein (1953) published the results of experimental cerebral infarction in monkeys and dogs and some observations on postmortem brains from stroke patients. They observed that haemorrhage into infarcted tissue was often worse when the occluded symptomatic artery remained occluded, and that the haemorrhage seemed to occur around the periphery of the infarct from collateral arterioles and postcapillary venules vasodilating to supply the ischaemic tissue and then leaking. They produced massive intracerebral haemorrhages in dogs by this means, although they noted differences between the species which seemed to depend on the adequacy of the collateral supply.

This alternative, but possibly equally attractive, hypothesis has been all but forgotten, although it probably deserves further attention.

There is debate about the effect of recanalisation. Until recently it was accepted that early recanalisation, such as might occur with spontaneous lysis of an embolus, increased the risk of haemorrhagic transformation. However, several recent studies have contradicted this, suggesting that haemorrhage is more common in infarcts where the artery remains occluded, as shown by catheter angiography (Ogata, 1989; Mori et al., 1990, 1992; Bozzao et al., 1992; Pessin et al., 1992). There are obviously many unanswered questions about the causes, associated factors and clinical significance of HTI.

5.5 The diagnosis of subarachnoid haemorrhage (SAH)

SAH refers to the spontaneous extravasation of blood into the subarachnoid space when a blood vessel near the surface of the brain leaks. It is a condition, not a disease, that can be produced by many causes (see Section 9.1). Although, as we have seen (see Section 5.3.1), the clinical distinction of stroke due to cerebral infarction and intracerebral haemorrhage is unreliable and we have to rely on imaging, the clinical features of SAH are reasonably distinct, and at least this type of stroke can be diagnosed clinically with reasonable confidence. However, confirmatory investigations are needed in almost all cases (see Section 5.5.3).

5.5.1 Clinical features

Blood in the subarachnoid space acts as a meningeal irritant and incites a typical clinical response, regardless of aetiology; patients usually complain of headache, photophobia, stiff neck and nausea, and they may also vomit. Confusion, restlessness and impaired consciousness are also frequent (Table 5.2).

Headache

Headache is the cardinal clinical feature of SAH and occurs in 85–100% of patients (Walton, 1956; Sarner & Rose, 1967; Kopitnik & Samson, 1993; Vestergaard et al., 1993; Kumral et al., 1995). In a consecutive series of 92 patients with SAH due a to ruptured aneurysm, in whom the onset of the headache was recorded, 62 had headache as the first symptom; the others were immediately unconscious (van Gijn et al., 1985). The headache arises suddenly, classically in a *split second*, 'like a blow on the head' or 'an explosion

Table 5.2 Diagnosis of subarachnoid haemorrhage (SAH).

Principal symptoms
Headache: sudden, maximal in seconds, unusually severe, usually
   occipital or retro-orbital. Duration: hours (possibly minutes, we
   do not know) to weeks
Nausea
Vomiting
Neck stiffness
Photophobia
Sudden loss of consciousness

Neurological signs
None (very often)
Meningism
Focal neurological signs: IIIrd nerve palsy (posterior
   communicating artery aneurysm), dysphasia, hemiparesis (AVM,
   intracerebral haematoma)
Subhyaloid haemorrhages in optic fundi
Fever
Raised blood pressure
Limitation of straight leg raising/Kernig's sign
Altered consciousness

inside the head', reaching a maximum within seconds. Of the 62 patients reported above, 54 (87%) had an explosive onset. In the other eight patients (13%) the headache came on more gradually, in minutes rather than seconds. Headache of gradual onset occurs more commonly in patients with non-aneurysmal perimesencephalic SAH (see Section 9.1.2), i.e. in about 20% of patients, compared with 13% with aneurysmal SAH (Rinkel *et al.*, 1991), but the predictive value of this feature is limited, because non-aneurysmal perimesencephalic SAH is about nine times less common than aneurysmal SAH. A biphasic headache may occur in patients whose SAH is due to dissection of a vertebral artery (see Section 9.1.3): first, a severe occipital headache radiating from the back of the neck, followed after an interval of hours of days by sudden exacerbation of the headache but of a more diffuse type.

The headache is generally diffuse and poorly localised but tends to spread over minutes to hours to the back of the head, neck and back as blood tracks down into the spinal subarachnoid space. Sometimes the headache is maximal behind the eyes. The headache is often described by patients as the most severe headache they have ever had, but it can occasionally be milder; it is the suddenness of onset which is most characteristic.

More often than not there is no obvious precipitating factor (Matsuda *et al.*, 1993). Amongst the 33 patients with SAH in the OCSP, six (18%) SAHs occurred whilst resting (none occurred whilst asleep), 13 (39%) during moderate activity and six (18%) during strenuous activity, such as

weight-lifting and sexual intercourse; the activity at onset was not known in the other eight patients (Wroe *et al.*, 1992). Similar proportions have been reported in other series (Ferro & Pinto, 1994). The headache usually lasts 1–2 weeks, but it may be longer. Perhaps it may last only a few hours, or even less, if there has been a small leak of blood, in which case there may be no other associated symptoms, such as neck stiffness. We do not know exactly how short in duration a headache may be and still be due to SAH. We have not come across anyone with a headache due to SAH that resolved within 1 hour, but it is still possible that this may occur, and so it is perhaps best to consider SAH in anyone with a sudden unusual severe headache, even if it resolves within minutes, particularly if there is any impairment of consciousness.

> *Consider subarachnoid haemorrhage whenever a patient complains of the sudden onset of 'the worst headache in my life'.*

It is not uncommon in clinical practice to encounter patients who describe having had a severe headache of sudden onset 3-weeks (or more) ago, sounding very much like an SAH, which resolved after a few hours or days. It is then extremely difficult to know what to do, because decisions about investigation for an aneurysm can only be based on the patient's history rather than the brain CT or CSF examination (see Section 9.4.5).

'Sentinel/warning' headache. A history of previous episodes of sudden headache is generally believed to be common in patients with aneurysmal SAH and to have been due to a 'warning' leak. Indeed, on specific questioning many patients do recall a previous episode of headache that was unusually severe, lasted several hours, and that was sometimes accompanied by transient loss of consciousness, transient focal deficits or neck stiffness (Duffy, 1983; Leblanc, 1987; Ostergaard, 1990; Juvela, 1992; Vesari *et al.*, 1993). One case–control study found that as many as 40% of patients admitted with SAH had previous episodes of severe headache, against only one of 20 patients admitted with cerebral infarction and none of 100 control patients admitted with a non-neurological disorder (Verweij *et al.*, 1988). Such episodes are either not reported to the family physician or they are misdiagnosed (Adams *et al.*, 1980). Many neurosurgeons and neurologists are therefore convinced that important advances in the overall management of aneurysmal SAH can be expected from early recognition of rupture on the very first occasion, followed by emergency clipping of the aneurysm.

A major difficulty with the notion of these 'warning leaks' or 'sentinel headaches' is that all studies have been hospital-based, most have been retrospective and even prospectively conducted and controlled studies may be biased by hindsight (i.e. recall bias). Recently, a prospective study has been completed amongst an expanding group of general practitioners in the Netherlands, who for a 5-year period recorded all instances of unusually severe and sudden headache that came to their attention (Linn *et al.*, 1994). Such episodes were recorded in 148 patients, 37 (25%) of whom had SAH (including four patients with a rapidly fatal course and no further investigations). Only two of the 37 patients with SAH had had previous episodes of sudden headache on systematic questioning by the general practitioner at the time of presentation for the headache. Also, the amount and distribution of extravasated blood on brain CT was similar to that in a previous hospital series of patients with SAH, at least for the 25 patients for whom CT scans were available for review. The notion of frequent 'minor leaks' was therefore not supported by radiological findings. Finally, the overall outcome in the 33 initial survivors was good in 23 patients and poor in 10, which again is not strikingly different from the outcome in hospital series (Linn *et al.*, 1994). Even in the 34 patients with sudden headache (of a total of 148) who were not referred or investigated, follow-up failed to disclose any haemorrhagic events that would necessitate reclassification of the original episode of 'benign sudden headache' as a 'warning leak'.

> *It is not clear how frequently patients with aneurysmal subarachnoid haemorrhage have had preceding and unrecognised 'warning leaks'. Whether this is frequent or not, doctors must be educated to consider subarachnoid haemorrhage in any patient who reports a sudden severe headache.*

On the basis of this single population study, the conclusion seems inevitable that the proportion of aneurysmal SAH patients with 'warning leaks' has been overestimated in the past. Indeed, it seems that the notion of 'warning leaks' is to a large extent an artificial result of close questioning of patients who are already aware that they have a dangerous brain disorder, an atmosphere that may easily lead to overinterpretation of minor and innocuous headaches in the recent past. Of course, there are patients with SAH who seek medical help but are misdiagnosed as, for instance, acute sinusitis, migraine or a strained neck (Adams *et al.*, 1980). However, such patients would probably, in better clinical circumstances, be diagnosed as 'classical' SAH.

Vomiting

Vomiting (and nausea) is common at the outset, in contrast to other differential diagnoses, such as migraine, in which vomiting more often comes after the headache starts.

Neck stiffness

Neck stiffness due to meningism is a painful resistance to voluntary or passive neck flexion because of cervical meningeal inflammation. It is a common symptom and a sign of blood in the subarachnoid space, but it does not occur immediately; it develops after some 3–12 hours and may not develop at all in deeply unconscious patients or in patients with small leaks (Vermeulen & van Gijn, 1990). Therefore, its absence can not be used to exclude the diagnosis of SAH in a patient with sudden headache. Brudzinski's sign (flexion at the hip and knee in response to forward flexion of the neck) is also due to blood in the subarachnoid space but is less reliable.

Pain and stiffness in the back and legs may follow SAH after some hours or days because blood irritates the lumbosacral nerve roots. Kernig's sign (passive extension of the knee with the hip flexed elicits pain in the back and leg and resistance to hamstring stretch) is a sign of inflammation or blood around the lumbosacral nerve roots, but is seldom present without obvious meningism.

Photophobia

Patients are often photophobic and irritable for several days after SAH, presumably due to meningeal irritation by the blood.

Loss of consciousness

Loss of consciousness occurred in 50% of patients with presumed aneurysmal SAH who were well enough to be entered into a clinical trial of medical treatment (Vermeulen *et al.*, 1984). As these figures do not include the 10% of patients with SAH who die at home or during transportation to hospital (Linn *et al.*, 1994) or another 20% who reach hospital and die within the first 24 hours (Hijdra & van Gijn, 1982), it is likely that at least 60% of all patients with SAH lose consciousness at, or soon after, onset. The patient may regain alertness and orientation or may remain with various degrees of lethargy, confusion, agitation or obtundation. Bizarre actions, which may be misinterpreted as psychological in origin, include grimacing, spitting, making sucking or kissing sounds, spluttering, singing, whistling, yelling and screaming. The altered level of consciousness may be due to a lot of blood in the subarachnoid space or to a complication of SAH, such as brain displacement by haematoma or hydrocephalus, reduced cerebral blood flow by the sudden increase in CSF pressure or a fall in systemic blood pressure or arterial oxygen concentration.

Epileptic seizures

Epileptic seizures (partial or generalised) may occur at onset or subsequently, as a result of irritation or damage to the cerebral cortex by the subarachnoid and any intracerebral blood. In the OCSP, two of the 33 patients (6%, 95% confidence interval (CI): 0–14%) with SAH had an epileptic seizure at onset, but neither of these patients had later seizures. A total of six patients with SAH (18%, 95% CI: 5–31%) had single or recurrent seizures after their SAH; the actuarial risk of experiencing a post-SAH seizure was 12% (95% CI: 0–30%) by the end of the first year, 28% (95% CI: 3–52%) by the second year and 44% (95% CI: 13–75%) by the third year (Burn *et al.*, 1996). This risk was higher than experienced by patients with ischaemic stroke and, of course, is likely to be influenced by subsequent events, such as rebleeding, cerebral infarction and operation. Data from other series indicate that about 10% of patients with SAH develop epileptic seizures, most occurring on the first day of the SAH but one-third not having their first seizure until 6-months later and one-third of those even more than 1-year later (Sarner & Rose, 1967; Hart *et al.*, 1981; Hasan *et al.*, 1993). The only independent predictors of epilepsy after SAH are a large amount of cisternal blood on brain CT and rebleeding (Hasan *et al.*, 1993).

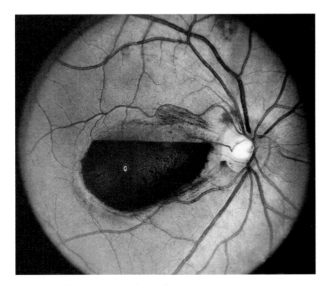

Figure 5.25 Ocular fundus of a patient with subhyaloid haemorrhage, appearing as sharply demarcated linear streaks of brick red-coloured blood or flame-shaped haemorrhage in the preretinal layer, adjacent to the optic disc and spreading out from the disc.

Intraocular haemorrhage

Intraocular haemorrhage develops in approximately 20% of patients with a ruptured aneurysm and may also complicate non-aneurysmal SAH, or intracranial haemorrhage in general (Manschot, 1954). The haemorrhage is caused by a sustained increase in the pressure of the CSF, with obstruction of the central retinal vein as it traverses the optic nerve sheath, in turn leading to congestion of the retinal veins (Manschot, 1954). Mostly, the haemorrhages appear at the time of aneurysmal rupture, but exceptionally later, without evidence of rebleeding. Linear streaks of blood or flame-shaped haemorrhages appear in the preretinal layer (subhyaloid), usually near the disc (Fig. 5.25); one-third lie at the periphery (Fahmy, 1973). If large, the preretinal haemorrhage may extend into the vitreous body. Patients may complain of large brown blobs obscuring their vision and, if the haemorrhages do not resolve spontaneously, vitrectomy may be required (see Section 13.10.4). Patients with ruptured aneurysms and preretinal subhyaloid haemorrhages have a worse outcome (see Section 13.10.4) than patients without (Manschot, 1954; Fahmy, 1973; Keane, 1979).

Focal neurological signs

Focal neurological signs at around SAH onset suggest an underlying intracerebral structural lesion such as an AVM, or an aneurysm which has compressed cranial nerves or has bled into the brain substance, causing an intracerebral haematoma. Sometimes, therefore, the clinical manifestations of a ruptured AVM or aneurysm may be indistinguishable from a stroke syndrome due to PICH or cerebral infarction, particularly if little or no blood has entered the subarachnoid space.

The classic cranial nerve palsy is an oculomotor (IIIrd) nerve palsy which frequently occurs with aneurysms at the origin of the posterior communicating artery from the internal carotid artery (Hyland & Barnett, 1954), and less frequently with aneurysms of the carotid bifurcation, the posterior cerebral artery, the basilar bifurcation (Watanabe *et al.*, 1982) and the superior cerebellar artery (Vincent & Zimmerman, 1980). Third nerve palsy may also occur with unruptured aneurysms (presumably by expansion of the wall of the unruptured aneurysm) or several days after the SAH, as a result of swelling of the ipsilateral cerebral hemisphere due to cerebral ischaemia induced by vasospasm. Most often the pupil is dilated and unreactive but in some patients it is spared (Kissel *et al.*, 1983; Nadeau & Trobe, 1983). Abducens (VIth) nerve palsies, frequently bilateral in the acute stage, may develop after SAH as a false localising sign of raised intracranial pressure, due to traction on the nerves against the petrous temporal bone, caused by downward transtentorial herniation of the diencephalon. Occasionally, posterior circulation aneurysms may cause a VIth nerve palsy due to direct compression (Fisher, 1975).

If a patient presents following a sudden, severe headache and is found to have a IIIrd nerve palsy, rupture of a posterior communicating artery aneurysm is highly likely.

If there are other signs of neurological involvement, such as motor or sensory deficits, visual field defects or aphasia, then it is likely that a haematoma is present, usually within the brain parenchyma, but occasionally in the subdural space, extrinsically compressing the brain. Cerebellar and brainstem signs can, however, be due to the ischaemic effects of vertebral artery dissection, if this is the cause of the SAH (see Section 9.1.3).

Systemic features

Fever, hypertension, albuminuria, glycosuria and electrocardiographic (ECG) changes may be present in the acute phase. Pyrexia rarely exceeds 38.5°C during the first 2–3 days, but thereafter it may rise to over 39°C, presumably due to accumulation of breakdown products of blood in the subarachnoid space (Rousseaux *et al.*, 1980).

The important distinguishing feature of pyrexia due to blood in the subarachnoid space and pyrexia due to intercurrent infection is the pulse rate; it remains disproportionately low in the former and rises with the latter.

About 20–25% of patients with SAH have a history of pre-existing hypertension, but following a SAH about 50% of patients have a markedly raised blood pressure (Artiola *et al.*, 1980; Vermeulen *et al.*, 1984). In most patients this is a reactive phenomenon, probably serving to counteract the decrease in cerebral perfusion resulting from increased CSF pressure and later vasospasm. Because the blood pressure returns to normal levels within a few days, antihypertensive drugs are usually not indicated if the patient was previously normotensive (see Section 9.3.4).

Cardiac arrhythmias and ECG abnormalities are common after SAH (see Section 13.10.2) (Wijdicks *et al.*, 1990). The most common are ST segment and T-wave changes, U-wave abnormalities, QT prolongation and sinus arrhythmias (Marion *et al.*, 1986; Stober *et al.*, 1988; Brouwers *et al.*, 1989). Life-threatening arrhythmias, such as ventricular fibrillation or 'torsade de pointe' may occur on 24-hour monitoring (Andreoli *et al.*, 1987), but these are extremely rare in most series (Carruth & Silverman, 1980; Hijdra *et al.*, 1987). In one series of patients investigated by serial ECGs,

at least one ECG was abnormal in every patient (Brouwers *et al.*, 1989). Virtually all ECG abnormalities changed to other ECG abnormalities, in no constant order, and then disappeared during the observation period of 10 days, without any significant consequences. In contrast, Estanol *et al.* (1979) found that runs of ventricular tachycardia occurred in 20% of those monitored, and prolonged QT intervals in 60%; the latter often represent delayed ventricular repolarisation and predispose to ventricular arrhythmias. The mechanism of these ECG changes is unexplained but is thought to be sustained sympathetic stimulation, perhaps caused by dysfunction of the insular cortex, which results in reversible structural neurogenic damage to the myocardium, such as contraction bands, focal myocardial necrosis and subendocardial ischaemia (Pollick *et al.*, 1988; Mayer *et al.*, 1994; Svigelj *et al.*, 1994). However, there is no correlation between plasma noradrenaline concentrations and ECG abnormalities after aneurysmal SAH (Brouwers *et al.*, 1995). The prognostic value of these ECG changes has not been resolved, but at any rate in patients with SAH they seem to be more important as indicators of intracranial disease than as predictors of potentially fatal heart disease (Brouwers *et al.*, 1989).

Sudden death

SAH is the major, if not only, stroke type to cause sudden death (within minutes). Sudden (or relatively sudden) death occurs in about 15% of patients, before they receive any medical attention (Bonita & Thomson, 1985; Schievink *et al.*, 1995). The features that tend to be associated with sudden death are ruptured posterior circulation aneurysms, intraventricular haemorrhage and acute pulmonary oedema (Schievink *et al.*, 1995). The cause of very sudden death is uncertain but could be the sudden rise in intracranial pressure in cases with large intracerebral haemorrhages and SAHs (it takes some time for SAH to cause raised intracranial pressure sufficient to be fatal unless there is an associated large intracerebral haematoma); intraventricular haemorrhage with acute expansion of the fourth ventricle; cardiac arrhythmia; and acute pulmonary oedema.

5.5.2 Differential diagnosis

The abrupt onset of a severe headache may not only be caused by SAH but also by several other conditions, such as meningitis or encephalitis, intracerebral haemorrhage (particularly posterior fossa haemorrhage), obstruction of the cerebral ventricles or a rapid rise in blood pressure (Table 5.3). The most discriminating feature of the headache of SAH is its sudden onset (maximal within seconds), but, even

Table 5.3 Differential diagnosis of sudden unexpected headache.

With neck rigidity
SAH
Acute painful neck conditions
Meningitis/encephalitis
Stroke: ischaemic or haemorrhagic; cerebellar or intraventricular
Recent head injury

Without neck rigidity
Migraine
Thunderclap headache
Pressor responses
Benign orgasmic cephalgia
Benign exertional headache
Reaction whilst on monoamine oxidase inhibitors
Phaeochromocytoma
Expanding intracranial aneurysm
Carotid or vertebral artery dissection
Intracranial venous thrombosis
Occipital neuralgia
Acute obstructive hydrocephalus

so, only about 25% of patients with sudden headache in general practice prove to have SAH (van Gijn, 1992). This is because a headache with a more common cause, such as migraine and tension headache, can also, on occasion, arise suddenly. Nonetheless, always be careful; missed SAH can be fatal.

> *Patients with rare manifestations of common headache syndromes (i.e. sudden onset of migraine) probably outnumber those with common manifestations of rare headache syndromes (i.e. sudden headache in subarachnoid haemorrhage). Therefore, although most people with a sudden severe headache have not had a subarachnoid haemorrhage, they must all be investigated to exclude this diagnosis.*

Acute painful neck conditions to be distinguished from meningism

Meningism refers to painful resistance to passive or voluntary neck flexion because of irritation of the cervical meninges by subarachnoid blood or inflammation. This can be elicited in the supine patient by placing both hands behind the patient's head and, as one attempts to lift the head up off the pillow the patient does not allow the neck to be flexed and so the examiner lifts the patient's head, neck and shoulders off the bed, as if the patient were like a board. In contrast, passive rotation of the neck is achieved with ease. Meningism may be a feature of SAH, meningitis, a posterior fossa mass and cerebellar tonsillar coning. However, it characteristically disappears as coma deepens.

Other causes of a painful or stiff neck include bony lesions (i.e. trauma or arthritis) and ligamentous strain in the neck, extrapyramidal rigidity, systemic infections, cervical lymphadenitis, parotitis, tonsillitis and upper-lobe pneumonia. However, it is usually quite easy to distinguish meningism from these other acute painful neck conditions. For example, pain arising from the cervical spine may not only be felt in the neck and back of the head but also in the shoulder and arm, it is often evoked or exacerbated by certain movements or positions of the neck other than flexion and there is usually tenderness to palpation over segments of the cervical spine.

Meningitis, encephalitis

Meningitis is an acute febrile illness that usually presents with the subacute onset over 1–2 days of generalised headache, meningism, photophobia and fever. But, it can be difficult to distinguish from SAH if the patient is found comatose, has neck rigidity and there is no available history. Clues to the diagnosis of meningitis include a high fever, tachycardia and a purpuric skin rash (meningococcal meningitis). If the patient is fully conscious and has no focal neurological signs and if meningitis is suspected, a lumbar puncture should be done immediately. But, if the patient is very ill, antibiotics should be given at once, before proceeding to brain CT and then, if indicated because there is no blood seen and no intracranial mass, a CSF examination.

Cerebellar stroke

Cerebellar stroke often gives rise to sudden severe headache, nausea and vomiting but is usually accompanied by neurological symptoms and signs, such as vertigo and unsteadiness, which help distinguish it from SAH (see Section 4.2.7). However, if the lesion is large, the patient may present in coma due to direct brainstem compression or obstruction of CSF flow from the fourth ventricle, causing hydrocephalus and raised intracranial pressure, or there may be meningism without signs of definite brainstem dysfunction. Urgent brain CT is required to confirm the diagnosis and lumbar puncture should certainly not be done; indeed, lumbar puncture should almost always be preceded by brain CT in unconscious patients, even if there are no focal signs of a mass lesion and no clinical evidence of raised intracranial pressure (such as papilloedema).

Intraventricular haemorrhage

Intraventricular haemorrhage, which may be primary (i.e. arising within the ventricles or from immediately beneath the ependymal lining) or secondary to an extension from a primary parenchymal haemorrhage (i.e. to a caudate haemorrhage or ruptured subependymal AVM with extension into the intraventricular system), may mimic SAH (see Section 9.1.5). Patients present with sudden severe headache, confusion, vomiting or collapse with loss of consciousness (Darby et al., 1988). Brain CT or MRI scan is required for diagnosis in vivo.

Migraine

Migraine headache can sometimes arise suddenly, be severe and prostrating, unilateral or generalised, and associated with photophobia, irritability, mild confusion, anorexia, mild fever, extraocular muscle palsy (ophthalmoplegic migraine) or symptoms of brainstem disturbance (basilar migraine) and thus be mistaken for SAH. However, migraineurs generally have a past or family history of migraine and the headache is commonly unilateral and throbbing, not so rapid in onset and of shorter duration, and follows the resolution of focal 'positive' neurological symptoms of the migraine aura that arose gradually and spread with intensification over several minutes (Lance, 1993). Vomiting tends to occur well into the migraine attack, in contrast to SAH, in which it commonly occurs soon after onset.

Thunderclap headache

Thunderclap headache is characterised by paroxysmal onset of severe, generalised pain in the head, sometimes with vomiting, and without obvious precipitant or known cause. It may last up to 1 day or so. Clinically, the syndrome can not be distinguished from SAH and so the diagnosis is made by exclusion; if both brain CT and CSF (performed within 2 weeks after onset (see Section 5.5.3)) are normal, the episode is attributed to an unusually explosive bout of 'ordinary' headache and not to SAH. The prognosis of thunderclap headache is much more benign than that of SAH; a 3-year follow-up study of 71 patients found identical recurrences in 12, again without evidence of SAH, whereas nearly 50% proceeded to episodes of more obvious migraine or tension headache (Wijdicks et al., 1988).

Idiopathic stabbing headache

Three specific varieties of sudden sharp stabbing headache have been described: ice-pick-like pains, 'jabs and jolts syndrome' and ophthalmodynia (Lance, 1993). As these pains are transient and lancinating, they are unlikely to be confused with the headache of SAH. The mechanism

is unknown but the quality of the pain resembles trigeminal neuralgia and suggests paroxysmal neuronal discharge.

Post-traumatic headache

Immediately after a head injury, there is often headache due to soft-tissue damage and, if the patient is concussed, intracranial vessels dilate, giving rise to a pulsating headache, which is made worse by head movement, jolting, coughing, sneezing and straining (Lance, 1993). Normally the headache gradually disappears as the tissue damage resolves. Tubbs and Potter (1970) found that only 83 of 200 patients admitted to hospital with head injury had a headache in the day or so after head injury, only 22 (11%) complained spontaneously (the remainder admitted to headache only on questioning) and only three required an analgesic.

The diagnosis of post-traumatic headache should not be confused with SAH if there is a history of head injury, but the patient may be amnesic and there may be no witness (see Section 9.1.4). If the CT is suggestive of spontaneous intracranial haemorrhage, the patient should be considered for cerebral angiography (see Section 5.5.3) (Sakas et al., 1995).

> If the circumstances of a traumatic head injury are unclear and a reasonable chance exists of a spontaneous intracranial haemorrhage as a cause of the accident and head injury, then brain CT should be done as soon as the patient's condition allows, regardless of the severity of the head injury.

Benign orgasmic cephalgia and benign exertional headache

Acute, severe, explosive occipital or generalised headache, usually occurring at the moment of sexual orgasm or during strenuous exercise (benign orgasmic cephalgia and benign exertional headache, respectively), may mimic SAH. The history of headache onset during sexual intercourse may not be forthcoming without specific and sensitive enquiry. Points in favour of the diagnosis are a history of previous sexual or exertional headaches, no alteration in consciousness, short duration of the headache (minutes to hours, although SAH may possibly cause short-duration headache too and we do not really know how brief headache due to SAH can be) and no signs of meningeal irritation, such as neck stiffness (or low back pain and sciatica in the ambulant patient) (Silbert et al., 1991). These headaches can occur at any time in life and do not necessarily occur every time the patient experiences orgasm or exercises strenuously. If patients present soon after their first-ever sudden orgasmic headache, it is not possible to exclude an SAH without brain CT and lumbar puncture.

Diagnostic difficulty also arises in distinguishing benign orgasmic cephalgia and benign exertional headache of sudden onset from the 'sentinel headache' of SAH, which may be due to stretching or haemorrhage into the aneurysm wall rather than a minor leak into the subarachnoid space (see Section 5.5.1) (Wijdicks *et al.*, 1988).

Reaction whilst on monoamine oxidase inhibitor drugs (MAOIs)

People taking classic MAOIs, such as phenelzine, may experience sudden severe headache after ingesting sympathomimetic agents, red wine or foods with a high tyramine content, such as mature cheese, pickled herrings, game and yeast extract. This is because MAOIs irreversibly block the ability of both monoamine oxidase (MAO) isoforms (A and B) to metabolise dietary tyramine in the liver (A) and gut wall (B). The combination of a classic MAOI and oral tyramine can provoke dangerous hypertension (see Section 8.3.1). The headache is often over the occipital region of the head and associated with a rapid rise in blood pressure. It can be relieved by the alpha noradrenergic blocking agent, phentolamine. Some cases of intracranial haemorrhage have occurred at the height of a pressor reaction (Lance, 1993).

Phaeochromocytoma

Patients with phaeochromocytoma experience acute pressor reactions and, in about 80% of attacks, they complain of headache (Thomas *et al.*, 1966). The headache is usually of sudden onset, bilateral, severe and throbbing and often associated with nausea and other symptoms of catecholamine release. It appears to be related to a rapid increase in blood pressure and lasts less than 1 hour in about 75% of patients, but it may last from a few minutes to a few hours. Some patients may collapse with loss of consciousness or develop focal neurological signs during the episode. Attacks may be provoked by exertion, straining, emotional upset, worry or excitement (Lance & Hinterberger, 1976).

The diagnosis depends on clinical suspicion being aroused when the history is first taken (which can be difficult because the condition is so rare) and is confirmed by finding increased excretion of catecholamines (metanephrine and vanillylmandelic acid) in three 24-hour specimens of urine, or raised plasma free metanephrine or normetanephrine levels during the attack (Lenders *et al.*, 1995). Care must be taken before the urine collection that the patient does not have chronic renal failure and has not been taking any substances which can interfere with the assay (such as methyldopa) or confuse the interpretation of finding catecholamines or catecholamine-like substances in the urine (such as sympathomimetic drugs, MAOIs or nasal decongestant sprays). Consuming bananas, coffee, tea or chocolate can also interfere with the assay by stimulating the secretion of catecholamines or producing metabolites similar to catecholamines. The blood sugar is usually raised at the time of the attack, a useful distinction from hypoglycaemic attacks, which may simulate phaeochromocytoma because of secondary release of adrenaline in response to low blood sugar. The tumour may arise at any point along the line of development of the sympathetic chain from the neck to the pelvis and scrotum and can be localised by CT and aortic angiography if present in the characteristic suprarenal site.

Expanding intracranial aneurysm

Unruptured aneurysms are not associated with migraine or other recurrent headaches (Lance, 1993), but in extremely rare cases they may cause a severe headache, even without focal cranial nerve signs; pressure on the IIIrd cranial nerve from a posterior communicating artery aneurysm causes pain behind the eye that can be of fairly sudden onset.

Carotid or vertebral artery dissection (see also Section 7.1)

Dissection of the wall of an internal carotid artery may cause a fairly distinctive headache syndrome, which is ipsilateral, involving the forehead, periorbital region, face, teeth or neck, and has a burning or throbbing quality. The headache may be associated with an ipsilateral Horner's syndrome or monocular blindness and contralateral focal neurological symptoms or signs (West *et al.*, 1976; Fisher, 1982; Mokri *et al.*, 1986; Bogousslavsky *et al.*, 1987). Dissection of the wall of a vertebral artery causes pain in the upper posterior neck and occiput, usually on one side, and may be associated with symptoms and signs of posterior circulation ischaemia, such as a lateral medullary syndrome (Caplan *et al.*, 1985). Vertebral artery dissection can also be a cause of SAH (see Section 9.1.3).

Intracranial venous thrombosis

Thrombosis of the cerebral veins or venous sinuses presents with headache in about 75% of patients (Bousser *et al.*, 1985). Nearly 50% of the patients have increased intracranial pressure, one-third have focal neurological signs, such as a hemiparesis or VIth nerve palsy, and one-third also have seizures. Usually the onset is less sudden than in SAH (although headache can arise suddenly without other neurological features), the clinical picture is more of a generalised encephalopathy, brain CT or MRI may show widespread venous infarcts and haemorrhages (see Sections 5.3.5 and 8.2.1) and the CSF is normal or contains a modest excess of white blood cells, red blood cells and protein.

Occipital neuralgia

Occipital neuralgia is characterised by an aching or paroxysmal jabbing pain in the posterior neck and occipital region in the distribution of the greater or lesser occipital nerves (Fig. 5.26). It may rarely present quite dramatically, like an SAH (Pascual-Leone & Pascual, 1992), but is usually characterised by diminished sensation or dysaesthesiae of the affected area (C2 distribution), focal tenderness over the point where the greater occipital nerve trunk crosses the superior nuchal line and a therapeutic response to infiltration of local anaesthetic near the tender area on the nerve trunk.

Acute obstructive hydrocephalus

Any acute obstruction of the flow of CSF causes a rapid increase in intracranial pressure and headache, which is commonly bilateral and exacerbated by coughing, sneezing, straining or head movement. Intermittent obstructive hydrocephalus may therefore cause severe paroxysmal headaches. Tumours in the vicinity of the third ventricle or within it, such as a colloid cyst, may also interfere intermittently with CSF outflow or perhaps with the function of the midbrain reticular formation, so that posture can not be maintatined

and the patient may fall heavily to the ground, due to loss of muscle tone. Brain CT or MRI usually identify the offending lesion (Fig. 5.27).

Multiple sclerosis

An isolated case report exists of a 27-year-old man who had been awakened by 'the worst headache' of his life and 2-days later developed an oculomotor nerve palsy, which was considered to be due to multiple sclerosis; initial CT, lumbar puncture and cerebral angiogram were unremarkable, but subsequent CSF examination revealed oligoclonal bands and MRI displayed multiple white-matter lesions (Galer *et al.*, 1990). It is difficult to be sure whether this patient had multiple sclerosis and whether demyelination was the cause of the symptoms, but the case is nevertheless salutary.

5.5.3 Investigations to confirm the diagnosis

Cranial CT

All patients presenting with a suspected recent SAH (i.e. within the last few days) should initially have urgent brain CT to determine whether there is blood in the subarachnoid space; the site of any SAH or intracerebral or intraventricular haemorrhage and therefore the likely cause (see Section 9.4.1); the presence of any complications, such as hydrocephalus; the presence of any contraindications to lumbar puncture (i.e. cerebral oedema or haematoma with brain shift, or a large cerebellar stroke) in case no blood is evident on CT; and whether there is any other intracranial pathology that may account for the symptoms and signs (Fig. 5.28).

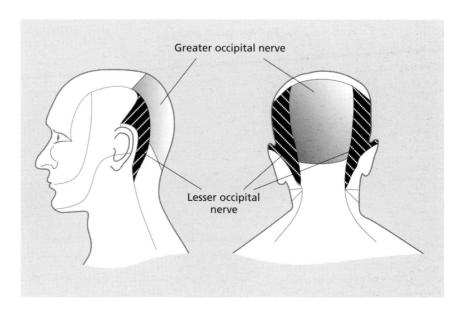

Figure 5.26 Diagram showing the anatomical distribution of the sensory innervation of the greater and lesser occipital nerves.

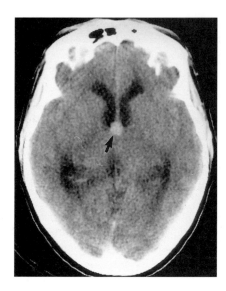

Figure 5.27 CT brain scan showing a tumour in the third ventricle (arrow) at the foramen of Monro, causing obstructive hydrocephalus.

Sensitivity of CT in SAH depends on the size of the SAH, the resolution of the scanner, the skills of the radiologist and the timing of the CT after symptom onset; the sensitivity is greatest in the first few days and falls thereafter, as blood in the subarachnoid space is resorbed. Of course, minute amounts of subarachnoid blood may be overlooked by the uninitiated (Fig. 5.29). Depending on the amount of blood in the cisterns and the delay before scanning, an 'absent' or 'missing' (isodense) cistern or absent cortical sulci may provide the only clue to the presence of subarachnoid blood (Fig. 5.30). Failure to detect SAH with brain CT is particularly likely

with an aneurysm of the posterior inferior cerebellar artery (Adams *et al.*, 1983; Ruelle *et al.*, 1988; Stone *et al.*, 1988). CT evidence of subarachnoid blood after rupture of an intracranial aneurysm can disappear very rapidly (Fig. 5.31). Therefore, the term 'resorption' may not always be appropriate to describe this process, diffusion and sedimentation being alternative explanations. After 3 days, the chance of finding subarachnoid blood on brain CT decreases sharply, to 50% on day 7, 20% on day 9 and almost nil after 10 days (van Gijn & van Dongen, 1982; Brouwers *et al.*, 1992).

> *If brain CT (third generation) is done within 1–2 days after rupture of an intracranial aneurysm, extravasated blood near the circle of Willis will be demonstrated in more than 95% of patients.*
>
> *If subarachnoid haemorrhage is suspected and yet the brain CT scan appears normal, look carefully at the interpeduncular cistern, ambient cisterns, quadrigeminal cistern, the region of the anterior communicating artery and posterior inferior cerebellar artery, the posterior horns of the lateral ventricles and the cortical sulci. If blood is present in these sites, it may be isodense or slightly hyperdense, and hence the normally hypodense cisterns and sulci may be difficult to see and seem 'absent'.*

Haemorrhage from an intracranial aneurysm can result not only in SAH but also in an intraparenchymal haematoma. Intraparenchymal blood is easily seen on plain CT and it persists for longer than subarachnoid blood, because the 'resorption' of intraparenchymal blood, as seen on CT, occurs over 2–4 weeks rather than a few days, which is the case for subarachnoid blood (van Gijn & van Dongen, 1982;

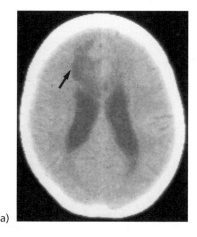

(a)

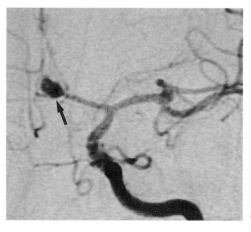

(b)

Figure 5.28 Brain CT scan (a) showing a 2–3-week-old intracerebral haemorrhage in the frontal lobes (arrow) of a patient who presented with an acute behavioural disorder and was misdiagnosed as being a hysterical alcoholic. Subsequent cerebral angiography (b) revealed an anterior communicating artery aneurysm (arrow) which had ruptured and bled into the frontal lobes.

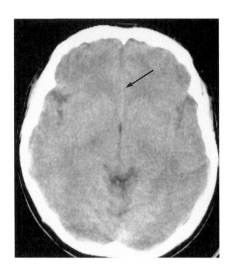

Figure 5.29 Brain CT scan within 24 hours of onset of SAH showing only a minute amount of blood in the subarachnoid space. There was a hint of increased density (blood) in the inferior part of the anterior interhemispheric fissure only (arrow).

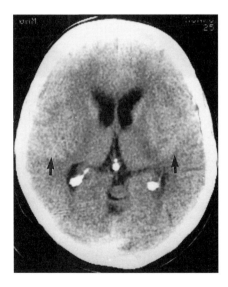

Figure 5.30 Brain CT scan of a patient with SAH showing isodense blood in the cortical sulci giving the appearance of 'absent' sulci. In particular, the Sylvian fissures are not seen because they are filled with just enough blood to raise the density of the CSF to that of brain parenchyma (arrows).

Brouwers *et al.*, 1992). The proportion of patients with a haematoma after aneurysmal haemorrhage varies amongst different series, because it depends on referral patterns. If patients are admitted to a general neurology service, there is usually little or no selection according to the clinical condition, and moribund patients are included. In these series, the proportion of patients with an intracerebral haematoma is around one-third of all patients with a ruptured aneurysm (van Gijn & van Dongen, 1982; Brouwers *et al.*, 1992).

A normal CT scan: false-negative or non-haemorrhagic 'thunderclap headache'? Some patients have a benign kind of headache but of sudden onset and of such severity that they are referred to hospital with a provisional diagnosis of SAH. This diagnosis is subsequently excluded by means of early CT and lumbar puncture. The true diagnosis in these patients is 'crash migraine'; a sudden exacerbation of tension headache (Pearce & Pearce, 1986; Wijdicks *et al.*, 1988); benign orgasmic cephalalgia (Lance, 1976; Porter & Jankovic, 1981); a vascular headache provoked by some other type of exertion (Paulson, 1983); or it remains unknown and is called thunderclap headache (see Section 5.5.2). Investigations are, of course, negative in all these categories of patients, but a CT scan and a lumbar puncture need to be done before the diagnosis can be made, although only on the first occasion in patients with orgasmic, exertional or other recurrent forms of explosive headache. A normal CT scan alone in such patients leaves a small risk of missing an SAH, or higher if more than 3 days have elapsed. In one consecutive series from the Netherlands, the negative predictive value of CT scanning performed within 12 hours of onset of sudden headache was 97% (95% CI: 88–99%). This means that, in this series, 97% of people with a sudden headache who had a normal CT scan (i.e. no subarachnoid blood) within 12 hours of onset of headache also had a normal CSF (i.e. negative spectrophotometric analysis of CSF for xanthochromia) more than 12 hours after the event, and therefore did not have an SAH (Table 5.4.) However, there was an important small minority (3%) with sudden headache and normal CT within 12 hours who *did* have xanthochromia in the CSF, and angiography subsequently confirmed a ruptured aneurysm. The chance that a lumbar puncture will show evidence of haemorrhage and xanthochromia despite a truly normal CT scan made within hours of a sudden episode of headache depends not only on this small number of early false-negative CT scans in SAH, but also on the relative proportion of patients with non-haemorrhagic, innocuous thunderclap headaches, which in turn depends on local referral patterns.

Always do a lumbar puncture if the history is suggestive of subarachnoid haemorrhage and the CT scan (performed early, within a few days) is normal. Frequently, the cerebrospinal fluid will be normal too, but occasionally in this setting an abnormal cerebrospinal fluid will be the only objective evidence for the diagnosis of subarachnoid haemorrhage.

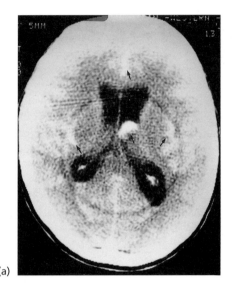 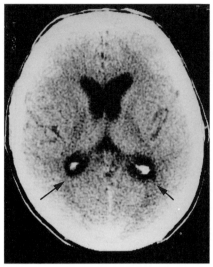

(a) (b)

Figure 5.31 Brain CT scan showing rapid clearance of evidence of SAH. (a) CT scan at 12 hours after the SAH shows extensive subarachnoid blood (hyperdensity—arrows) in all the cortical sulci and the lateral ventricles. (b) At 3 days after the SAH there is almost complete disappearance of the blood. There is only a tiny amount remaining in the occipital poles of the lateral ventricles (arrows).

Lumbar puncture

Lumbar puncture without prior brain CT is potentially dangerous in patients with an intracerebral haematoma (Duffy, 1982); brain herniation may occur even in patients without focal signs or a decreased level of consciousness (Hillman, 1986). If brain CT shows definite evidence of extravasated blood, a lumbar puncture will add no extra information. However, if the CT scan shows no evidence of SAH, then lumbar puncture must be done to examine the CSF for blood products; as stated above, in the presence of a negative CT scan, there is about a 3% chance that lumbar puncture

Table 5.4 Detection of SAH on early CT scan within 12 hours of sudden headache in 175 patients with a normal neurological examination. (From van der Wee *et al.*, 1995.)

	SAH		
	Yes	No	Total
CT scan positive*	117	0	117
CT scan negative†	2	56	58
Total	119	56	175

Sensitivity: 117/119 = 98% (95% CI: 94–99.8%)
Specificity: 56/56 = 100%
Positive predictive value: 117/117 = 100%
Negative predictive value: 56/58 = 97% (95% CI: 88–99.6%)

* CT scan shows subarachnoid blood.
† CT scan does not show subarachnoid blood.

will show evidence of SAH, at least within the first 3 days. After this period, the proportion of negative CT scans after SAH becomes increasingly larger, and the yield of lumbar puncture increasingly greater (for the first 2 weeks, at least).

A lumbar puncture should not be done until about 12 hours after headache onset, to enable a reliable distinction to be made between a traumatic tap and haemorrhage in the subarachnoid space. The reason is that it takes up to 12 hours for red cells to lyse and for haemoglobin to be broken down into oxyhaemoglobin, which after centrifugation of the CSF results in a yellowish colour of the supernatant (xanthochromia) (Vermeulen & van Gijn, 1990). Because xanthochromia is the only reliable proof that haemorrhagic spinal fluid has not resulted from the trauma of the puncture itself (Vermeulen & van Gijn, 1990), it is crucial that the CSF is not examined within 12 hours of onset of headache; no xanthochromia within 12 hours does not exclude SAH and a repeat CSF can not be performed at a later date, because it may not be able to distinguish xanthochromia due to SAH from that due to any trauma from the initial CSF tap (Table 5.5). Although a decrease in red blood cell concentration in serial samples taken at the same procedure occurs more often in traumatic punctures than in intracranial haemorrhage, this can still occur in patients with intracranial haemorrhage and, conversely, a constant number of red cells can be seen with traumatic taps (Buruma *et al.*, 1981; Vermeulen & van Gijn, 1990). So the time-honoured 'three-tube method' should be abandoned in favour of looking for xanthochromia.

Table 5.5 Indications for lumbar puncture in patients with suspected SAH but a negative brain CT. (Some data from Matthews & Frommeyer, 1955; Tourtelotte *et al.*, 1964.)

If the onset of sudden headache was less than 3 days before
1 Wait until at least 12 hours have elapsed since the onset of symptoms before doing a lumbar puncture
2 If the CSF is not only clear and colourless but also acellular (no more than a few red blood cells/mm³), a ruptured aneurysm has been excluded and there is no need for further investigation
3 If the CSF is bloodstained
  (a) Spin down the CSF immediately (if it contains red blood cells from a traumatic tap and is allowed to stand, oxyhaemoglobin will be formed *in vitro*, bilirubin will not, but its absence can not exclude SAH)
  (b) Perform spectrophotometric analysis of the supernatant for xanthochromia, unless the yellow colour is evident to the naked eye. If spectrophotometry has to be deferred for practical reasons, store the CSF wrapped in tin foil, because daylight may induce breakdown of bilirubin

If the onset of sudden headache was more than 3 days before
1 Do a lumber puncture immediately (after brain CT)
2 If the CSF is unequivocally xanthochromic (with or without red cells), no further CSF tests are necessary
3 If the CSF is clear, colourless and acellular, still do spectrophotometry: the red cells have been lysed and the presence of pigment may not be visible to the naked eye
4 If the interval is more than 2 weeks from headache onset, xanthochromia may still be detectable up until 4 weeks, but normal spectrophotometric testing can not exclude SAH

> *Lumbar puncture should be done only after at least 12 hours have elapsed since the onset of headache.*
>
> *It is a widely held myth that the distinction between xanthochromia and a traumatic 'bloody' tap can be made by collecting the cerebrospinal fluid in three consecutive test-tubes and counting the number of red cells in each tube.*

Oxyhaemoglobin and bilirubin are the main breakdown products of haemoglobin, at least *in vivo*, and on spectrophotometry they can be recognised by characteristic absorption bands (Barrows *et al.*, 1955). If the lumbar puncture is performed more than 12 hours after the onset of SAH, the yellow colour of the CSF should be visible with the naked eye. At 3 weeks after SAH, xanthochromia is still found but in only 70% of patients with SAH, and after 4 weeks in only 40% (Vermeulen *et al.*, 1983).

> *Xanthochromia is invariably found between 12 hours and 2 weeks after SAH.*

It is usually not difficult to make the clinical distinction between SAH and meningitis, because in most patients with SAH there is an adequate history of an abrupt onset of headache or unconsciousness. The difficulty mainly arises when a patient is found in a confused state with marked neck stiffness and moderate fever; in these cases a lumbar puncture should probably be done first, unless CT can be done very quickly. However, if the diagnosis of meningitis is not sustained and if the CSF is bloodstained, the patient must have an angiogram to exclude an aneurysm or other source of bleeding.

References

Adams HP, Jergenson DD, Kassell NF, Sahs AL (1980). Pitfalls in the recognition of subarachnoid haemorrhage. *J Am Med Assoc* 244: 794–6.

Adams HP, Kassell NF, Torner JC, Sahs AL (1983). CT and clinical correlations in recent aneurysmal subarachnoid haemorrhage: a preliminary report of the Cooperative Aneurysm Study. *Neurology* 33: 981–8.

Alberts MJ, Faulstich ME, Gray L (1992). Stroke with negative brain magnetic resonance imaging. *Stroke* 23: 663–7.

Allen CMC (1983). Clinical diagnosis of acute stroke syndrome. *Quatern J Med* 43: 515–23.

Ambrose J (1973). Computerised transverse axial scanning (tomography): part 2: clinical application. *Br J Radiol* 46: 1023–47.

American Nimodipine Study Group (1992). Clinical trial of nimodipine in acute ischemic stroke. *Stroke* 23: 3–8.

Anderson CS, Taylor BV, Hankey GJ, Stewart-Wynne E, Jamrozik KD (1994). Validation of a clinical classification for subtypes of acute cerebral infarction. *J Neurol Neurosurg Psychiatr* 57: 1173–9.

Andreoli A, di Pasquale G, Pinelli G, Grazi P, Tognetti F, Testa C (1987). Subarachnoid haemorrhage: frequency and severity of cardiac arhythmias. A survey of 70 cases studied in the acute phase. *Stroke* 18: 558–64.

Andrews RJ (1991). Transhemispheric diaschisis: a review and comment. *Stroke* 22: 943–9.

Angeloni U, Bozzao L, Fantozzi LM, Bastianello S, Kushner M, Fieschi C (1991). Internal borderzone infarctions following acute middle cerebral artery occlusion: proceedings of the XIV Symposium Neuroradiologicum 1990. *Neuroradiology* 33 (Suppl.): 232.

Artiola I, Fortuny L, Adams GBT, Briggs M (1980). Surgical mortality in an aneurysm population: effects of age, blood pressure and preoperative neurological state. *J Neurol Neurosurg Psychiatr* 43: 879–82.

Ashok PP, Radhakrishnan K, Sridharan R, El-Mangoush MA (1986). Incidence and pattern of cerebrovascular diseases in Benghazi, Libya. *J Neurol Neurosurg Psychiatr* 49: 519–23.

Baker LL, Kucharczyk J, Sevick RJ, Mintorovitsh J, Moseley ME (1991). Recent advances in MR imaging/spectroscopy of cerebral ischemia. *Am J Roentgenol* 156: 1133–43.

Bamford J (1992). Clinical examination in diagnosis and subclassification of stroke. *Lancet* 339: 400–2.

Bamford JM, Warlow CP (1988). Evolution and testing of the lacunar hypothesis. *Stroke* 19: 1074–82.

Bamford J, Sandercock PAG, Jones L, Warlow CP (1987). The natural history of lacunar infarction: the Oxfordshire Community Stroke Project. *Stroke* 18: 545–51.

Bamford J, Sandercock P, Dennis M, Burn J, Warlow C (1990). A prospective study of acute cerebrovascular disease in the community: the Oxfordshire Community Stroke Project—1981–86. 2. Incidence, case fatality rates and overall outcome at one year of cerebral infarction, primary intracerebral and subarachnoid haemorrhage. *J Neurol Neurosurg Psychiatr* 53: 16–22.

Bamford J, Sandercock P, Dennis M, Burn J, Warlow C (1991). Classification and natural history of clinically identifiable subtypes of cerebral infarction. *Lancet* 337: 1521–6.

Barrows LJ, Hunter FT, Banker BQ (1955). The nature and clinical significance of pigments in the cerebrospinal fluid. *Brain* 78: 59–80.

Bastianello S, Pierallini A, Colonnese C et al. (1991). Hyperdense middle cerebral artery CT sign. *Neuroradiology* 33: 207–11.

Becker H, Desch H, Hacker H, Pencz A (1979). CT fogging effect with ischaemic cerebral infarcts. *Neuroradiology* 18: 185.

Beghi E, Bogliun G, Cavalletti G et al. (1989). Haemorrhagic infarction: risk factors, clinical and tomographic features, and outcome. A case control study. *Acta Neurol Scand* 80: 226–31.

Besson G, Robert C, Hommel M, Perret J (1995). Is it clinically possible to distinguish non hemorrhagic infarct from hemorrhagic stroke? *Stroke* 26: 1205–9.

Bogousslavsky J, Regli F (1985). Anticoagulant-induced intracerebral bleeding in brain ischaemia. *Acta Neurol Scand* 71: 464–71.

Bogousslavsky J, Despland P-A, Regli F (1987). Spontaneous carotid dissection with acute stroke. *Arch Neurol* 44: 137–40.

Bogousslavsky J, Regli F, Uske A, Maeder P (1991). Early spontaneous haematoma in cerebral infarct. *Neurology* 41: 837–40.

Bonita R, Thomson S (1985). Subarachnoid haemorrhage: epidemiology, diagnosis, management and outcome. *Stroke* 16: 591–4.

Bonke B, Koudestaal PJ, Dijkstra G et al. (1989). Detection of lacunar infarction in brain CT scans: no evidence of bias from accompanying patient information. *Neuroradiology* 31: 170–3.

Bottomely PA (1989). Human *in vivo* NMR spectroscopy in diagnostic medicine: clinical tool or research probe? *Radiology* 170: 1–15.

Bousser M-G, Chiras J, Bories J, Castaigne P (1985). Cerebral venous thrombosis—a review of 38 cases. *Stroke* 16: 199–213.

Bowler JV, Wade MD, Jones BE et al. (1995). Contribution of diaschisis to the clinical deficit in human cerebral infarction. *Stroke* 26: 1000–6.

Bozzao L, Angeloni U, Bastianello S, Fantozzi LM, Pierallini A, Fieschi C (1992). Early angiographic and CT findings in patients with haemorrhagic infarction in the distribution. *Am J Neuroradiol* 12: 1115–21.

Bradley WG (1994). Haemorrhage and haemorrhagic infections in the brain. In: Hasso AN, Truwit CL, eds. *Neuroimaging Clinics of North America*, Vol. 4(4). Philidelphia:WB Saunders Co, 707–32.

Brant-Zawadski M, Pereira B, Bartkowski H et al. (1987). MR imaging and spectroscopy in clinical and experimental cerebral ischaemia: a review of the middle cerebral artery. *Am J Neuroradiol* 8: 39–45.

Broderick JP, Phillips SJ, Whisnant JP, O'Fallon WM, Bergstrahl EJ (1989). Incidence rates of stroke in the eighties: the end of the decline in stroke? *Stroke* 20: 577–82.

Brouwers PJAM, Westenberg HGM, van Gijn J (1995). Noradrenaline concentrations and electrocardiographic abnormalities after aneurysmal subarachnoid haemorrhage. *J Neurol Neurosurg Psychiatr* 58: 614–17.

Brouwers PJAM, Wijdicks EFM, van Gijn J (1992). Infarction after aneurysm rupture does not depend on the distribution or clearance rate of blood. *Stroke* 23: 374–9.

Brouwers PJAM, Wijdicks EFM, Hasan D et al. (1989). Serial electrocardiographic recording in aneurysmal subarachnoid haemorrhage. *Stroke* 20: 1162–7.

Bryan RN, Levy LM, Whitlow WD, Killian JM, Preziosi TJ, Rosario JA (1991). Diagnosis of acute cerebral infarction: comparison of CT and MR imaging. *Am J Neuroradiol* 12: 611–20.

Burn J, Dennis M, Bamford J, Sandercock P, Wade D, Warlow C (1996). Epileptic seizures after a first ever in a lifetime stroke: the Oxfordshire Community Stroke Project. *Br Med J* (in press).

Buruma OJS, Janson HLF, den Bergh FAJTM, Bots GTAM (1981). Blood-stained cerebrospinal fluid: traumatic puncture or haemorrhage? *J Neurol Neurosurg Psychiatr* 44: 144–7.

Cameron EW (1994). Transient ischaemic attacks due to meningoma—report of four cases. *Clin Radiol* 49: 416–18.

Campbell JK, Houser OW, Stevens JC, Wahner HL, Baker HL, Folger WN (1978). Computed tomography and radionuclide imaging in the evaluation of ischaemic stroke. *Radiology* 126: 695–702.

Caplan LR, Zarins CK, Hemmati M (1985). Spontaneous dissection of the extracranial vertebral arteries. *Stroke* 16: 1030–8.

Carruth JE, Silverman ME (1980). Torsade de pointe atypical ventricular tachycardia complicating subarachnoid haemorrhage. *Chest* 78: 886–93.

Celani MG, Ceravolo MG, Duca E et al. (1992). Was it infarction or haemorrhage? A clinical diagnosis by means of the Allen Score. *J Neurol* 239: 411–13.

Celani MG, Righetti E, Migliacci R et al. (1994). Comparability and validity of two clinical scores in the early diagnosis of stroke. *Br Med J* 308: 1674–6.

Chamorro A, Alday M, Vila N, Saiz A, Tolosa E (1994). Safety of anticoagulation following large cerebral infarction. *Neurology* 44: A287.

Chien D, Kwong KK, Gress DR, Buonanno FS, Buxton RB, Rosen BR (1992). MR diffusion imaging of cerebral infarction in humans. *Am J Neuroradiol* 13: 1097–102.

Clasen RA, Huckman MS, Von Roenn LA, Pandolfi S, Laing I, Clasen JR (1980). Time course of cerebral swelling in stroke: a correlative autopsy and CT study. *Adv Neurol* 28: 395–412.

Crepin-Leblond T, Moulin T, Ziegler F *et al.* (1994). A randomised trial of heparin therapy in acute ischaemic stroke: first results. *Cerebrovasc Dis* 4: 259.

Damasio H (1983). A computed tomographic guide to the identification of cerebral vascular territories. *Arch Neurol* 40: 138–42.

Darby DG, Donnan GA, Saling MA, Walsh KW, Bladin PF (1988). Primary intraventricular haemorrhage: clinical and neuropsychological findings in a prospective stroke series. *Neurology* 38: 68–75.

Davis KR, Ackerman RH, Kistler JP *et al.* (1977). Computed tomography of cerebral infarction: haemorrhage, contrast enhancement and time of appearance. *Comput Tomogr* 1: 71.

deBruine J, Limburg M, van Royen E, Hijdra A, Hill T, van der Schoot J (1990). SPET brain imaging with 201 diethyldithiocarbamate in acute ischaemic stroke. *Eur J Nuc Med* 17: 248–51.

Dennis MS, Bamford JM, Molyneux AJ, Warlow CP (1987). Rapid resolution of signs of primary intracerebral haemorrhage in computed tomograms of the brain. *Br Med J* 279: 379–81.

DeWitt D, Kistler P, Miller D, Richardson E, Buonanno F (1987). NMR–neuropathologic correlation in stroke. *Stroke* 18: 342–51.

Dickmann U, Voth E, Schicha H, Henze T, Prange H, Emrich D (1988). Heparin therapy, deep vein thrombosis and pulmonary embolism after intracerebral haemorrhage. *Klin Wochenschr* 66: 1182–3.

Dobkin JA, Mintun MA (1993). Clinical PET: Aesop's tortoise? *Radiology* 186: 13–15.

Donnan G, Tress B, Bladin P (1982). A prospective study of lacunar infarction using computerised tomography. *Neurology* 32: 49–56.

Donnan GA, Bladin PF, Berkovic SF, Longley WA, Saling MM (1991). The stroke syndrome of striatocapsular infarction. *Brain* 114: 51–70.

Dorman P, Sandercock PAG and the IST Collaborative Group (1996). Should patients with visible infarction on the admission CT scan be excluded from acute stroke trials? An analysis of data on 12 450 patients randomised in the IST. *J Neurol Neurosurg Psychiatr* (in press).

Dormont D, Anxionnat R, Evrad S, Louaille C, Chiras J, Marsault C (1994). MRI in cerebral venous thrombosis. *J Neuroradiol* 21: 81–99.

Duffy GP (1982). Lumbar puncture in spontaneous subarachnoid haemorrhage. *Br Med J* 285: 1163–4.

Duffy GP (1983). The warning leak in spontaneous subarachnoid haemorrhage. *Med J Aust* i: 514–16.

Ellis SJ (1993). Functional magnetic resonance: neurological enlightenment? *Lancet* 342: 882.

Elster AD (1992). MR contrast enhancement in the brainstem and deep cerebral infarction. *Am J Neuroradiol* 12: 1127–32.

Estanol BV, Dergal EB, Cesarman E *et al.* (1979). Cardiac arrhythmias associated with subarachnoid haemorrhage: a prospective study. *Neurosurgery* 5: 675–9.

Fahmy JA (1973). Fundal haemorrhages in ruptured intracranial aneurysms. 1. Material, frequency, and morphology. *Acta Ophthalmol* 51: 189–98.

Ferro JM, Pinto AN (1994). Sexual activity is a common precipitant of subarachnoid haemorrhage. *Cerebrovasc Dis* 4: 375.

Fisher CM (1975). Clinical syndromes in cerebral thrombosis, hypertensive haemorrhage, and ruptured saccular aneurysm. *Clin Neurosurg* 22: 117–47.

Fisher CM (1982). The headache and pain of spontaneous carotid dissection. *Headache* 22: 60–5.

Fisher M, Adams RD (1951). Observations on brain embolism with special reference to the mechanism of haemorrhagic infarction. *J Neuropathol Exp Neurol* 10: 92–4.

Fisher M, Sotak CH (1992). Diffusion weighted MR imaging and ischaemic stroke. *Am J Neuroradiol* 13: 1103–5.

Fisher M, Sotak CH, Minematsu K, Li L (1992). New magnetic resonance techniques for evaluation cerebrovascular disease. *Ann Neurol* 32: 115–22.

Fishman RA (1992). Cerebrospinal fluid in cerebrovascular disorders. In: Barnett HJM, Mohr JP, Stein BM, Yatsu FM, eds. *Stroke, Pathophysiology, Diagnosis and Management*, 2nd edn. Churchill Livingstone, 103–10.

Frackowiak RSJ (1985). *Studies of Energy Metabolism in Human Cerebrovascular Disease: New Brain Imaging Techniques in Cerebrovascular Diseases*. London: John Libbey Eurotext.

Francke CL, Ramos LMP, van Gijn J (1990). Development of multifocal haemorrhage in a cerebral infarct during computed tomography. *J Neurol Neurosurg Psychiatr* 53: 531–2.

Gacs G, Fox AJ, Barnett HJM, Vinuela F (1982). CT visualisation of intracranial arterial thromboembolism. *Stroke* 14: 756–62.

Galer BS, Lipton RB, Weinstein S, Bello L, Solomon S (1990). Apoplectic headache and oculomotor palsy: an unusual presentation of multiple sclerosis. *Neurology* 40: 1465–6.

Globus JH, Epstein JA (1953). Massive cerebral haemorrhage: spontaneous and experimentally induced. *J Neuropathol Exp Neurol* 12: 107–31.

Graeber MC, Jordan E, Mishra SK, Nadeau SE (1992). Watershed infarction on computed tomographic scan: an unreliable sign of hemodynamic stroke. *Arch Neurol* 49: 311–13.

Hacke W, Kaste M, Fieschi C *et al.* for the ECASS Study Group (1995). Intravenous thrombolysis with recombinant tissue plasminogen activator for acute hemispheric stroke: the European Cooperative Acute Stroke Study (ECASS). *J Am Med Assoc* 274: 1017–25.

Hakim AM, Ryder-Cooke A, Melanson D (1993). Sequential computerised tomographic appearance of strokes. *Stroke* 14: 893–7.

Hankey GJ, Khangure MS, Stewart-Wynne EG (1988). Detection of basilar artery thrombosis by computed tomography. *Clin Radiol* 39: 140–3.

Hart RG, Easton JD (1986). Haemorrhagic infarcts. *Stroke* 17: 586–9.

Hart RG, Byer JA, Slaughter JL, Hewett JE, Easton JD (1981). Occurrence and implications of seizures in subarachnoid haemorrhage due to ruptured intracranial aneurysms. *Neurosurgery* 8: 417–21.

Hasan D, Schonk RSM, Avezaat CJJ, Tanghe HLJ, van Gijn J, van der Lugt PJM (1993). Epileptic seizures after subarachnoid haemorrhage. *Ann Neurol* 33: 286–91.

Hasso AN, Stringer WA, Brown KD (1994). Cerebral ischaemia

and infarction. In: Hasso AN, Truwit CL, eds. *Neuroimaging Clinics of North America*, Vol. 4(4). Philadelphia: WB Saunders Co, 733–52.

Hawkins GC, Bonita R, Broad JB, Anderson NE (1995). Inadequacy of clinical scoring systems to differentiate stroke subtypes in population-based studies. *Stroke* 26: 1338–42.

Hayman A, Taber K, Ford J, Bryan R (1991). Mechanisms of MR signal alteration by acute intracerebral blood: old concepts and new theories. *Am J Neuroradiol* 12: 899–907.

Hayman AL, Taber KH, Jhingran SG, Killian SM, Carroll RG (1989). Cerebral infarction: diagnosis and assessment of prognosis by using 123IMP-SPECT and CT. *Am J Neuroradiol* 10: 557–62.

Hayman LA, Evans RA, Bastion FO, Hinck VC (1981). Delayed high dose contrast CT: identifying patients at risk of massive haemorrhagic infarction. *Am J Neuroradiol* 2: 139–46.

Heiss WD (1992). Experimental evidence of ischaemic thresholds and functional recovery. *Stroke* 23: 1668–72.

Heiss W-D, Huber M, Fink GR *et al.* (1992). Progressive derangement of periinfarct viable tissue in ischaemic stroke. *J Cer Bl Fl Metab* 12: 193–203.

Higano S, Uemura F, Shishido F *et al.* (1990). Evaluation of ischaemic threshold for the indication of thrombolytic therapy of embolic stroke in very acute phase. *Stroke* 21 (Suppl. 1): I-120.

Hijdra A, van Gijn J (1982). Early death from rupture of an intracranial aneurysm. *J Neurosurg* 57: 765–8.

Hijdra A, Vermeulen M, van Gijn J, van Crevel H (1987). Rerupture of intracranial aneurysms: a clinicoanatomic study. *J Neurosurg* 67: 29–33.

Hillman J (1986). Should computed tomography scanning replace lumbar puncture in the diagnostic process in suspected subarachnoid haemorrhage? *Surg Neurol* 26: 547–50.

Hommel M, Grand S, Devoulon P, Le Bas J-F (1994). New directions in magnetic resonance in acute cerebral ischemia. *Cerebrovasc Dis* 4: 3–11.

Hornig CR, Dorndorf W, Agnoli AL (1986). Haemorrhagic cerebral infarction—a prospective study. *Stroke* 17: 179–85.

Hornig CR, Bauer T, Simon C, Trittmacher S, Dorndorf W (1993) Haemorrhagic transformation in cardioembolic cerebral infarction. *Stroke* 24: 465–8.

Howe FA, Maxwell RJ, Saunders DE, Brown MM, Griffiths JR (1993). Proton spectroscopy *in vivo*. *Mag Reson Quart* 9: 31–9.

Huston J, Lewis BD, Wiebers DO, Meyer FB, Riederer SJ, Weaver AL (1993). Carotid artery: prospective blinded comparison of two-dimensional time-of-flight MR angiography with conventional angiography and duplex US. *Radiology* 186: 339–44.

Hyland HH, Barnett HJM (1954). The pathogenesis of cranial nerve palsies associated with intracranial aneurysms. *Proc Roy Soc Med* 47: 141–6.

Ida M, Mizunuma K, Tada S (1994). Subcortical low intensity in early cortical ischaemia. *Am J Neuroradiol* 15: 1387–93.

Infeld B, Davis SM, Lichtenstein M, Mitchell PJ, Hopper JL (1995). Crossed cerebellar diaschisis and brain recovery after stroke. *Stroke* 26: 90–5.

Inoue Y, Takemoto K, Miyamoto T (1980). Sequential computed tomography scans in acute cerebral infarction. *Radiology* 135: 655–62.

Juvela S (1992). Minor leak before rupture of an intracranial aneurysm and subarachnoid haemorrhage of unknown etiology. *Neurosurgery* 30: 7–11.

Kay R, Wong KS, Woo J (1994). Pilot study of low-molecular-weight heparin in the treatment of acute ischaemic stroke. *Stroke* 25: 684–5.

Keane JR (1979). Retinal haemorrhage: its significance in 110 patients with acute encephalopathy of unknown cause. *Arch Neurol* 36: 691–4.

Kendall BE, Pullicino P (1980). Intravascular contrast injection in ischaemic lesions II. Effect on prognosis. *Neuroradiology* 19: 241–4.

Kertesz A, Black SE, Nicholson L, Carr T (1987). The sensitivity and specificity of MRI in stroke. *Neurology* 37: 1580–5.

Kinkel WR, Jacobs L (1976). Computerised axial tomography in cerebrovascular disease. *Neurology* 26: 924–30.

Kissel JT, Burde RM, Klingele TG, Zeiger HE (1983). Pupil-sparing oculomotor palsies with internal carotid–posterior communicating artery aneurysms. *Ann Neurol* 13: 149–54.

Kistler JP, Hochberg FH, Brooks BR, Richardson EP, New PFJ, Schnur J (1975). Computerised axial tomography: clinicopathologic correlation. *Neurology* 25: 201–9.

Kittner SJ, Sharkness CM, Price TR *et al.* (1990). Infarcts with a cardiac source of embolism in the NINCDS Stroke Data Bank: historical features. *Neurology* 40: 281–4.

Kopitnik TA, Samson DS (1993). Management of subarachnoid haemorrhage. *J Neurol Neurosurg Psychiatr* 56: 947–59.

Kumral E, Bogousslavsky J, Van Melle G, Regli F, Pierre P (1995). Headache at stroke onset: the Lausanne Stroke Registry. *J Neurol Neurosurg Psychiatr* 58: 490–2.

Kwong KK (1995). Functional magnetic resonance imaging with echo planar imaging. *Mag Reson Quart* 11: 1–20.

Lance JW (1976). Headache related to sexual activity. *J Neurol Neurosurg Psychiatr* 39: 1226–30.

Lance JW (1993). *Mechanism and Management of Headache*, 5th edn. Cambridge: Butterworth-Heinemann, Cambridge University Press.

Lance JW, Hinterberger H (1976). Symptoms of phaeochromocytoma, with particular reference to headache, correlated with catecholamine production. *Arch Neurol* 33: 281–8.

Lang EW, Daffertshofer M, Daffershofer A, Wirth SB, Chesnut RM, Hennerici M (1995). Variability of vascular territory in stroke: pitfalls and failure of stroke pattern interpretation. *Stroke* 26: 942–5.

Leblanc R (1987). The minor leak preceding subarachnoid haemorrhage. *J Neurosurg* 66: 35–9.

Lee D, Vinuela F, Pelz D, Lau C, Donald A, Merskey H (1987). Interobserver variation in computed tomography of the brain. *Arch Neurol* 44: 30–1.

Lenders JW, Keiser HR, Goldstein DS *et al.* (1995). Plasma metanephrines in the diagnosis of phaeochromocytoma. *Ann Intern Med* 123: 101–9.

Leys D, Pruvo JP, Godefroy O, Rondepierre P, Leclerc X (1992).

Prevalence and significance of hyperdense middle cerebral artery in acute stroke. *Stroke* 23: 317–24.

Limburg M, Van Royen EA, Hijdra A, deBruine JF, Verbeeten BWJ (1990). Single photon emission computed tomography and early death in acute ischaemic stroke. *Stroke* 21: 1150–5.

Lindgren A, Norrving B, Rudling O, Johansson BO (1994). Comparison of clinical and neuroradiological findings in first-ever stroke: a population-based study. *Stroke* 25: 1371–7.

Lindley RI, Wardlaw JM, Ricci S, Celani M, Sandercock P, on behalf of the International Stroke Trial Group (1992). Haemorrhagic transformation of cerebral infarction in acute stroke patients in the International Stroke Trial Pilot. *Cerebrovasc Dis* 2: 234.

Linn FHH, Wijdicks EFM, van der Graaf Y, Weerdesteyn-van Vliet FAC, Bartelds AIM, van Gijn J (1994). Prospective study of sentinel headache in aneurysmal subarachnoid haemorrhage. *Lancet* 344: 590–3.

Lodder J (1984). CT detected haemorrhagic infarction: relation with size of infarct and the presence of midline shift. *Acta Neurol Scand* 70: 329–35.

Lodder J, Krijne-Kubat B, Broekman J (1986). Cerebral haemorrhagic infarction at autopsy: cardiac embolic causes and the relationship to the cause of death. *Stroke* 17: 626–9.

Madden K, Karanjia P, Marshfield WI, Adams H, Clarke W and the TOAST Investigators (1994). Accuracy of initial stroke subtype diagnosis in the TOAST trial. *Neurology* 44 (Suppl. 2): A271.

Manelfe C, Clanet M, Gigaud M, Bonafe A, Guiraud B, Rascol A (1981). Internal capsule: normal anatomy and ischaemic changes demonstrated by computed tomography. *Am J Neuroradiol* 2: 149–55.

Manschot WA (1954). Subarachnoid haemorrhage: intraocular symptoms and their pathogenesis. *Am J Ophthalmol* 38: 501–5.

Marion DW, Segal R, Thompson ME (1986). Subarachnoid haemorrhage and the heart. *Neurosurgery* 18: 101–6.

Masson M, Prier S, Desbleds MT, Colombani JM, Juliard JM (1984). Transformation d'un infarctus cérébral en hémorragie au cours d'un examen tomodensitométrique, chez un patient sous traitement anticoagulant. *Rev Neurol (Paris)* 140: 502–6.

Matsuda M, Ohashi M, Shiino A, Matsumura K, Handa J (1993). Circumstances precipitating aneurysmal subarachnoid haemorrhage. *Cerebrovasc Dis* 3: 285–8.

Matthews WF, Frommeyer WB (1955). The *in vitro* behaviour of erythrocytes in human cerebrospinal fluid. *J Lab Clin Med* 45: 508–15.

Mayer SA, Fink ME, Homma S et al. (1994). Cardiac injury associated with neurogenic pulmonary oedema following subarachnoid haemorrhage. *Neurology* 44: 815–20.

Merrick MV (1990). Cerebral perfusion studies. *Eur J Nucl Med* 17: 98.

Mohr JP, Biller J, Hilal SK et al. (1995). Magnetic resonance versus computed tomographic imaging in acute stroke. *Stroke* 26: 807–12.

Mokri B, Sundt TM, Houser OW, Piepgras DG (1986). Spontaneous dissection of the cervical internal carotid artery. *Ann Neurol* 19: 126–38.

Mori E, Tabuchi M, Ohsumi Y et al. (1990). Intraarterial urokinase infusion therapy in acute thromboembolic stroke. *Stroke* 21:

I-74.

Mori E, Yoneda Y, Tabuchi M et al. (1992). Intravenous recombinant tissue plasminogen activator in acute carotid artery territory stroke. *Neurology* 42: 976–82.

Morretti J-l, Defer G, Cinotti L et al. (1990). 'Luxury perfusion' with ^{99m}Tc-HMPAO and ^{123}I-IMP SPECT imaging during the subacute phase of stroke. *Eur J Nucl Med* 16: 17–22.

Multicentre Acute Stroke Trial—Italy (MAST-I) Group (1995). Randomised controlled trial of streptokinase, aspirin and combination of both in treatment of acute ischaemic stroke. *Lancet* 346: 1509–14.

Nadeau SE, Trobe JD (1983). Pupil sparing in oculomotor palsy: a brief review. *Ann Neurol* 13: 143–8.

Okada Y, Yamaguchi T, Minematsu K et al. (1989). Haemorrhagic transformation in cerebral embolism. *Stroke* 20: 598–603.

Ostergaard JR (1990). Warning leak in subarachnoid haemorrhage. *Br Med J* 301: 190–1.

Ott BR, Zamani A, Kleefield J, Funkenstein HH (1986). The clinical spectrum of haemorrhagic infarction. *Stroke* 17: 630–7.

Pascual-Leone A, Pascual AP (1992). Occipital neuralgia: another benign cause of 'thunderclap headache'. *J Neurol Neurosurg Psychiatr* 55: 411–15.

Paulson GW (1983). Weightlifter's headache. *Headache* 23: 193–4.

Paxton R, Ambrose J (1974). The EMI scanner: a brief review of the first 650 patients. *Br J Radiol* 47: 530.

Pearce JMS, Pearce SHS (1986). Benign paroxysmal cranial neuralgia or cephalgia fugax. *Br Med J* 292: 1015.

Perkin GD (1995). Cerebral venous thrombosis: developments in imaging and treatment. *J Neurol Neurosurg Psychiatr* 59: 1–3.

Pessin MS, Teal PA, Caplan LR (1992). Haemorrhagic transformation: guilt by association? *Am J Neuroradiol* 12: 1123–6.

Pfleger MD, Hardee EP, Contant CF, Hayman AL (1994). Sensitivity and specificity of fluid-blood levels for coagulopathy in acute intracerebral haematomas. *Am J Neuroradiol* 15: 217–23.

Pierce JN, Taber KH, Hayman LA (1994). Acute intracerebral haemorrhage secondary to thrombocytopenia: CT appearances unaffected by absence of clot retraction. *Am J Neuroradiol* 15: 213–15.

Pollick C, Cujec B, Parker S, Tator C (1988). Left ventricular wall motion abnormalities in subarachnoid haemorrhage: an echocardiographic study. *J Am Coll Cardiol* 12: 600–5.

Porter M, Jankovic J (1981). Benign coital cephalalgia—differential diagnosis and treatment. *Arch Neurol* 38: 710–12.

Pounguarin N, Viriyavejaku IA, Komontri C (1991). Siriraj stroke score and validation study to distinguish supratentorial intracerebral haemorrhage from infarction. *Br Med J* 302: 1565.

Pullicino P, Kendall BE (1980). Contrast enhancement in ischaemic lesions. I. Relationship to prognosis. *Neuroradiology* 19: 235–40.

Raynaud C, Rancurel G, Tzourio N et al. (1989). SPECT analysis of recent cerebral infarction. *Stroke* 20: 192–204.

Ricci S, Celani MG, LaRosa F et al. (1991). SEPIVAC: a community-based study of stroke incidence in Umbria, Italy. *J Neurol Neurosurg Psychiatr* 54: 695–8.

Rimdusid P, Wardlaw J, Lindley RI, Sandercock P, on behalf of the

International Stroke Trial Collaboration Group (1995). Haemorrhagic infarction in acute ischaemic stroke patients: International Stroke Trial Pilot Study. *Cerebrovasc Dis* 5: 264.

Rinkel GJE, Wijdicks EFM, Vermeulen M, Hasan D, Brouwers PJAM, van Gijn J (1991). The clinical course of perimesencephalic nonaneurysmal subarachnoid haemorrhage. *Ann Neurol* 29: 463–8.

Ross B, Michaelis T (1994). Clinical applications of magnetic resonance spectroscopy. *Mag Reson Quart* 10: 191–247.

Rother J, Guckel F, Neff W, Kuhnen J, Hennerici M, Schwartz A (1994). Assessment of cerebral blood volume in acute stroke using dynamic contrast-enhanced magnetic resonance imaging. *Neurology* 44: A182.

Rousseaux P, Scherpereel R, Bernard MH, Graftieaux JP, Guyot JF (1980). Fever and cerebral vasopsasm in ruptured intracranial aneurysms. *Surg Neurol* 14: 459–65.

Royal College of Radiologists (1995). *Making the Best Use of a Department of Clinical Radiology*, 3rd edn. London: Royal College of Radiologists.

Ruelle A, Cavazzani P, Andrioli G (1988). Extracranial posterior inferior cerebellar artery aneurysm causing isolated intraventricular haemorrhage: a case report. *Neurosurgery* 23: 774–7.

Sacco RL, Ellenberg JH, Mohr JP *et al.* (1989). Infarcts of undetermined cause: the NINDS Stroke Data Bank. *Ann Neurol* 25: 382–90.

Sage MR (1982). Blood–brain barrier: a phenomenon of increasing importance to the imaging clinician. *Am J Neuroradiol* 3: 127–38.

Saito I, Segawa H, Shiokawa Y, Taniguchi M, Tsutsumi K (1987). Middle cerebral artery occlusion: correlation of computed tomography and angiography with clinical outcome. *Stroke* 18: 863–8.

Sakas DE, Dias LS, Beale D (1995). Subarachnoid haemorrhage presenting as head injury. *Br Med J* 310: 1186–7.

Samuelsson M, Lindell D, Norrving B (1994). Gadolinium-enhanced magnetic resonance imaging in patients with presumed lacunar infarction. *Cerebrovasc Dis* 4: 12–19.

Sarner M, Rose FC (1967). Clinical presentation of ruptured intracranial aneurysm. *J Neurol Neurosurg Psychiatr* 30: 67–70.

Sato A, Takahashi S, Soma Y *et al.* (1991). Cerebral infarction: early detection by means of contrast enhanced cerebral arteries at MR imaging. *Radiology* 178: 433–9.

Saunders DE, Howe FA, van den Boogaart A, McLean MA, Griffiths JR, Brown MA (1995). Continuing ischaemic damage after acute middle cerebral artery infarction in humans demonstrated by short-echo proton spectroscopy. *Stroke* 26: 1007–13.

Savoiardo M (1986). CT scanning. In: Barnett HJM, Mohr JP, Stein BM, Yatsu FM, eds. *Stroke: Pathophysiology, Diagnosis and Management*. New York: Churchill Livingstone, 189–219.

Schievink WI, Wijdicks EFM, Parisi JE, Piepgras DG, Whisnant JP (1995). Sudden death from aneurysmal subarachnoid haemorrhage. *Neurology* 45: 871–4.

Shinar D, Gross CR, Hier DB *et al.* (1987). Interobserver reliability in the interpretation of computed tomographic scans of stroke patients. *Arch Neurol* 44: 149–55.

Silbert PL, Edis RH, Stewart-Wynne EG, Gubbay SS (1991). Benign vascular sexual headache and exertional headache: interrelationships and long term prognosis. *J Neurol Neurosurg Psychiatr* 54: 417–21.

Simmons Z, Biller J, Adams H, Dunn V, Jacoby C (1986). Cerebellar infarction: comparison of computed tomography and magnetic resonance imaging. *Ann Neurol* 19: 291–3.

Skriver EB, Olsen TS (1981). Transient disappearance of cerebral infarcts on CT scan, the so-called fogging effect. *Neuroradiology* 22: 61–5.

Skriver EB, Olsen TS, McNair P (1990). Mass effect and atrophy after stroke. *Acta Radiol* 31: 431–8.

Sotaniemi KA, Pyhtinen J, Myllylä VV (1990). Correlation of clinical and computed tomographic findings in stroke patients. *Stroke* 21: 1562–6.

Stober T, Anstatt Th, Sen S, Schimrig KK, Jager H (1988). Cardiac arrhythmias in subarachnoid haemorrhage. *Acta Neurochir* 93: 37–44.

Stone JL, Crowell RM, Gandhi YN, Jafar JJ (1988). Multiple intracranial aneurysms: magnetic resonance imaging for determination of the site of rupture—report of a case. *Neurosurgery* 23: 97–100.

Sung CY, Chu NS (1992). Late CT manifestation in spontaneous putaminal haemorrhage. *Neuroradiology* 34: 200–4.

Svigelj V, Grad A, Tekavcic I, Kiauta T (1994). Cardiac arrhythmia associated with reversible damage to insula in a patient with subarachnoid haemorrhage. *Stroke* 25: 1053–5.

Tanaka H, Ueda Y, Date C *et al.* (1981). Incidence of stroke in Shibata, Japan: 1976–1978. *Stroke* 12: 460–6.

Terent A, Ronquist G, Bergstrom K, Hallgren R, Aberg H (1981). Ischaemic oedema in stroke: a parallel study with computed tomography and cerebrospinal fluid markers of disturbed brain cell metabolism. *Stroke* 12: 33–40.

Thomas JE, Rooke E, Kvale WF (1966). The neurologist's experience with phaeochromocytoma: a review of 100 cases. *J Am Med Assoc* 197: 754–8.

Tomsick T, Brott T, Barsan W *et al.* (1990). Thrombus localisation with emergency cerebral computed tomography. *Stroke* 21: 180.

Tomura N, Uemura K, Inugami A, Fujita H, Higano S, Shishido F (1988). Early CT finding in cerebral infarction: obscuration of the lentiform nucleus. *Radiology* 168: 463–7.

Torigoe R, Harad K, Matsuo H (1990). Assessment of cerebral infarction by MRI—particularly fogging effect. *No-To-Shinkei* 42 (6): 547–52.

Torvik A (1984). The pathogenesis of watershed infarcts in the brain. *Stroke* 15: 221–3.

Tourtelotte WW, Metz LN, Bryan ER, DeJong RN (1964). Spontaneous subarachnoid hemorrhage: factors affecting the rate of clearing of cerebrospinal fluid. *Neurology* 14: 301–6.

Tourtellotte WW, Haerer AF, Heller GL *et al.* (1964). *Post-lumbar Puncture Headaches*. Springfield Ill: Charles C Thomas, 50.

Truwit CL, Barkovitch AJ, Gean-Marton A, Hibri N, Norman D (1990). Loss of the insular ribbon: another sign of acute middle cerebral artery infarction. *Radiology* 176: 801–6.

Tubbs ON, Potter JM (1970). Early post-concussional headache. *Lancet* ii: 128–9.

Ueda K, Omae T, Hirota Y *et al.* (1981). Decreasing trend in incidence and mortality from stroke in Hisayama residents, Japan. *Stroke* 12: 154–60.

van der Wee N, Rinkel GJE, Hasan D, Van Gijn J (1995). Detection of subarachnoid heamorrhage on early CT: is lumbar puncture still needed after a negative scan? *J Neurol Neurosurg Psychiatr* 58: 357–9.

van der Zwan A, Hillen B (1991). Review of the variability of the territories of the major cerebral arteries. *Stroke* 22: 1078–84.

van Gijn J (1992). Subarachnoid haemorrhage. *Lancet* 339: 653–5.

van Gijn J, van Dongen KJ (1982). The time course of aneurysmal haemorrhage on computed tomograms. *Neuroradiology* 23: 153–6.

van Gijn J, van Dongen KJ, Vermeulen M, Hijdra A (1985). Perimesencephalic haemorrhage: a nonaneurysmal and benign form of subarachnoid haemorrhage. *Neurology* 35: 493–7.

Vemmos KN, Mparmparesou M, Kontogianni M, Zis V, Stranjalis G, Moulopoulos S (1994). Haemorrhagic transformation in embolic stroke. *Cerebrovasc Dis* 4: 230.

Vermeulen M, van Gijn J (1990). The diagnosis of subarachnoid haemorrhage. *J Neurol Neurosurg Psychiatr* 53: 365–72.

Vermeulen M, van Gijn J, Blijenberg BG (1983). Spectrophotometric analysis of CSF after subarachnoid haemorrhage: limitations in the diagnosis of rebleeding. *Neurology* 33: 112–14.

Vermeulen M, Lindsay KW, Murray GD *et al.* (1984). Antifibrinolytic treatment in subarachnoid haemorrhage. *N Engl J Med* 311: 432–7.

Versari P, Bassi P, Limoni P *et al.* (1993). Unrecognised warning leak in ruptured intracranial aneurysm. *Cerebrovasc Dis* 3: 289–94.

Verweij RD, Wijdicks EFM, van Gijn J (1988). Warning headache in aneurysmal subarachnoid haemorrhage: a case-controlled study. *Arch Neurol* 45: 1019–20.

Vestergaard K, Andersen G, Nielsen MI, Jensen TS (1993). Headache in stroke. *Stroke* 24: 1621–4.

Vincent FM, Zimmerman JE (1980). Superior cerebellar artery aneurysm presenting as an oculomotor palsy in a child. *Neurosurgery* 6: 661–4.

Virapongse C, Cazenave C, Quisling R, Sarwar M, Hunter S (1987). The empty delta sign: frequence and significance in 76 cases of dural sinus thrombosis. *Radiology* 162: 779–85.

Vogl TJ, Bergman C, Villringer A, Einhaupl K, Lissner J, Felix R (1994). *Am J Roentgenol* 162: 1191–8.

von Kummer R, Meyding-Lamade U, Frosting M *et al.* (1994). Sensitivity and prognostic value of early CT in occlusion of the middle cerebral artery trunk. *Am J Neuroradiol* 15: 9–15.

Wall SD, Brant-Zawadzki M, Jeffrey RB, Barnes B (1982). High frequency CT findings within 24 hours after cerebral infarction. *Am J Roentgenol* 138: 307–11.

Walton JN (1956). *Subarachnoid Haemorrhage*. Edinburgh: Livingstone.

Warach S, Li W, Ronthal M, Edelman RR (1992). Acute cerebral ischaemia: evaluation with dynamic contrast enhanced MR imaging and MR angiography. *Radiology* 182: 41–7.

Warach S, Gaa J, Siewert B, Wielopolski P, Edelman RR (1995). Acute human stroke studied by whole brain echo planar

diffusion-weighted magnetic resonance imaging. *Ann Neurol* 37: 231–41.

Ward G, Jamrozik K, Stewart-Wynne E (1988). Incidence and outcome of cerebrovascular disease in Perth, Western Australia. *Stroke* 19: 1501–6.

Wardlaw J, Dennis MS, Lindley RI, Sellar RJ, Warlow CP (1996). The validity of a simple clinical classification of acute ischaemic stroke. *J Neurol* 243: 274–9.

Wardlaw JM, Sellar RJ (1994). A simple practical classification of cerebral infarcts on CT and its interobserver reliability. *Am J Neuroradiol* 15: 1933–9.

Wardlaw JM, Dennis MS, Lindley RI, Sellar RJ, Warlow CP (1993). How accurate is a simple clinical classification of predicting the site and extent of cerebral infarction in routine hospital practice. In: *Proceedings of Second International Conference on Stroke*, Geneva, 12–15 May, p. 64.

Watanabe A, Ishii R, Tanaka R, Tokiguchi S, Ito JC (1982). Relation of cranial nerve involvement to the location of intracranial aneurysms. *Neurol Medico-chirurg* 22: 910–16.

Weiller C, Ringelstein EB, Reiche W, Thron A, Buell U (1990). The large striatocapsular infarct: a clinical and pathological entity. *Arch Neurol* 47: 1085–91.

Weir CJ, Murray GD, Adams FG, Muir KW, Grossett DG, Lees KR (1994). Poor accuracy of scoring systems for differential clinical diagnosis of intracranial haemorrhage and infarction. *Lancet* 344: 999–1002.

West TET, Davies RJ, Kelly RE (1976). Horner's syndrome and headache due to carotid artery disease. *Br Med J* i: 818–21.

Wijdicks EFM, Kerkhoff H, van Gijn J (1988). Long-term follow-up of 71 patients with thunderclap headache mimicking subarachnoid haemorrhage. *Lancet* ii: 68–70.

Wijdicks EFM, Vermeulen M, Murray GD, Hijdra A, van Gijn J (1990). The effect of treating hypertension following aneurysmal subarachnoid haemorrhage. *Clin Neurol Neurosurg* 92: 111–17.

Wing SD, Norman D, Pollock JA, Newton TH (1976). Contrast enhancement of cerebral infarcts in computed tomography. *Radiology* 121: 89–92.

Witt J-P, Holl K, Heissler HE, Dietz H (1991). Stable xenon CT CBF: effects of blood flow alterations on CBF calculations during inhalation of 33% stable xenon. *Am J Neuroradiol* 12: 973–5.

Wroe SJ, Sandercock P, Bamford J, Dennis M, Slattery J, Warlow C (1992). Diurnal variation in incidence of stroke: Oxfordshire Community Stroke Project. *Br Med J* 304: 155–7.

Yang SS, Ryu SJ, Wu CL (1990). Early CT diagnosis of cerebral ischaemia. *Stroke* 21: I–121.

Yuh WTC, Crain MR, Loes DJ, Greene GM, Ryals TJ, Sato Y (1991). MR imaging of cerebral ischaemia: findings in the first 24 hours. *Am J Neuroradiol* 12: 621–9.

Yuh WTC, Simonson TM, Wang A *et al.* (1994). Venous occlusive disease: MR findings. *Am J Neuroradiol* 15: 309–16.

Zeumer H, Ringelstein EB (1987). Computed tomographic patterns of brain infarctions as a pathogenetic key. In: *New Trends in the Diagnosis and Management of Stroke*. Heidelberg: Springer Verlag, 75–85.

Zigun JR, Frank JA, Barrios FA *et al.* (1993). Measurement of brain activity with bolus administration of contrast agents and gradient echo MR imaging. *Radiology* 186: 353–6.

What caused this transient or persisting ischaemic event?

6

6.1   Introduction

Having established that a patient has had a stroke or transient ischaemic attack (TIA) (see Chapter 3), where the lesion is likely to be and its relationship to the vascular supply (see Chapter 4) and that the cause is ischaemia rather than haemorrhage (see Chapter 5), the next step is to define the cause of the ischaemia, i.e. what caused *this* ischaemic event? If, for whatever reason, it has been impossible to distinguish an ischaemic stroke from primary intracerebral haemorrhage (PICH), then the causes of the latter (see Chapter 8) must be considered as well. Naturally, how far one pursues 'the cause' must depend on how finding it will influence the subsequent management and, more importantly, the outcome of an individual patient with 'a stroke'.

So often physicians regard a stroke as a stroke, without realising that the cause may determine the immediate outcome (see Section 10.2), have a substantial impact on the risk of recurrence (see Section 16.1) and influence the choice of both the immediate (see Chapters 11 and 12) and long-term treatment (see Chapter 16). Moreover, discovering the cause may have unanticipated later relevance; for example, ischaemic stroke due to carotid dissection as a consequence of a car accident (rather than due to atherothrombosis as a consequence of hypertension and smoking) may lead to substantial compensation from an insurance company. Finding the cause is, therefore, important and may not be very difficult. Indeed, the hunt for the cause makes stroke patients more 'interesting', particularly to some neurologists. The first clue is the clinical syndrome (i.e. where and how big is

Table 6.1 What caused *this* ischaemic stroke?

A man of 70 years old suddenly developed a left hemiparesis which recovered in a few days. There was no visual field defect, nor was there any obvious sensory inattention or neglect. He was known to be hypertensive, discovered to be in atrial fibrillation, and his ECG showed an unsuspected but probably old anterior myocardial infarction. There was a loud right carotid bruit. The early brain CT was normal but MRI showed multiple presumed lacunar infarcts in the periventricular white matter of both cerebral hemispheres. Therefore, the stroke could have been due to one of the following:

Embolism from the heart (either from thrombus in the fibrillating left atrium or from thrombus in the left ventricle as a result of the myocardial infarction)

Embolism from atherothrombotic carotid stenosis

Low flow distal to severe atherothrombotic carotid stenosis or occlusion

Intracranial small vessel disease causing lacunar infarction (particularly as one can not be sure from the clinical syndrome whether there were any 'cortical' signs, such as constructional apraxia)

Without further investigation, something unusual, such as thrombocythaemia

CT, computerised tomography; ECG, electrocardiogram; MRI, magnetic resonance imaging.

the area of brain ischaemia or infarction?), but the general examination of the patient usually provides more information about the cause than an obsessional neurological examination, and a few well-targeted investigations should complete the picture. Of course, as we shall see, a patient may have several competing causes for an episode of cerebral ischaemia, making it impossible to know which one is *the* cause (Table 6.1). At the end of the day, however, focal cerebral or ocular ischaemia is always due to low or absent blood flow, and the question is: 'Why is, or *was*, the relevant blood vessel blocked or narrow?'

6.1.1 What to expect

There is no *qualitative* difference between an ischaemic stroke and a TIA; anything which causes an ischaemic stroke may, if less severe or less prolonged, cause a TIA, whilst anything which causes a TIA may, if more severe or more prolonged, cause an ischaemic stroke. The *quantitative* difference is arbitrary and is enshrined in the temporal distinction of symptoms lasting more or less than 24 hours (see Section 3.1.3). It is not surprising that imaging evidence of infarction becomes gradually more likely the longer the duration of the symptoms (Koudstaal *et al.*, 1992) and that

all types of ischaemic stroke are about equally likely to be preceded by TIAs (Table 6.2). Therefore, there is no great difference between searching for the cause of an ischaemic stroke and searching for the cause of a TIA.

> *Anything which causes an ischaemic stroke may, if less severe or less prolonged, cause a transient ischaemic attack, whilst anything which causes a transient ischaemic attack may, if more severe or more prolonged, cause an ischaemic stroke. There is no qualitative difference between the causes of transient ischaemic attack and ischaemic stroke.*

In *community*-based studies (i.e. without any selection bias), about 50% of all cerebral ischaemic events, whether permanent or transient, are due to the thrombotic and embolic complications of atheroma, which is a disorder of large and medium-sized arteries, about 25% are due to intracranial small vessel disease, about 20% to embolism from the heart and the rest to rarities (Fig. 6.1). Not surprisingly, where admission rates are low, hospital-referred stroke patients are rather less likely to have lacunar strokes (because they are milder and therefore more often looked after at home) and more likely to have something unusual, particularly if the hospital has a special interest in stroke or one of its causes (because of hospital referral bias; see Section 10.2.6). Age will colour one's expectations too: a 21-year-old female is hardly likely to have atheroma, whilst an 81-year-old male is very unlikely to have a rare cause of cerebral ischaemia, although this is still possible.

> *About 95% of ischaemic strokes and transient ischaemic attacks are due to the embolic or thrombotic consequences of atherothrombosis affecting large or medium-sized arteries, intracranial small vessel disease or embolism from the heart.*

In this chapter we will consider the nature of the three main causes of cerebral ischaemia: atherothromboem-

Table 6.2 The frequency of TIAs before various types of ischaemic stroke. (Unpublished data collected by Dr Claudio Sacks from the Oxfordshire Community Stroke Project.)

	Frequency of preceding TIAs (%)
All ischaemic strokes	14
Total anterior circulation infarction	16
Partial anterior circulation infarction	15
Lacunar infarction	12
Posterior circulation infarction	12
Presumed cardioembolic ischaemic stroke	16

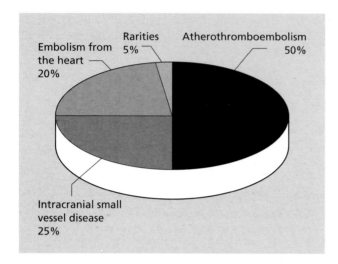

Figure 6.1 The approximate frequency of the main causes of ischaemic stroke and probably of TIAs as well.

bolism, intracranial small vessel disease and embolism from the heart. The more unusual causes will be mostly described in Chapter 7.

6.2   Atherothromboembolism

Atheroma is the most common, but far from the only, arterial disorder (Table 6.3). It seems to be almost universal in the elderly, even though it begins in children and young adults. When complicated by thrombosis or embolism, it is the most common, but not the only, cause of cerebral ischaemia and infarction.

6.2.1   The pattern of atheroma

Atheroma affects mainly the large (e.g. arch of the aorta) and medium-sized arteries, particularly at places of arterial branching (e.g. the carotid bifurcation), tortuosity (e.g. the carotid siphon) and confluence (e.g. the basilar artery) (Fig. 6.2) (Fisher, 1951, 1954; Hutchinson & Yates, 1957; Schwartz & Mitchell, 1961; Cornhill *et al.*, 1980; Ross *et al.*, 1988; Amarenco *et al.*, 1992). It is remarkable how free of atheroma some arterial sites can be—for example, the internal carotid artery (ICA) from just distal to the origin to the siphon and the main cerebral arteries distal to the circle of Willis; therefore, occlusion of the middle cerebral artery (MCA) is much more likely to be due to embolism than to local thrombosis on an atheromatous plaque (Lhermitte *et al.*, 1970; Miller & Cohen, 1987).

Atheroma affects large and medium-sized arteries, particularly at places of branching, tortuosity and confluence.

Presumably this distribution of atheroma is determined by sites of haemodynamic shear stress and endothelial trauma:

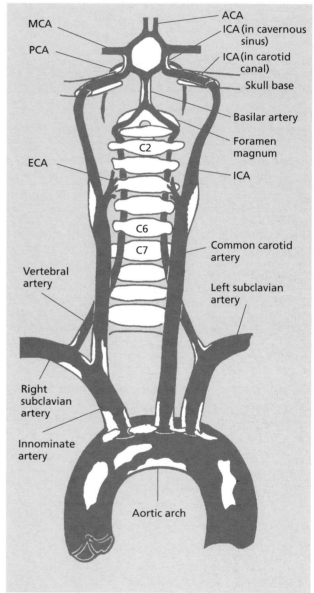

Figure 6.2 The distribution of atheroma (white identations of the arterial lumen) in the arteries supplying the brain and eye in Caucasians. Intracranial atheroma is relatively more frequent than extracranial atheroma in Japanese, Chinese and Afro-Caribbean populations. ACA, anterior cerebral artery; ECA, external carotid artery; ICA, internal carotid artery; MCA, middle cerebral artery; PCA, posterior cerebral artery.

Table 6.3 The causes of arterial disease affecting the circulation to the brain and eye.

ATHEROTHROMBOEMBOLISM (see Section 6.2)
Embolism (see Section 6.2.2)
Occlusive thrombosis (see Section 6.2.2)
Low flow (see Section 6.5.5)
Ectasia (see Section 6.2.2)

INTRACRANIAL SMALL VESSEL DISEASE (see Section 6.3)
Occlusive thrombosis
Rupture?

PRIMARY INFLAMMATORY VASCULAR DISORDER (see Section 7.2)
*Giant cell arteritis
Takayasu's arteritis
*Systemic lupus erythematosus
*Antiphospholipid antibody syndrome
Sneddon's syndrome
Systemic necrotising vasculitis
    Polyarteritis nodosa
    Churg–Strauss syndrome
    Wegener's granulomatosis
Rheumatoid arthritis
Sjögren's syndrome
Behçet's disease
Relapsing polychondritis
Progressive systemic sclerosis (scleroderma)
*Sarcoidosis
Isolated angiitis of the central nervous system
Malignant atrophic papulosis (Kohlmeier–Degos' disease)
Acute posterior multifocal placoid pigment epitheliopathy
Buerger's disease
Lymphomatoid granulomatosis

SECONDARY INFLAMMATORY VASCULAR DISORDER
Infections (see Section 7.8)
*Drugs (see Section 6.5.6)
Irradiation (see Section 7.9)
Inflammatory bowel disease (see Section 6.5.6)
Coeliac disease (see Section 6.5.6)

CONGENITAL
Fibromuscular dysplasia (see Section 7.3)
Arterial loops (see Section 7.3)
Ehlers–Danlos syndrome (see Section 7.3)
Pseudoxanthoma elasticum (see Section 7.3)
Marfan's syndrome (see Section 7.3)
Arteriovenous malformations (see Section 8.2.2)

*ARTERIAL DISSECTION
Trauma (see Section 7.1)
Atheroma (see Section 7.1)
Cystic medial necrosis (see Section 7.1)
Fibromuscular dysplasia (see Section 7.3)
Marfan's syndrome (see Section 7.3)

Ehlers–Danlos syndrome (see Section 7.3)
Pseudoxanthoma elasticum (see Section 7.3)
Inflammatory arterial disease (see Section 7.2)
Infective arterial disease (e.g. syphilis) (see Section 7.8)

TRAUMA
Penetrating neck injury (see Section 7.1)
    Neck laceration/surgery
    Missile wounds
    Oral trauma
    Tonsillectomy
    Cerebral catheter angiography
    Attempted jugular vein catheterisation
Non-penetrating (blunt) neck injury (see Section 7.1)
    Carotid compression
    Cervical manipulation
    Blow to the neck
    Cervical flexion–extension 'whiplash' injury
    Minor head movements?
    Cervical rib
    Fractured clavicle
    Head-banging
    Labour
    Epileptic seizures
    Yoga
    Attempted strangulation
    Atlanto-occipital instability
    Atlanto-axial dislocation
    Fractured base of skull
    Faulty posture of neck during general anaesthesia
    Vomiting

METABOLIC DISORDERS
Mitochondrial cytopathy (MELAS syndrome) (see Section 7.15)
Hypoglycaemia (see Section 6.5.6)
Homocystinuria (see Section 6.5.6)
Fabry's disease (see Section 6.5.7)
Oxalosis (see Section 6.4)

MISCELLANEOUS
Vasospasm (migraine)? (see Section 7.5)
*Leukoaraiosis (see Section 7.12)
Pregnancy/oral contraceptives/oestrogens (see Sections 7.10 and 7.11)
Snake bite (see Section 7.6)
Fat embolism (see Section 6.5.6)
Fibrocartilaginous embolism (see Section 7.1)
Cerebral autosomal dominant arteriopathy with subcortical infarcts and leucoencephalopathy (CADASIL) (see Section 6.5.6)
Tuberous sclerosis (see Section 6.5.7)
Neurofibromatosis (see Section 6.5.7)
Aneurysms (see Section 7.4)
Epidermal naevus syndrome (see Table 6.14)

* The most common 'rare' causes of arterial disease, i.e. well under 5% of all patients with ischaemic stroke/TIA.
MELAS, mitochondrial encephalopathy with lactic acidosis and stroke-like episodes.

Table 6.4 The prevalence of vascular risk factors and diseases in 244 patients with a first-ever in a lifetime ischaemic stroke. Data from the Oxfordshire Community Stroke Project. (From Sandercock *et al.*, 1989.)

	n	Per cent
Hypertension (blood pressure > 160/90 mmHg × 2 pre-stroke)	126	52
Angina and/or past myocardial infarction	92	38
Current smokers	66	27
Claudication and/or absent foot pulses	60	25
Major cardiac embolic source	50	20
TIA	35	14
Cervical arterial bruit	33	14
Diabetes mellitus	24	10
Any of the above	196	80

boundary-zone flow separation and blood stagnation; or of turbulence; all of which might promote thrombosis, which itself may be involved in the progression of atheroma (Hugh & Fox, 1970; Grady, 1984; Motomiya & Karino, 1984; McMillan, 1985; Reneman *et al.*, 1985). Interestingly, in some individuals there can be very severe atherothrombotic stenosis at a particular site on one side of the body, but none at all at the mirror-image site on the other side of the body, perhaps reflecting intra-individual geometric differences in arterial anatomy (Fisher & Fieman, 1990). Alternatively, maybe once an atheromatous plaque is established, its growth becomes self-promoting as a result of some sort of positive feedback loop, either biochemical or haemodynamic. On the whole, however, individuals with atheroma affecting one artery tend to have it affecting many others, subclinically if not clinically, so that patients with cerebral ischaemia often have (Table 6.4) or develop (see Section 16.1.1) angina, myocardial infarction and claudication (Mitchell & Schwartz, 1962; Hertzer *et al.*, 1985; Di Pasquale *et al.*, 1986; Miller & Cohen, 1987; Craven *et al.*, 1990). Presumably there are certain genetically predisposed individuals who are likely to develop atheroma, or to have particularly extensive or severe atheroma when exposed to causal risk factors such as hypertension, whilst the arterial anatomy determines where the lesion occurs in such individuals. It is, however, notable that black and Oriental races tend to have more intracranial and less extracranial atheroma (see Section 6.2.3).

> *Individuals with atheroma affecting one artery almost always have atheroma affecting several other arteries, with or without clinical manifestations.*

6.2.2 The nature and progression of atheroma

Atheroma begins as intimal fatty streaks in children (Fig. 6.3). Over many years, arterial smooth muscle cells proliferate and the intima is invaded by macrophages, fibrosis occurs, and intra- and extracellular cholesterol and other lipids are deposited to form fibrolipid plaques (Ross, 1986; Mitchinson & Ball, 1987). These plaques invade the media and spread around and along the arterial wall, and so the wall thickens and the lumen narrows. Later the plaques become necrotic and calcified. From an early stage, or perhaps even from the very first stage, atheromatous plaques are complicated by platelet adhesion, activation and aggregation, which initiate blood coagulation and thus mural thrombosis (Imparato *et al.*, 1979; Gower *et al.*, 1987; Fuster *et al.*, 1992; Ware & Heistad, 1993). Thrombus is incorporated into the plaque which re-endothelialises and so 'heals'. The atherothrombotic plaque may grow to obstruct the arterial lumen, and then intraluminal thrombus propagates proximally or distally, or the thrombotic part may be lysed by fibrinolytic mechanisms in the vessel wall and blood, or it may embolise—in whole or in part—to obstruct a smaller distal artery, perhaps the same one on several occasions. Therefore, emboli consist of any combination of cholesterol debris, platelet aggregates and fibrin. Depending on their size, composition, consistency and age, emboli may be lysed, fragment or remain to occlude the distal artery and perhaps promote local antero- and retrograde thrombosis. Presumably the pattern and velocity of local blood flow to some extent determines the fate of obstructing emboli (Gunning *et al.*, 1964; Castaigne *et al.*, 1970; Hutchinson, 1972; Whisnant, 1982; Norris & Bornstein, 1986). Whether brain infarction then occurs or not depends on the adequacy of any collateral blood supply (Harrison & Marshall, 1988; see Section 11.1.3).

Emboli are transmitted to the brain or eye via their normal arterial supply, which itself varies in distribution between individuals (see Section 4.3). So an embolus from the origin of the ICA usually goes to the eye or the anterior two-thirds of the cerebral hemisphere, but on occasion it may go to the occipital cortex if the blood in the posterior communicating artery (PCoA) is flowing from the ICA to the PCoA. However, if an artery is occluded, then an embolus may impact in a surprising place; for example, with severe vertebral arterial disease and therefore poor flow distally into the basilar artery, an embolus from the ICA origin may reach the basilar artery via the circle of Willis. With ICA occlusion, it is possible to have an ipsilateral MCA distribution cerebral infarct due to an embolus travelling from the contralateral ICA origin via the anterior communicating artery; from the blind stump of the proximal ipsilateral ICA

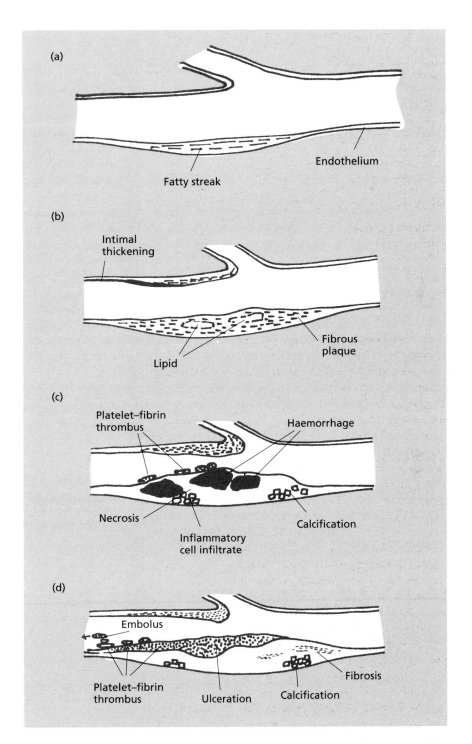

Figure 6.3 The growth, progression and complications of atheromatous plaques: (a) early deposition of lipid in the artery wall; (b) further build-up of fibrous and lipid material; (c) necrosis, inflammatory cell infiltrate, calcification and new vessel formation, haemorrhage leading to; (d) ulceration and platelet–fibrin thrombus formation on the plaque surface.

or from disease of the ipsilateral external carotid artery (ECA) via orbital collaterals; or from the tail of thrombus in the ICA distal to the occlusion. Finally, ischaemic stroke ipsilateral to an ICA occlusion may be due to low flow in its normal territory of supply, or within a boundary zone (see Section 6.5.5), particularly if the collateral blood supply is poor (Finklestein *et al.*, 1980; Countee *et al.*, 1981; Bogous-slavsky & Regli, 1986a; Ryan & Day, 1987; Hankey & Warlow, 1991a; Kleiser *et al.*, 1991). Curiously, emboli from the neck arteries (or from the heart) seldom seem to enter the small perforating arteries of the brain to cause lacunar infarction (see Section 6.3).

> *Atherothrombosis affects large and medium-sized arteries and causes about 50% of ischaemic strokes and transient ischaemic attacks, as a result of embolism to the brain, acute thrombotic arterial occlusion or low flow distal to a severely narrowed or occluded artery.*

It seems likely that at least the complications of atherothromboembolism, if not atheroma itself, can be regarded as an acute-on-chronic disorder, because TIAs tend to cluster, stroke tends to occur early after a TIA and affect the same arterial territory (see Section 16.1.1), the risk of ischaemic stroke ipsilateral to severe carotid stenosis is highest soon after symptomatic presentation and then declines (see Section 16.7.5), presumed artery-to-artery embolic strokes tend to recur early (see Section 16.1.3) and emboli detected with transcranial Doppler (TCD) sonography are more likely if a stenosis is severe or has been recently symptomatic (Babikian *et al.*, 1994; Siebler *et al.*, 1994; Ries *et al.*, 1995). This may be because an atheromatous plaque becomes 'active' from time to time, as a result of: fissuring, cracking or rupture of the fibrous cap covering the rather rigid lesion; of ulceration perhaps; or sometimes of haemorrhage within the plaque. Any of these events exposes the thrombogenic centre of the plaque to flowing blood and so could cause complicating thrombosis. Even severe stenosis alone may be sufficient to cause thrombosis, with or without embolism. At other times, the plaque is static and quiescent, or slowly growing, without causing any clinical symptoms (Constantinides, 1967; Harrison & Marshall, 1977; Fisher *et al.*, 1987; Svindland & Torvik, 1988; Richardson *et al.*, 1989; Torvik *et al.*, 1989; Gomez, 1990; Ogata *et al.*, 1990, 1994). Whatever else, increasing severity of stenosis, at least at the origin of the ICA, is undoubtedly a most powerful predictor of ischaemic stroke ipsilateral to the lesion (see Section 16.7.5 and Fig. 16.23).

> *Atherothromboembolism is an acute-on-chronic disease. Although the formation of atherothrombotic plaque is a long and chronic process over many years, the clinical manifestations usually occur acutely (e.g. an ischaemic stroke) and tend to cluster in time (e.g. stroke tends to occur sooner rather than later after a transient ischaemic attack) as a result of the sudden breakdown and 'activation' of an atherothrombotic plaque.*

Dilatation and ectasia of atheromatous cerebral arteries are unusual; such vessels often contain thrombus which may embolise or occlude the origin of small branch arteries of the ectatic vessel. Cranial nerve and brainstem compression are

other occasional complications (see Section 4.3.3; Schwartz *et al.*, 1993).

6.2.3 The causes of atheroma

The current view is that atheroma is initiated by some sort of endothelial injury, which, perhaps in genetically susceptible individuals, is then amplified by factors such as hypertension, cigarette-smoking and hypercholesterolaemia (Ross, 1986). Thrombosis certainly complicates atheroma and may even be involved in its very beginnings (Duguid, 1976). Evidence comes from animal models of atheroma (none of which is entirely satisfactory), pathological examination of human arteries and epidemiological studies of 'risk factors', which may be as much risk factors for the complicating thrombosis as for the underlying atheroma itself (if, indeed, the two processes can be separated). Whatever the exact mechanisms, it is quite clear that there are certain individual and population characteristics (risk factors) which make the *clinical* consequences of atheroma (i.e. ischaemic stroke, myocardial infarction, etc.) more likely (Table 6.5). In some,

Table 6.5 Factors associated with an increased risk of occlusive vascular disorders (i.e. ischaemic stroke, myocardial infarction, claudication, etc.).

Definite
Age
Male sex
High blood pressure
Cigarette-smoking
Diabetes mellitus
High plasma fibrinogen
Blood lipids (definite for myocardial infarction but not for cerebral ischaemia)

*Possible**
High plasma factor VII coagulant activity
Low blood fibrinolytic activity
Raised tissue plasminogen activator antigen
Physical inactivity
Raised haematocrit
Obesity
Diet (salt, antioxidants, coffee, etc.)
Alcohol (none, or heavy drinking)
Race
Social deprivation

See also Table 6.8

---

* Somewhat or very uncertain association with stroke, because any association is weak, because any association has been under-researched in comparison with coronary heart disease, or because any association has been examined in relation to all stroke rather than just one pathological type of stroke, such as ischaemic stroke or PICH.

Table 6.6 Relative risk and relative odds.

Calculation of relative risk, relative odds and absolute risk difference in a longitudinal study of a cohort of individuals, some of whom have a risk factor for stroke ($a + b$), and some of whom develop a stroke during follow-up ($a + c$)

Stroke during follow-up

		Yes	No
Risk factor present at baseline	Yes	a	b
	No	c	d

The risk of stroke in those with the risk factor ($R+$) is $\dfrac{a}{a + b}$

The risk of stroke in those without the risk factor ($R-$) is $\dfrac{c}{c + d}$

∴ The relative risk $= \dfrac{R+}{R-}$ i.e. $\dfrac{a}{a + b} \times \dfrac{c + d}{c} = \dfrac{ac + ad}{ac + bc}$

and the absolute risk difference is $(R+) - (R-)$

The odds of stroke in those with the risk factor ($O+$) is $\dfrac{a}{b}$

The odds of stroke in those without the risk factor ($O-$) is $\dfrac{c}{d}$

∴ The relative odds (or odds ratio) $= \dfrac{O+}{O-}$ i.e. $\dfrac{ad}{bc}$

Note: when stroke is rare (i.e. a and c are small compared with b and d), then the relative risk and relative odds are about the same value

In a case–control study, patients with stroke ($a + c$) and controls from the same population without a stroke ($b + d$) are identified and the exposure to the risk factor compared using the odds ratio

Stroke and no-stroke control patients identified at one point in time

		Yes	No
Risk factor present	Yes	a	b
	No	c	d

The odds of a stroke patient having the risk factor are $\dfrac{a}{c}$

The odds of a control patient having the risk factor are $\dfrac{b}{d}$

∴ The relative odds (or odds ratio) $= \dfrac{a}{c} \div \dfrac{b}{d} = \dfrac{ad}{bc}$

high relative risk or odds); consistency of association across several studies; a dose–response relationship (i.e. the greater the exposure to the risk factor, the greater the risk of the disease); independence from confounding variables (Fig. 6.4); a clear temporal sequence of exposure to the risk factor *before* disease onset; biological and epidemiological plausibility, although there is no end to human ingenuity in constructing plausible hypotheses to explain the natural world; and, most convincing of all but not always feasible, demonstration that attenuation of the risk factor leads to a fall in disease inci-

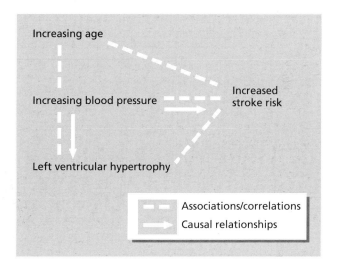

Figure 6.4 'Confounding' in observational studies of aetiology which attempt to relate a risk factor to a disease such as stroke. In this example, increasing age is associated with both increasing blood pressure and increasing risk of stroke. In fact, age and blood pressure are independent of the confounding effect of one on the other; in other words, for a population of a given age there is an increasing risk of stroke with increasing blood pressure, and for a population of a given blood pressure there is an increasing risk of stroke with increasing age. Therefore, in some way independent of ageing, increasing blood pressure is strongly associated with stroke risk and this is in fact a causal relationship (see Section 6.2.3). Also, increasing age is associated with increasing stroke risk, not because age and blood pressure are associated, which they are, but because of something else (perhaps increasing prevalence of atrial fibrillation with age, etc.). On the other hand, although left-ventricular hypertrophy is associated with increasing stroke risk, this association more or less disappears if blood pressure is controlled for, because, presumably, the association is explained mostly by the fact that increasing blood pressure causes *both* stroke *and* left-ventricular hypertrophy. So hypertension is a confounding factor and explains the left-ventricular hypertrophy/stroke relationship. Unfortunately, it is not possible to adjust for confounding factors if they are not suspected or measured and, even when they are, statistical adjustment is not always easy, or even possible, so that some associations said to be unconfounded may not be as real as they seem. (From Davey Smith *et al.*, 1992; Datta, 1993; Phillips & Davey Smith, 1993; Leon, 1993.)

but by no means all, instances, there is a plausible biological explanation for the connection between a risk factor, through atherothrombotic arterial disease, to the clinical syndrome. It is, however, important to be clear that a risk factor indicates an *association* between that factor and the disease of interest (Table 6.6). A *causal* relationship between a risk factor and a disease is supported if there is a strong association between the risk factor and the disease (i.e. a dence, preferably by means of a randomised controlled trial (Glynn, 1993). However, even if a risk factor is associated with a high relative risk of stroke, and even if the relationship is causal, the factor may have very little impact on overall stroke incidence if that particular risk factor is rarely present in the population (e.g. *rheumatic* atrial fibrillation (AF) in developed countries) and/or if the baseline risk of stroke is very low in the population where the risk factor is acting (e.g. oral contraceptives in young women). In other words, the impact of a risk factor is very low if the proportion of stroke cases attributable to that risk factor is very low (low population-attributable risk). On the other hand, a causal risk factor with a rather modest relative risk may be of major importance in determining stroke incidence if it is very prevalent (e.g. hypertension) and/or the background risk of stroke in the population is high (e.g. in elderly people) so that the population-attributable risk is then high.

This epidemiological approach to defining risk factors, and possible causation, has tended to lump all strokes together, more so in cohort than in case–control studies, so the heterogeneous nature of the pathology and causes of stroke may obscure the relationship between a particular risk factor and, for example, a particular type of stroke, such as PICH rather than infarction, or a lacunar infarct (LACI) rather than a cardioembolic infarct. Furthermore, stroke itself may change some risk factors (e.g. blood pressure and blood glucose increase temporarily after acute stroke (see Section 15.7), whilst plasma cholesterol falls (see Section 6.6.1)); make information of past activities impossible to obtain (because of confusion, aphasia); lead to bias in recording risk factors (because it is impossible to blind assessors to stroke or control status); and require treatment which modifies risk factors (e.g. stopping smoking or lowering blood pressure). Therefore, case–control studies based on stroke survivors are fraught with difficulty, even more so if only hospital-admitted patients are studied so excluding mild cases or those that die before admission. Using TIA patients as a surrogate for ischaemic stroke and extracting information from medical records *before* any stroke or TIA could avoid some of these problems.

The tendency to lump strokes together might also, in part, explain the curious quantitative differences between stroke and coronary heart disease (CHD) risk factors, although qualitatively they are the same: why is it that smoking, raised cholesterol and male sex are far stronger risk factors for myocardial infarction whilst hypertension is a far stronger risk factor for stroke? Could it be that some types of stroke are not to do with cholesterol, smokers and male sex and, if such types could be identified and removed from the analysis, would ischaemic strokes have a more similar risk factor profile to CHD, which, it seems, is less heterogeneous

than stroke and mostly to do with atherothrombosis? As can be seen in Table 6.4, the vast majority of ischaemic stroke patients (taken as a group) have one or more of the definite vascular risk factors, which will be discussed below.

> *It is curious that some risk factors are so much stronger for stroke (e.g. increasing blood pressure) and yet others so much stronger for coronary heart disease (e.g. plasma cholesterol, cigarette-smoking, male sex) if the underlying vascular pathology (atheroma) is the same.*

An alternative approach, which defines cases in terms of carotid disease displayed by non-invasive ultrasound, perhaps gets closer to risk factors for 'atheroma' (or rather atherothrombosis, because ultrasound can not separate atheroma from complicating thrombus), but so far there are very few longitudinal studies and the cross-sectional case–control studies are rather small (Hennerici & Steinke, 1991; Fabris *et al.*, 1994). Furthermore, progression or regression of arterial stenosis may be as much to do with changes in any complicating thrombus (such as lysis) as with growth or resolution in atheroma in the vessel wall, or due to temporary changes in the plaque, such as haemorrhage.

Age

Age is the strongest risk factor for TIAs and ischaemic stroke overall, and almost certainly for the various subcategories of ischaemic stroke (Fig. 6.5). For example, an 80 year old has about 30 times the risk of ischaemic stroke as a 50 year old (Bamford *et al.*, 1988, 1990).

Sex

There is much less of an excess of ischaemic strokes and TIAs in men than in women compared with CHD. What excess there is does not apply in young adults and in the very elderly (Lerner & Kannel, 1986) (Fig. 6.6). Notwithstanding popular dogma, this changing relationship between age and gender in the elderly is probably not explained by the menopause (Colditz *et al.*, 1987).

Blood pressure

Increasing blood pressure is strongly associated, independently of age, with stroke risk, probably involving all the main pathological types of stroke, including ischaemic stroke and TIA (Whelton, 1994). The relationship between usual diastolic blood pressure and subsequent stroke is log-linear throughout the normal range and there is no threshold below which the stroke risk becomes stable, at least not within the 'normal' range of blood pressure which has been

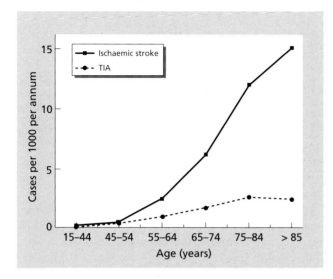

Figure 6.5 The incidence of first-ever in a lifetime ischaemic stroke and of TIA in the Oxfordshire Community Stroke Project. The flattening of TIA incidence in old age may be because cases did not come to medical attention or, when they did, they were not diagnosed. (From Dennis *et al.*, 1989; Bamford *et al.*, 1990.)

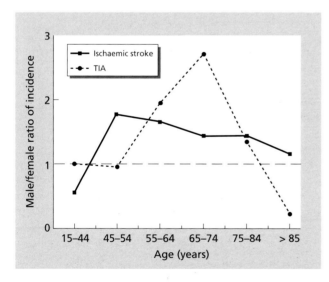

Figure 6.6 The ratio of male-to-female incidence of first-ever in a lifetime ischaemic stroke and of TIA in the Oxfordshire Community Stroke Project. (From Dennis *et al.*, 1989; Bamford *et al.*, 1990.)

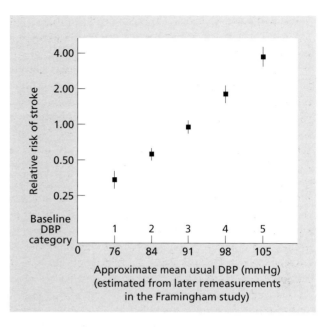

Figure 6.7 The relative risk of stroke related to the usual diastolic blood pressure in five categories defined by usual baseline blood pressure, from an overview analysis of seven prospective observational studies. Solid squares represent stroke risks relative to risk in the whole study population; their size is proportional to the number of strokes in each blood-pressure category and the vertical lines represent 95% confidence intervals. (Reproduced with permission from MacMahon *et al.*, 1990.)

studied, from 70 to 110 mmHg diastolic (Fig. 6.7). The proportional increase in stroke risk associated with a given increase in blood pressure is similar, in males and females, at all levels of blood pressure, and almost doubles with each 7.5-mmHg increase in usual diastolic blood pressure (Collins & MacMahon, 1994). However, the association is attenuated with increasing age, although of course the absolute risk of stroke in the elderly is far higher than in the young (Prospective Studies Collaboration, 1995). The relationship between stroke and systolic blood pressure is possibly stronger, and even 'isolated' systolic hypertension with a 'normal' diastolic blood pressure is associated with increased stroke risk (Kannel *et al.*, 1981; Rowe, 1983; Shaper *et al.*, 1991; Keli *et al.*, 1992). There is no doubt that, as emphasised by the results of randomised controlled trials, the relationship between increasing blood pressure and stroke risk is causal, although, it must be admitted, it is not clear which types of strokes are prevented by reducing the blood pressure, largely because in the clinical trials all stroke outcomes have been lumped together (MacMahon & Rodgers, 1993, 1994; Collins & McMahon, 1994; Mulrow *et al.*, 1994; see Section 16.3.1). It is also not clear whether hypertension is still a risk factor in the *very* elderly, where stroke risk may be associated with low blood pressures, perhaps because low pressures reflect pre-existing cardiovascular disease; however, studies have been small and a systematic overview is clearly required to clarify this issue (Evans, 1987; Langer *et al.*, 1991).

Hypertension seems to increase the risk of ischaemic stroke by increasing the extent and severity of atheroma and intracranial small vessel disease (Russell, 1975; Chobanian, 1983; Lusiani *et al.*, 1987; Reed *et al.*, 1988; Homer *et al.*, 1991; Sutton-Tyrell *et al.*, 1993; Fine-Edelstein *et al.*, 1994). Furthermore, progression of large vessel stenosis can be slowed by treating hypertension (Sutton-Tyrell *et al.*, 1994).

Cigarette-smoking

Cigarette-smoking undoubtedly has an association with stroke, with a relative risk of about 1.5, but this seems to become weaker in the elderly. Males and females are equally affected, and there is even some association with passive smoking (Shinton & Beevers, 1989; Donnan *et al.*, 1993a). The relationship is present not just for 'all strokes' but also separately for ischaemic stroke, where the relative risk is about 2.0. The risk declines after stopping smoking, so supporting a causal relationship, even though it has proved impossible to do a satisfactory randomised controlled trial (Donnan *et al.*, 1989; Shinton & Beevers, 1989; Rose & Colwell, 1992; Kawachi *et al.*, 1993). Most of the ultrasound and angiogram studies show an association between carotid disease and smoking (Haapanen *et al.*, 1989; O'Leary *et al.*, 1992; Fine-Edelstein *et al.*, 1994). There are not enough data to know whether there is a connection between pipe- and cigar-smoking and stroke.

Diabetes mellitus

Diabetes mellitus about doubles the risk of ischaemic stroke, independently of any confounding association between diabetes and hypertension (Barrett-Connor & Khaw, 1988; Rosengren *et al.*, 1989; Manson *et al.*, 1991; Burchfiel *et al.*, 1994). Diabetics also have thicker carotid arterial walls, presumably due to early atheroma (Folsom *et al.*, 1994). However, the relationship between diabetes and carotid stenosis assessed by ultrasound is unclear (Fine-Edelstein *et al.*, 1994). Any studies based on only *fatal* strokes will exaggerate the association with diabetes, because diabetics are more likely to die of stroke than non-diabetics (Jorgensen *et al.*, 1994c; see Sections 10.2.7 and 15.18.3).

Blood lipids

Increasing total plasma cholesterol, increasing low-density lipoprotein-cholesterol and decreasing levels of high-density lipoprotein-cholesterol are strong risk, and indeed in some way causal, factors for CHD, more in the middle-aged than the elderly. A long-term reduction of plasma cholesterol of 0.6 mmol/L should reduce the risk of CHD events by about 25%, more in the young and less in the elderly (Law *et al.*, 1994a; Thompson, 1994). The relationship with stroke is much less certain; there is some association in case–control studies, in cohort studies and in the attempts to relate carotid stenosis with blood lipids (Reed *et al.*, 1988; Homer *et al.*, 1991; Qizilbash *et al.*, 1991; Woo *et al.*, 1991; Benfante *et al.*, 1994; Fine-Edelstein *et al.*, 1994; Lindenstrom *et al.*, 1994). However, a recent systematic review of the cohort studies revealed no association between all stroke types combined and increasing plasma total cholesterol at baseline, except perhaps in populations under the age of 45 years at screening (Prospective Studies Collaboration, 1995). Furthermore, any effect of cholesterol-lowering on subsequent risk of strokes is marginal at best (Scandinavian Simvastatin Survival Study Group, 1994: Herbert *et al.*, 1995). This contrast between CHD and ischaemic stroke is striking, and may in part be explained by the seemingly negative association between increasing plasma cholesterol and intracranial haemorrhage, which could obscure a positive association with ischaemic stroke if the pathological type of stroke is not accounted for (Law *et al.*, 1994b); the fact that stroke occurs at a later age than myocardial infarction, so that relatively few strokes have yet occurred to be analysed in the large cohort studies and randomised trials; the relatively narrow range of cholesterol levels examined in many studies; the loss of stroke-susceptible individuals from the population by prior death from CHD; uncertainties about the effect of stroke itself on lipid levels in case–control studies; and perhaps by not differentiating ischaemic strokes likely to be due to intracranial small vessel disease from those due to large vessel atherothrombosis (Pedro-Botet *et al.*, 1992). The role of plasma triglyceride as a predictive factor, or cause, of CHD and ischaemic stroke is unclear (Garber & Avins, 1994).

Plasma fibrinogen

Plasma fibrinogen has a strong and consistent positive association with stroke, but not perhaps with carotid stenosis. Cigarette-smoking is a confounding variable, so it may be that the effect of cigarette-smoking is mediated, at least in part, by increasing the fibrinogen level and thus accelerating thrombosis. Less important but still confusing confounding factors include age, hypertension, diabetes, hyperlipidaemia, lack of exercise, social class, social activity, season of the year, alcohol consumption and stress. It is not yet certain, therefore, whether plasma fibrinogen really is a causal factor and, if so, whether it acts by increasing plasma viscosity or through promoting thrombosis. The confusion is compounded because there is no standard method for measuring plasma fibrinogen, it tends to rise after acute events, including infections, it is not easy to lower fibrinogen and no satisfactory randomised controlled trials have been reported (Meade *et al.*, 1987; Cook & Ubben, 1990; Rosengren *et al.*, 1990; Ernst & Resch, 1993; Fine-Edelstein *et al.*, 1994; Woodhouse *et al.*, 1994).

Raised plasma factor VII coagulant activity and low blood fibrinolytic activity

Raised plasma factor VII coagulant activity and low blood fibrinolytic activity seem to be independent risk factors for CHD, but there are no good data for stroke (Meade *et al.*, 1993). Raised *tissue plasminogen activator antigen* is associated with both coronary and stroke risk, perhaps because it is a marker of endogenous fibrinolytic activation (Ridker *et al.*, 1994), and there is also evidence that raised *von Willebrand factor antigen* is a risk factor for ischaemic stroke (N. Qizilbash *et al.*, personal communication, 1996). Although many attempts have been made to find them, there are no consistent associations between other coagulation and platelet parameters with vascular disease. Coagulation parameters are altered by acute stroke so often that case–control studies are invalidated and it has not been practical to do very many long-term cohort studies.

Physical exercise

Physical exercise somewhat reduces blood pressure, plasma cholesterol, plasma fibrinogen and the risk of non-insulin-dependent diabetes mellitus. So, not surprisingly, lack of exercise is associated with CHD (*Lancet*, 1990; Berlin & Colditz, 1990; Arroll & Beaglehole, 1992; Connelly *et al.*, 1992; Manson *et al.*, 1992). There is now increasing evidence that lack of exercise is also associated with an increased risk of stroke, in both cohort and case–control studies (Wannamethee & Shaper, 1992; Shinton & Sagar, 1993; Lindenstrom *et al.*, 1993). So far there is insufficient evidence from randomised trials to be sure that deliberately increasing exercise leads to a reduction in the risk of vascular events, although it should (O'Connor *et al.*, 1989; Gloag, 1992; see Section 16.3.5).

Raised haematocrit

Raised haematocrit is a weak risk factor for stroke, but this issue is confounded by the fact that cigarette-smoking, blood pressure and plasma fibrinogen are all positively associated with haematocrit (Welin *et al.*, 1987).

Obesity

Obesity has seldom been studied as a risk factor for stroke, whilst the explanation for the known association between obesity and CHD is controversial (Abbott *et al.*, 1994). There is confounding by cigarette-smoking, because smokers are lighter than non-smokers. Obesity is associated with hypertension, diabetes, hypercholesterolaemia and lack of exercise, which may explain any increased risk of stroke. Raised waist-to-hip ratio, as a measure of central obesity, and change in body weight may be stronger risk factors than the traditional measure of obesity based on weight compared with height (Welin *et al.*, 1987; Wannamethee & Shaper, 1989; Lee & Paffenbarger, 1992; Folsom *et al.*, 1994).

Dietary constituents

The only dietary constituent which definitely increases stroke risk is salt, probably by increasing the systemic blood pressure (Law *et al.*, 1991a,b; Frost *et al.*, 1991). Diets low in potassium (Khaw & Barrett-Connor, 1987), fresh fruit and vegetables (Acheson & Williams, 1983), fish (Keli *et al.*, 1994; Ascherio *et al.*, 1995), vitamin E (Steinberg, 1993; Hennekens *et al.*, 1994); vitamin C (Bulpitt, 1995; Gale *et al.*, 1995), betacarotene (Kardinaal *et al.*, 1993), flavonoids (Hertog *et al.*, 1993) and selenium (Virtamo *et al.*, 1985) may or may not increase the risk of arterial disease. If there is any adverse effect at all of coffee consumption on vascular disease, it may be working through the rather small (and perhaps negligible) hyperlipidaemic effect of boiled coffee, or because coffee-drinkers are more likely to be smokers (Thelle, 1991; Kawachi *et al.*, 1994).

Alcohol

The relationship between alcohol, ischaemic stroke and carotid stenosis is unclear (van Gijn *et al.*, 1993; see also Section 8.5.2). Whilst heavy alcohol consumption may be an independent, and perhaps causal, risk factor, it seems that modest consumption is protective (Camargo, 1989; Marmot & Brunner, 1991; Shinton *et al.*, 1993; Doll *et al.*, 1994; Kiechl *et al.*, 1994; Kiyohara *et al.*, 1995). 'Binge' drinking does not unequivocally cause stroke (Gorelick, 1987). Much of this confusion is because of: the difficulty of measuring alcohol consumption accurately, particularly over time; different types of alcohol drinks may have different effects; variation in the temporal patterns of drinking behaviour; including ex-drinkers with lifetime non-drinkers in the analysis; taking non-drinkers as a group, including some people who have given up drinking because of symptoms of vascular or other diseases; the biases inherent in case–control studies; publication bias; small numbers; confounding with cigarette-smoking, which is positively related, and exercise, which is negatively related to alcohol consumption, as well as the possibility of unknown confounders which might link no drinking or heavy drinking with an excess risk of vascular disease; lumping ischaemic together with haemorrhagic strokes; and the lack of systematic overviews of all the evidence (Ben-Shlomo *et al.*, 1992). Also, heavy alcohol consumption almost certainly increases the blood pressure and may cause AF as well as a cardiomyopathy, so leading to embolism from the heart to the brain (*Lancet*, 1985; MacMahon & Norton, 1986; Puddey *et al.*, 1987; Marmot *et al.*, 1994; Kaplan, 1995). It seems most unlikely that a randomised trial of modest alcohol consumption, or of quitting heavy consumption, to reduce the risk of vascular disorders without increasing the risk of other disorders, will ever be feasible, so we are left trying to interpret, with difficulty, the available observational data.

Race

Stroke in general is more common in Afro-Caribbeans than Caucasians (Gillum, 1988; Balarajan, 1991; Howard *et al.*, 1994), but it is not clear whether this applies to both ischaemic stroke and intracranial haemorrhage and, even if it does, whether the relationship is due to the higher prevalence of hypertension, diabetes, sickle cell trait and social deprivation in Afro-Caribbeans. South Asian populations in the UK have a high stroke mortality (Balarajan, 1991) and, indeed, a high prevalence of CHD, central obesity (high waist-to-hip ratio), insulin resistance and diabetes mellitus (McKeigre *et al.*, 1991); this may in part be because they are genetically more at risk than Caucasian populations by virtue of their higher serum lipoprotein (a) concentrations (Bhatnagar *et al.*, 1995). The *pattern* of atheroma also appears to differ between racial groups; for example, there is less extracranial but more intracranial atheroma in Afro-Caribbeans, Japanese and perhaps Chinese compared with Caucasian populations (Caplan *et al.*, 1986; Feldmann *et al.*, 1990; Leung *et al.*, 1993).

Social deprivation

Social deprivation is certainly associated with increased stroke mortality (Pocock *et al.*, 1980; Carstairs & Morris, 1990), perhaps because stroke is more common in the unemployed (Franks *et al.*, 1991), low-income groups (Lynch *et al.*, 1994), those who are depressed (see below), those who have a poor diet (see below), lower social classes (Acheson & Williams, 1983; Shaper *et al.*, 1991; Hannaford *et al.*, 1994) and, it has been suggested as well as refuted, those who had

poor *in utero* or infant health and nutrition (Barker, 1995; Paneth & Susser, 1995). Also, there are clearly social class differences in health risk behaviours, such as smoking, diet and exercise (Marmot *et al.*, 1991).

Vascular disease elsewhere

Because atheroma in one place is likely to be accompanied by atheroma in others (see Section 6.2.1) and because embolism from the heart is a common cause of ischaemic stroke (see Section 6.4), it is not surprising that non-stroke vascular disorders of various kinds are associated with, i.e. are risk factors for, ischaemic stroke and TIA (Table 6.7).

CHD (e.g. angina or myocardial infarction) is clearly associated with an increased risk of stroke in postmortem studies (Kagan, 1976; Stemmermann *et al.*, 1984), case–control studies (Friedman *et al.*, 1968; Herman *et al.*, 1983; Woo *et al.*, 1991) and cohort studies (Harmsen *et al.*, 1990; Shaper *et al.*, 1991; Wolf *et al.*, 1991). In part this association reflects not just the fact that patients with coronary atheroma are also likely to have atheroma of the arteries supplying the brain, but that embolism can occur from left-ventricular thrombus complicating myocardial infarction (Dexter *et al.*, 1987). It is not surprising that electrocardiogram (ECG) abnormalities and cardiac failure, because they both reflect CHD and hypertension, are associated with increased risk of stroke, as is left-ventricular hypertrophy (Kagan *et al.*, 1980; Kannel *et al.*, 1983; Knutsen *et al.*, 1988; Levy *et al.*, 1990; Shaper *et al.*, 1991). AF is considered later (see Section 6.4).

Cervical bruits (carotid or supraclavicular) are usually caused by stenosis of the underlying arteries (see Section 6.5.7), mostly due to atheroma, and so become more common with age; about 5% of asymptomatic people over the age of 75 years have bruits (Sandok *et al.*, 1982; Ricci *et al.*, 1991; O'Leary *et al.*, 1992). Bruits are clearly a risk factor for stroke, but not necessarily in the same arterial territory as the bruit, and also of coronary events, because atheroma of one artery is likely to be accompanied by atheroma of other arteries in the same predisposed individual (Wiebers

Table 6.7 Evidence of degenerative vascular disease outside the head is associated with an increased risk of ischaemic stroke and TIA.

Myocardial infarction/angina/coronary artery surgery
Cardiac failure
Left-ventricular hypertrophy
AF
Cervical arterial bruit/stenosis
Peripheral vascular disease

et al., 1990). The risk of these various vascular events increases with severity of the carotid stenosis (see Section 16.12.2).

Atheroma affecting the leg arteries is associated with cerebrovascular disease so often that it is hardly surprising that claudicants have an increased risk of stroke (Harmsen *et al.*, 1990; Smith *et al.*, 1990; Ogren *et al.*, 1995). Little seems to be known about the prevalence of abdominal aortic aneurysms in ischaemic stroke/TIA patients, but it is presumably quite high—about 10–20%, depending on the selection of the patients and the definition of an aneurysm (Carty *et al.*, 1993; Karanjia *et al.*, 1994).

Other risk factors

Various other associations with CHD, if not with ischaemic stroke, have been described, and some of the 246 counted in

Table 6.8 Miscellaneous possible risk factors for vascular disease, particularly ischaemic stroke.

Possible risk factor	Reference
Snoring and sleep apnoea	Waller & Bhopal, 1989; Spriggs *et al.*, 1992
Corneal arcus	Chambless *et al.*, 1990; Menotti *et al.*, 1993
Hyperhomocysteinaemia	Lindgren *et al.*, 1995; Perry *et al.*, 1995; Stampfer & Malinow, 1995
Raised white blood cell count, but this is probably because smokers have higher counts than non-smokers	Yarnell *et al.*, 1991; Kannel *et al.*, 1992
Large platelets	O'Malley *et al.*, 1995
Recent infection	Grau *et al.*, 1995
Plasma viscosity, which is largely determined by plasma fibrinogen	Yarnell *et al.*, 1991
Type A behaviour	Johnston, 1993
Severely threatening life events	House *et al.*, 1990; Rosengren *et al.*, 1993
Phobic anxiety	Haines *et al.*, 1987
Depression and hopelessness	Anda *et al.*, 1993
Psychotropic drugs	Thorogood *et al.*, 1992
Psychological stress	Harmsen *et al.*, 1990
Family history of stroke	Welin *et al.*, 1987; Kiely *et al.*, 1993
Low serum albumin	Phillips *et al.*, 1989
High body iron stores	Ascherio & Willett, 1994
Impaired ventilatory function	Strachan, 1991; Menotti *et al.*, 1993
Dental disease	De Stefano *et al.*, 1993
Low bone density	Browner *et al.*, 1993
Blood group	Whincup *et al.*, 1990
Serum sialic acid	Lindberg *et al.*, 1991
Diagonal ear-lobe crease	Patel *et al.*, 1992

1981 (Hopkins & Williams, 1981) and others described since may or may not be important (Table 6.8).

> *The most important risk factors for ischaemic stroke and transient ischaemic attack are age, blood pressure, plasma fibrinogen, diabetes mellitus and cigarette-smoking. Of these, raised blood pressure is definitely causal.*

6.3 Intracranial small vessel disease

LACIs, and indeed lacunar TIAs, make up about 25% of cerebral ischaemic events (Bamford *et al.*, 1987; Hankey & Warlow, 1991b). It is likely that most are due to a specific vascular pathology affecting the small (40–800 µm diameter) perforating arteries of the brain, i.e. the lenticulostriate perforating branches of the MCA, the thalamoperforating branches of the proximal posterior cerebral artery and the perforating branches of the basilar artery to the brainstem (Bamford & Warlow, 1988; Orgogozo & Bogousslavsky, 1989; Besson *et al.*, 1991; see Section 4.4.6). However, this hypothesis is not accepted by everyone (Millikan & Futrell, 1990; Horowitz *et al.*, 1992). What may be the same small vessel disease is variously called lipohyalinosis, microatheroma, fibrinoid necrosis, hyalinosis and angionecrosis (Fisher, 1969, 1979, 1991). But, the vascular pathology is not well described, because the case fatality of lacunar stroke is so low and because it is technically so difficult to track down the tiny relevant artery to the small infarct in postmortem material and then relate the findings to the clinical details of the preceding stroke. It appears that the muscle and elastin in the arterial wall are replaced by collagen, there is subintimal hyalinisation and the vessel becomes tortuous. It is conceivable that the same microvascular pathology leads to arterial rupture and intracerebral haemorrhage, perhaps due to microaneurysm formation (so-called Charcot–Bouchard aneurysms), although these may be artefacts of the pathological specimens (Fisher, 1972; Besson *et al.*, 1991; Challa *et al.*, 1992; see Section 8.2.1).

To go along with the lacunar hypothesis (i.e. that *most* LACIs are caused by intracranial small vessel disease), patients with lacunar ischaemic strokes and TIAs have a much lower frequency of cardiac and large vessel embolic sources than those with cortical strokes and TIAs which are more likely to be due to embolism from large arteries or the heart (Fig. 6.8; Olsen *et al.*, 1985; Kappelle & van Gijn, 1986; Kappelle *et al.*, 1988; Norrving & Cronqvist, 1989; Lodder *et al.*, 1990; Boiten & Lodder, 1991; Hankey & Warlow, 1991b; Tegeler *et al.*, 1991; Landi *et al.*, 1993; Mast *et al.*, 1994). Moreover, emboli are rarely if ever detected in the MCA or common carotid artery (CCA) by

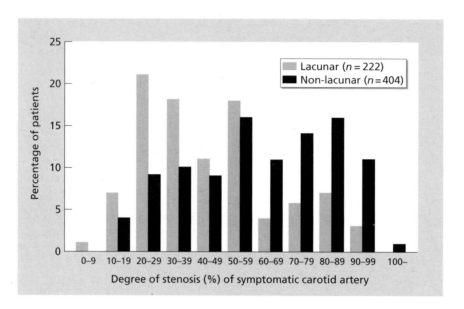

Figure 6.8 The relationship between the degree of stenosis of the recently symptomatic carotid artery with the likelihood of a non-LACI (territorial) and of an LACI on computerised tomography scan in patients at the time of randomisation in the European Carotid Surgery Trial. Patients with lesser degrees of stenosis tended to have LACIs whilst those with more severe stenosis tended to have non-LACI (territorial). (From Boiten *et al.*, 1996.)

Doppler ultrasound (Grosset *et al.*, 1994; Tegeler *et al.*, 1995). However, 'cortical' and 'lacunar' patients otherwise have a very similar risk factor profile, including a similar prevalence of hypertension (Adams *et al.*, 1989; Lodder *et al.*, 1990; Sacco *et al.*, 1991; Boiten & Lodder, 1993; You *et al.*, 1995). It is conceivable, therefore, that the same type of individuals (i.e. hypertensive, diabetic, etc.) develop *either* intracranial small vessel disease and so LACI *or* large vessel atherothromboembolism and so cortical infarction; *or* they may have these different ischaemic stroke types at different times; *or* perhaps the lacunar hypothesis is wrong, which we do not believe, and the small vessel angiopathy is really the result of embolisation from proximal sites.

> *Intracranial small vessel disease causes about 25% of ischaemic strokes and transient ischaemic attacks. Usually the clinical syndrome is 'lacunar'.*

One question that has never been answered is whether there is a similar small vessel disease which affects the blood supply to the optic nerve and retina; are there, therefore, 'lacunar' ocular syndromes equivalent to lacunar cerebral syndromes? What is clear is that a high proportion of patients with ischaemic amaurosis fugax, retinal infarction and acute ischaemic optic neuropathy do not have any detectable and likely proximal source of embolism (or of low flow) in the heart or in the arterial supply to the eye, and perhaps it is these patients who have symptomatic small vessel disease like patients with cerebral LACI (Hayreh, 1981;

Guyer *et al.*, 1985; Bruno *et al.*, 1990; Hankey *et al.*, 1991).

6.4 Embolism from the heart

Embolism of material from the heart to the brain, as well as to other organs, is undisputed, but not all cardiac sources of embolism pose equal threats: for example, a mechanical prosthetic valve is much more likely to cause embolism than mitral valve prolapse (MVP) (Cerebral Embolism Task Force, 1989; Hart, 1992). However, there are two practical problems: (i) as technology advances, more and more *potential* cardiac sources of embolism are being identified (Table 6.9), although non-rheumatic AF is by far the most common in developed countries, where there is a low incidence of rheumatic fever (Table 6.10); (ii) patients may have two or more competing causes of cerebral ischaemia, such as carotid stenosis *and* AF, so one can not be sure which is *the* cause in an individual patient (De Bono & Warlow, 1981; Bogousslavsky *et al.*, 1986a, 1990). As far as one can tell, cardiac embolism probably causes *about* 20% of ischaemic stroke and TIAs (see Fig. 6.1; Nishide *et al.*, 1983; Cerebral Embolism Task Force, 1989; Kittner *et al.*, 1991; Broderick *et al.*, 1992). Of course, not all emboli are either the same size or made of the same thing (fibrin, platelets, calcium, infected vegetations, tumour, etc.); some are large and impact permanently in the trunk of the MCA to cause a major stroke (i.e. a total anterior circulation infarct (TACI), others impact in a more distal branch of a cerebral artery (to cause a partial anterior circulation infarct (PACI), others merely cause a TIA and still others are asymptomatic

Table 6.9 Cardiac sources of embolism in anatomical sequence.

Right-to-left shunt (paradoxical emboli from the venous system) via
Patent foramen ovale
Atrial septal defect
Ventricular septal defect
Pulmonary arteriovenous malformation

Left atrium
Thrombus
    AF*
    Sinoatrial disease (sick sinus syndrome)
    Atrial septal aneurysm
Myxoma and other tumours*

Mitral valve
Rheumatic endocarditis (stenosis* or regurgitation)
Infective endocarditis*
Mitral annulus calcification
Mitral valve prolapse
Non-bacterial thrombotic (marantic) endocarditis
Libman–Sacks endocarditis
Anticardiolipin antibody syndrome
Prosthetic heart valve*
Papillary fibroelastoma

Left ventricle
Mural thrombus
    Acute myocardial infarction (within previous few weeks)*
    Left-ventricular aneurysm or akinetic segment
    Dilated cardiomyopathy*
    Mechanical 'artificial' heart*
    Blunt chest injury (myocardial contusion)
Myxoma and other tumours*
Hydatid cyst
Primary oxalosis

Aortic valve
Rheumatic endocarditis (stenosis or regurgitation)
Infective endocarditis*
Syphilis
Non-infective thrombotic (marantic) endocarditis
Libman–Sacks endocarditis
Anticardiolipin antibody syndrome
Prosthetic heart valve*
Calcific stenosis/sclerosis/calcification

CHD (particularly with right-to-left shunt)

Cardiac manipulation/surgery/catheterisation/valvuloplasty/ angioplasty

* Substantial risk of embolism.

Table 6.10 Prevalence of potential cardiac sources of embolism in 244 patients with a first-ever in a lifetime ischaemic stroke in the Oxfordshire Community Stroke Project. (From Sandercock *et al.*, 1989.)

	n	%
Any AF	31	13
Without rheumatic heart disease	28	11
With rheumatic heart disease	3	1
Mitral regurgitation	15	6
Recent (<6 weeks) myocardial infarction	12	5
Prosthetic valve	3	1
Mitral stenosis	2	1
Paradoxical embolism	1	1
Any of the above	50	20
Other sources of uncertain significance (aortic stenosis/ sclerosis; mitral annulus calcification, mitral valve prolapse, etc.)	28	11

(Kempster *et al.*, 1988; Caplan, 1993). Emboli may also occlude the basilar artery and its branches and even the ICA in the neck (Castaigne *et al.*, 1973; Caplan, 1993). TIAs are just as common before a presumed cardioembolic stroke as before any other (see Table 6.2), so supporting the hypothesis that there is no qualitative difference between TIA and ischaemic stroke: embolism from the heart can cause an ischaemic stroke or a TIA at different times.

> *Embolism from the heart causes about 20% of ischaemic strokes and transient ischaemic attacks. The most substantial embolic threats are non-rheumatic or rheumatic atrial fibrillation, infective endocarditis, prosthetic heart valve, recent myocardial infarction, dilated cardiomyopathy, intracardiac tumours and rheumatic mitral stenosis.*

Atrial fibrillation

Although AF is by far the most common cause of cardioembolic stroke, it can not be the cause of more than about 20%, since it is present in less than this proportion of all patients with a stroke (Sandercock *et al.*, 1992). The average absolute risk of stroke in unanticoagulated non-rheumatic AF people randomised in the recent primary prevention trials was about 5%/year, six times greater than in those in sinus rhythm (Hart & Halperin, 1994; see Section 16.5.1). However, AF may be responsible for a greater proportion of ischaemic strokes in the *very* elderly, where its frequency in the population is highest (Wolf *et al.*, 1991).

> *Non-rheumatic atrial fibrillation is the most common cause of embolism from the heart to the brain.*

In fibrillating stroke patients the AF can not *always* be causal, because some patients have had a PICH, although it is conceivable that this has been confused with haemorrhagic transformation of an infarct on computerised tomography (CT) (see Section 5.4); in a few, the AF is caused by the stroke; about 20% have other possible causes, such as carotid stenosis; and yet others have lacunar (presumed non-embolic) syndromes (Weinberger *et al.*, 1988; Bogousslavsky *et al.*, 1990; Sandercock *et al.*, 1992; Vingerhoets *et al.*, 1993; Kanter *et al.*, 1994). Also, AF is often caused by either CHD or hypertensive heart disease, both of which may be associated with stroke by mechanisms other than embolism from the left atrium, such as carotid stenosis or hypertensive intracerebral haemorrhage (Davies & Pomerance, 1972). Furthermore, 'only' about 13% of non-rheumatic fibrillating patients have detectable (by transoesphageal echocardiography) thrombus in the left atrium (although, of course, some thrombi may have completely embolised or be too small to be detected), and it is not known for sure whether these patients have a higher stroke risk than those without detectable thrombi (Daniel, 1993). Nonetheless, AF is clearly *the* cause of ischaemic stroke in many patients, as supported by pathological evidence (Aberg, 1969; Hinton *et al.*, 1977; Britton & Gustafsson, 1985); case–control studies (Friedman *et al.*, 1968); most but not all cohort studies (Wolf *et al.*, 1978; Davis *et al.*, 1987; Flegel *et al.*, 1987; Harmsen *et al.*, 1990); and the lower prevalence of AF in lacunar ischaemic stroke probably due to small vessel disease (Sandercock *et al.* 1992). The effective prevention of stroke by anticoagulating fibrillating patients (see Section 16.5.1) is not a good supporting argument, because conceivably anticoagulation may prevent artery-to-artery as well as heart-to-artery embolic events and *in situ* arterial thrombosis.

Within the fibrillating population, there must be some individuals at particularly high risk and others at particularly low risk of embolisation: for example, those with no other detectable cardiac disease (so-called lone AF) have a very low relative and absolute risk of stroke, whilst those with rheumatic mitral valve disease have a much higher risk (Wolf *et al.*, 1978; Close *et al.*, 1979; Kopecky *et al.*, 1987). Other risk factors include a previous embolic event, increasing age, hypertension and diabetes, as well as perhaps left-ventricular dysfunction and enlarged left atrium defined by echocardiography (Stroke Prevention in Atrial Fibrillation Investigators, 1992; Atrial Fibrillation Investigators, 1994; Benjamin *et al.*, 1995; van Latum *et al.*, 1995). Spontaneous echo contrast in the left atrium, probably a consequence of blood stasis, is associated with an increased risk of embolism (Daniel *et al.*, 1988; Chimowitz *et al.*, 1993a), as perhaps

are left-atrial thrombi, left-atrial appendage size and dysfunction and various haemostatic variables (Gustafsson *et al.*, 1990; Di Pasquale *et al.*, 1995). It is still not clear whether stroke risk is importantly different in those with recent-onset AF, paroxysmal AF and thyrotoxic AF (Petersen, 1990).

Coronary heart disease

Embolism from left-ventricular mural thrombus complicating acute myocardial infarction is considered later (see Section 7.7). A chronic left-ventricular aneurysm after myocardial infarction does often contain thrombus, but embolisation does not apper to be very common (Meltzer *et al.*, 1986).

Prosthetic heart valves

Prosthetic heart valves, particularly mechanical rather than tissue ones, have long been known to be complicated by thrombosis, followed sometimes by embolism. Furthermore, infective endocarditis is a potential risk for any type of prosthetic valve. It seems that asymptomatic emboli, at least as detected by TCD, are surprisingly frequent, but these may be gaseous bubbles rather than solid fragments of thrombi (Georgiadis *et al.*, 1994; Sliwka *et al.*, 1995). There is little difference in stroke risk between the different types of mechanical valve, but those in the mitral position are more prone to thrombosis than those in the aortic position (De Bono, 1982). For all valves, the overall risk of embolism is about 2%/year, provided patients with mechanical valves are on anticoagulants (Bloomfield *et al.*, 1991; Hammermeister *et al.*, 1993). Some Bjork–Shiley tilting disc valves have disintegrated with not just serious cardiac consequences but also embolisation of their components to the cerebral circulation (Fig. 6.9).

Rheumatic valvular disease

Rheumatic valvular disease, particularly mitral, is a well-recognised cause of embolism from the left atrium to the brain. Even when the patient is in sinus rhythm, and there is no thrombus in the left atrium, degenerate and sometimes calcific fragments of valve can be discharged into the circulation. Of course, infective endocarditis (see blow) and intracerebral haemorrhage due to anticoagulation (see Section 8.4.1) are other causes of stroke in these patients (Daley *et al.*, 1951; Coulshed *et al.*, 1970).

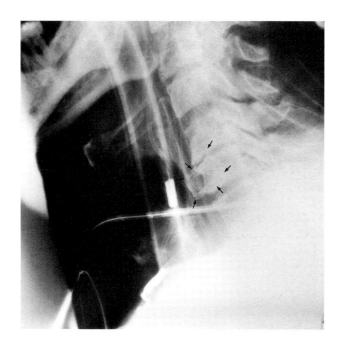

Figure 6.9 Lateral neck X-ray of a patient whose mechanical heart valve had disintegrated. Part of the valve (arrows) has impacted in the carotid artery.

Non-rheumatic sclerosis and particularly calcification of the aortic and mitral valves

Non-rheumatic sclerosis and particularly calcification of the aortic and mitral valves may also be a source of embolism in some patients but are both so common in normal elderly people that a cause-and-effect relationship is difficult to be sure of in an individual unless calcific emboli are seen in the retina or on brain CT (Penner & Font, 1969; Swash & Earl, 1970; Stein *et al.*, 1977; De Bono & Warlow, 1979; Brockmeier *et al.*, 1981; Nestico *et al.*, 1984; Benjamin *et al.*, 1992; O'Donoghue *et al.*, 1993).

Infective endocarditis

Infective endocarditis, acute or subacute, is complicated by ischaemic stroke or TIA in about 20% of cases, as a result of embolism of infected vegetations. Cerebrovascular symptoms can be the first, but they more often occur in the context of someone who is already ill, perhaps in hospital, and before the infection has been controlled (Jones & Siekert, 1989; Hart *et al.*, 1990; Salgado, 1991). Haemorrhagic transformation of an infarct, possibly as a consequence of the unwise use of anticoagulation, seems to be fairly common. Primarily haemorrhagic strokes, intracerebral or, rarely, subarachnoid, are as or more commonly due to a pyogenic vasculitis as the more well-known mycotic aneurysms,

which can be single or multiple and most often affect the distal branches of the MCA (Fig. 6.10; Masuda *et al.*, 1992; see Section 8.2.8). These aneurysms do not always rupture and they tend to resolve with time, so that, on balance, cerebral angiography to detect unruptured aneurysms with a view to surgery is unnecessary, and so is surgical repair of any asymptomatic aneurysm found after a ruptured aneurysm has been repaired (van der Meulen *et al.*, 1992). Other neurological complications of infective endocarditis include meningitis, a diffuse encephalopathy perhaps due to showers of small emboli, discitis and headache (Kanter & Hart, 1991).

It is important to realise that fever, cardiac murmur and vegetations seen on echocardiography are not invariable. Therefore, in an otherwise unexplained ischaemic or haemorrhagic stroke, blood cultures are indicated, particularly if the erythrocyte sedimentation rate (ESR) is raised, with a mild anaemia and neutrophil leucocytosis. The cerebrospinal fluid (CSF) can be normal but more than 100 polymorphs/mm^3 is said to suggest endocarditis; however, as high or higher counts have been described in PICH and in haemorrhagic transformation of an infarct, but not in cerebral infarction (Sornas *et al.*, 1972; Powers, 1986).

In infective endocarditis the blood cultures can be negative and the echocardiogram normal.

Non-bacterial thrombotic (marantic) endocarditis

Small sterile vegetations, consisting of fibrin and platelets, appear on the cardiac valves in cachectic and debilitated patients as a result of cancer (usually adenocarcinomas) and sometimes of disseminated intravascular coagulation, burns and septicaemia, usually but not only in elderly people. These vegetations are friable and may embolise to cause ischaemic stroke (and sometimes global encephalopathy due

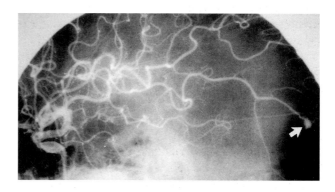

Figure 6.10 Carotid angiogram (lateral) showing a mycotic cerebral aneurysm on a distal branch of the MCA (arrow).

to multiple emboli), ischaemia in other organs and pulmonary embolism. The vegetations are so small that they are all but impossible to diagnose during life. The diagnosis should be suspected in an ischaemic stroke/TIA patient who is cachectic and who may have additional evidence of systemic embolisation without any other cause being found (Graus *et al.*, 1985; Lopez *et al.*, 1987). Similar vegetations are found in systemic lupus erythematosus and the antiphospholipid antibody syndrome (see Section 7.2).

Non-ischaemic 'primary' cardiomyopathies

Non-ischaemic 'primary' cardiomyopathies are well known to be complicated by intracardiac thrombus, particularly if they are of the dilated type rather than hypertrophic subaortic stenosis. Many are familial (Fuster *et al.*, 1981; Rice *et al.*, 1981; Meltzer *et al.*, 1986; Kelly & Strauss, 1994).

Sinoatrial disease (sick sinus syndrome)

Sinoatrial disease (sick sinus syndrome) can be associated with intracardiac thrombus and embolism, particularly if bradycardia alternates with tachycardia or the patient is in AF. This can be familial (Bathen *et al.*, 1978; Fisher *et al.*, 1988; Pierre *et al.*, 1993).

Atrial septal aneurysm

Atrial septal aneurysm is rare but may be complicated by thrombus, embolism and so cerebral ischaemia. Very often it is associated with a patent foramen ovale (PFO) and so with the potential for paradoxical embolism from the venous system (Silver & Dorsey, 1978; Nater *et al.*, 1992; Cabanes *et al.*, 1993).

Mitral valve (or leaflet) prolapse

MVP (or mitral leaflet prolapse) is so common in normal people and the diagnostic criteria are so variable that it is impossible to pin it down as the likely cause of an ischaemic stroke or TIA in an individual, unless there is complicating infective endocarditis, AF, gross mitral regurgitation or thrombus in the left atrium (Levy & Savage, 1987; Devereux *et al.*, 1987). MVP can be familial and associated with various inherited disorders of connective tissue (see Section 7.3; Devereux *et al.*, 1982). Although MVP is more common than expected in young TIA patients (Barnett *et al.*, 1980), it is odd, if the relationship really is causal, that thrombus on the valve cusps has been so rarely seen (Geyer & Franzini, 1979; Chesler *et al.*, 1983) and that embolism to anywhere other than the brain or eye has never been described.

Moreover, MVP does not appear to be more frequent than expected in ischaemic stroke (Cabanes *et al.*, 1993; Marini *et al.*, 1993) and there is no excess risk of first-ever stroke or recurrent stroke in patients with uncomplicated MVP (Orencia *et al.*, 1995a, b). Therefore, in an individual patient we would *not* regard uncomplicated MVP as a *definite* cause for ischaemic stroke/TIA, even if no other cause can be found.

> *Uncomplicated mitral valve prolapse should no longer be considered a cause of embolism from the heart to the brain.*

Paradoxical embolism

Paradoxical embolism from the venous system or the right atrium has for decades been a well-accepted concept, based on a number of convincing autopsy examples (Fig. 6.11). The conduits for such emboli from the right to the left side of the heart are a PFO, which is found in about 25% of unselected postmortems and in a similar proportion of normal people using transoesophageal echocardiography; an atrial septal defect; or, rarely, a ventriculoseptal defect (Jeanrenaud & Kappenberger, 1991; Gautier *et al.*, 1991; Cabanes *et al.*, 1993). Although bubbles can be shown to move from the right to the left side of the heart so frequently, it must be very rare for thrombus to do so, or at least to be able to make a certain diagnosis of such an event during life (see Section 6.7.3). Another, but very unusual, route for emboli to reach the brain via the venous system is through or from a pulmonary arterial venous malformation, either isolated or as part of hereditary haemorrhagic telangiectasia; clues are clubbing, cyanosis, haemoptysis, bruit over the chest and a 'coin lesion' on the chest X-ray (Fig. 6.12; Dennis, 1985).

> *Although a patent foramen ovale is common in normal individuals, it is most unusual for cerebral ischaemia to be due to paradoxical embolism from the right heart to the left atrium and so to the brain.*

Intracardiac tumours

Myxomas, found in the left atrium much more often than in any other cardiac chamber, are the most common intracardiac tumour but are still extremely rare; some are familial (Joynt *et al.*, 1965; Chalmers & Campbell, 1987; Markel *et al.*, 1987; Kasarkis *et al.*, 1988; Knepper *et al.*, 1988; Mattle *et al.*, 1995). Tumour or complicating thrombus may embolise to the brain, eye and elsewhere. Myxomatous emboli cause not just focal cerebral ischaemia but also fusiform and irregular aneurysmal dilatations at the sites of

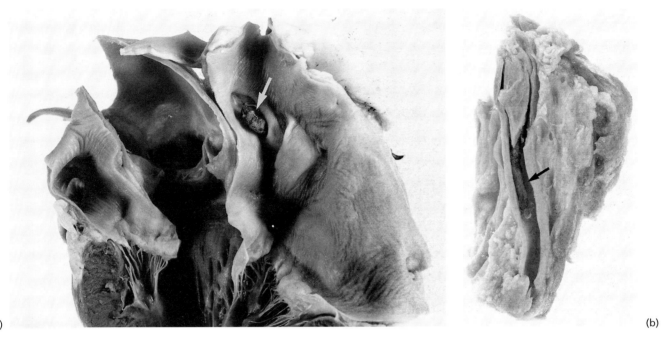

(a)

(b)

Figure 6.11 Paradoxical embolism. A postmortem specimen showing: (a) a venous thrombus (arrow) protruding through a PFO into the left atrium; (b) part of the same thrombus (arrow) in the right CCA. (Courtesy of Dr John Webb.)

Figure 6.12 Pulmonary arteriovenous malformation: (a) chest X-ray showing pulmonary arteriovenous malformations (arrows); (b) pulmonary angiogram showing more clearly the arteriovenous malformation on the left (arrow). (Courtesy of Dr John Reid, Royal Infirmary, Edinburgh, UK.)

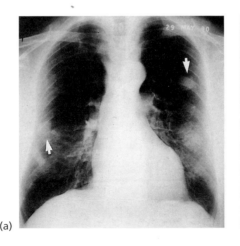

(a)

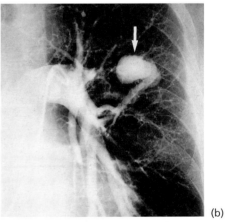

(b)

earlier symptomatic or even asymptomatic embolic occlusions, and these can rupture to cause PICH or subarachnoid haemorrhage (Roeltgen *et al.*, 1981; Fig. 6.13). Cardiac tumours may also cause cardiac symptoms (such as shortness of breath, palpitations, syncope, etc.) and myxomas are often associated with consitutional problems, such as malaise, weight loss, anaemia, raised ESR and hypergammaglobulinaemia. Myocardial *hydatid cysts* and intracardiac calcification due to *primary oxalosis* are even rarer causes of

embolism to the brain, the former with the subsequent development of intracranial cysts (Di Pasquale *et al.*, 1989; Benomar *et al.*, 1994).

Myocardial contusion

Myocardial contusion as a result of blunt chest injury can be associated with left-ventricular thombus; rare cases of embolisation have been described (Dugani *et al.*, 1984).

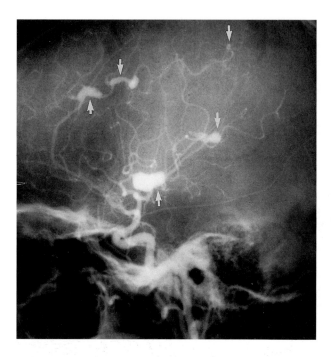

Figure 6.13 Angiogram showing multiple aneurysmal dilatations of cerebral arteries (arrows) as a result of embolism from a cardiac myxoma. (Courtesy of Professor Alastair Compston.)

6.5 From history and signs to cause

As already emphasised in Chapter 3, the diagnosis of stroke (versus not stroke) and TIA (versus not TIA) depends essentially on the history and to a lesser extent on the examination of the nervous system and brain imaging. The clinical syndrome, based simply again on the history and examination, predicts the site and size of the lesion, which, if ischaemic as diagnosed on early CT, takes one quite a long way towards determining the likely cause of the ischaemic event (Fig. 6.14; see Chapter 4; Bogousslavsky *et al.*, 1993a; Lindgren *et al.*, 1994a,b; Martin & Bogousslavsky, 1995). Of course, this is easier when the patient has had a stroke with physical signs and comes quickly to medical attention, rather than a TIA with no signs and which occurred some time in the past. Using brain CT or magnetic resonance imaging (MRI) to define the site and size of the brain lesion early after stroke or TIA onset and so to classify the site and size of the infarct is rather unhelpful, because ischaemic stroke subtype classification may need to be done so fast, once acute treatment becomes available, that there is no time for imaging (see Chapter 11); MRI and, particularly, CT may be normal even in clinically definite stroke (see Section 5.3.7); and CT and, particularly, MRI may not be immediately available or even practicable in very ill stroke patients. Morever, any scheme

of early classification for routine clinical use must be applicable to all or, at least, most patients and this again rules out any 'test' which is not quickly and generally available (Bamford, 1992). Brain imaging, however, may *confirm and refine* the site and size of the ischaemic lesion predicted clinically and so help one towards the likely cause. For example, although most pure motor strokes are due to small vessel disease, in a few the CT or MRI scan shows striatocapsular infarction, which is likely to be due to MCA occlusion or to infarction in the territory of the anterior choroidal artery (Bogousslavsky, 1991; Donnan *et al.*, 1993b).

6.5.1 Total anterior circulation infarction (TACI)

The acute stroke clinical syndrome of a TACI (hemiparesis, with or without hemisensory loss, involving two out of face, upper and lower limbs; homonymous hemianopia; and a new cortical deficit such as aphasia or neglect (see Section 4.4.8)) is a reasonable predictor of infarction of most of the MCA territory on brain CT, as a consequence of occlusion of either the MCA trunk (or proximal large branch) or the ICA in the neck (Olsen *et al.*, 1985; Saito *et al.*, 1987; Angeloni *et al.*, 1990; Naylor *et al.*, 1993; Anderson *et al.*, 1994; Wardlaw *et al.*, 1996) The *cause* of the arterial occlusion therefore lies in the heart (e.g. embolism as a consequence of AF, recent myocardial infarction, etc.) or is atherothrombosis (complicated by embolism or occasionally propagating thrombosis) of the ICA and sometimes the aortic arch or on the right of the innominate artery, or it is something unusual affecting the carotid artery, such as dissection. If, therefore, the heart is clinically normal (history, examination, chest X-ray and ECG) and if there is no evidence of arterial disease in the neck (bruits, palpation perhaps, but mainly duplex sonography), then it is important to consider rarities, such as infective endocarditis, PFO (echocardiogram, blood cultures) and carotid dissection (angiogram, possibly, but check for past history of neck trauma). Although TCD may confirm an MCA occlusion (but not if the MCA has already recanalised), this will not help in the search for a cause, whereas an angiogram *might*, if it could be justified on the basis of changing the patient's management (e.g. traumatic carotid dissection could lead to later litigation, fibromuscular dysplasia could stop the search for other explanations, a giant aneurysm with contained thrombus might be surgically treatable or anticoagulants could be given, etc. (see Section 6.6.4)). Of course, increasingly MRI and MR angiography (MRA) are able to replace catheter angiography to show lesions such as dissection, aneurysms, etc., but this is not always easily available or particularly practicable in patients in the acute stage of stroke (see Sections 6.6.3 and 6.6.4).

6.5.2 Partial anterior circulation infarction (PACI)

PACI is a more restricted clinical syndrome, with only two out of the three components of the TACI syndrome, a new isolated cortical dysfunction, such as dysphasia, a predominantly proprioceptive deficit in one limb or a motor/sensory deficit restricted to one body area or part of one body area (e.g. one leg, one hand, etc.) (see Section 4.4.9). This syndrome is reasonably predictive of a restricted cortical infarct due to occlusion of a branch of the MCA or, much less commonly, of the trunk of the anterior cerebral artery, as a result of embolism from the heart or from proximal sites of atherothrombosis (usually the carotid bifurcation) or to any other cause of the TACI syndrome (Olsen et al., 1985; Saito

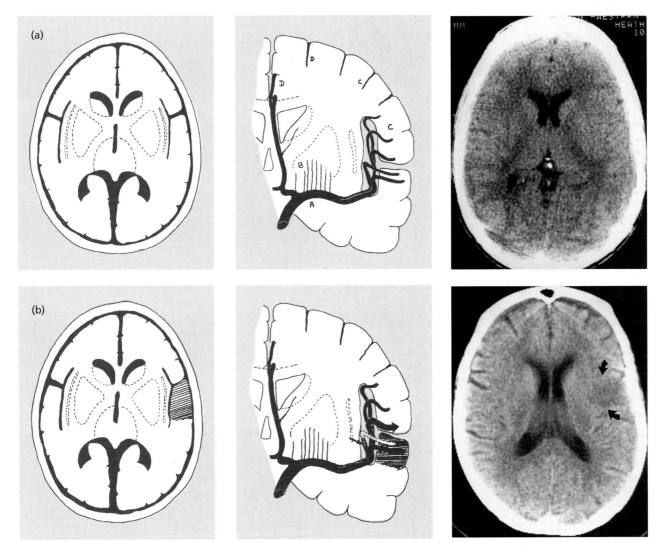

Figure 6.14 Various patterns of arterial occlusion causing different types of cerebral infarction. Left-hand column, diagram of CT brain scan through the level of the basal ganglia; middle column, diagram of the MCA and anterior cerebral arteries on a coronal brain section; right-hand column, corresponding CT brain scan. A, main trunk of MCA; B, lenticulostriate perforating branches of the MCA; C, cortical branches of the MCA; D, cortical branches of the anterior cerebral arteries. (a) Normal arterial anatomy and CT scan; (b) occlusion (usually embolic—arrow—from heart, aorta or ICA) of a cortical branch of the MCA and restricted cortical infarct on CT (arrows); (c) occlusion (usually embolus—arrow—as in (b) above) of MCA trunk to cause infarction of entire MCA territory (arrows); (d) occlusion of one lenticulostriate artery to cause an LACI (arrow); note that the patient has an old LACI in the opposite hemisphere; (e) occlusion of the MCA trunk but with good cortical collaterals from the anterior and posterior cerebral arteries to cause a striatocapsular infarct (arrows).

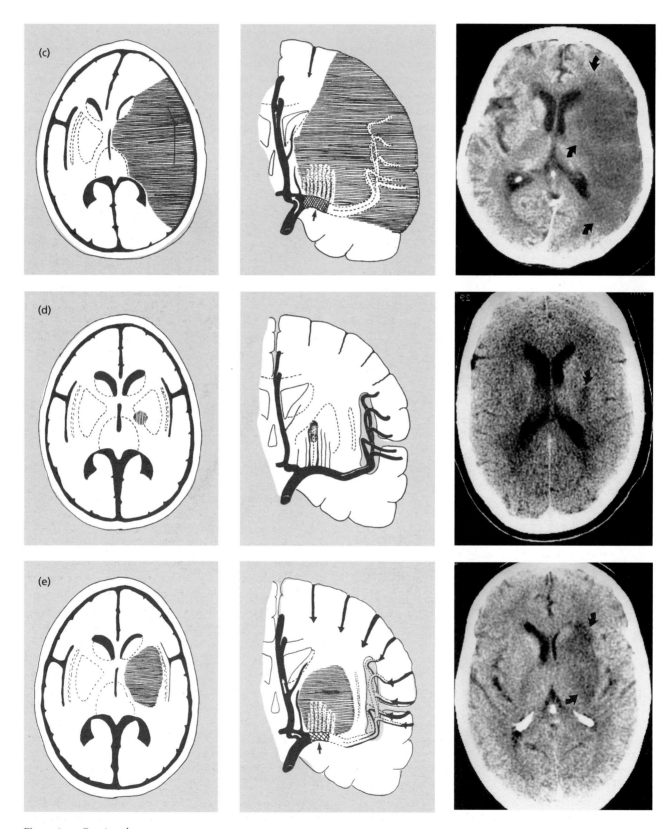

Figure 6.14 *Continued.*

et al., 1987; Angeloni *et al.*, 1990; Kazui *et al.*, 1993; Naylor *et al.*, 1993; Anderson *et al.*, 1994; Wardlaw *et al.*, 1996). Investigation is therefore the same as for the patient with a TACI, except it is usually easier, because the patient is fully conscious and less impaired. Investigation must be quicker, because of the higher risk of early recurrence (see Section 16.1.2) and because the patient has more to lose from a recurrence, which might, next time, be a TACI. Therefore, one has to keep in mind the potential for secondary prevention, particularly eligibility for carotid endarterectomy, which will require early duplex sonography and perhaps cerebral angiography, sooner rather than later (see Section 6.6.4). TCD is unlikely to demonstrate the blocked cerebral artery because this will almost always be distal to the MCA trunk, at a point where TCD is not particularly sensitive. Occasionally, however, patients with a large PACI, but falling short of the full definition of a TACI, do have MCA trunk occlusion, presumably because good collateral flow to the margins of the central infarcted area of brain restricts the clinical syndrome. This is particularly likely with striato-capsular infarction, which usually presents as a PACI (see Section 4.3.2; Donnan *et al.*, 1991). Some PACI syndromes are due to infarction in the centrum ovale (Bogousslavsky & Regli, 1992) and in boundary zones (see Section 6.5.5). Anterior choroidal artery infarcts may also present as a PACI (or LACI) syndrome and seem to be due to either embolism from proximal sites or intracranial small vessel disease (Hupperts *et al.*, 1994; Leys *et al.*, 1994).

> *Total and partial anterior circulation infarction/transient ischaemic attack is usually caused by occlusion of the main stem or a branch of the middle cerebral artery, by occlusion of the anterior cerebral artery or by occlusion of the internal carotid artery. This is usually due to embolism from the heart, to embolism from proximal arterial sites of atherothombosis (the internal carotid artery origin, the aortic arch, etc.) or sometimes to thrombotic occlusion of severe internal carotid artery stenosis.*

6.5.3 Lacunar infarction (LACI)

Lacunar syndromes, the vast majority of which are due to infarction rather than haemorrhage, as defined by early CT, are almost always due to small deep infarcts, which are more likely to be seen on MRI than on CT (Donnan *et al.*, 1982, 1995; Anzalone & Landi, 1989; Hommel *et al.*, 1990; Lindgren *et al.*, 1994a,b; Lodder *et al.*, 1994; see Section 4.4.6). These small deep infarcts are mostly *not* caused by embolism from proximal sources, because the heart and extracranial arteries are far more likely to be normal than in patients with TACIs or PACIs; because emboli are rarely if

ever observed in the MCA by TCD; and because what has been found in the very small number of pathology studies is small vessel disease within the brain (particularly in the internal capsule, basal ganglia or pons) or atheroma at the origin of a single perforating artery (Bogousslavsky *et al.*, 1991; see Section 6.3). There is not, therefore, the same urgency or pressure to rule out a cardiac source of embolism or carotid stenosis. There is, however, a slight concern that prevention with antithrombotic drugs *might* be counterproductive if the same underlying arterial disease which causes LACIs may, in the future, cause PICH (see Section 8.2.1; Besson *et al.*, 1993). However, this is no more than speculation, because the randomised trials did not differentiate different types of vascular pathology at randomisation, nor did they categorise the ischaemic stroke outcomes by clinical subtype (see Chapter 16).

The *capsular warning syndrome* is a rather characteristic clustering, over hours or a few days, of TIAs, consisting usually of weakness down the whole of one side of the body without, if one can be sure, any cognitive or language deficit (i.e. lacunar TIAs), followed within hours or days by a LACI in the internal capsule. Presumably this syndrome is because of intermittent closure of a single lenticulostriate or other perforating artery, followed by complete occlusion, and one is unlikely to find a proximal arterial or cardiac cause, as in any other type of LACI (Donnan *et al.*, 1993c).

6.5.4 Posterior circulation infarction (POCI)

Ischaemia and infarction in the brainstem and/or occipital region is aetiologically more heterogeneous than the other three main clinical syndromes (Castaigne *et al.*, 1973; Caplan & Tettenborn, 1992; Bogousslavsky *et al.*, 1993b; see Section 4.4.7). Emboli from the heart may reach a small artery supplying the brainstem (e.g. superior cerebellar artery) to cause a fairly restricted deficit, block the basilar artery to produce a major brainstem stroke, or travel on to block one or both posterior cerebral arteries to cause a homonymous hemianopia or cortical blindness. Of course, a shower of emboli from the heart could produce any combination of these deficits. Similarly, embolism from the vertebral artery (because of atherothrombosis usually, but sometimes another disorder, such as dissection) or from atherothrombosis of the basilar artery, aortic arch or innominate or subclavian arteries could and does produce exactly the same clinical features as embolism from the heart (Caplan, 1993). Even thromboembolism within the carotid territory can, in some individuals, cause occlusion of the posterior cerebral artery (Gasecki *et al.*, 1994). Basilar occlusion, usually as a result of severe atherothrombotic stenosis, is likely to produce massive brainstem infarction.

Obstruction, usually by atheroma at the origin of the small arteries arising from the basilar artery or by small vessel disease within the brainstem, may produce restricted brainstem syndromes, and certainly some patients with a lacunar syndrome have a small infarct in the brainstem (Nighoghossian *et al.*, 1993; Bogousslavsky *et al.*, 1994). A POCI does not, therefore, provide much of a clue to the cause of the ischaemic event, at least not just from the syndromic identification. An exception is the patient with simultaneous brainstem signs *and* a homonymous hemianopia, where embolism from the heart or a proximal artery must be the likely cause, not small vessel disease.

> *Posterior circulation infarction/transient ischaemic attack can be caused by almost any cause of cerebral ischaemia, which makes it very difficult to be certain of the exact cause in an individual patient.*

Cerebellar ischaemic strokes (see Section 4.3.3) are mostly due to embolism from the heart, vertebral and basilar arteries or to atherothrombotic occlusion at the origin of the cerebellar arteries; and some are said to be due to low flow (Amarenco & Caplan, 1993; Tohgi *et al.*, 1993).

Thalamic infarcts (see Section 4.3.3) can be caused by intracranial small vessel disease affecting one of the small perforating arteries; atheromatous occlusion of these same arteries as they arise from the posterior cerebral and other medium-sized arteries; and embolic occlusion (from the heart, basilar, vertebral and other proximal arterial sites) of these arteries (Castaigne *et al.*, 1981; Bogousslavsky & Caplan, 1993).

6.5.5 Low flow

Most TIAs and ischaemic strokes are caused, we believe, by sudden embolic or sometimes thrombotic occlusion of an artery. However, focal ischaemia could conceivably be due to low flow alone (i.e. without acute vessel occlusion) but usually only distal to a highly stenosed or occluded ICA or other artery, where the vascular bed may be maximally dilated and therefore where the brain is particularly vulnerable to any further fall in perfusion pressure (particularly if arteries carrying collateral blood flow are also diseased). Under these circumstances, a small drop in systemic blood pressure might cause symptoms of focal ischaemia without any acute occlusive event. Of course, under *normal* circumstances quite large falls in systemic blood pressure do not cause cerebral symptoms, because of autoregulation of cerebral blood flow (see Section 11.1.2). Indeed, the pressure gradient across and blood flow through large arteries is not affected until the diameter stenosis is reduced by more than 50% of the original lumen, and often by much more (Brice *et al.*, 1964; De-

Weese *et al.*, 1970; Archie & Feldman, 1981). Even then, cerebral blood flow is usually normal, because of the considerable potential for collateral supply via the circle of Willis and other channels distal to severe disease of one or more of the two carotid and two vertebral arteries (see Section 4.3). But, eventually, as stenosis becomes even more severe, cerebral vasodilatation can not compensate for any further fall in perfusion pressure, particularly if the collateral circulation is also compromised, and this point can be identified when positron emission tomography (PET) shows that the cerebral perfusion reserve is exhausted (i.e. when the ratio of cerebral blood flow to cerebral blood volume falls below about 6.0 and the oxygen extraction fraction starts to rise) (see Section 11.1.2; Gibbs *et al.*, 1984; Powers *et al.*, 1987). Using TCD to demonstrate impaired cerebrovascular reactivity is an indirect but a more practical alternative to PET (see Section 6.6.4), as may be isotopic measurement of the mean cerebral transit time (Naylor *et al.*, 1994), gradient echo MRI (Kleinschmidt *et al.*, 1995) and MRA (Mandai *et al.*, 1994).

Most ischaemic strokes and TIAs occur 'out of the blue' with no previous precipitating activity. However, transient falls in systemic blood pressure should be suspected if TIAs or ischaemic stroke occurs on standing or sitting up quickly; after a heavy meal; in very hot weather; after a hot bath or on warming the face; on exercise; during a Valsalva manoeuvre; during a clinically obvious episode of cardiac arrhythmia (chest pain, palpitations, etc.); during operative hypotension (see Section 7.14); or if the patient has recently been started on, or increased the dose of, any drug likely to cause hypotension, such as calcium blockers or vasodilators. In addition, there is usually very obvious evidence of severe arterial disease in the neck, i.e. bruits and/or absent pulsations (Caplan & Sergay, 1976; Pantin & Young, 1980; Raymond *et al.*, 1980; Nobile-Orazio & Sterzi, 1981; Ruff *et al.*, 1981; Russell & Page, 1983; Stark & Wodak, 1983; Hankey & Gubbay, 1987; Russell, 1988; Kamata *et al.*, 1994; Gironell *et al.*, 1995). The TIAs themselves may be atypical in the sense that they develop over minutes rather than seconds; consist of regular jerking and shaking of one arm and/or leg contralateral to the cerebral ischaemia; or there is monocular or binocular visual blurring, dimming, fragmentation or bleaching, often just in bright light (see Section 3.2.2). There may be additional non-focal features, such as faintness or even loss of consciousness (Furlan *et al.*, 1979; Yanagihara *et al.*, 1985; Wiebers *et al.*, 1989; Tatemichi *et al.*, 1990). Of course, these clinical guidelines to 'low-flow' ischaemic episodes can not be validated against a 'low-flow' gold standard (versus acute arterial occlusion), because at present there is no such gold standard. It is thus conceivable that low flow is a more frequent cause of cerebral ischaemia, or less frequent, than we currently believe.

At the moment, from the treatment point of view, it makes little difference if low-flow TIAs are recognised as such, because, unless the precipitating factor(s) can be avoided or reversed, treatment is surgical to relieve any obstruction to blood flow if it is practical and safe to do so (i.e. carotid endarterectomy (see Section 16.7)); this is exactly the same as the treatment would be if the attacks were due to embolism from severe carotid stenosis. One simply has to acknowledge that, in patients with ischaemic stroke or TIAs and severe disease of the relevant supplying artery, an unknown proportion are due to low flow rather than embolism, and even perhaps that different attacks at different times in the same patient could be caused by different mechanisms. If the large arteries are not severely diseased, a transient fall in blood pressure will cause not focal but non-focal symptoms, such as faintness or loss of consciousness (see Section 3.3.4; Kendell & Marshall, 1963).

Boundary-zone infarction (see Section 4.3.4)

If cerebral infarction occurs as a result of low flow, it is said to be likely to do so not within major arterial territories, but between these territories in the so-called boundary (or border) zones (Fig. 6.15). The alternative term of watershed infarction is a misnomer based on geographical ignorance; a watershed is the line separating the water flowing *into* differ-ent river basins (e.g. the narrow elevated ground *between* two drainage areas), which is the opposite of the pattern of arterial supply, where the flow is from larger to smaller vessels. Sudden, profound and relatively prolonged hypotension (e.g. as a result of cardiac arrest, or cardiac surgery) often seems to cause infarction bilaterally in the so-called posterior boundary zones between the supply territories of the MCA and the posterior cerebral artery in the parieto-occipital regions; so the clinical features include cortical blindness, visual disorientation and agnosia, and amnesia. Low-flow infarction distal to severe ICA stenosis or occlusion tends to cause unilateral infarction in the so-called anterior boundary zone between the supply territories of the MCA and the anterior cerebral artery in the frontoparasagit-tal region; this causes contralateral weakness of the leg more than the arm and sparing the face, some impaired sensation in the same distribution, and aphasia if in the dominant hemisphere. Unilateral posterior boundary-zone infarction causes contralateral hemianopia, cortical sensory loss and, if in the dominant hemisphere, aphasia. Curiously, unilateral boundary-zone infarcts can develop and progress over days and weeks. Finally, there is an internal boundary zone in the corona radiata and centrum ovale, lateral and/or above the lateral ventricle, between the supply of the small perforating branches of the MCA and the medullary arteries, which arise from the cortical branches of the MCA and the anterior

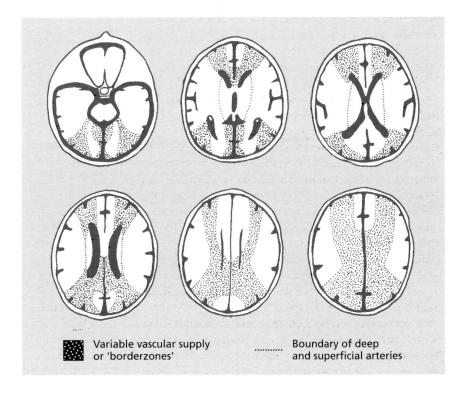

Figure 6.15 Boundary zones between the territories of the MCA, anterior and posterior cerebral arteries. The maximum extent of these variable zones is shown on CT templates (see also Figs 4.29, 4.33, 4.38 & 4.40). (Adapted from van der Zwan *et al.*, 1992.)

Variable vascular supply or 'borderzones'

Boundary of deep and superficial arteries

and perhaps posterior cerebral arteries. Infarction can occur within this internal boundary zone (Torvik, 1984; Bogousslavsky & Regli, 1986a,b; Yanagihara *et al.*, 1988; Bladin & Chambers, 1993).

Diagnosis

The diagnosis of cerebral infarction caused by low flow is far from easy. Essentially, it comes more from the circumstances at the onset of the stroke (see above) than from the clinical syndrome (which can be a TACI or PACI if low flow is affecting the whole or part of the MCA territory, or a PACI or LACI if low flow is affecting a boundary zone), or from the brain CT/MRI-defined site and size of infarction. This is because there is such a large variation between individuals in *where* the boundary zones are and they may even change with time in the same individual in response to changes in peripheral resistance, as a consequence of disease of the major cerebral arteries (Fig. 6.15; van der Zwan *et al.*, 1992, 1993). Moreover, however a boundary zone is defined on CT/MRI, there is little difference between 'boundary-zone' and 'territorial' infarcts from the point of view of demographic characteristics, vascular risk factors and even the prevalence of severe arterial disease in the neck; therefore, some but by no means all 'boundary-zone' infarcts as defined by CT or MRI have a probable haemodynamic (i.e. low-flow) cause, but others could well be due to embolism or acute occlusive thrombosis (Angeloni *et al.*, 1990; Hupperts *et al.*, 1993, 1996).

Perhaps the whole boundary-zone concept is flawed, because of the following.

1 The position of this zone is so variable between and within individuals it can not be defined anatomically on CT/MRI.
2 Even when it is (uncertainly) defined, the cause of ischaemia within it may be *either* low flow *or* acute arterial occlusion.
3 In a sense any arterial territory *has* to have a vulnerable (to ischaemia) terminal zone, which forms a boundary with adjacent territories, and there is no reason to suppose that this zone is more susceptible to ischaemia caused by low flow as a result of a drop of perfusion pressure without acute arterial occlusion than as a result of acute arterial occlusion.
4 Just because cerebral blood flow may be compromised in patients with so-called boundary-zone infarcts, defined by CT/MRI, does not mean such infarcts were *not* due to acute arterial occlusion.
5 What matters clinically is not *where* the brain lesion is but why it occurred, and this depends not so much on imaging as on points in the clinical history and examination which suggest low flow as a consequence of a sudden fall in systemic blood pressure, or of perfusion pressure, distal to a very stenotic or occluded artery.
6 Finally, the management of the patient is not much influenced *whatever* the cause of focal cerebral ischaemia; in a patient with severe arterial disease, a symptomatic severe carotid stenosis should usually be treated surgically if it is technically possible to do so, risk factors are minimised (without causing symptomatic hypotension by overtreating hypertension) and antithrombotic drugs are prescribed (see Chapter 16).

> *The exact site of boundary zones between the territories of supply of the major cerebral arteries is so variable between, and even within, individuals that the diagnosis of an infarct in a boundary zone based on CT/MRI becomes all but impossible.*

6.5.6 Clues from the history

The vast majority of TIAs and ischaemic strokes start suddenly without any obvious provocation and there are few if any symptoms other than those of a focal neurological or ocular deficit. Sometimes, however, there are clues to the cause in the history, even if they require some tenacity to recognise (Table 6.11).

Table 6.11 Important clues from the history which may suggest the cause of an ischaemic stroke or TIA, or that the diagnosis of cerebrovascular disease should be reconsidered.

Gradual onset
Low flow (see Section 6.5.5)
Migraine (see Section 7.5)
Structural intracranial lesion (see Sections 3.3.2 and 3.5.2)
Multiple sclerosis (see Sections 3.3.2 and 3.5.7)

Precipitating factors
Suspected systemic hypotension (standing up quickly, heavy meal, hot weather, hot bath, warming the face, exercise, Valsalva manoeuvre, chest symptoms such as pain or palpitations, starting or changing blood pressure-lowering drugs) (see Section 6.5.5)
Head-turning (see Section 6.5.6)
Hypoglycaemia (see Section 6.5.6)
Valsalva manoeuvre (see Section 6.5.6)

Recent headache
Carotid/vertebral dissection (see Section 7.1)
Migrainous stroke/TIA (see Sections 3.3.2 and 7.5)
Intracranial venous thrombosis (see Section 8.2.5)
Giant cell arteritis (or other primary inflammatory vascular disorders) (see Section 7.2)
Structural intracranial lesion (see Sections 3.3.2 and 3.5.2)

Continued

Table 6.11 *Continued.*

Epileptic seizures
Intracranial venous thrombosis (see Section 8.2.5)
Mitochondrial cytopathy (see Section 7.15)
Non-vascular intracranial lesion (see Sections 3.3.2 and 3.5.2)

Malaise
Inflammatory arterial disorders (see Section 7.2)
Infective endocarditis (see Section 6.4)
Cardiac myxoma (see Section 6.4)
Cancer (see Section 7.9)
Thrombotic thrombocytopenic purpura (see Section 7.6)
Sarcoidosis (see Section 7.2)

Associated vascular disease or risk factors
Heart disease (see Section 6.4)
Claudication (see Section 6.2.3)
Hypertension (see Section 6.2.3)
Smoking (see Section 6.2.3)

Drugs
Oral contraceptives (see Section 7.10)
Oestrogens in men (see Section 7.10)
Blood pressure-lowering/vasodilators (see Section 6.5.5)
Hypoglycaemic drugs (see Section 6.5.6)
Cocaine (see Section 6.5.6)
Amphetamines (see Section 6.5.6)
Ephedrine (see Section 6.5.6)
Phenylpropanolamine (see Section 6.5.6)
Ecstasy (see Section 6.5.6)
Allopurinol (see Section 6.5.6)
Interleukin 2 (see Section 6.5.6)
Deoxycoformycin (see Section 6.5.6)
L-Asparaginase (see Section 7.6)

Injury to head or neck
Chronic subdural haematoma
Vertebral/carotid artery dissection (see Section 7.1)
See also Table 6.3

Self-audible bruits
ICA stenosis (distal) (see Section 6.5.6)
Dural arteriovenous fistula (see Section 8.2.7)
Glomus tumour
Caroticocavernous fistula (see Section 8.2.11)

Past medical history
Inflammatory bowel disease (see Section 6.5.6)
Coeliac disease (see Section 6.5.6)
Homocystinuria (see Section 6.5.6)
Irradiation of the head or neck (see Section 7.9)
Recurrent deep venous thrombosis
Recurrent miscarriages

Family history
See Table 6.12

Gradual onset

Gradual onset of ischaemic stroke or TIA over hours or days, rather than seconds or minutes, is unusual (see Section 3.2.1). If the onset is gradual and stroke or TIA is not likely to be due to low flow (see Section 6.5.5) or migraine (see Section 7.5), then the diagnosis should be rethought and a structural intracranial lesion looked for again, or for the first time if brain CT/MRI has not already been done (e.g. intracranial tumour, chronic subdural haematoma, cerebral abscess, etc.). Under the age of 50 years, multiple sclerosis should also be considered. However, a priori, focal neurological deficits which develop over hours, and even 1–2 days, in an *elderly* patient are still more likely to be due to a vascular than a non-vascular cause, because the former is so much more common than the latter; it is only when progression occurs over a longer period that the likelihood of a non-vascular cause (such as chronic subdural haematoma) starts to rise.

Precipitating factors

The *exact* activity and *time* of onset may both be important. Anything to suggest a drop in blood pressure may be relevant (see Section 6.5.5), as are *pregnancy* (see Section 7.11) and any *operative procedure* (see Section 7.14). *Turning the head* is a rare cause of *symptomatic* vertebral artery occlusion against a spondylotic spur of bone, and so brainstem ischaemic stroke or TIA, and has seldom been demonstrated for certain (Mapstone & Spetzler, 1982; Sakai *et al.*, 1988; Rosengart *et al.*, 1993; Sturzenegger *et al.*, 1994); of course, non-specific 'dizziness' or 'light-headedness' during neck extension or head turning is common in the elderly, but the exact cause is very uncertain and may lie in the peripheral vestibular apparatus, as it does in benign positional vertigo. Unusual or forced neck turning or manipulation may cause arterial dissection (see Section 7.1). Recurrent attacks occurring first thing in the morning, or during exercise, suggest *hypoglycaemia*, which is easy to diagnose in a diabetic patient on hypoglycaemic drugs but more difficult if there is a less obvious cause of hypoglycaemia, such as the very rare insulinoma or drugs, such as pentamidine (see Section 3.3.2). Hypoglycaemic focal neurological episodes tend to be transient rather than persisting and consist more often of right- than left-sided weakness. Also, curiously, consciousness is unimpaired and there seldom seem to be any of the usual systemic manifestations of hypoglycaemia (Illangasekera, 1981; Malouf & Brust, 1985; Wallis *et al.*, 1985; Foster & Hart, 1987; Pell & Frier, 1990; Rother *et al.*, 1992; Shintani *et al.*, 1993). Onset during a Valsalva manoeuvre (e.g. lifting a heavy object) suggests a low-flow ischaemic stroke (see

Section 6.5.5) or paradoxical embolism, and so may set off a search for a deep venous thrombosis (DVT) if there is evidence on echocardiography of a PFO (see Sections 6.4 and 6.7.3).

Headache

Headache at around the onset of ischaemic stroke or TIA is not uncommon (about 25% of patients with stroke), is usually mild and, if localised at all, tends to be related to the site of the brain/eye lesion (see Sections 3.2.3 and 15.9). Headache is more common with vertebrobasilar than carotid distribution ischaemia, and less common with lacunar ischaemia (Nichols *et al.*, 1990; Koudstaal *et al.*, 1991a; Vestergaard *et al.*, 1993; Jorgensen *et al.*, 1994a; Kumral *et al.*, 1995). Severe pain unilaterally in the head, face, neck or eye at around the time of stroke onset is highly suggestive of carotid dissection, whilst vertebral dissection tends to cause unilateral or sometimes bilateral occipital pain (see Section 7.1). *Migrainous stroke* may be accompanied by headache (see Section 7.5), and in the context of the differential diagnosis of TIAs migraine should be fairly obvious, unless there is no headache (see Section 3.3.2). Although *intracranial venous thrombosis* causes either a benign intracranial hypertension syndrome or a subacute encephalopathy, sometimes a focal onset does occur and headache can be a clue (see Section 8.2.5; Bousser *et al.*, 1985; Enevoldson & Russell, 1990). Finally, stroke or TIA in the context of a patient who has had a headache for days or weeks previously must raise the possibility of *giant cell arteritis* and other primary inflammatory vascular disorders (see Section 7.2). Pain in the jaw muscles with chewing, and which resolves with rest, strongly suggests claudication, which is due to ECA disease as a result of giant cell arteritis far more often than as a result of atherothrombosis.

Epileptic seizures

Epileptic seizures, partial or generalised, within hours of stroke onset are distinctly unusual in adults (<5%), but are rather more common in childhood stroke. They are more likely with haemorrhagic than ischaemic strokes and if the infarct is extensive and involves the cerebral cortex (Davalos *et al.*, 1992; Lancman *et al.*, 1993; Burn *et al.*, 1996). They are also likely with *venous infarction* and *mitochondrial cytopathy* (see Section 7.15). Of course, partial motor seizures can be confused with limb-shaking TIAs, but the former are more clonic and the jerking spreads in a typical Jacksonian way from one body part to another (see Sections 3.2.2 and 6.5.5). Very rarely, transient focal ischaemia seems to cause a partial epileptic seizure, but proving a causal rela-

tionship is seldom possible (Kaplan, 1993). One might also be mistaken with the diagnosis of stroke and a tumour on CT misinterpreted as an infarct (often because contrast enhancement can look similar to an infarct (see Section 5.3.5)); partial seizures after a 'stroke' should always make one re-examine the diagnosis. Also, seizures in the presence of a history of a few days' malaise, headache and fever should make one very alert to encephalitis and the need for an electroencephalogram (EEG) (to show bilateral diffuse rather than focal slow waves) and CSF examination (raised white cell count, but this can also occur in stroke (see Section 6.4)).

Malaise

Stroke occurring in the context of a patient who has been generally unwell for days, weeks or months should make one consider an inflammatory arterial disorder, particularly giant cell arteritis (see Section 7.2), infective endocarditis (see Section 6.4), cardiac myxoma (see Section 6.4), cancer (see Section 7.9), thrombotic thrombocytopenic purpura (see Section 7.6) or even sarcoidosis (see Section 7.2).

Vascular risk factors

Vascular risk factors (see Section 6.2.3) and diseases should obviously be sought. It is most unusual for an ischaemic stroke or TIA to occur in someone with *no* vascular risk factors, unless they are very old, or young with some unusual cause of stroke (see Table 6.4). *Heart disease* of any sort may be relevant (source of embolism to the brain, arrhythmias causing low-flow ischaemia, etc.) and symptoms should be specifically sought in the history: angina, shortness of breath, palpitations, etc.

Drugs

Drugs may well be relevant: oral contraceptives in women and oestrogens in men (see Section 7.10), anything which may lower the blood pressure (see Section 6.5.5), hypoglycaemic agents (see above) and drugs of abuse, which seem to be a more common problem in the US than elsewhere (Caplan *et al.*, 1982; Caplan, 1994a). At present, the most commonly implicated *drug of abuse* is *cocaine* (and its 'crack' form), which, within hours of administration, can cause ischaemic stroke, TIA, PICH and subarachnoid haemorrhage (Cregler & Mark, 1986; Levine *et al.*, 1990; Libman *et al.*, 1993). Although a cocaine vasculitis has been described (see Section 8.5.4; Krendel *et al.*, 1990; Fredericks *et al.*, 1991), more likely explanations are an acute rise of systemic blood pressure causing rupture of an unsuspected arteriovenous malformation or aneurysm; cardiac arrhythmia, myocardial infarction or cardiomyopathy and so cerebral embolism; and possibly vasoconstriction and complicating thrombosis (Daras *et al.*, 1991; Konzen *et al.*, 1995; see Section 9.1.4). *Amphetamines* seem to cause a small vessel vasculopathy, leading to intracranial haemorrhage, but acute hypertension is another possible mechanism; ischaemic stroke is less common (Harrington *et al.*, 1983; Isner *et al.*, 1986; Rothrock *et al.*, 1988; Sauer, 1991; see Section 8.5.3). Other sympathomimetic drugs, such as *ephedrine, phenylpropanolamine* and '*Ecstasy*' (methylene dioxymethylamphetamine) may cause stroke in similar ways (Delaney & Estes, 1980; Glick *et al.*, 1987; Kase *et al.*, 1987; Harries & de Silva, 1992; Bruno *et al.*, 1993). Other causes of stroke or stroke-like syndromes in drug-abusers should not be forgotten: infective endocarditis (see Section 6.4), head or neck trauma (see Section 7.1), embolisation of injected particulate foreign matter contaminating drugs and human immunodeficiency virus (HIV) infection (see Section 7.8).

Various therapeutic drugs have been implicated, with varying levels of proof, in hypersensitivity reactions which may include a cerebral vasculitis, e.g. *allopurinol* (Mills, 1971), *interleukin 2* and *deoxycoformycin* (Steinmetz *et al.*, 1989). *L-Asparaginase* is also said to cause stroke (see Section 7.6).

Injury

Injury in the days and weeks before ischaemic stroke or TIA onset is crucial information. A head injury might have caused a *chronic subdural haematoma* (highly unlikely if more than 3 months previously), but this should have been considered earlier at the stroke versus not-stroke stage (see Section 3.5.2). Of possible relevance is an injury to the neck in the hours, days or possibly a few weeks before onset, because this may cause *carotid or vertebral dissection* (see Section 7.1). After long-bone fracture fat embolism may cause a generalised encephalopathy, but just occasionally there are additional focal features (Jacobson *et al.*, 1986). It is therefore essential to *ask* about any injury, strangulation, car crash, unusual yoga exercises, neck manipulation, etc. (see Table 6.3).

Self-audible bruits

Self-audible bruits, often but not always audible to the examiner as well, are very unlikely to be due to carotid bifurcation atherothrombosis where the source of the sound is too far from the ear. Pulsatile bruits (differentiated from tinnitus by being in time with the pulse) are much more likely to indicate *distal* ICA stenosis (dissection or, rarely, atherothrombosis), a dural arteriovenous malformation near the petrous temporal bone, a glomus tumour, a caroticocavernous fistula or just heightened awareness of one's own pulse (Thie *et al.*, 1993).

Past medical history

Past medical history may be important. Other than heart disease (see above), *inflammatory bowel disease* could be relevant: both *ulcerative* and *Crohn's colitis* can be complicated by cerebral arterial occlusion and intracranial venous thrombosis (Johns, 1991; Jorens *et al.*, 1991; Jackson *et al.*, 1993; Lossos *et al.*, 1995). The bowel disease is not necessarily active at the time of stroke and the association has been related to thrombocytosis, hypercoagulability, immobility, paradoxical embolism from the legs, vasculitis and dehydration. Cerebral vasculitis has also been described with *coeliac disease* (Rush *et al.*, 1986). *Homocystinuria*, an autosomal recessive inborn error of metabolism, is complicated by cerebral arterial and intracranial venous thrombosis and may be suspected if there is mental retardation, Marfanoid habitus, osteoporosis, high myopia and dislocated lenses; the arterial vascular pathology appears to differ from atheroma (Schimke *et al.*, 1965; Mudd *et al.*, 1985; Visy *et al.*, 1991; Rubba *et al.*, 1994). *Irradiation* of the head and neck cause, months or years later, stenotic and sometimes apparently atherothrombotic lesions, with fibrosis of the arterial wall and aneurysm formation (see Section 7.9). Recurrent DVT suggests *protein C, protein S* or *antithrombin III deficiency*, particularly if there is a family history (see Section 7.6), and the antiphospholipid antibody syndrome (see Section 7.2). Of course, *any* reason for a recent DVT (e.g. a long air journey) should raise the question of paradoxical embolism (see Sections 6.4 and 6.7.3). Recurrent miscarriage suggests the antiphospholipid antibody syndrome (see Section 7.2).

> If a patient has had, or has, deep venous thrombosis in the legs, then think about paradoxical embolism to the brain, a familial clotting factor problem or the antiphospholipid antibody syndrome.

Previous strokes and/or transient ischaemic attacks

Previous strokes and/or TIAs going back months or more make certain causes unlikely (e.g. infective endocarditis, arterial dissection).

Family history

Several rare conditions are familial and can cause cerebral

Table 6.12 Identifiable causes of familial stroke (including intracranial haemorrhage) and TIA. (See also Natowicz & Kelly, 1987; DeGraba & Penix, 1995.)

Connective-tissue disorders
Ehlers–Danlos syndrome (see Section 7.3)
Pseudoxanthoma elasticum (see Section 7.3)
Marfan's syndrome (see Section 7.3)
Fibromuscular dysplasia (see Section 7.3)
Familial MVP (see Section 6.4)

Haematological disorders
Sickle cell disease/trait (see Section 7.6)
Antithrombin III deficiency (see Section 7.6)
Protein C deficiency (see Section 7.6)
Protein S deficiency (see Section 7.6)
Plasminogen abnormality/deficiency (see Section 7.6)
Dysfibrinogenaemia (see Section 7.6)
Haemophilia and other inherited coagulation factor deficiencies (see Section 8.4.4)

Others
Familial hypercholesterolaemia
Neurofibromatosis (see Section 6.5.7)
Homocystinuria (see Section 6.5.6)
Fabry's disease (see Section 6.5.7)
Dutch and Icelandic cerebral amyloid angiopathy (see Section 8.2.3)
Migraine (see Section 7.5)
Familial cardiac myxoma (see Section 6.4)
Familial cardiomyopathies (see Section 6.4)
Mitochondrial cytopathy (see Section 7.1.5)
CADASIL (cerebral autosomal dominant arteriopathy with subcortical infarcts and leucoencephalopathy) (see Section 6.5.6)
Sneddon's syndrome (see Section 7.2)
Arteriovenous malformations (see Section 8.2.2)
Intracranial saccular aneurysms (see Sections 8.2.4 and 9.1.1)

infarction and ischaemia (Table 6.12), and genetic factors play at least some part in the development of stroke risk factors, such as hypertension and diabetes. In addition, an autosomal dominantly inherited small vessel vasculopathy has been reported, with migraine, recurrent lacunar more often than cortical ischaemic strokes and TIAs, starting in middle age and merging with later dementia, so-called 'CADASIL' (cerebral autosomal dominant arteriopathy with subcortical infarcts and leucoencephalopathy). On CT, and more obviously on MRI, there are focal, diffuse and confluent lesions in the cerebral white matter, which are probably due to the arteriopathy causing ischaemia. The cause is unknown but in some families a genetic locus has been identified on chromosome region 19_q12 (Chabriat *et al.*, 1995; Ragno *et al.*, 1995; Sabbadini *et al.*, 1995).

6.5.7 Clues from the examination

Neurological examination

Neurological examination is *primarily* to localise the brain lesion, although in patients with TIAs, or those seen some days after a minor stroke, there will probably be no signs at all. Just sometimes, however, there may be a clue to the cause: a Horner's syndrome ipsilateral to a TACI or PACI (i.e. not part of a brainstem stroke, where it might be expected) suggests dissection of the ICA, or sometimes atherothrombotic occlusion (see Section 7.1); lower cranial nerve lesions ipsilateral to a TACI or PACI can also occur in a carotid dissection and, like the Horner's syndrome, are due to stretching and bulging of the arterial wall in relation to the affected nerves (Panisset & Eidelman, 1990); IIIrd, IVth and VIth nerve palsies have been described ipsilateral to ICA occlusion, presumably due to ischaemia of the nerve trunks (Kapoor *et al.*, 1991).

In a TACI or brainstem stroke one would expect some drowsiness, but with more restricted infarcts consciousness is normal. Therefore, if consciousness is impaired and yet the 'stroke' itself seems mild, it is important to reconsider the differential diagnosis (particularly chronic subdural haematoma); to consider the diffuse encephalopathic disorders which have focal features and which may masquerade as stroke, e.g. cerebral vasculitis of some sort (see Section 7.2), non-bacterial thrombotic endocarditis (see Section 6.4), intracranial venous thrombosis (see Section 8.2.5), mitochondrial cytopathy (see Section 7.15), thrombotic thrombocytopenic purpura (see Section 7.6), etc.; and to remember that co-morbidity, such as pneumonia, sedative drugs, infection and hypoglycaemia, may make the neurological deficit seem worse than it really is (see Section 15.4, severe versus not so severe stroke).

> *If the neurological deficit is mild and yet the patient is drowsy, then consider chronic subdural haematoma, cerebral vasculitis, non-bacterial thrombotic endocarditis, intracranial venous thrombosis, mitochondrial cytopathy, thrombotic thrombocytopenic purpura, sedative drugs, hypoglycaemia or co-morbidity, such as pneumonia or infection.*

Eyes

The eyes may provide general clues to the cause of a stroke (e.g. diabetic or hypertensive retinopathy) or may reveal papilloedema, which would make the diagnosis of ischaemic stroke, or even intracerebral haemorrhage, most unlikely. In addition, it is worth searching thoroughly for evidence of emboli (Arruga & Sanders, 1982; see Section 3.2.6).

Fibrin–platelet emboli are rarely observed, perhaps because they are likely to move through the retinal circulation and disperse and are dull greyish white plugs; they suggest embolism from the heart or proximal sources of athero-thrombosis. On the other hand, cholesterol emboli seem to be more permanent and therefore are quite commonly seen as glittering orange or yellow bodies which lodge at arterio-lar branching points, usually without obstructing the blood flow, and they reflect the ophthalmoscope light; obviously these strongly suggest embolisation from proximal arterial sources of atheroma, but they are often asymptomatic. 'Calcific' retinal emboli appear as solid, white and non-reflective bodies and tend to lodge on, or near the edge of, the optic disc; they suggest embolism from aortic or mitral valve calcification. Localised areas of periarteriolar sheathing, seen as opaque white obliteration of segments of the retinal arterioles, suggest embolism, usually cholesterol, in the past. Roth spots in the retina are very suggestive of infective endo-carditis; dislocated lenses should make one think about Marfan's syndrome or homocystinuria; angioid streaks of the retina about pseudoxanthoma elasticum; and in hyper-viscosity syndromes there is a characteristic retinopathy (see Section 7.6).

Dilated episcleral vessels may be a clue to functional anas-tamoses between branches of the ECA and orbital branches of the ICA distal to severe ICA disease. With very severe dis-ease of the ICA, usually accompanied by severe disease of the ipsilateral ECA as well, the eye may become so ischaemic that ischaemic oculopathy develops (see Section 3.2.6 and Fig. 3.8). Here there are haemorrhages scattered around the retina, microaneurysms, dilatation of the retinal veins and irregular arteries and veins. The retinal blood flow is extremely impaired, and this can be demonstrated by lightly compressing the eye with one finger whilst observing the fun-dus and noting collapse of the central retinal artery. Later features include impaired visual acuity, eye pain, rubeosis of the iris (dilated blood vessels), fixed dilated pupil, neovas-cular glaucoma, cataract and corneal oedema (Sturrock & Mueller, 1984; Russell & Ikeda, 1986).

Arterial pulses

It is *always* worth feeling *both* radial pulses simultaneously, because any inequality in timing or volume suggests subcla-vian or innominate stenosis or occlusion, and this is further supported if there is an ipsilateral supraclavicular bruit or lower blood pressure in the arm with the weak or delayed pulse. Normally, the ICA is too deep and rostral to be felt in the neck, so any loss of the 'carotid' pulsation reflects CCA or innominate occlusion or severe stenosis, both rather rare situations.

The arterial pulse felt in the neck comes from the common, not the internal carotid artery.

The superficial temporal pulses should be easily felt and symmetrical: if there is unilateral absence or delay, this sug-gests ECA or CCA disease. Of course, tenderness of *any* of the branches of the ECA (occipital, facial, superficial tempo-ral) points towards giant cell arteritis. Tenderness of the carotid artery in the neck (i.e. the CCA) can occur in acute carotid occlusion but is more likely to be a sign of dissection or possibly arteritis.

Absence of several neck and arm pulses in a young person suggests Takayasu's arteritis (see Section 7.2), whilst delayed or absent leg pulses suggests coarctation of the aorta. Other causes of widespread disease of the aortic arch are atheroma, giant cell arteritis, syphilis, subintimal fibrosis, arterial dis-section and trauma (Ross & McKusick, 1953; Dalal et al., 1971; Wickremasinghe et al., 1978).

The foot and femoral pulses (and femoral bruits) should never be forgotten: because peripheral vascular disease is so common in patients with TIA and ischaemic stroke (see Section 6.2.1) and it is an important predictor of future seri-ous vascular events (see Section 16.1); because the state of the femoral artery is important to assess before cerebral angiography via the femoral route (see Section 6.6.4); and because, if after angiography the leg pulses disappear, then one can know whether this was a result of the angiography. Obviously, any evidence of systemic embolism would direct the search towards a source of embolism in the heart.

Finally, when the hand is on the abdomen a brief thought about an aortic aneurysm is in order whilst searching for any masses or hepatosplenomegaly; although the prevalence of aortic aneurysm in these patients is unknown, it could well be quite high, particularly if the patient has carotid stenosis (Carty et al., 1993; Karanjia et al., 1994).

Cervical bruits (Table 6.13 & Fig. 6.16)

Listening to the neck is a favourite occupation for inquisitive physicians and acquisitive surgeons and can lead to some useful information. A local bruit, occasionally palpable, over the carotid bifurcation (i.e. high up under the jaw) is predic-tive of some degree of carotid stenosis (>25% by the European Carotid Surgery Trial (ECST) method), but very tight stenosis (or occlusion) may not cause a bruit at all (Hankey & Warlow, 1990; Fig. 6.17). External carotid stenosis can also cause a bruit. As a sensitive and specific test for severe internal carotid stenosis, a bruit is not, therefore, particularly useful. Bruits transmitted from the heart become attenuated as one listens further up the neck towards the angle of the jaw, thyroid bruits are bilateral and more obvi-

Table 6.13 The source of neck bruits.

Carotid bifurcation arterial bruit
ICA origin stenosis
ECA origin stenosis

Supraclavicular arterial bruit
Subclavian artery stenosis
Vertebral artery origin stenosis
Can be normal in young adults

Diffuse neck bruit
Thyrotoxicosis
Hyperdynamic circulation (pregnancy, anaemia, fever, haemodialysis)

Transmitted bruit from the heart and great vessels
Aortic stenosis/regurgitation
Mitral regurgitation
Patent ductus arteriosus
Coarctation of the aorta

Venous hum

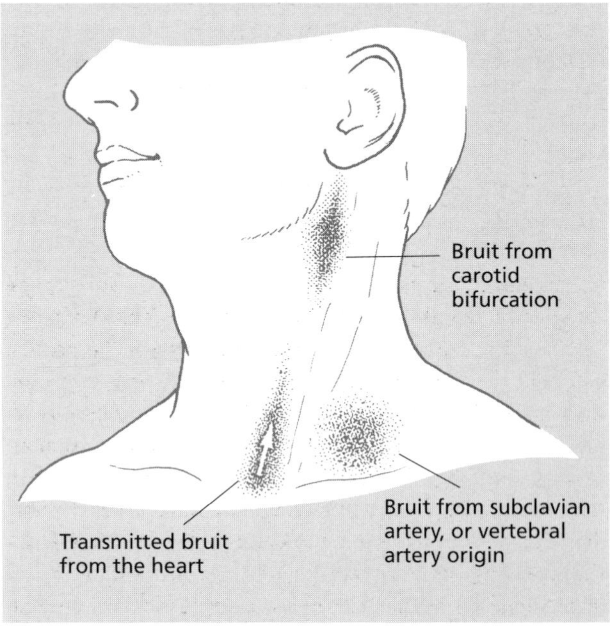

ously over the gland, a hyperdynamic circulation tends to cause a diffuse bruit, if any, and venous hums are more continuous and roaring and in any event are obliterated by light pressure over the ipsilateral jugular vein (Sandok *et al.*, 1982). An arterial bruit in the supraclavicular fossa suggests either subclavian or proximal vertebral arterial disease, but a transmitted bruit from aortic stenosis must also be considered. Normal young adults quite often have a short supraclavicuiar bruit; the reason is unknown.

> *Carotid bruits are neither specific nor sensitive in the diagnosis of carotid stenosis of sufficient severity to make surgery worthwhile.*

Cardiac examination

Cardiac examination is important, particularly to look for any cardiac source of embolism. If physicians feel underconfident about their cardiological abilities, then they should get properly trained or a cardiologist will have to be consulted. AF will already have been suspected from the radial pulse, left-ventricular hypertrophy suggests hypertension or aortic stenosis and most *major* cardiac sources of embolism are fairly obvious clinically (e.g. AF, mitral stenosis, prosthetic heart valve).

Fever

Fever is distinctly unusual in the first hours after stroke

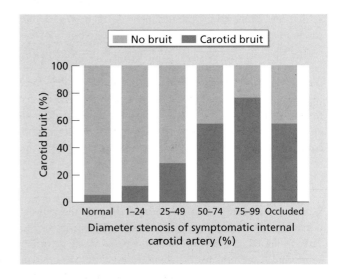

Figure 6.16 The sites of various cervical bruits. Note that a bruit arising from the carotid bifurcation is high up under the angle of the jaw and that localised supraclavicular bruits are due to either subclavian or vertebral origin artery stenosis. (From Warlow, 1995; reproduced with permission from the *Oxford Textbook of Medicine*, Oxford University Press.)

Figure 6.17 The percentage of patients with a localised bruit over the symptomatic carotid bifurcation for various degrees of ICA origin stenoses as estimated (using the ECST method) from 298 carotid angiograms. (Adapted with permission from Hankey & Warlow, 1990.)

Table 6.14 Clues to the cause of ischaemic stroke/TIA from examination of the skin and nails.

Finger-clubbing	Right-to-left intracardiac shunt (see Section 6.4) Cancer (see Section 7.9) Pulmonary arterial venous malformation (see Section 6.4) Infective endocarditis (see Section 6.4) Inflammatory bowel disease (see Section 6.5.6)
Splinter haemorrhages	Infective endocarditis (see Section 6.4) Cholesterol embolisation syndrome (see Section 7.16) Vasculitis (see Section 7.2)
Scleroderma	Systemic sclerosis (see Section 7.2)
Livedo reticularis	Sneddon's syndrome (see Section 7.2) Systemic lupus erythematosus (see Section 7.2) Polyarteritis nodosa (see Section 7.2) Cholesterol embolisation syndrome (see Section 7.16)
Lax skin	Ehlers–Danlos syndrome (see Section 7.3) Pseudoxanthoma elasticum (see Section 7.3)
Skin colour	Anaemia (see Section 7.6) Polycythaemia (see Section 7.6) Cyanosis (right-to-left intracardiac shunt, pulmonary arterial venous malformation) (see Section 6.4)
Porcelain-white papules/scars	Kohlmeier–Degos' disease (see Section 7.2)
Skin scars	Ehlers–Danlos syndrome (see Section 7.3)
Petechiae/purpura/bruising	Thrombotic thrombocytopenic purpura (see Section 7.6) Fat embolism (see Section 6.5.6) Cholesterol embolisation syndrome (see Section 7.16) Ehlers–Danlos syndrome (see Section 7.3)
Orogenital ulceration	Behçet's disease (see Section 7.2)
Rash	Fabry's disease (see Section 6.5.7)
Epidermal naevi	Epidermal naevus syndrome (Dobyns & Garg, 1991)
Café-au-lait patches	Neurofibromatosis (see Section 6.5.7)
Thrombosed veins, needle marks	Intravenous drug abuse (see Section 6.5.6)

onset. Any raised temperature at this time must, therefore, be taken seriously and endocarditis or other infections, inflammatory vascular disorders or cardiac myxoma considered. Later on, fever is quite common and usually reflects some complication of stroke (see Section 15.12).

Skin and nails

The skin and nails occasionally provide clues to the cause of ischaemic stroke or TIA (Table 6.14). *Fabry's disease* is a rare sex-linked recessive disorder in which there is a deficiency of alpha-galactosidase A, which results in the accumulation of glycosphingolipids in vascular endothelial and other cells. Ischaemic stroke, mostly due to occlusion of small blood vessels, is a common complication (Grewal, 1994). The patients are young males (very occasionaly heterozygote females) and usually already have skin angiokeratomas in the bathing-trunks area, as well as burning pain and paraesthesia in the hands and feet (but seldom any signs) due to a small fibre neuropathy. Corneal dystrophy, renal failure and secondary hypertension, and myocardial ischaemia are additional complications. *Tuberous sclerosis* may possibly be complicated by cerebral emboli from a cardiac tumour (rhabdomyoma) (Kandt *et al.*, 1985). *Neurofibromatosis* may also be complicated by similar tumours and also by irradiation (for optic nerve glioma) induced distal carotid occlusion, causing the moyamoya syndrome (see Section 7.13), intracranial aneurysms or tumour compression of intracranial arteries (Rizzo & Lessell, 1994).

Getting to the bottom of the cause of an ischaemic stroke or transient ischaemic attack requires much more than just neurological skills. Stroke medicine, like neurology, is part of general internal medicine.

6.6 Investigation

Investigation has little or nothing to do with the diagnosis of stroke (versus not stroke) or of TIA (versus not TIA), which are both revealed largely by the history (see Chapter 3). Any investigations are mainly to help unravel the pathological type of stroke (cerebral infarction versus intracerebral haemorrhage versus subarachnoid haemorrhage (see Chapter 5)) and then the cause of cerebral ischaemia (or intracranial haemorrhage (see Chapters 8 and 9)), particularly one that can be treated. The site of any infarct, on brain CT/MRI, relevant to the symptoms may help distinguish carotid from vertebrobasilar distribution attacks when the clinical distinction is difficult (e.g. transient hemiparesis in a patient who does not attempt to speak *could* be due to a cortical, internal capsule or pontine lesion). Investigation may also provide relevant prognostic information, e.g. left-ventricular hypertrophy on the ECG, severe carotid stenosis on angiography, etc. (see Section 16.1). In addition, patients with angina or other cardiac symptoms, claudication or suspected aortic aneurysm may need specific investigations directed at *these* problems with a view to appropriate treatment (Adams, 1991; Donnan, 1992; Hankey & Warlow, 1992).

> *Ideally, any investigation should be accurate, non-invasive, accessible, inexpensive and, most importantly, informative, in the sense that the result (positive or negative, high or low, etc.) will influence patient management and outcome.*

6.6.1 Routine investigations for all, or almost all, patients

Although there are no absolute rules, it is reasonable that all ischaemic stroke/TIA patients, unless they are already heavily dependent or institutionalised, should have a basic non-invasive screen of first-line investigations within 24 hours of presentation, none of which requires hospital admission (Table 6.15). The chance of picking up a relevant abnormality (yield) may be very low for the full blood count, ESR and syphilis serology, but these tests are cheap and the consequences of missing a treatable disorder, such as giant cell arteritis, syphilis or thrombocythaemia, are serious. There is a higher chance of picking up a treatable abnormality with the blood glucose, urine analysis and ECG. Depending on the definition, many or even most patients are hypercholesterolaemic, but whether that is acted on or not is discussed later (see Section 16.3.2); immediately after stroke, but probably not TIA, there is a transient fall in plasma cholesterol, which will lead to an

Table 6.15 First-line investigations for ischaemic stroke/TIA.

Investigation	Disorders suggested	Yield* (%)
Full blood count	Anaemia, polycythaemia, leukaemia, thrombocythaemia, heparin-associated thrombocytopenia with thrombosis, infections	1
ESR	Vasculitis, infections, cardiac myxoma, hyperviscosity, cholesterol embolisation syndrome, marantic endocarditis	2
Plasma glucose	Diabetes mellitus, hypoglycaemia	5
Plasma cholesterol	Hypercholesterolaemia	45
Syphilis serology	Syphilis, anticardiolipin antibody syndrome	<1†
Urinalysis	Diabetes, renal disease, infective endocarditis, systemic vasculitis	5
ECG	Arrhythmia, left-ventricular hypertrophy, silent myocardial infarction	17

* For any one investigation, the yield represents the proportion of patients in whom a positive test result may lead to a useful change in management (e.g. the diagnosis of diabetes in a previously undiagnosed case). The figures assume that *all* ischaemic stroke/TIA patients have the investigations and data have been taken from various more or less reliable sources but should not be regarded as precise statements of some universal truth.
† In the Oxfordshire Community Stroke Project, eight of 675 first-ever in a lifetime strokes had positive syphilis serology (VDRL and/or TPHA), of which one turned out to have previously undiagnosed secondary syphilis (see also Kelley *et al.*, 1989). TPHA, *Treponema pallidum* haemagglutination test; VDRL, Venereal Disease Reference Laboratory.

underestimate of the usual level (Mendez *et al.*, 1987; Woo *et al.*, 1990). Some very reasonably argue that plasma urea and electrolytes should be more or less routine, because so many TIA/stroke patients are hypertensive or on diuretics, a stroke patient may be dehydrated, and just occasionally electrolyte disturbance can mimic cerebral ischaemia. If almost all stroke patients have the basic tests and if the results are in their records and acted on, then that may well do more good than ordering, inappropriately, a huge range of further tests and missing some crucial clue from one of the routine investigations (such as an ESR of 100 mm in the first hour).

> *All patients should have a full blood count, erythrocyte sedimentation rate, plasma glucose and cholesterol, syphilis serology, urine analysis and ECG.*

6.6.2 Second-line investigations for some patients

Second-line investigations (Table 6.16) are mostly more costly and/or invasive and/or dangerous, so they need to be targeted on patients most likely to gain from a useful change in management as a consequence of an abnormal (or normal) result. The likelihood of a positive result (i.e. the yield) depends on the selection of patients for the investigation, and a balance has to be struck between overinvestigation (high cost, possibly high risk, low yield, false-positive results leading to even more overinvestigation) and underinvestigation (low cost, low risk, high yield but occasional missed diagnosis). This balance will depend on the management consequences of missing, or not, a particular diagnosis. For example, missing severe carotid stenosis would be more harmful, because carotid endarterectomy reduces the risk of stroke, than missing the lupus anticoagulant, because the relevance of that finding is unknown and the effect of any treatment is uncertain. Also, the balance will be affected by a reasonable tendency to search for a cause, particularly an unusual cause, in patients whose ischaemic event is unlikely to be due to atherothromboembolism (see Section 6.7.1), intracranial small vessel disease (see Section 6.7.2) or embolism from the heart (see Section 6.7.3), i.e. a patient with no vascular risk factors or obvious non-stroke vascular disease and who is under the age of about 50 years.

The main indications for the second-line investigations and the disorders likely to be detected are listed in Table 6.16. These will be discussed in further detail in other sections of this chapter and in Chapter 7, although at this stage it will be helpful to discuss imaging the brain and the cerebral circulation.

6.6.3 Imaging the brain

CT scanning

CT scanning of the brain almost belongs in the category of routine investigation, because, amongst confirmed strokes, it is the key to distinguishing ischaemic stroke from PICH (see Section 5.3.4). This fundamental distinction between ischaemia and haemorrhage determines the strategy for looking for the cause of a stroke; it is crucial to decisions about continuing, stopping or starting antithrombotic treatment, such as anticoagulants or aspirin; it is also crucial in any decision which may have to be made about carotid endarterectomy later. The limited, but important, role for CT in excluding intracranial structural lesions that can occasionally present as a TIA or stroke has already been discussed (see Section 3.3.3). Transient monocular blindness is one type of TIA after which a brain CT is not really neces-

sary, because examining the eye clinically will exclude any structural causes of the symptoms.

It can not be overemphasised that early brain CT is *not* to demonstrate infarcts. Within the first few hours of stroke onset, the main thrust of management and research into acute treatment is, once PICH has been excluded, to *prevent* the appearance of infarction on CT and so, one hopes, to reduce stroke mortality and disability. There is, therefore, no point at all in delaying CT until, or in the hope that, any infarct becomes visible, nor, indeed, is there much point in repeating CT in the hope of demonstrating an infarct after an early normal scan; a *clinically* definite stroke with a normal CT can be assumed to be due to an infarct and the clinical syndrome is predictive enough of the site and size of the brain lesion (see Section 4.4) and so to some extent of its likely cause (see Sections 6.5.1–6.5.4). In any case, it may not be possible to pinpoint the relevant infarct, because some patients have so much periventricular low density (leukoaraiosis (see Section 7.12)) or so many small infarcts or cortical atrophy that a small recently symptomatic infarct will simply not be distinguished (see Section 5.3.5).

Sometimes, on an unenhanced CT scan done within hours of stroke onset, the MCA or basilar artery is hyperdense, particularly if thin slices are obtained (Fig. 6.18; see also Section 5.3.5). This is probably due to a blood clot (acute embolus or secondary thrombus) in the arterial lumen and is, therefore, a pointer towards embolism either from the heart or from the extracranial arteries. The abnormal density disappears within days, unlike the persistence of calcified

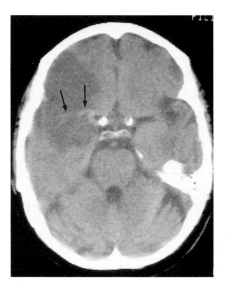

Figure 6.18 Hyperdense MCA (arrows) on an unenhanced CT brain scan within hours of the onset of a cerebral TACI.

Table 6.16 Second-line investigations for selected ischaemic stroke/TIA patients.

Investigation	Indications	Disorders suggested
Blood		
Urea and electrolytes	Hypertension, diuretic therapy, generally ill patient, dehydration	Diuretic-induced hypokalaemia, renal impairment, hyponatraemia
Liver function	Fever, malaise, raised ESR, suspected malignancy	Giant cell arteritis and other inflammatory arterial disorders, infective endocarditis, non-bacterial thrombotic endocarditis
Calcium	Recurrent focal neurological symptoms very rarely due to hypercalcaemia	Hypercalcaemia
Thyroid function tests	AF	Thyrotoxicosis
Activated partial thromboplastin time Dilute Russell's viper venom time Anticardiolipin antibody* Antinuclear and other autoantibodies	Young (<50 years) and no other cause found, past history or family history of venous thrombosis, especially if unusual sites (cerebral, mesenteric, hepatic veins), recurrent miscarriages, thrombocytopenia, cardiac valve vegetations, livedo reticularis, raised ESR, malaise, etc., positive Venereal Disease Research Laboratory (VDRL) test	Antiphospholipid antibody syndrome, systemic vasculitis, systemic lupus erythematosus
Serum proteins Serum protein electrophoresis Plasma viscosity	Elevated ESR	Paraproteinaemias, nephrotic syndrome, cardiac myxoma
Haemoglobin electrophoresis	Afro-Caribbean patients	Sickle cell trait or disease, and other haemoglobinopathies
Protein C and S, antithrombin III, activated protein C resistance, thrombin time†	Personal or family history of thrombosis (usually venous, particularly in unusual sites such as hepatic vein) at unusually young age	Deficiency states
Blood cultures	Fever, cardiac murmur, haematuria, deranged liver function, raised ESR, malaise, unexplained stroke	Infective endocarditis
HIV serology	Young (<40 years), drug addict, homosexual, blood products/transfusion, systemically unwell, lymphadenopathy, pneumonia, CMV retinitis, etc.	HIV infection
Lipoprotein fractionation	Elevated cholesterol or strong family history	Hyperlipoproteinaemia
Serum homocysteine (after methionine load)	Marfanoid habitus, high myopia, dislocated lenses, osteoporosis, mental retardation, young patient	Homocystinuria
Leucocyte alpha-galactosidase A	Corneal opacities, cutaneous angiokeratomas, paraesthesias and pain, renal failure	Fabry's disease
Blood/CSF lactate	Young pateint, basal ganglia calcification, epilepsy, parieto-occipital ischaemia	MELAS/mitochondiral cytopathy
Serum fluorescent treponemal antibody absorption test (FTA)	Positive blood VDRL or TPHA	Meningovascular syphilis
Cardiac enzymes	History or ECG evidence of recent myocardial infarction	Recent myocardial infarction
Drug screen	Young patient, no other obvious cause	Cocaine/amphetamine, etc.-induced ischaemic stroke
Urine		
Amino acids	Marfanoid habitus, high myopia, dislocated lenses, osteoporosis, mental retardation, young patient	Homocystinuria
Drug screen	Young patient, no other obvious cause	Cocaine/amphetamine, etc.-induced ischaemic stroke

Continued

Table 6.16 *Continued.*

Investigation	Indications	Disorders suggested
Imaging		
Chest X-ray (CXR)	Hypertension, finger-clubbing, cardiac murmur or abnormal ECG, young patient, ill patient	Calcified heart valves, enlarged heart, pulmonary arteriovenous malformation (AVM), baseline in ill patients
Brain CT scan	Continuing carotid TIAs of the brain, carotid endarterectomy being considered, thrombolysis being considered, taking or due to take anticoagulants or perhaps antiplatelet drugs, deteriorating stroke patient	Structural intracranial lesion, intracerebral haemorrhage
MRI	Suggestion of arterial dissection, uncertain diagnosis of stroke	Arterial dissection, loss of flow voids, multiple sclerosis
Carotid ultrasound with a view to carotid angiography	Carotid TIA or mild ischaemic stroke	Extracranial carotid stenosis
Cerebral angiography	Carotid ultrasound suggests about >50% stenosis of recently symptomatic ICA and patient fit and willing for surgery (see Fig. 6.24), suspected arterial dissection, arteritis, AVM or aneurysm	Arterial dissection, arteritis, AVM
Arch aortography	Symptoms of subclavian steal and unequal brachial pulses and blood pressures	Subclavian or innominate stenosis
Cardiac		
Echocardiography (transthoracic or transoesophageal)	Possible cardiac source of embolism and young (<50 years), or clinical, ECG or CXR evidence of embologenic heart disease, aortic arch dissection	Cardiac source of embolism, aortic arch atheroma or dissection
24-hour ECG	Palpitations or loss of consciousness during a suspected TIA, suspicious resting ECG	Intermittent AF or heart block
Others		
EEG	Doubt about diagnosis of TIA or stroke: ?epilepsy, ?generalised encephalopathy	Seizure disorder, structural lesion, encephalitis, diffuse encephalopathy due to inflammatory vascular disorders, Creutzfeldt-Jakob disease
CSF (up to 100 white cells/mm³ seen in cerebral infarction)	Positive blood VDRL or TPHA, young patient, ?infective endocarditis, possibility of multiple sclerosis	Vasculitis, meningovascular syphilis, syphilis, multiple sclerosis, infective endocarditis
Body red cell mass	Raised haematocrit	Primary polycythaemia
Temporal artery biopsy	Older (>60 years), jaw claudication, headache, polymyalgia, malaise, anaemia, raised ESR	Giant cell arteritis

* Repeat to ensure persistently raised.
† Transient falls occur after stroke so any low level must be repeated and family members investigated.
CMV, cytomegalovirus; FTA, fluorescent *Treponema* antigen; MELAS, mitochondrial encephalomyopathy with lactic acidosis and stroke-like episodes; TPHA, *Treponema pallidum* haemagglutination test.

emboli or calcified arterial wall, both of which may cause confusion on an early CT (Leys *et al.*, 1992). In routine clinical practice, this radiological feature has little impact on determining the cause of cerebral ischaemia, the clinical syndrome being as good a predictor, or a better predictor, of the likely site and size of any infarct, and so of which arterial territory is involved, and of prognosis.

The problem of reliably detecting boundary-zone infarction has been addressed earlier, and it is looking increasingly likely that many so-called boundary-zone infarcts on CT (or MRI) may not be due to low flow but to acute arterial occlusion. This confusion is because of the present uncertainty about exactly where the boundary zones are in individual patients (see Section 6.5.5).

In general, therefore, brain CT has little role in determining the *cause* of an ischaemic event, because if one needs to know within hours of the onset the scan will probably be normal anyway, whilst later on the scan can still be normal and any infarct already reasonably well predicted, both in site and size, on the basis of the neurological symptoms and signs (see Section 4.4; Bogousslavsky *et al.*, 1993a). However, if there *is* an anatomically relevant infarct slightly inappropriate to the clinical syndrome (i.e. it is in the correct general area of the brain, such as an LACI on CT/MRI in a patient who appears to have a PACI clinical syndrome), it is probably best to keep all options open and investigate the patient as though he or she has both types of infarct; another possibility might be venous infarction (see Section 5.3.5). It follows that repeat CT scanning, with or without intravenous contrast enhancement, is unnecessary in the search for the *cause* of an ischaemic event, but it may be needed if there is uncertainty that the patient has had a stroke at all (or even a TIA in some circumstances) or if the patient deteriorates (see Section 15.5).

> The results of brain CT and MRI do not reliably guide early (within hours) decisions in the management of *acute* ischaemic stroke, but the site and size of any infarct which does eventually appear may, in some cases, help in finding the cause of the infarct.

MRI

MRI of the brain, using T1- and T2-weighted sequences, is more sensitive than CT and will therefore display smaller infarcts, especially in the brainstem and cerebellum, and becomes even more sensitive after gadolinium enhancement, which may indicate which of several lesions on an unenhanced scan is the recently symptomatic one, even LACIs sometimes (see Section 5.3.6). Also, T1- and T2-weighted images may reveal the changes of infarction earlier than CT, but not always (Miyashita *et al.*, 1988; Shuaib *et al.*, 1992; Edelman & Warach, 1993; Regli *et al.*, 1993; Hommel *et al.*, 1994; Samuelsson *et al.*, 1994; Mohr *et al.*, 1995). MRI is also better than CT at demonstrating small amounts of blood clot, e.g. petechial haemorrhages at the borders of an infarct, but it is not known whether this has any practical impact on stroke management or whether MRI is just demonstrating what in general is already known from postmortem studies.

It is still possible to have the clinical syndrome of a stroke, and certainly of a TIA, and yet no relevant lesion on routine MRI, or at least any relevant lesion that can be differentiated from diffuse or multiple periventricular high-signal areas (Salgado *et al.*, 1986; Alberts *et al.*, 1992; Lindgren *et al.*,

1994a). There are, however, a number of more complex MRI techniques, such as diffusion-weighted imaging, which can demonstrate very early ischaemic lesions, but as yet these have no clinical relevance in influencing patient management (see Section 5.3.8).

MRI has surprisingly little impact on determining the *cause* of the ischaemic stroke (or TIA, where lesions are also more often seen that on CT), but it can be helpful in two ways: (i) the loss of flow void in a major cerebral vessel may provide direct information about exactly which artery (or vein) is blocked and where; and (ii) it may be possible to visualise the widening of the arterial wall in cases of dissection, particularly if the neck, as well as the brain is imaged, so making invasive angiography unnecessary (see Section 7.1). MRI may also demonstrate arterial ectasia (Aichner *et al.*, 1993; see Section 6.2.2). Finally, the MRI may come up with surprises, such as the features of multiple sclerosis, which can be clinically confused with stroke in young adults and with small focal infarcts in the cerebellum in some patients with 'isolated vertigo', who in previous times would have been diagnosed as 'acute labyrinthitis', because the less sensitive CT was normal (see Section 4.2.7).

MRI is considerably less practical than CT in acutely ill, confused stroke patients, particularly those requiring some form of monitoring, so it is likely that CT will remain the first-line brain imaging investigation for acute stroke for the foreseeable future, reserving MRI for more complicated cases.

'Silent infarction'

Unexpected focal low-density areas are often seen on brain CT or MRI in patients with TIA or stroke in areas of the brain that are *clearly irrelevant* to the presenting or any past clinical event; distal to asymptomatic carotid stenosis; in patients with CHD; and even in apparently normal elderly people (Dennis *et al.*, 1990; Tanaka *et al.*, 1993; Caplan, 1994b; Boon *et al.*, 1994; Brott *et al.*, 1994). These asymptomatic lesions are usually small and deep, rather than large and cortical. The assumption is too often made that they are due to previous subclinical infarction, or perhaps intracerebral haemorrhage, or that the patient had not recognised or had simply forgotten a previous symptomatic event. 'Silent infarctions' seem to have no clinical relevance and in any event the frequency of such lesions varies enormously, depending on the precise definition of the radiological abnormality, the imaging technique used, how the patients are selected, whether the observer is blind to any presenting clinical syndrome and the demographic characteristics of the patients (Herderschee *et al.*, 1992; Jorgensen *et al.*, 1994b).

'Silent' cerebral infarctions on CT/MRI are quite common, but it is unclear whether they have any influence on patient prognosis or management.

6.6.4 Imaging the cerebral circulation

It would obviously be of interest to image the cerebral circulation in everyone with an ischaemic stroke or TIA to try and find out which artery is blocked, where any embolus may have originated and how quickly recanalisation occurs. However, at present all this information rarely influences the clinical management and should not be sought routinely, because of the risk and cost (of catheter angiography), or it simply can not be sought at all, because the technology is either not available (e.g. MRA) or difficult to use accurately (e.g. ultrasound). In practice, imaging the cerebral circulation must be very carefully directed to answer the relevant clinical question and the answer must be likely to influence the patient's management (Hankey & Warlow, 1992; Sellar, 1995). The main indications for imaging the cerebral circulation are as follows.

1 The patient is a potential candidate for carotid surgery (see Section 16.7).
2 Frequent vertebrobasilar TIAs, particularly with subclavian steal (see Section 16.10).
3 Possibility of traumatic arterial dissection (see Section 7.1).
4 Young patient under some circumstances (see Section 7.17, and also below).

Selection for carotid surgery

Selection for carotid surgery is discussed in detail later (see Section 16.7). The critical imaging question is whether the patient has severe stenosis at the origin of the ICA ipsilateral to the cerebral or ocular ischaemia. The most cost-effective way to do this at present is by using duplex sonography, followed by intra-arterial X-ray angiography if the duplex suggests stenosis or occlusion of the symptomatic ICA (Hankey & Warlow, 1990). Merely doing an angiogram in patients with a carotid bifurcation bruit will miss some patients with severe stenosis and subject too many with mild or moderate stenosis, with nothing to gain from carotid surgery, to the hazards of angiography (see Fig. 6.17).

Duplex sonography combines real-time ultrasound imaging to demonstrate the arterial anatomy with pulsed Doppler flow analysis at any point of interest in the vessel lumen. Its accuracy is enhanced, and it is technically easier to do, if the Doppler signals are colour-coded to show the direction of blood flow and its velocity (Fig. 6.19; Humphrey *et al.*, 1990; Bray & Glatt, 1995). The amount of luminal stenosis is calculated not just from the real-time ultrasound image, which can be inaccurate when the lesion is echolucent or calcification scatters the ultrasound beam, but from the blood flow velocities derived from the Doppler signal. If colour Doppler is not available but only grey-scale duplex, it is usually helpful to first insonate the supraorbital artery with a simple continuous-wave Doppler probe, because *inward*

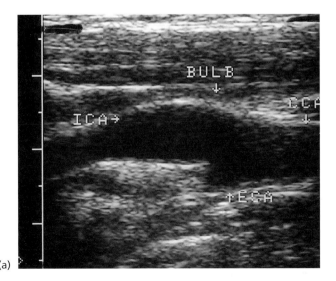 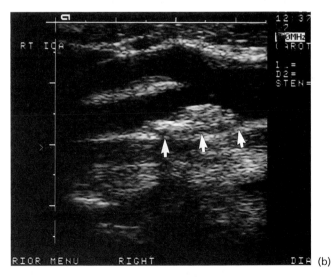

(a)　　　　(b)

Figure 6.19 Duplex sonography: (a) normal bifurcation; (b) stenosis of ICA origin (arrows).

flow of blood strongly suggests severe ICA stenosis or occlusion, although not necessarily at the origin.

Although duplex sonography is non-invasive and now reasonably widely available, there are problems: it requires skill, training, considerable experience and constant audit of the results against any subsequent angiography to be sure of accurate measurements of stenosis and avoidance of pitfalls, such as confusing the ECA for the ICA; it may be difficult to interpret, particularly if there is severe plaque or periarterial calcification; it is not completely reliable in distinguishing very tight (>90%) stenosis (which is operable) from occlusion (which is not), unless perhaps colour Doppler is used and interpreted using very stringent criteria (Gortler *et al.*, 1994; Young *et al.*, 1994; Berman *et al.*, 1995; Blakeley *et al.*, 1995); it is not completely sensitive and specific for severe (70–99%) ICA stenosis; different machines vary in their accuracy in measuring carotid stenosis (Howard *et al.*, 1991); and it provides little information about the proximal arterial anatomy, which, as it happens, is seldom affected by disease relevant to the surgeon, or about distal anatomy, but how often these are really important problems is not at all clear (e.g. the upper limit of the stenotic lesion, stenosis of the carotid siphon and asymptomatic intracranial aneurysms may not be visible). Duplex sonography is still, therefore, a screening test to select patients likely to have severe ICA origin stenosis, or who *seem* to have ICA occlusion, and who *then* mostly require catheter angiography. Whether ultrasound characteristics of the plaque (soft, hard, calcified, etc.) are important predictors of ipsilateral ischaemic stroke (see Section 16.7.8), and therefore of relevance to the selection of patients for carotid surgery, is much debated but still uncertain, largely because the appropriate natural history studies have never been done and now probably never can be, at least not in symptomatic patients who mostly require endarterectomy if they have severe ICA stenosis.

> *Screening with* reliable *duplex sonography, usually followed by selective safe catheter angiography, is at present the most cost-effective way to diagnose carotid stenosis that is severe enough to make carotid endarterectomy worthwhile.*

Bearing these limitations in mind, it is a quick and simple investigation in experienced hands and it is neither unpleasant nor risky. Very rarely, the pressure of the Doppler probe on the carotid bifurcation can dislodge thrombus or cause enough carotid sinus stimulation to lead to bradycardia or hypotension (Rosario *et al.*, 1987; Friedman, 1990). The same complication applies to the various arterial compression manoeuvres which may be carried out during TCD or extracranial Doppler sonography, and these should be avoided in patients who may have carotid bifurcation disease (Khaffaf *et al.*, 1994).

Spiral CT angiography is a recently developed and still evolving non-invasive method of imaging the carotid arteries, but it requires a large dose of intravenous contrast material to outline the arterial lumen, it gives only a limited view of a short segment of the neck arteries, with no intracranial information, the images obtained depend on the proficiency of the operator in their selection, and so far it has not been well evaluated against the gold standard of selective catheter angiography. However, it does provide multiple viewing angles, three-dimensional reconstruction and imaging of calcium deposits separately from the vessel lumen outlined by the contrast (Heiken *et al.*, 1993; Cumming & Morrow, 1994; Fig. 6.20).

Carotid angiography is invasive, uncomfortable, costly, carries a risk and normally requires hospital admission. About 4% of patients have a TIA or stroke, 25% of them permanent, as a result of angiography, and more if the patient has *severe* carotid disease, which, with duplex sonography, is now *precisely* the sort of patient selected to have angiography (Hankey *et al.*, 1990a,b; Davies & Humphrey, 1993). TIAs and strokes occur because the catheter may dislodge atheromatous plaque or dissect the arterial wall, thrombus may form at the tip or thrombus may form in blood contaminating the contrast-containing syringe. In addition, there are systemic and allergic adverse effects, particularly during intravenous digital subtraction angiography (they are less likely with intra-arterial contrast injections), where large quantities of contrast are used (bradycardia, hypotension, angina, shortness of breath, nausea, vomiting, headache, epileptic seizures, transient blindness, periorbital oedema, urticaria, bronchospasm and renal failure). Some patients develop a haematoma, aneurysm or nerve injury at the site of arterial puncture (which is usually into the femoral artery in the groin), and the occasional patient develops *de novo*, or has worsened symptoms of, peripheral vascular disease in the leg distal to the puncture site, sometimes leading even to amputation. The cholesterol embolisation syndrome is very rare, but it can be fatal (see Section 7.16).

Compared with conventional selective catheter angiography, *intra-arterial digital subtraction angiography* is quicker, less contrast is used and the images are easier to manipulate and store, but the spatial resolution is less and there is no evidence that it is much safer (Fig. 6.21). Neither *intravenous digital subtraction* nor *arch aortography* is a satisfactory alternative to selective conventional or intra-arterial digital angiography, because so often the images are poor and stenoses impossible to measure, vessels may over-

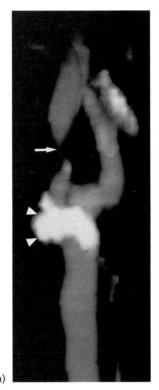
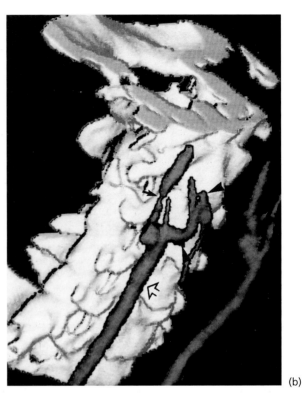

Figure 6.20 Spiral CT of the carotid bifurcation. (a) Two-dimensional reconstruction to show the tight stenosis at the origin of the ICA (arrow) as well as areas of calcification at the distal end of the CCA (arrowheads). (b) Three-dimensional reconstruction of the same artery to show the relationship with the cervical vertebrae. CCA (open arrow), ICA stenosis (arrow), ECA and branches (arrowheads).

(a)

(b)

Figure 6.21 Intra-arterial digital carotid angiogram to show a stenosis (arrow) at the origin of the ICA (the ICA can be differentiated easily from the ECA—arrowhead—because the ICA has no branches in the neck).

lap, there is insufficient information about intracranial vessels and the techniques are not necessarily safer (Pelz *et al.*, 1985). For all these reasons, therefore, very urgent efforts are needed to develop safe but accurate alternatives to intra-arterial catheter angiography, perhaps a combination of colour Doppler of the carotid bifurcation with MRA of all the extra- and intracranial vessels (Young *et al.*, 1994; Siewert *et al.*, 1995), but, as yet, this combination has not been properly compared with the 'gold standard' of intra-arterial angiography (a gold standard that we have to accept, whether we like it or not, because it was based on this technique that the effectiveness of carotid endarterectomy was evaluated) (Rothwell & Warlow, 1996).

MRA alone is unlikely to be acceptable, at least at the present stage of development, because the pictures are not always adequate to allow measurement of the carotid stenosis (movement and swallowing artefacts are particular problems); the severity of the stenosis tends to be overestimated; there may be a flow gap distal to a stenosis of only 60%, making precise measurement impossible, and even in the posterior part of the carotid bulb, in both cases probably due to loss of laminar flow and increased residence times of the blood; and severe stenosis can be confused with occlusion (Heiserman *et al.*, 1992; Riles *et al.*, 1992; Sitzer *et al.*, 1993;

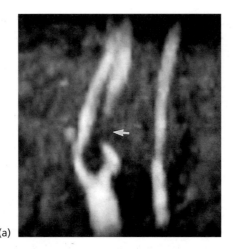 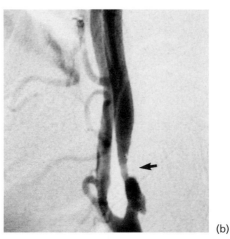

(a)   (b)

Figure 6.22 (a) MRA (three-dimensional time of flight) of severe internal carotid stenosis. Whilst the stenosis is clearly 'severe', it is not possible to measure its exact extent because of the 'flow gap' (arrow) distal to the lesion. On the other hand, conventional angiography (b) shows the lesion clearly (arrow) so that a stenosis of 82% (by the ECST or common carotid (CC) method) or 71% (by the North American Symptomatic Carotid Endosterectomy Trial (NASCET) method) can be measured. The marked irregularity of the surface of the stenosis is also clearly visible, whereas that feature was lost on the MRA.

Mittl *et al.*, 1994; Young *et al.*, 1994; Blakeley *et al.*, 1995; Siewert *et al.*, 1995; Fig. 6.22). So far, there have not been enough methodologically sound comparisons of MRA with intra-arterial angiography in a large number of patients, with a wide range of stenoses and occlusion, without excluding images which are difficult to measure, and using appropriate statistical methodology to distinguish between bias and imprecision over the whole range of stenoses (Rothwell & Warlow, 1996). Anyway, at present, MRA is expensive, not readily available and claustrophobic for some people, requires the patient to lie still for several minutes, and may be contraindicated if there is any metal in the body (see Section 5.3.6).

Measuring the severity of carotid stenosis. Biplanar, but better triplanar (Jeans *et al.*, 1986), views of the carotid bifurcation are required by selective intra-arterial catheter angiography (digital or conventional) so that the residual lumen can be seen without overlap of other vessels, measured at the narrowest point and then compared with a suitable denominator to derive the percentage diameter stenosis, which is the measurement on which decisions concerning carotid endarterectomy have to be made (because this is what the randomised controlled trials used (see Section 16.7.5)). Using the residual lumen *alone* is unsatisfactory, because normal arteries vary in size, and there is also variation in the magnification factor between different centres (Barnett & Warlow, 1993).

> *The severity of any carotid stenosis must be measured as accurately as possible; guesswork is unacceptable.*

There are *three* possible denominators that can be used (Fig. 6.23). Using the distal ICA (the North American Symptomatic Carotid Endarterectomy Trial (NASCET) method) tends to underestimate the extent of any stenosis at the origin of the ICA, because the normal carotid bulb is wider than the distal ICA and also because distal to severe stenosis the ICA tends to collapse, increasingly so from a European Carotid Surgery Trial (ECST) measured stenosis of about 50% upwards; on the other hand, at least the denominator to be measured can be seen (Fox, 1993). The *estimated* diameter at the site of the stenosis, which is usually, but not always, at the carotid bulb, measures the lesion at the right place but does require some guesswork to imagine where the original arterial lumen *was* (the ECST method). There is least observer variability using the diameter of the normal CCA (the common carotid (CC) method), which is almost always seen on selective angiograms, does not change in size very much along the portion proximal by 1–2 cm to the carotid bifurcation, is seldom affected by disease so much that a normal part can not be found, and bears a reasonably constant relationship to the diameter of the normal carotid bulb and distal ICA. All three methods predict equally well the risk of ipsilateral ischaemic stroke and are, therefore, valid in this sense (Rothwell *et al.*, 1994b). Fortunately, it is easy to convert the measurement by one method to either

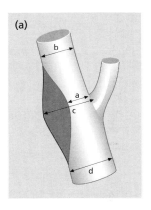

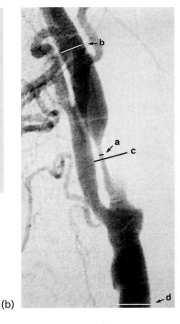

Figure 6.23 (a) Three methods of measuring percentage diameter stenosis at the origin of the ICA in the neck. All use as the numerator the minimum residual lumen where the stenosis is most severe (a). However, the denominator differs. In the ECST, it is an *estimate* (c) of the normal lumen diameter at the site of the stenosis (whether this is at the bifurcation, more distal in the ICA or in the distal CCA); in the North American Symptomatic Carotid Endarterectomy Trial (NASCET) method, it is the diameter of the ICA lumen when it becomes normal and free of disease, usually well beyond the bulb (b), and in the cases of near occlusion of the ICA an arbitrary 95% stenosis is assigned; in the common carotid (CC) method, it is the diameter of the CCA proximal to the bifurcation, where it is free of disease and the diameter is fairly constant (d). (b) An illustrative example from a carotid angiogram in which (a)–(d) correspond with the measurements described in (a) above. The stenosis measures 89% by the ECST method, 88% by the CC method and 85% by the NASCET method.

of the other two methods because they are all linearly related, at least within the moderate and severe stenosis range (Rothwell *et al.*, 1994a). The ECST and CC method give essentially identical results and can be converted to the NASCET measurement by the formula:

NASCET per cent stenosis

$$= \frac{(\text{ECST or CC stenosis per cent} - 40)}{0.6}$$

One might imagine that *ulceration of an atherothrombotic plaque* suggests a particularly high risk of active thrombosis, embolism and therefore of what really matters, i.e. ipsilateral ischaemic stroke. Unfortunately, this is difficult to show in practice, because angiography tends to underesti-

mate the ulceration described by vascular surgeons and pathologists; it is not clear what the gold standard of ulceration is supposed to be, either at postmortem or by imaging; there is considerable interobserver variability in the angiographic diagnosis of 'ulceration'; and so far there is only one satisfactory observational study, which showed that, for the same degree of stenosis, 'ulceration' (on angiography) increases the risk of ipsilateral ischaemic stroke. What effect the demonstration of a 'floating thrombus' has on the risk of stroke is also unknown (O'Leary *et al.*, 1987; Ricotta *et al.*, 1987; Wechsler, 1988; Estol *et al.*, 1991; Martin *et al.*, 1992; Eliaziw *et al.*, 1994; Streifler *et al.*, 1994). At present, therefore, the only agreed and reliable angiographic criterion for the prediction of ipsilateral ischaemic stroke is percentage diameter stenosis and it is, therefore, mainly on this measurement that the carotid endarterectomy surgery decision is made (see Section 16.7.5).

Present policy. At present, we use selective intra-arterial digital angiography of the symptomatic ICA(s) *only* in recently symptomatic patients who are fit for and willing to consider carotid endarterectomy and who have stenosis or possible occlusion of that artery on duplex sonography (Fig. 6.24). Late views are important if there is difficulty distinguishing occlusion from extreme ICA stenosis, when contrast may eventually be seen to pass up to the head (Fig. 6.25). We do not think that angiography of the contralateral ICA, if asymptomatic, vertebral arteries or aortic arch is very useful, and in any event this increases the risk of the whole procedure. However, many vascular surgeons do seem to want this extra information. Perhaps a compromise is at least to have duplex sonography or MRA of the asymptomatic ICA. Angiography should be timed so that any necessary surgery can be scheduled within days or 1–2 weeks. So it should be done within days of presentation after a TIA and, in patients with ischaemic stroke, within 1–2 weeks of neurological stabilisation; any further delay is unacceptable, because of the particularly high risk (preventable by surgery) of stroke early after a symptomatic carotid ischaemic event (see Section 16.1.1).

At the moment, non-invasive imaging (ultrasound, MRA, spiral CT) is not sufficiently accurate to replace selective intra-arterial catheter angiography for the definitive detection and evaluation of carotid stenosis, prior to carotid endarterectomy.

Frequent vertebrobasilar transient ischaemic attacks

Frequent vertebrobasilar TIAs, thought to be due to atherothromboembolism and unresponsive to antiplatelet

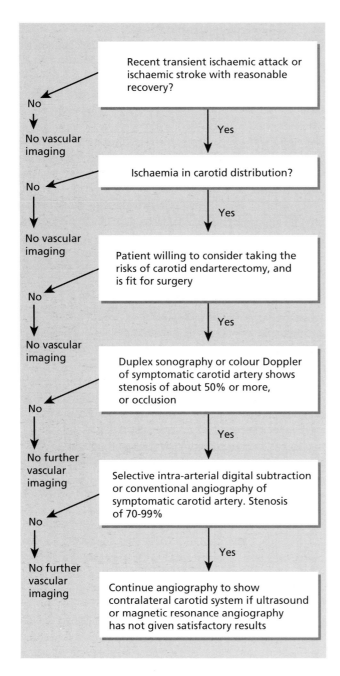

Figure 6.24 Carotid artery imaging strategy for patients with ischaemic events to select those suitable for carotid endarterectomy.

than in the carotid circulation (particularly without colour Doppler), it may be necessary to use intra-arterial digital subtraction aortography followed by selective catheterisation of the vertebral arteries, with intracranial as well as neck views. However, this policy may change with improvements in ultrasound and MRI technology. Depending on the surgical approach proposed, it may also be necessary to image the carotid arteries. Although asymptomatic *subclavian steal* is quite common, *symptomatic* subclavian steal is rare. The clinical syndrome is quite easily recognised by unequal blood pressures between the two arms, a supraclavicular bruit and vertebrobasilar TIAs, which may or may not be brought on by exercise of the arm ipsilateral to the subclavian stenosis or occlusion (see Section 16.10). It is only this sort of patient who may require surgery and therefore who have to accept the risk of the preceding angiography.

Traumatic arterial dissection

Traumatic arterial dissection tends to heal without any treatment, although many physicians use anticoagulants. It is not, therefore, absolutely necessary to diagnose, unless doing so aborts unnecessary further investigation to look for the cause of an ischaemic stroke or TIA; there are medicolegal issues such as litigation against some assailant or other person responsible for the trauma; or the patient is being entered into a randomised trial. The gold standard is intra-arterial angiography, because ultrasound is neither specific

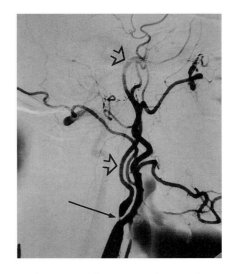

Figure 6.25 Selective carotid angiogram showing almost complete occlusion of the ICA (arrow) with poor flow distal to the lesion (open arrows) and delayed filling of the carotid siphon. Normally the carotid siphon fills well before the branches of the ECA.

drugs or anticoagulants, are unusual. It is not clear that vascular surgery has much to offer other than in the rather special situation of subclavian steal (see Section 16.10). There is seldom, therefore, a need to visualise the vertebral and basilar arteries. Where this is necessary, ultrasound should be used in the first instance, but, because it is more difficult nor sensitive enough to rely on. However, there is increasing evidence that MRI, to show thrombus within and widening of the vessel wall, and MRA, to show narrowing of the vessel lumen, may be sufficient, and clearly this is the safest option (see Section 7.1).

Young patients with ischaemic stroke or transient ischaemic attack

Young patients with ischaemic stroke or TIA very seldom have atheromatous stenosis of their extra- or intracranial arteries and are not, therefore, usually candidates for carotid endarterectomy or any other sort of vascular surgery. Indeed, severe ICA origin stenosis can be excluded by duplex sonography. What possible reasons are there, therefore, for intra-arterial catheter angiography unless there is suspicion of traumatic arterial dissection (see above)? This issue is hotly debated and may be resolved, at least the safety aspects, by the further development of MRI, MRA and spiral CT. Reasons to want to know the state of the intra- or extracranial circulation are very rare, or would not change management, or both. Possibilities include the following.

1 An unsuspected aneurysm of the extra- or intracranial circulation large enough to contain thrombus which might embolise to the brain or eye. This is very rare, but surgery may be required to clip or remove an aneurysm, or perhaps anticoagulation might be indicated (see Section 7.4).

2 Fibromuscular dysplasia is sometimes found, but whether and how it should be treated is not at all clear (see Section 7.3).

3 The beading and narrowing of cerebral arteries seen in some cases of cerebral vasculitis is neither specific nor sensitive, and this diagnosis is better made by serological tests or by meningeal/cortical biopsy, if clinically justifiable (see Section 7.2).

4 Moyamoya syndrome is exceedingly rare and any treatment possibilities are severely limited (see Section 7.13).

Of course, in most acute ischaemic strokes there must be, or must have been, an occluded blood vessel, but knowing which one and where has no bearing on management, *unless* it turns out that thrombolysis is an effective treatment when a major cerebral artery is occluded but dangerous when open (we are unlikely to know this in the near future, because current randomised trials mostly do not make the distinction (see Section 11.5)). Anyway, as far as the MCA trunk is concerned, TCD provides reasonably accurate information on whether the artery is occluded, stenosed or normal (see below). Also, perforating arteries are too small to be visualised by any method at present.

Transcranial Doppler sonography

TCD is non-invasive, repeatable on demand, can be done at the bedside, inexpensive and it is not too difficult to perform accurately. Essentially, it provides information on velocity blood flow, and its direction in relation to the ultrasound probe, in major intracranial arteries at the base of the brain, and so whether such arteries are occluded or stenosed (Fig. 6.26). However, the patient has to keep reasonably still; the examination can take as long as an hour; the skull is impervious to ultrasound in about 5–10% of cases, more so with increasing age and in females, but this may soon be solved by the use of intravenous echo contrast (Otis et al., 1995); exact vessel identification may be difficult, but colour-flow real-time imaging makes this easier; diagnostic criteria vary; and the technique is not always accurate in comparison with cerebral angiography (Ley-Pozo & Ringelstein, 1990; Petty et al., 1990; Naylor, 1992; Bornstein & Norris, 1994; Wechsler & Babikian, 1994; Rother et al., 1994). Certainly TCD can display occlusion or stenosis of the MCA trunk, flow in the anterior cerebral artery and, less easily, occlusion or stenosis of the basilar artery. However, at present, this information is of little *clinical* relevance and so TCD is essentially a research tool.

What may soon become of clinical relevance is the increasing realisation that emboli can be detected by TCD as high-intensity transient signals (HITS) on the sonogram (Tegeler, 1994; Fig. 6.27). However, there is still considerable controversy surrounding the interpretation of HITS and difficulty excluding artefact, distinguishing gaseous from solid material and being sure of the exact nature of the latter. Also, the methods and criteria for HITS detection are not yet standardised (Markus, 1993; Grosset et al., 1993; Babikian et al., 1994). HITS may help in distinguishing cardiac from artery-to-artery emboli, because the former should be detected in several arterial distributions and the latter in just the one arterial distribution distal to the supposed embolic source (Grosset et al., 1994; Markus et al., 1994). However, the frequency of HITS can be so frustratingly low that their detection requires prolonged monitoring or automation (Markus & Brown, 1993). Conceivably, HITS detection might help distinguish organic from hysterical events, and be used to monitor treatment, surgical or medical. TCD may also have a role in detecting paradoxical embolism (see Section 6.4).

Finally, TCD can be used to assess cerebrovascular reserve, i.e. the capacity for intracranial vasodilatation in response to acetazolamide, carbon dioxide inhalation or breath-holding (Bishop et al., 1986; Markus & Harrison, 1992; Chimowitz et al., 1993b; see also Section 11.1.2). There is however, still debate about exactly how to stan-

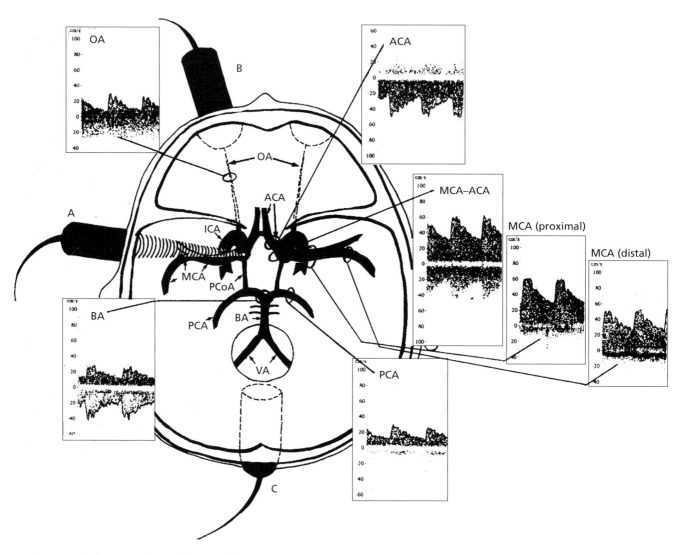

Figure 6.26 Techniques of TCD. Diagram of the head looked at from above (eyes at the top of the diagram) to illustrate the cranial sonographic windows (A, temporal; B, orbital; C, foramen magnum) and typical waveforms obtained from the major intracranial arteries. Note that the power output of the transducer must be reduced to 10% of the maximum for the transorbital approach to avoid damage to the eyes. BA, basilar artery; OA, ophthalmic artery; PCA, posterior cerebral artery; PCoA, posterior communicating artery; VA, vertebral artery.

dardise this test (what exactly is 'abnormal'?) and it is not routinely used. It may even be important to recognise normal variation during the day (Ameriso *et al.*, 1994). Interestingly, impaired reactivity may have some prognostic significance for identifying individual patients at particularly high risk of stroke from amongst patients with ICA occlusion and in identifying stroke patients with so-called boundary-zone infarction, although with time, and presumably collaterali-sation, the reactivity can return to normal (Kleiser *et al.*, 1991; Weiller *et al.*, 1991; Kleiser & Widder, 1992; Widder *et al.*, 1994). Whether this high risk of stroke or of bound-ary-zone infarction is due to low flow, or to embolism from

diseased arteries providing collateral blood supply or from the distal end of an ICA occlusion is not clear.

> *The assessment of cerebrovascular reserve is still not standardised and so far it is unclear whether this measurement has any clinical relevance.*

6.6.5 Imaging the coronary circulation

Symptomatic coronary heart disease (CHD) is common in TIA and ischaemic stroke patients (about one-third have angina or have had a myocardial infarction) and requires the

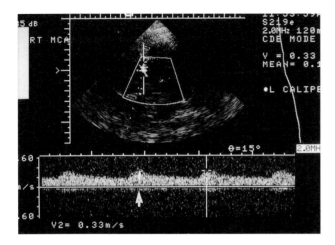

Figure 6.27 TCD from the MCA. Arrow shows the HITS of an embolus. Note that the embolic signal does not extend beyond the Doppler trace and is of higher intensity (brightness) than the rest of the Doppler signal.

usual cardiological investigations and treatment. In addition, a substantial proportion of patients *without* symptomatic CHD have evidence of subclinical coronary artery lesions, the exact figure depending on how intensively the patients are investigated (Chimowitz & Mancini, 1992; Love *et al.*, 1992). Therefore, it is hardly surprising that the future risk of serious coronary events is high (see Section 16.1.1). However, the detection of *asymptomatic* coronary artery disease does not at present influence management, because risk factors will be treated and antithrombotic drugs used anyway, and it is uncertain whether coronary artery surgery has any impact on the long-term prognosis. There is no indication, therefore, for exercise ECG testing, thallium-201 dipyridamole scintigraphy or coronary angiography, unless the patient has cardiac symptoms or other reasons, such as an abnormal resting ECG, to suggest coronary artery disease requiring treatment.

6.6.6 Cost-effectiveness

Not everyone will agree with our views on the investigation of ischaemic stroke/TIA patients and there is considerable variation in practice between and within countries (UK-TIA Study Group, 1983; Hopkins *et al.*, 1989). We must emphasise that our criteria for *any* investigation include neither academic interest nor financial profit, but simply whether the result will usefully influence the patient's management without unacceptable risk. Of course, what is meant by 'unacceptable' must depend on the balance of the risk of investigation and the risk of *not* doing the investigation and so prejudicing a patient's outcome; this balance will surely

change as new and safer investigations are developed. Thus, in this sense we are minimalist and should, as a result, be cost-effective, although we would be the first to acknowledge that the precise *cost* of most investigations is rarely known, although the *charges* may be (the charges, of course, do not necessarily reflect the costs, but rather whether the charger wishes to make a profit or is prepared to stand a loss, and also what the market will bear). However, even our minimalist approach could be challenged if, for example, it was decided that carotid endarterectomy was not cost-effective in stroke prevention (see Section 18.5), in which case duplex sonography and cerebral angiography would hardly ever be needed.

What would probably improve cost-effectiveness more than anything else is a quick and efficient method to actually do the routine investigations and to get the results into the patients' notes without having to repeat tests which go 'missing', as well as minimising, or even abolishing, hospital stay. Just one unnecessary day in hospital, because an angiogram has been postponed, could pay for hundreds of full blood counts or serological tests for syphilis. The efficient use of the resources we do have is likely to be more productive and achievable than complaining about resources we do not have, at least up to a point. A counterexample would be that, without having duplex technology, which is somewhat costly, we would either have to angiogram all patients potentially suitable for carotid endarterectomy, at considerable risk, or angiogram none of them, which would deny stroke prevention to at least some individuals; therefore, without duplex sonography, one could not possibly have a cost-effective carotid endarterectomy service.

At the end of the day, the debate about cost-effectiveness should concentrate on expensive investigations (such as MRA) and not on inexpensive investigations (such as the ESR) which, even if done in extremely large numbers, will have a negligible impact on the overall investigation budget. Moreover, the cost of investigation must be seen within the context of the total hospital costs of stroke; even in a specialist neuroscience unit, the investigation cost is only about 12% of the budget, whilst in general internal medical and geriatric units, where the vast majority of strokes are managed, the proportion is less than 2% (see Section 17.7).

6.7 Identifying the three most common causes of ischaemic stroke or transient ischaemic attack (TIA)

About 95% of ischaemic strokes and TIAs are caused by atherothromboembolism, intracranial small vessel disease or embolism from the heart (see Fig. 6.1). The rarities may or

Table 6.17 Non-atheromatous, non-cardioembolic conditions predisposing to ischaemic stroke amongst 244 cases of first-ever in a lifetime ischaemic stroke in the Oxfordshire Community Stroke Project. (Adapted from Sandercock *et al.*, 1989.)

	Total number	Per cent	95% confidence interval
Arteritis	9	4	1.7–6.9
Migraine	7	3	1.2–5.8
Major operation	3	1	0.2–3.6
Inflammatory bowel disease	3	1	0.2–3.6
Neck trauma	2	1	0.1–2.9
Carcinoma of the thyroid	1	<1	0.0–2.3
Autoimmune disease*	1	<1	0.0–2.3
Leukaemia	1	<1	0.0–2.3
Oral contraceptive use (in the past)	1	<1	0.0–2.3
Total	28†	12	7.8–16.1

* One patient with rheumatoid arthritis, glomerulonephritis and myasthenia gravis.
† Eighteen of these 28 patients also had one or more vascular risk factors (hypertension, heart disease, peripheral vascular disease, cervical bruit, diabetes mellitus, etc.), making the exact cause of ischaemic stroke uncertain. Non-atheromatous, non-embolic conditions seemed to be the only predisposing factors in 10 of the 244 patients (4%, 95% confidence interval: 2–7%).

may not be reasonably obvious from the clinical history, examination and routine investigations and should be looked for particularly assiduously, with further investigations, where they are most likely to be present, i.e. in patients under the age of 50 years or if there is no positive evidence of one of three main causes of cerebral ischaemia. Of course, there is the familiar problem of two, three or even four competing causes for cerebral ischaemia in an individual patient (see Table 6.1), but this is not always the case and, when it does occur, one must, as usual, concentrate on the treatable. For example, if a patient definitely has giant cell arteritis, then that should be treated, whether or not the patient has a prosthetic heart valve. As the giant cell arteritis is coming under control, one should, of course, consider whether the valve is functioning normally or likely to be a source of embolism and whether any anticoagulation is sufficient. Something like 10% of patients have evidence of both atherothrombosis *and* a cardiac source of embolism (De Bono & Warlow, 1981; Bogousslavsky *et al.*, 1986a,b), whilst about 50% of the patients with an identifiable rare cause of cerebral ischaemia also have one or more of the common vascular risk factors (Table 6.17).

In the first minutes, or even hours, of the first medical contact, all one has available is the clinical syndrome and this can take one a long way towards the cause (see Section 6.5). In the next few days, during which further investigation can be done, a more precise idea of the cause may be found which, although useless for influencing the acute treatment, may well help in modifying further management. The stroke syndrome is not very helpful in deciding *between* competing causes, although LACI/TIA is *unlikely* to be due to carotid stenosis or embolism from the heart, even if one or both embolic sources are present. Nonetheless, many physicians do feel that severe ICA stenosis should be operated on and non-rheumatic AF should be anticoagulated, even if the patient has had a recent lacunar syndrome (see Section 16.7.8).

Our guidelines to distinguish the three main causes of ischaemic stroke/TIA are based on common sense and the scientific literature, as far as it goes, but have not and can not be thoroughly validated, because there is no gold standard to define the cause in *every* case, and even for those who die the autopsy can leave uncertainties. Apart from minor details, these guidelines are similar to those independently put forward by Adams *et al.* in 1993. In clinical *research*, one often has to accept uncertainty and use rigid rules, and so it is not surprising that a large proportion of ischaemic strokes in this context are of unknown cause (40% in the study by Adams *et al.*, 1993). However, in clinical *practice*, the exact cause is less important than deciding what to do next, i.e. what is the treatment for *this* particular case? For example, one would not anticoagulate a fibrillating stroke patient if he/she were an elderly alcoholic, so it really does not matter whether the infarct was lacunar due to intracranial small vessel disease, and so perhaps nothing to do with the AF, or cortical and more likely to be due to embolism from the heart; in this case, although one is not sure whether the AF caused the stroke, at least one is sure that anticoagulation is unwise. If a patient has a patent foramen ovale (PFO) and no other cause of cerebral ischaemia, then paradoxical embolism *might* have been responsible, but because we have no idea what the risk of recurrence is or whether antithrombotic drugs or surgical closure of the defect influences this risk, then in a sense the PFO is a *clinical* irrelevance. However, it would be of great *scientific* interest if a large number of similar patients were followed up to answer these questions concerned with the risk of recurrence, so that, in the future, clinical practice could be improved. There are numerous other examples of the general principle, which can be expressed as 'keep your eye on the (clinical) ball and base management decisions on serious evidence and not a whim.'

It is all but impossible to be sure of the actual cause of ischaemic stroke or transient ischaemic attack if several potential causes are present in the same individual.

6.7.1 Is the ischaemic stroke or TIA due to atherothromboembolism?

Although atherothromboembolism is the most common cause of ischaemic stroke/TIA, about 50% of patients have other causes, and so one can not just assume that all cases are due to this admittedly common vascular disorder. More positive evidence, if possible, is required. As usual, it is not possible to be precise in every individual, but there are at least some criteria which make atherothromboembolism more, or less, likely (Table 6.18). This problem is more difficult when one is dealing with vertebrobasilar, rather than carotid ischaemia, because there are so many causal possibilities and because it is difficult to image the vertebral circulation non-invasively (see Section 6.5.4); however, a large infarct in the cerebellum or in the territory of the posterior cerebral artery is likely to be atherothromboembolic if there is no cardiac source of embolism. It is worth making a positive diagnosis of atherothromboembolism, because this stops the fruitless search for alternatives if clinical assessment and routine investigations fail to identify anything else; it directs attention to defining the degree of any symptomatic ICA stenosis and therefore the need for carotid endarterectomy (see Section 16.7); and it emphasises the

control of vascular risk factors (see Section 16.3) and the use of aspirin as an antithrombotic drug (see Section 16.4). As mentioned earlier, one can not be absolutely precise about whether an event was due to acute arterial occlusion or low flow, or either mechanism at different times; fortunately, this difficulty seldom affects clinical management (see Section 6.5.5).

6.7.2 Is the ischaemic stroke or TIA due to intracranial small vessel disease?

This is highly likely if the clinical syndrome is lacunar (easier in stroke than TIA patients to be certain about) and particularly so if there is no cardiac source of embolism clinically, no clinical or ultrasound evidence of arterial disease in the neck and no reasonably obvious rare cause of stroke clinically or on the routine investigations (see Section 6.5.3; Table 6.19; Chimowitz *et al.*, 1991). It is very likely that there will be vascular risk factors present and, apart from recent myocardial infarction and AF, these are about as likely as in non-lacunar ischaemic stroke (Lodder *et al.*, 1990; Landi *et al.*, 1992a; see Section 6.3). From the *management* point of view, a positive diagnosis of intracranial small vessel disease does reduce the urgency for the detection of severe carotid stenosis, which, if found, is difficult to interpret: is it really the cause of the LACI by embolism or low flow (in which case carotid endarterectomy may be indicated) or is it 'asymptomatic', in which case it ought to be left alone? Our view is that, even if the syndrome is lacunar we would often recommend carotid endaterectomy if the patient has severe (>70%) carotid stenosis on the symptomatic side, but we would also admit that others may not feel the same way (see Section 16.7.8). Similarly, we would anticoagulate a lacunar patient in AF, even though we recognise that the AF *might* not be relevant; however, at least we could reassure ourselves that worthwhile *primary* stroke prevention is achieved by anticoagulation of AF patients (see Section 16.5), which is

Table 6.18 When atherothromboembolism is more, or less, likely to be the cause of ischaemic stroke or TIA.

More likely if
TACI or PACI/ischaemia (clinical syndrome ± CT/MRI evidence)
Cerebellar infarction/ischaemia
Posterior cerebral artery territorial infarction/ischaemia
Boundary-zone infarction/ischaemia (clinical syndrome ± CT/MRI evidence)
Carotid, subclavian, vertebral bruit/absent carotid pulses/unequal radial pulses
Duplex sonography or angiography shows arterial stenosis of more than 50%, or occlusion, of the symptomatic artery
Evidence of clinical complications of atherothrombosis elsewhere: angina, past myocardial infarction, claudication, femoral bruits, absent foot pulses
Patient age greater than 60 years
Cholesterol emboli in the retina

Less likely if
Patient age less than 40 years
LACI/TIA (clinical syndrome ± CT/MRI evidence)
Definite cardiac embolic source
Clear evidence or alternative mechanism (e.g. migrainous stroke, high ESR and giant cell arteritis, arterial dissection, etc.)
No vascular bruits, normal pulses
No arterial stenosis on duplex sonography or angiography
No evidence of atherothrombosis elsewhere

Table 6.19 When intracranial small vessel disease is likely to be the cause of ischaemic stroke or TIA.

Lacunar syndrome (clinically defined)
CT/MRI shows a small deep and relevant infarct in internal capsule/basal ganglia area, cerebral peduncle or pons, or is normal
No clinical (cervical bruits) or ultrasonographic/angiographic evidence of arterial stenosis >50%, or occlusion of, the symptomatic artery in the neck
No evidence of a cardiac embolic source
Vascular risk factors present, particularly hypertension or diabetes

probably more than can be said for carotid endarterectomy (see Section 16.12).

6.7.3 Is the ischaemic stroke or TIA due to embolism from the heart?

Clearly, the diagnosis can only be considered at all if there is an identifiable cardioembolic source (Table 6.20), which is the case in about 30% of ischaemic stroke/TIA patients (Cerebral Embolism Task Force, 1989; see Tables 6.9 & 6.10), and more in recent studies using transoesophageal echocardiography (Mast *et al.*, 1994). However, in maybe one-third, the cardiac source is irrelevant, because there is another, perhaps more likely, cause of cerebral ischaemia, such as carotid stenosis (see Section 6.4).

Fortunately, the majority of cardiac lesions of substantial embolic relevance can be suspected, and even definitively diagnosed, on the basis of a competent clinical examination, ECG and chest X-ray (Burnett *et al.*, 1984; Shapiro *et al.*, 1985). *Transthoracic* echocardiography may be indicated to refine the clinical diagnosis and guide the management of any suspected lesions (e.g. mitral stenosis, atrial myxoma). *Transoesphageal* echocardiography, with intravenous echo contrast, whilst somewhat invasive, occasionally risky (cardiac arrhythmias, vocal cord paresis, bacteraemia, oesophageal perforation and, exceptionally, endocarditis) and perhaps difficult to do in acute stroke, provides even more information if required (e.g. PFO, thrombus in the left atrium) and displays atheromatous plaques in the aortic arch, which could be relevant, but so far not directly treatable, sources of emboli (Tegeler & Downes, 1991; Bartzokis *et al.*, 1991; Black *et al.*, 1991; Tunick *et al.*, 1991; Hart, 1992; De Rook *et al.*, 1992; Donnan & Jones, 1995; Stollberger *et al.*, 1995). The advantages of transthoracic versus transoesphageal echocardiography are listed in Table 6.21.

> *It is not clear that transoesophageal echocardiography provides much more information for clinical decision-making than transthoracic echocardiography, although it certainly provides more anatomical information.*

Routine transthoracic or transoesophageal echocardiography is hardly justifiable, because the yield in *unselected* patients is extremely low, particularly in the sense of changing management (Burnett *et al.*, 1984; Good *et al.*, 1986; Cerebral Embolism Task Force, 1989; Cujec *et al.*, 1991; Voyce *et al.*, 1992). However, it may well be indicated if a cardiac source of embolism is suspected on the basis of the history (past rheumatic fever, ischaemic events in more than one vascular territory, etc.), cardiac examination (murmurs, etc.) ECG (AF, recent myocardial infarction) or chest X-ray (enlarged left atrium, valvular calcification), *particularly* if there is no reasonable alternative cause (such as severe symp-

Table 6.20 Embolism from the heart to the brain or eye.

Evidence in favour
Identified cardiac source of embolism, particularly one with a substantial embolic risk (see Table 6.9)
Ischaemic events in more than one arterial territory, particularly if more than one organ is involved
No evidence clinically (bruits, palpation), on ultrasound or by angiography of arterial disease (>50% stenosis) in the neck
Calcific emboli in the retina (very rare)
Calcific emboli on brain CT (even rarer)
No vascular risk factors
Age less than 50 years
No other explanation for the stroke

Evidence against
Lacunar syndrome (clinical syndrome ± CT/MRI evidence)
Boundary-zone infarction/ischaemia (clinical syndrome ± possibly CT/MRI evidence)

Uncertain evidence one way or the other
Haemorrhagic transformation of the infarct
Speed of symptom onset
Past TIA

Table 6.21 Comparison of transthoracic versus transoesophageal echocardiography for detecting potential cardiac sources of embolism. These comparisons are changing as more experience is being gained. (Adapted from Adams & Love, 1995; Daniel & Mugge, 1995.)

Transthoracic echocardiography preferred	Transoesophageal echocardiography preferred
Left-ventricular thrombus	Atrial thrombus
Left-ventricular dyskinesis	Atrial appendage thrombus
Mitral stenosis	Spontaneous echo contrast
Mitral annulus calcification	Intracardiac tumours
Aortic stenosis	*Atrial septal defect
	Atrial septal aneurysm
	*PFO
	Mitral and aortic valve vegetations
	Prosthetic heart valve malfunction
	Aortic arch atherothrombosis/dissection
	MVP?

* TCD detection of intravenously injected air bubbles is less invasive, more specific, but not quite so sensitive (Di Tullio *et al.*, 1993); galactose particle suspension increases sensitivity (Jauss *et al.*, 1994; Klotzsch *et al.*, 1994).

tomatic carotid stenosis, giant cell arteritis, etc.). In young patients (<40 years, perhaps) with no detectable cause of cerebral ischaemia, it is justifiable to examine the heart in considerable detail, at least as far as transoesophageal echocardiography, which is particularly useful for detecting left-atrial thrombus and examining the aortic arch for atheroma or dissection (see Section 7.1). However, the detection of intracardiac thrombus is not *necessarily* relevant, because not all such thrombi embolise, and the lack of intracardiac thrombus may not be relevant, either because it may be too small to be detected or perhaps it has all embolised already.

> *The presence of intracardiac thrombus does not necessarily mean that embolism has occurred, whilst the absence of intracardiac thrombus does not necessarily mean that embolism has not occurred. In either case, embolism may recur sooner or later.*

The decision whether an identified *potential* embolic source in the heart was *the* cause of the ischaemic stroke or TIA can be quite easy if most of the criteria in Table 6.20 are fulfilled — for example, if the patient is aged 30 years, has a prosthetic heart valve and no vascular disorder or risk factors. Also, some cardiac lesions are much more substantial causes of embolism than others (see Table 6.9). On the other hand, it can be impossible, e.g. if the patient is 70 years old and has both AF *and* severe ICA stenosis ipsilateral to a PACI; in this situation one might be tempted (correctly perhaps) to recommend anticoagulation as well as carotid endarterectomy. Also, some cardiac lesions are so common in the normal stroke-free population (e.g. PFO, MVP) that their relevance in an individual ischaemic stroke patient is unassessable without additional evidence of embolism (see Table 6.20). Once again, one comes back to treating what is treatable (to prevent stroke recurrence), *provided* the risks are not thought to outweigh the potential benefits *and* the patient is prepared to accept the risk of treatment(s), as well as the benefit. Whether emboli detection with TCD becomes helpful in sorting out the origin of emboli remains to be seen (see Section 6.6.4). Other than lacunar syndromes (which are seldom due to cardiac embolism), the clinical or brain CT/MRI features of any cerebral ischaemic event do not reliably distinguish a cardioembolic from some other cause of ischaemic stroke (Bogousslavsky *et al.*, 1986b; Kittner *et al.*, 1991, 1992).

Long-term monitoring of the ECG

The frequency of cardiac arrhythmias in TIA patients is similar to the frequency in the normal population of the same age (De Bono & Warlow, 1981). Therefore, unless an arrhythmia can be shown to *coincide* with a cerebral ischaemic event (which is unlikely to happen unless the events are occurring, if not daily, at least several times a week), its relevance (in the sense of causing hypotension and focal cerebral ischaemia) to any neurological symptoms is profoundly uncertain. Hypotensive *focal* cerebral ischaemic events are uncommon anyway (see Section 6.5.5), unless there is also severe arterial disease in the neck. We only monitor the ECG if the ischaemic events are occurring frequently enough to be captured on the tape, and particularly if no other cause is likely and if the focal neurological symptoms are accompanied by faintness, chest pain, shortness of breath or palpitations. Treatment of the arrhythmia should then reduce the risk of recurrence of neurological symptoms. Other indications are a patient in sinus rhythm, who *might* have paroxysmal AF (history of palpitations or possibly irregular pulse, etc.) and so require anticoagulation (see Section 16.5), or to check that any treatment to return the patient to sinus rhythm has been effective.

Venography

Venography, or some reliable non-invasive method to detect DVT of the legs, may be required if paradoxical embolism is suspected, but this is a very rare event. Criteria to suspect paradoxical embolism include an ischaemic event occuring in the context of a Valsalva manoeuvre (lifting, straining, coughing, etc.) or anything else likely to increase right-atrial pressure and so encourage blood flow from the right to the left atrium; a PFO identified with contrast echocardiography; perhaps clot in the right atrium or across the interatrial septum, possibly from a central venous line; a reason for DVT (e.g. recent surgery or air travel) and no other more likely cause (Mas, 1991; Ranoux *et al.*, 1993; Brogno *et al.*, 1994). Of course, any venography must be done early (within 48 hours at most) because DVT is so common as a *consequence* of stroke, particularly in a paralysed leg (see Section 15.13; Warlow, 1978; Landi *et al.*, 1992b).

References

Abbott RD, Behrens GR, Sharp DS *et al.* (1994). Body mass index and thromboembolic stroke in nonsmoking men in older middle age: the Honolulu Heart Program. *Stroke* 25: 2370–6.

Aberg H (1969). Atrial fibrillation. I. A study of atrial thrombosis and systemic embolism in a necropsy material. *Acta Med Scand* 185: 373–9.

Acheson RM, Williams DRR (1983). Does consumption of fruit and vegetables protect against stroke? *Lancet* i: 1191–3.

Adams HP Jr (1991). Investigation of the patient with ischaemic stroke. *Cerebrovasc Dis* 1 (Suppl. 1): 54–60.

Adams HP Jr, Love BB (1995). Transesophageal echocardiography in the evaluation of young adults with ischaemic stroke: promises and concerns. *Cerebrovasc Dis* 5: 323–7.

Adams HP Jr, Bendixen BH, Kappelle LJ *et al.* (1993). Classification of subtype of acute ischaemic stroke: definitions for use in a multicentre clinical trial. *Stroke* 24: 35–41.

Adams RJ, Carroll RM, Nichols FT *et al.* (1989). Plasma lipoproteins in cortical versus lacunar infarction. *Stroke* 20: 448–52.

Aichner FT, Felber SR, Birbamer GG, Posch A (1993). Magnetic resonance imaging and magnetic resonance angiography of vertebrobasilar dolichoectasia. *Cerebrovasc Dis* 3: 280–4.

Alberts MJ, Faulstich ME, Gray L (1992). Stroke with negative brain magnetic resonance imaging. *Stroke* 23: 663–7.

Amarenco P, Caplan LR (1993). Vertebrobasilar occlusive disease: review of selected aspects. 3. Mechanisms of cerebellar infarctions. *Cerebrovasc Dis* 3: 66–73.

Amarenco P, Duyckaerts C, Tzourio C, Henin D, Bousser M-G, Hauw J-J (1992). The prevalence of ulcerated plaques in the aortic arch in patients with stroke. *N Engl J Med* 326: 221–5.

Ameriso SF, Mohler JG, Suarez M, Fisher M (1994). Morning reduction of cerebral vasomotor reactivity. *Neurology* 44: 1907–9.

Anda R, Williamson D, Jones D *et al.* (1993). Depressed affect, hopelessness, and the risk of ischaemic heart disease in a cohort of US adults. *Epidemiology* 4: 285–94.

Anderson CS, Taylor BV, Hankey GJ, Stewart-Wynne EG, Jamrozik KD (1994). Validation of a clinical classification for subtypes of acute cerebral infarction. *J Neurol Neurosurg Psychiatr* 57: 1173–9.

Angeloni U, Bozzao L, Fantozzi L, Bastianello S, Kushner M, Fieschi C (1990). Internal borderzone infarction following acute middle cerebral artery occlusion. *Neurology* 40: 1196–8.

Anzalone N, Landi G (1989). Non ischaemic causes of lacunar syndromes: prevalence and clinical findings. *J Neurol Neurosurg Psychiatr* 52: 1188–90.

Archie JP, Feldman RW (1981). Critical stenosis of the internal carotid artery. *Surgery* 89: 67–70.

Arroll B, Beaglehole R (1992). Does physical activity lower blood pressure? A critical review of the clinical trials. *J Clin Epidemiol* 45: 439–47.

Arruga J, Sanders MD (1982). Ophthalmologic findings in 70 patients with evidence of retinal embolism. *Ophthalmology* 89: 1336–47.

Ascherio A, Willett WC (1994). Are body iron stores related to the risk of coronary heart disease? *N Engl J Med* 330: 1119–24.

Ascherio A, Rimm EB, Stampfer MJ, Giovannucci EL, Willett WC (1995). Dietary intake of marine n-3 fatty acids, fish intake, and the risk of coronary disease among men. *N Engl J Med* 332: 977–82.

Atrial Fibrillation Investigators (1994). Risk factors for stroke and efficacy of antithrombotic therapy in atrial fibrillation. *Arch Intern Med* 154: 1449–57.

Babikian VL, Hyde C, Pochay V, Winter MR (1994). Clinical correlates of high-intensity transient signals detected on transcranial Doppler sonography in patients with cerebrovascular disease. *Stroke* 25: 1570–3.

Balarajan R (1991). Ethnic differences in mortality from ischaemic heart disease and cerebrovascular disease in England and Wales. *Br Med J* 302: 560–4.

Bamford J (1992). Clinical examination in diagnosis and subclassification of stroke. *Lancet* 339: 400–2.

Bamford J, Sandercock P, Jones L, Warlow C (1987). The natural history of lacunar infarction: the Oxfordshire Community Stroke Project. *Stroke* 18: 545–51.

Bamford J, Sandercock P, Dennis M, Burn J, Warlow C (1990). A prospective study of acute cerebrovascular disease in the community: the Oxfordshire Community Stroke Project, 1981–86. 2. Incidence, case fatality rates and overall outcome at one year of cerebral infarction, primary intracerebral and subarachnoid haemorrhage. *J Neurol Neurosurg Psychiatr* 53: 16–22.

Bamford J, Sandercock P, Dennis M *et al.* (1988). A prospective study of acute cerebrovascular disease in the community: the Oxfordshire Cummunity Stroke Project 1981–86. 1. Methodology, demography and incident cases of first ever stroke. *J Neurol Neurosurg Psychiatr* 51: 1373–80.

Bamford JM, Warlow CP (1988). Evolution and testing of the lacunar hypothesis. *Stroke* 19: 1074–82.

Barker DJP (1995). Fetal origins of coronary heart disease. *Br Med J* 311: 171–4.

Barnett HJM, Warlow CP (1993). Carotid endarterectomy and the measurement of stenosis. *Stroke* 24: 1281–4.

Barnett HJM, Boughner DR, Taylor DW, Cooper PE, Kostuk WJ, Nichol PM (1980). Further evidence relating mitral-valve prolapse to cerebral ischaemic events. *N Engl J Med* 302: 139–44.

Barrett-Connor E, Khaw K-T (1988). Diabetes mellitus: an independent risk factor for stroke? *Am J Epidemiol* 128: 116–23.

Bartzokis T, Lee R, Yeok TK, Grogin H, Schnittger (1991). Transeosophageal echo Doppler echocardiographic assessment of pulmonary venous flow patterns. *J Am Soc Echocardiogr* 4: 457–64.

Bathen J, Sparr S, Rokseth R (1978). Embolism in sinoatrial disease. *Acta Med Scand* 203: 7–11.

Benfante R, Yano K, Hwang L-J, Curb JD, Kagan A, Ross W (1994). Elevated serum cholesterol is a risk factor for both coronary heart disease and thromboembolic stroke in Hawaiian Japanese men: implications of shared risk. *Stroke* 25: 814–20.

Benjamin EJ, D'Agostino RB, Belanger AJ, Wolf PA, Levy D (1995). Left atrial size and the risk of stroke and death. *Circulation* 92: 835–41.

Benjamin EJ, Plehn JF, D'Agostino RB *et al.* (1992). Mitral annular calcification and the risk of stroke in an elderly cohort. *N Engl J Med* 327: 374–9.

Benomar A, Yahyaoui M, Birouk N, Vidailhet M, Chkili T (1994). Middle cerebral artery occlusion due to hydatid cysts of myocardial and intraventricular cavity cardiac origin: two cases. *Stroke* 25: 886–8.

Ben-Shlomo Y, Markowe H, Shipley M, Marmot MG (1992).

Stroke risk from alcohol consumption using different control groups. *Stroke* 23: 1093–8.

Berlin JA, Colditz GA (1990). A meta-analysis of physical activity in the prevention of coronary heart disease. *Am J Epidemiol* 132: 612–28.

Berman SS, Devine JJ, Erdoes LS, Hunter GC (1995). Distinguishing carotid artery pseudo-occlusion with color-flow Doppler. *Stroke* 26: 434–8.

Besson G, Hommel M, Perret J (1991). Historical aspects of the lacunar concept. *Cerebrovasc Dis* 1: 306–10.

Besson G, Clavier I, Hommel M, Perret J (1993). Co-existence of lacunar infarcts and intracranial haemorrhages. *Rev Neurol* 149: 55–7.

Bhatnagar D, Anand IS, Durrington PN *et al.* (1995). Coronary risk factors in people from the Indian subcontinent living in West London and their siblings in India. *Lancet* 345: 405–9.

Bishop CCR, Powell S, Insall M, Rutt D, Browse NL (1986). Effect of internal carotid artery occlusion on middle cerebral artery blood flow at rest and in response to hypercapnia. *Lancet* i: 710–12.

Black IW, Hopkins AP, Lee LCL, Walsh WF, Jacobson BM (1991). Left atrial spontaneous echo contrast: a clinical and echocardiographic analysis. *J Am Coll Cardiol* 18: 398–404.

Bladin CF, Chambers BR (1993). Clinical features, pathogenesis, and computed tomographic characteristics of internal watershed infarction. *Stroke* 24: 1925–32.

Blakeley DD, Oddone EZ, Hasselblad V, Simel DL, Matchar DB (1995). Noninvasive carotid artery testing: a meta-analytic review. *Ann Intern Med* 122: 360–7.

Bloomfield P, Wheatley DJ, Prescott RJ, Miller HC (1991). Twelve-year comparison of a Bjork–Shiley mechanical heart valve with porcine bioprostheses. *N Engl J Med* 324: 573–9.

Bogousslavsky J (1991). Topographic patterns of cerebral infarcts: correlation with aetiology. *Cerebrovasc Dis* 1 (Suppl. 1): 61–8.

Bogousslavsky J, Caplan LR (1993). Vertebrobasilar occlusive disease: review of selected aspects. 3. Thalamic infarcts. *Cerebrovasc Dis* 3: 193–205.

Bogousslavsky J, Regli F (1986a). Borderzone infarctions distal to internal carotid artery occlusion: prognostic implications. *Ann Neurol* 20: 346–50.

Bogousslavsky J, Regli F (1986b). Unilateral watershed cerebral infarcts. *Neurology* 36: 373–7.

Bogousslavsky J, Regli F (1992). Centrum ovale infarcts: subcortical infarction in the superficial territory of the middle cerebral artery. *Neurology* 42: 1992–8.

Bogousslavsky J, Regli F, Maeder P (1991). Intracranial large-artery disease and 'lacunar' infarction. *Cerebrovasc Dis* 1: 154–9.

Bogousslavsky J, Maeder P, Regli F, Meuli R (1994). Pure midbrain infarction: clinical syndromes, MRI, and aetiologic patterns. *Neurology* 44: 2032–40.

Bogousslavsky J, van Melle G, Regli F, Kappenberger L (1990). Pathogenesis of anterior circulation stroke in patients with nonvalvular atrial fibrillations: the Lausanne Stroke Registry. *Neurology* 40: 1046–50.

Bogousslavsky J, Regli F, Besson G, Pinho e Melo T, Nater B (1993a). Early clinical diagnosis of stroke subtype. *Cerebrovasc Dis* 3: 39–44.

Bogousslavsky J, Regli F, Maeder P, Meuli R, Nader J (1993b). The aetiology of posterior circulation infarcts: a prospective study using magnetic resonance imaging and magnetic resonance angiography. *Neurology* 43: 1528–33.

Bogousslavsky J, Hachinski VC, Boughner DR, Fox AJ, Vinuela F, Barnett HJM (1986a). Cardiac and arterial lesions in carotid transient ischaemic attacks. *Arch Neurol* 43: 223–8.

Bogousslavsky J, Hachinski VC, Boughner DR, Fox AR, Vinuela F, Barnett HJM (1986b). Clinical predictors of cardiac and arterial lesions in carotid ischaemic attacks. *Arch Neurol* 43: 229–33.

Boiten J, Lodder J (1991). Lacunar infarcts: pathogenesis and validity of the clinical syndromes. *Stroke* 22: 1374–8.

Boiten J, Lodder J (1993). Prognosis for survival, handicap and recurrence of stroke in lacunar and superficial infarction. *Cerebrovasc Dis* 3: 221–6.

Boiten J, Rothwell PM, Slattery J, Warlow CP, for the European Carotid Surgery Trialists' Collaborative Group (1996). Ischaemic lacunar stroke in the European Carotid Surgery Trial: risk factors, distribution of carotid stenosis, effect of surgery and type of recurrent stroke. *Cerebrovasc Dis* (in press.)

Boon A, Lodder J, Heuts-van Raak L, Kessels F (1994). Silent brain infarcts in 755 consecutive patients with a first-ever supratentorial ischaemic stroke: relationship with index-stroke subtype, vascular risk factors, and mortality. *Stroke* 25: 2384–90.

Bornstein NM, Norris JW (1994). Transcranial Doppler sonography is at present of limited clinical value. *Arch Neurol* 51: 1057–9.

Bousser M-G, Chiras J, Bories J, Castaigne P (1985). Cerebral venous thrombosis—a review of 38 cases. *Stroke* 16: 199–213.

Bray JM, Glatt B (1995). Quantification of atheromatous stenosis in the extracranial internal carotid artery. *Cerebrovasc Dis* 5: 414–26.

Brice JG, Dowsett DJ, Lowe RD (1964). Haemodynamic effects of carotid artery stenosis. *Br Med J* 2: 1363–6.

Britton M, Gustafsson C (1985). Non-rheumatic atrial fibrillation as a risk factor for stroke. *Stroke* 16: 182–8.

Brockmeier LB, Adolph RJ, Gustin BW, Holmes JC, Sacks JG (1981). Calcium emboli to the retinal artery in calcific aortic stenosis. *Am Heart J* 101: 32–7.

Broderick JP, Phillips SJ, O'Fallon M, Frye RL, Whisnant JP (1992). Relationship of cardiac disease to stroke occurence, recurrence and mortality. *Stroke* 23: 1250–6.

Brogno D, Lancaster G, Rosenbaum M (1994). Embolism interruptus. *N Engl J Med* 330: 1761–2.

Brott T, Tomsick T, Feinberg W *et al.* for the Asymptomatic Carotid Atherosclerosis Study Investigators (1994). Baseline silent cerebral infarction in the asymptomatic carotid atherosclerosis study. *Stroke* 25: 1122–9.

Browner WS, Pressman AR, Nevitt MC, Cauley JA, Cummings SR, for the Study of Osteoporotic Fractures Research Group (1993). Association between low bone density and stroke in elderly women: the study of osteoporotic fractures. *Stroke* 24: 940–6.

Bruno A, Corbett JJ, Biller J, Adams HP, Qualls C (1990). Transient monocular visual loss patterns and associated vascular abnormalities. *Stroke* 21: 34–9.

Bruno A, Nolte KB, Chapin J (1993). Stroke associated with ephedrine use. *Neurology* 43: 1313–16.

Bulpitt CJ (1995). Vitamin C and vascular disease: be cautious about the association until large randomised trials have been done. *Br Med J* 310: 1548–9.

Burchfiel CM, Curb JD, Rodriguez BL, Abbott RD, Chiu D, Yano K (1994). Glucose intolerance and 22 year stroke incidence: the Honolulu Heart Program. *Stroke* 25: 951–7.

Burn J, Dennis M, Bamford J, Sandercock P, Wade D, Warlow C (1996). Epileptic seizures after a first ever in a lifetime stroke: the Oxfordshire Community Stroke Project. *Br Med J* (in press).

Burnett PJ, Milne JR, Greenwood R, Giles MR, Camm J (1984). The role of echocardiography in the investigation of focal cerebral ischaemia. *Postgrad Med J* 60: 116–19.

Cabanes L, Mas JL, Cohen A *et al.* (1993). Atrial septal aneurysm and patent foramen ovale as risk factors for cryptogenic stroke in patients less than 55 years of age: a study using transoesophageal echocardiography. *Stroke* 24: 1865–73.

Camargo CA (1989). Moderate alcohol consumption and stroke: the epidemiologic evidence. *Stroke* 20: 1611–26.

Caplan LR (1993). Brain embolism, revisited. *Neurology* 43: 1281–7.

Caplan LR (1994a). Drugs. In: Kase CS, Caplan LR, eds. *Intracerebral Haemorrhage*. Boston: Butterworth Heinemann, 201–20.

Caplan LR (1994b). Silent brain infarcts. *Cerebrovasc Dis* 4 (Suppl. 1): 32–9.

Caplan LR, Sergay S (1976). Positional cerebral ischaemia. *J Neurol Neurosurg Psychiatr* 39: 385–91.

Caplan LR, Tettenborn B (1992). Vertebrobasilar occlusive disease: review of selected aspects. 2. Posterior circulation embolism. *Cerebrovasc Dis* 2: 320–6.

Caplan LR, Gorelick PB, Hier DB (1986). Race, sex and occlusive cerebrovascular disease: a review. *Stroke* 17: 648–55.

Caplan LR, Hier DB, Banks G (1982). Current concepts of cerebrovascular disease—stroke: stroke and drug abuse. *Stroke* 13: 869–72.

Carstairs V, Morris R (1990). Deprivation and health in Scotland. *Health Bull* 48: 162–9.

Carty GA, Nachtigal T, Magyar R, Herzler G, Bays R (1993). Abdominal duplex ultrasound screening for occult aortic aneurysm during carotid arterial evaluation. *J Vasc Surg* 17: 696–702.

Castaigne P, Lhermitte F, Gautier J-C, Escourolle R, Derouesne C (1970). Internal carotid artery occlusion: a study of 61 instances in 50 patients with post-mortem data. *Brain* 93: 231–58.

Castaigne P, Lhermitte F, Buge A, Escourolle R, Hauw JJ, Lyon-Caen O (1981). Paramedian thalamic and midbrain infarcts: clinical and neuropathological study. *Ann Neurol* 10: 127–48.

Castaigne P, Lhermitte F, Gautier JC *et al.* (1973). Arterial occlusions in the vertebrobasilar system: a study of 44 patients with post mortem data. *Brain* 96: 133–54.

Cerebral Embolism Task Force (1989). Cardiogenic brain embolism: the second report of the Cerebral Embolism Task Force. *Arch Neurol* 46: 727–43.

Chabriat H, Vahedi K, Iba-Zizen MT *et al.* (1995). Clinical spectrum of CADASIL: a study of 7 families. *Lancet* 346: 934–9.

Challa VR, Moody DM, Bell MA (1992). The Charcot–Bouchard aneurysm controversy: impact of a new histologic technique. *J Neuropathol Exp Neurol* 51: 264–71.

Chalmers N, Campbell IW (1987). Left atrial metastasis presenting as recurrent embolic strokes. *Br Heart J* 58: 170–2.

Chambless LE, Fuchs FD, Linn S *et al.* (1990). The association of corneal arcus with coronary heart disease and cardiovascular disease mortality in the Lipid Research Clinics Mortality Follow-up Study. *Am J Pub Health* 80: 1200–4.

Chesler E, King RA, Edwards JE (1983). The myxomatous mitral valve and sudden death. *Circulation* 67: 632–9.

Chimowitz MI, Mancini J (1992). Asymptomatic coronary artery disease in patients with stroke: prevalence, prognosis, diagnosis, and treatment. *Stroke* 23: 433–6.

Chimowitz MI, Furlan AJ, Sila CA, Paranandi L, Beck GJ (1991). Aetiology of motor or sensory stroke: a prospective study of the predictive value of clinical and radiological features. *Ann Neurol* 30: 519–25.

Chimowitz MI, DeGeorgia MA, Poole RM, Hepner A, Armstrong WM (1993a). Left atrial spontaneous echo contrast is highly associated with previous stroke in patients with atrial fibrillation or mitral stenosis. *Stroke* 24: 1015–19.

Chimowitz MI, Furlan AJ, Jones SC *et al.* (1993b). Transcranial Doppler assessment of cerebral perfusion reserve in patients with carotid occlusive disease and no evidence of cerebral infarction. *Neurology* 43: 353–7.

Chobanian AV (1983). The influence of hypertension and other haemodynamic factors in atherogenesis. *Progr Cardiovasc Dis* 26: 177–96.

Close JB, Evans DW, Bailey SM (1979). Persistent lone atrial fibrillation—its prognosis after clinical diagnosis. *J Roy Coll Gen Practit* 29: 547–9.

Colditz GA, Willett WC, Stampfer MJ, Rosner B, Speizer FE, Hennekens CH (1987). Menopause and the risk of coronary heart disease in women. *N Engl J Med* 316: 1105–10.

Collins R, MacMahon S (1994). Blood pressure, antihypertensive drug treatment and the risks of stroke and of coronary heart disease. *Br Med Bull* 50: 272–98.

Connelly JB, Cooper JA, Meade TW (1992). Strenuous exercise, plasma fibrinogen, and factor VII activity. *Br Heart J* 67: 351–4.

Constantinides P (1967). Pathogenesis of cerebral artery thrombosis in man. *Arch Pathol* 83: 422–8.

Cook NS, Ubben D (1990). Fibrinogen as a major risk factor in cardiovascular disease. *Trends Pharmacol Sci* 11: 444–51.

Cornhill JF, Akins D, Hutson M, Chandler A (1980). Localisation of atherosclerotic lesions in the human basilar artery. *Atherosclerosis* 35, 77–86.

Coulshed N, Epstein EJ, McKendrick CS, Galloway RW, Walker E

(1970). Systemic embolism in mitral valve disease. *Br Heart J* 32: 26–34.

Countee RW, Vijayanathan T, Chavis P (1981). Recurrent retinal ischaemia beyond cervical carotid occlusions: clinical–angiographic correlations and therapeutic implications. *J Neurosurg* 55: 532–42.

Craven TE, Ryu JE, Espeland MA *et al.* (1990). Evaluation of the associations between carotid artery atherosclerosis and coronary artery stenosis: a case–control study. *Circulation* 82: 1230–42.

Cregler LL, Mark H (1986). Special report: medical complications of cocaine abuse. *N Engl J Med* 315: 1495–500.

Cujec B, Polasek P, Voll C, Shuaib A (1991). Transesophageal echocardiography in the detection of potential cardiac source of embolism in stroke patients. *Stroke* 22: 727–33.

Cumming MJ, Morrow IM (1994). Carotid artery stenosis: a prospective comparison of CT angiography and conventional angiography. *Am J Radiol* 163: 517–23.

Dalal PM, Deshpande CK, Daftary SG (1971). Aortic arch syndrome. *Neurology* 19: 155–71.

Daley R, Mattingly TW, Holt CL, Bland EF, White PD (1951). Systemic arterial embolism in rheumatic heart disease. *Am Heart J* 42: 566–81.

Daniel WG (1993). Should transesophageal echocardiography be used to guide cardioversion? *N Engl J Med* 328: 803–4.

Daniel WG, Mugge A (1995). Transesophageal echocardiography. *N Engl J Med* 332: 1268–79.

Daniel WG, Nellessen U, Schroeder E *et al.* (1988). Left atrial spontaneous contrast in mitral valve disease: an indicator for increased thrombembolic risk. *J Am Coll Cardiol* 11: 1204–11.

Daras M, Tuchman AJ, Marks S (1991). Central nervous system infarction related to cocaine abuse. *Stroke* 22: 1320–5.

Datta M (1993). You cannot exclude the explanation you have not considered. *Lancet* 342: 345–7.

Davalos A, de Cendra E, Molins A, Ferrandiz M, Lopez-Pousa S, Genis D (1992). Epileptic seizures at the onset of stroke. *Cerebrovasc Dis* 2: 327–31.

Davey Smith G, Phillips AN, Neaton JD (1992). Smoking as an 'independent' risk factor for suicide: illustration of an artifact from observational epidemiology? *Lancet* 340: 709–12.

Davies KN, Humphrey PR (1993). Complications of cerebral angiography in patients with symptomatic carotid territory ischaemia screened by carotid ultrasound. *J Neurol Neurosurg Psychiatr* 56: 967–72.

Davies MJ, Pomerance A (1972). Pathology of atrial fibrillation in man. *Br Heart J* 34: 520–5.

Davis PH, Dambrosia JM, Schoenberg BS *et al.* (1987). Risk factors for ischaemic stroke: a prospective study in Rochester, Minnesota. *Ann Neurol* 22: 319–27.

De Bono DP (1982). Cardiac causes of transient neurologic disturbances. In: Warlow CP, Morris PS, eds. *Transient Ischaemic Attacks*. New York: Dekker, 99–124.

De Bono DP, Warlow CP (1979). Mitral-annulus calcification and cerebral or retinal ischaemia. *Lancet* ii: 383–5.

De Bono DP, Warlow CP (1981). Potential sources of emboli in patients with presumed transient cerebral or retinal ischaemia. *Lancet* i: 343–6.

DeGraba TJ, Penix L (1995). Genetics of ischaemic stroke. *Curr Opin Neurol* 8: 24–9.

Delaney P, Estes M (1980). Intracranial haemorrhage with amphetamine abuse. *Neurology* 30: 1125–8.

Dennis M (1985). Neurological complications of pulmonary arteriovenous malformations. *Br Med J* 289: 1392–3.

Dennis M, Bamford J, Sandercock P, Warlow C (1989). Incidence of transient ischaemic attacks in Oxfordshire, England. *Stroke* 20: 333–9.

Dennis M, Bamford J, Sandercock P, Molyneux A, Warlow C (1990). Computed tomography in patients with transient ischaemic attacks: when is a transient ischaemic attack not a transient ischaemic attack but a stroke? *J Neurol* 237: 257–61.

De Rook FA, Comess KA, Albers GW, Popp RL (1992). Transoesophageal echocardiography in the evaluation of stroke. *Ann Intern Med* 117: 922–32.

De Stefano F, Anda RF, Kahn HS, Williamson DF, Russell CM (1993). Dental disease and risk of coronary heart disease and mortality. *Br Med J* 306: 688–91.

Devereux RB, Brown T, Kramer-Fox R, Sachs I (1982). Inheritance of mitral valve prolapse: effect of age and sex on gene expression. *Ann Intern Med* 97: 826–32.

Devereux RB, Kramer-Fox R, Shear K, Kligfield P, Pini R, Savage DD (1987). Diagnosis and classification of severity of mitral valve prolapse: methodologic, biologic, and prognostic considerations. *Am Heart J* 113: 1265–79.

DeWeese JA, May AG, Lipchik EO, Rob CG (1970). Anatomic and haemodynamic correlations in carotid artery stenosis. *Stroke* 1: 149–57.

Dexter DD, Whisnant JP, Connolly DC, O'Fallon WM (1987). The association of stroke and coronary heart disease; a population study. *Mayo Clin Proc* 62: 1077–83.

Di Pasquale G, Andreoli A, Pinelli *et al.* (1986). Cerebral ischaemia and asymptomatic coronary artery disease: a prospective study of 83 patients. *Stroke* 17: 1098–101.

Di Pasquale G, Ribani M, Andreoli A, Zampa GA, Pinelli G (1989). Cardioembolic stroke in primary oxalosis with cardiac involvement. *Stroke* 20: 1403–6.

Di Pasquale G, Urbinati S, Pinelli G (1995). New echocardiographic markers of embolic risk in atrial fibrillation. *Cerebrovasc Dis* 5: 315–22.

Di Tullio M, Sacco RL, Venketasubrammanian N, Sherman D, Mohr JP, Homma S (1993). Comparison of diagnostic techniques for the detection of a patent foramen ovale in stroke patients. *Stroke* 24: 1020–4.

Dobyns WB, Garg BP (1991) Vascular abnormalities in epidermal nevus syndrome. *Neurology* 41: 276–8.

Doll R, Peto R, Hall E, Wheatley K, Gray R (1994). Mortality in relation to consumption of alcohol: 13 years' observations on male British doctors. *Br Med J* 309: 911–18.

Donnan GA (1992). Investigation of patients with stroke and transient ischaemic attacks. *Lancet* 339: 473–7.

Donnan GA, Jones EF (1995). Aortic arch atheroma and stroke.

Cerebrovasc Dis 5: 10–13.

Donnan GA, Tress BM, Bladin PF (1982). A prospective study of lacunar infarction using computerized tomography. *Neurology* 32: 49–55.

Donnan GA, You R, Thrift A, McNeil JJ (1993a). Smoking as a risk factor for stroke. *Cerebrovasc Dis* 3: 129–38.

Donnan GA, Norrving B, Bamford J, Bogousslavsky J (1993b). Subcortical infarction: classification and terminology. *Cerebrovasc Dis* 3: 248–51.

Donnan GA, Norrving B, Bamford JM, Bogousslavsky J (1995). *Lacunar and Other Subcortical Infarctions*. Oxford: Oxford University Press.

Donnan GA, Bladin PF, Berkovic SF, Longley WA, Saling MM (1991). The stroke syndrome of striatocapsular infarction. *Brain* 114: 51–70.

Donnan GA, O'Malley HM, Quang L, Hurley S, Bladin PF (1993c). The capsular warning syndrome: pathogenesis and clinical features. *Neurology* 43: 957–62.

Donnan GA, McNeil JJ, Adena MA, Doyle AE, O'Malley HM, Neill GC (1989). Smoking as a risk factor for cerebral ischaemia. *Lancet* ii: 643–7.

Dugani BV, Higginson LAJ, Beanlands DS, Akyurekli Y (1984). Recurrent systemic emboli following myocardial contusion. *Am Heart J* 108: 1354–7.

Duguid JB (1976). *The Dynamics of Atherosclerosis*. Aberdeen University Press.

Edelman RR, Warach S (1993). Magnetic resonance imaging (first of two parts). *N Engl J Med* 328: 708–16.

Eliaziw M, Streifler JY, Fox AJ, Hachinski VC, Ferguson GG, Barnett HJM, for the North American Symptomatic Carotid Endarterectomy Trial (1994). Significance of plaque ulceration in symptomatic patients with high-grade carotid stenosis. *Stroke* 25: 304–8.

Enevoldson TP, Russell RWR (1990). Cerebral venous thrombosis: new causes for an old syndrome? *Quart J Med* 77: 1255–75.

Ernst E, Resch KL (1993). Fibrinogen as a cardiovascular risk factor: a meta-analysis and review of the literature. *Ann Intern Med* 118: 956–63.

Estol C, Claassen D, Hirsch W, Wechsler L, Moossy J (1991). Correlative angiographic and pathologic findings in the diagnosis of ulcerated plaques in the carotid artery. *Arch Neurol* 48: 692–4.

European Carotid Surgery Trialists' Collaborative Group (1995). Risk of stroke in the distribution of an asymptomatic carotid artery. *Lancet* 345: 209–12.

Evans JG (1987). Blood pressure and stroke in an elderly English population. *J Epidemiol Commun Health* 41: 275–82.

Fabris F, Zanocchi M, Bo M *et al.* (1994). Carotid plaque, ageing, and risk factors: a study of 457 subjects. *Stroke* 25: 1133–40.

Feldmann E, Daneault N, Kwan E *et al.* (1990). Chinese–white differences in the distribution of occlusive cerebrovascular disease. *Neurology* 40: 1541–5.

Fine-Edelstein JS, Wolf PA, O'Leary DH *et al.* (1994). Precursors of extracranial carotid atherosclerosis in the Framingham Study. *Neurology* 44: 1046–50.

Finklestein S, Kleinman GM, Guneo R, Baringer JR (1980). Delayed stroke following carotid occlusion. *Neurology* 30: 84–8.

Fisher CM (1951). Occlusion of the internal carotid artery. *Arch Neurol Psychiatr* 65: 346–77.

Fisher CM (1954). Occlusion of the carotid arteries. *Arch Neurol Psychiatr* 72: 187–204.

Fisher CM (1969). The arterial lesions underlying lacunes. *Acta Neuropathol* 12: 1–15.

Fisher CM (1972). Cerebral miliary aneurysms in hypertension. *Am J Pathol* 66: 313–30.

Fisher CM (1979). Capsular infarcts—the underlying vascular lesions. *Arch Neurol* 36: 65–73.

Fisher CM (1991). Lacunar infarcts—a review. *Cerebrovasc Dis* 1: 311–20.

Fisher M, Fieman S (1990). Geometric factors of the bifurcation in carotid atherogenesis. *Stroke* 21: 267–71.

Fisher M, Sacoolidge JC, Taylor CR (1987). Patterns of fibrin deposits in carotid artery plaques. *Angiology* 38: 393–9.

Fisher M, Kase CS, Stelle B, Mills RM (1988). Ischaemic stroke after cardiac pacemaker implantation in sick sinus syndrome. *Stroke* 19: 712–15.

Flegel KM, Shipley MJ, Rose G (1987). Risk of stroke in non-rheumatic atrial fibrillation. *Lancet* i: 526–9.

Folsom AR, Prineas RJ, Kaye SA, Munger RG (1990). Incidence of hypertension and stroke in relation to body fat distribution and other risk factors in older women. *Stroke* 21: 701–6.

Folsom AR, Eckfeldt JH, Weitzman S *et al.* for the Atherosclerosis Risk in Communities (ARIC) Study Investigators (1994). Relation of carotid artery wall thickness to diabetes mellitus, fasting glucose and insulin, body size, and physical activity. *Stroke* 25: 66–73.

Foster JW, Hart RG (1987). Hypoglycaemic hemiplegia: two cases and a clinical review. *Stroke* 18: 944–6.

Fox AJ (1993). How to measure carotid stenosis. *Radiology* 186: 316–18.

Franks PJ, Adamson C, Bulpitt PF, Bulpitt CJ (1991). Stroke death and unemployment in London. *J Epidemiol Commun Health* 45: 16–18.

Fredericks RK, Lefkowitz DS, Challa VR, Troost BT (1991). Cerebral vasculitis associated with cocaine abuse. *Stroke* 22: 1437–9.

Friedman GD, Loveland DB, Ehrlich SP (1968). Relationship of stroke to other cardiovascular disease. *Circulation* 38: 533–41.

Friedman SG (1990). Transient ischaemic attacks resulting from carotid duplex imaging. *Surgery* 107: 153–5.

Frost CD, Law MR, Wald NJ (1991). By how much does dietary salt reduction lower blood pressure? II—analysis of observational data within populations. *Br Med J* 302: 815–18.

Furlan AJ, Whisnant JP, Kearns TP (1979). Unilateral visual loss in bright light: an unusual symptom of carotid artery occlusive disease. *Arch Neurol* 36: 675–6.

Fuster V, Badimon L, Badimon JJ, Chesebro JH (1992). The pathogenesis of coronary artery disease and the acute coronary syndromes. *N Engl J Med* 326: 242–50.

Fuster V, Gersh BJ, Giuliani ER, Tajik AJ, Brandenburg RO, Frye

RL (1981). The natural history of idiopathic dilated cardiomyopathy. *Am J Cardiol* 47: 525–31.

Gale CR, Martyn CN, Winter PD, Cooper C (1995). Vitamin C and risk of death from stroke and coronary heart disease in cohort of elderly people. *Br Med J* 310: 1563–6.

Garber AM, Avins AL (1994). Triglyceride concentration and coronary heart disease. *Br Med J* 309: 2–3.

Gasecki AP, Fox AJ, Lebrun LH, Daneault N, for the Collaborators of the North American Carotid Endarterectomy Trial (NASCET) (1994). Bilateral occipital infarctions associated with carotid stenosis in a patient with persistent trigeminal artery. *Stroke* 25: 1520–3.

Gautier JC, Durr A, Koussa S, Lascault G, Grosgogeat Y (1991). Paradoxical cerebral embolism with a patent foramen ovale: a report of 29 patients. *Cerebrovasc Dis* 1: 193–202.

Georgiadis D, Grosset DG, Kelman A, Faichney A, Lees KR (1994). Prevalence and characteristics of intracranial microemboli signals in patients with different types of prosthetic cardiac valves. *Stroke* 25: 587–92.

Geyer SJ, Franzini DA (1979). Myxomatous degeneration of the mitral valve complicated by nonbacterial thrombotic endocarditis with systemic embolisation. *Am J Clin Pathol* 72: 489–92.

Gibbs JM, Wise RJS, Leenders KL, Jones T (1984). Evaluation of cerebral perfusion reserve in patients with carotid-artery occlusion. *Lancet* i: 310–14.

Gillum RF (1988). Stroke in blacks. *Stroke* 16: 1–9.

Gironell A, Rey A, Marti-Vilalta JL (1995). Positional cerebral ischaemia. *Cerebrovasc Dis* 5: 313–14.

Glick R, Hoying J, Cerullo L, Perlman S (1987). Phenylpropanolamine: an over-the-counter drug causing central nervous system vasculitis and intracerebral haemorrhage. Case report and review. *Neurosurgery* 20: 969–74.

Gloag D (1992). Exercise, fitness, and health: people need to be more active more often. *Br Med J* 305: 377–8.

Glynn JR (1993). A question of attribution. *Lancet* 342: 530–2.

Gomez CR (1990). Carotid plaque morphology and risk for stroke. *Stroke* 21: 148–51.

Good DC, Frank S, Verhulst S, Sharma B (1986). Cardiac abnormalities in stroke patients with negative arteriograms. *Stroke* 17: 6–11.

Gorelick PB (1987). Alcohol and stroke. *Stroke* 18: 268–71.

Gortler M, Niethammer R, Widner B (1994). Differentiating subtotal carotid artery stenoses from occlusions by colour-coded duplex sonography. *J Neurol* 241: 301–5.

Gower DJ, Lewis JC, McWhorter JM, Davis CH (1987). Carotid plaque as a source of emboli in humans: a scanning electron microscopic study. *Neurosurgery* 20: 362–8.

Grady PA (1984). Pathophysiology of extracranial cerebral arterial stenosis—a critical review. *Stroke* 15: 224–36.

Grau AJ, Buggle F, Heindl S *et al.* (1995). Recent infection as a risk factor for cerebrovascular ischaemia. *Stroke* 26: 373–9.

Graus P, Rogers LR, Posner JB (1985). Cerebrovascular complications in patients with cancer. *Medicine* 64: 16–35.

Grewal RP (1994). Stroke in Fabry's disease. *J Neurol* 241: 153–6.

Grosset DG, Georgiadis D, Kelman AW, Lees KR (1993). Quantification of ultrasound emboli signals in patients with cardiac and carotid disease. *Stroke* 24: 1922–4.

Grosset DG, Georgiadis D, Abdullah I, Bone I, Lees KR (1994). Doppler emboli signals vary according to stroke subtype. *Stroke* 25: 382–4.

Gunning AJ, Pickering GW, Robb-Smith AHT, Russell RR (1964). Mural thrombosis of the internal carotid artery and subsequent embolism. *Quart J Med* 33: 155–95.

Gustafsson C, Blomback M, Britton M, Hamsten A, Svensson J (1990). Coagulation factors and the increased risk of stroke in nonvalvular atrial fibrillation. *Stroke* 21: 47–51.

Guyer DR, Miller NR, Auer CL, Fine SL (1985). The risk of cerebrovascular and cardiovascular disease in patients with anterior ischaemic optic neuropathy. *Arch Ophthalmol* 103: 1136–42.

Haapanen A, Koskenvou M, Kaprio J, Kesaniemi YA, Heikkila K (1989). Carotid arteriosclerosis in identical twins discordant for cigarette smoking. *Circulation* 80: 10–16.

Haines AP, Imeson JD, Meade TW (1987). Phobic anxiety and ischaemic heart disease. *Br Med J* 295: 297–9.

Hammermeister KE, Sethi GK, Henderson WG, Oprian C, Kim T, Rahimtoola S, for the Veterans Affairs Cooperative Study on Valvular Heart Disease (1993). A comparison of outcomes in men 11 years after heart-valve replacement with a mechanical valve or bioprosthesis. *N Engl J Med* 328: 1289–96.

Hankey GJ, Gubbay SS (1987). Focal cerebral ischaemia and infarction due to antihypertensive therapy. *Med J Austr* 146: 412–14.

Hankey GJ, Warlow CP (1990). Symptomatic carotid ischaemic events: safest and most cost effective way of selecting patients for angiography, before carotid endarterectomy. *Br Med J* 300: 1485–91.

Hankey GJ, Warlow CP (1991a). Prognosis of symptomatic carotid artery occlusion: an overview. *Cerebrovasc Dis* 1: 245–56.

Hankey GJ, Warlow CP (1991b). Lacunar transient ischaemic attacks: a clinically useful concept? *Lancet* 337: 335–8.

Hankey G, Warlow CP (1992). Cost-effective investigation of patients with suspected transient ischaemic attacks. *J Neurol Neurosurg Psychiatr* 55: 171–6.

Hankey GJ, Slattery J, Warlow CP (1991). Prognosis and prognostic factors of retinal infarction: a prospective cohort study. *Br Med J* 302: 499–504.

Hankey GJ, Warlow CP, Molyneux AJ (1990a). Complications of cerebral angiography for patients with mild carotid territory ischaemia being considered for cartotid endarterectomy. *J Neurol Neurosurg Psychiatr* 53: 542–8.

Hankey GJ, Warlow CP, Sellar RJ (1990b). Cerebral angiographic risk in mild cerebrovascular disease. *Stroke* 21: 209–22.

Hannaford PC, Croft PR, Kay CR (1994). Oral contraception and stroke: evidence from the Royal College of General Practitioners' Oral Contraception Study. *Stroke* 25: 935–42.

Harmsen P, Rosengren A, Tsipogianni A, Wilhelmsen L (1990).

Risk factors for stroke in middle-aged men in Goteborg, Sweden. *Stroke* 21: 223–9.

Harries DP, de Silva R (1992). 'Ecstasy' and intracerebral haemorrhage. *Scot Med J* 37: 150–2.

Harrington H, Heller A, Dawson D, Caplan L, Rumbaugh C (1983). Intracerebral haemorrhage and oral amphetamine. *Arch Neurol* 40: 503–7.

Harrison MJG, Marshall J (1977). The finding of thrombus at carotid endarterectomy and its relationship to the timing of surgery. *Br J Surg* 64: 511–12.

Harrison MJG, Marshall J (1988). The variable clinical and CT findings after carotid occlusion: the role of collateral blood supply. *J Neurol Neurosurg Psychiatr* 51: 269–72.

Hart RG (1992). Cardiogenic embolism to the brain. *Lancet* 339: 589–94.

Hart RG, Halperin JL (1994). Atrial fibrillation and stroke: revisiting the dilemmas. *Stroke* 25: 1337–41.

Hart RG, Foster JW, Luther MF, Kanter MC (1990). Stroke in infective endocarditis. *Stroke* 21: 695–700.

Hayreh SS (1981). Anterior ischaemic optic neuropathy. *Arch Neurol* 38: 675–8.

Hebert PR, Gaziano JM, Hennekens CH (1995). An overview of trials of cholesterol lowering and risk of stroke. *Arch Intern Med* 155: 50–5.

Heiken JP, Brink JA, Vannier MW (1993). Spiral (helical) CT. *Radiology* 189: 647–56.

Heiserman JE, Drayer BP, Fram EK *et al.* (1992). Carotid artery stenosis: clinical efficacy of two-dimensional time-of-flight MR angiography. *Radiology* 182: 761–8.

Hennekens CH, Buring JE, Peto R (1994). Antioxidant vitamins— benefits not yet proved. *N Engl J Med* 330: 1080–1.

Hennerici M, Steinke W (1991). Carotid plaque developments: aspects of haemodynamic and vessel wall–platelet interaction. *Cerebrovasc Dis* 1: 142–8.

Herderschee D, Hijdra A, Algra A, Koudstaal PJ, Kappelle LJ, van Gijn J, for the Dutch TIA Study Group (1992). Silent stroke in patients with transient ischaemic attack or minor ischaemic stroke. *Stroke* 23: 1220–4.

Herman B, Schmitz PIM, Leyten ACM *et al.* (1983). Multivariate logistic analysis of risk factors for stroke in Tilburg, The Netherlands. *Am J Epidemiol* 118: 514–25.

Hertog MGL, Feskens EJM, Hollman PCH, Katan MB, Kromhout D (1993). Dietary antioxidant flavonoids and risk of coronary heart disease: the Zutphen Elderly Study. *Lancet* 342: 1007–11.

Hertzer NR, Young JR, Beven EG *et al.* (1985). Coronary angiography in 506 patients with extracranial cerebrovascular disease. *Arch Intern Med* 145: 849–52.

Hinton RC, Kistler JP, Fallon JT, Friedlich AL, Fisher CM (1977). Influence of etiology of atrial fibrillation on incidence of systemic embolism. *Am J Cardiol* 40: 509–13.

Homer D, Ingall TJ, Baker HL, O'Fallon WM, Kottke BA, Whisnant JP (1991). Serum lipids and lipoproteins are less powerful predictors of extracranial carotid artery atherosclerosis than are cigarette smoking and hypertension. *Mayo Clin Proc* 66:

259–67.

Hommel M, Besson G, Le Bas JF *et al.* (1990). Prospective study of lacunar infarction using magnetic resonance imaging. *Stroke* 21: 546–54.

Hommel M, Grand S, Devoulon P, Le Bas J-F (1994). New directions in magnetic resonance in acute cerebral ischaemia. *Cerebrovasc Dis* 4: 3–11.

Hopkins A, Menken M, DeFriese GH, Feldman RG (1989). Differences in strategies for the diagnosis and treatment of neurologic disease among British and American neurologists. *Arch Neurol* 46: 1142–8.

Hopkins PN, Williams RR (1981). A survey of 246 suggested coronary risk factors. *Atherosclerosis* 40: 1–52.

Horowitz DR, Tuhrim S, Weinberger JM, Rudolp SH (1992). Mechanisms in lacunar infarction. *Stroke* 23: 325–7.

House A, Dennis M, Mogridge L, Hawton K, Warlow C (1990). Life events and difficulties preceding stroke. *J Neurol Neurosurg Psychiatr* 53: 1024–8.

Howard G, Anderson R, Sorlie P, Andrews V, Backlund E, Burke GL (1994). Ethnic differences in stroke mortality between non-Hispanic whites, Hispanic whites, and blacks: the national longitudinal mortality study. *Stroke* 25: 2120–5.

Howard G, Chambless LE, Baker WH *et al.* (1991). A multicentre validation study of Doppler ultrasound versus angiography. *J Stroke Cerebrovasc Dis* 1: 166–73.

Hugh AE, Fox JA (1970). The precise localisation of atheroma and its association with stasis at the origin of the internal carotid artery—a radiographic investigation. *Br J Radiol* 43: 377–83.

Humphrey P, Sandercock P, Slattery J (1990). A simple method to improve the accuracy of non-invasive ultrasound in selecting TIA patients for cerebral angiography. *J Neurol Neurosurg Psychiatr* 53: 966–71.

Hupperts RMM, Lodder J, Heuts-van Raak EPM, Kessels F (1994). Infarcts in the anterior choroidal artery territory: anatomical distribution, clinical syndromes, presumed pathogenesis and early outcome. *Brain* 117: 825–34.

Hupperts RMM, Lodder J, Wilmink J, Boiten J, Heuts-van Raak EPM (1993). Haemodynamic mechanism in small subcortical borderzone infarcts? *Cerebrovasc Dis* 3: 231–5.

Hupperts RMM, Lodder J, Heits-van Raak EPM, Wilmink JT, Kessels AGH (1996). Borderzone brain infarction on CT taking into account the variability in vascular supply artery. *Cerebrovasc Dis* (in press).

Hutchinson EC (1972). Lesions in cerebrovascular disease and their clinical implications. *Br Med J* 1: 89–91.

Hutchinson EC, Yates PO (1957). Carotico-vertebral stenosis. *Lancet* i: 2–8.

Illangasekera VLU (1981). Insulinoma masquerading as carotid transient ischaemic attacks. *Postgrad Med J* 57: 232–4.

Imparato AM, Riles TS, Gorstein F (1979). The carotid bifurcation plaque: pathologic findings associated with cerebral ischaemia. *Stroke* 10: 238–45.

Isner JM, Estes, NA, Thompson PD *et al.* (1986). Acute cardiac events temporally related to cocaine abuse. *N Engl J Med* 315:

1438–43.

Jackson M, Lennox G, Jaspan T, Lowe J (1993). Cerebral venous and systemic thrombosis in resolving ulcerative colitis. *Cerebrovasc Dis* 3: 178–9.

Jacobson DM, Terrence CF, Reinmuth OM (1986). The neurologic manifestations of fat embolism. *Neurology* 36: 847–51.

Jauss M, Kaps M, Keberle M, Haberbosch W, Dorndorf W (1994). A comparison of transoesophageal echocardiography and transcranial Doppler sonography with contrast medium for detection of patent foramen ovale. *Stroke* 25: 1265–7.

Jeanrenaud X, Kappenberger L (1991). Patent foramen ovale and stroke of unknown origin. *Cerebrovasc Dis* 1: 184–92.

Jeans WD, Mackenzie S, Baird RN (1986). Angiography in transient cerebral ischaemia using three views of the carotid bifurcation. *Br J Radiol* 59: 135–42.

Johns DR (1991). Cerebrovascular complications of inflammatory bowel disease. *Am J Gastroenterol* 86: 367–70.

Johnston DW (1993). The current status of the coronary prone behaviour pattern. *J Roy Soc Med* 86: 406–9.

Jones HR, Siekert RG (1989). Neurological manifestations of infective endocarditis. *Brain* 112: 1295–315.

Jorens PG, Delvigne CR, Hermans CR, Haber I, Holvoet J, De Deyn PP (1991). Cerebral arterial thrombosis preceding ulcerative colitis. *Stroke* 22: 1212.

Jorgensen HS, Nakayama H, Raaschou HO, Olsen TS (1994c). Stroke in patients with diabetes: the Copenhagen Stroke Study. *Stroke* 25: 1977–84.

Jorgensen HS, Jespersen HF, Nakayama H, Raaschou HO, Olsen TS (1994a). Headache in stroke: the Copenhagen Stroke Study. *Neurology* 44: 1793–7.

Jorgensen HS, Nakayama H, Raaschou HO, Gam J, Olsen TS (1994b). Silent infarction in acute stroke patients: prevalence, localisation, risk factors and clinical significance: the Copenhagen Stroke Study. *Stroke* 25: 97–104.

Joynt RJ, Zimmerman G, Khalifeh R (1965). Cerebral emboli from cardiac tumours. *Arch Neurol* 12: 84–91.

Kagan A, Popper JS, Rhoads GG (1980). Factors related to stroke incidence in Hawaii Japanese men: the Honolulu Heart Study. *Stroke* 11: 14–21.

Kagan AR (1976). Atherosclerosis and myocardial lesions in subjects dying from fresh cerebrovascular disease. *Bull World Heath Org* 53: 597–600.

Kamata T, Yokata T, Furukawa T, Tsukagoshi H (1994). Cerebral ischaemic attack caused by postprandial hypotension. *Stroke* 25: 511–13.

Kandt RS, Gebarski SS, Goetting MG (1985). Tuberous sclerosis with cardiogenic cerebral embolism: magnetic resonance imaging. *Neurology* 35: 1223–5.

Kannel WB, Anderson K, Wilson PWF (1992). White blood cell count and cardiovascular disease: insights from the Framingham Study. *J Am Med Assoc* 267: 1253–6.

Kannel WB, Wolf PA, Verter J (1983). Manifestations of coronary disease predisposing to stroke: the Framingham Study. *J Am Med Assoc* 250: 2942–6.

Kannel WB, Wolf PA, McGee DL, Dawber TR, McNamara P, Castelli WP (1981). Systolic blood pressure, arterial rigidity, and risk of stroke: the Framingham Study. *J Am Med Assoc* 245: 1225–9.

Kanter MC, Hart RG (1991). Neurologic complications of infective endocarditis. *Neurology* 41: 1015–20.

Kanter MC, Tegeler CH, Pearce LA *et al.* on behalf of the Stroke Prevention in Atrial Fibrillation Investigators (1994). Carotid stenosis in patients with atrial fibrillation. *Arch Intern Med* 154: 1372–7.

Kaplan NM (1995). Alcohol and hypertension. *Lancet* 345: 1588–9.

Kaplan PW (1993). Focal seizures resembling transient ischaemic attacks due to subclinical ischaemia. *Cerebrovasc Dis* 3: 241–3.

Kapoor R, Kendall BE, Harrison MJG (1991). Permanent oculomotor palsy with occlusion of the internal carotid artery. *J Neurol Neurosurg Psychiatr* 54: 745–6.

Kappelle LJ, van Gijn J (1986). Lacunar infarcts. *Clin Neurol Neurosurg* 88: 3–17.

Kappelle LJ, Koudstaal PJ, van Gijn J, Ramos LMP, Keunen JEE (1988). Carotid angiography in patients with lacunar infarction: a prospective study. *Stroke* 19: 1093–6.

Karanjia PN, Madden KP, Lobner S (1994). Co-existence of abdominal aortic aneurysm in patients with carotid stenosis. *Stroke* 25: 627–30.

Kardinaal AFM, Kok FJ, Ringstad J *et al.* (1993). Antioxidants in adipose tissue and risk of myocardial infarction: the EURAMIC Study. *Lancet* 342: 1379–84.

Kasarskis EJ, O'Connor W, Earle G (1988). Embolic stroke from cardiac papillary fibroelastomas. *Stroke* 19: 1171–3.

Kase CS, Foster TE, Reed JE, Spatz EL, Girgis GN (1987). Intracerebral haemorrhage and phenylpropanolamine use. *Neurology* 37: 399–404.

Kawachi I, Colditz GA, Stampfer MJ *et al.* (1993). Smoking cessation and decreased risk of stroke in women. *J Am Med Assoc* 269: 232–6.

Kawachi I, Colditz GA, Stone CB (1994). Does coffee drinking increase the risk of coronary heart disease? Results from a meta-analysis. *Br Heart J* 72: 269–75.

Kazui S, Sawada T, Naritomi H, Kuriyama Y, Yamaguchi T (1993). Angiographic evaluation of brain infraction limited to the anterior cerebral artery territory. *Stroke* 24: 549–53.

Keli S, Bloemberg B, Kromhout D (1992). Predictive value of repeated systolic blood pressure measurements for stroke risk: the Zutphen Study. *Stroke* 23: 347–51.

Keli SO, Feskens EJM, Kromhout D (1994). Fish consumption and risk of stroke: the Zutphen study. *Stroke* 25: 328–32.

Kelley RE, Bell L, Kelley SE, Lee S-C (1989). Syphilis detection in cerebrovascular disease. *Stroke* 20: 230–4.

Kelly DP, Strauss AW (1994). Inherited cardiomyopathies. *N Engl J Med* 330: 913–19.

Kempster PA, Gerraty RP, Gates PC (1988). Asymptomatic cerebral infarction in patients with chronic atrial fibrillation. *Stroke* 19: 955–7.

Kendell RE, Marshall J (1963). Role of hypotension in the genesis of transient focal cerebral ischaemic attacks. *Br Med J* 2: 344–8.

Khaffaf N, Karnik R, Winker W-B, Valentin A, Slany J (1994). Embolic stroke by compression manoeuvre during transcranial Doppler sonography. *Stroke* 25: 1056–7.

Khaw K-T, Barrett-Connor E (1987). Dietary potassium and stroke-associated mortality: a 12-year prospective population study. *N Engl J Med* 316: 235–40.

Kiechl S, Willeit J, Egger G, Oberhollenzer M, Aichner F (1994). Alcohol consumption and carotid atherosclerosis: evidence of dose-dependent atherogenic and antiatherogenic effects. Results from the Bruneck Study. *Stroke* 25: 1593–8.

Kiely DK, Wolf PA, Cupples LA, Beiser AS, Myers RH (1993). Familial aggregation of stroke: the Framingham Study. *Stroke* 24: 1366–71.

Kittner SJ, Sharkness CM, Price TR *et al.* (1991). Infarcts with a cardiac source of embolism in the NINCDS Stroke Data Bank: historical features. *Neurology* 40: 281–4.

Kittner SJ, Sharkness CM, Sloan MA *et al.* (1992). Features on initial computed tomography scan of infarcts with a cardiac source of embolism in the NINDS stroke data bank. *Stroke* 23: 1748–51.

Kiyohara Y, Kato I, Iwamoto H, Nakayama K, Fujishima M (1995). The impact of alcohol and hypertension on stroke incidence in a general Japanese population: the Hisayama study. *Stroke* 26: 368–72.

Kleinschmidt A, Steinmetz H, Sitzer M, Merboldt K-D, Frahm J (1995). Magnetic resonance imaging of regional cerebral blood oxygenation changes under acetazolamide in carotid occlusive disease. *Stroke* 26: 106–10.

Kleiser B, Widder B (1992). Course of carotid artery occlusions with impaired cerebrovascular reactivity. *Stroke* 23: 171–4.

Kleiser B, Krapf H, Widder B (1991). Carbon dioxide reactivity and patterns of cerebral infarction in patients with carotid artery occlusion. *J Neurol* 238: 392–4.

Klotzsch C, Janssen G, Berlit P (1994). Transesophageal echocardiography and contrast-TCD in the detection of a patent foramen ovale: experiences with 111 patients. *Neurology* 44: 1603–6.

Knepper LE, Biller J, Adams HP, Bruno A (1988). Neurologic manifestations of atrial myxoma: a 12-year experience and review. *Stroke* 19: 1435–40.

Knutsen R, Knutsen SF, Curb JD, Reed DM, Kautz JA, Yano K (1988). Predictive value of resting electrocardiograms for 12-year incidence of stroke in the Honolulu Heart Program. *Stroke* 19: 555–9.

Konzen JP, Steven SR, Garcia JH (1995). Vasospasm and thrombus formation as possible mechanisms of stroke related to alkaloidal cocaine. *Stroke* 26: 1114–18.

Kopecky SJ, Gersh BJ, McGoon MD *et al.* (1987). The natural history of lone atrial fibrillation: a population-based study over three decades. *N Engl J Med* 317: 669–74.

Koudstaal PJ, van Gijn J, Kappelle LJ, for the Dutch TIA Study Group (1991a). Headache in transient or permanent cerebral ischaemia. *Stroke* 22: 754–9.

Koudstaal PJ, van Gijn J, Frenken CWGM *et al.* for the Dutch TIA Study Group (1992). TIA, RIND, minor stroke: a continuum, or different subgroups? *J Neurol Neurosurg Psychiatr* 95: 71–4.

Koudstaal PJ, van Gijn J, Lodder J *et al.* for the Dutch TIA Study Group (1991b). Transient ischaemic attacks with and without a relevant infarct on computed tomographic scans cannot be distinguished clinically. *Arch Neurol* 48: 916–20.

Krendel DA, Ditter SM, Frankel MR, Ross WK (1990). Biopsy-proven cerebral vasculitis associated with cocaine abuse. *Neurology* 40: 1092–4.

Kumral E, Bogousslavsky J, van Melle G, Regli F, Pierre P (1995). Headache at stroke onset: the Lausanne Stroke Registry. *J Neurol Neurosurg Psychiatr* 58: 490–2.

Lancet (1985). Alcohol and atrial fibrillation. *Lancet* i: 1374.

Lancet (1990). Who's for tennis? *Lancet* 336: 1157–8.

Lancman ME, Golimstok A, Norscini J, Granillo R (1993). Risk factors for developing seizures after a stroke. *Epilepsia* 34: 141–3.

Landi G, Cella E, Boccardi E, Musicco M (1992a). Lacunar versus non-lacunar infarcts: pathogenetic and prognostic differences. *J Neurol Neurosurg Psychiatr* 55: 441–5.

Landi G, D'Angelo A, Boccardi E *et al.* (1992b). Venous thromboembolism in acute stroke: prognostic importance of hypercoagulability. *Arch Neurol* 49: 279–83.

Landi G, Motto C, Cella E *et al.* (1993). Pathogenetic and prognostic features of lacunar transient ischaemic attack syndromes. *J Neurol Neurosurg Psychiatr* 56: 1265–70.

Langer RD, Ganiats TG, Barrett-Connor E (1991). Factors associated with paradoxical survival at higher blood pressures in the very old. *Am J Epidemiol* 134: 29–38.

Law MR, Frost CD, Wald NJ (1991a). By how much does dietary salt reduction lower blood pressure? I—analysis of observational data among populations. *Br Med J* 302: 811–15.

Law MR, Frost CD, Wald NJ (1991b). By how much does dietary salt reduction lower blood pressure? III—analysis of data from trials of salt reduction. *Br Med J* 302: 819–24.

Law MR, Thompson SG, Wald NJ (1994b). Assessing possible hazards of reducing serum cholesterol. *Br Med J* 308: 373–9.

Law MR, Wald NJ, Thompson SG (1994a). By how much and how quickly does reduction in serum cholesterol concentration lower risk of ischaemic heart disease? *Br Med J* 308: 367–73.

Lee I-M, Paffenbarger RS (1992). Change in body weight and longevity. *J Am Med Assoc* 268: 2045–9.

Leon DA (1993). Failed or misleading adjustment for confounding. *Lancet* 342: 479–81.

Lerner DJ, Kannel WB (1986). Patterns of coronary heart disease morbidity and mortality in the sexes: a 26 year follow up of the Framingham population. *Am Heart J* 111: 383–90.

Leung SY, Ng THK, Yuen ST, Lauder IJ, Ho FCS (1993). Pattern of cerebral atherosclerosis in Hong Kong Chinese: severity in intracranial and extracranial vessels. *Stroke* 24: 779–86.

Levine S, Brust JCM, Futrell N *et al.* (1990). Cerebrovascular complications of the use of the 'crack' form of alkaloidal cocaine. *N Engl J Med* 323: 699–704.

Levy D, Savage D (1987). Prevalence and clinical features of mitral valve prolapse. *Am Heart J* 113: 1281–90.

Levy D, Garrison RJ, Savage DD, Kannel WB, Castelli WP (1990). Prognostic implications of echocardiographically determined left ventricular mass in the Framingham Heart Study. *N Engl J Med* 322: 1561–6.

Ley-Pozo J, Ringelstein EB (1990). Noninvasive detection of occlusive disease of the carotid siphon and middle cerebral artery. *Ann Neurol* 28: 640–7.

Leys D, Pruvo JP, Godefroy O, Rondepierre Ph, Leclerc X (1992). Prevalence and significance of hyperdense middle cerebral artery in acute stroke. *Stroke* 23: 317–24.

Leys D, Mounier-Vehier F, Lavenue I, Rondepierre Ph, Pruvo JP (1994). Anterior choroidal artery territory infarcts: study of presumed mechanisms. *Stroke* 25: 837–42.

Lhermitte F, Gautier JC, Derouesne C (1970). Nature of occlusions of the middle cerebral artery. *Neurology* 20: 82–8.

Libman RB, Masters SR, de Paola A, Mohr JP (1993). Transient monocular blindness associated with cocaine abuse. *Neurology* 43: 228–9.

Lindberg G, Eklund GA, Gullberg B, Rastam L (1991). Serum sialic acid concentration and cardiovascular mortality. *Br Med J* 302: 143–6.

Lindenstrom E, Boysen G, Nyboe J (1993). Lifestyle factors and risk of cerebrovascular disease in women: the Copenhagen City Heart Study. *Stroke* 24: 1468–72.

Lindenstrom E, Boysen G, Nyboe J (1994). Influence of total cholesterol, high density lipoprotein cholesterol, and triglycerides on risk of cerebrovascular disease: the Copenhagen City Heart Study. *Br Med J* 309: 11–15.

Lindgren A, Norrving B, Rudling O, Johansson BB (1994a). Comparison of clincal and neuroradiological findings in first-ever stroke: a population-based study. *Stroke* 25: 1371–7.

Lindgren A, Brattstrom L, Norrving B, Hultberg B, Andersson A, Johansson BB (1995). Plasma homocysteine in the acute and convalescent phase after stroke. *Stroke* 26: 795–800.

Lindgren A, Roijer A, Norrving B, Wallin L, Eskilsson J, Johansson BB (1994b). Carotid artery and heart disease in subtypes of cerebral infarction. *Stroke* 25: 2356–62.

Lodder J, Bamford J, Kappelle J, Boiten J (1994). What causes false clinical prediction of small deep infarcts? *Stroke* 25: 86–91.

Lodder J, Bamford JM, Sandercock PAG, Jones LN, Warlow CP (1990). Are hypertension or cardiac embolism likely cause of lacunar infarction? *Stroke* 21: 375–81.

Lopez JA, Ross RS, Fishbein MC, Siegel RJ (1987). Nonbacterial thrombotic endocarditis: a review. *Am Heart J* 113: 773–84.

Lossos A, River Y, Eliakim A, Steiner I (1995). Neurological aspects of inflammatory bowel disease. *Neurology* 45: 416–21.

Love BB, Grover-McKay M, Biller J, Rezai K, McKay CR (1992). Coronary artery disease and cardiac events with asymptomatic and symptomatic cerebrovascular disease. *Stroke* 23: 939–45.

Lusiani L, Visona A, Castellani V et al. (1987). Prevalence of atherosclerotic involvement of the internal carotid artery in hypertensive patients. *Int J Cardiol* 17: 51–6.

Lynch JW, Kaplan GA, Cohen RD et al. (1994). Childhood and adult socioeconomic status as predictors of mortality in Finland.

Lancet 343: 524–7.

McKeigre PM, Shah B, Marmot MG (1991). Relation of central obesity and insulin resistance with high diabetes prevalence and cardiovascular risk in South Asians. *Lancet* i: 337, 382–6.

MacMahon SW, Norton RN (1986). Alcohol and hypertension: implications for prevention and treatment. *Ann Intern Med* 105: 124–6.

MacMahon S, Rodgers A (1993). The effects of blood pressure reduction in older patients: an overview of five randomised controlled trials in elderly hypertensives. *Clin Exp Hyperten* 15 (6): 967–78.

MacMahon S, Rodgers A (1994). Antihypertensive agents and stroke prevention. *Cerebrovasc Dis* 4 (Suppl. 1): 11–15.

MacMahon S, Peto R, Cutler J et al. (1990). Blood pressure, stroke, and coronary heart disease. Part 1. Prolonged differences in blood pressure: prospective observational studies corrected for the regression dilution bias. *Lancet* 335: 765–74.

McMillan DE (1985). Blood flow and the localization of atherosclerotic plaques. *Stroke* 16: 582–7.

Malouf R, Brust JCM (1985). Hypoglycaemia: causes, neurological manifestations, and outcome. *Ann Neurol* 17: 421–30.

Mandai K, Sueyoshi K, Fukunaga R et al. (1994). Evaluation of cerebral vasoreactivity by three-dimensional time-of-flight magnetic resonance angiography. *Stroke* 25: 1807–11.

Manson JE, Colditz GA, Stampfer MJ et al. (1991). A prospective study of maturity-onset diabetes mellitus and risk of coronary heart disease and stroke in women. *Arch Intern Med* 151: 1141–7.

Manson JE, Nathan DM, Krolewski AS, Stampfer MJ, Willett WC, Hennekens CH (1992). A prospective study of exercise and incidence of diabetes among US male physicians. *J Am Med Assoc* 268: 63–7.

Mapstone T, Spetzler RF (1982). Vertebrobasilar insufficiency secondary to vertebral artery occlusion from a fibrous band: case report. *J Neurosurg* 56: 581–3.

Marini C, Carolei A, Roberts RS et al. (1993). Focal cerebral ischaemia in young adults: a collaborative case–control study. *Neuroepidemiology* 12: 70–81.

Markel ML, Waller BF, Armstrong WF (1987). Cardiac myxoma: a review. *Medicine* 66: 114–25.

Markus HS (1993). Transcranial Doppler detection of circulating cerebral emboli: a review. *Stroke* 24: 1246–50.

Markus HS, Brown MM (1993). Differentiation between different pathological cerebral embolic materials using transcranial Doppler in an *in vitro* model. *Stroke* 24: 1–5.

Markus HS, Harrison MJG (1992). The estimation of cerebrovascular reactivity using transcranial Doppler, including the use of breath-holding as the vasodilatory stimulus. *Stroke* 23: 668–73.

Markus HS, Droste DW, Brown MM (1994). Detection of asymptomatic cerebral embolic signals with Doppler ultrasound. *Lancet* 343: 1011–12.

Marmot M, Brunner E (1991). Alcohol and cardiovascular diseases: the status of the U shaped curve. *Br Med J* 303: 565–8.

Marmot MG, Davey Smith G, Stansfeld S *et al.* (1991). Health inequalities among British civil servants: the Whitehall II study. *Lancet* 337: 1387–93.

Marmot MG, Elliott P, Shipley MJ *et al.* (1994). Alcohol and blood pressure: the INTERSALT study. *Br Med J* 308: 1263–7.

Martin R, Bogousslavsky J (1995). Embolic versus nonembolic causes of ischaemic stroke. *Cerebrovasc Dis* 5: 70–4.

Martin R, Bogousslavsky J, Miklossy J *et al.* (1992). Floating thrombus in the innominate artery as a cause of cerebral infarction in young adults. *Cerebrovasc Dis* 2: 177–81.

Mas JL (1991). Patent foramen ovale, stroke and paradoxical embolism. *Cerebrovasc Dis* 1: 181–3.

Mast H, Thompson JLP, Voller H, Mohr JP, Marx P (1994). Cardiac sources of embolism in patients with pial artery infarcts and lacunar lesions. *Stroke* 25: 776–81.

Masuda J, Yutani C, Waki R, Ogata J, Kuriyama Y, Yamaguchi T (1992). Histopathological analysis of the mechanisms of intracranial haemorrhage complicating infective endocarditis. *Stroke* 23: 843–50.

Mattle HP, Maurer D, Sturzenegger M, Ozdoba C, Baumgartner RW, Schroth G (1995). Cardiac myxomas: a long term study. *J Neurol* 242: 689–94.

Meade TW, Imeson J, Stirling Y (1987). Effects of changes in smoking and other characteristics on clotting factors and the risk of ischaemic heart disease. *Lancet* ii: 986–90.

Meade TW, Ruddock V, Stirling Y, Chakrabarti R, Miller GJ (1993). Fibrinolytic activity, clotting factors, and long-term incidence of ischaemic heart disease in the Northwick Park Heart Study. *Lancet* 342: 1076–9.

Meltzer RS, Visser CA, Fuster V (1986). Intracardiac thrombi and systemic embolization. *Ann Intern Med* 104: 689–98.

Mendez I, Hachinski V, Wolfe B (1987). Serum lipids after stroke. *Neurology* 37: 507–11.

Menotti A, Lanti M, Seccareccia F, Giampaoli S, Dima F (1993). Multivariate prediction of the first major cerebrovascular event in an Italian population sample of middle-aged men followed up for 25 years. *Stroke* 24: 42–8.

Miller VT, Cohen BA (1987). Angiographic comparison of carotid arteries in unilateral cerebral ischaemia. *Neurology* 37: 1027–30.

Millikan C, Futrell N (1990). The fallacy of the lacune hypothesis. *Stroke* 21: 1251–7.

Mills RM (1971). Severe hypersensitivity reactions associated with Allopurinol. *J Am Med Assoc* 216: 799–802.

Mitchell JRA, Schwartz CJ (1962). Relationship between arterial disease in different sites: a study of the aorta and coronary, carotid and iliac arteries. *Br Med J* 1: 1293–301.

Mitchinson MJ, Ball RY (1987). Macrophages and atherogenesis *Lancet* ii: 146–8.

Mittl RL, Broderick M, Carpenter JP *et al.* (1994). Blinded-reader comparison of magnetic resonance angiography and Duplex ultrasonography for carotid artery bifurcation stenosis. *Stroke* 25: 4–10.

Miyashita K, Naritomi H, Sawada T *et al.* (1988). Identification of recent lacunar lesions in cases of multiple small infarctions by magnetic resonance imaging. *Stroke* 19: 834–9.

Mohr JP, Biller J, Hilal SK *et al.* (1995). Magnetic resonance versus computed tomographic imaging in acute stroke. *Stroke* 26: 807–12.

Motomiya M, Karino T (1984). Flow patterns in the human carotid artery bifurcation. *Stroke* 15: 50–5.

Mudd SH, Skovby F, Levy HL *et al.* (1985). The natural history of homocystinuria due to cystathionine beta-synthase deficiency. *Am J Hum Genet* 37: 1–31.

Mulrow CD, Cornell JA, Herrera CR, Kadri A, Farnett L, Aguilar C (1994). Hypertension in the elderly: implications and generalizability of randomised trials. *J Am Med Assoc* 272: 1932–8.

Nater B, Bogousslavksy J, Regli F, Stauffer J-C (1992). Stroke patterns with atrial septal aneurysm. *Cerebrovasc Dis* 2: 342–6.

Natowicz M, Kelly RI (1987). Mendelian aetiologies of stroke. *Ann Neurol* 22: 175–92.

Naylor AR (1992). Transcranial Doppler sonography. In: Miller JD, Teasdale G, eds. *Current Neurosurgery*. Edinburgh: Churchill Livingstone, 77–100.

Naylor AR, Sandercock PAG, Sellar RJ, Warlow CP (1993). Patterns of vascular pathology in acute, first-ever cerebral infarction. *Scot Med J* 38: 41–4.

Naylor AR, Merrick MV, Gillespie I *et al.* (1994). Prevalence of impaired cerebrovascular reserve in patients with symptomatic carotid artery disease. *Br J Surg* 81: 45–8.

Nestico PF, Depace NL, Morganroth J, Kotler MN, Ross J (1984). Mitral annular calcification: clinical, pathophysiology, and echocardiographic review. *Am Heart J* 107: 989–96.

Nichols FT, Mawad M, Mohr JP, Stein B, Hilal S, Michelsen WJ (1990). Focal headache during balloon inflation in the internal carotid and middle cerebral arteries. *Stroke* 21: 555–9.

Nighoghossian N, Ryvlin P, Trouillas P, Laharotte JC, Froment JC (1993). Pontine versus capsular pure motor hemiparesis. *Neurology* 43: 2197–201.

Nishide M, Irino T, Gotoh M, Naka M, Tsuji K (1983). Cardiac abnormalities in ischaemic cerebrovascular disease studied by two-dimensional echocardiography. *Stroke* 14: 541–5.

Nobile-Orazio E, Sterzi R (1981). Cerebral ischaemia after nifedipine treatment. *Br Med J* 283: 948.

Norris JW, Bornstein NM (1986). Progression and regression of carotid stenosis. *Stroke* 17: 755–7.

Norrving B, Cronqvist S (1989). Clinical and radiologic features of lacunar versus nonlacunar minor stroke. *Stroke* 20: 59–64.

O'Connor GT, Buring JE, Yusuf S *et al.* (1989). An overview of randomised trials of rehabilitation with exercise after myocardial infarction. *Circulation* 80: 234–44.

O'Donoghue ME, Dangond F, Burger AJ, Suojanen JN, Zarich S, Tarsy D (1993). Spontaneous calcific embolization to the supraclinoid internal carotid artery from a regurgitant bicuspid aortic valve. *Neurology* 43: 2715–17.

Ogata J, Masuda J, Yutani C, Yamaguchi T (1990). Rupture of atheromatous plaque as a cause of thrombotic occlusion of stenotic internal carotid artery. *Stroke* 21: 1740–5.

Ogata J, Masuda J, Yutani C, Yamaguchi T (1994). Mechanisms

of cerebral artery thrombosis: a histopathological analysis on eight necropsy cases. *J Neurol Neurosurg Psychiatr* 57: 17–21.

Ogren M, Hedblad B, Isacsson S-O, Janzon L, Jungquist G, Lindell S-E (1995). Ten year cerebrovascular morbidity and mortality in 68 year old men with asymptomatic carotid stenosis. *Br Med J* 310: 1294–8.

O'Leary DH, Bryan FA, Goodison MW *et al.* (1987). Measurement variability of carotid atherosclerosis: real-time (B-mode) ultrasonography and angiography. *Stroke* 18: 1011–17.

O'Leary DH, Polak JF, Kronmal RA *et al.* on behalf of the CHS Collaborative Research Group (1992). Distribution and correlates of sonographically detected carotid artery disease in the Cardiovascular Health Study. *Stroke* 23: 1752–60.

Olsen TS, Skriver EB, Herning M (1985). Cause of cerebral infarction in the carotid territory: its relation to the size and the location of the infarct and to the underlying vascular lesion. *Stroke* 16: 459–66.

O'Malley T, Langhorne P, Elton RA, Stewart C (1995). Platelet size in stroke patients. *Stroke* 26: 995–9.

Orencia AJ, Petty GW, Khandheria BK, O'Fallon WM, Whisnant JP (1995b). Mitral valve prolapse and the risk of stroke after initial cerebral ischaemia. *Neurology* 45: 1083–6.

Orencia AJ, Petty GW, Khandheria BK *et al.* (1995a). Risk of stroke with mitral valve prolapse in population-based cohort study. *Stroke* 26: 7–13.

Orgogozo JM, Bogousslavsky J (1989). Lacunar syndromes. In: Vinken PJ, Bruyn GW, Klawans HL, eds. *Handbook of Clinical Neurology*, Vol. 10. Amsterdam: Elsevier Science Publishers, 235–69.

Otis S, Rush M, Boyajian R (1995). Contrast-enhanced transcranial imaging: results of an American phase-two study. *Stroke* 26: 203–9.

Paneth N, Susser M (1995). Early origin of coronary heart disease (the 'Barker hypothesis'): hypotheses, no matter how intriguing, need rigorous attempts at refutation. *Br Med J* 310: 411–12.

Panisset M, Eidelman BH (1990). Multiple cranial neuropathy as a feature of internal carotid artery dissection. *Stroke* 21: 141–7.

Pantin CFA, Young RAL (1980). Postprandial blindness. *Br Med J* 281: 1686.

Patel V, Champ C, Andrews PS, Gostelow BE, Gunasekara NPR, Davidson AR (1992). Diagonal earlobe creases and atheromatous disease: a postmortem study. *J Roy Coll Phys Lond* 26: 274–7.

Pedro-Botet J, Senti M, Nogues X *et al.* (1992). Lipoprotein and apolipoprotein profile in men with ischaemic stroke: role of lipoprotein (a), triglyceride-rich lipoproteins, and apolopoprotein E polymorphism. *Stroke* 23: 1556–62.

Pell ACH, Frier BM (1990). Restoration of perception of hypoglycaemia after hemiparesis in an insulin dependent diabetic patient. *Br Med J* 300: 369–70.

Pelz DM, Fox AJ, Vinuela F (1985). Digital subtraction angiography: current clinical applications. *Stroke* 16: 528–36.

Penner R, Font RL (1969). Retinal embolism from calcified vegetations of aortic valve. *Arch Ophthalmol* 81: 565–8.

Perry IJ, Refsum H, Morris RW, Ebrahim SB, Weland PM, Shaper AG (1995). Prospective study of serum total homocysteine concentration and risk of stroke in middle-aged British men. *Lancet* 346: 1395–8.

Petersen P (1990). Thromboembolic complications in atrial fibrillation. *Stroke* 21: 4–13.

Petty GW, Wiebers WO, Meissner I (1990). Transcranial Doppler ultrasonography: clinical applications in cerebrovascular disease. *Mayo Clin Proc* 65: 1350–64.

Phillips A, Shaper AG, Whincup PH (1989). Association between serum albumin and mortality from cardiovascular disease, cancer, and other causes. *Lancet* ii: 1434–6.

Phillips AN, Davey Smith G (1993). Confounding in epidemiological studies. *Br Med J* 306: 142–3.

Pierre Ph, Bogousslavsky J, Menetrey R, Regli F, Kappenberger L (1993). Familial sick sinus disease: another Mendelian aetiology of stroke. *Cerebrovasc Dis* 3: 120–2.

Pocock SJ, Shaper AG, Cook DG *et al.* (1980). British Regional Heart Study: geographic variations in cardiovascular mortality, and the role of water quality. *Br Med J* 280: 1243–9.

Powers WJ (1986). Should lumbar puncture be part of the routine evaluation of patients with cerebral ischaemia? *Stroke* 17: 332–3.

Powers WJ, Press GA, Grubb RL, Gado M, Raichle ME (1987). The effect of hemodynamically significant carotid artery disease on the hemodynamic status of the cerebral circulation. *Ann Intern Med* 106: 27–35.

Prospective Studies Collaboration (1995). Cholesterol, diastolic blood pressure and stroke: 13 000 strokes in 450 000 people in 45 prospective cohorts. *Lancet* 346: 1647–53.

Puddey IB, Beilin LJ, Vandongen R (1987). Regular alcohol use raises blood pressure in treated hypertensive subjects: a randomised controlled trial. *Lancet* i: 647–51.

Qizilbash N, Jones L, Warlow C, Mann J (1991). Fibrinogen and lipids as risk factors for transient ischaemic attacks and minor ischaemic strokes. *Br Med J* 303: 605–9.

Ragno M, Tournier-Lasserve E, Fiori MG *et al.* (1995). An Italian kindred with cerebral autosomal dominant arteriopathy with subcortical infarcts and leukoencephalopathy (CADASIL). *Ann Neurol* 38: 231–6.

Ranoux D, Cohen A, Cabanes L, Amarenco P, Bousser M-G, Mas JL (1993). Patent foramen ovale: is stroke due to paradoxical embolism? *Stroke* 24: 31–4.

Raymond LA, Sacks JG, Choromokos E, Khodadad G (1980). Short posterior ciliary artery insufficiency with hyperthermia (Uhthoff's symptom). *Am J Ophthalmol* 90: 619–23.

Reed DM, Resch JA, Hayashi T, MacLean C, Yano K (1988). A prospective study of cerebral artery atherosclerosis. *Stroke* 19: 820–5.

Regli L, Regli F, Maeder P, Bogousslavsky J (1993). Magnetic resonance imaging with gadolinium contrast agent in small deep (lacunar) cerebral infarcts. *Arch Neurol* 50: 175–80.

Reneman RS, van Merode T, Hick P, Hoeks APG (1985). Flow velocity patterns in and distensibility of the carotid artery bulb in subjects of various ages. *Circulation* 71: 500–9.

Ricci S, Flamini FO, Celani MG *et al.* (1991). Prevalence of internal carotid-artery stenosis in subjects older than 49 years: a population study. *Cerebrovasc Dis* 1: 16–19.

Rice GPA, Ebers GC, Newland F, Wysocki GP (1981). Recurrent cerebral embolism in cardiac amyloidosis. *Neurology* 31: 904–6.

Richardson PD, Davies MJ, Born GVR (1989). Influence of plaque configuration and stress distribution on fissuring of coronary atherosclerotic plaques. *Lancet* ii: 941–4.

Ricotta JJ, Schenk EA, Ekholm SE, DeWeese JA (1987). Angiographic and pathologic correlates in carotid artery disease. *Surgery* 99: 284–92.

Ridker PM, Hennekens CH, Stampfer MJ, Manson JE, Vaughan DE (1994). Prospective study of endogenous tissue plasminogen activator and risk of stroke. *Lancet* 343: 940–3.

Ries S, Schminke U, Daffertshofer M, Schindlmayr C, Hennerici M (1995). High intensity transient signals and carotid artery disease. *Cerebrovasc Dis* 5: 124–7.

Riles TS, Eidelman EM, Litt AW, Pinto RS, Oldford F, Schwartzenberg GWST (1992). Comparison of magnetic resonance angiography, conventional angiography, and Duplex scanning. *Stroke* 23: 341–6.

Rizzo JF, Lessel S (1994). Cerebrovascular abnormalities in neurofibromatosis type 1. *Neurology* 44: 1000–2.

Roederer GO, Langlois YE, Jager KA *et al.* (1984). The natural history of carotid arterial disease in asymptomatic patients with cervical bruits. *Stroke* 15: 605–13.

Roeltgen DP, Weimer GR, Patterson LF (1981). Delayed neurologic complications of left atrial myxoma. *Neurology* 31: 8–13.

Rosario JA, Hachinski VA, Lee DH, Fox AJ (1987). Adverse reactions to Duplex scanning. *Lancet* ii: 1023.

Rose G, Colwell L (1992). Randomised controlled trial of anti-smoking advice: final (20 year) results. *J Epidemiol Commun Health* 46: 75–7.

Rosengart A, Hedges TR, Teal PA *et al.* (1993). Intermittent downbeat nystagmus due to vertebral artery compression. *Neurology* 43: 216–18.

Rosengren A, Orth-Gomer K, Wedel H, Wilhelmsen L (1993). Stressful life events, social support, and mortality in men born in 1933. *Br Med J* 307: 1102–5.

Rosengren A, Welin L, Tsipogianni A, Wilhelmsen L (1989). Impact of cardiovascular risk factors on coronary heart disease and mortality among middle aged diabetic men: a general population study. *Br Med J* 299: 1127–31.

Rosengren A, Wilhelmsen L, Welin L, Tsipogianni A, Teger-Nilsson A-C, Wedel H (1990). Social influences and cardiovascular risk factors as determinants of plasma fibrinogen concentration in a general population sample of middle aged men. *Br Med J* 300: 634–8.

Ross R (1986). The pathogenesis of atherosclerosis—an update. *N Engl J Med* 314: 488–500.

Ross RS, McKusick VA (1953). Aortic arch syndromes: diminished or absent pulses in arteries arising from arch of aorta. *Arch Intern Med* 92: 701–40.

Ross RT, Morrow IM, Cheang MS (1988). The relationship of brachiocephalic vessel atheroma to transient ischaemia of the brain and retina. *Quart J Med* 67: 487–95.

Rother J, Schreiner A, Wentz K-U, Hennerici M (1992). Hypoglycemia presenting as basilar artery thrombosis. *Stroke* 23: 112–13.

Rother J, Schwartz A, Wentz KU, Rautenberg W, Hennerici M (1994). Middle cerebral artery stenoses: assessment by magnetic resonance angiography and transcranial Doppler ultrasound. *Cerebrovasc Dis* 4: 273–9.

Rothrock JF, Rubenstein R, Lyden PD (1988). Ischaemic stroke associated with methamphetamine inhalation. *Neurology* 38: 589–92.

Rothewell PM, Warlow CP (1996). Making sense of the measurement of carotid stenosis. *Cerebrovasc Dis* 6: 54–8.

Rothwell PM, Gibson RJ, Slattery J, Warlow CP, for the European Carotid Surgery Trialists' Collaborative Group (1994b). The prognostic value and reproducibility of measurements of carotid stenosis: a comparison of three methods on 1001 angiograms. *Stroke* 25: 2440–4.

Rothwell PM, Gibson RJ, Slattery J, Sellar RJ Warlow CP, for the European Carotid Surgery Trialists' Collaborative Group (1994a). The equivalence of measurements of carotid stenosis: a comparison of three methods on 1001 angiograms. *Stroke* 25: 2435–9.

Rowe JW (1983). Systolic hypertension in the elderly. *N Engl J Med* 309: 1246–7.

Rubba P, Mercuri M, Faccenda F *et al.* (1994). Premature carotid atherosclerosis: dose it occur in both familial hypercholesterolemia and homocystinuria: ultrasound assessment of arterial intima–media thickness and blood flow velocity. *Stroke* 25: 943–50.

Ruff RL, Talman WT, Petito F (1981). Transient ischaemic attacks associated with hypotension in hypertensive patients with carotid artery stenosis. *Stroke* 12: 353–5.

Rush PJ, Inman R, Bernstein M, Carlen P, Resch L (1986). Isolated vasculitis of the central nervous system in a patient with coeliac disease. *Am J Med* 81: 1092–4.

Russell RWR (1975). How does blood-pressure cause stroke? *Lancet* ii: 1283–5.

Russell RWR (1988). Cause and treatment of insufficiency in the cerebral circulation. *Clin Neurol Neurosurg* 90: 19–24.

Russell RWR, Ikeda H (1986). Clinical and electrophysiological observations in patients with low pressure retinopathy. *Br J Ophthalmol* 70: 651–6.

Russell RWR, Page NGR (1983). Critical perfusion of brain and retina. *Brain* 106: 419–34.

Ryan PG, Day AL (1987). Stump embolization from an occluded internal carotid artery: case report. *J Neurosurg* 67: 609–11.

Sabbadini G, Francia A, Calandriello L *et al.* (1995). Cerebral autosomal dominant arteriopathy with subcortical infarcts and leucoencephalopathy (CADASIL): clinical, neuroimaging, pathological and genetic study of a large Italian family. *Brain* 118: 207–15.

Sacco SE, Whisnant JP, Broderick JP, Phillips SJ, O'Fallon WM (1991). Epidemiological characteristics of lacunar infarcts in a population. *Stroke* 22: 1236–41.

Saito I, Segawa H, Shiokawa Y, Taniguchi M, Tsutsumi K (1987). Middle cerebral artery occlusion: correlation of computed tomography and angiography with clinical outcome. *Stroke* 18: 863–8.

Sakai F, Ishii K, Ingarashi H *et al.* (1988). Regional cerebral blood flow during an attack of vertebrobasilar insufficiency. *Stroke* 19: 1426–30.

Salgado AV (1991). Central nervous system complications of infective endocarditis. *Stroke* 22: 1461–3.

Salgado ED, Weinstein M, Furlan AJ *et al.* (1986). Proton magnetic resonance imaging in ischaemic cerebrovascular disease. *Ann Neurol* 20: 502–7.

Samuelsson M, Lindell D, Norrving B (1994). Gadolinium-enhanced magnetic resonance imaging in patients with presumed lacunar infarcts. *Cerebrovasc Dis* 4: 12–19.

Sandercock PAG, Warlow CP, Jones LN, Starkey IR (1989). Predisposing factors for cerebral infarction: the Oxfordshire Community Stroke Project. *Br Med J* 298: 75–80.

Sandercock PAG, Bamford J, Dennis M *et al.* (1992). Atrial fibrillation and stroke: prevalence in different stroke types and influence on early and long term prognosis (Oxfordshire Community Stroke Project). *Br Med J* 305: 1460–5.

Sandok BA, Whisnant JP, Furlan AJ, Mickell JL (1982). Carotid artery bruits: prevalence survey and differential diagnosis. *Mayo Clin Proc* 57: 227–30.

Sauer CM (1991). Recurrent embolic stroke and cocaine-related cardiomyopathy. *Stroke* 22: 1203–5.

Scandinavian Simvastatin Survival Study Group (1994). Randomised trial of cholesterol lowering in 4444 patients with coronary heart disease: the Scandinavian Simvastatin Survival Study (4S). *Lancet* 344: 1383–9.

Schimke RN, McKusick VA, Huang T, Pollack AD (1965). Homocystinuria: studies of 20 families with 38 affected members. *J Am Med Assoc* 193: 87–95.

Schwartz A, Rautenberg W, Hennerici M (1993). Dolichoectatic intracranial arteries: review of selected aspects. *Cerebrovasc Dis* 3: 273–9.

Schwartz CJ, Mitchell JRA (1961). Atheroma of the carotid and vertebral arterial systems. *Br Med J* 2: 1057–63.

Sellar RJ (1995). Imaging blood vessels of the head and neck. *J Neurol Neurosurg Psychiatr* 59: 225–37.

Shaper AG, Phillips AN, Pocock SJ, Walker M, Macfarlane PW (1991). Risk factors for stroke in middle aged British men. *Br Med J* 302: 1111–15.

Shapiro LM, Westgate GJ, Shine K, Donaldson R (1985). Is cardiac ultrasound mandatory in patients with transient ischaemic attacks? *Br Med J* 291: 786–7.

Shintani S, Tsuruoka S, Shiigai T (1993). Hypoglycaemic hemiplegia: a repeat SPECT study. *J Neurol Neurosurg Psychiatr* 56: 700–1.

Shinton R, Beevers G (1989). Meta-analysis of relation between cigarette smoking and stroke. *Br Med J* 298: 789–94.

Shinton R, Sagar G (1993). Lifelong exercise and stroke. *Br Med J* 307: 231–4.

Shinton R, Sagar G, Beervers G (1993). The relation of alcohol consumption to cardiovascular risk factors and stroke: the West Birmingham Stroke Project. *J Neurol Neurosurg Psychiatr* 56: 458–62.

Shuaib A, Lee D, Pelz D, Fox A, Hachinski VC (1992). The impact of magnetic resonance imaging on the management of acute ischaemic stroke. *Neurology* 42: 816–18.

Siebler M, Kleinschmidt A, Sitzer M, Steinmetz H, Freund H-J (1994). Cerebral microembolism in symptomatic and asymptomatic high-grade internal carotid artery stenosis. *Neurology* 44: 615–18.

Siewert B, Patel MR, Warach S (1995). Magnetic resonance angiography. *Neurologist* 1: 167–84.

Silver MD, Dorsey JS (1978). Aneurysms of the septum primum in adults. *Arch Pathol Lab Med* 102: 62–5.

Sitzer M, Furst G, Fischer H *et al.* (1993). Between-method correlation in quantifying internal carotid stenosis. *Stroke* 24: 1513–8.

Sliwka U, Diehl RR, Meyer B, Schondube F, Noth J (1995). Transcranial Doppler 'high intensity transient signals' in the acute phase and long-term follow-up of mechanical heart valve implantation. *J Stroke Cerebrovasc Dis* 5: 139–46.

Smith G, Shipley MJ, Rose G (1990). Intermittent claudication, heart disease risk factors, and mortality: the Whitehall study. *Circulation* 82: 1925–31.

Sornas R, Ostlund H, Muller R (1972). Cerebrospinal fluid cytology after stroke. *Arch Neurol* 26: 489–501.

Spriggs DA, French JM, Murdy JM, Curless RH, Bates D, James OFW (1992). Snoring increases the risk of stroke and adversely affects prognosis. *Quart J Med* 84: 555–62.

Stampfer MJ, Malinow MR (1995). Can lowering homocysteine levels reduce cardiovascular risk? *N Engl J Med* 332: 328–9.

Stark RJ, Wodak J (1983). Primary orthostatic cerebral ischaemia. *J Neurol Neurosurg Psychiatr* 46: 883–91.

Stein PD, Sabbah HN, Pitha JV (1977). Continuing disease process of calcific aortic stenosis: role of microthrombi and turbulent flow. *Am J Cardiol* 39: 159–63.

Steinberg D (1993). Antioxidant vitamins and coronary heart disease. *N Engl J Med* 328: 1487–9.

Steinmetz JC, DeConti R, Ginsburg R (1989). Hypersensitivity vasculitis associated with 2-deoxycoformycin and allopurinol therapy. *Am J Med* 86: 498–9.

Stemmermann GN, Hayashi T, Resch JA, Chung CS, Reed DM, Rhoads GG (1984). Risk factors related to ischaemic and haemorrhagic cerebrovascular disease at autopsy: the Honolulu Heart Study. *Stroke* 15: 23–8.

Stollberger C, Brainin M, Abzieher F, Slany J (1995). Embolic stroke and transoesophageal echocardiography: can clinical parameters predict the diagnostic yield? *J Neurol* 242: 437–42.

Strachan DP (1991). Ventilatory function as a predictor of fatal stroke. *Br Med J* 302: 84–7.

Streifler JY, Eliaziw M, Fox AJ *et al.* for the North American Symptomatic Carotid Endarterectomy Trial (1994). Angiographic detection of carotid plaque ulceration: comparison with surgical observations in a multicenter study. *Stroke* 25: 1130–2.

Stroke Prevention in Atrial Fibrillation Investigators (1992). Predictors of thromboembolism in atrial fibrillation: II. Echocardiographic features of patients at risk. *Ann Intern Med* 116: 6–12.

Sturrock GD, Mueller HR (1984). Chronic ocular ischaemia. *Br J Ophthalmol* 68: 716–23.

Sturzenegger M, Newell DW, Douville C, Byrd S, Schoonover K (1994). Dynamic transcranial Doppler assessment of positional vertebrobasilar ischaemia. *Stroke* 25: 1776–83.

Sutton-Tyrell K, Alcorn HG, Wolfson SK, Kelsey SF, Kuller LH (1993). Predictors of carotid stenosis in older adults with and without isolated systolic hypertension. *Stroke* 24: 355–61.

Sutton-Tyrell K, Wolfson SK, Kuller LH (1994). Blood pressure treatment slows the progression of carotid stenosis in patients with isolated systolic hypertension. *Stroke* 25: 44–50.

Svindland A, Torvik A (1988). Atherosclerotic carotid disease in asymptomatic individuals. *Acta Neurol Scand* 78: 506–17.

Swash M, Earl CJ (1970). Transient visual obscurations in chronic rheumatic heart-disease. *Lancet* ii: 323–6.

Tanaka H, Sueyoshi K, Nishino M, Ishida M, Fukunaga R, Abe H (1993). Silent brain infarction and coronary artery disease in Japanese patients. *Arch Neurol* 50: 706–9.

Tatemichi TK, Young WL, Prohovnik I, Gitelman DR, Correll JW, Mohr JP (1990). Perfusion insufficiency in limb-shaking transient ischaemic attacks. *Stroke* 21: 341–7.

Tegeler CH (1994). High-intensity transient signals detected by Doppler ultrasonography: searching for answers. *Cerebrovasc Dis* 4: 379–82.

Tegeler CH, Downes TR (1991). Cardiac imaging in stroke. *Stroke* 22: 1206–11.

Tegeler CH, Shi F, Morgan T (1991). Carotid stenosis in lacunar stroke. *Stroke* 22: 1124–8.

Tegeler CH, Knappertz VA, Nagaraja D, Mooney M, Dalley GM (1995). Relationships of common carotid artery high intensity transient signals in patients with ischaemic stroke to white matter versus territorial infarct pattern on brain CT scan. *Cerebrovasc Dis* 5: 128–32.

Thelle DS (1991). Coffee, cholesterol, and coronary heart disease. *Br Med J* 302: 804.

Thie A, Goossens-Merkt H, Freitag J, Spitzer K, Zeumer H, Kunze K (1993). Pulsatile tinnitus: clinical and angiological evaluation. *Cerebrovasc Dis* 3: 160–7.

Thompson SG (1994). Why sources of heterogeneity in meta-analysis should be investigated. *Br Med J* 309: 1351–5.

Thorogood M, Cowen P, Mann J, Murphy M, Vessey M (1992). Fatal myocardial infarction and use of psychotropic drugs in young women. *Lancet* 340: 1067–8.

Tohgi H, Takahashi S, Chiba K, Hirata Y, for the Tohoku Cerebellar Infarction Study Group (1993). Cerebellar infarction: clinical and neuroimaging analysis in 293 patients. *Stroke* 24: 1697–701.

Torvik A (1984). The pathogenesis of watershed infarcts in the brain. *Stroke* 15: 221–3.

Torvik A, Svindland A, Lindboe CF (1989). Pathogenesis of carotid thrombosis. *Stroke* 20: 1477–83.

Tunick PA, Perez JL, Kronzon I (1991). Protruding atheromas in the thoracic aorta and systemic embolization. *Ann Intern Med* 115: 423–7.

UK-TIA Study Group (1983). Variation in the use of angiography and carotid endarterectomy by neurologists in the UK-TIA Aspirin Trial. *Br Med J* 286: 514–17.

van der Meulen JHP, Weststrate W, van Gijn J, Habbema JDF (1992). Is cerebral angiography indicated in infective endocarditis? *Stroke* 23: 1662–7.

van der Zwan A, Hillen B, Tulleken CAF, Dujovny M, Dragovic L (1992). Variability of the territories of the major cerebral arteries. *J Neurosurg* 77: 927–40.

van der Zwan A, Hillen B, Tulleken CAF, Dujovny M (1993). A quantitative investigation of the variability of the major cerebral arterial territories. *Stroke* 24: 1951–9.

van Gijn J, Stampfer MJ, Wolfe C, Algra A (1993). The association between alcohol and stroke. In: Verschuren PM, ed. *Health Issues Related to Alcohol Consumption*. Washington: ILSI Press, 44–79.

van Latum JC, Koudstaal PJ, Venables GS, van Gijn J, Kappelle LJ, Algra A, for the European Atrial Fibrillation Trial (EAFT) Study Group (1995). Predictors of major vascular events in patients with a transient ischaemic attack or minor ischaemic stroke and with nonrheumatic atrial fibrillation. *Stroke* 16: 801–6.

Vestergaard K, Andersen G, Nielsen MI, Jensen TS (1993). Headache in stroke. *Stroke* 24: 1621–4.

Vingerhoets F, Bogousslavsky J, Regli F, van Melle G (1993). Atrial fibrillation after acute stroke. *Stroke* 24: 26–30.

Virtamo J, Valkeila E, Alfthan G, Punsar S, Huttunen JK, Karvonen MJ (1985). Serum selenium and the risk of coronary heart disease and stroke. *Am J Epidemiol* 122: 276–82.

Visy JM, Le Coz P, Chadefaux B *et al.* (1991). Homocystinuria due to 5,10-methylenetetrahydrofolate reductase deficiency revealed by stroke in adult siblings. *Neurology* 41: 1313–15.

Voyce SJ, Aurigemma GP, Dahlberg S *et al.* (1992). A comparison to two dimensional echocardiography vs carotid duplex scanning in older patients with cerebral ischaemia. *Arch Intern Med* 152: 2089–93.

Waller PC, Bhopal RS (1989). Is snoring a cause of vascular disease? An epidemiological review. *Lancet* i: 143–6.

Wallis WE, Donaldson I, Scott RS, Wilson J (1985). Hypoglycaemia masquerading as cerebrovascular disease (hypoglycaemic hemiplegia). *Ann Neurol* 18: 510–12.

Wannamethee G, Shaper AG (1989). Body weight and mortality in middle aged British men: impact of smoking. *Br Med J* 299: 1497–502.

Wannamethee G, Shaper AG (1992). Physical activity and stroke in British middle aged men. *Br Med J* 304: 597–601.

Wardlaw JM, Merrick MV, Ferrington CM *et al.* (1996). Comparison of a simple isotope method of predicting likely middle cerebral artery occlusion with transcranial Doppler ultrasound in acute ischaemic stroke. *Cerebrovasc Dis* 6: 32–9.

Ware JA, Heistad DD (1993). Platelet–endothelium interactions. *N Engl J Med* 328: 628–35.

Warlow CP (1978). Venous thromboembolism after stroke. *Am Heart J* 96: 283–5.

Warlow CP (1995). *Oxford Textbook of Medicine*, Vol. 3. Oxford: Oxford University Press, 3946–64.

Wechsler LR (1988). Ulceration and carotid artery disease. *Stroke* 19: 650–3.

Wechsler LR, Babikian VL (1994). Transcranial Doppler sonography clinically useful. *Arch Neurol* 51: 1054–6.

Weiller C, Ringelstein EB, Reiche W, Buell U (1991). Clinical and haemodynamic aspects of low-flow infarcts. *Stroke* 22: 1117–23.

Weinberger J, Rothlauf E, Materese E, Halperin J (1988). Noninvasive evaluation of the extracranial carotid arteries in patients with cerebrovascular events and atrial fibrillations. *Arch Intern Med* 148: 1785–8.

Welin L, Svardsudd K, Wilhelmsen L, Larsson B, Tibblin G (1987). Analysis of risk factors for stroke in a cohort of men born in 1913. *N Engl J Med* 317: 521–6.

Whelton PK (1994). Epidemiology of hypertension. *Lancet* 344: 101–6.

Whincup PH, Cook DG, Phillips AN, Shaper AG (1990). ABO blood group and ischaemic heart disease in British men. *Br Med J* 300: 1679–82.

Whisnant JP (1982). Multiple particles injected may all go to the same cerebral artery branch. *Stroke* 13: 720.

Wickremasinghe HR, Peiris JB, Thenabadu PN, Sheriffdeen AH (1978). Transient embologenic aortoarteritis. *Arch Neurol* 35: 416–22.

Widder B, Kleiser B, Krapf H (1994). Course of cerebrovascular reactivity in patients with carotid artery occlusions. *Stroke* 25: 1963–7.

Wiebers DO, Swanson JW, Cascino TL, Whisnant JP (1989). Bilateral loss of vision in bright light. *Stroke* 20: 554–8.

Wiebers DO, Whisnant JP, Sandok BA, O'Fallon WM (1990). Prospective comparison of a cohort with asymptomatic carotid bruit and a population-based cohort without carotid bruit. *Stroke* 21: 984–8.

Wolf PA, Abbott RD, Kannel WB (1991). Atrial fibrillation as an independent risk factor for stroke: the Framingham Study. *Stroke* 22: 983–8.

Wolf PA, Dawber TR, Thomas E, Kannel WB (1978). Epidemiologic assessment of chronic atrial fibrillation and risk of stroke: the Framingham Study. *Neurology* 28: 973–7.

Woo J, Lam CWK, Kay R, Wong HY, Teoh R, Nicholls G (1990). Acute and long term changes in serum lipids after acute stroke. *Stroke* 21: 1407–11.

Woo J, Lau E, Lam CW et al. (1991). Hypertension, lipoprotein (a), and apoliprotein A-I as risk factors for stroke in the Chinese. *Stroke* 22: 203–8.

Woodhouse PR, Khaw KT, Plummer M, Foley A, Meade TW (1994). Seasonal variations of plasma fibrinogen and factor VII activity in the elderly; winter infections and death from cardiovascular disease. *Lancet* 343: 435–9.

Yanagihara T, Piepgras DG, Klass DW (1985). Repetitive involuntary movement association with episodic cerebral ischaemia. *Ann Neurol* 18: 244–50.

Yanagihara T, Sundt TM, Piepgras DG (1988). Weakness of the lower extremity in carotid occlusive disease. *Arch Neurol* 45: 297–301.

Yarnell JWG, Baker IA, Sweetnam PM et al. (1991). Fibrinogen, viscosity, and white blood cell count are major risk factors for ischaemic heart disease: the Caerphilly and Speedwell Collaborative Heart Disease Studies. *Circulation* 83: 836–44.

You R, McNeil JJ, O'Malley HM, Davis SM, Donnan GA (1995). Risk factors for lacunar infarction syndromes. *Neurology* 45: 1483–7.

Young GR, Humphrey PRD, Shaw MDM, Nixon TE, Smith ETS (1994). Comparison of magnetic resonance angiography, duplex ultrasound, and digital subtraction angiography in assessment of extracranial internal carotid artery stenosis. *J Neurol Neurosurg Psychiatr* 57: 1466–78.

Unusual causes of ischaemic stroke and transient ischaemic attack

7

Most textbooks devote 95% of the discussion of causes of ischaemic stroke and transient ischaemic attacks (TIAs) to 5% of cases with a rare or unusual cause. Although we will not be quite so unbalanced, it is not unreasonable to discuss rare disorders in detail if their diagnosis leads to a specific early treatment or the prevention of stroke recurrence. Also, many unusual causes are confusing and require explanation.

7.1   Arterial trauma and dissection

Ischaemic strokes and TIAs, particularly in young and middle-aged patients, are increasingly being found to be due to arterial trauma and dissection, perhaps because physicians are more attuned to the possibility—and so ask the right questions—or, possibly, because of improved diagnostic technology.

Penetrating neck injuries

Penetrating neck injuries are more likely to damage the carotid than the better-protected vertebral arteries (see Table 6.3). Such trauma causes laceration, dissection and intimal tears, which may be complicated by thrombosis occluding the artery, or non-occlusive thrombosis with embolism to the brain or eye within hours, days, or possibly even weeks after the injury. Years later, ischaemic stroke or TIA can be the result of the gradual formation of a traumatic aneurysm with contained thrombus which then embolises (see Section 7.4; Davis & Zimmerman, 1983).

Non-penetrating (blunt) neck injuries

Non-penetrating (blunt) neck injuries (see Table 6.3) are more subtle causes of ischaemic stroke and TIA, because the injury may have seemed rather trivial at the time or the cerebrovascular symptoms are overshadowed by more substantial injuries, or any stroke occurs days or weeks later. Blunt trauma usually causes intimal tearing or dissection with complicating thrombosis or embolism, whilst traumatic rupture of an atheromatous plaque, vasospasm and delayed aneurysm formation are all exceptionally rare (Davis & Zimmerman, 1983). The internal carotid artery (ICA) and, very rarely, the common carotid artery are more vulnerable to a direct blow to the neck or to compression, whereas the vertebral arteries are more prone to rotational and hyperextension injuries at the level of the atlas and axis (Hughes & Brownell, 1968; Sherman et al., 1981; Hilton-Jones & Warlow, 1985a; Pozzati et al., 1989; Frisoni & Anzola, 1991; Thie et al., 1993; Tulyapronchote et al., 1994; de Recondo et al., 1995). The subclavian artery can be damaged distal to the vertebral artery origin by a fractured clavicle or cervical rib, to cause mural thrombosis and then embolisation retrogradely during the reversal of subclavian artery blood flow in diastole and so up the vertebral artery, or up the right common carotid artery (Prior et al., 1979). The same haemodynamic mechanism could also presumably cause embolism to the brain of atherothrombotic material in the distal subclavian arteries and in the aortic arch.

Cervical arterial dissection

Cervical arterial dissection is usually traumatic or coincides with an apparently trivial neck movement, but it can be truly spontaneous, at least in patients with atheroma, cystic medial necrosis, fibromuscular dysplasia (FMD), Marfan's syndrome and other arterial disorders (see Section 7.3 and Table 6.3). Blood enters into and splits the arterial wall to form an intramural haematoma of variable length. There may be one or more intimal tears so that the false and true lumen are in communication (Fig. 7.1). Ischaemic stroke or TIA is caused by the true lumen being occluded by the dissection; complicating occlusive and perhaps propagating thrombosis within the true lumen; or embolism from non-occlusive thrombosis within the true lumen (O'Connell et al., 1985). Usually only one artery is affected, but sometimes two or more arteries appear to be affected more or less simultaneously.

Helpful clues to the diagnosis, other than any history of preceding neck trauma (see Table 6.3), are: pain in the face, around the eye, in the neck or side of the head ipsilateral to ICA dissection, or occipitally and in the back of the neck—usually unilaterally—for vertebral dissection; a Horner's syndrome due to damage to the sympathetic fibres around the ICA; a self-audible bruit, because carotid dissection tends to spread distally to the base of the skull, or just be present distally; and, occasionally, unilateral lower cranial nerve palsies, particularly hypoglossal, as a result of pressure from the expanded ICA wall at the base of the skull, or perhaps ischaemia. Oculomotor nerve palsy ipsilateral to an ICA dissection has been rarely described. These features very often precede, as well as accompany, the onset of cerebral ischaemia by hours or days (Mokri et al., 1986, 1988; Pozzati et al., 1990; Vighetto et al., 1990; Hinse et al., 1991; Caplan & Tettenborn, 1992; Sturzenegger & Huber, 1993; Schievink et al., 1993a; Biousse et al., 1995; Silbert et al., 1995).

> Cervical arterial dissection is diagnosed by first asking the right question: 'In the last few days or weeks have you had any injury or damaged your neck, a car crash, or done anything to twist your neck?' and then by ordering the correct investigations before the dissection heals: duplex ultrasound, magnetic resonance imaging of the neck and, if necessary, selective catheter angiography.

Although ICA (but less often vertebral) dissection can be suspected on duplex sonography (which is occasionally diagnostic), the definitive investigation is cerebral angiography; nowadays magnetic resonance imaging (MRI) combined with MR angiography may suffice if the images are characteristic and can even be diagnostic when a conventional angiogram is normal (Rother et al., 1995; Sturzenegger, 1995; Sturzenegger et al., 1995; Fig. 7.2). If the carotid is completely occluded by the dissection, imaging may be nonspecific, because a similar appearance could arise from any cause of ICA occlusion. Imaging must be done within days of symptom onset, because dissection often resolves spontaneously (Mullges et al., 1992; Sturzenegger et al., 1993; Steinke et al., 1994).

Recurrence of dissection, in the same or a different artery, seems to be distinctly unusual, but there is uncertainty because there have been so few large, prospective community-based follow-up studies (Schievink et al., 1993b, 1994b; Leys et al., 1995).

Intracranial arterial dissection

Intracranial arterial dissection is much rarer and more likely to present with subarachnoid haemorrhage, due to rupture of pseudoaneurysmal bulging of the arterial adventitia and the lack of external elastic lamina in the intradural section of the vessel, than with cerebral ischaemia (see Section 9.1.3). Basilar dissection usually causes a massive brainstem infarct (Farrell et al., 1985; Caplan & Tettenborn, 1992).

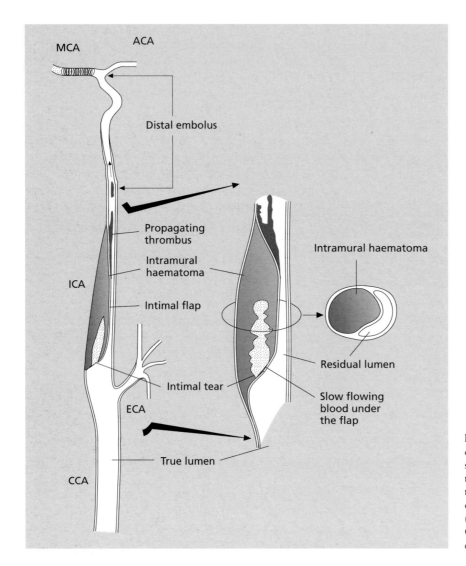

Figure 7.1 Diagram of an arterial dissection at the origin of the ICA showing: intramural thrombus; intimal tears; complicating non-occlusive thrombosis; and embolism with distal occlusion of the middle cerebral artery (MCA). ACA, anterior cerebral artery; CCA, common carotid artery; ECA, external carotid artery.

Aortic dissection

Aortic dissection causes *focal* cerebral ischaemia (i.e. ischaemic stroke or TIA) only if the dissection blocks or extends up one of the neck arteries to cause occlusion or mural thrombosis and embolism. More often, any cerebral ischaemia is generalised, perhaps causing low-flow infarction as a result of systemic hypotension. Clues to the diagnosis are anterior chest pain and/or interscapular pain; diminished, unequal or absent arterial pulses in the arms, neck and sometimes legs; acute aortic regurgitation; simultaneous or sequential ischaemia in carotid, vertebral, spinal, coronary and other aortic branches if the dissection extends over several centimetres; a normal electrocardiogram (ECG) unless there is complicating acute myocardial infarction (MI); and mediastinal widening and left pleural effusion on

the chest X-ray. Intra-arterial aortography is diagnostic and allows full evaluation of the extent of the lesion, but transoesophageal echocardiography and dynamic computerised tomography (CT), or MRI, of the aortic arch are safer and perhaps quicker if the expertise is available locally, although they give less information about coronary patency (Gerber *et al.*, 1986; DeSanctis *et al.*, 1987; Carrel *et al.*, 1991; Veyssier-Belot *et al.*, 1993; Banning *et al.*, 1995).

Fibrocartilaginous embolism

Fibrocartilaginous embolism is extraordinarily rare. Embolic material from a disrupted intervertebral disc, perhaps as a result of trauma, can somehow reach the circulation of the spinal cord, rarely of the brain (Bots *et al.*, 1981; Toro-Gonzalez *et al.*, 1993).

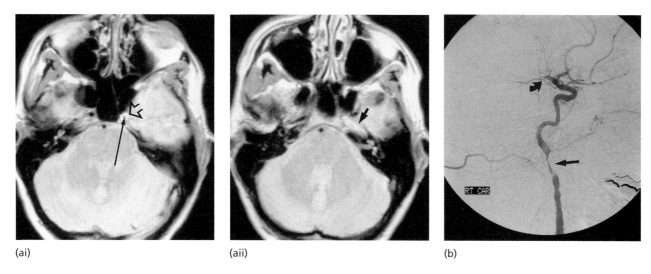

(ai)   (aii)   (b)

Figure 7.2 (a) Carotid dissection on MRI. Expansion of the arterial wall by blood clot is diagnostic but is *not* seen in every case, because the lesion may be too small, the MRI cuts are not through the relevant part of the artery, there is intraluminal thrombus which can not be differentiated from intramural haematoma, or perhaps the clot is so fresh that there is not enough methaemoglobin to enhance the signal on T1-weighted images. The true lumen is seen as an eccentric signal void on T1- and T2-weighted axial images and is surrounded by semilunar hyperintensity, corresponding with the intramural haematoma, but the signal intensity does depend on the age of the haematoma and the pulse sequence selected (Kitanaka *et al.*, 1994; Zuber *et al.*, 1994). In the example shown (proton density-weighted axial MRI), the dissected distal ICA is seen passing through the skull base in the carotid canal (i) (arrow). The high signal of the intramural thrombus (open arrow) and central flow void (thin arrow) are clearly seen ((ii)—slice immediately craniad of (i)). (b) Carotid dissection on angiography. The diagnostic features include an elongated and tapering stenosis (arrow), often irregular and possibly with complete occlusion of the lumen. Sometimes there is aneurysmal bulging of the adventitial wall to the false lumen, an intimal flap, a floating thrombus or an obviously double lumen. Unlike carotid atheroma, dissection is usually well distal to the internal carotid orgin and also it seldom reaches beyond the base of the skull. Vertebral dissection is usually at the C1/C2 vertebral level. There may be intracranial distal branch occlusions, presumably due to embolism (curved arrow).

7.2   Primary inflammatory vascular disorders

Most of the autoimmune or collagen vascular and related disorders, such as systemic lupus erythematosus (SLE) (see Table 6.3) can be complicated by, or occasionally present with, various neurological syndromes, including strokes and TIAs (Moore & Cupps, 1983; Sigal, 1987; Berlit *et al.*, 1993; Moore, 1995). Usually there is an acute, subacute or chronic inflammatory reaction in the arterial and/or venous wall, with or without granuloma formation. The cellular proliferation, necrosis and subsequent fibrosis may be sufficient to occlude the vessel lumen; precipitate thrombosis, which may be complicated by embolism; and promote aneurysm formation, dissection or even wall rupture. Therefore, these changes may cause not just focal and generalised cerebral ischaemia, either due to arterial or venous occlusion, but also intracranial haemorrhage. In addition, non-neurological complications (such as hypertension due to renal involvement) and adverse effects of treatment (opportunistic meningeal and cerebral infections due to immunosuppression) may lead to cerebral ischaemia or haemorrhage.

> *Vasculitic disorders affecting the central nervous system may cause not just thrombosis within arteries but also rupture of any affected arteries, to cause subarachnoid or intracerebral haemorrhage and intracranial venous thrombosis.*

Amongst patients *presenting* with stroke there are very, very few who are already known to have, or who are discovered to have, a primary inflammatory vascular disorder. In fact, patients with these disorders are more likely to present with a generalised encephalopathy, with or without focal features, which does not really fit with the 'typical stroke patient' and even less with the 'typical TIA patient'. Nonetheless, these disorders are well worth looking out for, even in stroke and TIA patients, because their presence will require a detailed general evaluation of the patient in terms of renal function, joint problems, etc., they will certainly change the way the patient is managed and they often require specific treatment.

Clues to the diagnosis of a primary inflammatory disorder, unless it is already known, are: systemic features, such as weight loss, headache, malaise, facial rash, livedo reticularis, arthropathy, renal failure and fever; the lack of any other obvious and more common cause of stroke; a raised erythrocyte sedimentation rate (ESR), or anaemia, in the routine screening tests; and, when diagnostic suspicion is aroused, more specific immunological tests, such as serum anticardiolipin antibodies, double-stranded deoxyribonucleic acid (DNA) antibodies or antineutrophil cytoplasmic antibodies (ANCA) (Charles & Maini, 1993), and biopsy of the superficial temporal artery, meninges, cerebral cortex, skin, kidney, etc. There are no *specific* angiographic criteria for cerebral 'vasculitis': focal narrowing, dilatation and beading of small cerebral arteries, sometimes with aneurysm formation, are occasionally seen, but so they are with malignant meningitis, meningovascular syphilis and other chronic meningeal infections, drug abuse, irradiation, puerperal angiopathy, herpes zoster vasculitis and malignant hypertension, and as a result of 'vasospasm' after subarachnoid haemorrhage (Fig. 7.3); moreover, angiography is often normal in biopsy-proved vasculitis. Tumour emboli may also cause focal arterial dilatations and stenoses (see Fig. 6.13). Brain CT, and the more sensitive MRI, may show areas of presumed infarction, and sometimes haemorrhage, in both cerebral grey and white matter, along with diffuse meningeal and subependymal involvement (Fig. 7.4) (cf. multiple sclerosis lesions being confined to the periventricular white matter, but the distinction is impossible in many cases (Wechsler *et al.*, 1993; Alhalabi & Moore, 1994)). Oligoclonal banding of immunoglobulin G (IgG) may be

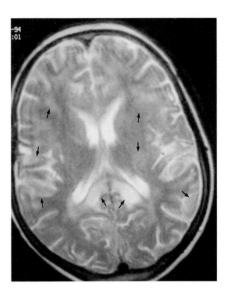

Figure 7.4 MRI (T2-weighted) of cerebral vasculitis: note the lesions affect grey as well as white matter (arrows), unlike in multiple sclerosis.

found in the cerebrospinal fluid (CSF) and does not really help in differentiating vasculitic disorders from multiple sclerosis (McLean *et al.*, 1995). The electroencephalogram (EEG) may help in the sense that bilateral diffuse slowing in a patient with a single focal lesion clinically would suggest a diffuse encephalopathic process of some sort, in this context vasculitic.

> *'Beading' of intracranial arteries is neither a specific nor a sensitive sign of cerebral vasculitis, which can not be diagnosed reliably without meningeal or cerebral histopathology.*

Giant cell arteritis

Giant cell arteritis (temporal arteritis) is probably the most common 'vasculitic' cause of ischaemic stroke and *should* be easily enough diagnosed because of the almost invariable accompanying or preceding malaise, polymyalgia and other general symptoms, and—almost always—an ESR raised well over 50, and often over 100. The patients are always elderly, seldom under the age of 60 years and never under the age of 50 years. There is frequently a mild normochromic normocytic anaemia, a raised platelet count and somewhat disturbed liver function. *Any* medium or large artery may be affected (carotid, vertebral, coronary, femoral, aorta, etc.). Although the most commonly involved arteries are the branches of the external carotid artery (ECA) (superficial temporal, occipital, facial), which causes the headache and facial pain, scalp tenderness and sometimes jaw claudica-

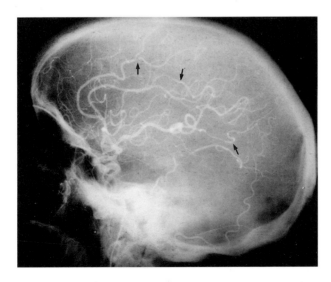

Figure 7.3 Cerebral angiogram in a patient with cerebral vasculitis to show focal dilatations and constrictions (i.e. beading) of branches of the middle and anterior cerebral arteries (arrows). (The figure was supplied by Dr Evelyn Teasdale, Institute of Neurological Sciences, Glasgow, UK.)

tion, it is the involvement of the extradural vertebral artery and ICA and the ophthalmic, posterior ciliary and central retinal arteries which are responsible for the brain and eye symptoms (Fig. 7.5); i.e. cerebral infarction, TIAs and infarction of the optic nerve (anterior ischaemic optic neuropathy (see Section 3.4.3)) more commonly than of the retina (see Fig. 3.17). Curiously, the anterior, middle and posterior cerebral and basilar arteries and their branches are seldom affected.

Biopsy of an affected artery is the definitive investigation to show giant cells and other evidence of chronic inflammation in the vessel wall and destruction of the internal elastic lamina. A clinical diagnosis *alone* is not enough to commit elderly patients to months or years of the dangers of corticosteroids, nor are ultrasound abnormalities of the branches of the ECA (Puechal *et al.*, 1995); the knowledge that a biopsy was positive is immensely reassuring if steroid complications occur many months after the start of treatment. To maximise the chance of a positive result, it is best to biopsy an extracranial artery that is *tender*, if possible. Otherwise, at least 2 cm of the superficial temporal artery should be taken and, if negative and the case is still a puzzle, the other super-

ficial temporal artery should be biopsied. Unfortunately, a negative biopsy does not rule out the diagnosis, because the arterial lesions can be patchy, so one may *have* to accept the clinical diagnosis, backed up, hopefully, by the complete resolution of the general symptoms (polymyalgia, headache, etc.) within 24–48 hours of starting corticosteroids, and a normal ESR within about 1 month. If there is diagnostic doubt, corticosteroids should be slowly withdrawn and, if any symptoms recur or the ESR rises, the diagnostic process must be started again (Wilkinson & Russell, 1972; Jonasson *et al.*, 1979; Huston & Hunder, 1980; Hall *et al.*, 1983; Caselli *et al.*, 1988).

> *If a patient presents with cerebral or ocular ischaemia and is aged over 50 years, and there is a recent history of malaise and headache, then an erythrocyte sedimentation rate must be done urgently and high doses of corticosteroids started, even before the results of any temporal artery biopsy are known.*

Takayasu's arteritis

Takayasu's arteritis (pulseless disease) is histologically identical to giant cell arteritis but affects preferentially the aorta and the large arteries arising from it, to cause multiple regions of smooth stenosis, irregularity, occlusion and aneurysmal bulging, mainly but not exclusively in young Oriental women (Fig. 7.6). Like giant cell arteritis, there are often systemic features, such as malaise, fever, weight loss, anaemia and raised ESR, at least in the early stages of the illness. The neurological features reflect the gradually increasing global, and focal, cerebral and ocular ischaemia, as the arteries become stenosed and occluded: claudication of jaw muscles; headache; ischaemic oculopathy (see Section 6.5.7); syncope, particularly on sitting or standing up; seizures; confusion; and low-flow cerebral ischaemia with, sometimes, focal ischaemic strokes and TIAs. There may also be ischaemic necrosis of the lips, nasal septum and palate. The arms and hands may become ischaemic, as may the kidneys, to cause hypertension (which can be difficult to diagnose if the upper-limb arteries are involved), and sometimes the legs. Aortic regurgitation and coronary artery occlusion are further complications (Lupi-Herrera *et al.*, 1977; Hall *et al.*, 1985).

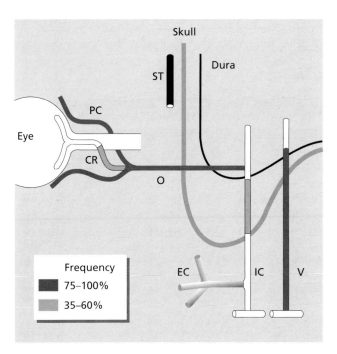

Figure 7.5 Diagram showing the distribution of giant cell arteritis in the arteries of the head and neck. The most frequently affected arteries are the ophthalmic (O), posterior ciliary (PC), superficial temporal (ST) and vertebral (V). Less often affected are the central retinal (CR), distal internal carotid (IC) and other external carotid (EC) artery branches. (Adapted with permission from Wilkinson & Russell, 1972.)

Systemic lupus erythematosus

SLE more often causes a generalised subacute or chronic encephalopathy than focal ischaemic (or sometimes) haemorrhagic cerebral episodes. Scattered cerebral infarcts and haemorrhages, of varying size, are found in some but by no

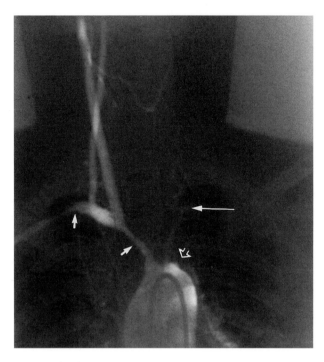

Figure 7.6 Arch aortogram showing the typical changes of Takayasu's arteritis. There are long sections of smoothly narrowed lumen affecting several of the major arteries of the neck (arrows), the left subclavian artery is completely occluded (open arrow) and the left common carotid artery ends in collaterals (long arrow). (The figure was supplied by Professor Takenori Yamaguchi, National Cardiovascular Centre, Osaka, Japan.)

means all cases. If any cerebrovascular pathology at all *is* found, it is *not* a vasculitis but rather bland intimal proliferation involving small vessels. Why the occasional patient has large artery occlusion is unknown, but embolism from the heart is obviously one possibility. Indeed, embolism from cardiac valvular vegetations, some of which are due to Libman–Sacks endocarditis, is more common than previously thought.

The vast majority of patients have circulating antinuclear antibodies of various sorts, as well as non-neurological features of SLE, such as arthropathy. A high proportion have anticardiolipin antibodies (see below), which seem to be particularly associated with cardiac valvular vegetations and arterial thrombosis (Bennett *et al.*, 1972; Haas, 1982; Devinsky *et al.*, 1988; Khamashta *et al.*, 1990; Kitagawa *et al.*, 1990; Mills, 1994; Mitsias & Levine, 1994; Hama & Boumpas, 1995).

Antiphospholipid syndrome

Depending on the selection of patients, the timing of the blood sample after the onset of cerebral ischaemia, the labo-

ratory methods and what level is deemed 'normal', from 1 to 40% or so of ischaemic stroke/TIA patients have raised circulating IgG or IgM anticardiolipin antibodies and/or the lupus anticoagulant, the latter detected by the activated partial thromboplastin time, Russell's viper venom time or some other functional clotting assay (Drenkard *et al.*, 1989; Antiphospholipid Antibodies in Stroke Study Group, 1990, 1993; Bick, 1993; Montalban *et al.*, 1994; Muir *et al.*, 1994). However, only a few of these patients have some or all of the constellation of features known as the antiphospholipid antibody syndrome (APS): recurrent miscarriages, arterial and venous thrombosis in any sized vessel, livedo reticularis, heart valve vegetations, migraine-like headaches, thrombocytopenia and false-positive syphilis serology (Coull & Goodnight, 1990; Hughes, 1993; Feldmann & Levine, 1995). Therefore, anticardiolipin antibodies are not specific to the APS, particularly if they are not present in high titres on repeated testing. They can be found in some normal individuals and also in SLE and other collagen vascular disorders, malignancy and human immunodeficiency virus (HIV) infection, and as a result of a variety of drugs, such as chlorpromazine, hydrallazine, phenytoin, valproate, procainamide and quinidine. The cause of thrombosis in the APS, the natural history, the nature of the relationship and overlap with SLE, and what any treatment should be (aspirin, anticoagulants or immunosuppression (see Section 11.9)) are all uncertain (Babikian & Levine, 1992; Levine *et al.*, 1995).

> *The antiphospholipid antibody syndrome can not be diagnosed on the basis of a single raised titre of anticardiolipin in the serum. The titre must be substantially raised on several occasions and associated not just with cerebral ischaemia but also with some combination of deep venous thrombosis, recurrent miscarriage, livedo reticularis, cardiac valvular vegetations, thrombocytopenia and migraine.*

Sneddon's syndrome

Sneddon's syndrome is the combination of widespread and prominent livedo reticularis with ischaemic strokes/TIAs, and often some of the immunological abnormalities of SLE (particularly anticardiolipin antibodies and the lupus anticoagulant), if not the full-blown syndrome. Clearly, this may in some way be one type of APS, which itself may be part of the spectrum of SLE, although meningeal granulomatous changes have been described (Burton, 1988; Stockhammer *et al.*, 1993; Kalashnikova *et al.*, 1994; Boortz-Marx *et al.*, 1995; Geschwind *et al.*, 1995).

Systemic necrotising vasculitis

Systemic necrotising vasculitis is a group of related disorders, including polyarteritis nodosa, Wegener's granulomatosis, the Churg–Strauss syndrome and various hypersensitivity vasculitides (see Table 6.3). They have similar cerebrovascular complications to those of SLE; ischaemia and haemorrhage may affect the brain, spinal cord, eye and almost any other organ. However, in contrast, the vascular pathology is a necrotising vasculitis affecting small and medium-sized arteries. One is less likely to find the serum antibodies characteristic of SLE and more likely to find eosinophilia, ANCA and haematuria (Ford & Siekert, 1965; Moore & Fauci, 1981; Nishino *et al.*, 1993).

Rheumatoid disease

Rheumatoid disease is very rarely complicated by a systemic and cerebral necrotising vasculitis (see above). Atlanto-occipital dislocation may cause symptomatic vertebral artery compression with posterior circulation ischaemia (Watson *et al.*, 1977; Beck & Corbett, 1983; Howell & Molyneux, 1988).

Sjögren's syndrome

Sjögren's syndrome can also be complicated by a systemic and cerebral necrotising vasculitis (see above), the latter causing transient or permanent focal neurological deficits, aseptic meningitis and global encephalopathy (Alexander *et al.*, 1982; de la Monte *et al.*, 1983; Bragoni *et al.*, 1994).

Behçet's disease

Behçet's disease (International Study Group for Behçet's Disease, 1990) can be complicated by a chronic meningitis and occlusion of extra- and intracranial arteries, perhaps more often those supplying the brainstem, to cause ischaemic stroke/TIA and primary intracerebral haemorrhage (PICH). How frequently this vasculopathy is due to an inflammatory arteritis is not known, but florid necrotising vasculitis appears to be distinctly unusual. Intracranial venous thrombosis also occurs. The neurological complications tend to coincide with flare-ups of the mucocutaneo-ocular symptoms but can antedate them (Kawakita *et al.*, 1967; Iragui & Maravi, 1986; Altinors *et al.*, 1987; Serdaroglu *et al.*, 1989; Wechsler *et al.*, 1992, 1993).

Relapsing polychondritis

Relapsing polychondritis is sometimes complicated by a sys-

temic and cerebral necrotising vasculitis (see above) (Stewart *et al.*, 1988).

Progressive systemic sclerosis

Progressive systemic sclerosis is hardly ever complicated by stroke, but a carotid and cerebral arteritis has been described (Lee & Haynes, 1967; Pathak & Gabor, 1991; Hietaharju *et al.*, 1993).

Sarcoid angiitis

Sarcoid angiitis can affect the small arteries and veins of the meninges and brain, usually causing cranial nerve palsies, aseptic meningtis and sometimes a global encephalopathy. Focal cerebral ischaemia and haemorrhage do very rarely occur. The diagnosis should be reasonably obvious from the non-neurological features, such as hilar lymphadenopathy, uveitis, etc. (Matthews, 1979; Caplan *et al.*, 1983; Stern *et al.*, 1985; Sethi *et al.*, 1986; Brown *et al.*, 1989).

Isolated angiitis of the central nervous system (CNS)

Isolated angiitis of the CNS is a very rare disorder indeed. A granulomatous angiitis, similar to sarcoid, affects the small leptomeningeal, cortical and spinal cord blood vessels to cause a subacute encephalopathy, with or without stroke-like episodes due to ischaemia or sometimes haemorrhage, and sometimes a myelopathy. Systemic symptoms are uncommon, but sometimes there is fever, headache, raised ESR, and a raised CSF protein with lymphocytosis. The diagnosis can only really be made from meningeal/cortical biopsy, which may well be helpful to stop the continuing search for an alternative diagnosis and for specific immunosuppressive treatment, although this is not always particularly successful (Hankey, 1991; Vollmer *et al.*, 1993).

Malignant atrophic papulosis

Malignant atrophic papulosis (Kohlmeier–Degos disease) is another very rare syndrome. There are crops of painless, pinkish papules on the trunk, which heal to form distinctive, circular, porcelain-white scars. Intimal endothelial proliferation and thrombosis in small arteries can cause ischaemia in the brain, spinal cord and gut (Scully *et al.*, 1980; Sotrel *et al.*, 1983; Burton, 1988).

Acute posterior multifocal placoid pigment epitheliopathy

Acute posterior multifocal placoid pigment epitheliopathy is a well-defined but rare ocular disorder with rapidly deteriorating central vision. This can occasionally be complicated by a systemic, including cerebral, vasculitis (Wilson *et al.*, 1988; Bewermeyer *et al.*, 1993).

Buerger's disease (thromboangiitis obliterans)

Buerger's disease (thromboangiitis obliterans) is a rare, but it seems real, inflammatory disorder of mainly distal small and medium arteries and veins, in the lower and upper limbs, to cause gangrene, much more often in men than women, and in smokers. It is often associated with migrating thrombophlebitis and Raynaud's phenomenon but not with the systemic or laboratory disturbances so often seen in the other forms of vasculitis. Cerebrovascular complications have very occasionally been described (Biller *et al.*, 1981; Drake, 1982; Berlit *et al.*, 1984; Lie, 1986).

Lymphomatoid granulomatosis

Lymphomatoid granulomatosis is a rare disorder, possibly lymphomatous, which affects the lungs, skin, CNS and peripheral nervous system as a result of vascular infiltration by abnormal lymphocytes and plasmacytoid cells. The vessel walls become necrotic. The clinical neurological syndrome is of a subacute encephalopathy, cranial neuropathies, seizures and stroke (Leibow, 1973; Schmidt *et al.*, 1984).

7.3   Congenital arterial anomalies

There are several rather unusual anomalies of the arteries which are probably congenital, some being familial, and which may be an occasional cause of cerebral and ocular ischaemia.

Fibromuscular dysplasia

FMD is an uncommon segmental disorder of small and medium-sized arteries (Mettinger, 1982; Luscher *et al.*, 1987). It is found at any age, more in females than males, and usually affects more than one artery in an individual. It can be familial. The renal arteries are the most commonly involved, to cause hypertension. In the neck, the mid to high cervical portion of the ICA and the vertebral artery at the level of the first two cervical vertebrae are the most common sites, i.e. well away from the usual sites of atheroma. The arterial wall is fibrosed and thickened in segments, alternating with atrophy, so that the typical angiographic appearance is of a 'string of beads' (Fig. 7.7). Sometimes there is smooth concentric tubular narrowing of the affected segment or a 'web' at the proximal ICA, which looks more regu-

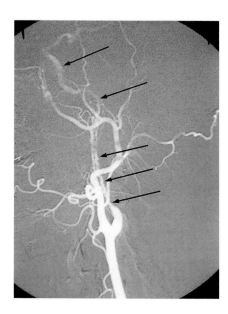

Figure 7.7 Angiogram showing FMD of the ICA. Note the irregular 'beaded' outline of the artery (arrows). (The figure was supplied by Dr Evelyn Teasdale, Institute of Neurological Sciences, Glasgow, UK.)

lar than typical atherothrombotic stenosis (Morgenlander & Goldstein, 1991). FMD seems to be associated with intracranial saccular aneurysms and vascular malformations and itself can be complicated by aneurysm formation, dissection and arteriovenous fistulae. How often and even whether FMD is complicated by thrombosis and embolism is unknown and so, when it is found, one can seldom be sure that it is relevant to any neurological symptoms. Therefore, it is uncertain whether either antithrombotic drugs or angioplasty are sensible treatments, particularly as the natural history is not really known.

Hypoplastic carotid arteries

Hypoplastic, or even absent, carotid arteries have been described. Presumably this situation renders the brain more likely to become ischaemic, although this does not seem to have been described (Schlenska, 1986). A hypoplastic, or absent, vertebral artery is quite common, and usually the other vertebral artery is enlarged to compensate.

Internal carotid artery loops

ICA loops are probably congenital and of no consequence unless complicated by aneurysmal swelling (see Section 7.4), hypoglossal nerve palsy or possibly pulsatile tinnitus. Focal ischaemia on head movement must be extraordinarily rare

(Sarkari *et al.*, 1970; Desai & Toole, 1975). An association with carotid dissection has been suggested (Barbour *et al.*, 1994). Some degree of kinking, buckling and tortuosity of the ICA is quite common, becomes commoner with age and is likely to be due to atheroma or FMD, but it can be congenital (Metz *et al.*, 1961).

Ehlers–Danlos syndrome, pseudoxanthoma elasticum and Marfan's syndrome

Ehlers–Danlos syndrome, pseudoxanthoma elasticum and Marfan's syndrome are all inherited disorders of connective tissue which can be complicated by, or present with: arterial dissection or even rupture, aneurysm formation and caroticocavernous fistula (Bowen *et al.*, 1987; Schievink *et al.*, 1990, 1994a, b; Mayer *et al.*, 1994).

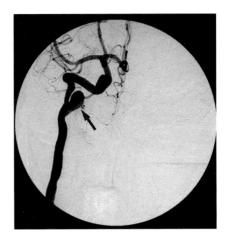

Figure 7.8 Angiogram showing an extracranial aneurysm (traumatic) of the ICA (arrow). (The figure was supplied by Dr Evelyn Teasdale, Institute of Neurological Sciences, Glasgow, UK.)

7.4 Embolisation from arterial aneurysms

Aneurysms may contain thrombus, which can then embolise distally, although it is difficult to be certain about this mechanism unless there is no other more likely cause of cerebral ischaemia and no possibility of vasospasm complicating rupture of an intracranial aneurysm (Maruyama *et al.*, 1989). This situation has been occasionally described with intracranial saccular and fusiform aneurysms (Fisher *et al.*, 1980; Sakaki *et al.*, 1980; Steinberger *et al.*, 1984) and with extracranial ICA or vertebral aneurysms, which are due to blunt or penetrating trauma, infection, carotid surgery, irradiation, atheroma, FMD or inherited disorders of connective tissue, such as Marfan's syndrome (Schwartz *et al.*, 1962; Nesbit *et al.*, 1979; Mokri & Piepgras, 1981; Catala *et al.*, 1993). The diagnosis is made by angiography (Fig. 7.8). Thrombus in the aneurysm may be seen on CT, MRI or angiography. Extracranial aneurysms should also be suspected if there is a pulsatile swelling in the neck or pharynx, dysphagia, a Horner's syndrome or compression of the lower cranial nerves at the base of skull; compression of the spinal cord or roots is exceptional (Dubard *et al.*, 1994).

7.5 Migraine

A *migrainous* stroke should not be a diagnosis of desperation when no other cause for ischaemic stroke can be found, but a *positive* statement to describe a rather characteristic clinical syndrome (see also Section 3.2.1). The occasional patient, from thousands who have previously had migrainous auras (with or without headache), may one day, for no

known reason, experience their typical aura, which then persists as a focal neurological deficit. To make the diagnosis, there should be, in addition, no reason to suspect that the stroke has been caused by anything else, particularly anything which can be associated or confused with migraine, such as cervical arterial dissection (see Section 7.1), APS (see Section 7.2), mitochondrial cytopathy (see Section 7.15) or even an arteriovenous malformation (see Section 8.2.2; Bousser *et al.*, 1985; Shuaib, 1991). Most often, a migrainous stroke causes a homonymous hemianopia (reflecting the most common transient features of migrainous auras), seldom seems to cause persisting and severe disability and perhaps does not recur very often, although data are sparse (Henrich *et al.*, 1986; Broderick & Swanson, 1987). Arterial occlusion has very rarely been demonstrated and it is not clear why it occurs, although 'vasospasm' is often postulated and is said to have been observed in the retinal circulation during transient monocular blindness in a few patients (Winterkorn *et al.*, 1993). Of course, migrainous auras lasting the usual 20–30 minutes can be confused with TIAs, a problem which has been discussed earlier (see Section 3.3.2). Finally, migraine has very rarely been blamed for PICH (see Section 8.3.2).

Migraine is probably not a risk factor for ischaemic stroke in general, but it may be in young women (Marini *et al.*, 1993; Buring *et al.*, 1995; Tzourio *et al.*, 1995). If so, it is not clear if the migraine attack itself causes stroke in some way, whether factors associated with migraine cause stroke (i.e. vasospasm, platelet hyperaggregability, etc.) or whether both migraine and stroke are a reflection of some shared underlying factor, possibly genetic.

> *A migrainous stroke is a well-defined clinical syndrome.*
> *It is a diagnosis neither of exclusion nor of desperation.*

However, a 'normal' stroke (caused, say, by embolism from severe carotid stenosis) can start during the course a typical migrainous episode for that particular individual and so appear to have been provoked by migraine. Sometimes, a normal stroke, or even otherwise asymptomatic low cerebral blood flow, can provoke migrainous episodes with an aura typical for that particular patient or, occasionally, be followed by typical migraine with an aura which has never been previously experienced (Olesen *et al.*, 1993). The potential for confusion in this field is clearly immense. It is not always easy to sort out the exact chronological, let alone the exact aetiological, relationship between migraine and stroke in a particular case, but, at the end of the day, it is feasible, given a careful history, to recognise 'migrainous' strokes.

7.6 Haematological disorders

Just occasionally, ischaemic strokes and TIAs represent a complication of an underlying haematological disorder, which itself may be quite common (such as sickle cell disease) or extremely rare (such as protein S deficiency) (Table 7.1; Grotta *et al.*, 1986; Hart & Kanter, 1990; Greaves, 1993). The diagnosis is not difficult, because the routine first-line investigations will pick up most of the disorders (full blood count, platelet count and ESR) and, if there is no obvious other cause, fairly standard haematological tests will pick up the rest (see Table 6.16). As with cardiac embolism, it can be difficult to know if a diagnosed haematological disorder is *the* cause of an ischaemic stroke if there is a competing cause, but, as often as not, the haematological disorder needs treating in its own right anyway, so that management decisions are usually fairly straightforward. Of course, a haematological disorder may exacerbate any ischaemia caused by co-existent atherothromboembolism or by any other cause of cerebral ischaemia.

Polycythaemia

Polycythaemia is conventionally defined as a haematocrit above 0.50 in males and 0.47 in females, provided the patient is rested and normally hydrated and the blood has been taken without venous occlusion. Above this level, the diagnosis should usually be pursued further by measuring the red cell mass.

Polycythaemia rubra vera (primary polycythaemia) may be complicated by TIAs, cerebral infarction or intracranial

Table 7.1 Haematological disorders that may cause or predispose to cerebral and ocular ischaemia.

Quantitative abnormalities of formed blood elements

Erythrocytes	Polycythaemia rubra vera, anaemia (severe)
Leucocytes	Leukaemia
Platelets	Essential thrombocythaemia

Qualitative abnormalities of formed blood elements

Erythrocytes	Haemoglobinopathies (e.g. sickle cell disease, haemoglobin SC disease, thalassaemia), paroxysmal nocturnal haemoglobinuria
Platelets	Abnormalities of secretion, adhesion, aggregation?

Coagulation disorders

Hereditary deficiency of coagulation inhibitors	Antithrombin III, protein C, protein S, activated protein C resistance
Hereditary abnormalities of fibrinolysis	Plasminogen deficiency and/or abnormality?
Elevated concentrations of coagulation factors	Factors II, VII (see Section 6.2.3)
Antifibrinolytic drugs	

Hyperviscosity

Erythrocytes	Polycythaemia
Immunoglobulins	Waldenström's macroglobulinaemia, multiple myeloma, cryoglobulinaemia

Immunological disorders
APS (see Section 7.2)

Prothrombotic states of uncertain cause
Thrombotic thrombocytopenic purpura and haemolytic–uraemic syndrome
Cancer (see Section 7.9)
Disseminated intravascular coagulation
Pregnancy and the puerperium (see Section 7.11)
Oral contraceptives (see Section 7.10)
Heparin-associated thrombocytopenia with thrombosis (see Section 7.14)
L-Asparaginase therapy
Nephrotic syndrome
Snake bite
Desmopressin
Intravenous immunoglobulin

venous thrombosis (Silverstein *et al.*, 1962; Wetherley-Mein *et al.*, 1987). The increased thrombotic tendency is not just due to the increased whole-blood viscosity but also because the platelet count is raised, and platelet activity may be enhanced as well. Curiously, there can be a haemostatic defect as a result of defective platelet function, so causing intracranial haemorrhage.

Relative polycythaemia is due to reduced plasma volume (diuretics, alcohol, dehydration, hypertension, obesity) and *secondary polycythaemia* to a raised red cell mass (chronic hypoxia, smoking, cerebellar haemangioblastoma, renal tumour, etc.). Whether the raised haematocrit of relative and secondary polycythaemia is a risk factor for stroke is unclear (see Section 6.2.3). A causal relationship is rather unlikely, although some possible cases have been reported (Doll & Greenberg, 1985). Also, increased whole-blood viscosity might have a particularly adverse effect in the microcirculation of a cerebral infarct caused by something else, e.g. embolism from the heart.

Essential thrombocythaemia

Essential thrombocythaemia (idiopathic primary thrombocytosis) (platelet count >500 × 10^9/L) causes arterial and venous thrombosis. Occasionally, paradoxically, there is a bleeding tendency, because platelet function is defective. Headache and transient focal and non-focal neurological disturbances are the most common neurological symptoms (Preston *et al.*, 1979; Jabaily *et al.*, 1983; Murphy *et al.*, 1983; Michiels *et al.*, 1993). Before making this diagnosis, other causes of thrombocytosis should be excluded: malignancy, splenectomy or hyposplenism, surgery and other trauma, haemorrhage, iron deficiency, infections, polycythaemia rubra vera, myelofibrosis and leukaemia.

Leukaemia

Leukaemia is more often the cause of intracranial haemorrhage (because of the haemostatic defect or CNS leukaemic infiltration (see Section 8.4.5)) than cerebral arterial or venous occlusion, which occurs, it is thought, because of the increased whole-blood viscosity (Graus *et al.*, 1985; Davies-Jones, 1995). *Malignant angioendotheliosis*, an intravascular form of lymphoma, can present like a stroke, but the neurological involvement soon becomes diffuse and progressive (Lennox *et al.*, 1989). L-Asparaginase treatment for leukaemia can cause both cerebral ischaemia and haemorrhage (Feinberg & Swenson, 1988).

Sickle cell disease

Homozygotic children and young adults often develop ischaemic stroke and, sometimes, intracranial haemorrhage (Wood, 1978; Adams *et al.*, 1988; Pavlakis *et al.*, 1988). Stroke is much rarer in heterozygotic adults, if it occurs at all, except perhaps in the context of a hypoxia-provoked sickle cell crisis (Greenberg & Massey, 1985; Feldenzer *et al.*, 1987). Small and large arteries and veins are occluded by thrombi as a result of the rigid red blood cells, raised whole-blood viscosity, thrombocytosis, impaired fibrinolytic activity and arterial stenosis due to fibrous proliferation of the intima; the last can be detected in the middle cerebral artery with transcranial Doppler and is predictive of stroke (Adams *et al.*, 1992).

Stroke may also complicate *haemoglobin SC disease* (Fabian & Peters, 1984) but has not been convincingly associated with *thalassaemia*, and when it has occurred was perhaps due to the associated thrombocythaemia (Wong *et al.*, 1990).

Iron-deficiency anaemia

Iron-deficiency anaemia (and presumably other types of anaemia), if severe, may provoke TIAs if there is already severe arterial disease. It probably does not cause ischaemic stroke, and it is much more likely to cause non-specific neurological symptoms, such as generalised weakness, poor concentration and faintness (Siekert *et al.*, 1960; Shahar & Sadeh, 1991).

The paraproteinaemias

Waldenström's macroglobulinaemia, multiple myeloma and perhaps cryoglobulinaemia can be complicated by arterial or venous cerebral infarction as a result of occlusion of vessels with acidophilic material, thought to be precipitants of the abnormal plasma proteins. Intracranial haemorrhage also occurs due to the reduced number and impaired reactivity of platelets, perhaps as a result of uraemia. More often, however, the patients have neither strokes nor TIAs, but the 'hyperviscosity syndrome', which presents as a global encephalopathy, of rather uncertain pathology: headache, ataxia, diplopia, dysarthria, lethargy, poor concentration, drowsiness and coma, visual blurring and deafness; the retina shows dilatation and tortuosity of the veins, venous occlusions, papilloedema and haemorrhages. Similar symptoms may also be due to uraemia, hypercalcaemia or lymphoma complicating the paraproteinaemia (Abramsky & Slavin, 1974; Preston *et al.*, 1978; Scheithauer *et al.*, 1984; Davies-Jones, 1995).

Paroxysmal nocturnal haemoglobinuria

Paroxysmal nocturnal haemoglobinuria is exceedingly rare, and cerebral arterial thrombosis is a less frequent complication than intracranial venous thrombosis. Almost always, the patients are anaemic at neurological presentation, and there may be a history of abdominal pain, recurrent deep venous thrombosis, dark urine, haemolysis and a low platelet and granulocyte count (Al-Hakim *et al.*, 1993).

Thrombotic thrombocytopenic purpura (TTP)

TTP is a rare acute or subacute disease, rather similar to, or perhaps the same as, the *haemolytic–uraemic syndrome.* Platelet microthrombi cause infarcts in many organs, including the brain, leading to a fluctuating encephalopathic illness, with confusion and epileptic seizures, with or without focal features, rather than a simple stroke syndrome. Brain CT may be normal or show infarcts and, occasionally, intracerebral haemorrhage, possibly due to therapeutic heparinisation rather than the TTP itself. The patient is ill, with malaise, fever, skin purpura, renal failure, proteinuria and haematuria. The blood film shows thrombocytopenia, haemolytic anaemia and fragmented red blood cells (Silverstein, 1968; Ridolfi & Bell, 1981; Sheth *et al.*, 1986; Kay *et al.*, 1991; Moake, 1994; Neild, 1994; Oberlander *et al.*, 1995).

Disseminated intravascular coagulation (DIC)

DIC tends to cause an acute or subacute global encephalopathy rather than stroke-like episodes. There are widespread haemorrhagic cerebral infarcts and intracranial haemorrhages. The diagnosis is confirmed by the low platelet count, low plasma fibrinogen, raised fibrin degradation products and raised D-dimer. However, because the patients are so often critically ill as a result of their primary disease, it can be very difficult to disentangle any *added* effect of DIC on the brain (Schwartzman & Hill, 1982).

Hypercoagulability

There are a few rare conditions in which spontaneous and recurrent venous thrombosis (usually in the legs but sometimes in the head) and seldom, if ever, arterial thromboses are presenting or complicating features (Greaves, 1993; Schafer, 1994). These conditions are usually familial: *antithrombin III deficiency* (Arima *et al.*, 1992), *protein S deficiency* (Koelman *et al.*, 1992; Rich *et al.*, 1993; Nighoghossian *et al.*, 1994), *protein C deficiency* (Vieregge *et al.*, 1989; Kazui *et al.*, 1993; Confavreux *et al.*, 1994; van Kuijck *et al.*, 1994), *activated protein C resistance* (Simioni *et al.*, 1995) and *plasminogen abnormality or deficiency* (Schutta *et al.*, 1991; Nagayama *et al.*, 1993).

This whole area is very difficult. Although familial deficiency of antithrombin III, protein C and protein S can cause venous thrombosis, there are far more asymptomatic people with the same deficiency. Therefore, in patients with these coagulation abnormalities, it is conceivable that the cause of any stroke is something quite different (e.g. arterial dissection), so that the patient must be properly investigated. Also,

paradoxical embolism from the venous system must be considered and excluded, as far as it is possible to do so (see Section 6.7.3), before *arterial* thrombosis is postulated. Moreover, acute stroke itself and anticoagulants cause a reduction in the level of these coagulation factors, so that to make the diagnosis of deficiency the tests must be repeated on several later occasions and, to make the diagnosis of familial deficiency, the family members must be tested. Finally, the risk of recurrence and what any treatment should be are quite unknown. Therefore, just how relevant low levels of these natural anticoagulants really are in quite a high proportion of ischaemic stroke patients with 'no other cause' is uncertain (Martinez *et al.*, 1993; Barinagarrementeria *et al.*, 1994; Forsyth & Dolan, 1995).

The *nephrotic syndrome* can be complicated by ischaemic stroke, perhaps due to 'hypercoagulability' (Chaturvedi, 1993), and at least one reason for cerebral ischaemia in the *APS* could be hypercoagulability (see Section 7.2). *Desmopressin* and *intravenous immunoglobulin* are other possible causes of hypercoagulability (Steg & Lefkowitz, 1994; Grunwald & Sather, 1995). Defibrination and bleeding is a much more likely consequence of *snake bite*, but ischaemic stroke has been described (Bashir & Jinkins, 1985).

Despite many attempts to relate quantitative abnormalities of platelet behaviour, impaired fibrinolysis and an increase in coagulation factors to ischaemic stroke and TIA in general, no definite cause-and-effect relationship has ever been demonstrated (see also Section 6.2.3). In most cases, any changes in these haematological variables are a consequence rather than a cause of the cerebral ischaemic event.

7.7 Stroke in association with acute myocardial infarction (MI)

Coronary and cerebral arterial atheroma are so often both present in the same individual patient that it is hardly surprising that there is a past history of MI or current angina in about 20% of ischaemic stroke and TIA patients (see Table 6.4) or that MI occurs so frequently during their long-term follow-up (see Section 16.1.1). However, if a stroke (or TIA) occurs within hours or days of an acute MI, it is tempting, and often correct, to suspect a cause-and-effect relationship (Table 7.2).

In the pre-thrombolytic era, left-ventricular mural thrombus, diagnosed by echocardiography, occurred within days of an acute MI in about 20% of patients, mostly in those with anterior infarcts, large infarcts or a dyskinetic wall segment. Such thrombi may embolise, particularly if protruding or mobile, but most of them seem to do little harm, since

Table 7.2 Causes of stroke within hours or days of acute MI.

Cerebral infarction/TIA	Embolism from left-ventricular mural thrombus
	Instrumentation of the aorta/coronary arteries
	Low-flow infarcts due to hypotension/cardiac arrest
	Atrial fibrillation and embolism from the left atrium
Intracerebral haemorrhage	Thrombolytic drugs
	Anticoagulants
	Antiplatelet drugs
Both MI and stroke caused by the same disorder	Giant cell arteritis
	Infective endocarditis
	Aortic arch dissection
	Embolism from the heart to both cerebral and coronary arteries (e.g. atrial myxoma)

clinically evident systemic embolism occurs in less than 5% of acute MIs (Kinney, 1985; Meltzer *et al.*, 1986; Lancet, 1990; Sloan & Gore, 1992; Vaitkus & Barnathan, 1993). Of course, one can not assume any stroke is ischaemic unless brain CT has excluded PICH, which is a very real possibility in the present age of thrombolytic treatment and was so, to some extent, even before, as a consequence of anticoagulants or aspirin (see Sections 8.4.1–8.4.3; Sloan & Gore, 1992; Fibrinolytic Therapy Trialists' (FTT) Collaborative Group, 1994). Moreover, ischaemic stroke after an acute MI could have other causes, such as emboli occurring during coronary angiography or angioplasty or low-flow infarction due to systemic hypotension; rarely, some non-atheromatous pathological mechanism may cause more or less simultaneous brain and heart ischaemia (e.g. giant cell arteritis (see Section 7.2)).

> *Stroke complicating acute myocardial infarction is not necessarily due to embolism from the heart or hypotension; it may be due to intracerebral haemorrhage. Brain CT scan is always required.*

After the acute period, the risk of stroke is much lower, about 1% in the first year, perhaps higher if there is persisting left-ventricular thrombus (Stratton & Resnick, 1987; Tanne *et al.*, 1993; Bodenheimer *et al.*, 1994). Of course, not all such strokes are due to embolism from the heart, because many of these patients also have disease of their extra- and intracranial arteries and other non-cardiac causes of stroke (Martin *et al.*, 1993).

Just occasionally, MI can be clinically 'silent', in which case the only diagnostic clues may be raised cardiac enzymes

routinely measured in an ischaemic stroke patient (but these may be unreliable, as an increase can occur as a result of the stroke) or a routine ECG showing recent ischaemic changes, such as ST elevation, *particularly* if the changes evolve typically for acute MI over time (see Section 15.2.3; Chin *et al.*, 1977; von Arbin *et al.*, 1982). If still in doubt, echocardiography may show the typical dyskinetic segment of an acute MI.

7.8 Infections

Ischaemic stroke has long been known to complicate those infections of the meninges which cause inflammation and secondary thrombosis of arteries and veins traversing the meninges to enter the brain. Therefore, sudden focal or multifocal ischaemic events in patients with *tuberculous, fungal or syphilitic meningitis* are not unexpected (Table 7.3; Dalal & Dalal, 1989). Occasionally, acute *bacterial meningitis* can be similarly complicated (Igarashi *et al.*, 1984). Some viruses, particularly *herpes zoster*, cause periarterial inflammation and thrombosis: middle cerebral artery occlusion with cerebral infarction has been quite often described a few weeks after the onset of ophthalmic zoster (Bourdette *et al.*, 1983; Sigal, 1987) and sometimes chickenpox (Leopold,

Table 7.3 Infections causing ischaemic stroke and TIAs.

Chronic meningitis	Tuberculosis
	Syphilis
	Fungal (*Cryptococcus*, *Candida*, *Aspergillus*, mucormycosis)
Acute bacterial meningitis	Meningococcal
	Pneumococcal
	Haemophilus
	Borrelia
	Leptospirosis
Viral	Herpes zoster
	Human immunodeficiency virus (HIV)
	Cytomegalovirus
Mycoplasma	
Worms	Neurotrichinosis
	Cysticercosis
Cat-scratch disease	
Carotid inflammation	Pharyngitis
	Tonsillitis
	Lymphadenitis
Infective endocarditis (see Section 6.4)	

Table 7.4 Causes of stroke in AIDS.

Intracranial haemorrhage	Thrombocytopenia
Cerebral infarction	Chronic fungal meningitis
	Herpes zoster vasculopathy
	Non-bacterial thrombotic (marantic) endocarditis
	Irradiation
	HIV vasculopathy?

Table 7.5 Possible causes of stroke in patients with cancer.

Non-bacterial thrombotic (marantic) endocarditis with embolism to the brain (see Section 6.4)
Tumour embolism, sometimes with aneurysm formation and rupture to cause intracranial haemorrhage
Opportunistic meningeal infections (herpes zoster, fungi)
Haemorrhage into primary tumours
   Malignant astrocytoma
   Oligodendroglioma
   Medulloblastoma
   Haemangioblastoma
Haemorrhage into metastases
   Melanoma
   Bronchus
   Germ cell tumours
   Hypernephroma
   Choriocarcinoma
Coagulopathy/thrombocytopenia and intracranial haemorrhage
'Hypercoagulability'
Neoplastic compression of extra- or intracranial arteries
Irradiation damage to extra- or intracranial arteries (atheroma, fibrosis, aneurysm)
Intracranial venous thrombosis due to tumour infiltration or compression, hypercoagulability, etc.
Drugs
   L-Asparaginase
   + Any causing haemostatic defect

1993). Acquired immune deficiency syndrome (AIDS) can be complicated by stroke in a variety of ways (Park *et al.*, 1990; Kieburtz *et al.*, 1993; Table 7.4). *Neurotrichinosis* (Fourestie *et al.*, 1993), *cysticercosis* (Del Brutto, 1992), *mycoplasma* (Mulder & Spierings, 1987), *cat-scratch disease* (Selby & Walker, 1979) and *Borrelia* (Reik, 1993) are also occasionally complicated by stroke. *Infective endocarditis* has been discussed earlier (see Section 6.4).

Finally, inflammation of the ICA in the neck, with secondary thrombosis, can very occasionally complicate pharyngitis, tonsillitis and lymphadenitis, particularly in children (Bickerstaff, 1964).

7.9 Cancer and irradiation

Stroke and cancer are both so common that any association may be no more than coincidence. Also, because patients may not be fully investigated because of the poor prognosis from their cancer, it may be unclear what the exact cause of any stroke was. However, there are some causal possibilities (Table 7.5) to be at least considered in cancer patients, although in most cases knowing the exact cause of any complicating stroke makes little if any difference to the stroke outcome, the risk of recurrence or the overall prognosis (Hickey *et al.*, 1982; Graus *et al.*, 1985; Lefkovitz *et al.*, 1986).

Excessive irradiation of the head or neck, almost always to treat tumours of some sort, can cause damage not just to the microvasculature but to intra- and extracranial large and medium-sized arteries as well (Fig. 7.9). Months, or more often years, after irradiation, a localised, stenotic and accelerated atheromatous lesion in the radiation field may

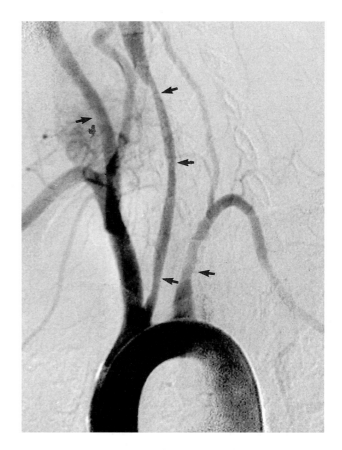

Figure 7.9 Arch aortogram showing narrowing (arrows) of the large arteries in the neck 20 years after irradiation of the cervical lymph nodes affected by Hodgkin's disease.

become symptomatic to cause ischaemic stroke or TIA, perhaps more likely if the plasma cholesterol is raised, and irradiation is one cause of the moyamoya syndrome (see Section 7.13). Fibrosis of the arterial wall and aneurysm formation with rupture have also been described. Ascribing any stroke to the irradiation can be difficult, unless the arterial lesion is in an unusual place for atheroma (e.g. terminal carotid artery) or an aneurysm (e.g. well away from the circle of Willis) and directly within the radiation field, and there is no other more likely cause (Murros & Toole, 1989; Scodary *et al.*, 1990; Bowen & Paulsen, 1992; Zuber *et al.*, 1993).

7.10 Female sex hormones

High-dose *exogenous oestrogen* given to men increases their risk of vascular death and presumably stroke and non-fatal vascular events (Coronary Drug Project Research Group, 1970; Henriksson & Edhag, 1986; Bayar & Corle, 1988). *Oral contraceptives* given to young women about triples their risk of stroke (probably less for haemorrhagic than ischaemic stroke), but exactly how they do so is unknown (Stadel, 1981a,b; Royal College of General Practitioners' Oral Contraception Study, 1983; Vessey *et al.*, 1984). The excess risk probably declines rapidly on stopping oral contraceptives (Stampfer *et al.*, 1988). Although it was hoped that the newer oral contraceptives with a lower oestrogen content would have a neglible risk, this may not be so; there is still about a doubling of risk of ischaemic stroke for 30–40 mg oestrogen pills, but perhaps no excess risk for intracranial haemorhage and no risk at all for the progestogen-only pill (Thorogood *et al.*, 1992; Lidegaard, 1993). Fortunately, the absolute risk of stroke in young women is so low that increasing it by a factor of even three makes little difference, unless their background risk is raised as a result of smoking or hypertension or by being over the age of about 30 years (Croft & Hannaford, 1989).

There are endless arguments about the balance of risks and benefits of *postmenopausal oestrogen replacements*, along with considerable commercial pressure to prescribe, which will never be properly resolved until the appropriate randomised trials are done. As far as vascular disorders are concerned, it seems that there is no excess risk and perhaps some protection from oestrogens, although the effect of adding progestogens is not known (Grady *et al.*, 1992; Belchetz, 1994). On balance, oestrogen replacement, with or without progestogen, is associated with a favourable lipid (higher serum high-density lipoprotein and lower low-density lipoprotein cholesterol) and haemostatic (lower fibrinogen) profile (Nabulsi *et al.*, 1993; Writing Group for the PEPI Trial, 1996). However, so far, these conclusions are based only on observational studies, which are easily subject to various forms of bias, particularly because hormone replacement therapy may be more likely to be given to women without rather than with vascular risk factors (Posthuma *et al.*, 1994). Also, any advantage with respect to vascular disease might be outweighed by an increased risk of certain forms of cancer of the breast and uterus (Davidson, 1995). At least in young women who have had a bilateral oophorectomy, there is good reason to prescribe hormone replacement therapy to reduce the excess risk of coronary heart disease, and perhaps of stroke too (Colditz *et al.*, 1987).

7.11 Pregnancy and the puerperium

Stroke complicating pregnancy or the puerperium is so rare in developed countries—perhaps a frequency of only about 1 or 2 per 10 000 deliveries—that it is all but impossible to estimate the exact risk, and even any excess risk over and above that in non-pregnant females of childbearing age (Grosset *et al.*, 1995; Sharshar *et al.*, 1995). It seems more common in India (Srinivasan, 1983).

Amongst the usual causes of strokes in young women, there are some which may be particularly associated with pregnancy: intracranial venous thrombosis, most often in the puerperium (Cantu & Barinagarrementeria, 1993); acute middle cerebral artery or other large cerebral artery occlusion, perhaps due to paradoxical embolism from the legs or pelvic veins; cervical arterial dissection during labour; low-flow infarction or DIC complicating obstetric disasters; ergot-type and other vasoconstricting drugs can cause postpartum cerebral segmental vasoconstriction, with headache, seizures and focal infarcts, but this may also occur spontaneously and possibly as a result of bromocriptine, so-called puerperal angiopathy; infective endocarditis; peripartum cardiomyopathy; sickle cell crisis; and intracranial haemorrhage due to eclampsia, anticoagulants or rupture of an aneurysm or vascular malformation (Wiebers, 1985; Wiebers & Mokri, 1985; Richards *et al.*, 1988; Donaldson, 1989; Raroque *et al.*, 1993; Dyken & Biller, 1994; Janssens *et al.*, 1995). Eclampsia usually causes a more global encephalopathic syndrome, with seizures, cortical blindness and impaired consciousness (i.e. essentially hypertensive encephalopathy), and should not be confused with focal cerebral infarction or haemorrhage or with intracranial venous thrombosis. Haemorrhagic choriocarcinoma metastases can look exactly like multiple PICH, the diagnostic test being a raised serum human chorionic gonadotrophin level (see Section 5.3.4). There is a curious tendency for migraine auras without headache to occur in pregnancy, and clearly these should be differentiated from TIAs (see Section 3.3.2).

In general, therefore, stroke in pregnancy should be investigated in the same way as any other stroke in a young, otherwise healthy, female, but bearing in mind excess fetal exposure to diagnostic irradiation. The risk of stroke recurrence in any future pregnancy is unknown, but presumably must be fairly low.

7.12 Leukoaraiosis

Leukoaraiosis (Binswanger's disease, chronic progressive subcortical encephalopathy, subcortical arteriosclerotic encephalopathy, periventricular leucoencephalopathy) is not the *cause* of anything. It is a radiological diagnosis with, perhaps, a defined vascular and brain pathology. It is defined as a brain CT scan appearance of more or less symmetrical periventricular and subcortical hypodensity in the cerebral white matter, with or without ventricular dilatation and focal hypodensities, and is commonly seen in elderly people (Fig. 7.10). The same features are seen even better as high-signal areas on T2-weighted MRI. These radiological appearances can be found in apparently normal elderly people but are also associated with gradual dementia, unsteadiness of gait and recurrent ischaemic—particularly lacunar— or, occasionally, haemorrhagic strokes, more frequently in patients with hypertension, other vascular risk factors, atherosclerosis and cerebral atrophy (Bogousslavsky *et al.*, 1987; Cadelo *et al.*, 1991; van Swieten *et al.*, 1991a; Leys *et al.*, 1992; Bots *et al.*, 1993; Breteler *et al.*, 1994). The underlying brain pathology is demyelination, axonal loss and glio-

sis, probably due to anoxia as a result of sclerotic changes in the long perforating arteries of the periventricular white matter, rather than any atheroma of the large arteries, which is variable in extent and severity (Caplan & Schoene, 1978; van Swieten *et al.*, 1991b; Chimowitz *et al.*, 1992; Streifler *et al.*, 1995).

> *Leukoaraiosis is neither a disease nor a definite cause of anything. Nowadays it is a radiologically defined appearance on CT or MRI which is associated with ageing, dementia, unsteadiness of gait and lacunar ischaemic strokes. However, it can also be found in apparently normal people.*

This condition does, therefore, arise as an *additional* diagnostic possibility in patients persisting with an ischaemic (usually lacunar) or haemorrhagic stroke. Preceding hypertension, unsteady gait and dementia and the characteristic brain CT/MRI would suggest that the underlying vascular and brain pathology of leukoaraiosis is present. However, this does not change the management of the TIA or stroke, whatever its cause turns out to be.

7.13 Moyamoya syndrome

This syndrome is as rare as the name is memorable. It is a *radiologically* defined syndrome, not a disease, of severe stenosis or occlusion of one, or more often both, *distal* ICAs, frequently with additional involvement of parts of the circle of Willis and sometimes of the proximal cerebral and basilar arteries. As a result, numerous tiny collaterals develop from the lenticulostriate, thalamoperforating and pial arteries at

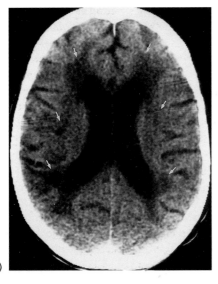

(a)

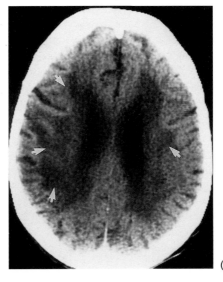

(b)

Figure 7.10 Brain CT scan showing leucoaraiosis ((a) and (b) show two adjacent slices through the lateral ventricles). Note numerous patchy areas of hypodensity in the periventricular white matter (arrows).

the base of the brain; orbital and ethmoidal branches of the ECA; leptomeningeal collaterals from the posterior cerebral artery; and transdural vessels from branches of the ECA. This pattern of collaterals looks like a puff of smoke (moyamoya in Japanese) in the basal ganglia region on the cerebral angiogram (Fig. 7.11). Sometimes there are associated intracranial aneurysms (Bruno *et al.*, 1988; Chen *et al.*, 1988; Ikeda, 1991; Herreman *et al.*, 1994; Bitzer & Topka, 1995).

> *The moyamoya syndrome is a radiological appearance defined on cerebral angiography. There are various causes for the occlusion of arteries at the base of the brain, but often there is no explanation.*

This pattern of arterial disease is almost, but not entirely, confined to the Japanese and other Asians. It can be familial or congenital, and various acquired causes of the occlusion of the arteries at the base of the brain have been suggested: a generalised fibrous disorder of arteries; basal meningeal or nasopharyngeal infection; vasculitis; irradiation; trauma; fibromuscular dysplasia (FMD); sickle cell disease; and neurofibromatosis. Atheroma is very rarely responsible, perhaps because it is not usually distributed so distally in the ICA (Steinke *et al.*, 1992). In most cases, however, no cause is found.

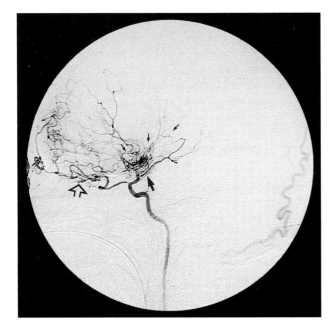

Figure 7.11 Carotid angiogram (lateral) from a patient with the moyamoya syndrome. The ICA ends in numerous small dilated lenticulostriate arteries (thin arrows) and meningeal and ophthalmic artery collaterals (fat arrows and open arrows, respectively). (The figure was supplied by Professor Takenori Yamaguchi, National Cardiovascular Centre, Osaka, Japan.)

The syndrome presents in children with recurrent cerebral ischaemia and infarction, mental retardation, headache, seizures and occasionally involuntary movements, all of which presumably reflect the consequences of low cerebral blood flow. Adults more often present with subarachnoid, PICH or ventricular haemorrhage due to rupture of the collaterals or aneurysms (see Section 8.2.9).

7.14 Perioperative stroke

Cardiac surgery

Cardiac surgery is complicated by stroke in about 2% of cases, the risk being greater for valve than for coronary artery surgery (*Lancet*, 1989). A more diffuse neurological syndrome, with postoperative confusion, soft neurological signs and neuropsychological impairments, is much more common than a focal stroke, but it mostly resolves in days or weeks, perhaps coinciding with the reversible brain swelling which has been demonstrated immediately postoperatively (Shaw *et al.*, 1986; Harris *et al.*, 1993; Barbut *et al.*, 1994; Pugsley *et al.*, 1994). Bilateral ischaemic optic neuropathy must be distinguished from bilateral occipital infarction causing postoperative blindness (*Lancet*, 1984). Possible mechanisms for these complications include embolisation during surgery (of platelet aggregates, fibrin, calcific debris from the aortic or mitral valves, intracardiac thrombus, endocarditis, atheromatous debris from the aorta, fat, air, silicone or particulate matter from the pump–oxygenator system); embolism after surgery from thrombus on suture lines or on prosthetic material, complicating MI, atrial fibrillation or infective endocarditis; global hypoperfusion and ischaemia, due to perioperative hypotension; haemodilution during surgery; a simultaneous carotid endarterectomy under the same anaesthetic to relieve severe carotid stenosis; the cholesterol embolisation syndrome (see Section 7.16); thrombosis associated with heparin-induced thrombocytopenia (Aster, 1995); and intracranial haemorrhage due to thrombocytopenia or antithrombotic drugs. Possible risk factors for these complications include increasing age, intraoperative hypotension, severe aortic atheroma and lengthy extracorporeal circulation. Whether carotid bruits or stenosis influence the risk of perioperative stroke or not is uncertain, but the absolute risk is low, unless the carotid lesion is symptomatic, when the risk may be quite high (Reed *et al.*, 1988; Gerraty *et al.*, 1993; see Section 16.12.2).

Instrumentation of the coronary arteries and aorta may occasionally dislodge valvular or atheromatous debris and thrombus to cause cerebral ischaemia (Ayas & Wijdicks,

1995). Thrombus may also form on an intra-arterial catheter tip, a fragment of catheter may break off and embolise or there may be systemic hypotension. Finally, the cholesterol embolisation syndrome is a rare complication (see Section 7.16) (Galbreath *et al.*, 1986).

General surgery

General surgery is less frequently complicated by stroke than cardiac surgery. There are numerous possible mechanisms, including intra- or postoperative hypotension, causing low-flow infarction perhaps, particularly if there are stenotic or occluded arteries supplying the brain; a haemostatic defect due to antithrombotic drugs or DIC, causing intracranial haemorrhage; positional trauma and dissection of neck arteries during general anaesthesia; paradoxical embolism from postoperative deep venous thrombosis; neck artery penetrating trauma due to attempted venous catheterisation or neck surgery; perioperative MI or atrial fibrillation; infective endocarditis; or the rather nebulous concept of postoperative 'hypercoagulability' (Hart & Hindman, 1982; Tettenborn *et al.*, 1993). Sometimes, any stroke would have happened anyway, particularly in elderly people with multiple vascular risk factors, who increasingly are having surgery as anaesthesia becomes safer.

7.15   Mitochondrial cytopathy

A large family of multisystem disorders is associated with structural abnormalities of mitochondria and biochemical defects in the respiratory chain (Petty *et al.*, 1986; Hilton-Jones *et al.*, 1995; Jackson *et al.*, 1995). Many are now known to be due to various deletions, duplications and specific mutations in mitochondrial DNA, where inheritance is usually through the maternal line. There are a number of rather characteristic, but often overlapping, clinical phenotypes, one of which is characterised by stroke: mitochondrial encephalopathy, lactic acidosis and strokes (MELAS).

MELAS patients present as children or young or middle-aged adults with recurrent focal cerebral ischaemic episodes, usually first affecting the occipital lobes, with infarcts not necessarily corresponding with the territories of distribution of the main cerebral arteries (Ciafaloni *et al.*, 1992). These ischaemic episodes tend to be complicated in the acute stage, or later, by partial and secondary generalised epileptic seizures. Eventually the patients become demented and usually cortically blind. The cause of the infarcts is uncertain; they are due either to a defect in brain oxidative metabolism or to the structural changes that can be seen in small cerebral blood vessels (Ohama *et al.*, 1987). MELAS patients are

often rather short, with sensorineural deafness, migraine, episodic vomiting, diabetes mellitus and some learning disability. There may be additional features more characteristic of other mitochondrial syndromes, such as proximal muscle weakness, exercise intolerance, progressive external ophthalmoplegia, pigmentary retinopathy, myoclonus, ataxia, cardiomyopathy and ovarian and testicular failure.

The diagnosis of MELAS should be suspected in a young patient with an ischaemic stroke, particularly if it is in the occipital lobe and complicated by epilepsy and if there is no other fairly obvious cause (e.g. embolism from the heart). CT of the brain frequently shows basal ganglia calcification and areas of low density in the cerebral hemisphere, reflecting the infarcts, which, at least to begin with, may disappear, and eventually atrophy (Hasuo *et al.*, 1987). The fasting plasma and, particularly, the CSF lactate are raised, usually at rest but, if not, after exercise, although this may be difficult to achieve in disabled patients; CSF lactate may, however, be raised for some days after epileptic seizures, subarachnoid haemorrhage, meningitis and stroke. In most, but not all, patients, muscle biopsy shows ragged red fibres on Gomori trichrome staining and, with electron microscopy, large numbers of abnormal mitchondria are seen. Finally, the point mutation in mitochondrial DNA (at base pair (bp) 3243 in the leucine transfer ribonucleic acid (tRNA)) can be demonstrated in white blood cells, but sometimes only in muscle. However, not all MELAS patients have this mutation and also it can be found in other mitochondrial clinical syndromes, in relatives of MELAS patients who may or may not be symptomatic and in some normal people (Hammans *et al.*, 1991, 1995; Koo *et al.*, 1993). At present, there are no specific treatment possibilities.

7.16   The cholesterol embolisation syndrome

This is a rare syndrome seen in patients with widespread atheromatous disease. It can be spontaneous but is more often a complication of instrumentation or surgery of large atheromatous arteries, such as the aorta, and possibly of anticoagulants or thrombolytic therapy, which releases atheromatous debris and cholesterol crystals into the circulation. Cholesterol emboli are found occluding the microcirculation throughout the body, including the brain and spinal cord.

Hours or days after instrumentation or surgery, a subacute syndrome develops which can look similar to systemic vasculitis or infective endocarditis, with malaise, fever, proteinuria, haematuria and renal failure, abdominal pain, drowsiness and confusion, skin petechiae, splinter haemorrhages, livedo reticularis, cyanosis of fingers and toes, peripheral gangrene, raised ESR, anaemia, neutrophil leucocytosis and eosinophilia, hypocomplementaemia and thrombocytopenia. In this context, there may be additional strokes, but these may not necessarily be due to focal manifestations of cholesterol embolisation in the brain but coincidental, because these patients have such widespread vascular disease. The diagnosis is made by finding cholesterol debris in the microcirculation of biopsy material from kidney, skin or muscle; however, the specificity of this finding is uncertain, because such emboli can be found in people without the syndrome, albeit rarely, at least in unselected postmortems (Coppeto *et al.*, 1984; Cosio *et al.*, 1985; Fine *et al.*, 1987; Cross, 1991; Pochmalicki *et al.*, 1992).

7.17 The young patient

There is nothing very different about the young compared with the old ischaemic stroke or TIA patient; the range of causes is similar — it is just that under the age of about 40 years neither atherothromboembolism nor intracranial small vessel disease is at all likely (but they are still not impossible), whereas over the age of 60 years these disorders become almost overwhelmingly more likely than anything else, other than embolism from the heart. But young patients attract more than their fair share of sympathy and tend to get more intensively investigated, which is not unreasonable because the proportion with an unusual (and treatable) cause is higher than in the old.

Innumerable series of 'young stroke patients' (young being defined as anything from less than 30 to less than 50 years) have been reported; the mix of causes and the proportion with 'no cause' depend on referral bias, as well as investigation intensity, diagnostic criteria differences and biases, and all these can change as the years go by and as more causes are discovered (van den Berg & Limburg, 1993). Three series are shown in Table 7.6.

7.18 The case with no cause

Even after taking an exhaustive history, examining the patient obsessionally and undertaking numerous investigations, there are still patients in whom no reasonable explanation for their stroke can be found or in whom any putative cause might be regarded as somewhat marginal (e.g. mild mitral leaflet prolapse with no complications, oral contraceptives, a rather uncertain diagnosis of migrainous stroke, etc.). Naturally, the intensity of any search for a cause must depend on the previous level of dependency and the age of the patient, the severity of the stroke (aggressive investiga-

Table 7.6 The causes of ischaemic stroke or TIA in hospital-referred young adults.

	Hilton-Jones & Warlow (1985b) (n = 60)	Carolei et al. (1993) (n = 333)	Adams et al. (1995) (n = 329)
Arterial disease	*42 (67%)*	*119 (36%)*	*154 (47%)*
'Atherosclerosis'	7	110	58
Trauma	13		7
Dissection		1	20
Mechanical arterial compression			1
Migraine	10	4	13
Moyamoya syndrome			14
Intracranial arterial aneurysm			2
FMD		2	4
'Vasculitis'	1	2	10
SLE			5
Ulcerative colitis	1		1
Neck malignancy			1
Drug abuse			7
Alcohol abuse			5
Postoperative coarctation of aorta			1
Microangiopathy			2
Infections			3
Embolism from the heart	*5 (8%)*	*64 (19%)*	*58 (18%)*
'Haematological' disorders	*5 (8%)*	*18 (5%)*	*19 (6%)*
Severe anaemia		3	1
Thrombocytosis			
Platelet abnormality	2	1	1
Sickle cell disease			1
Antithrombin III deficiency			1
Protein C deficiency			1
Protein S deficiency			1
Oral contraception	3	13	
Pregnancy/post-partum		1	7
Undetermined and other	*9 (13%)*	*132 (40%)*	*98 (30%)*

tion is reasonable in milder strokes, where there is more to lose from a disabling recurrence), and the consequences of missing the diagnosis (at any age, infective endocarditis must not be missed, whereas traumatic arterial dissection without any medicolegal consequences is not so important, because there is no generally accepted treatment and recurrence is unlikely).

In a puzzling case, it is important to go over the history and examination again, and to check not only that the appropriate investigations have been ordered but that the results have been discussed and are actually available in the medical records. It may turn out that the diagnosis of stroke or TIA has to be revised, which takes one back to be 'stroke' versus 'not stroke' issues discussed in Chapter 3. For example, it is surprising how often, in young people, multiple sclerosis can be confused with stroke, in elderly patients how the pseudobulbar palsy of motor neurone disease can be called a stroke, or at any age how migraine aura without headache can be confused with TIA. So 'no cause for a stroke' may simply mean that the patient has not had a stroke in the first place.

> If there is no obvious cause for a stroke or transient ischaemic attack, it is important to retake the history, re-examine the patient and check not only that all the relevant investigations have been done but that the results have been seen and discussed.

If the stroke diagnosis is secure and all the relevant investigations are negative, then there is little one can do except await events and hope that any recurrence does not bring to light a diagnostic clue which should have led to an effective treatment at the time of the first stroke. In general, the problem is seldom the lack of a key investigation but more often the lack of a good clinical history. Therefore, other than checking out all the possible investigations in Tables 6.13 and 6.14, we think it best to retake the history, re-examine the patient and follow-up the patient carefully. Fortunately, strokes with *truly* no cause seldom seem to recur.

References

Abramsky O, Slavin S (1974). Neurologic manifestations in patients with mixed cryoglobulinaemia. *Neurology* 24: 245–9.

Adams HP, Kappelle LJ, Biller J *et al.* (1995). Ischemic stroke in young adults. *Arch Neurol* 52: 491–5.

Adams RJ, Nichols FT, McKie V, McKie K, Milner P, Gammal TE (1988). Cerebral infarction in sickle cell anemia: mechanism based on CT and MRI. *Neurology* 38: 1012–17.

Adams R, McKie V, Nichols F *et al.* (1992). The use of transcranial ultrasonography to predict stroke in sickle cell disease. *N Engl J Med* 326: 605–10.

Alexander EL, Provost TT, Stevens MB, Alexander GE (1982). Neurologic complications of primary Sjögren's syndrome. *Medicine* 61: 247–57.

Al-Hakim M, Katirji B, Osorio I, Weisman R (1993). Cerebral venous thrombosis in paroxysmal nocturnal hemoglobinuria: report of two cases. *Neurology* 43: 742–6.

Alhalabi M, Moore PM (1994). Serial angiography in isolated angiitis of the central nervous system. *Neurology* 44: 1221–6.

Altinors N, Senveli E, Arda N *et al.* (1987). Intracerebral haemorrhage and haematoma in Behçet's disease: case report. *Neurosurgery* 21: 582–3.

Antiphospholipid Antibodies in Stroke Study Group (1990). Clinical and laboratory findings in patients with antiphospholipid antibodies and cerebral ischaemia. *Stroke* 21: 1268–73.

Antiphospholipid Antibodies in Stroke Study (APASS) Group (1993). Anticardiolipin antibodies are an independent risk factor for first ischaemic stroke. *Neurology* 43: 2069–73.

Arima T, Motomura M, Nishiura Y *et al.* (1992). Cerebral infarction in a heterozygote with variant antithrombin III. *Stroke* 23: 1822–5.

Aster RH (1995). Heparin-induced thrombocytopenia and thrombosis. *N Engl J Med* 332: 1374–6.

Ayas N, Wijdicks EFM (1995). Cardiac catheterization complicated by stroke: 14 patients. *Cerebrovasc Dis* 5: 304–7.

Babikian VL, Levine SR (1992). Therapeutic considerations for stroke patients with antiphospholipid antibodies. *Stroke* 23 (Suppl. I): I-33–I-37.

Banning AP, Ruttley MST, Musumeci F, Fraser AG (1995). Acute dissection of the thoracic aorta. Transoesophageal echocardiography is the investigation of choice. *Br Med J* 310: 72–3.

Barbour PJ, Castaldo JE, Rae-Grant AD (1994). Internal carotid artery redundancy is significantly associated with dissection. *Stroke* 25: 1201–6.

Barbut D, Hinton RB, Szatrowski TP *et al.* (1994). Cerebral emboli detected during bypass surgery are associated with clamp removal. *Stroke* 25: 2398–402.

Barinagarrementeria F, Cantu-Brito C, de la Pena A, Izaguirre R (1994). Prothombotic states in young people with idiopathic stroke: a prospective study. *Stroke* 25: 287–90.

Bashir R, Jinkins J (1985). Cerebral infarction in a young female following snake bite. *Stroke* 16: 328–30.

Bayar DP, Corle DK (1988). Hormone therapy for prostate cancer: results of the Veterans Administration Cooperative Urological Research Group Studies. *NCI Monogr* 7: 165–70.

Beck DO, Corbett JJ (1983). Seizures due to central nervous system rheumatoid meningovasculitis. *Neurology* 33: 1058–61.

Belchetz PE (1994). Hormonal treatment of postmenopausal women. *N Engl J Med* 330: 1062–71.

Bennett R, Hughes GRV, Bywaters EGL, Holt PJL (1972). Neuropsychiatric problems in systemic lupus erythematosus. *Br Med J* 4: 342–5.

Berlit P, Kessler C, Reuther R, Krause K-H (1984). New aspects of thromboangiitis obliterans (von Winiwarter–Buerger's disease). *Eur Neurol* 23: 394–9.

Berlit P, Moore PM, Bluestein HG (1993). Vasculitis, rheumatic disease and the neurologist: the pathophysiology and diagnosis of neurologic problems in systemic disease. *Cerebrovasc Dis* 3: 139–45.

Bewermeyer H, Nelles G, Huber M, Althaus C, Neuen-Jacob E, Assheuer J (1993). Pontine infarction in acute posterior multifocal placoid pigment epitheliopathy. *J Neurol* 241: 22–6.

Bick RL (1993). The antiphospholipid–thrombosis syndromes: fact, fiction, confusion, and controversy. *Am J Clin Pathol* 100: 477–80.

Bickerstaff ER (1964). Aetiology of acute hemiplegia in childhood. *Br Med J* 2: 82–7.

Biller J, Asconape J, Challa VR, Toole JF, Mclean WT (1981). A case for cerebral thromboangiitis obliterans. *Stroke* 12: 686–9.

Biousse V, d'Anglejan-Chatillon J, Touboul P-J, Amarenco P, Bousser M-G (1995). Time course of symptoms in extracranial carotid artery dissections: a series of 80 patients. *Stroke* 26: 235–9.

Bitzer M, Topka H (1995). Progressive cerebral occlusive disease after radiation therapy. *Stroke* 26: 131–6.

Bodenheimer MM, Sauer D, Shareef B, Brown MW, Fleiss JL, Moss AJ (1994). Relation between myocardial infarct location and stroke. *J Am Coll Cardiol* 24: 61–6.

Bogousslavsky J, Regli F, Uske A (1987). Leukoencephalopathy in patients with ischaemic stroke. *Stroke* 18: 896–9.

Boortz-Marx RL, Clark HB, Taylor S, Wesa KM, Anderson DC (1995). Sneddon's syndrome with granulomatous leptomeningeal infiltration. *Stroke* 26: 492–5.

Bots GTAM, Wattendorff AR, Buruma OJS, Roos RAC, Endtz LJ (1981). Acute myelopathy caused by fibrocartilaginous emboli. *Neurology* 31: 1250–6.

Bots ML, van Swieten JC, Breteler MMB *et al.* (1993). Cerebral white matter lesions and atherosclerosis in the Rotterdam study. *Lancet* 341: 1232–7.

Bourdette DN, Rosenberg NL, Yatsu FM (1983). Herpes zoster ophthalmicus and delayed ipsilateral cerebral infarction. *Neurology* 33: 1428–32.

Bousser M-G, Baron JC, Chiras J (1985). Ischaemic strokes and migraine. *Neuroradiology* 27: 583–7.

Bowen J, Paulsen CA (1992). Stroke after pituitary irradiation. *Stroke* 23: 908–11.

Bowen J, Boudoulas H, Wooley CF (1987). Cardiovascular disease of connective tissue origin. *Am J Med* 82: 481–8.

Bragoni M, Di Piero V, Priori R, Valesini G, Lenzi GL (1994). Sjögren's syndrome presenting as ischaemic stroke. *Stroke* 25: 2276–9.

Breteler MMB, van Amerongen NM, van Swieten JC *et al.* (1994). Cognitive correlates of ventricular enlargement and cerebral white matter lesions on magnetic resonance imaging: the Rotterdam Study. *Stroke* 25: 1109–15.

Broderick JP, Swanson JW (1987). Migraine-related strokes: clinical profile and prognosis in 20 patients. *Arch Neurol* 44: 868–71.

Brown MM, Thompson AJ, Wedzicha JA, Swash M (1989). Sarcoidosis presenting with stroke. *Stroke* 20: 400–5.

Bruno A, Adams HP, Biller J, Rezai K, Cornell S, Aschenbrener CA (1988). Cerebral infarction due to moyamoya disease in young adults. *Stroke* 19: 826–33.

Buring JE, Hebert P, Romero J *et al.* (1995). Migraine and subsequent risk of stroke in the Physicians' Health Study. *Arch*

Neurol 52: 129–34.

Burton JL (1988). Livedo reticularis, porcelain-white scars, and cerebral thromboses. *Lancet* i: 1263–5.

Cadelo M, Inzitari D, Pracucci G, Mascalchi M (1991). Predictors of leukoaraiosis in elderly neurological patients. *Cerebrovasc Dis* 1: 345–51.

Cantu C, Barinagarrementeria F (1993). Cerebral venous thrombosis associated with pregnancy and puerperium: review of 67 cases. *Stroke* 24: 1880–4.

Caplan LR (1995). Binswanger's disease—revisited. *Neurology* 45: 626–33.

Caplan LR, Schoene WC (1978). Clinical features of subcortical arteriosclerotic encephalopathy (Binswanger disease). *Neurology* 28: 1206–15.

Caplan LR, Tettenborn B (1992). Vertebrobasilar occlusive disease: review of selected aspects. 1. Spontaneous dissection of extracranial and intracranial posterior circulation arteries. *Cerebrovasc Dis* 2: 256–65.

Caplan L, Corbett J, Goodwin J, Shenker TD, Schatz N (1983). Neuro-ophthalmologic signs in the angiitic form of neurosarcoidosis. *Neurology* 33: 1130–5.

Carolei A, Marini C, Ferranti E *et al.* (1993). A prospective study of cerebral ischaemia in the young: analysis of pathogenic determinants. *Stroke* 24: 362–7.

Carrel T, Laske A, Jenny R, von Segesser L, Turina M (1991). Neurological complications associated with acute aortic dissection: is there a place for a surgical approach? *Cerebrovasc Dis* 1: 296–301.

Caselli RJ, Hunder GG, Whisnant JP (1988). Neurologic disease in biopsy-proved giant cell (temporal) arteritis. *Neurology* 38: 352–9.

Catala M, Rancurel G, Koskas F, Martin-Delassalle E, Kieffer E (1993). Ischaemic stroke due to spontaneous extracranial vertebral giant aneurysm. *Cerebrovasc Dis* 3: 322–6.

Charles PJ, Maini RN (1993). The clinical implications of autoantibody detection in rheumatology. *J Roy Coll Phys Lond* 27: 358–62.

Chaturvedi S (1993). Fulminant cerebral infarctions with membranous nephropathy. *Stroke* 24: 473–5.

Chen ST, Liu YH, Hsu CY, Hogan EL, Ryu SJ (1988). Moyamoya disease in Taiwan. *Stroke* 19: 53–9.

Chimowitz MI, Estes ML, Furlan AJ, Awad IA (1992). Further observations on the pathology of subcortical lesions identified on magnetic resonance imaging. *Arch Neurol* 49: 747–52.

Chin PL, Kaminski J, Rout M (1977). Myocardial infarction coincident with cerebrovascular accidents in the elderly. *Age Ageing* 6: 29–37.

Ciafaloni E, Ricci E, Shanske S, *et al.* (1992). MELAS: clinical features, biochemistry and molecular genetics. *Ann Neurol* 31: 391–8.

Colditz GA, Willett WC, Stampfer MJ, Rosner B, Speizer, FE, Hennekens CH (1987). Menopause and the risk of coronary heart disease in women. *N Engl J Med* 316: 1105–10.

Confavreux C, Brunet P, Petiot P, Berruyer M, Trillet M, Aimard G (1994). Congenital protein C deficiency and superior sagittal sinus thrombosis causing isolated intracranial hypertension. *J Neurol Neurosurg Psychiatr* 57: 655–7.

Coppeto JR, Lessell S, Lessell IM, Greco TP, Eisenberg MS (1984). Diffuse disseminated atheroembolism: three cases with neuro-ophthalmic manifestation. *Arch Ophthalmol* 102: 225–8.

Coronary Drug Project Research Group (1970). The coronary drug project: initial findings leading to modifications of its research protocol. *J Am Med Assoc* 214: 1303–13.

Cosio FG, Zager RA, Sharma HM (1985). Atheroembolic renal disease causes hypocomplementaemia. *Lancet* i: 118–21.

Coull BM, Goodnight SH (1990). Antiphospholipid antibodies, prethrombotic states, and stroke. *Stroke* 25: 13–18.

Croft P, Hannaford PC (1989). Risk factors for acute myocardial infarction in women: evidence from the Royal College of General Practitioners' oral contraception study. *Br Med J* 298: 165–8.

Cross SS (1991). How common is cholesterol embolism? *J Clin Pathol* 44: 859–61.

Dalal PM, Dalal KP (1989). Cerebrovascular manifestations of infectious disease. In: Vinken PJ, Bruyn GW, Klawans HL, eds. *Handbook of Clinical Neurology*, Vol. II: *Vascular Diseases*, Part III. Amsterdam: Elsevier, 411–41.

Davidson NE (1995). Hormone-replacement therapy—breast versus heart versus bone. *N Engl J Med* 332: 1638–9.

Davies-Jones GAB (1995). Neurological manifestations of haematological disorders. In: Aminoff MJ, ed. *Neurology and General Medicine*, 2nd edn. New York: Churchill Livingstone, 219–45.

Davis JM, Zimmerman RA (1983). Injury of the carotid and vertebral arteries. *Neuroradiology* 25: 55–69.

de la Monte SM, Hutchins GM, Gupta PK (1983). Polymorphous meningitis with atypical mononuclear cells in Sjögren's syndrome. *Ann Neurol* 14: 455–61.

Del Brutto OH (1992). Cysticercosis and cerebrovascular disease: a review. *J Neurol Neurosurg Psychiatr* 55: 252–4.

de Recondo A, Woimant F, Ille O, Rougemont D, Guichard JP (1995). Post traumatic common carotid artery dissection. *Stroke* 26: 705–6.

Desai B, Toole JF (1975). Kinks, coils, and carotids: a review. *Stroke* 6: 649–53.

DeSanctis RW, Doroghazi RM, Austen WG, Buckley MJ (1987). Aortic dissection. *N Engl J Med* 317: 1060–7.

Devinsky O, Petito CK, Alonso DR (1988). Clinical and neuropathological findings in systemic lupus erythematosus: the role of vasculitis, heart emboli, and thrombotic thrombocytopenic purpura. *Ann Neurol* 23: 380–4.

Doll DC, Greenberg BR (1985). Cerebral thrombosis in smokers' polycythemia. *Ann Intern Med* 102: 786–7.

Donaldson JO (1989). *Neurology of Pregnancy*. London: WB Saunders.

Drake ME (1982). Winiwarter–Buerger disease ('tromboangiitis obliterans') with cerebral involvement. *J Am Med Assoc* 248: 1870–2.

Drenkard C, Sanchez-Guerrero J, Alarcon-Segovia D (1989). Fall in antiphospholipid antibody at time of thromboocclusive episodes

in systemic lupus erythematosus. *J Rheumatol* 16: 614–17.

Dubard T, Pouchot J, Lamy C, Hier C, Caplan LR, Mas JL (1994). Upper limb peripheral motor deficits due to extracranial vertebral artery dissection. *Cerebrovasc Dis* 4: 88–91.

Dyken ME, Biller J (1994). Peripartum cardiomyopathy and stroke. *Cerebrovasc Dis* 4: 325–8.

Fabian RH, Peters BH (1984). Neurological complications of haemoglobin SC disease. *Arch Neurol* 41: 289–92.

Farrell MA, Gilbert JJ, Kaufmann JCE (1985). Fatal intracranial arterial dissection: clinical pathological correlation. *J Neurol Neurosurg Psychiatr* 48: 111–21.

Feinberg WM, Swenson MR (1988). Cerebrovascular complications of L-asparaginase therapy. *Neurology* 38: 127–33.

Feldenzer JA, Bueche MJ, Venes JL, Gebarski SS (1987). Superior sagittal sinus thombosis with infarction in sickle cell trait. *Stroke* 18: 656–60.

Feldmann E, Levine SR (1995). Cerebrovascular disease with antiphospholipid antibodies: immune mechanisms, significance, and therapeutic options. *Ann Neurol* 37 (S1): S114–S130.

Fibrinolytic Therapy Trialists' (FTT) Collaborative Group (1994). Indications for fibrinolytic therapy in suspected acute myocardial infarction: collaborative overview of early mortality and major morbidity results from all randomised trials of more than 1000 patients. *Lancet* 343: 311–22.

Fine MJ, Kapoor W, Falanga V (1987). Cholesterol crystal embolisation: a review of 221 cases in the English literature. *Angiology* 38: 769–84.

Fisher M, Davidson RI, Marcus EM (1980). Transient focal cerebral ischaemia as a presenting manifestation of unruptured cerebral aneurysms. *Ann Neurol* 8: 367–72.

Ford RG, Siekert RG (1965). Central nervous system manifestations of periarteritis nodosa. *Neurology* 15: 114–22.

Forsyth PD, Dolan G (1995). Activated protein C resistance in cases of cerebral infarction. *Lancet* 345: 795.

Fourestie V, Douceron H, Brugieres P, Ancelle T, Lejonc JL, Gherardi RK (1993). Neurotrichinosis: a cerebrovascular disease associated with myocardial injury and hypereosinophilia. *Brain* 116: 603–16.

Frisoni GB, Anzola GP (1991). Vertebrobasilar ischaemia after neck motion. *Stroke* 22: 1452–60.

Galbreath C, Salgado ED, Furlan AJ, Hollman J (1986). Central nervous system complications of percutaneous transluminal coronary angioplasty. *Stroke* 17: 616–19.

Gerber O, Heyer EJ, Vieux U (1986). Painless dissections of the aorta presenting as acute neurologic syndromes. *Stroke* 17: 644–7.

Gerraty RP, Gates PC, Doyle JC (1993). Carotid stenosis and perioperative stroke risk in symptomatic and asymptomatic patients undergoing vascular or coronary surgery. *Stroke* 24: 1115–18.

Geschwind DH, FitzPatrick M, Mischel PS, Cummings JL (1995). Sneddon's syndrome is a thrombotic vasculopathy: neuropathologic and neuroradiologic evidence. *Neurology* 45:

557–60.

Grady D, Rubin SM, Petitti DB et al. (1992). Hormone therapy to prevent disease and prolong life in postmenopasual women. Ann Intern Med 117: 1016–37.

Graus F, Rogers LR, Posner JB (1985). Cerebrovascular complications in patients with cancer. Medicine 64: 16–35.

Greaves M (1993). Coagulation abnormalities and cerebral infarction. J Neurol Neurosurg Psychiatr 56: 433–9.

Greenberg J, Massey EW (1985). Cerebral infarction in sickle cell trait. Ann Neurol 18: 354–5.

Grosset DG, Ebrahim S, Bone I, Warlow C (1995). Stroke in pregnancy and the puerperium: what magnitude of risk? J Neurol Neurosurg Psychiatr 58: 129–31.

Grotta JC, Manner C, Pettigrew LC, Yatsu FM (1986). Red blood cell disorders and stroke. Stroke 17: 811–17.

Grunwald Z, Sather SDC (1995). Intraoperative cerebral infarction after desmopressin administration in infants in end-stage renal disease. Lancet 345: 1364–5.

Haas LF (1982). Stroke as an early manifestation of systemic lupus erythematosus. J Neurol Neurosurg Psychiatr 45: 554–6.

Hall S, Barr W, Lie JT, Stanson AW, Kazmier FJ, Hunder GG (1985). Takayasu arteritis: a study of 32 North American patients. Medicine 64: 89–99.

Hall S, Persellin S, Lie JT, O'Brien PC, Kurland LT, Hunder GG (1983). The therapeutic impact of temporal artery biopsy. Lancet ii: 1217–20.

Hama N, Boumpas DT (1995). Cerebral lupus erythematosus: diagnosis and rational drug treatment. CNS Drugs 3 (6): 416–26.

Hammans SR, Sweeney MG, Brockington M, Morgan-Hughes JA, Harding AE (1991). Mitochondrial encephalopathies: molecular genetic diagnosis from blood samples. Lancet 337: 1311–13.

Hammans SR, Sweeney MG, Hanna MG, Brockington M, Morgan-Hughes JA, Harding AE (1995). The mitochondrial DNA transfer RNA Leu(UUR) A→G (3243) mutation: a clinical and genetic study. Brain 118: 721–34.

Hankey GJ (1991). Isolated angiitis/angiopathy of the central nervous system. Cerebrovasc Dis 1: 2–15.

Harris DNF, Bailey SM, Smith PLC, Taylor KM, Oatridge A, Bydder GM (1993). Brain swelling in first hour after coronary artery bypass surgery. Lancet 342: 586–7.

Hart R, Hindman B (1982). Mechanisms of perioperative cerebral infarction. Stroke 13: 766–73.

Hart RG, Kanter MC (1990). Haematologic disorders and ischaemic stroke: a selective review. Stroke 21: 1111–21.

Hasuo K, Tamura S, Yasumori K et al. (1987). Computed tomography and angiography in MELAS (mitochondrial myopathy, encephalopathy, lactic acidosis and stroke-like episodes): report of 3 cases. Neuroradiology 29: 393–7.

Henrich JB, Sandercock PAG, Warlow CP, Jones LN (1986). Stroke and migraine in the Oxfordshire Community Stroke Project. J Neurol 233: 257–62.

Henriksson P, Edhag O (1986). Orchidectomy versus oestrogen for prostatic cancer: cardiovascular effects. Br Med J 293: 413–15.

Herreman F, Nathal E, Yasui N, Yonekawa Y (1994). Intracranial aneurysms in moyamoya disease: report of ten cases and review of the literature. Cerebrovasc Dis 4: 329–36.

Hickey WF, Garnick MB, Henderson IC, Dawson DM (1982). Primary cerebral venous thrombosis in patients with cancer—a rarely diagnosed paraneoplastic syndrome. Am J Med 73: 740–50.

Hietaharju A, Jaaskelainen S, Hietarinta M, Frey H (1993). Central nervous system involvement and psychiatric manifestations in systemic sclerosis (scleroderma): clinical and neurophysiological evaluation. Acta Neurol Scand 87: 382–7.

Hilton-Jones D, Warlow CP (1985a). Non-penetrating arterial trauma and cerebral infarction in the young. Lancet i: 1435–8.

Hilton-Jones D, Warlow CP (1985b). The causes of stroke in the young. J Neurol 232: 137–43.

Hilton-Jones D, Squier MV, Taylor D, Matthews PM (1995). Metabolic Myopathies. London: Saunders.

Hinse P, Thie A, Lachenmayer L (1991). Dissection of the extracranial vertebral artery: report of four cases and review of the literature. J Neurol Neurosurg Psychiatr 54: 868–9.

Howell SJL, Molyneux AJ (1988). Vertebrobasilar insufficiency in rheumatoid atlanto-axial subluxation: a case report with angiographic demostration of left vertebral artery occlusion. J Neurol 235: 189–90.

Hughes GRV (1993). The antiphospholipid syndrome: ten years on. Lancet 342: 341–4.

Hughes JT, Brownell B (1968). Traumatic thrombosis of the internal carotid artery in the neck. J Neurol Neurosurg Psychiatr 31: 307–14.

Huston KA, Hunder GG (1980). Giant cell (cranial) arteritis: a clinical review. Am Heart J 100: 99–107.

Igarashi M, Gilmartin RC, Gerald B, Wilburn F, Jabbour JT (1984). Cerebral arteritis and bacterial meningitis. Arch Neurol 41: 531–5.

Ikeda E (1991). Systemic vascular changes in spontaneous occlusion of the circle of Willis. Stroke 22: 1358–62.

International Study Group for Behçet's Disease (1990). Criteria for diagnosis of Behçet's disease. Lancet 335: 1078–80.

Iragui VJ, Maravi E (1986). Behçet syndrome presenting as cerebrovascular disease. J Neurol Neurosurg Psychiatr 49: 838–40.

Jabaily J, Iland HJ, Laszlo J et al. (1983). Neurologic manifestations of essential thrombocythaemia. Ann Intern Med 99: 513–18.

Jackson MJ, Schaefer JA, Johnson MA, Morris AAM, Turnbull DM, Bindoff LA (1995). Presentation and clinical investigation of mitochondrial respiratory chain disease: a study of 51 patients. Brain 118: 339–57.

Janssens E, Hommel M, Mounier-Vehier F, Leclerc X, Guerin du Magenet B, Leys D (1995). Postpartum cerebral angiopathy possibly due to bromocriptine therapy. Stroke 26: 128–30.

Jonasson F, Cullen JF, Elton RA (1979). Temporal arteritis: a 14-year epidemiological, clinical and prognostic study. Scot Med J 24: 111–17.

Kalashnikova LA, Nasonov EL, Stoyanovich LZ, Kovalyov VU, Kocheleva NM, Reshetnyak TM (1994). Sneddon's syndrome and the primary antiphospholipid syndrome. Cerebrovasc Dis 4:

76–82.

Kawakita H, Nishimura M, Satoh Y, Shibata N (1967). Neurological aspects of Behçet's disease: a case report and clinico-pathological review of the literature in Japan. *J Neurol Sci* 5: 417–39.

Kay AC, Solberg LA, Nichols DA, Petitt RM (1991). Prognostic significance of computed tomography of the brain in thrombotic thrombocytopenic purpura. *Mayo Clin Proc* 66: 602–7.

Kazui S, Kuriyama Y, Sakata T, Hiroki M, Miyashita K, Sawada T (1993). Accelerated brain infarction in hypertension complicated by hereditary heterozygous protein C deficiency. *Stroke* 24: 2097–103.

Khamashta MA, Cervera R, Asherson RA *et al.* (1990). Association of antibodies against phopholipids with heart valve disease in systemic lupus erythematosus. *Lancet* 335: 1541–4.

Kieburtz KD, Eskin TA, Ketonen L, Tuite MJ (1993). Opportunistic cerebral vasculopathy and stroke in patients with the acquired immunodeficiency syndrome. *Arch Neurol* 50: 430–2.

Kinney EL (1985). The significance of left ventricular thrombi in patients with coronary heart disease: a retrospective analysis of pooled data. *Am Heart J* 109: 191–4.

Kitagawa Y, Gotoh F, Koto A, Okayasu H (1990). Stroke in systemic lupus erythematosus. *Stroke* 21: 1533–9.

Kitanaka C, Tanaka J, Kuwahara M, Teraoka A (1994). Magnetic resonance imaging study of intracranial vertebrobasilar artery dissections. *Stroke* 25: 571–5.

Koelman JHTM, Bakker CM, Plandsoen WCG, Peeters FLM, Barth PG (1992). Hereditary protein S deficiency presenting with cerebral sinus thrombosis in an adolescent girl. *J Neurol* 239: 105–6.

Koo B, Becker LE, Chuang S *et al.* (1993). Mitochondrial encephalopathy, lactic acidosis, stroke-like episodes (MELAS): clinical, radiological, pathological, and genetic observations. *Ann Neurol* 34: 25–32.

Lancet (1984). Ischaemia of the optic disc. *Lancet* i: 1391–2.

Lancet (1989). Brain damage and open-heart surgery. *Lancet* ii: 364–6.

Lancet (1990). Left ventricular thrombosis and stroke following myocardial infarction. *Lancet* 335: 759–60.

Lee JE, Haynes JM (1967). Carotid arteritis and cerebral infarction due to scleroderma. *Neurology* 17: 18–22.

Lefkovitz NW, Roessmann U, Kori SH (1986). Major cerebral infarction from tumor embolus. *Stroke* 17: 555–7.

Leibow AA (1973). The J Burns Amberson Lecture—pulmonary angiitis and granulomatosis. *Am Rev Respir Dis* 108: 1–18.

Lennox IM, Zeeh J, Currie N, Martin G, Adams JH (1989). Malignant angioendotheliosis—an unusual cause of stroke. *Scot Med J* 34: 407–8.

Leopold NA (1993). Chickenpox stroke in an adult. *Neurology* 43: 1852–3.

Levine SR, Brey RL, Kara L *et al.* (1995). Recurrent stroke and thrombo-occlusive events in the antiphospholipid syndrome. *Ann Neurol* 38: 119–24.

Leys D, Moulin T, Stojkovic T, Begey S, Chavot D, Donald

investigators (1995). Follow-up of patients with history of cervical artery dissection. *Cerebrovasc Dis* 5: 43–9.

Leys D, Pruvo JP, Scheltens Ph *et al.* (1992). Leuko-araiosis: relationship with the types of focal lesions occurring in acute cerebrovascular disoders. *Cerebrovasc Dis* 2: 169–76.

Lidegaard O (1993). Oral contraception and risk of a cerebral thromboembolic attack: results of a case–control study. *Br Med J* 306: 956–63.

Lie JT (1986). Thromboangiitis obliterans (Buerger's disease) in women. *Medicine* 65: 65–72.

Lupi-Herrera E, Sanchez-Torres G, Marcushamer J, Mispireta J, Horwitz S, Vela JE (1977). Takayasu's arteritis: clinical study of 107 cases. *Am Heart J* 93: 94–103.

Luscher TF, Lie JT, Stanson AW, Houser OW, Hollier LH, Sheps SG (1987). Arterial fibromuscular dysplasia. *Mayo Clin Proc* 62: 931–52.

McLean BN, Miller D, Thompson EJ (1995). Oligoconal banding of IgG in CSF, blood–brain barrier function, and MRI findings in patients with sarcoidosis, systemic lupus erythematosus, and Behçet's disease involving the nervous system. *J Neurol Neurosurg Psychiatr* 58: 548–54.

Marini C, Carolei A, Roberts RS *et al.* (1993). Focal cerebral ischaemia in young adults: a collaborative case–control study. *Neuroepidemiology* 12: 70–81.

Martin R, Bogousslavsky J, for the Lausanne Stroke Registry Group (1993). Mechanisms of late stroke after myocardial infarct: the Lausanne Stroke Registry. *J Neurol Neurosurg Psychiatr* 56: 760–4.

Martinez HR, Rangel-Guerra RA, Marfil LJ (1993). Ischaemic stroke due to deficiency of coagulation inhibitors: report of 10 young adults. *Stroke* 24: 19–25.

Maruyama M, Asai T, Kuriyama Y *et al.* (1989). Positive platelet scintigram of a vertebral aneurysm presenting thromboembolic transient ischaemic attacks. *Stroke* 20: 687–90.

Matthews WB (1979). Neurosarcoidosis. In: Vinken PJ, Bruyn GW, eds. *Handbook of Clinical Neurology*: Vol. 38, *Neurological Manifestations of Systemic Disease*, Part 1. Amsterdam: North-Holland Publishing Company, 521–42.

Mayer SA, Tatemichi TK, Spitz JL, Desmond DW, Gamboa ET, Gropen TI (1994). Recurrent ischaemic events and diffuse white matter disease in patients with pseudoxanthoma elasticum. *Cerebrovasc Dis* 4: 294–7.

Meltzer RS, Visser CA, Fuster V (1986). Intracardiac thrombi and systemic embolization. *Ann Intern Med* 104: 689–98.

Mettinger KL (1982). Fibromuscular dysplasia and the brain. II. Current concept of the disease. *Stroke* 13: 53–8.

Metz H, Murray-Leslie RM, Bannister RG, Bull JWD, Marshall J (1961). Kinking of the internal carotid artery in relation to cerebrovascular disease. *Lancet* i: 424–6.

Michiels JJ, Koudstaal PJ, Mulder AH, van Vliet HHDM (1993). Transient neurologic and ocular manifestations in primary thrombocythemia. *Neurology* 43: 1107–10.

Mills JA (1994). Systemic lupus erythematosus. *N Engl J Med* 330: 1871–9.

Mitsias P, Levine SR (1994). Large cerebral vessel occlusive disease in systemic lupus erythematosus. *Neurology* 44: 385–93.

Moake JL (1994). Haemolytic–uraemic syndrome: basic science. *Lancet* 343: 393–7.

Mokri B, Piepgras DG (1981). Cervical internal carotid artery aneurysm with calcific embolism to the retina. *Neurology* 31: 211–14.

Mokri B, Houser OW, Sandok BA, Piepgras DG (1988). Spontaneous dissections of the vertebral arteries. *Neurology* 38: 880–5.

Mokri B, Sundt TM, Houser OW, Piepgras DG (1986). Spontaneous dissection of the cervical internal carotid artery. *Ann Neurol* 19: 126–38.

Montalban J, Rio J, Khamastha M *et al.* (1994). Value of immunologic testing in stroke patients: a prospective multicentre study. *Stroke* 25: 2412–15.

Moore PM (1995). Neurological manifestation of vasculitis: update on immunopathogenic mechanisms and clinical features. *Ann Neurol* 37 (S1): S131–S141.

Moore PM, Cupps TR (1983). Neurological complications of vasculitis. *Ann Neurol* 14: 155–67.

Moore PM, Fauci AS (1981). Neurological manifestations of systemic vasculitis: a retrospective and prospective study of the clinicopathologic features and responses to therapy in 25 patients. *Am J Med* 71: 517–24.

Morgenlander JC, Goldstein LB (1991). Recurrent transient ischaemic attacks and stroke in association with an internal carotid artery web. *Stroke* 22: 94–8.

Muir KW, Squire IB, Alwan W, Lees KR (1994). Anticardiolipin antibodies in an unselected stroke population. *Lancet* 344: 452–6.

Mulder LJMM, Spierings ELH (1987). Stroke due to intravascular coagulation in *Mycoplasma pneumoniae* infection. *Lancet* ii: 1152–3.

Mullges W, Ringelstein EB, Leibold M (1992). Non-invasive diagnosis of internal carotid artery dissections. *J Neurol Neurosurg Psychiatr* 55: 98–104.

Murphy MF, Clarke CRA, Brearley RL (1983). Superior sagittal sinus thrombosis and essential thrombocythaemia. *Br Med J* 287: 1344.

Murros KE, Toole JF (1989). The effect of radiation on carotid arteries: a review article. *Arch Neurol* 46: 449–55.

Nabulsi AA, Folsom AR, White A *et al.* for the Atherosclerosis Risk in Communities Study Investigators (1993). Association of hormone-replacement therapy with various cardiovascular risk factors in postmenopausal women. *N Engl J Med* 328: 1069–75.

Nagayama T, Shinohara Y, Nagayama M, Tsuda M, Yamamura M (1993). Congenitally abnormal plasminogen in juvenile ischaemic cerebrovascular disease. *Stroke* 24: 2104–7.

Neild GH (1994). Haemolytic–uraemic syndrome in practice. *Lancet* 343: 398–401.

Nesbit RR, Neistadt A, May AG (1979). Bilateral internal carotid artery aneurysms. *Arch Surg* 114: 293–5.

Nighoghossian N, Berruyer M, Getenet J-C, Trouillas P (1994). Free protein S spectrum in young patients with stroke.

Cerebrovasc Dis 4: 304–8.

Nishino H, Rubino FA, DeRemee RA, Swanson JW, Parisi JE (1993). Neurological involvement in Wegener's granulomatosis: an analysis of 324 consecutive patients at the Mayo Clinic. *Ann Neurol* 33: 4–9.

Oberlander DA, Biller J, McCarthy LJ (1995). Thrombotic thrombocytopenic purpura: a neurological perspective. *J Stroke Cerebrovasc Dis* 5: 175–9.

O'Connell BK, Towfighi J, Brennan RW *et al.* (1985). Dissecting aneurysms of head and neck. *Neurology* 35: 993–7.

Ohama E, Ohara S, Ikuta F, Tanaka K, Nishizawa M, Miyatake T (1987). Mitochondrial angiopathy in cerebral blood vessels of mitochondrial encephalomyopathy. *Acta Neuropathol* 74: 226–33.

Olesen J, Friberg L, Olsen TS *et al.* (1993). Ischaemia-induced (symptomatic) migraine attacks may be more frequent than migraine-induced ischaemic insults. *Brain* 116: 187–202.

Park YD, Belman AL, Kim T-S *et al.* (1990). Stroke in pediatric acquired immunodeficiency syndrome. *Ann Neurol* 28: 303–11.

Pathak R, Gabor AJ (1991). Scleroderma and central nervous system vasculitis. *Stroke* 22: 410–13.

Pavlakis SG, Bello J, Prohovnik I *et al.* (1988). Brain infarction in sickle cell anaemia: magnetic resonance imaging correlates. *Ann Neurol* 23: 125–30.

Petty RKH, Harding AE, Morgan-Hughes JA (1986). The clinical features of mitochondrial myopathy. *Brain* 109: 915–38.

Pochmalicki G, Feldman L, Meunier P, Rougeot C, Weschler J, Jan F (1992). Cholesterol embolisation syndrome after thrombolytic therapy for myocardial infarction. *Lancet* 339: 58–9.

Posthuma WFM, Westendorp RGJ, Vandenbroucke JP (1994). Cardioprotective effect of hormone replacement therapy in postmenopausal women: is the evidence biased? *Br Med J* 308: 1268–9.

Pozzati E, Giuliani G, Acciarri N, Nuzzo G (1990). Long-term follow-up of occlusive cervical carotid dissection. *Stroke* 21: 528–31.

Pozzati E, Giuliani G, Poppi M, Faenza A (1989). Blunt traumatic carotid dissection with delayed symptoms. *Stroke* 20: 412–16.

Preston FE, Cooke KB, Foster ME, Winfield DA, Lee D (1978). Myelomatosis and the hyperviscosity syndrome. *Br J Haematol* 38: 517–30.

Preston FE, Martin JF, Stewart RM, Davies-Jones GAB (1979). Thrombocytosis, circulating platelet aggregates, and neurological dysfunction. *Br Med J* 2: 1561–3.

Prior AL, Wilson LA, Gosling RG, Yates AK, Russell RWR (1979). Retrograde cerebral embolism. *Lancet* ii: 1044–7.

Puechal X, Chauveau M, Menkes CJ (1995). Temporal Doppler-flow studies for suspected giant-cell arteritis. *Lancet* 345: 1437–8.

Pugsley W, Klinger L, Paschalis C, Treasure T, Harrison M, Newman S (1994). The impact of microemboli during cardiopulmonary bypass on neuropsychological functioning. *Stroke* 25: 1393–9.

Raroque HG, Tesfa G, Purdy P (1993). Postpartum cerebral angiopathy: is there a role for sympathomimetic drugs? *Stroke*

24: 2108–10.

Reed GL, Singer DE, Picard EH, DeSanctis RW (1988). Stroke following coronary-artery bypass surgery: a case–control estimate of the risk from carotid bruits. *N Engl J Med* 319: 1246–50.

Reik L (1993). Stroke due to Lyme disease. *Neurology* 43: 2705–7.

Rich C, Gill JC, Wernick S, Konkol RJ (1993). An unusual cause of cerebral venous thrombosis in a four-year-old child. *Stroke* 24: 603–5.

Richards A, Graham D, Bullock R (1988). Clinicopathological study of neurological complications due to hypertensive disorders of pregnancy. *J Neurol Neurosurg Psychiatr* 51: 416–21.

Ridolfi RL, Bell WR (1981). Thrombotic thrombocytopenic purpura: report of 25 cases and review of the literature. *Medicine* 60: 413–28.

Rother J, Schwartz A, Rautenberg W, Hennerici M (1995). Magnetic resonance angiography of spontaneous vertebral artery dissection suspected on Doppler ultrasonography. *J Neurol* 242: 430–6.

Royal College of General Practitioners' Oral Contraception Study (1983). Incidence of arterial disease among oral contraceptive users. *J Roy Coll Gen Practit* 33: 75–82.

Sakaki T, Kinugawa K, Tanigake T, Miyamoto S, Kyoi K, Utsumi S (1980). Embolism from intracranial aneurysms. *J Neurosurg* 53: 300–4.

Sarkari NBS, Holmes JM, Bickerstaff ER (1970). Neurological manifestations associated with internal carotid loops and kinks in children. *J Neurol Neurosurg Psychiatr* 33: 194–200.

Schafer AI (1994). Hypercoagulable states: molecular genetics to clinical practice. *Lancet* 344: 1739–42.

Scheithauer BW, Rubinstein LJ, Herman MM (1984). Leukoencephalpathy in Waldenström's macroglobulinemia: immunohistochemical and electron microscopic observations. *J Neuropathol Exp Neurol* 43: 408–25.

Schievink WI, Bjornsson J, Piepgras DG (1994a). Coexistence of fibromuscular dysplasia and cystic medial necrosis in a patient with Marfan's syndrome and bilateral carotid artery dissections. *Stroke* 25: 2492–6.

Schievink WI, Mokri B, O'Fallon WM (1994b). Recurrent spontaneous cerevical artery dissection. *N Engl J Med* 330: 393–7.

Schievink WI, Mokri B, Whisnant JP (1993b). Internal carotid artery dissection in a community: Rochester, Minnesota, 1987–1992. *Stroke* 24: 1678–80.

Schievink WI, Limburg M, Oorthuys JWE, Fleury P, Pope FM (1990). Cerebrovascular disease in Ehlers–Danlos syndrome Type IV. *Stroke* 21: 626–32.

Schievink WI, Mokri B, Garrity JA, Nichols DA, Piepgras DG (1993a). Ocluar motor nerve palsies in spontaneous dissections of the cervical internal carotid artery. *Neurology* 43: 1938–41.

Schlenska GK (1986). Absence of both internal carotid arteries. *J Neurol* 233: 263–6.

Schmidt BJ, Meagher-Villemore IT, Del Carpio J (1984).

Lymphomatoid granulomatosis with isolated involvement of the brain. *Ann Neurol* 15: 478–81.

Schutta HS, Williams EC, Baranski BG, Sutula TP (1991). Cerebral venous thrombosis with plasminogen deficiency. *Stroke* 22: 401–5.

Schwartz CJ, Mitchell JRA, Hughes JT (1962). Transient recurrent cerebral episodes and aneurysm of carotid sinus. *Br Med J* 1: 770–1.

Schwartzman RJ, Hill JB (1982). Neurologic complications of dissesminated intravascular coagulation. *Neurology* 32: 791–7.

Scodary DJ, Tew JM, Thomas GM, Tomsick T, Liwnicz BH (1990). Radiation-induced cerebral aneurysms. *Acta Neurochirurg* 102: 141–4.

Scully RE, Galdabini JJ, McNeely BU (1980). Case records of the Massachusetts General Hospital: weekly clinicopathological exercises. *N Engl J Med* 303: 1103–11.

Selby G, Walker GL (1979). Cerebral arteritis in cat-scratch disease. *Neurology* 29: 1413–18.

Serdaroglu P, Yazici H, Ozdemir C, Yurdakul S, Bahar S, Aktin E (1989). Neurologic involvement in Behçet's syndrome. *Arch Neurol* 46: 265–9.

Sethi KD, El Gammal T, Patel BR, Swift TR (1986). Dural sarcoidosis presenting with transient neurologic symptoms. *Arch Neurol* 43: 595–7.

Shahar A, Sadeh M (1991). Severe anaemia associated with transient neurological deficits. *Stroke* 22: 1201–2.

Sharshar T, Lamy C, Mas JL, for the Stroke in Pregnancy Study Group (1995). Incidence and causes of strokes associated with pregnancy and puerperium: a study in public hospitals of Ile de France. *Stroke* 26: 930–6.

Shaw PJ, Bates D, Cartlidge NEF *et al.* (1986). Neurological complications of coronary artery bypass graft surgery: six month follow-up study. *Br Med J* 293: 165–7.

Sherman DG, Hart RG, Easton JD (1981). Abrupt change in head position and cerebral infarction. *Stroke* 12: 2–6.

Sheth KJ, Swick HM, Haworth N (1986). Neurological involvement in haemolytic–uraemic syndrome. *Ann Neurol* 19: 90–3.

Shuaib A (1991). Stroke from other etiologies masquerading as migraine-stroke. *Stroke* 22: 1068–74.

Siekert RG, Whisnant JP, Millikan CH (1960). Anaemia and intermittent focal cerebral arterial insufficiency. *Arch Neurol* 3: 386–90.

Sigal LH (1987). The neurologic presentation of vasculitic and rheumatologic syndromes. *Medicine* 66: 157–80.

Silbert PL, Mokri B, Schievink WI (1995). Headache and neck pain in spontaneous internal carotid and vertebral artery dissections. *Neurology* 45: 1517–22.

Silverstein A (1968). Thrombotic thrombocytopenic purpura: the initial neurologic manifestations. *Arch Neurol* 18: 358–62.

Silverstein A, Gilbert H, Wasserman LR (1962). Neurologic complications of polycythaemia. *Ann Intern Med* 57: 909–16.

Simioni P, de Ronde H, Prandoni P, Saladini M, Bertina RM, Girolami A (1995). Ischaemic stroke in young patients with activated protein C resistance: a report of three cases belonging to three different kindreds. *Stroke* 26: 885–90.

Sloan MA, Gore JM (1992). Ischaemic stroke and intracranial haemorrhage following thrombolytic therapy for acute myocardial infarction: a risk–benefit analysis. *Am J Cardiol* 69: 21A–38A.

Sotrel A, Lacson AG, Huff KR (1983). Childhood Kohlmeier–Degos disease with atypical skin lesions. *Neurology* 33: 1146–51.

Srinivasan K (1983). Cerebral venous and arterial thrombosis in pregnancy and puerperium: a study of 135 patients. *Angiology* 34: 731–46.

Stadel BV (1981a). Oral contraceptives and cardiovascular disease. Part I. *N Engl J Med* 305: 612–18.

Stadel BV (1981b). Oral contraceptives and cardiovascular disease. Part II. *N Engl J Med* 305: 672–7.

Stampfer MJ, Willett WC, Colditz GA, Speizer FE, Hennekens CH (1988). A prospective study of past use of oral contraceptive agents and risk of cardiovascular diseases. *N Engl J Med* 319: 1313–17.

Steg RE, Lefkowitz DM (1994). Cerebral infarction following intravenous immunoglobulin therapy for myasthenia gravis. *Neurology* 44: 1180–1.

Steinberger A, Ganti SR, McMurtry JG, Hilal SK (1984). Transient neurological deficits secondary to saccular vertebrobasilar aneurysms. *J Neurosurg* 60: 410–13.

Steinke W, Rautenberg W, Schwartz A, Hennerici M (1994). Noninvasive monitoring of internal carotid artery dissection. *Stroke* 25: 998–1005.

Steinke W, Tatemichi TK, Mohr JP, Massaro A, Prohovnik I, Solomon RA (1992). Caudate haemorrhage with moyamoya-like vasculopathy from atherosclerotic disease. *Stroke* 23: 1360–3.

Stern BJ, Krumholz A, Johns C, Scott P, Nissim J (1985). Sarcoidosis and its neurological manifestations. *Arch Neurol* 42: 909–17.

Stewart SS, Ashizawa T, Dudley AW, Goldberg JW, Lidsky MD (1988). Cerebral vasculitis in relapsing polychondritis. *Neurology* 38: 150–2.

Stockhammer G, Felber SR, Zelger B et al. (1993). Sneddon's syndrome: diagnosis by skin biopsy and MRI in 17 patients. *Stroke* 24: 685–90.

Stratton JR, Resnick AD (1987). Increased embolic risk in patients with left ventricular thrombi. *Circulation* 75: 1004–11.

Streifler JY, Eliasziw M, Benavente OR et al. (1995). Lack of relationship between leukoaraiosis and carotid artery disease. *Arch Neurol* 52: 21–4.

Sturzenegger M (1995). Spontaneous internal carotid artery dissection: early diagnosis and management in 44 patients. *J Neurol* 242: 231–8.

Sturzenegger M, Huber P (1993). Cranial nerve palsies in spontaneous carotid artery dissection. *J Neurol Neurosurg Psychiatr* 56: 1191–9.

Sturzenegger M, Mattle HP, Rivoir A, Baumgartner RW (1995). Ultrasound findings in carotid artery dissection: analysis of 43 patients. *Neurology* 45: 691–8.

Sturzenegger M, Mattle HP, Rivoir A, Rihs F, Schmid C (1993).

Ultrasound findings in spontaneous extracranial vertebral artery dissection. *Stroke* 24: 1910–21.

Tanne D, Goldbourt U, Zion M et al. (1993). Frequency and prognosis of stroke/TIA among 4808 survivors of acute myocardial infarction. *Stroke* 24: 1490–5.

Tettenborn B, Caplan LR, Sloan MA et al. (1993). Postoperative brainstem and cerebellar infarcts. *Neurology* 43: 471–7.

Thie A, Hellner D, Lachenmayer L, Janzen RWC, Kunze K (1993). Bilateral blunt traumatic dissections of the extracranial internal carotid artery: report of eleven cases and review of the literature. *Cerebrovasc Dis* 3: 295–303.

Thorogood M, Mann J, Murphy M, Vessey M (1992). Fatal stroke and use of oral contraceptives: findings from a case–control study. *Am J Epidemiol* 136: 35–45.

Toro-Gonzalez G, Navarro-Roman L, Roman GC et al. (1993). Acute ischaemic stroke from fibrocartilaginous embolism to the middle cerebral artery. *Stroke* 24: 738–40.

Tulyapronchote R, Selhorst JB, Malkoff MD, Gomez CR (1994). Delayed sequelae of vertebral artery dissection and occult cervical fractures. *Neurology* 44: 1397–9.

Tzourio C, Tehindrazanarivelo A, Iglesias S et al. (1995). Case–control study of migraine and risk of ischaemic stroke in young women. *Br Med J* 310: 830–3.

Vaitkus PT, Barnathan ES (1993). Embolic potential, prevention and management of mural thrombus complicating anterior myocardial infarction: a meta-analysis. *J Am Coll Cardiol* 22: 1004–9.

van den Berg JSP, Limburg M (1993). Ischaemic stroke in the young: influence of diagnostic criteria. *Cerebrovasc Dis* 3: 227–30.

van Kuijck MAP, Rotteveel JJ, van Oostrom CG, Novakova I (1994). Neurological complications in children with protein C deficiency. *Neuropaediatrics* 25: 16–19.

van Swieten JC, van den Hout JHW, van Ketel BA, Hijdra A, Wokke JHJ, van Gijn J (1991b). Periventricular lesions in the white matter on magnetic resonance imaging in the elderly: a morphometric correlation with arteriolosclerosis and dilated perivascular spaces. *Brain* 114: 761–74.

van Swieten JC, Geyskes GG, Derix MMA et al. (1991a). Hypertension in the elderly is associated with white matter lesions and with cognitive decline. *Ann Neurol* 30: 825–30.

Vessey MP, Lawless M, Yeates D (1984). Oral contraceptives and stroke: findings in a large prospective study. *Br Med J* 289: 530–1.

Veyssier-Belot C, Cohen A, Rougemont D, Levy C, Amarenco P, Bousser M-G (1993). Cerebral infarction due to painless thoracic aortic and common carotid artery dissections. *Stroke* 24: 2111–13.

Vieregge P, Schwider G, Kompf D (1989). Cerebral venous thrombosis in hereditary protein C deficiency. *J Neurol Neurosurg Psychiatr* 52: 135–7.

Vighetto A, Lisovoski F, Revol A, Trillet M, Aimard G (1990). Internal carotid artery dissection and ipsilateral hypoglossal nerve palsy. *J Neurol Neurosurg Psychiatr* 53: 530–1.

Vollmer TL, Guarnaccia J, Harrington W, Pacia SV, Petroff OAC

(1993). Idiopathic granulomatous angiitis of the central nervous system: diagnostic challenges. *Arch Neurol* 50: 925–30.

von Arbin M, Britton M, de Faire U, Helmers C, Miah K, Murray V (1982). Myocardial infarction in patients with acute cerebrovascular disease. *Eur Heart J* 3: 136–41.

Watson P, Fekete J, Deck J (1977). Central nervous system vasculitis in rheumatoid arthritis. *Can J Neurol Sci* 4: 269–72.

Wechsler B, Dell'Isola B, Vidailhet M *et al.* (1993) MRI in 31 patient with Behçet's disease and neurological involvement: prospective study with clinical correlation. *J Neurol Neurosurg Psychiatr* 56: 793–8.

Wechsler B, Vidailhet M, Piette JC *et al.* (1992). Cerebral venous thrombosis in Behçet's disease: clinical study and long-term follow-up of 25 cases. *Neurology* 42: 614–18.

Wetherley-Mein G, Pearson TC, Burney PGJ, Morris RW (1987). Polycythaemia study: a project of the Royal College of Physicians Research Unit. 1. Objectives, background and design. *J Roy Coll Phys Lond* 21: 7–16.

Wiebers DO (1985). Ischaemic cerebrovascular complications of pregnancy. *Arch Neurol* 42: 1106–13.

Wiebers DO, Mokri B (1985). Internal carotid artery dissection after childbirth. *Stroke* 16: 956–9.

Wilkinson IMS, Russell RWR (1972). Arteries of the head and neck in giant cell arteritis. *Arch Neurol* 27: 378–91.

Wilson CA, Choromokos EA, Sheppard R (1988). Acute posterior multifocal placoid pigment epitheliopathy and cerebral vasculitis. *Arch Ophthalmol* 106: 796–800.

Winterkorn JMS, Kupersmith MJ, Wirtschafter JD, Forman S (1993). Brief report: treatment of vasospastic amaurosis fugax with calcium-channel blockers. *N Engl J Med* 329: 396–8.

Wong V, Yu YL, Liang RHS, Tso WK, Li AMC, Chan TK (1990). Cerebral thrombosis in β-thalassemia/haemoglobin E disease. *Stroke* 21: 812–16.

Wood DH (1978). Cerebrovascular complications of sickle cell anaemia. *Stroke* 9: 73–5.

Writing Group for the PEPI Trial (1996). Effects of hormone replacement therapy on endometrial histology in postmenopausal women. The Postmenopausal Estrogen/Progestin Interventions (PEPI) Trial. *J Am Med Assoc* 275: 370–5.

Zuber M, Khoubesserian P, Meder JF, Mas JL (1993). A 34-year delay and focal postirradiation intracranial vasculopathy. *Cerebrovasc Dis* 3: 181–2.

Zuber M, Meary E, Meder J-F, Mas J-L (1994). Magnetic resonance imaging and dynamic CT scan in cervical artery dissections. *Stroke* 25: 576–81.

What caused this intracerebral haemorrhage?

8

8.1   Introduction

As a rule, there is no single cause for primary intracerebral haemorrhage (PICH) but a network of interacting factors. Take the classical example of a so-called hypertensive haemorrhage: a haematoma developing in the region of the basal ganglia, in an elderly patient on anticoagulants for chronic atrial fibrillation and for an even longer period on antihyper-tensive drugs. Should hypertension or anticoagulants be considered *the* cause of the PICH? The weight of each of these two factors depends on the degree of damage to the small arteries in the brain as a result of previously raised blood pressure (unknown), on the actual blood pressure immediately before the onset of the haemorrhage (also unknown) and probably also on the degree of anticoagulation. Even a combination of recognised 'causes', such as that of hyperten-

287

sion and anticoagulants, does not invariably lead to intracerebral haemorrhage. Apparently, the presence or absence of other factors, of minor importance by themselves, can be decisive. Possible examples of such additional factors are diet, smoking, head trauma and the plasma cholesterol. Not uncommonly, a combination of minor factors may lead to PICH, as some patients seem to lack even a single one of the major 'causes'. In general, therefore, we are dealing with a combination of causal factors, rather than with single causes, and even for the major factors the relationship with subsequent PICH is neither sufficient nor necessary (Wulff, 1995).

The major causal factors can be broadly distinguished into three categories (Table 8.1): anatomical factors (lesions or malformations of the vasculature in the brain), haemodynamic factors (blood pressure) and haemostatic factors (to do with platelet function or with the coagulation system). Abnormalities of the vascular system account for the vast majority of haemorrhages. The type of underlying

Table 8.1 Causal factors in PICH.

Anatomical factors: changes or malformations of the cerebral blood vessels
Lipohyalinosis and microaneurysms in small, penetrating vessels (see Section 8.2.1)
Cerebral arteriovenous malformations (see Section 8.2.2)
Amyloid angiopathy (see Section 8.2.3)
Saccular aneurysms (see Section 8.2.4)
Intracranial venous thrombosis (see Section 8.2.5)
Microangiomas (see Section 8.2.6)
Dural arteriovenous malformations (see Section 8.2.7)
Septic arteritis and mycotic aneurysms (see Section 8.2.8)
Moyamoya syndrome (see Section 8.2.9)
Arterial dissection (see Section 8.2.10)
Caroticocavernous fistula (see Section 8.2.11)

Haemodynamic factors
Arterial hypertension (see Section 8.3.1)
Migraine (see Section 8.3.2)

Haemostatic factors
Anticoagulants (see Section 8.4.1)
Antiplatelet drugs (see Section 8.4.2)
Thrombolytic treatment (see Section 8.4.3)
Haemophilia (see Section 8.4.4)
Leukaemia and thrombocytopenia (see Section 8.4.5)

Other factors
Intracerebral tumours (see Section 8.5.1)
Alcohol (see Section 8.5.2)
Amphetamines (see Section 8.5.3)
Cocaine and other smpathomimetic drugs (see Section 8.5.4)
Vasculitis (see Section 8.5.5)

---

abnormality varies with age: below the age of 40 years arteriovenous malformations (AVMs) or microangiomas are the most common single cause of intracerebral haemorrhage, whereas between 40 and 70 years the most frequent lesions are deep haemorrhages from rupture of small perforating arteries, and in the elderly one also finds haemorrhages in the white matter ('lobar' haemorrhages), commonly attributed to amyloid angiopathy (Schutz *et al.*, 1990). These a priori probabilities are discussed in more detail in Section 8.6, in relation to the site of the haemorrhage.

8.2 Anatomical factors

8.2.1 Lipohyalinosis and microaneurysms

When Charcot and Bouchard (1868) examined the brains of patients who had died from intracerebral haemorrhage and immersed them in running water to remove not only unclotted blood but also most of the brain tissue, they found multiple, minute outpouchings of small blood vessels, which they called miliary aneurysms. Such miliary aneurysms were most frequent in the thalamus and corpus striatum, and less often in the pons, cerebellum and cerebral white matter (Fig. 8.1). Their view that these microaneurysms were commonly the source of primary bleeding was generally accepted until the beginning of the 20th century, when the lesions they had seen were attributed to nothing more than perivascular collections of blood clot (Ellis, 1909; Adams & vander Eecken, 1953). Other explanations gained ascendancy, particularly an older theory that haemorrhages were in fact secondary to previous brain infarction. In 1963, Ross Russell not only rediscovered the existence of microaneurysms, but also established a close relationship between these abnormalities and hypertension (Ross Russell, 1963). He performed postmortem studies of the brains of hypertensive and normotensive elderly, by injecting barium sulphate into the basal arteries of the brain and by examining brain slices after fixation. Microaneurysms were found in 15 of 16 brains from hypertensive patients and in only 10 of 38 brains from normotensives; more than 10 microaneurysms were found only in previously hypertensive patients, with one dubious exception in the control group. The microaneurysms measured 300–900 μm in diameter and were found on small arteries 100–300 μm in diameter, commonly branches of the lateral lenticulostriate arteries in the region of the basal ganglia (Fig. 8.2). On microscopical study, the walls of the aneurysm consisted of connective tissue only, the muscle layer of the parent vessel being interrupted at the origin of the aneurysm. Some aneurysms were thrombosed, others showed evidence

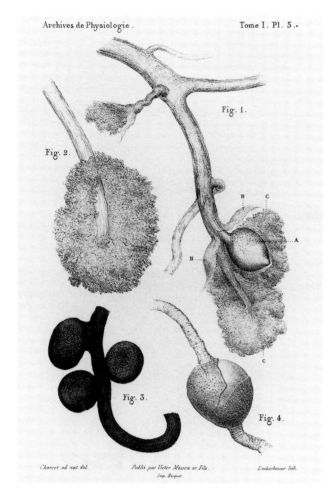

Archives de Physiologie .   Tome I. Pl. 5 ..

Fig. 1.

Fig. 2.

B   c

A

B

c

Fig. 3.

Fig. 4.

Charcot ad nat. del.   Publié par Victor Masson et Fils .   Zuckerbauer lith.
Imp. Becquet.

Figure 8.1 'Miliary aneurysms' (Charcot & Bouchard, 1868). (Fig. 1) A microaneurysm within a clot; (Fig. 2) a clot only; (Fig. 3) and (Fig. 4) microaneurysms without surrounding clot.

of previous leakage in the form of iron-laden macrophages, and occasionally a thin-walled aneurysm had ruptured whilst the contrast agent was being injected. These findings were confirmed and expanded in a larger study, by Cole and Yates (1967b), of the brains of 100 normotensive patients, seven of whom had microaneurysms, and of 100 hypertensive patients, with microaneurysms in 46 cases. Most microaneurysms occurred on vessels below 250 μm in diameter. Twenty of the 100 hypertensive patients and one normotensive patient had died from massive intracerebral haemorrhage, but because of the disruption of brain tissue it was possible on only one occasion to trace the haemorrhage to a specific aneurysm. In 13 of the 46 brains of those hypertensive patients who had microaneurysms, there were also small haemorrhages in the white matter of the cerebral hemi-

spheres, the basal ganglia and the internal capsule; in only four cases were there massive haemorrhages (Cole & Yates, 1967a). Apart from hypertension, age was found to be an important determinant for the occurrence of microaneurysms: even in severely hypertensive patients, these lesions were rare under the age of 50 years. The distribution of microaneurysms through the brain paralleled that of small perforating vessels: most densely in the region of the thalamus, basal ganglia and internal capsule, and more sparsely in the pons, cerebellum and cerebral white matter (Fig. 8.3). Cole and Yates (1967c) also described two types of pseudoaneurysms, both of which were thought to be the result rather than the cause of intracerebral haemorrhage. One type consisted of globular, often laminated, clots at the site of rupture of an arteriole, sizes varying between 1 mm and 1 cm. These occlusive thrombi strikingly resembled some of the more ragged aneurysms described by Charcot and Bouchard (1868), and were identical to the 'fibrin globes' reported by Fisher a few years later (Fig. 8.4) (Fisher, 1971). The second type consisted of the haemorrhage extending into a short section of the perivascular space of an arteriole, before it entered the main bulk of the haematoma; in this way, the arteriole was covered with an irregular, bullous mantle of clotted blood. These two types of pseudoaneurysms were also found in patients under 40 years with haemorrhages from saccular aneurysms or other specific sources, subjects in whom true microaneurysms are extremely rare.

It is questionable whether microaneurysms are the single and only source of haemorrhage from small perforating vessels. Fisher (1971) microscopically examined the border region of the haematoma in two patients with putaminal haemorrhage and in one patient with a pontine haemorrhage. In all three cases, he found not single but multiple points of bleeding, which were identified as 'fibrin globes', in the margin of the haematoma (Fig. 8.4); the core of each 'fibrin globe' consisted of a plug of platelets, which occluded the lumen of a small artery. In the putaminal haemorrhages, he also found the primary source of the haemorrhage, in the form of a clot in the ruptured wall of a relatively large artery. Fisher proposed that rupture of a single small artery might subsequently lead to damage and rupture of other vessels, thus causing an 'avalanche' of secondary haemorrhages. The degenerative changes he found in the walls of the small perforating vessels, consisting of a segmental process of fatty changes and fibrinoid necrosis (so-called lipohyalinosis (see also Section 6.3)), were associated with local thinning; these weak spots might well be vulnerable to microtrauma in the form of an adjacent haemorrhage. Others also found fibrinoid necrosis of the walls of these small vessels as an almost invariable phenomenon in patients with PICH (Ooneda *et al.*, 1973). Fisher's emphasis on degenerative changes other

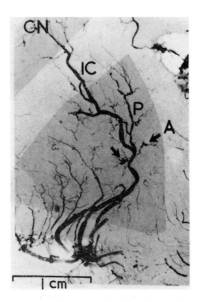

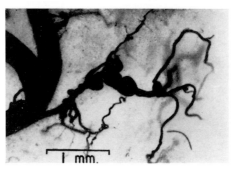

Figure 8.2 Microaneurysms. Left: X-ray of striate arteries in coronal section of basal ganglia from elderly hypertensive subject; barium sulphate had been injected in the arterial tree before formalin fixation of the brain. Irregularity of main trunks, attenuation of small arteries and number of microaneurysms (arrows). Right: enlarged view of area showing multiple aneurysms. (From Ross Russell, 1963; by kind permission of the author and *Brain*.)

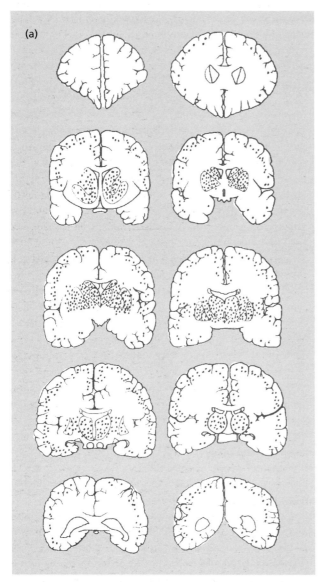

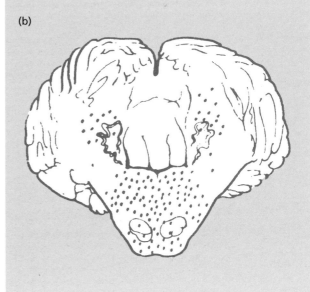

Figure 8.3 (a) Sites of all microaneurysms discovered in the cerebral hemispheres of 53 patients (46/100 with hypertension and 7/100 normotensives). Successive front-to-back sections, from top to bottom and left to right. (b) Sites of microaneurysms in the hind brains of 53 patients, represented in a single section. (From Cole & Yates, 1967b; by kind permission of the authors and the *Journal of Pathology and Bacteriology*.)

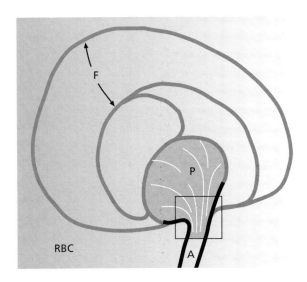

Figure 8.4 Schematic representation of an occlusive thrombus at the site of rupture in a small perforating artery. A, ruptured artery; F, fibrin; P, platelets; RBC, red blood cells. (From Fisher, 1971; by kind permission of the author and Charles C. Thomas, publisher.)

than microaneurysms was also confirmed by an electron-microscopic study of specimens obtained at autopsy or emergency surgery, which showed the most common site of rupture to be at distal bifurcations of lenticulostriate arteries, and rarely in the wall of a microaneurysm (Takebayashi & Kaneko, 1983). The arteries in question were affected by atrophy and fragmentation of smooth-muscle cells. In autopsied cases, the ruptured perforators mostly measured 500–700 μm, in contrast to the smaller size of the arteries previously reported to form microaneurysms. Also, in fatal cases there were invariably multiple sites of rupture, two to 11 in number. Rapid expansion of intracerebral haematomas has repeatedly been documented (Kelley *et al.*, 1982; Chen *et al.*, 1989; Bae *et al.*, 1992). Further support for the 'avalanche' theory comes from systematic studies of patients with PICH in whom the first computerised tomography (CT) scan was performed within 24 hours of the first symptoms and a second CT scan 1-day later, showing an increase in size in 10–14% of patients; expansion occurred most often in patients admitted within a few hours, in patients with large or irregularly shaped haematomas and in patients with liver failure (Fujii *et al.*, 1994; Mayer *et al.*, 1994).

It seems, therefore, that perforating vessels can tear without preceding aneurysmal dilatation, and that microaneurysms are perhaps as much a marker of degenerative changes in small-calibre arteries as a necessary source of bleeding. The relative proportions are unknown. Some maintain that even the microaneurysms demonstrated by

contemporary studies are artefacts caused by the injection technique or misinterpretations of arteriolar coils (Challa *et al.*, 1992).

'Hypertensive' intracerebral haemorrhage results from degenerative changes in small perforating vessels, most of which are found in deep regions: basal ganglia, cerebellum and brainstem. Microaneurysms occur on these vessels but are not necessarily the site of rupture.

Recurrent bleeding has been documented after bleeding in the basal ganglia (Fig. 8.5) or cerebellum, presumably from degenerative arteriolar disease (Lee *et al.*, 1990), but such recurrences are distinctly less common than with haemorrhages at the border between white and grey matter, presumably caused by amyloid angiopathy (see Section 8.2.3) (Passero *et al.*, 1995).

8.2.2 Cerebral arteriovenous malformations (AVMs)

Although demonstrable AVMs are the most common single cause of PICH in the young, they underlie not more than about one-third of all cases, at least in a series of 72 patients aged under 45 years referred to a university hospital (Toffol *et al.*, 1987). AVMs are conglomerates of dilated arteries and veins, without a capillary network between them, and are embedded in a stroma devoid of normal brain tissue. On angiography, they are recognisable by the large feeding arteries and the rapid shunting of blood to veins that are enlarged and tortuous, often with a central tangle of dilated vessels, between arteries and veins (see Chapter 14). According to the classification of McCormick (1966), AVMs should be anatomically distinguished from four other types of vascular anomalies: venous angiomas, cavernous angiomas, telangiectasias and varices. The first three of these four types will be further discussed below, under the heading of microangiomas, together with small AVMs (see Section 8.2.6). Multiple AVMs are extremely rare: in only 4% of cases if there is no underlying systemic disorder, such as hereditary haemorrhagic telangiectasia or Rendu–Osler–Weber syndrome (Willinsky *et al.*, 1990). Familial occurrence of AVMs has been reported but is very uncommon (Yokoyama *et al.*, 1991).

The larger supratentorial AVMs, about one-third of the total, receive feeding arteries from different arterial systems, from two or all three major supratentorial arteries (Parkinson & Bachers, 1980). In 10–20%, they are associated with thin-walled saccular aneurysms on feeding arteries, different from the classical sites of saccular aneurysms at the circle of Willis (see Section 9.1.1). These associated aneurysms are likely sources of bleeding and, with AVMs in

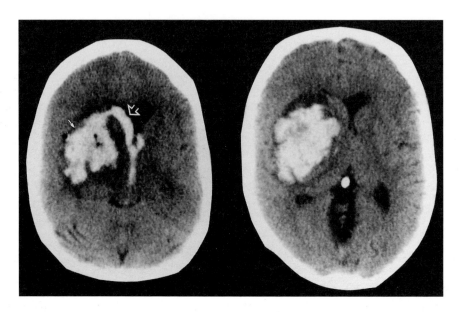

Figure 8.5 Rebleeding in a 40-year-old woman with 'hypertensive' intracerebral haemorrahge. Left: large haematoma in the right basal ganglia (arrow), with rupture into the frontal horn of the right lateral ventricle (open arrow); the haematoma was surgically removed on the same day, because of progressive deterioration of consciousness. Right: fresh haematoma, indicated by sudden deterioration, 4 weeks after the initial episode; angiography was normal.

which one or more aneurysms have formed, the annual risk of rebleeding is as high as 7%, against the usual rate of 2–3%/year for AVMs without associated aneurysm, regardless of whether previous rupture has occurred (Aminoff, 1987; Heros & Tu, 1987; Brown *et al.*, 1990; Ondra *et al.*, 1990; Marks *et al.*, 1992). AVMs are believed to increase in size over the years, but this has rarely been documented (Waltimo, 1973; Mendelow *et al.*, 1987; Minakawa *et al.*, 1989). Spontaneous regression through thrombosis does also occur, mostly in patients over 30 years, with AVMs under 2 cm in size and with single feeders (Wakai *et al.*, 1983; Minakawa *et al.*, 1989). Spontaneous thrombosis of an AVM is usually preceded by an episode of haemorrhage, although exceptions have been reported (Wharen *et al.*, 1982; Guazzo & Xuereb, 1994).

Aneurysms are often found on the feeding arteries to arteriovenous malformations, when the risk of bleeding, or rebleeding, is about double the risk in patients without such aneurysms.

Haemorrhages from AVMs are mostly in the white matter ('lobar'), but they also occur in the deep nuclei of the cerebral hemisphere (Toffol *et al.*, 1987). Subarachnoid haemorrhage (SAH) results if the haematoma reaches the surface of the brain, but SAH from an AVM without a parenchymal haematoma is rare — in only 4% (Aoki, 1991). If an AVM does rupture, it is mostly on the venous side of the malforma-

tion. This is in accordance with the finding that in unruptured AVMs the risk of future bleeding is relatively great if there is only a single draining vein, and even greater if venous drainage is impaired or confined to the deep venous system (Miyasaka *et al.*, 1992). Rupture of a vein would also explain the often slower onset of the clinical deficits with haemorrhages from AVMs than with haematomas from ruptured small arteries or from saccular aneurysms.

8.2.3 Amyloid angiopathy

This disorder has only been recognised as a cause of PICH, particularly of lobar haemorrhages, in the last few decades. Although case reports started to appear at the beginning of this century (Fischer, 1910; Vinters, 1987), the first series of patients were not reported until the 1970s (Torack, 1975; Jellinger, 1977). Interestingly, in the first reports, the condition was usually associated with dementia of the Alzheimer type, characterised by the presence of amyloid plaques in the brain, but it is now well established that amyloid angiopathy may occur without clinical evidence of dementia and also without amyloid plaques or any of the other hallmarks of Alzheimer's disease necessarily being present in the brain parenchyma (Gilbert & Vinters, 1983; Kalyan Raman & Kalyan Raman, 1984). In amyloid angiopathy, the underlying abnormality consists of patchy deposits of amyloid in the muscle layer of small and medium-sized arteries (Fig. 8.6) in the leptomeninges, the cerebral cortex and the subcortical white matter (Vinters, 1987). In unselected autopsies, these abnormalities also occur in subjects without a history of haemorrhage, the proportion increasing with age, from 5 to 10% in those aged between 60 and 69 years, approximately 25% between ages 70 and 79 years, 40% between 80 and 89 years, to more than 50% for those over 90 years (Tomonaga, 1981; Vinters & Gilbert, 1983; Masuda *et al.*, 1988). Arteries in the occipital, parietal and frontal lobes are most often involved. The amyloid deposits occur only in cerebral vessels and are therefore not part of a process of generalised amyloidosis.

What evidence is there to attribute the occurrence of haemorrhages in the white matter to amyloid angiopathy, given that it is so common in the brain of elderly subjects? The morphological difference between amyloid angiopathy with haemorrhages and amyloid angiopathy without haemorrhages is the greater extent of the amyloid deposits and the presence of secondary fibrinoid necrosis of the wall of cortical arteries of those with PICH, sometimes leading to the for-

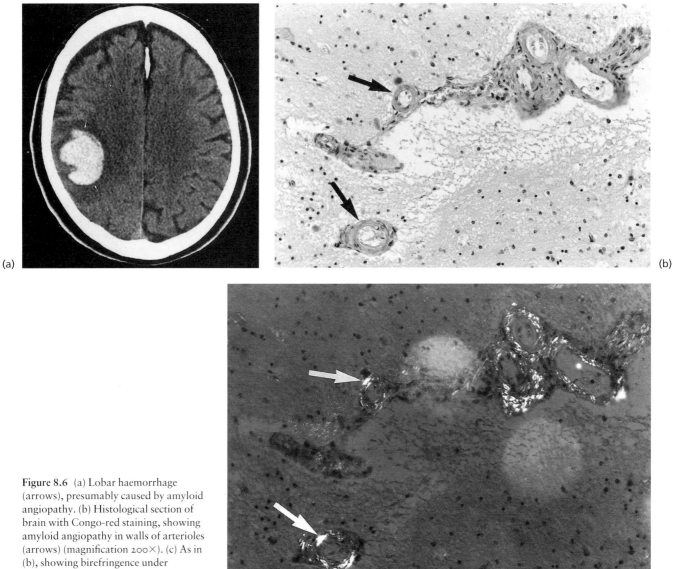

(a)

(b)

(c)

Figure 8.6 (a) Lobar haemorrhage (arrows), presumably caused by amyloid angiopathy. (b) Histological section of brain with Congo-red staining, showing amyloid angiopathy in walls of arterioles (arrows) (magnification 200×). (c) As in (b), showing birefringence under polarised light (arrows) (see also Fig. 5.8).

mation of aneurysms (Vonsattel *et al.*, 1991; Maeda *et al.*, 1993). Such secondary changes are rare in meningeal vessels affected by amyloid angiopathy, which bleed only rarely (Yamada *et al.*, 1993). The site of haemorrhages associated with amyloid angiopathy is almost exclusively lobar, conforming to the distribution of amyloid angiopathy; cerebellar haemorrhages associated with amyloid angiopathy are less common (Masuda *et al.*, 1988; Itoh *et al.*, 1993). The site of rupture occurs at the border zone between the white and grey matter and may enter the subarachnoid space; pure SAHs from rupture of leptomeningeal vessels have not been reported (Yamada *et al.*, 1993).

The proportion of haemorrhages in general that are related to amyloid angiopathy is probably fairly constant, at least above the age of 50 years, because the steep rise in the incidence of PICH with increasing age applies to deep haemorrhages (including those in the cerebellum and pons), at least as much as to lobar haemorrhages (Broderick *et al.*, 1993a). Given that lobar haemorrhage accounts for approximately 25–40% of all PICH in community studies (Broderick *et al.*, 1993a; Anderson *et al.*, 1994) and that in large autopsy series 30% of lobar haemorrhages are attributable to amyloid angiopathy (Itoh *et al.*, 1993), the proportion of amyloid-related lobar haemorrhages amongst all PICH would be about 10%, a rate that was confirmed in a small autopsy series (7/60) from a hospital for chronic care (Ishii *et al.*, 1984). With a single lobar haemorrhage detected on CT scanning, it is impossible to distinguish between one associated with amyloid angiopathy and one with arteriolar degeneration; magnetic resonance imaging (MRI) may give a clue to the diagnosis of amyloid angiopathy by showing evidence of previous punctate haemorrhages (Hendricks *et al.*, 1990). If surgery is indicated (see Chapter 12), the diagnosis can usually be made from immunohistochemical study of biopsy specimens (Yong *et al.*, 1992). In amyloid angiopathy, the vessels may be so brittle that even mild head trauma precipitates a haemorrhage (Kalyan Raman & Kalyan Raman, 1984). One of our own patients was an old woman who bled in both hemispheres when she tripped getting off a bus, without any direct head injury. Intracranial haemorrhage distant from the site of a previous neurosurgical intervention may also have to be attributed to amyloid angiopathy (Waga *et al.*, 1983). Thrombolytic therapy for myocardial infarction can be another precipitating factor (see Section 8.4.3).

Multiple haemorrhages, either at the same time or separated only by days, is a fairly typical, although not unique, characteristic of haemorrhages associated with amyloid angiopathy (Finelli *et al.*, 1984; Gilles *et al.*, 1984; Passero *et al.*, 1995). Other causes of multiple PICH are listed in Table 8.2 and range from occult head injury to sepsis and diffuse intravascular coagulation (Wijdicks *et al.*, 1994). Multiple

haemorrhages are rare (< 1%) in patients with PICH and a history of hypertension, in whom the most likely source of haemorrhage is lipohyalinosis and microaneurysms (Weisberg, 1981). Recurrent haemorrhages of the 'hypertensive' type have been reported but are much less common than with amyloid angiopathy (Lee *et al.*, 1990). In the case of simultaneous haemorrhage, it is assumed that the arteries affected by amyloidosis are so fragile that another tear is induced by the initial haemorrhage, even in a distant part of the brain.

> Haemorrhages into the white matter ('lobar' haemorrhages) are most often caused by the same type of 'hypertensive' arteriolar disease that is associated with deep haemorrhages, but in those aged over 70 years cerebral amyloid angiopathy is also a common underlying condition, in approximately 30%. Amyloid angiopathy can be more specifically suspected with multiple or recurrent haemorrhages, preceding episodes of transient deficits or, rarely, a family history of intracerebral haemorrhage.

Hereditary forms of amyloid angiopathy with intracerebral haemorrhages have been reported from the Netherlands (Luyendijk *et al.*, 1988; Wattendorff *et al.*, 1995; see Fig. 8.18) and Iceland (Gudmundsson *et al.*, 1972). In the Dutch variety, the amyloid has been identified as a beta-protein antigenically related to amyloid plaques in Alzheimer's disease (van Duinen *et al.*, 1987). The same applies to the sporadic variety of amyloid angiopathy, with or without haemorrhages (Coria *et al.*, 1987; Maruyama *et al.*, 1990). In the Icelandic form, however, the amyloid is antigenically different, and is of the cystatin-C type; the onset of the haemorrhages occurs at a median age of 30 years, compared with 55 years in the Dutch type of hereditary cerebral haemorrhage with amyloidosis (Jensson *et al.*, 1987).

Two clinical manifestations of cerebral amyloid angiopathy other than haemorrhages should be mentioned briefly. One consists of recurrent, transient episodes of focal weak-

Table 8.2 Causes of multiple haemorrhages in the brain parenchyma.

Amyloid angiopathy (see Sections 5.3.4 and 8.2.3)
Intracranial venous thrombosis (see Sections 5.3.5 and 8.2.5)
Thrombolytic treatment (see Section 8.4.3)
Metastases (melanoma, bronchial carcinoma, renal carcinoma, choriocarcinoma (see Section 8.5.1)
Cerebral vasculitis (see Section 7.2)
Diffuse intravascular coagulation (see Sections 7.6 and 8.4.5)
Haemostatic disorder (see Sections 8.4.3 and 8.4.4)
Leukaemia (see Section 8.4.5)
Occult head injury

---

ness, paraesthesias, numbness with spread and, less often, visual distortion. These attacks may be due to transient ischaemia (Smith *et al.*, 1985; Yong *et al.*, 1992). The occurrence of a large cerebral haemorrhage in an area of the brain implicated by the earlier recurrent spells raises the possibility that partial seizures or small haemorrhages or a combination of these two may have heralded the larger one (Greenberg *et al.*, 1993). Conversely, the occurrence of new-onset, focal seizures followed by PICH in the same area of the brain suggests not only an AVM but also amyloid angiopathy as a possible underlying cause (Cocito *et al.*, 1994). The other non-haemorrhagic clinical syndrome is a subacute dementia; the underlying lesions may not only consist of multiple haemorrhages (Greenberg *et al.*, 1993), but also diffuse demyelination of the subcortical white matter similar to that in Binswanger's disease (see Section 7.12) (Gray *et al.*, 1985). In both these conditions—Binswanger's disease and diffuse demyelination associated with amyloid angiopathy—the final common pathway is chronic ischaemia, as a result of narrowing of the arterioles supplying the white matter. In the former case the lumen decreases as a result of hypertrophy of the medial layer of arterioles (van Swieten *et al.*, 1991) and in the latter through deposits of beta-protein and secondary fibrinoid necrosis (Gray *et al.*, 1985). MRI scanning is a sensitive but not a specific method for diagnosing this type of leucoencephalopathy during life (Loes *et al.*, 1990) and also in familial cases of amyloid angiopathy (Haan *et al.*, 1990).

8.2.4 Saccular aneurysms

In the neurology/neurosurgery service of a large community hospital, approximately one-third of the patients with the clinical syndrome of SAH have an intracerebral haematoma on CT scanning (van Gijn & van Dongen, 1982). Patients with large haematomas often die early, so highly specialised referral centres will see a smaller proportion of haematomas associated with aneurysmal haemorrhages. There is no study available, at least not from the CT era, which directly compares the frequency of haematomas from ruptured saccular aneurysms with that of primary intracerebral haematomas. An educated guess can be made from the overall annual incidence rates (per 100 000 in a Western European population): for first-ever in a lifetime strokes the number is approximately 200 (Bamford *et al.*, 1988), some 12% or 24 consisting of PICH; for SAH the annual incidence rate is about six to eight per 100 000 (Herman *et al.*, 1982; Bamford *et al.*, 1990; Ricci *et al.*, 1991; Broderick *et al.*, 1993b). Given that two out of every seven patients with SAH have a haematoma, as against 24 patients with PICH from the same population, approximately one in 13 of all intrac-

erebral haematomas is secondary to rupture of a saccular aneurysm. However, this is the ratio for all ages combined. Below age 65 years, SAH and PICH are about equally common, in which case the proportion of haematomas from aneurysmal haemorrhage would be around one in seven (Broderick *et al.*, 1993b).

About one in 13 of all intracerebral haematomas are due to a ruptured saccular aneurysm, but more like two in 13 under the age of 65 years.

Haematomas from aneurysmal haemorrhage can be fairly reliably diagnosed on the basis of at least one of two characteristics: the association with cisternal haemorrhage and the typical location (see Section 9.4.1; Hayward & O'Reilly, 1976; van Gijn & van Dongen, 1980; Laissy *et al.*, 1991). Aneurysms of the anterior cerebral artery cause haematomas either in the frontal lobe, paramedially or sometimes more laterally, but always converging towards the midline, or else characteristically in the septum pellucidum or in the subarachnoid space between the frontal horns. Haematomas from ruptured aneurysms at the origin of the posterior communicating artery from the internal carotid artery involve the medial part of the temporal lobe; more rarely, aneurysms of the internal carotid artery are found at the terminal bifurcation into the middle and anterior cerebral arteries, and these may bleed upward and cause haematomas in the basal ganglia, particularly in the head of the caudate nucleus (Hayward & O'Reilly, 1976). Haematomas from middle cerebral artery aneurysms often follow the course of the Sylvian fissure, or at least extend as far laterally as the junction between the skull vault and the sphenoid ridge (see Figs 9.9 & 9.10). If doubt remains in a deteriorating patient, where rapid evacuation of the haematoma seems indicated, (spiral) CT scanning with infusion of contrast may show—or to some extent exclude—an aneurysm (Le Roux *et al.*, 1993). It is important to distinguish between a parenchymal haematoma from a ruptured aneurysm and PICH, whether deep or lobar, because a patient with a ruptured aneurysm may require more urgent treatment, medical or surgical (see Section 13.3.1).

If the location of an intracerebral haematoma is compatible with a ruptured aneurysm, the patient should be urgently transferred to a neurosurgical facility for surgery to at least be considered, even if the patient's clinical condition is poor.

Subdural haematomas may also be associated with aneurysm rupture. As a rule, this is associated with a tell-tale extravasation of blood in the subarachnoid space (see Section 9.4.1), but occasionally the subdural haematoma is the only manifestation (see Section 8.10).

8.2.5 Intracranial venous thrombosis

There are many causes of intracranial venous thrombosis (Table 8.3). Extensive haemorrhages occur in only a minority of patients, although the precise proportion depends on referral patterns and also on the assiduity with which the diagnosis is pursued in patients with the syndrome of benign intracranial hypertension. Haemorrhages are most often secondary to infarction caused by obstruction of cortical veins ('venous infarction'; Fig. 8.7). Therefore, the haemorrhage is usually preceded by an ischaemic phase, manifested by focal deficits, seizures or a global encephalopathy, without radiological evidence of extravasation of blood, the interval being hours or days. A haemorrhagic infarct in the parasagittal region, particularly if bilateral, should raise the possibility of intracranial venous thrombosis. Sometimes rupture of a thrombosed vein causes haemorrhage without previous infarction (Krücke, 1971). Whether anticoagulation in intracranial venous thrombosis is safe and effective is still a controversial issue (see also Section 5.3.5).

> *Intracranial venous thrombosis is an underdiagnosed condition. Apart from other presentations (headache, visual symptoms relating to papilloedema, ischaemic neurological deficits), it should be included in the differential diagnosis of primary intracerebral haemorrhage. The diagnosis should be strongly suspected if the patient is a young woman, if the haemorrhage has been preceded by some of the other manifestations and if the haemorrhage is in the parasagittal region. In the case of bilateral parasagittal haemorrhages, the diagnosis should be assumed until proved otherwise.*

8.2.6 Microangiomas

Microangiomas are defined not only by their small size but also by not showing up on angiograms (Ogilvy *et al.*, 1988). In patients under 45 years, in whom lipohyalinosis and amyloid angiopathy are rare, microangiomas may well account for most of the haemorrhages for which angiography shows no cause, particularly if outside the region of the basal ganglia; in one large series, the proportion of these unexplained haemorrhages was around 25% (Toffol *et al.*, 1987). Intraventricular haemorrhages without parenchymal haematoma may be caused by AVMs (see Section 9.1.5). If angiography is negative, primary intraventricular haemorrhages are often attributed to microangiomas, although with little proof. Microangiomas occur disproportionately often in the brainstem (Abe *et al.*, 1989). They were originally termed 'cryptic malformations', because only specimens

Table 8.3 Causal or contributing factors in intracranial venous thrombosis. (From Ameri & Bousser, 1992.)

INFECTIOUS FACTORS

Local
Penetrating injury
Intracranial infection: bacterial or fungal abscess, empyema, meningitis
Regional infection: otitis, tonsillitis, sinusitis, stomatitis, dermatitis

General
Bacterial: septicaemia, endocarditis, typhoid, tuberculosis
Viral: measles, hepatitis, encephalitis, herpes, HIV, cytomegalovirus
Fungal: aspergillosis

NON-INFECTIOUS FACTORS

Local
Head injury (with or without fracture, open or closed)
Neurosurgical procedures
Cerebral infarction or haemorrhage
Tumours (meningioma, metastasis, glomus tumour)
Porencephaly, arachnoid cysts
Infusions into the internal jugular vein

General
Any surgical procedure, with or without deep venous thrombosis
Hormonal
    Pregnancy or puerperium
    Oral contraceptives (oestrogens or progestogens)
Medical
    Cardiac: congenital heart disease, cardiac failure, pacemaker
    Tumours: any visceral carcinoma, lymphoma, leukaemia, carcinoid, L-asparaginase therapy
    Red blood cell disorders: polycythaemia, post-haemorrhagic anaemia, sickle cell disease, paroxysmal nocturnal haemoglobinuria
    Thrombocythaemia
    Coagulation disorders: deficiency of antithrombin III, protein C or circulating anticoagulants; disseminated intravascular coagulation, heparin- or heparinoid-induced thrombocytopenia, treatment with antifibrinolytic agents
    Severe dehydration of any cause (including myelography or angiography)
    Digestive system: cirrhosis, Crohn's disease, ulcerative colitis
    Connective-tissue disease: systemic lupus erythematosus, giant cell arteritis, Wegener's granulomatosis
    Various: Behçet's disease, sarcoidosis, nephrotic syndrome, neonatal asphyxia, parenteral injections, androgen therapy

HIV, human immunodeficiency virus.

taken at surgery or autopsy could identify the vascular lesion (Crawford & Russell, 1956). Apart from small AVMs, three other histological types of vascular anomalies have been distinguished under the general heading of 'microangiomas'. Sometimes these other types are large enough to be identified on angiograms, but most are below their spatial resolution.

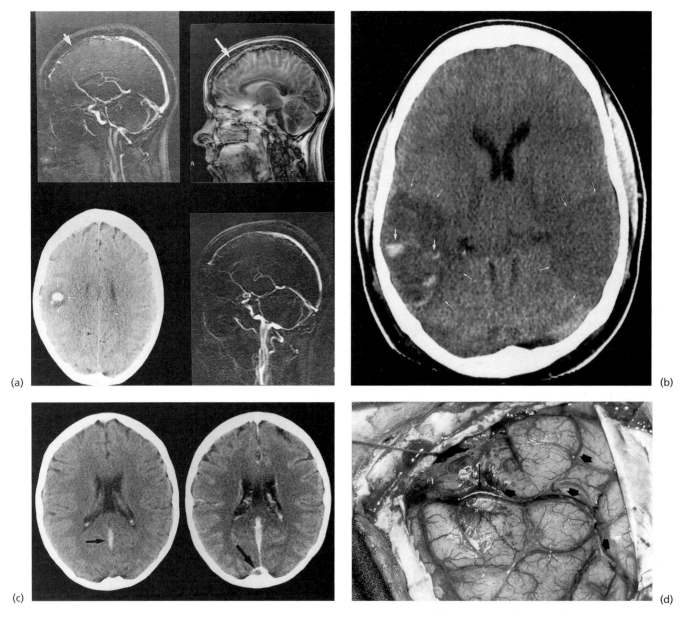

Figure 8.7 Intracranial venous thrombosis. (a) MRI and CT images of 27-year-old woman with intracranial venous thrombosis, manifested by a generalised seizure, 2 weeks after confinement. Top, left: MRI venogram (midline sagittal section) showing impaired filling of the anterior part of the superior sagittal sinus (arrow). Top, right: MRI of brain (T2-weighted midline sagittal section) shows abnormal hyperintensity in the corresponding part of the superior sagittal sinus caused by the thrombus (arrow). Bottom, left: CT scan (non-contrast) showing a haemorrhagic infarct in the right parietal lobe (arrows). Bottom, right: MRI venogram, 6 months after the episode; the anterior part of the superior sagittal sinus is now patent. (b) CT brain scan (without contrast) showing bilateral venous infarcts (thin arrows) resulting from thrombosis of the superior sagittal sinus and cortical veins; the infarct on the right side is haemorrhagic (thick arrows). (c) CT scans of 46-year-old woman with intracranial venous thrombosis. Left: unenhanced scan, showing abnormal hyperdensity in the straight sinus (arrow) due to thrombus. Right: same slice after contrast enhancement, with non-filling area in the posterior end of the superior sagittal sinus ('empty delta-sign'; arrow) due to the thrombus surrounded by enhanced blood. (d) Cortical vein thrombosis. Photograph taken during operation for removal of an intracerebral haematoma, in the pre-CT era; a number of veins show a string of light spots (short, broad arrows) over a large part of their course, indicating thrombus. The bright white band (long, thin arrow) is caused by reflected light.

Small arteriovenous malformations

Not only the malformations themselves but also the haemorrhages are smaller than with AVMs that do show up on conventional angiography (Lobato *et al.*, 1992). Figure 8.8 shows an example of a small lobar haemorrhage in a young, non-hypertensive patient, where neither angiography nor MRI could detect the source.

Cavernous angiomas

Cavernous angiomas consist of sharply demarcated areas with widely dilated and thin-walled vascular channels, without intervening brain tissue (Fig. 8.9). They are often asymptomatic and are encountered in 0.5% of routine autopsies (Otten *et al.*, 1989). If clinical manifestations occur at all,

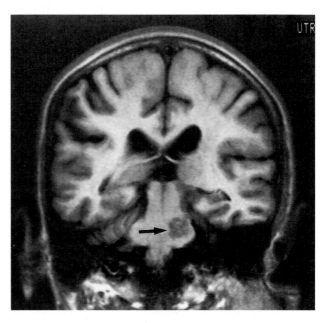

Figure 8.9 Probable cavernous angioma of the brainstem. MRI scan (T1-weighted scan in the coronal plane) of a 48-year-old woman who had experienced an attack, lasting several hours, of vertigo, tinnitus, a burning feeling around the nose, and pins and needles of the right body half below the face. The marginated but rather sharply demarcated border of the abnormality in the left half of the pons and middle cerebellar peduncle in the absence of space-occupying effect suggests a cavernous angioma (arrow). Left vertebral angiography was normal. Three years later, the lesion had not changed.

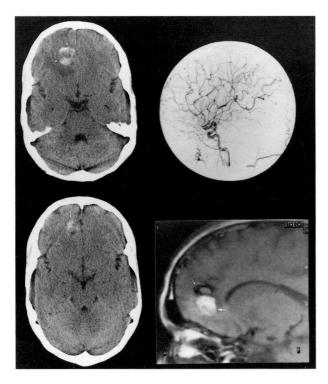

Figure 8.8 Suspected but angiographically occult 'microangioma', in a 25-year-old woman. Top, left; CT brain scan showing a parasagittal haemorrhage (arrow) in the right frontal lobe (clinically manifested by sudden headache, followed by a seizure). Top, right: normal right carotid angiogram (the left carotid angiogram was also normal). Bottom, left: CT scan, 3 months after the event; residual lesion with calcification (arrow) and a region of hypodensity. Bottom, right: sagittal MRI scan (T1-weighted), 4 months after the event; sharply demarcated, hypodense lesion (cavernous angioma?—thin arrow), with residual, hyperintense region (haemosiderin) at its ventral border (thick arrow).

they are more often due to epileptic seizures than to haemorrhage, at least if the cavernoma is in a cerebral hemisphere (Simard *et al.*, 1986). In the posterior fossa, any symptoms are those of a mass lesion, usually in the brainstem, in some cases later followed by haemorrhage (Zimmerman *et al.*, 1991). After a first rupture, rebleeding is not uncommon (Tung *et al.*, 1990). A familial form of the disorder has been detected in Mexican–American families (Rigamonti *et al.*, 1988; Kattapong *et al.*, 1995), and recently also in a family from Germany (van Schayck *et al.*, 1994).

Venous angiomas

Venous angiomas consist of several dilated veins, without an abnormal input on the arterial side, converging into a single abnormal vein, which in turn drains into the venous system on the surface of the brain or, less commonly, into the deep venous system. The radial orientation of the peripheral veins creates the impression of a *caput medusae* (Fig. 8.10). Venous angiomas are the most common vascular anomaly incidentally encountered at autopsy: in a series of over 4000 consecutive autopsies, 4% of all brains harboured one or more vascular malformations, 63% of which were venous angiomas (Sarwar & McCormick, 1978). Most occur in the frontal lobes, followed by the parietal lobes and the cerebellum (Garner *et al.*, 1991). Rupture of venous angiomas is extremely rare, and if these lesions are ever symptomatic the most common manifestations are seizures or transient focal deficits (Garner *et al.*, 1991). If venous angiomas do bleed, one should beware of an associated abnormality, such as a cavernous angioma, an AVM or a tumour (Rigamonti *et al.*, 1990; Meyer *et al.*, 1995).

Telangiectasias

Telangiectasias are small lesions in which the vessels resemble capillaries but have a widened lumen (20–500 μm), separated by normal brain tissue; they occur most often in the pons. They are mere curiosities, noted in less than 1% of autopsies, constituting 17% of all vascular anomalies (Sarwar & McCormick, 1978). They have a very low potential for bleeding unless they are multiple, in which case other organs are often affected as well (Rendu–Osler–Weber disease) (Román *et al.*, 1978). Two patients with pontine haemorrhage and telangiectasias were described many decades ago (Teilmann, 1953). Occasionally telangiectasias give rise to brainstem deficits without haemorrhage (Farrell & Forno, 1970).

The 'cryptic' nature of microangiomas has had to yield to a great extent to the recent advances in brain imaging techniques. To start with, repetition of the 'old-fashioned' catheter angiogram may show a vascular malformation that was not visible initially, perhaps through compression by the adjacent haematoma. The yield of a second angiogram in patients with negative studies in the acute stage is in the order of 10–20%, i.e. after exclusion of patients in whom age or the location of the haemorrhage strongly favours degenerative arteriolar disease or amyloid angiopathy (see Section 8.6) (Willinsky *et al.*, 1993; Halpin *et al.*, 1994). Soon after the advent of CT scanning, it became clear that this technique was more sensitive than angiography in the detection of microangiomas, even without contrast enhancement (Becker *et al.*, 1979). MRI scanning shows angiomas as low-intensity lesions on T2-weighted images and has the additional potential of distinguishing cavernous angiomas from AVMs and venous angiomas, on the basis of their regular margins (Imakita *et al.*, 1989). Cavernous angiomas are further suggested on T2-weighted MRI by a central focus of high intensity, surrounded by a rim of low intensity that represents the paramagnetic effect of haemosiderin, but this pattern is not absolutely pathognomonic, as it may occasionally be seen in an AVM (Rapacki *et al.*, 1990).

8.2.7 Dural arteriovenous fistulas

Dural arteriovenous fistulas are fed by meningeal branches, most often from the middle meningeal or occipital branches of the external carotid artery, more rarely from the internal

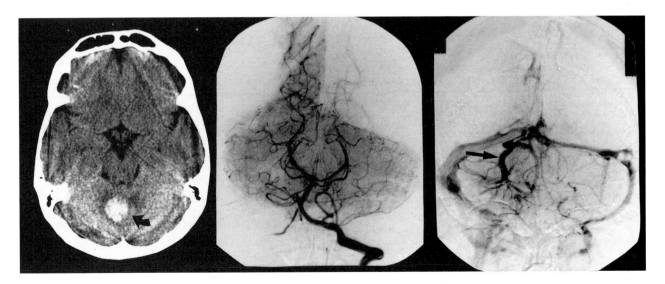

Figure 8.10 Venous angioma. Left: CT scan, showing haematoma in the vermis of the cerebellum (arrow). Middle: left vertebral angiogram, showing normal arterial phase. Right: left vertebral angiogram in the venous phase showing the venous angioma, with abnormal venous structures converging towards a single draining vein (*caput medusae*, arrow).

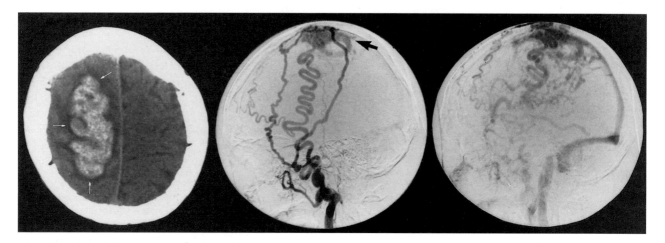

Figure 8.11 Dural fistula with intraparenchymal haemorrhage. Left: CT scan showing a marginated haemorrhage at the convexity of the right hemisphere (arrows); the clinical deficit, a left hemiparesis, had developed gradually, over about 1 hour. Middle: right external carotid angiogram (arterial phase), showing abnormally large meningeal branches, converging towards the dural fistula (arrow). Right: right external carotid angiogram (venous phase) showing filling of abnormal dilated intracranial veins.

carotid or vertebral artery (Aminoff, 1973). As a rule, drainage is directly into dural sinuses, most often the transverse or sigmoid sinus, less commonly the superior sagittal or cavernous sinus (Fig. 8.11). Only in exceptional cases does the anomaly communicate with superficial veins of the cerebral convexity or the cerebellum, or with perimesencephalic veins (Aminoff, 1973; Obrador *et al.*, 1975). It is especially with drainage through superficial veins that haemorrhage is the presenting event, occurring in the subarachnoid space (see Section 9.1.4) or into the brain parenchyma (Malik *et al.*, 1984). The most common manifestations are pulsatile tinnitus (if the dural arteriovenous fistula is near the temporal bone), headache or visual symptoms from papilloedema (obscurations, inferior nasal field defects or concentric field constriction, and eventually impaired acuity) (Wall & George, 1987), the papilloedema reflecting increased pressure of the cerebrospinal fluid through increased pressure in the superior sagittal sinus. Head injury, with or without skull fracture, may cause a dural arteriovenous fistula, presumably through thrombosis of the dural sinus in question (Chaudhary *et al.*, 1982), but in not more than approximately one in 20 cases of dural fistula (Obrador *et al.*, 1975).

8.2.8 Septic arteritis and mycotic aneurysms

Intracranial haemorrhage complicates infective endocarditis in about 5% of cases (see Chapter 6; Kanter & Hart, 1991). It most commonly results not from mycotic aneurysms but from acute, pyogenic necrosis of the arterial wall early in the disease, usually before effective treatment with antibiotics and with virulent organisms such as *Staphylococcus aureus* (Hart *et al.*, 1987, 1990; Masuda *et al.*, 1992). Mycotic aneurysms may develop and rupture later, during antimicrobial therapy or with less virulent bacteria, such as *Streptococcus viridans*, *Strep. sanguis* or *Staph. epidermidis*. Haemorrhages from mycotic aneurysms occur in the cortex and in the underlying white matter, or occasionally only in the subarachnoid space at the convexity of the brain, because the septic emboli tend to lodge at the periphery of the arterial tree (Masuda *et al.*, 1992). Only around 10% of mycotic aneurysms associated with infective endocarditis are located proximally on the middle or anterior cerebral arteries, with patterns of haemorrhage resembling those from 'ordinary' saccular aneurysms (Brust *et al.*, 1990).

> *Most mycotic aneurysms are located superficially in the cerebral hemisphere, in the cortex or underlying white matter.*

In general, a lobar haemorrhage is only exceptionally associated with endocarditis if a patient has no history of heart disease, recent cerebral ischaemia, recent malaise, fever or loss of weight. This is because the prevalence of 'hypertensive' microangiopathy and amyloid angiopathy is vastly greater than that of infective endocarditis. In addition, more than 80% of patients with PICH from septic emboli have a history of heart disease or intravenous drug abuse, or have had prodromal episodes suggesting embolisation, or both (Hart *et al.*, 1987; Salgado *et al.*, 1987).

The combined case fatality of PICH and the underlying endocarditis is in the order of 25–50%, higher than that of

PICH alone in the corresponding age groups (Hart *et al.*, 1987; Monsuez *et al.*, 1989).

8.2.9 Moyamoya syndrome

Intracerebral, SAH or, occasionally, ventricular haemorrhage is the most common manifestation of the moyamoya syndrome in adults (Nijdam *et al.*, 1986), whereas in children it is more often encountered as a cause of cerebral infarction (see Section 7.13; Bruno *et al.*, 1988). The bleeding is caused by rupture of one of the widened perforating vessels, or sometimes of an associated dissecting aneurysm (Yamashita *et al.*, 1983). Therefore, most haemorrhages occur in the basal ganglia. Without the angiographic diagnosis of the primarily occlusive disorder, these can not be distinguished from the much more common 'hypertensive' haemorrhages, as a result of small vessel lipohyalinosis.

8.2.10 Arterial dissection (see also Section 7.1)

Haemorrhage is an uncommon complication of arterial dissection, and any extravasation is almost invariably confined to the subarachnoid space (see Chapter 9). It occurs when a subadventitial dissection of an intracranial artery, usually the vertebral artery, extends as far as the intradural space, where there is no adventitial layer or external elastic lamina. A single patient has been reported in whom haemorrhage in the parietal lobe was the presenting feature of carotid dissection in the neck; the initial cerebral lesion may have been ischaemic, but this remains speculative (Kitanaka & Teraoka, 1993).

8.2.11 Caroticocavernous fistula

Pulsating exophthalmos is the most common manifestation of a fistula created by a ruptured aneurysm of the internal carotid artery within the cavernous sinus. Rarely, rupture of one of the dilated and tortuous veins that drain into the cavernous sinus occurs, resulting in an intraparenchymal haematoma (d'Angelo *et al.*, 1988).

8.3 Haemodynamic factors

8.3.1 Arterial hypertension

Chronically raised blood pressure

Chronically raised blood pressure is by far the most powerful risk factor for stroke in general, whether ischaemic or

haemorrhagic (see Section 6.2.3). In many cases, it is chronic hypertension that underlies the degenerative change in small perforating arteries (lipohyalinosis and microaneurysms (see Section 8.2.1)) and ultimately leads to rupture, constituting the most common cause of intracerebral haemorrhage, mostly in the basal ganglia, cerebellum or brainstem, less often in the subcortical white matter. In fact, few studies have assessed the risk of increasing blood pressure for haemorrhagic stroke separately from ischaemic stroke. In a case–control study, the relative risk for patients with hypertension (140/90 or higher) of suffering PICH was 3.9 (95% confidence interval: 2.7–5.7); if the definition of hypertension included evidence of hypertrophy of the left ventricle on the electrocardiogram (ECG) or of cardiomegaly on the chest X-ray, the relative risk was 5.4, with a 95% confidence interval of 3.7–7.9 (Brott *et al.*, 1986). Nevertheless, as pointed out in the introduction to this chapter, hypertension is neither a sufficient nor a necessary cause of PICH. Brott *et al.* (1986) analysed the determinants in a consecutive, hospital-based series of patients with PICH and found hypertension (as determined by history) in only 45%; this rate was similar for haemorrhages in the thalamus and basal ganglia, where causes other than lipohyalinosis and microaneurysms are unlikely. The proportion of hypertensive patients increased to 56% by adding those with evidence of left-ventricular hypertrophy on the chest X-ray or the ECG (Brott *et al.*, 1986). In a large and prospective hospital series from the Netherlands, 59% of the patients with PICH had a history of hypertension (Franke *et al.*, 1992). Similarly, a controlled study of patients who had died from PICH showed that only 46% of these fatal cases had been hypertensive, at least judged from mean heart weight (Bahemuka, 1987). All these pieces of evidence from different sources seem to suggest that, strictly speaking, the term 'hypertensive intracerebral haemorrhage' is a misnomer. On the other hand, the 'normotensive' patients in these series may have had mild degrees of hypertension, without signs of ventricular hypertrophy or end-organ damage. After all, in any disorder, 'high-risk' patients make up only a small proportion of the patients with that disorder, and the majority are patients with moderate risk of the disorder (Rose, 1992).

> *Factors other than hypertension must contribute to the rupture of small perforating vessels, because this occurs in some, but not all, subjects with hypertension, and sometimes even without hypertension.*

Acutely raised blood pressure

Acutely raised blood pressure can definitely precipitate PICH, particularly in previously normotensive individuals

(Caplan, 1988). The rapid increase in pressure is transmitted to the wall of small arterioles, which is not relatively protected by previous hypertrophy, as occurs in long-standing hypertension. Examples of acutely raised blood pressure as a cause of intracerebral haemorrhage are renal failure, even after transplantation (Adams *et al.*, 1986); eclampsia (Richards *et al.*, 1988); exposure to severe cold weather (Caplan *et al.*, 1984); certain drugs which cause acute hypertension, such as monoamine oxidase inhibitors; and pain induced by dental procedures (Barbas *et al.*, 1987). After carotid endarterectomy for severe stenosis, there may be relative hypertension in a previously underperfused hemisphere, in some cases resulting in intracerebral haemorrhage (see Section 16.7.3). Transient but steep rises in blood pressure may also account for at least some of the supratentorial haemorrhages that may occur during or shortly after operations in the posterior fossa, such as microvascular decompression of the Vth cranial nerve in patients with trigeminal neuralgia (Haines *et al.*, 1978).

8.3.2 Migraine

Migraine may theoretically be associated with intracerebral haemorrhage in an indirect fashion, through the presence of an AVM, because the presence of such malformations may precipitate migraine attacks, which disappear after their removal (Weiskrantz *et al.*, 1974; Troost *et al.*, 1979), and also directly. Three women (45–61 years) with a long history of migraine attacks suffered lobar haemorrhages after an unusually severe attack, with tenderness of the carotid artery in the neck and evidence of ipsilateral vasospasm on angiography; the density and compactness of the haemorrhages on brain CT did not suggest that the haemorrhages were secondary to infarction (Cole & Aubé, 1990). Surgical specimens in two of these patients had evidence of necrosis in the walls of intracranial vessels, probably as a result of ischaemia, with secondary inflammatory changes. Although extremely rare, migraine should perhaps be suspected as a cause of lobar haemorrhage if a severe episode of headache preceded rather than accompanied the stroke.

8.4 Haemostatic factors

8.4.1 Anticoagulants

The anatomical distribution of PICH associated with anticoagulant drugs is similar to that with lipohyalinosis and microaneurysms (see Section 8.2.7; Kase *et al.*, 1985; Franke *et al.*, 1990). During anticoagulant treatment, the risk of PICH, compared with age-matched control subjects not on anticoagulant drugs, is increased by a factor that lies between 7 and 11 (Wintzen *et al.*, 1984; Franke *et al.*, 1990; Fogelholm *et al.*, 1992). However, it is unknown what proportion of this excess risk should be attributed to the treatment itself and how much to arteriolar degeneration associated with the vascular condition for which the treatment was given (i.e. confounding by indication). The risk increases with the intensity of anticoagulation: in prospective studies, the risk of PICH was highest with international normalised ratio (INR) values exceeding 5.0 (Cannegieter *et al.*, 1995; European Atrial Fibrillation Trial Study Group, 1995). Nevertheless, many patients with anticoagulant-associated PICH are not deeply anticoagulated: the intensity of anticoagulation commonly exceeded the therapeutic range in only one study (Kase *et al.*, 1985), rarely in four larger studies (Wintzen *et al.*, 1984; Franke *et al.*, 1990; Rådberg *et al.*, 1991; Fogelholm *et al.*, 1992). The disproportionate rate of PICH in the first year of anticoagulant treatment, reported in all these four large studies, leads to the view that anticoagulant-related PICH in many patients is due to a low-threshold phenomenon in patients predisposed by underlying lipohyalinosis or microaneurysms. Similarly, the main risk factors for PICH in a cohort of patients on anticoagulant drugs for a single indication (lower-limb ischaemia) were systolic hypertension and insulin-dependent diabetes; an excessive level of anticoagulation could explain, at most, only 50% of the haemorrhages (Dawson *et al.*, 1993).

> *The risk of intracranial haemorrhage in patients on oral anticoagulants increases with the intensity of anticoagulation (especially with international normalised ratio values above 5.0), but in most patients with anticoagulant-related intracerebral haemorrhage the international normalised ratio values are within appropriate limits.*

A remarkable feature in PICH precipitated by anticoagulants is the gradual progression of the clinical deficits, observed in as many as 58% in the only series that systematically addressed this issue (Kase *et al.*, 1985). Also, the average volume of the haemorrhage is larger than in PICH not associated with anticoagulant drugs, according to studies in which the comparison was not confounded by sampling bias (Franke *et al.*, 1990; Rådberg *et al.*, 1991). A fluid-blood level within the haematoma (Fig. 8.12), i.e. a horizontal interface between unclotted serum (hypodense) and sedimented red cells (hyperdense), occurs in 60% of anticoagulant-related intracerebral haemorrhages, and only rarely otherwise (specificity 98%) (Pfleger *et al.*, 1994).

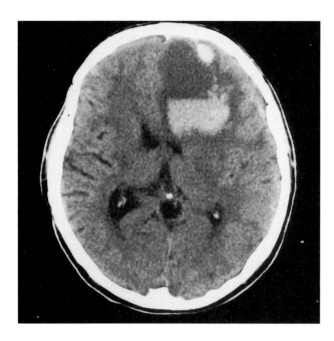

Figure 8.12 CT scan showing a haematoma in the left frontal lobe, with a horizontal border representing the interface between sedimented red cells and supernatant plasma, indicating impaired coagulation. There is also distortion of the ventricle and loss of sulci, indicating mass effect.

8.4.2 Antiplatelet therapy

In a complete overview, up to 1991, of all the randomised trials of antiplatelet therapy (mostly aspirin), for any indication, in which at least one haemorrhagic stroke had been recorded, the risk of intracranial haemorrhage over an average of 2 years was 0.3% in treated patients, versus 0.2% in controls (Antiplatelet Trialists' Collaboration, 1994a,b). Although this represents a relative risk of 1.5 (95% confidence interval: 1.1–2.1), the absolute risk is extremely low and can be expressed as one extra haemorrhage for every 1000 treated patients, in a period that was around 2 years for most of the trials.

> *Antiplatelet therapy is probably only a relatively minor contributory factor in the pathogenesis of primary intracerebral haemorrhage against a background of much more powerful determinants, most often lipohyalinosis and microaneurysms.*

The dose of aspirin is not an important factor with regard to the rate of PICH, at least not according to the few studies in which different doses were directly compared: 300 versus 1200 mg (Farrell *et al.*, 1991) and 30 versus 283 mg (Dutch TIA Trial Study Group, 1991). On the other hand, the confidence intervals in these comparisons are wide, as they are in trials comparing different antiplatelet agents.

8.4.3 Thrombolytic treatment

Intracerebral haemorrhage is a serious and often fatal complication of thrombolytic therapy for acute myocardial infarction, which occurs in 0.7–0.8% of patients (Carlson *et al.*, 1988; Gore *et al.*, 1991; Uglietta *et al.*, 1991), and usually within 24 hours (Kase *et al.*, 1990; Uglietta *et al.*, 1991; Wijdicks & Jack, 1993). Factors associated with increased risk are age over 65 years, body weight below 70 kg (in other words, a relatively high dose of the thrombolytic drug), hypertension on admission to hospital and administration of tissue plasminogen activator rather than streptokinase (Simoons *et al.*, 1993).

Several clues incriminate amyloid angiopathy as the most frequent anatomical abnormality underlying this complication. First, a disproportionate number of PICHs after thrombolysis occur in the white matter of the cerebral hemispheres, and multiple haematomas occur in about one-third (Kase *et al.*, 1990; Uglietta *et al.*, 1991; Wijdicks & Jack, 1993; Sloan *et al.*, 1995). Second, in a few operated patients, the brain tissue showed amyloid changes in blood vessels (Pendlebury *et al.*, 1991; Wijdicks & Jack, 1993; Sloan *et al.*, 1995).

A state of systemically enhanced thrombolysis from these drugs adversely affects the process of haemostasis in the brain, as reflected by fluid levels in lobar haematomas (Fig. 8.12; Wijdicks & Jack, 1993) and by a high case fatality within the first 3 days: 60–80% after thrombolytic therapy (Kase *et al.*, 1990; Uglietta *et al.*, 1991; Wijdicks & Jack, 1993) versus about 24% after intracerebral haemorrhage in general (Franke *et al.*, 1992).

8.4.4 Haemophilia

Intracranial bleeding in haemophilia occurs only with severe factor VIII deficiency and usually follows head injury, although the interval may be as long as several days (Martinowitz *et al.*, 1986). The mortality is high. Acquired immune deficiency syndrome (AIDS) is sometimes a contributory factor, because factor VIII replacement therapy may be delayed by a patient's impaired judgement (Andes & Wulff, 1990).

8.4.5 Leukaemia and thrombocytopenia
(see also Section 7.6)

Myeloid leukaemia may precipitate PICH, whereas this complication is exceptional in chronic lymphatic leukaemia or in hairy cell leukaemia (Ng *et al.*, 1991). Intracranial haemorrhage with leukaemia is usually multifocal and part of a generalised bleeding tendency, but occasionally it occurs as an isolated event (Kelly *et al.*, 1985). The pathogenesis is diverse. Most often, the direct cause is the formation of aggregates of tumour cells, which obstruct arterioles or capillaries in the cortex or subcortical white matter, and this is followed by local proliferation of white cells, with erosion of the vessel wall. Another cause is disseminated intravascular coagulation and consumption coagulopathy. Finally, the underlying cause may be thrombocytopenia, from infiltration of the bone marrow, after transplantation of bone marrow or liver (Pomeranz *et al.*, 1994; Wijdicks *et al.*, 1995), or as a side effect of chemotherapy. PICH should not be attributed to thrombocytopenia if the platelet count is above 20 × 10⁹/L, because above this limit the bleeding time is normal (provided platelet function is intact).

Thrombocytopenia as a cause of PICH may also be associated with myelofibrosis (Markel *et al.*, 1986), aplastic anaemia, diffuse intravascular coagulation with conditions other than leukaemia, and idiopathic thrombocytopenic purpura (Werlhof's disease).

8.5 Other factors

8.5.1 Intracerebral tumours

Haemorrhage into an intracerebral tumour accounts for approximately 5% of all PICH (Little *et al.*, 1979). The diagnosis is not too difficult if the patient is already known to have an intracerebral tumour, and it should also come readily to mind in case of a known extracranial tumour, but it may be delayed if intracerebral haemorrhage is the first manifestation of the tumour, which is the case in approximately 50% of all tumour haemorrhages (Little *et al.*, 1979). There are various causes for the haemorrhage. Most common is rupture of a fragile vessel in a hypervascular tumour or necrosis of part of the tumour. An exceptional cause is erosion of normal blood vessels by the tumour, which is characteristic of metastatic choriocarcinoma (van den Doel *et al.*, 1985).

On brain CT, several features suggest an underlying tumour (Kase, 1986, 1994). These include: a location of the haemorrhage that is unusual for PICH, the corpus callosum being an obvious example, at least if not associated with SAH; an irregular, mottled appearance of the haematoma, for instance with a low-density area in the centre of the haemorrhage, suggesting necrosis (Fig. 8.13); occurrence of multiple haemorrhages (a feature shared with some other types of haemorrhage; see Table 8.2); a disproportionate degree of surrounding oedema or mass effect; and nodular enhancement of surrounding tissue after intravenous contrast, other than the ring enhancement that represents the inflammatory response to the haemorrhage (see also Section 5.3.4). On MRI the diagnosis of tumorous haemorrhage is based on similar characteristics, with the addition that a tumour is less likely (but far from excluded) if haemosiderin is demonstrated, in the form of a hypodense rim on T2-

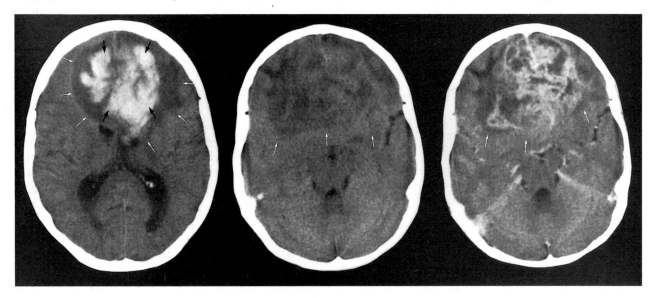

Figure 8.13 Haemorrhage caused by tumour, in a 71-year-old woman. Left: CT scan 1 day after sudden loss of consciousness, showing a bifrontal haematoma (thick arrows) with irregular shape and disproportionate oedema (hypodense margin around the haematoma—thin arrows). Middle: CT scan 3-months later, after a gradual recovery had been followed by secondary deterioration; diffuse oedema in both frontal lobes with considerable mass effect (arrows). Right: after injection of intravenous contrast a grossly irregular tumour emerges (glioblastoma).

weighted images (Destian *et al.*, 1989). When doubt remains, e.g. when tumour markers in the serum are negative, as well as investigations of the chest and abdomen, the issue is often decided by a second or third brain scan after an interval of several weeks or months (Fig. 8.13). If one can not wait so long, an angiogram of the intracerebral circulation may be helpful by showing pathological vessels.

Metastases are the most common tumours that cause intracerebral haemorrhage, melanoma and bronchial carcinoma being frequent primary tumours, followed by renal carcinoma and choriocarcinoma (Maiuri *et al.*, 1985). The last type of tumour is most often associated with pregnancy, but may also originate from the testis and subsequently lead to intracerebral haemorrhage from a metastasis (Timothy *et al.*, 1994). Gliomas and particularly glioblastomas are the next most common group of tumours to bleed. Rarer sources of intracerebral haemorrhage are pituitary adenomas, meningiomas and chondromas (Modesti *et al.*, 1976).

8.5.2 Alcohol

Massive intracerebral haemorrhages may occur in alcoholics who have evidence of liver damage, low platelet count and abnormalities of the clotting system (Weisberg, 1988). The haemorrhages may be so extensive that there are no focal deficits but a clinical syndrome suggesting a metabolic encephalopathy. Whether brief spells of excessive drinking ('binge drinking') can precipitate PICH, SAH or even stroke in general is controversial, as most of the case–control studies that addressed this issue were subject to bias (van Gijn *et al.*, 1993). A regular intake of three or more units of alcohol per day, however, is consistently associated with an increased risk of PICH as well as of SAH (Camargo, 1989; van Gijn *et al.*, 1993). This effect may be related to the antiplatelet action of alcohol, at least in part (Jakubowski *et al.*, 1988).

8.5.3 Amphetamines

Intracerebral haemorrhages can follow ingestion of amphetamine or methamphetamine, less often dextroamphetamine, with any route of administration and after doses as low as 20 mg (Harrington *et al.*, 1983; Caplan, 1994). The interval between ingestion and haemorrhage can be as short as a few minutes. Most of these haemorrhages are lobar, in the subcortical white matter (Caplan, 1994). Angiography shows scattered segments of narrowing and dilatation ('beading') or occlusion. At necropsy, the lesions correspond with areas of fibrinoid necrosis in small and medium-sized vessels, in the brain as well as in other organs (Citron *et al.*, 1970). There may be underlying anatomical abnormalities, such as

an AVM, but this is exceptional (Lukes, 1983; Caplan, 1994).

8.5.4 Cocaine and other sympathomimetic drugs

As with amphetamines, cocaine-associated haemorrhage may occur after oral ingestion, intravenous injection or inhalation, but relatively more often after inhalation of 'crack' cocaine, a mixture of cocaine hydrochloride and ammonia or baking soda (Levine *et al.*, 1991). These haemorrhages occur mostly in the white matter of the cerebral hemispheres. But, unlike with amphetamines, the rate of underlying vascular abnormalities is high, in the order of 80%, at least in patients with adequate angiographic or necropsy studies (Caplan, 1994). Arterial hypertension is another predisposing factor (Kibayashi *et al.*, 1995). PICH has also been reported in association with the use of ephedrine (Bruno *et al.*, 1993).

8.5.5 Vasculitis

Isolated angiitis of the central nervous system is by definition not associated with any systemic involvement. The causes are obscure, and it is uncertain whether the condition is a nosological entity (Hankey, 1991). Presenting features include chronic headache, mental deterioration, seizures and focal ischaemia. Occasionally, PICH may be the first clinical manifestation (Biller *et al.*, 1987). Other vasculitic disorders affecting the brain can sometimes present with, or be complicated by, intracerebral haemorrhage (see Section 7.2).

8.6 Relative frequency of causes

We have pointed out in the introduction to this chapter that age is an important factor in determining the a priori probability of a particular cause of a haemorrhage in an individual patient. AVMs are the leading cause in the young and degenerative small vessel disease (lipohyalinosis and microangiomas) in the middle-aged and the aged, whilst amyloid angiopathy is another important cause to consider in the aged. Some refinements of this global rule of thumb are possible, not only by taking into account the less common causes than these three, but also by considering factors other than age, particularly the location of the haematoma. Table 8.4 lists the different causes of PICH according to frequency by age group and by location (basal ganglia or thalamus, lobar haemorrhages in the cortex or white matter of the cerebral hemispheres, and cerebellum or brainstem). This rank order of the different causes is based partly on a large hospital

Table 8.4 A priori probabilities for structural causes of PICH (coagulopathies and haemodynamic factors excluded), according to the patients' age and the location of the haematoma.

Age (years)	Basal ganglia/thalamus	Lobar	Cerebellum/brainstem
Below 50	1 AVM or microangioma 2 Lipohyalinosis or microaneurysm 3 Moyamoya syndrome (4) Amphetamines/cocaine	1 AVM or microangioma 2 Saccular aneurysm* 3 Tumour 4 Intracranial venous thrombosis† (5) Amphetamines/cocaine 6 Infective endocarditis‡	1 AVM or microangioma 2 Lipohyalinosis or microaneurysm 3 Tumour
50–69	1 Lipohyalinosis or microaneurysm 2 AVM or microangioma 3 Atherosclerotic 'moyamoya syndrome'	1 Lipohyalinosis or microaneurysm 2 AMV or microangioma 3 Saccular aneurysm* (4) Tumour (5) Amyloid angiopathy 6 Intracranial venous thrombosis† 7 Infective endocarditis‡	1 Lipohyalinosis or microaneurysm 2 AVM or microangioma (3) Tumour (4) Amyloid angiopathy
70 or over	1 Lipohyalinosis or microaneurysm (2) Tumour (3) AVM or microangioma	1 Lipohyalinosis or microaneurysm 2 Amyloid angiopathy 3 Saccular aneurysm* 4 Tumour 5 AVM or microangioma 6 Intracranial venous thrombosis† 7 Infective endocarditis‡	1 Lipohyalinosis or microaneurysm 2 Amyloid angiopathy 3 Tumour 4 AVM or microangioma

* Haematomas in specific locations (see text).
† Haematoma usually in parasagittal area.
‡ With history of valvular heart disease.
Numbers in parentheses, rank order not certain.

series of young adults (15–45 years) with PICH (Toffol *et al.*, 1987), partly on a large surgical series of lobar haemorrhages with negative angiography, in which thorough histological study of the specimens was done (Wakai *et al.*, 1992), and finally—where nothing else is available—on guesswork. The relative importance of some causes depends also on geographical location, for instance drug abuse or endocarditis; the order given here reflects the relative frequencies in Europe and should be adjusted where necessary for cultural and geographical differences.

> *Arteriovenous malformations are the most common cause of primary intracerebral haemorrhage in the young, degenerative small vessel deficit in middle and old age, and amyloid angiopathy in old age.*

8.7 Clues from the history

The cause of intracerebral haemorrhage may occasionally be identified from clues in the history. Previous epileptic seizures should raise suspicions about the presence of an AVM, a tumour or, if focal and of recent onset, amyloid angiopathy (Greenberg *et al.*, 1993; Cocito *et al.*, 1994). A record of long-standing *hypertension* indicates lipohyalinosis or microaneurysms as the most probable underlying condition in a patient with a haematoma in the basal ganglia or in the posterior fossa; on the other hand, hypertension is so common that it may co-exist with other conditions. If the patient is known to have had cancer, especially melanoma, bronchial carcinoma or renal carcinoma, haemorrhage into a brain metastasis is a strong possibility.

The presence of *valvular heart disease* in a patient with PICH must raise the suspicion of septic embolism, although this will not be the cause in the vast majority of cases, because infective endocarditis is a rare disease, much rarer than the other causes of PICH, such as amyloid angiopathy. If *haemorrhages at other sites*, such as in the skin, have preceded the haemorrhagic stroke, a disorder of haemostasis is almost too obvious to be missed.

The use of *oral anticoagulant drugs* is a vital piece of information in patients with PICH, because, in consultation with the cardiologists, their action should probably be neutralised as soon as possible by intravenous injection of prothrombin complex concentrate and vitamin K (see Section 12.2.4). It is equally important to know about the use of *recreational drugs*, particularly cocaine and amphetamines. Finally, the circumstances preceding PICH may contribute to identifying its cause: an earlier phase of the illness with a dense neurological deficit (*haemorrhagic transformation of an infarct*), *puerperium* (intracranial venous thrombosis, choriocarcinoma), *neck trauma* (dissection of the vertebral or carotid artery) and *migrainous headache* (vasospasm). In any patient with *haemophilia*, a 'stroke', unexplained sudden coma or severe headache signifies intracranial bleeding until proved otherwise.

8.8 Clues from the examination

8.8.1 General examination

The general examination will provide few clues to the cause of an intracerebral haemorrhage, with the exception of *petechiae* or bruising, indicating a generalised haemostatic disorder, signs of malignant disease such as cutaneous melanoma, a collapsed lung or enlargement of the liver or spleen, or telangiectasias in the skin and mucous membranes. Auscultating the skull for detecting AVMs is useful for impressing naïve readers of textbooks as well as medical students and patients, but is not really rewarding (we offer a free copy of this book to anyone who has no other clues and only by auscultation diagnosed an AVM in an adult). Finding *hypertension* on admission is the rule, but only in about 50% of these patients is this a contributing factor (see Section 8.3.1) and in the others it is merely a reactive phenomenon (see Section 15.7). Signs of *hypertensive vascular changes in the retina* or *enlargement of the heart on percussion* will allow the identification of hypertension as a contributing factor, but absence of arteriolar thickening on fundoscopy does not exclude it. *Subhyaloid haemorrhages* indicate intracranial bleeding in general, most often SAH (Keane, 1979). *Heart murmurs* may be coincidental but should at least raise the possibility of infective endocarditis as a cause of PICH, as should the finding of needle marks in possible drug addicts.

8.8.2 Neurological examination

The clinical manifestations of intracerebral haemorrhage almost always include focal deficits, with or without a decreased level of consciousness. Coma or a lesser degree of obtundation in general is a non-localising feature, except with haemorrhages in the posterior fossa.

A *decreased level of consciousness* is one of the classic features of PICH as taught to medical students, but it is absent in a sizeable proportion of patients (see Section 5.3.1). A secondary decrease in the level of consciousness after admission, which occurs in about one-third of all patients, may result from actual enlargement of the haematoma, but also from the formation of oedema around an already large haematoma, from obstructive hydrocephalus with posterior fossa haematoma or from a medical complication (Fujii *et al.*, 1994; Mayer *et al.*, 1994).

The *focal deficits* in PICH are of course determined by the site and size of the haematoma. The pace at which these negative symptoms develop is usually a matter of seconds or minutes, rarely of hours. Table 8.5 lists the different combinations of motor, sensory, visual and oculomotor syndromes according to location. Some further comments are appropriate. With thalamic haemorrhages, the nature of the deficits depends on the location within the thalamus, as this conglomerate of nuclei has connections with almost every part of the cerebral cortex. Caudate haemorrhages produce few focal deficits but a predominance of general symptoms (headache, vomiting and a decrease in the level of consciousness) by rapid extension of the bleed into the ventricular system; these features may mimic SAH (Stein *et al.*, 1984). All haemorrhages in the posterior fossa may be complicated by obstructive hydrocephalus, whether in the cerebellum (Gerritsen van der Hoop *et al.*, 1988), midbrain (Sand *et al.*, 1986) or pons (Masiyama *et al.*, 1985). The prognosis of haemorrhages in the pons is not always as bleak as was believed before the CT scan era, when the diagnosis was made only in fatal cases; in prospective series from primary referral centres, the rate of survival is around 40% (Kushner & Bressman, 1985; Masiyama *et al.*, 1985). In fact, small haemorrhages in the pons, midbrain, thalamus and internal capsule may cause the well-known 'lacunar syndromes', here being caused by small deep haemorrhages rather than small deep infarcts (see Section 4.4.6; Kim *et al.*, 1994).

The relative probabilities of PICH occurring in the locations shown in Table 8.5 are estimated in Table 8.6. The proportions in this table are only an approximation of the truth, for two reasons. The first is that population studies, although unbiased, contain a small proportion of haemorrhages, in which subdivisions are subject to chance effects. Large hospital series, on the other hand, suffer from bias in that referral is less often considered in the case of moribund patients or, at the other extreme, with patients who have only very mild deficits.

Table 8.5 Focal deficits in PICH, according to the site of the lesion.

Site of PICH (with references)	Hemiparesis	Hemisensory loss	Hemianopia	Oculomotor disorders	Other deficits
Internal capsule (Mori *et al.*, 1985; Kim *et al.*, 1994)		+	[+]		[Cerebellar ataxia, contralateral]
Thalamus (Barraquer Bordas *et al.*, 1981; Kawahara *et al.*, 1986; Weisberg, 1986c; Kim *et al.*, 1994)	[+]	[+] (with anterolateral lesions)	[+] (with posterolateral lesions)	Small, unreactive pupils (medial or posterolateral lesions) Upward-gaze palsy (medial lesions) Hyperconvergence Dysconjugate gaze ('pseudo-sixth') Skew deviation Conjugate deviation, towards lesion or away from lesion ('wrong-way eyes')	Dysphasia (with left and dorsal lesions) Spatial disorientation (with right and dorsal lesions) Drowsiness (also with small lesions, if medial or posterolateral) Apathy (with anterolateral lesions) Amnesia
Caudate nucleus (Weisberg, 1984; Stein *et al.*, 1984; Waga *et al.*, 1986)		[+]	[+]	[Conjugate deviation, towards lesion]	Miosis, ipsilateral
Putamen (Hier *et al.*, 1977; Koba *et al.*, 1977)	+	[+]	[+]		Dysphasia (with dominant-hemisphere lesions) Spatial disorientation (with right lesions)
White matter of hemisphere (Ropper & Davis, 1980)	[+] (frontal lesions)	[+] (parietal lesions)	[+] (occipital lesions)	[Conjugate deviation, towards lesion]	Dysphasia, with good repetition (dominant temporal lesions) Ataxic hemiparesis (below motor cortex)
Cerebellum (Ott *et al.*, 1974; Dunne *et al.*, 1987; Gerritsen van der Hoop *et al.*, 1988; Kim *et al.*, 1994)				Small, reactive pupils [Conjugate deviation, away from the lesion]	Intense vertigo Inability to stand or sit Dysarthria Hemiataxia Decreased level of consciousness
Midbrain (Weisberg, 1986a; Sand *et al.*, 1986; Getenet *et al.*, 1994; Kim *et al.*, 1994)				Fixed, dilated pupils (with pretectal lesions) Bilateral IIIrd nerve palsy Horner's syndrome (with tegmental lesions) IVth nerve palsy (lesions of inferior colliculus)	Hemiataxia (lesions of middle cerebellar peduncle) Coma (tegmental lesions, bilateral)
Pons (Nakajima, 1983; Kushner & Bressman, 1985; Masiyama *et al.*, 1985; Weisberg, 1986b; Chung & Park, 1992; Kim *et al.*, 1994)	[+] (with basal lesions) (tetraparesis with bilateral lesions)	[+] (with tegmental lesions)		Pinpoint pupils (with bilateral tegmental lesions) Conjugate deviation, away from lesion (with tegmental lesions) Internuclear ophthalmoplegia	Hemiataxia, ipsilateral (with lesions of middle cerebellar peduncle) Ataxic hemiparesis, contralateral (with basal lesions, unilateral) VIIth nerve palsy, ipsilateral (with tegmental lesions) Coma (with tegmental lesions, bilateral)

Continued

Table 8.5 *Continued*.

Site of PICH (with references)	Hemiparesis	Hemisensory loss	Hemianopia	Oculomotor disorders	Other deficits
				If together with conjugate deviation: 'one-and-a-half syndrome' (Fisher, 1967; Nakajima, 1983)	Visual hallucinations
Medulla (Barinagarrementeria & Cantú, 1994)	[+] (with ventral lesions)	[+] (with medial lesions)		Rotatory nystagmus Vertigo (with lateral lesions)	Palatal weakness, hiccups (with lateral tegmental lesions) Facial numbness, ipsilateral (with lateral lesions) Hemianaesthesia of trunk and limbs, contralateral (with lateral lesions) Hemiataxia, ipsilateral (with lesions of inferior cerebellar peduncle) Horner's syndrome (with lateral lesions) XIIth nerve palsy, ipsilateral (with medial tegmental lesions)

+, present; [+], sometimes present.

Table 8.6 Approximate frequency of the different locations of PICH.

Entire basal ganglia region	5%
Putamen or internal capsule	30%
Lobar*	30%
Thalamus†	15%
Caudate nucleus‡	5%
Cerebellum	10%
Pons§ or midbrain	5%

* Anderson *et al.*, 1994.
† Kawahara *et al.*, 1986.
‡ Stein *et al.*, 1984.
§ Nakajima, 1983.
Other sources were the following, all being large (≥100) and consecutive hospital series: Waga & Yamamoto, 1983; Schütz, 1988; Kase *et al.*, 1992.

8.9 Investigations

8.9.1 Laboratory studies

Routine laboratory investigations (see Section 6.6.1) should not be forgotten from the point of view of general medical management, but they will seldom uncover the cause of PICH (e.g. massive liver damage).

Abnormalities of haemostasis may have contributed to the development of PICH, although it should be reiterated that identified and possible causes are not necessarily the only or even the true cause. Yet, haemostatic factors should be considered in every patient with PICH. Sometimes the relationship is obvious, e.g. if the patient is on anticoagulants. But, in other instances the relationship may be more indirect, such as the haemostatic defect in renal failure. If an intracerebral haemorrhage is related to a disorder of haemostasis, this is usually because of impaired clotting, that is, the secondary phase of haemostasis, which is dependent on adequate levels of coagulation factors. Abnormalities of primary haemostasis have to do with defects of platelet aggregation, from thrombocytopenia or platelet function defects; most commonly these result in haemorrhages in the skin and mucous membranes, and much more rarely in haemorrhages in organs such as the brain. The overview of the Antiplatelet Trialists' Collaboration, discussed earlier in Section 8.4.2, found an increased rate of intracerebral haemorrhages in patients on antiplatelet therapy, but in absolute terms the excess risk is very small (Antiplatelet Trialists' Collaboration, 1994a).

The most important screening test of primary haemostatic function is the platelet count. Thrombocytopenia precipitates PICH only with values under 20×10^9/L. A normal platelet count is reassuring only if platelet function is normal, and if this is uncertain, for example with renal failure or the presence of autoantibodies, the bleeding time should be determined as well. The clotting system (coagulation factors) can be assessed with the partial thromboplastin time (PTT), the prothrombin time (PT), the thrombin time (TT) or, preferably, the INR. Circulating antibodies which impair coagulation factor activity (inhibitor syndromes) may develop not only in patients with autoimmune diseases, but also in patients being treated with penicillin or streptomycin, and in haemophiliacs who have been treated with multiple plasma infusions. Appropriate tests can uncover these autoantibodies.

If infective endocarditis is suspected, the diagnosis may be strengthened by finding a high erythrocyte sedimentation rate or C reactive protein, and of course in that case blood cultures should be taken as well.

8.9.2 Brain CT scanning

This is the most important single investigation in patients with suspected intracranial haematomas. The location of the haematoma may to some extent indicate the underlying cause (Figs 8.14–8.17; see Table 8.4). The presence of a fluid-blood level strongly suggests an underlying coagulopathy, either iatrogenic or as a result of haematological disease (Pfleger *et al.*, 1994); a clot with a flat top may falsely suggest a disorder of coagulation, a problem which can be resolved by repositioning the patient. If *multiple or recurrent haemorrhages* are identified on CT scanning (see Table 8.2), this

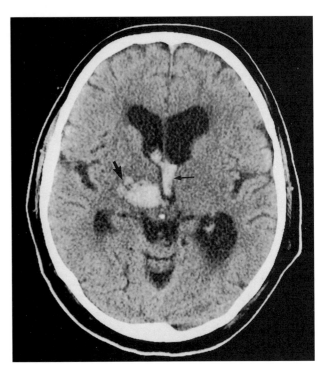

Figure 8.15 CT scan showing a haemorrhage in the right thalamus (thick arrow), with rupture into the third ventricle (thin arrow), resulting in obstructive hydrocephalus.

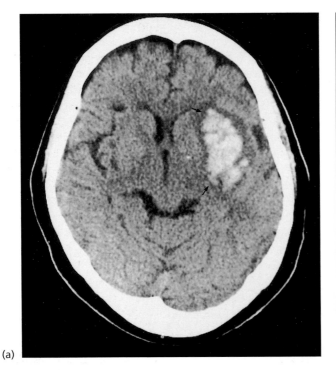

(a)

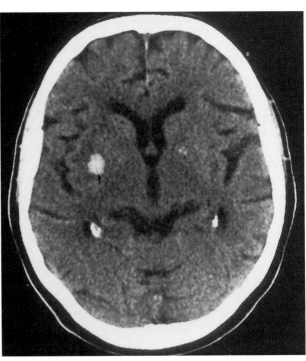

(b)

Figure 8.14 (a) CT scan showing a large haemorrhage in the left basal ganglia (arrows). (b) CT scan showing a small haemorrhage in the right internal capsule (arrow).

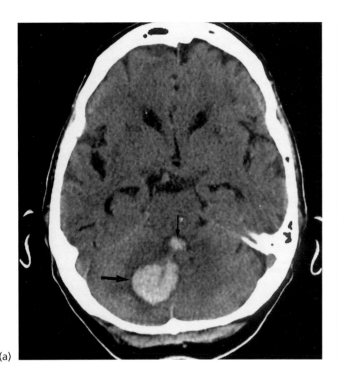
(a)

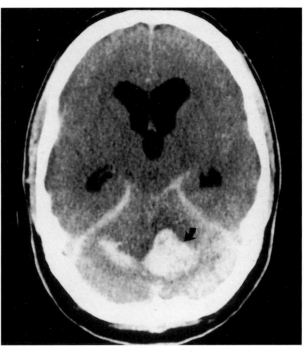
(b)

Figure 8.16 (a) CT scan showing a haemorrhage in right cerebellar hemisphere (thick arrow), with rupture into the fourth ventricle (thin arrow). (b) CT scan showing a large haemorrhage in left cerebellar hemisphere (arrow) and vermis (and smaller haemorrhage in right cerebellar hemisphere), with compression of the fourth ventricle and obstructive hydrocephalus.

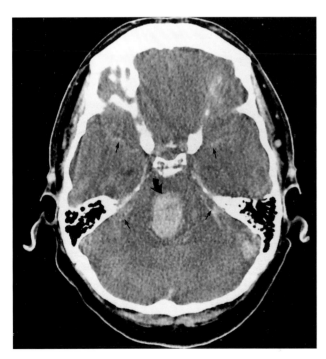

Figure 8.17 CT scan showing a primary haemorrhage in the pons (thick arrow), with some blood being visible in the subarachnoid space (thin arrows) through rupture into the fourth ventricle (not visible).

should raise the possibility of amyloid angiopathy in the case of lobar haemorrhages in an elderly patient (Fig. 8.18); of intracranial venous thrombosis if the irregular shape and parasagittal location suggests infarction as a result of venous congestion, with haemorrhagic transformation (see Fig. 8.7b); or of metastases if there is a history of malignant disease. Other important unenhanced CT scan signs in the diagnosis of intracranial venous thrombosis are marked hyperdensity of the straight sinus or transverse or sigmoid sinuses (see Fig. 8.7c) and—a less specific sign—a central filling defect in axial cuts of the superior sagittal sinus after injection of contrast, the so-called empty delta-sign (Ameri & Bousser, 1992).

Repeat brain CT with injection of contrast may be essential for picking up underlying lesions, such as tumours, AVMs or microangiomas. These can be most easily identified at a stage when the haemorrhage has resolved, at least partially.

8.9.3 MRI

It is especially for the demonstration of associated vascular anomalies that MRI scanning is useful in patients with PICH (see also Section 5.3.6). As flowing blood is not sus-

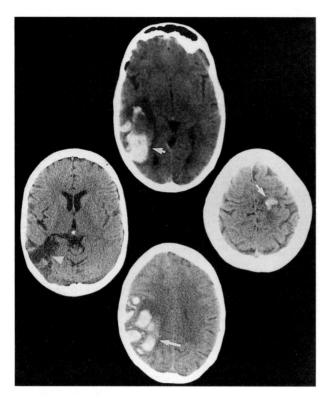

Figure 8.18 Multiple haemorrhages from familial amyloid angiopathy (CT scans). Top: haemorrhage in right temporal lobe (arrow), at age 51 years. Left and right: small haemorrhage (arrow) at the convexity of the left hemisphere, at age 54 years; the previous haemorrhage has left a hypodense scar (arrowhead). Bottom: haemorrhage in right parietal lobe (arrow), at age 55 years. The patient died after a fourth episode at the age of 56 years.

ceptible in the same way as brain tissue to the changes induced by strong magnetic fields, vascular channels appear as strongly hypointense 'empty' regions ('signal voids'), representing flowing blood (Fig. 8.19). MRI scanning may in this way identify AVMs, microangiomas and sometimes even saccular aneurysms. Signs of congestion of pial vessels may suggest a dural fistula draining into cortical veins, although most such anomalies communicate with dural sinuses (see Section 8.2.7; Willinsky *et al.*, 1994). Dedicated techniques for demonstrating moving blood (MR angiography (MRA)) are still more sensitive for the detection of vascular lesions than MR techniques used for brain imaging (for aneurysms, see Section 9.4.3) (Edelman *et al.*, 1990a,b). The developments of this technique are so rapid that eventually it may replace catheter angiography.

If intracranial venous thrombosis is suspected as a cause of

intracerebral haemorrhage, MRI is a useful tool in showing evidence of *thrombi within dural sinuses*, but again the abnormalities are time-dependent (Isensee *et al.*, 1994). In the acute stage (days 1–5), the thrombus appears isointense on T1-weighted images and strongly hypointense on T2-weighted images, in the subacute stage (up to day 15) the thrombus signal is strongly hyperintense on T1- as well as on T2-weighted images, and after the third week the thrombus signal is decreased in all sequences, until the restitution of normal blood flow (see Fig. 8.7a).

8.9.4 Cerebral angiography

Introducing a catheter into a peripheral (usually the femoral) artery and guiding it through the aorta to the extracranial vessels and then injecting radio-opaque fluids is not without risk, at least not in patients with ischaemic cerebrovascular disease (see Section 6.6.4) (Hankey *et al.*, 1990). Arterial dissection and contrast hypersensitivity are amongst the greatest dangers. In patients with intracerebral haemorrhage, this investigation is still often indicated to detect underlying vascular lesions that are amenable to specific treatment, particularly AVMs, saccular aneurysms and intracranial venous thrombosis (in the last case, only if MRI studies are inconclusive). This applies essentially to all patients under 50 years with PICH, provided they are fit for surgery. Angiography is especially indicated if the pattern of haemorrhage is compatible with a saccular aneurysm (in that situation, the angiogram should be performed as quickly as possible) or if MRI scanning shows 'flow void' phenomena consistent with AVMs.

> In any patient with intracerebral haemorrhage who is fit for surgery, one should at least consider cerebral angiography, with a view to detecting surgically treatable lesions, particularly saccular aneurysms and arteriovenous malformations. The indication is stronger if the patient is under the age of 50 years, if the haemorrhage is not in the deep regions of the brain and if the patient is not hypertensive.

The indications for angiography are less clear in patients without any clues to indicate a treatable lesion. It has often been assumed that the probability of finding such a lesion is low in patients over 65 years and in patients with pre-existing hypertension or with haemorrhages in the basal ganglia or the posterior fossa. A unique and prospective study assessed the value of angiography in 42 such 'low-risk' patients, and came up with a surprising number of lesions: eight AVMs and two aneurysms (24%; 95% confidence interval: 12–40%) (Halpin *et al.*, 1994). The rate of an angiographically demonstrable lesion was much higher

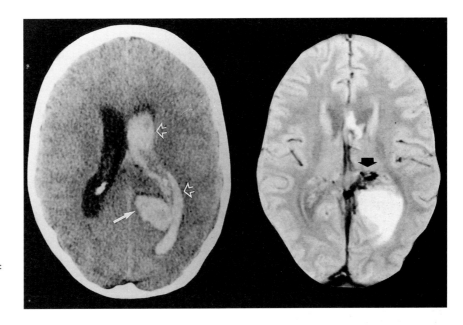

Figure 8.19 Intracerebral haemorrhage from AVM. Left: CT scan showing a haematoma in the medial part of the left occipital lobe (arrow), with rupture into the lateral ventricle (open arrows). Right: MRI scan (T1-weighted image) shows signal void (black, see arrow) from malformation and large draining vein.

(84%) in a parallel group of 38 patients with lobar haemorrhage who were also relatively young (below a mean of 46 years) and not hypertensive, but conversely there was still a fair proportion of positive angiograms in the presence of any of three 'negative predictors': 31% in patients above the mean age of 46 years; 13% for hypertension, and it had been as high as 36% in a previous study of fatal cases; 31% of patients with haemorrhage in the basal ganglia; and 18% of those with posterior fossa haemorrhage (McCormick & Rosenfield, 1973). Even the combination of high blood pressure and age above the mean was still associated with a structural lesion on angiography in 12% (Halpin *et al.*, 1994).

Angiography in search of a vascular anomaly rarely needs to be urgent, because with most lesions rebleeding occurs only after months or years, if at all. The only and important exception is when a saccular aneurysm is suspected. As the sensitivity of MRA increases, the need for catheter angiography may disappear, at least for this particular indication. Repeating angiography after a negative first study may still uncover small AVMs in 10–20%, presumably because at the initial study the lesion was being compressed by mass effect from the haematoma (Willinsky *et al.*, 1993; Halpin *et al.*, 1994).

8.10   Primary subdural haematoma

Subdural haematomas without attendant haemorrhage in the subarachnoid space or in the brain parenchyma are traditionally associated with trauma, but they can also occur 'spontaneously' (or, one might speculate, with trauma that is too slight to be remembered). Although these haematomas are not intraparenchymal, they are still included in this chapter because most of their many possible causes overlap with those of PICH (Table 8.7). Anticoagulant treatment is the most common precipitant, in urbanised areas of Western Europe accounting for approximately 25% of all subdural haematomas and 50% of those without obvious trauma (Wintzen & Tijssen, 1982). In anticoagulant-associated subdural haematoma, the onset may be very acute and even

Table 8.7 Causes of spontaneous subdural haematomas.*

Rupture of a small pial artery (McDermott *et al.*, 1984; Stephenson & Gibson, 1989; Bongioanni *et al.*, 1991; Borzone *et al.*, 1993; Yasui *et al.*, 1995)
Saccular aneurysm of major intracerebral artery (Williams *et al.*, 1983; O'Leary & Sweeny, 1986; Kondziolka *et al.*, 1988; Ragland *et al.*, 1993)
AVM (Oikawa *et al.*, 1993)
Intracavernous aneurysm of the carotid artery (Hodes *et al.*, 1988)
Aneurysm of middle meningeal artery (Korosue *et al.*, 1988)
Moyamoya syndrome (Oppenheim *et al.*, 1991)
Anticoagulant treatment (Wintzen & Tijssen, 1982)
Thrombolytic treatment (Gore *et al.*, 1991; Uglietta *et al.*, 1991)
Coagulation defects, also in children (Shih *et al.*, 1993)
Dural metastasis (Rothschild & Maxeiner, 1990); this may also cause *epi*dural haematoma (Anegawa *et al.*, 1989)
Lumbar puncture (Hart *et al.*, 1988; Vos *et al.*, 1991)

* Without associated intracerebral haemorrhage or SAH.

lethal (Wintzen, 1980). In those cases, rapid correction of the coagulation status is mandatory (see Section 8.4.1), usually followed by craniotomy. A ruptured small pial artery is probably the next most common cause, and sometimes angiography shows the extravasation from a small artery at the surface of the brain into the subdural space (Yasui *et al.*, 1995).

If the level of consciousness remains normal, spontaneous resolution may occur, even with an acute onset (Aoki, 1990; Kulah *et al.*, 1992). On the other hand, in patients in whom the onset of symptoms is measured in days or weeks, the haematoma presumably originating from a bridging vein (Wintzen, 1980), may deteriorate rather studdenly (Aoki & Tsutsumi, 1990). Some chronic subdural haematomas may present with acute headache, mimicking SAH (Kotwica & Brzezinski, 1985). Most spontaneous subdural haematomas occur over the convexity of the cerebral hemisphere, but subdural haematomas may also be found in the interhemispheric fissure, as a rule with aneurysms (Friedman & Brant Zawadzki, 1983; Houtteville *et al.*, 1988), or in the posterior fossa (Kanter *et al.*, 1984).

A subdural haematoma may also occur, together with an intraparenchymal haematoma, from degenerative arteriolar disease (Arai, 1983; Avis, 1993) or an AVM (Ezura & Kagawa, 1992), or with SAH, in which case the aneurysmal origin should be obvious (see Section 9.4.1).

References

Abe M, Kjellberg RN, Adams RD (1989). Clinical presentations of vascular malformations of the brain stem: comparison of angiographically positive and negative types. *J Neurol Neurosurg Psychiatr* 52: 167–75.

Adams HP Jr, Dawson G, Coffman TJ, Corry RJ (1986). Stroke in renal transplant recipients. *Arch Neurol* 43: 113–15.

Adams RD, vander Eecken HM (1953). Vascular diseases of the brain. *Ann Rev Med* 4: 213–52.

Ameri A, Bousser MG (1992). Cerebral venous thrombosis. *Neurol Clin* 10: 87–111.

Aminoff MJ (1973). Vascular anomalies in the intracranial dura mater. *Brain* 96: 601–12.

Aminoff MJ (1987). Treatment of unruptured cerebral arteriovenous malformations. *Neurology* 37: 815–19.

Anderson CS, Chakera TM, Stewart Wynne EG, Jamrozik KD (1994). Spectrum of primary intracerebral haemorrhage in Perth, Western Australia, 1989–90: incidence and outcome. *J Neurol Neurosurg Psychiatr* 57: 936–40.

Andes WA, Wulff K (1990). Intracranial hemorrhage in hemophiliacs with AIDS [letter]. *Thromb Haemost* 63: 326.

Anegawa S, Hirohata S, Tokutomi T, Kuramoto S (1989). Spontaneous epidural hematoma secondary to dural metastasis from an ovarian carcinoma—case report. *Neurol Med Chir Tokyo* 29: 854–6.

Antiplatelet Trialists' Collaboration (1994a). Collaborative overview of randomised trials of antiplatelet therapy—I: prevention of death, myocardial infarction, and stroke by prolonged antiplatelet therapy in various categories of patients. *Br Med J* 308: 81–106.

Antiplatelet Trialists' Collaboration (1994b). Collaborative overview of randomised trials of antiplatelet therapy–II: maintenance of vascular graft or arterial patency by antiplatelet therapy. *Br Med J* 308: 159–68.

Aoki N (1990). Acute subdural haematoma with rapid resolution. *Acta Neurochir Wien* 103: 76–8.

Aoki N (1991). Do intracranial arteriovenous malformations cause subarachnoid haemorrhage? Review of computed tomography features of ruptured arteriovenous malformations in the acute stage. *Acta Neurochir Wien* 112: 92–5.

Aoki N, Tsutsumi K (1990). Symptomatic subacute subdural haematoma following spontaneous acute subdural haematoma. *Acta Neurochir Wien* 102: 149–51.

Arai H (1983). Acute hypertensive subdural hematoma from arterial rupture shortly after the onset of cerebral subcortical hemorrhage: leakage of contrast medium during angiography. *Stroke* 14: 281–5.

Avis SP (1993). Nontraumatic acute subdural hematoma: a case report and review of the literature. *Am J Forensic Med Pathol* 14: 130–4.

Bae HG, Lee KS, Yun IG *et al.* (1992). Rapid expansion of hypertensive intracerebral hemorrhage. *Neurosurgery* 31: 35–41.

Bahemuka M (1987). Primary intracerebral hemorrhage and heart weight: a clinicopathologic case–control review of 218 patients. *Stroke* 18: 531–6.

Bamford J, Sandercock P, Dennis M, Burn J, Warlow C (1990). A prospective study of acute cerebrovascular disease in the community: the Oxfordshire Community Stroke Project—1981–86. 2. Incidence, case fatality rates and overall outcome at one year of cerebral infarction, primary intracerebral and subarachnoid haemorrhage. *J Neurol Neurosurg Psychiatr* 53: 16–22.

Bamford J, Sandercock P, Dennis M *et al.* (1988). A prospective study of acute cerebrovascular disease in the community: the Oxfordshire Community Stroke Project 1981–86. 1. Methodology, demography and incident cases of first-ever stroke. *J Neurol Neurosurg Psychiatr* 51: 1373–80.

Barbas N, Caplan L, Baquis G, Adelman L, Moskowitz M (1987). Dental chair intracerebral hemorrhage. *Neurology* 37: 511–12.

Barinagarrementeria F, Cantú C (1994). Primary medullary hemorrhage: report of four cases and review of the literature. *Stroke* 25: 1684–7.

Barraquer Bordas L, Illa I, Escartin A, Ruscalleda J, Marti Vilalta JL (1981). Thalamic hemorrhage: a study of 23 patients with diagnosis by computed tomography. *Stroke* 12: 524–7.

Becker DH, Townsend JJ, Kramer RA, Newton TH (1979). Occult cerebrovascular malformations: a series of 18 histologically verified cases with negative angiography. *Brain* 102: 249–87.

Biller J, Loftus CM, Moore SA, Schelper RL, Danks KR, Cornell SH (1987). Isolated central nervous system angiitis first presenting as spontaneous intracranial hemorrhage. *Neurosurgery* 20: 310–15.

Bongioanni F, Ramadan A, Kostli A, Berney J (1991). [Acute subdural hematoma of arteriolar origin. Traumatic or spontaneous?] L'hématome sous-dural aigu d'origine artériolaire. Traumatique ou spontane? *Neurochirurgie* 37: 26–31.

Borzone M, Altomonte M, Baldini M, Rivano C (1993). Pure subdural haematomas of arteriolar origin. *Acta Neurochir Wien* 121: 109–12.

Broderick J, Brott T, Tomsick T, Leach A (1993a). Lobar hemorrhage in the elderly: the undiminishing importance of hypertension. *Stroke* 24: 49–51.

Broderick JP, Brott T, Tomsick T, Miller R, Huster G (1993b). Intracerebral hemorrhage more than twice as common as subarachnoid hemorrhage. *J Neurosurg* 78: 188–91.

Brott T, Thalinger K, Hertzberg V (1986). Hypertension as a risk factor for spontaneous intracerebral hemorrhage. *Stroke* 17: 1078–83.

Brown RD Jr, Wiebers DO, Forbes GS (1990). Unruptured intracranial aneurysms and arteriovenous malformations: frequency of intracranial hemorrhage and relationship of lesions. *J Neurosurg* 73: 859–63.

Bruno A, Adams HP Jr, Biller J, Rezai K, Cornell S, Aschenbrener CA (1988). Cerebral infarction due to moyamoya disease in young adults. *Stroke* 19: 826–33.

Bruno A, Nolte KB, Chapin J (1993). Stroke associated with ephedrine use. *Neurology* 43: 1313–16.

Brust JC, Dickinson PC, Hughes JE, Holtzman RN (1990). The diagnosis and treatment of cerebral mycotic aneurysms. *Ann Neurol* 27: 238–46.

Camargo CA Jr (1989). Moderate alcohol consumption and stroke: the epidemiologic evidence. *Stroke* 20: 1611–26.

Cannegieter SC, Rosendaal FR, Wintzen AR, Van der Meer FJM, Vandenbroucke JP, Briët E (1995). Optimal oral anticoagulant therapy in patients with mechanical heart valves. *N Engl J Med* 333: 11–17.

Caplan L (1988). Intracerebral hemorrhage revisited. *Neurology* 38: 624–7.

Caplan LR (1994). Drugs. In: Kase CS, Caplan LR, eds. *Intracerebral Hemorrhage.* Boston: Butterworth-Heinemann, 201–20.

Caplan LR, Neely S, Gorelick P (1984). Cold-related intracerebral hemorrhage. *Arch Neurol* 41: 227.

Carlson SE, Aldrich MS, Greenberg HS, Topol EJ (1988). Intracerebral hemorrhage complicating intravenous tissue plasminogen activator treatment. *Arch Neurol* 45: 1070–3.

Challa VL, Moody DM, Bell MA (1992). The Charcot–Bouchard aneurysm controversy: impact of a new histologic technique. *J Neuropathol Exp Neurol* 51: 264–71.

Charcot JM, Bouchard C (1868). Nouvelles recherches sur la pathogénie de l'hémorrhagie cérébrale. *Arch Physiol Norm Pathol* 1: 110–27, 643–65, 725–34.

Chaudhary MY, Sachdev VP, Cho SH, Weitzner I Jr, Puljic S, Huang YP (1982). Dural arteriovenous malformation of the major venous sinuses: an acquired lesion. *Am J Neuroradiol* 3: 13–19.

Chen ST, Chen SD, Hsu CY, Hogan EL (1989). Progression of hypertensive intracerebral hemorrhage. *Neurology* 39: 1509–14.

Chung CS, Park CH (1992). Primary pontine hemorrhage: a new CT classification. *Neurology* 42: 830–4.

Citron BP, Halpern M, McCarron M et al. (1970). Necrotizing angiitis associated with drug abuse. *N Engl J Med* 283: 1003–11.

Cocito L, Nizzo R, Bisio N, Favale E (1994). Epileptic seizures heralding intracerebral hemorrhage [letter]. *Stroke* 25: 2292–3.

Cole AJ, Aubé M (1990). Migraine with vasospasm and delayed intracerebral hemorrhage. *Arch Neurol* 47: 53–6.

Cole FM, Yates P (1967a). Intracerebral microaneurysms and small cerebrovascular lesions. *Brain* 90: 759–68.

Cole FM, Yates PO (1967b). The occurrence and significance of intracerebral micro-aneurysms. *J Pathol Bacteriol* 93: 393–411.

Cole FM, Yates PO (1967c). Pseudo-aneurysms in relation to massive cerebral haemorrhage. *J Neurol Neurosurg Psychiatr* 30: 61–6.

Coria F, Castano EM, Frangione B (1987). Brain amyloid in normal aging and cerebral amyloid angiopathy is antigenically related to Alzheimer's disease beta-protein. *Am J Pathol* 129: 422–8.

Crawford JV, Russell DS (1956). Cryptic arteriovenous and venous hamartomas of the brain. *J Neurol Neurosurg Psychiatr* 19: 1–11.

d'Angelo VA, Monte V, Scialfa G, Fiumara E, Scotti G (1988). Intracerebral venous hemorrhage in 'high-risk' carotid–cavernous fistula. *Surg Neurol* 30: 387–90.

Dawson I, van Bockel JH, Ferrari MD, van der Meer FJ, Brand R, Terpstra JL (1993). Ischemic and hemorrhagic stroke in patients on oral anticoagulants after reconstruction for chronic lower limb ischemia. *Stroke* 24: 1655–63.

Destian S, Sze G, Krol G, Zimmerman RD, Deck MD (1989). MR imaging of hemorrhagic intracranial neoplasms. *Am J Roentgenol* 152: 137–44.

Dunne JW, Chakera T, Kermode S (1987). Cerebellar haemorrhage —diagnosis and treatment: a study of 75 consecutive cases. *Quart J Med* 64: 739–54.

Dutch TIA Trial Study Group (1991). A comparison of two doses of aspirin (30 mg vs. 283 mg a day) in patients after a transient ischemic attack or minor ischemic stroke. *N Engl J Med* 325: 1261–6.

Edelman RR, Mattle HP, Atkinson DJ, Hoogewoud HM (1990a). MR angiography. *Am J Roentgenol* 154: 937–46.

Edelman RR, Mattle HP, O'Reilly GV, Wentz KU, Liu C, Zhao B (1990b). Magnetic resonance imaging of flow dynamics in the circle of Willis. *Stroke* 21: 56–65.

Ellis AG (1909). The pathogenesis of spontaneous intracerebral hemorrhage. *Proc Pathol Soc Philadelphia* 12: 197–235.

European Atrial Fibrillation Trial Study Group (1995). Optimal oral anticoagulant therapy in patients with nonrheumatic atrial fibrillation and recent cerebral ischemia. *N Engl J Med* 333: 5–10.

Ezura M, Kagawa S (1992). Spontaneous disappearance of a huge cerebral arteriovenous malformation: case report. *Neurosurgery* 30: 595–9.

Farrell B, Godwin J, Richards S, Warlow C (1991). The United Kingdom transient ischaemic attack (UK-TIA) aspirin trial: final results. *J Neurol Neurosurg Psychiatr* 54: 1044–54.

Farrell DF, Forno LS (1970). Symptomatic capillary teleangiectasis of the brainstem without hemorrhage: report of an unusual case. *Neurology* 20: 341–6.

Finelli PF, Kessimian N, Bernstein PW (1984). Cerebral amyloid angiopathy manifesting as recurrent intracerebral hemorrhage. *Arch Neurol* 41: 330–3.

Fischer O (1910). Die presbyophren Demenz, deren anatomische Grundlage und klinische Abgrenzung. *Z gesamte Neurol Psychiatr* 3: 371–471.

Fisher CM (1967). Some neuro-ophthalmological observations. *J Neurol Neurosurg Psychiatr* 30: 383–92.

Fisher CM (1971). Pathological observations in hypertensive cerebral hemorrhage. *J Neuropathol Exp Neurol* 30: 536–50.

Fogelholm R, Eskola K, Kiminkinen T, Kunnamo I (1992). Anticoagulant treatment as a risk factor for primary intracerebral haemorrhage. *J Neurol Neurosurg Psychiatr* 55: 1121–4.

Franke CL, de Jonge J, van Swieten JC, Op de Coul AAW, Van Gijn J (1990). Intracerebral hematomas during anticoagulant treatment. *Stroke* 21: 726–30.

Franke CL, van Swieten JC, Algra A, Van Gijn J (1992). Prognostic factors in patients with intracerebral haematoma. *J Neurol Neurosurg Psychiatr* 55: 653–7.

Friedman MB, Brant Zawadzki M (1983). Interhemispheric subdural hematoma from ruptured aneurysm. *Comput Radiol* 7: 129–34.

Fujii Y, Tanaka R, Takeuchi S, Koike T, Minakawa T, Sasaki O (1994). Hematoma enlargement in spontaneous intracerebral hemorrhage. *J Neurosurg* 80: 51–7.

Garner TB, Del Curling O Jr, Kelly DL Jr, Laster DW (1991). The natural history of intracranial venous angiomas. *J Neurosurg* 75: 715–22.

Gerritsen van der Hoop R, Vermeulen M, Van Gijn J (1988). Cerebellar hemorrhage: diagnosis and treatment. *Surg Neurol* 29: 6–10.

Getenet JC, Vighetto A, Nighoghossian N, Trouillas P (1994). Isolated bilateral third nerve palsy caused by a mesencephalic hematoma. *Neurology* 44: 981–2.

Gilbert JJ, Vinters HV (1983). Cerebral amyloid angiopathy: incidence and complications in the aging brain. I. Cerebral hemorrhage. *Stroke* 14: 915–23.

Gilles C, Brucher JM, Khoubesserian P, Vanderhaeghen JJ (1984). Cerebral amyloid angiopathy as a cause of multiple intracerebral hemorrhages. *Neurology* 34: 730–5.

Gore JM, Sloan M, Price TR *et al.* (1991). Intracerebral hemorrhage, cerebral infarction, and subdural hematoma after acute myocardial infarction and thrombolytic therapy in the Thrombolysis in Myocardial Infarction Study. Thrombolysis in Myocardial Infarction, Phase II, pilot and clinical trial. *Circulation* 83: 448–59

Gray F, Dubas F, Roullet E, Escourolle R (1985). Leukoencephalopathy in diffuse hemorrhagic cerebral amyloid angiopaphy. *Ann Neurol* 18: 54–9.

Greenberg SM, Vonsattel JP, Stakes JW, Gruber M, Finklestein SP (1993). The clinical spectrum of cerebral amyloid angiopathy: presentations without lobar hemorrhage. *Neurology* 43: 2073–9.

Guazzo EP, Xuereb JH (1994). Spontaneous thrombosis of an arteriovenous malformation. *J Neurol Neurosurg Psychiatr* 57: 1410–12.

Gudmundsson G, Hallgrimsson J, Jonasson TA, Bjarnason O (1972). Hereditary cerebral haemorrhage with amyloidosis. *Brain* 95: 387–404.

Haan J, Roos RA, Algra PR, Lanser JB, Bots GT, Vegter van der Vlis M (1990). Hereditary cerebral haemorrhage with amyloidosis—Dutch type: magnetic resonance imaging findings in 7 cases. *Brain* 113: 1251–67.

Haines SJ, Maroon JC, Jannetta PJ (1978). Supratentorial intracerebral hemorrhage following posterior fossa surgery. *J Neurosurg* 49: 881–6.

Halpin SF, Britton JA, Byrne JV, Clifton A, Hart G, Moore A (1994). Prospective evaluation of cerebral angiography and computed tomography in cerebral haematoma. *J Neurol Neurosurg Psychiatr* 57: 1180–6.

Hankey GJ (1991). Isolated angiitis/angiopathy of the central nervous system. *Cerebrovasc Dis* 1: 2–15.

Hankey GJ, Warlow CP, Sellar RJ (1990). Cerebral angiographic risk in mild cerebrovascular disease. *Stroke* 21: 209–22.

Harrington H, Heller HA, Dawson D, Caplan L, Rumbaugh C (1983). Intracerebral hemorrhage and oral amphetamine. *Arch Neurol* 40: 503–7.

Hart IK, Bone I, Hadley DM (1988). Development of neurological problems after lumbar puncture. *Br Med J* 296: 51–2.

Hart RG, Kagan Hallet K, Joerns SE (1987). Mechanisms of intracranial hemorrhage in infective endocarditis. *Stroke* 18: 1048–56.

Hart RG, Foster JW, Luther MF, Kanter MC (1990). Stroke in infective endocarditis. *Stroke* 21: 695–700.

Hayward RD, O'Reilly GV (1976). Intracerebral haemorrhage: accuracy of computerised transverse axial scanning in predicting the underlying aetiology. *Lancet* i: 1–4.

Hendricks HT, Franke CL, Theunissen PH (1990). Cerebral amyloid angiopathy: diagnosis by MRI and brain biopsy. *Neurology* 40: 1308–10.

Herman B, Leyten ACM, van Luijk JH, Frenken CWGM, Op de Coul AAW, Schulte BPM (1982). Epidemiology of stroke in Tilburg, the Netherlands. The population-based stroke incidence register: 2. Incidence, initial clinical picture and medical care, and three-week case fatality. *Stroke* 13: 629–34.

Heros RC, Tu YK (1987). Is surgical therapy needed for unruptured arteriovenous malformations? *Neurology* 37: 279–86.

Hier DB, Davis KR, Richardson EP Jr, Mohr JP (1977). Hypertensive putaminal hemorrhage. *Ann Neurol* 1: 152–9.

Hodes JE, Fletcher WA, Goodman DF, Hoyt WF (1988). Rupture of cavernous carotid artery aneurysm causing subdural hematoma and death: case report. *J Neurosurg* 69: 617–19.

Houtteville JP, Toumi K, Theron J, Derlon JM, Benazza A, Hubert P (1988). Interhemispheric subdural haematomas: seven cases and review of the literature. *Br J Neurosurg* 2: 357–67.

Imakita S, Nishimura T, Yamada N et al. (1989). Cerebral vascular malformations: applications of magnetic resonance imaging to differential diagnosis. *Neuroradiology* 31: 320–5.

Isensee C, Reul J, Thron A (1994). Magnetic resonance imaging of thrombosed dural sinuses. *Stroke* 25: 29–34.

Ishii N, Nishihara Y, Horie A (1984). Amyloid angiopathy and lobar cerebral haemorrhage. *J Neurol Neurosurg Psychiatr* 47: 1203–10.

Itoh Y, Yamada M, Hayakawa M, Otomo E, Miyatake T (1993). Cerebral amyloid angiopathy: a significant cause of cerebellar as well as lobar cerebral hemorrhage in the elderly. *J Neurol Sci* 116: 135–41.

Jakubowski JA, Vaillancourt R, Deykin D (1988). Interaction of ethanol, prostacyclin, and aspirin in determining human platelet reactivity *in vitro*. *Arteriosclerosis* 8: 346–41.

Jansen C, Sprengers AM, Moll FL et al. (1994). Prediction of intracerebral haemorrhage after carotid endarterectomy by clinical criteria and intraoperative transcranial Doppler monitoring. *Eur J Vasc Surg* 8: 303–8.

Jellinger K (1977). Cerebrovascular amyloidosis with cerebral hemorrhage. *J Neurol* 214: 195–206.

Jensson O, Gudmundsson G, Arnason A et al. (1987). Hereditary cystatin C (gamma-trace) amyloid angiopathy of the CNS causing cerebral hemorrhage. *Acta Neurol Scand* 76: 102–14.

Kalyan Raman UP, Kalyan Raman K (1984). Cerebral amyloid angiopathy causing intracranial hemorrhage. *Ann Neurol* 16: 321–9.

Kanter MC, Hart RG (1991). Neurologic complications of infective endocarditis. *Neurology* 41: 1015–20.

Kanter R, Kanter M, Kirsch W, Rosenberg G (1984). Spontaneous posterior fossa subdural hematoma as a complication of anticoagulation. *Neurosurgery* 15: 241–2.

Kase CS (1986). Intracerebral hemorrhage: non-hypertensive causes. *Stroke* 17: 590–5.

Kase CS (1994). Intracranial tumors. In: Kase CS, Caplan LR, eds. *Intracerebral Hemorrhage*. Boston: Butterworth-Heinemann, 243–61.

Kase CS, Mohr JP, Caplan LR (1992). Intracerebral hemorrhage. In: Barnett HJM, Mohr JP, Stein BM, Yatsu FM, eds. *Stroke— Pathophysiology, Diagnosis, and Management*. New York: Churchill Livingstone, 561–616.

Kase CS, O'Neal AM, Fisher M, Girgis GN, Ordia JI (1990). Intracranial hemorrhage after use of tissue plasminogen activator for coronary thrombolysis. *Ann Intern Med* 112: 17–21.

Kase CS, Robinson RK, Stein RW et al. (1985). Anticoagulant-related intracerebral hemorrhage. *Neurology* 35: 943–8.

Kattapong VJ, Hart BL, Davis LE (1995). Familial cerebral cavernous angiomas: clinical and radiologic studies. *Neurology* 45: 492–7.

Kawahara N, Sato K, Muraki M, Tanaka K, Kaneko M, Uemura K (1986). CT classification of small thalamic hemorrhages and their clinical implications. *Neurology* 36: 165–72.

Keane JR (1979). Retinal hemorrhages: its significance in 100 patients with acute encephalopathy of unknown cause. *Arch Neurol* 36: 691–4.

Kelley RE, Berger JR, Scheinberg P, Stokes N (1982). Active bleeding in hypertensive intracerebral hemorrhage: computed tomography. *Neurology* 32: 852–6.

Kelly JK, Lazo A, Metes J, Wilner HI, Watts FB Jr (1985). Intracerebral hemorrhagic dissemination of acute myelocytic leukemia. *Am J Neuroradiol* 6: 113–14.

Kibayashi K, Mastri AR, Hirsch CS (1995). Cocaine induced intracerebral hemorrhage: analysis of predisposing factors and mechanisms causing hemorrhagic strokes. *Hum Pathol* 26: 659–63.

Kim JS, Lee JH, Lee MC (1994). Small primary intracerebral hemorrhage: clinical presentation of 28 cases. *Stroke* 25: 1500–6.

Kitanaka C, Teraoka A (1993). Spontaneous cervical internal carotid dissection presenting with intracerebral hematoma [letter]. *Stroke* 24: 1420–1.

Koba T, Yokoyama T, Kaneko M (1977). Correlation between the location of hematoma and its clinical symptoms in the lateral type of hypertensive intracerebral hemorrhage: observations on Pantopaque radiography of the hematoma cavity in cases of early surgical treatment. *Stroke* 8: 676–80.

Kondziolka D, Bernstein M, ter Brugge K, Schutz H (1988). Acute subdural hematoma from ruptured posterior communicating artery aneurysm. *Neurosurgery* 22: 151–4.

Korosue K, Kondoh T, Ishikawa Y, Nagao T, Tamaki N, Matsumoto S (1988). Acute subdural hematoma associated with nontraumatic middle meningeal artery aneurysm: case report. *Neurosurgery* 22: 411–13.

Kotwica Z, Brzezinski J (1985). Chronic subdural hematoma presenting as spontaneous subarachnoid hemorrhage: report of six cases. *J Neurosurg* 63: 691–2.

Krücke W (1971). [Pathology of cerebral vein and sinus thromboses] Pathologie der cerebralen Venen- und Sinusthrombosen. *Radiologe* 11: 370–7.

Kulah A, Tasdemir N, Fiskeci C (1992). Acute spontaneous subdural hematoma in a teenager. *Child Nerv Syst* 8: 343–6.

Kushner MJ, Bressman SB (1985). The clinical manifestations of pontine hemorrhage. *Neurology* 35: 637–43.

Laissy JP, Normand G, Monroc M, Duchateau C, Alibert F, Thiebot J (1991). Spontaneous intracerebral hematomas from vascular causes: predictive value of CT compared with angiography. *Neuroradiology* 33: 291–5.

Lee KS, Bae HG, Yun IG (1990). Recurrent intracerebral hemorrhage due to hypertension. *Neurosurgery* 26: 586–90.

Le Roux PD, Dailey AT, Newell DW, Grady MS, Winn HR (1993). Emergent aneurysm clipping without angiography in the moribund patient with intracerebral hemorrhage: the use of infusion computed tomography scans. *Neurosurgery* 33: 189–97.

Levine SR, Brust JC, Futrell et al. (1991). A comparative study of the cerebrovascular complications of cocaine: alkaloidal versus hydrochloride—a review. *Neurology* 41: 1173–7.

Little JR, Dial B, Belanger G, Carpenter S (1979). Brain hemorrhage from intracranial tumor. *Stroke* 10: 283–8.

Lobato RD, Rivas JJ, Gomez PA, Cabrera A, Sarabia R, Lamas E (1992). Comparison of the clinical presentation of symptomatic arteriovenous malformations (angiographically visualized) and occult vascular malformations. *Neurosurgery* 31: 391–6.

Loes DJ, Biller J, Yuh WT *et al.* (1990). Leukoencephalopathy in cerebral amyloid angiopathy: MR imaging in four cases. *Am J Neuroradiol* 11: 485–8.

Lukes SA (1983). Intracerebral hemorrhage from an arteriovenous malformation after amphetamine injection. *Arch Neurol* 40: 60–1.

Luyendijk W, Bots GT, Vegter van der Vlis M, Went LN, Frangione B (1988). Hereditary cerebral haemorrhage caused by cortical amyloid angiopathy. *J Neurol Sci* 85: 267–80.

McCormick WF (1966). The pathology of vascular ('arteriovenous') malformations. *J Neurosurg* 24: 807–16.

McCormick WF, Rosenfield DB (1973). Massive brain hemorrhage: a review of 144 cases and an examination of their causes. *Stroke* 4: 946–54.

McDermott M, Fleming JF, Vanderlinden RG, Tucker WS (1984). Spontaneous arterial subdural hematoma. *Neurosurgery* 14: 13–18.

MacMahon S, Peto R, Cutler J *et al.* (1990). Blood pressure, stroke, and coronary heart disease. Part 1, prolonged differences in blood pressure: prospective observational studies corrected for the regression dilution bias. *Lancet* 335: 765–74.

Maeda A, Yamada M, Itoh Y, Otomo E, Hayakawa M, Miyatake T (1993). Computer-assisted three-dimensional image analysis of cerebral amyloid angiopathy. *Stroke* 24: 1857–64.

Maiuri F, D'Andrea F, Gallicchio B, Carandente M (1985). Intracranial hemorrhages in metastatic brain tumors. *J Neurosurg Sci* 29: 37–41.

Malik GM, Pearce JE, Ausman JI, Mehta B (1984). Dural arteriovenous malformations and intracranial haemorrhage. *Neurosurgery* 15: 333–9.

Markel A, Nagler A, Yoffe G, Aboud L, Brook GJ (1986). Acute myelofibrosis with associated intracerebral haemorrhage. *Acta Haematol Basel* 75: 38–9.

Marks MP, Lane B, Steinberg GK, Snipes GJ (1992). Intranidal aneurysms in cerebral arteriovenous malformations: evaluation and endovascular treatment. *Radiology* 183: 355–60.

Marmot MG, Poulter NR (1992). Primary prevention of stroke. *Lancet* 339: 344–7.

Martinowitz U, Heim M, Tadmor R *et al.* (1986). Intracranial hemorrhage in patients with hemophilia. *Neurosurgery* 18: 538–41.

Maruyama K, Ikeda S, Ishihara T, Allsop D, Yanagisawa N (1990). Immunohistochemical characterization of cerebrovascular amyloid in 46 autopsied cases using antibodies to beta protein and cystatin C. *Stroke* 21: 397–403.

Masiyama S, Niizuma H, Suzuki J (1985). Pontine haemorrhage: a clinical analysis of 26 cases. *J Neurol Neurosurg Psychiatr* 48: 658–62.

Masuda J, Tanaka K, Ueda K, Omae T (1988). Autopsy study of incidence and distribution of cerebral amyloid angiopathy in Hisayama, Japan. *Stroke* 19: 205–10.

Masuda J, Yutani C, Waki R, Ogata J, Kuriyama Y, Yamaguchi T (1992). Histopathological analysis of the mechanisms of intracranial hemorrhage complicating infective endocarditis. *Stroke* 23: 843–50.

Mayer SA, Sacco RL, Shi T, Mohr JP (1994). Neurologic deterioration in noncomatose patients with supratentorial intracerebral hemorrhage. *Neurology* 44: 1379–84.

Mendelow AD, Erfurth A, Grossart K, Macpherson P (1987). Do cerebral arteriovenous malformations increase in size? *J Neurol Neurosurg Psychiatr* 50: 980–7.

Meyer B, Stangl AP, Schramm J (1995). Association of venous and true arteriovenous malformation: a rare entity among mixed vascular malformations of the brain. Case report. *J Neurosurg* 83: 141–4.

Minakawa T, Tanaka R, Koike T, Takeuchi S, Sasaki O (1989). Angiographic follow-up study of cerebral arteriovenous malformations with reference to their enlargement and regression. *Neurosurgery* 24: 68–74.

Miyasaka Y, Yada K, Ohwada T, Kitahara T, Kurata A, Irikura K (1992). An analysis of the venous drainage system as a factor in hemorrhage from arteriovenous malformations. *J Neurosurg* 76: 239–43.

Modesti LM, Binet EF, Collins GH (1976). Meningiomas causing spontaneous intracranial hematomas. *J Neurosurg* 45: 437–41.

Monsuez JJ, Vittecoq D, Rosenbaum A *et al.* (1989). Prognosis of ruptured intracranial mycotic aneurysms: a review of 12 cases. *Eur Heart J* 10: 821–5.

Mori E, Tabuchi M, Yamadori A (1985). Lacunar syndrome due to intracerebral hemorrhage. *Stroke* 16: 454–9.

Nakajima K (1983). Clinicopathological study of pontine hemorrhage. *Stroke* 14: 485–93.

Ng MH, Tsang SS, Ng HK, Sriskandavarman V, Feng CS (1991). An unusual case of hairy cell leukemia: death due to leukostasis and intracerebral hemorrhage. *Hum Pathol* 22: 1298–302.

Nijdam JR, Luijten JA, Van Gijn J (1986). Cerebral haemorrhage associated with unilateral Moyamoya syndrome. *Clin Neurol Neurosurg* 88: 49–51.

Obrador S, Soto M, Silvela J (1975). Clinical syndromes of arteriovenous malformations of the transverse-sigmoid sinus. *J Neurol Neurosurg Psychiatr* 38: 436–51.

Ogilvy CS, Heros RC, Ojemann RG, New PF (1988). Angiographically occult arteriovenous malformations. *J Neurosurg* 69: 350–5.

Oikawa A, Aoki N, Sakai T (1993). Arteriovenous malformation presenting as acute subdural haematoma. *Neurol Res* 15: 353–5.

O'Leary PM, Sweeny PJ (1986). Ruptured intracerebral aneurysm resulting in a subdural hematoma. *Ann Emerg Med* 15: 944–6.

Ondra SL, Troupp H, George ED, Schwab K (1990). The natural history of symptomatic arteriovenous malformations of the brain: a 24-year follow-up assessment. *J Neurosurg* 73: 387–91.

Ooneda G, Yoshida Y, Suzuki K, Sekiguchi T (1973). Morphogenesis of plasmatic arterionecrosis as the cause of hypertensive intracerebral hemorrhage. *Virchows Arch A Pathol Anat* 361: 31–8.

Oppenheim JS, Gennuso R, Sacher M, Hollis P (1991). Acute atraumatic subdural hematoma associated with moyamoya disease in an African-American. *Neurosurgery* 28: 616–18.

Ott KH, Kase CS, Ojemann RG, Mohr JP (1974). Cerebellar hemorrhage: diagnosis and treatment. A review of 56 cases. *Arch Neurol* 31: 160–7.

Otten P, Pizzolato GP, Rilliet B, Berney J (1989). [131 cases of cavernous angioma (cavernomas) of the CNS, discovered by retrospective analysis of 24 535 autopsies] A propos de 131 cas d'angiomes caverneux (cavernomes) du s.n.c., répérés par l'analyse rétrospective de 24 535 autopsies. *Neurochirurgie* 35: 82–3, 128–31.

Parkinson D, Bachers G (1980). Arteriovenous malformations: summary of 100 consecutive supratentorial cases. *J Neurosurg* 53: 285–99.

Passero S, Burgalassi L, D'Andrea P, Battistini N (1995). Recurrence of bleeding in patients with primary intracerebral hemorrhage. *Stroke* 26: 1189–92.

Pendlebury WW, Iole ED, Tracy RP, Dill BA (1991). Intracerebral hemorrhage related to cerebral amyloid angiopathy and t-PA treatment. *Ann Neurol* 29: 210–13.

Pfleger MJ, Hardee EP, Contant CF Jr, Hayman LA (1994). Sensitivity and specificity of fluid-blood levels for coagulopathy in acute intracerebral hematomas. *An J Neuroradiol* 15: 217–23.

Pomeranz S, Naparstek E, Ashkenazi E *et al.* (1994). Intracranial haematomas following bone marrow transplantation. *J Neurol* 241: 252–6.

Rådberg JA, Olsson JE, Rådberg CT (1991). Prognostic parameters in spontaneous intracerebral hematomas with special reference to anticoagulant treatment. *Stroke* 22: 571–6.

Ragland RL, Gelber ND, Wilkinson HA, Knorr JR, Tran AA (1993). Anterior communicating artery aneurysm rupture: an unusual cause of acute subdural hemorrhage. *Surg Neurol* 40: 400–2.

Rapacki TF, Brantley MJ, Furlow TW Jr, Geyer CA, Toro VE, George ED (1990). Heterogeneity of cerebral cavernous hemangiomas diagnosed by MR imaging. *J Comput Assist Tomogr* 14: 18–25.

Ricci S, Celani MG, La Rosa F *et al.* (1991). SEPIVAC: a community-based study of stroke incidence in Umbria, Italy. *J Neurol Neurosurg Psychiatr* 54: 695–8.

Richards A, Graham D, Bullock R (1988). Clinicopathological study of neurological complications due to hypertensive disorders of pregnancy. *J Neurol Neurosurg Psychiatr* 51: 416–21.

Rigamonti D, Hadley MN, Drayer BP *et al.* (1988). Cerebral cavernous malformations: incidence and familial occurrence. *N Engl J Med* 319: 343–7.

Rigamonti D, Spetzler RF, Medina M, Rigamonti K, Geckle DS, Pappas C (1990). Cerebral venous malformations. *J Neurosurg* 73: 560–4.

Román G, Fisher M, Perl DP, Poser CM (1978). Neurological manifestations of hereditary hemorrhagic teleangiectasis

(Rendu–Osler–Weber disease): report of two cases and review of the literature. *Ann Neurol* 4: 130–44.

Ropper AH, Davis KR (1980). Lobar cerebral hemorrhages: acute clinical syndromes in 26 cases. *Ann Neurol* 8: 141–7.

Rose G (1992). *The Strategy of Preventive Medicine*. Oxford: Oxford Medical Publications.

Ross Russell RW (1963). Observations on intracerebral aneurysms. *Brain* 86: 425–42.

Rothschild MA, Maxeiner H (1990). [Spontaneous subdural hemorrhage of natural cause in metastatic renal cell carcinoma] Spontane Subduralblutung aus natürlicher Ursache bei metastasierendem Nierenzellcarcinom. *Beitr Gerichtl Med* 48: 223–7.

Salgado AV, Furlan AJ, Keys TF (1987). Mycotic aneurysm, subarachnoid hemorrhage, and indications for cerebral angiography in infective endocarditis. *Stroke* 18: 1057–60.

Sand JJ, Biller J, Corbett JJ, Adams HP Jr, Dunn V (1986). Partial dorsal mesencephalic hemorrhages: report of three cases. *Neurology* 36: 529–33.

Sarwar M, McCormick WF (1978). Intracerebral venous angioma: case report and review. *Arch Neurol* 35: 323–5.

Schutz H, Bodeker RH, Damian M, Krack P, Dorndorf W (1990). Age-related spontaneous intracerebral hematoma in a German community. *Stroke* 21: 1412–18.

Schütz J (1988). *Spontane intrazerebrale Hämatome— Pathophysiologie, Klinik und Therapie*. Berlin and Heidelberg: Springer.

Shih SL, Lin JC, Liang DC, Huang JK (1993). Computed tomography of spontaneous intracranial haemorrhage due to haemostatic disorders in children. *Neuroradiology* 35: 619–21.

Simard JM, Garcia Bengochea F, Ballinger WE Jr, Mickle JP, Quisling RG (1986). Cavernous angioma: a review of 126 collected and 12 new clinical cases. *Neurosurgery* 18: 162–72.

Simoons ML, Maggioni AP, Knatterud G *et al.* (1993). Individual risk assessment for intracranial haemorrhage during thrombolytic therapy. *Lancet* 342: 1523–8.

Sloan MA, Price TR, Petito CK *et al.* (1995). Clinical features and pathogenesis of intracerebral hemorrhage after rt-PA and heparin therapy for acute myocardial infarction: the Thrombolysis in Myocardial Infarction (TIMI) II pilot and randomized clinical trial combined experience. *Neurology* 45: 649–58.

Smith DB, Hitchcock M, Philpott PJ (1985). Cerebral amyloid angiopathy presenting as transient ischemic attacks: case report. *J Neurosurg* 63: 963–4.

Stein RW, Kase CS, Hier DB *et al.* (1984). Caudate hemorrhage. *Neurology* 34: 1549–54.

Stephenson G, Gibson RM (1989). Acute spontaneous subdural haematoma of arterial origin. *Br J Neurosurg* 3: 225–8.

Takebayashi S, Kaneko M (1983). Electron microscopic studies of ruptured arteries in hypertensive intracerebral hemorrhage. *Stroke* 14: 28–36.

Teilmann K (1953). Hemangiomas of the pons. *Arch Neurol Psychiatr* 69: 208–23.

Timothy J, Sofat A, Sharr M, Doshi B (1994). Unusual presentation of a germ cell neoplasm [letter]. *J Neurol Neurosurg Psychiatr*

57: 1278–9.

Toffol GJ, Biller J, Adams HP Jr, (1987). Nontraumatic intracerebral hemorrhage in young adults. *Arch Neurol* 44: 483–5.

Tomonaga M (1981). Cerebral amyloid angiopathy in the elderly. *J Am Geriatr Soc* 28: 151–7.

Torack RM (1975). Congophilic angiopathy complicated by surgery and massive hemorrhage: a light and electron microscopic study. *Am J Pathol* 81: 349–65.

Troost BT, Mark LE, Maroon JC (1979). Resolution of classic migraine after removal of an occipital lobe AVM. *Ann Neurol* 5: 199–201.

Tung H, Giannotta SL, Chandrasoma PT, Zee CS (1990). Recurrent intraparenchymal hemorrhages from angiographically occult vascular malformations. *J Neurosurg* 73: 174–80.

Uglietta JP, O'Connor CM, Boyko OB, Aldrich H, Massey EW, Heinz ER (1991). CT patterns of intracranial hemorrhage complicating thrombolytic therapy for acute myocardial infarction. *Radiology* 181: 555–9.

van den Doel EM, van Merrienboer FJ, Tulleken CA (1985). Cerebral hemorrhage from unsuspected choriocarcinoma. *Clin Neurol Neurosurg* 87: 287–90.

van Duinen SG, Castano EM, Prelli F, Bots GT, Luyendijk W, Frangione B (1987). Hereditary cerebral hemorrhage with amyloidosis in patients of Dutch origin is related to Alzheimer disease. *Proc Natl Acad Sci USA* 84: 5991–4.

Van Gijn J, van Dongen KJ (1980). Computed tomography in the diagnosis of subarachnoid haemorrhage and ruptured aneurysm. *Clin Neurol Neurosurg* 82: 11–24.

Van Gijn J, van Dongen KJ (1982). The time course of aneurysmal haemorrhage on computed tomograms. *Neuroradiology* 23: 153–6.

Van Gijn J, Stampfer MJ, Wolfe CDA, Algra A (1993). The association between alcohol and stroke. In: Verschuren PM, ed. *Health Issues Related to Alcohol Consumption*. Washington: ILSI Press, 43–79.

van Schayck R, Pantel J, Faiss J, Kloss T, Keidel M, Diener HD (1994). Hereditary cavernous angiomas of the brain in a German family. *Cerebrovasc Dis* 4: 226 (abstract).

van Swieten JC, van den Hout JH, van Ketel BA, Hijdra A, Wokke JHJ, Van Gijn J (1991). Periventricular lesions in the white matter on magnetic resonance imaging in the elderly: a morphometric correlation with arteriolosclerosis and dilated perivascular spaces. *Brain* 114: 761–74.

Vinters HV (1987). Cerebral amyloid angiopathy: a critical review. *Stroke* 18: 311–24.

Vinters HV, Gilbert JJ (1983). Cerebral amyloid angiopathy: incidence and complications in the aging brain. II. The distribution of amyloid vascular changes. *Stroke* 14: 924–8.

Vonsattel JP, Myers RH, Hedley Whyte ET, Ropper AH, Bird ED, Richardson EP Jr (1991). Cerebral amyloid angiopathy without and with cerebral hemorrhages: a comparative histological study. *Ann Neurol* 30: 637–49.

Vos PE, de Boer WA, Wurzer JA, Van Gijn J (1991). Subdural hematoma after lumbar puncture: two case reports and review of the literature. *Clin Neurol Neurosurg* 93: 127–32.

Waga S, Yamamoto Y (1983). Hypertensive putaminal hemorrhage: treatment and results. Is surgical treatment superior to a conservative one? *Stroke* 14: 480–5.

Waga S, Shimosaka S, Sakakura M (1983). Intracerebral hemorrhage remote from the site of the initial neurosurgical procedure. *Neurosurgery* 13: 662–5.

Waga S, Fujimoto K, Okada M, Miyazaki M, Tanaka, Y (1986). Caudate hemorrhage. *Neurosurgery* 18: 445–50.

Wakai S, Chen CH, Wu KY, Chiu CW (1983). Spontaneous regression of a cerebral arteriovenous malformation: report of a case and review of the literature. *Arch Neurol* 40: 377–80.

Wakai S, Kumakura N, Nagai M (1992). Lobar intracerebral hemorrhage: a clinical, radiographic, and pathological study of 29 consecutive operated cases with negative angiography. *J Neurosurg* 76: 231–8.

Wall M, George D (1987). Visual loss in pseudotumor cerebri—incidence and defects related to visual field strategy. *Arch Neurol* 44: 170–5.

Waltimo O (1973). The change in size of intracranial arteriovenous malformations. *J Neurol Sci* 19: 21–7.

Wattendorff AR, Frangione B, Luyendijk W, Bots GTAM (1995). Hereditary cerebral haemorrhage with amyloidosis, Dutch type (HCHWA-D): clinicopathological studies. *J Neurol Neurosurg Psychiatr* 58: 699–705.

Weisberg L (1981). Multiple spontaneous intracerebral hematomas: clinical and computed tomographic correlations. *Neurology* 31: 897–900.

Weisberg LA (1984). Caudate hemorrhage. *Arch Neurol* 41: 971–4.

Weisberg LA (1986a). Mesencephalic hemorrhages: clinical and computed tomographic correlations. *Neurology* 36: 713–16.

Weisberg LA (1986b). Primary pontine haemorrhage: clinical and computed tomographic correlations. *J Neurol Neurosurg Psychiatr* 49: 346–52.

Weisberg LA (1986c). Thalamic hemorrhage: clinical–CT correlations. *Neurology* 36: 1382–6.

Weisberg LA (1988). Alcoholic intracerebral hemorrhage. *Stroke* 19: 1565–9.

Weiskrantz L, Warrington EK, Sanders MD, Marshall J (1974). Visual capacity in the hemianopic field following a restricted occipital ablation. *Brain* 97: 709–28.

Wharen RE, Scheithauer BW, Laws ER (1982). Thrombosed arteriovenous malformations of the brain: an important entity in the differential diagnosis of intractable focal seizure disorders. *J Neurosurg* 57: 520–6.

Wijdicks EFM, Jack CR Jr (1993). Intracerebral hemorrhage after fibrinolytic therapy for acute myocardial infarction. *Stroke* 24: 554–7.

Wijdicks EFM, De Groen PC, Wiesner RH, Krom RAF (1995). Intracerebral hemorrhage in liver transplant recipients. *Mayo Clin Proc* 70: 443–6.

Wijdicks EFM, Silbert PL, Jack CR, Parisi JE (1994). Subcortical hemorrhage in disseminated intravascular coagulation associated with sepsis. *Am J Neuroradiol* 15: 763–5.

Williams JP, Joslyn JN, White JL, Dean DF (1983). Subdural hematoma secondary to ruptured intracranial aneurysm: computed tomographic diagnosis. *J Comput Tomogr* 7: 142–53.

Willinsky RA, Lasjaunias P, Terbrugge K, Burrows P (1990). Multiple cerebral arteriovenous malformations (AVMs): review of our experience from 203 patients with cerebral vascular lesions. *Neuroradiology* 32: 207–10.

Willinsky RA, Fitzgerald M, Terbrugge K, Montanera W, Wallace M (1993). Delayed angiography in the investigation of intracerebral hematomas caused by small arteriovenous malformations. *Neuroradiology* 35: 307–11.

Willinsky RA, Terbrugge K, Montanera W, Mikulis D, Wallace MC (1994). Venous congestion: an MR finding in dural arteriovenous malformations with cortical venous drainage. *Am J Neuroradiol* 15: 1501–7.

Wintzen AR (1980). The clinical course of subdural haematoma: a retrospective study of aetiological, chronological, and pathological features in 212 patients and a proposed classification. *Brain* 103: 855–67.

Wintzen AR, Tijssen JG (1982). Subdural hematoma and oral anticoagulant therapy. *Arch Neurol* 39: 69–72.

Wintzen AR, de Jonge H, Loeliger EA, Bots GT (1984). The risk of intracerebral hemorrhage during oral anticoagulant treatment: a population study. *Ann Neurol* 16: 553–8.

Wulff HR (1995). *Rational Diagnosis and Treatment—an Introduction to Clinical Decision-making*, 2nd edn. Oxford: Blackwell Science.

Yamada M, Itoh Y, Otomo E, Hayakawa M, Miyatake T (1993). Subarachnoid haemorrhage in the elderly: a necropsy study of the association with cerebral amyloid angiopathy. *J Neurol Neurosurg Psychiatr* 56: 543–7.

Yamashita M, Tanaka K, Matsuo T, Yokoyama K, Fujii T, Sakamoto H (1983). Cerebral dissecting aneurysms in patients with moyamoya disease: report of two cases. *J Neurosurg* 58: 120–5.

Yasui T, Komiyama M, Kishi H et al. (1995). Angiographic extravasation of contrast medium in acute 'spontaneous' subdural hematoma. *Surg Neurol* 43: 61–7.

Yokoyama K, Asano Y, Murakawa T et al. (1991). Familial occurrence of arteriovenous malformation of the brain. *J Neurosurg* 74: 585–9.

Yong WH, Robert ME, Secor DL, Kleikamp TJ, Vinters HV (1992). Cerebral hemorrhage with biopsy-proved amyloid angiopathy. *Arch Neurol* 49: 51–8.

Zimmerman RS, Spetzler RF, Lee KS, Zabramski JM, Hargraves RW (1991). Cavernous malformations of the brain stem. *J Neurosurg* 75: 32–9.

What caused this subarachnoid haemorrhage?

9

9.1   Causes of subarachnoid haemorrhage (SAH)

Approximately 85% of all spontaneous haemorrhages into the subarachnoid space arise from rupture of saccular aneurysms at the base of the brain. This is a serious disorder, not only as a result of the initial haemorrhage, but also because of the potential complications (see Chapter 13). In unselected hospital series, the case fatality after 3 months is about 50% (Hijdra *et al.*, 1987). Specialised neurosurgical centres tend to publish more optimistic figures, because few patients in poor condition ever reach them (Fig. 9.1) (Whisnant *et al.*, 1993). Ten per cent of all SAHs are in patients with non-aneurysmal, perimesencephalic haemorrhage. This is an entirely benign but somewhat mysterious condition: the centre of the haemorrhage is somewhere around the midbrain, usually ventral to it, the angiogram is normal and the patients recover and, without exception, go

on to live a normal life. It is precisely for this reason that the pathology is so far unknown, but, for reasons explained below, the source of bleeding is not likely to be arterial and is probably a ruptured vein, perhaps a varicose vein. A small fraction of SAHs are due to arterial dissections or a variety of rare conditions, listed in Table 9.1. In the next sections, we shall separately discuss aneurysms, perimesencephalic haemorrhages, arterial dissections and the rare causes.

> *About 85% of all spontaneous subarachnoid haemorrhages are due to the rupture of an intracranial saccular aneurysm, 10% to non-aneurysmal perimesencephalic haemorrhage and 5% to rarities.*

The presenting features of all these different causes are often indistinguishable: a severe headache of sudden onset, which may be accompanied by focal deficits, a depressed level of consciousness or both (see Section 5.5). The only exception is perimesencephalic non-aneurysmal haemor-

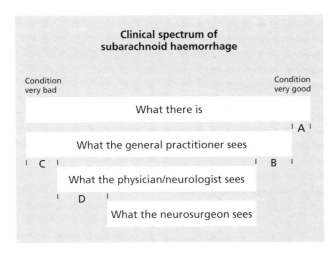

Clinical spectrum of subarachnoid haemorrhage

Condition very bad | | Condition very good

What there is

What the general practitioner sees | A

C | What the physician/neurologist sees | B

D | What the neurosurgeon sees

Figure 9.1 Referral bias in SAH. Patients can fail to reach specialised centres because: (A) they do not consult their general practitioner; (B) the diagnosis is missed; (C) they die before reaching hospital; (D) it is assumed that no treatment is possible. (From van Gijn, 1992; courtesy of the *Lancet*.)

Table 9.1 Specific causes of spontaneous SAH.

Saccular aneurysms (85%) (see Section 9.1.1)
Non-aneurysmal perimesencephalic haemorrhage (10%) (see Section 9.1.2)
Arterial dissection (see Section 9.1.3)
Rare conditions
  Cerebral arteriovenous malformation (see Section 8.2.2)
  Dural arteriovenous fistula (see Section 8.2.7)
  Spinal arteriovenous malformation (see Section 9.1.4)
  Saccular aneurysm of a spinal artery (see Section 9.1.4)
  Head trauma (see Section 9.1.4)
  Mycotic aneurysms (see Section 9.1.4)
  Metastasis of cardiac myxoma (see Section 9.1.4)
  Cocaine abuse (see Section 8.5.4)
  Sickle cell disease (see Section 9.1.4)
  Coagulation disorders (see Section 9.1.4)
  Pituitary apoplexy (see Section 9.1.4)
  Spinal meningioma (see Section 9.1.4)
  Rupture of circumferential artery of the brainstem (see Section 9.1.4)

rhage, where explosive headache is invariably the only symptom at onset. In the following sections about the pathological and pathophysiological background of all these causes, we shall occasionally run ahead of the story by mentioning the findings on computerised tomography (CT) scanning, as this technique, now readily available in many centres as an early adjunct to the history and examination, provides an *in vivo* picture of the pathology.

9.1.1 Saccular aneurysms

Although some textbooks for medical students still refer to aneurysms of the cerebral vessels as being 'congenital', this is wrong: they develop during the course of life. Aneurysms are almost never found in neonates and they are also rare in children (Riggs & Rupp, 1943; Housepian & Pool, 1958; Stehbens, 1963). Moreover, in those exceptional childhood aneurysms there is usually an underlying condition, such as trauma, infection or connective-tissue disorder (Table 9.2; Ferry *et al.*, 1974; Stehbens, 1982). The aneurysms arise at sites of arterial branching, usually at the base of the brain, either on the circle of Willis itself or at a nearby branching site (Fig. 9.2; Table 9.3). According to autopsy studies, the proportion of patients with aneurysms increases with age, but the absolute frequencies to some degree depend on whether fatal cases of SAH have been included and also on the diligence with which the search for unruptured aneurysms has been performed (McCormick, 1971). On the basis of autopsy series, estimates of the overall frequency of unruptured aneurysms in adults were as low as 0.3% in a review of eight routine series before 1970 (Bannerman *et al.*, 1970), but as high as 3%, 8% and 9% in three studies specifically dedicated to the question of aneurysms (Chason & Hindman, 1958; Stehbens, 1963; McCormick & Nofzinger, 1965). In angiography series, the obvious confounding factor is the underlying disease which prompted the investigation, such as ischaemic stroke or intracerebral haemorrhage,

Table 9.2 Conditions associated with saccular aneurysms.

Disorders of connective tissue
Marfan's syndrome (Finney *et al.*, 1976)
Ehlers—Danlos syndrome type IV (Schievink *et al.*, 1990)
Pseudoxanthoma elasticum (Munyer & Margulis, 1981)
Alpha$_1$-antitrypsin deficiency (Schievink *et al.*, 1994a)
Neurofibromatosis (Muhonen *et al.*, 1991)

Disorders of angiogenesis
Hereditary haemorrhagic telangiectasia (Román *et al.*, 1978)

Associated hypertension
Coarctation of the aorta (Wright, 1949; Robinson, 1967)
Polycystic kidney disease* (Chapman *et al.*, 1992)

Haemodynamic stress
Anomalies of the circle of Willis (Kayembe *et al.*, 1984)
Arteriovenous malformations (Okamoto *et al.*, 1984; Brown *et al.*, 1990)
Moyamoya syndrome (Nagamine *et al.*, 1981)

* In polycystic kidney disease, not only hypertension but also developmental factors contribute to the formation of intracranial aneurysms.

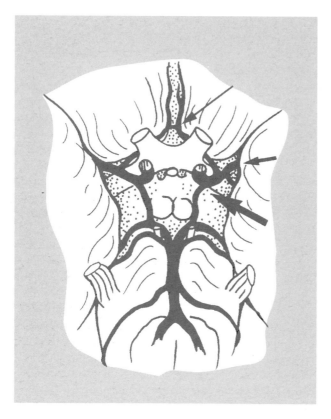

Figure 9.2 Schematic drawing of the circle of Willis in the suprasellar cistern at the base of the brain; the medial parts of the temporal lobes have been slightly retracted, to allow a better view. The anterior communicating artery is at the top of the drawing (long thin arrow), the origin of the posterior communicating artery from the carotid artery is at the lateral border of the suprasellar cistern (thick arrow) and the terminal bifurcation of the basilar artery is found in the most dorsal part of the suprasellar cisterns (bottom part of dotted area), in the interpeduncular fossa. The middle cerebral artery courses laterally, in the horizontal part of the Sylvian fissure (short arrow); aneurysms of this artery are found at the lateral end of the fissure (not visible), where it meets at right angles with the lateral part of the Sylvian fissure and where the artery trifurcates. (From Vermeulen *et al.*, 1992; courtesy of WB Saunders.)

which share hypertension as a risk factor with aneurysmal SAH (Sacco *et al.*, 1984; Knekt *et al.*, 1991). On the other hand, aneurysms may be missed on angiograms done for other purposes. With these qualifications, the proportion of incidental aneurysms in a recently published series of 1612 angiograms performed for other conditions was 2.7% for all patients, 3.7% for 974 patients aged 40 years or over and 6.2% for 273 patients aged 60 years or over (Ujiie *et al.*, 1993). A remarkable study in Japan reported the results of vascular imaging in 361 subjects without a family history of SAH, aged 39–71 years, who volunteered to undergo

catheter angiography or, in relatively few cases, magnetic resonance angiography (MRA) (Nakagawa & Hashi, 1994). Nineteen of them had aneurysms (5%), against an even greater proportion (seven of 39 or 18%) in subjects with affected relatives.

The rate at which aneurysms increase in size is often assumed to be gradual, but rapid expansion has been documented and may contribute to the risk of rupture (Barth & De Tribolet, 1994).

The notion of 'weak spots'

It is largely unknown why only some adults develop aneurysms at arterial bifurcations and most do not, except in specific but rare underlying conditions (see Table 9.2). The once popular notion of a congenital defect in the muscle layer of the wall (tunica media) being a weak spot through which the inner layers of the arterial wall would bulge has been largely dispelled by a number of contradictory observations. First, gaps in the muscle layer of intracerebral arteries are equally common in patients with and without aneurysms

Table 9.3 Site of ruptured aneurysms, in 326 consecutive patients. (From Vermeulen *et al.*, 1984.)*

Site of aneurysm	Number	Per cent
Anterior communicating artery complex†	134	41
Internal carotid artery‡	101	31
Middle cerebral artery§	60	18
Posterior circulation¶	31	10

* Half the patients were admitted to a general neurology unit and half to a department of neurosurgery; of the 326 aneurysms, 285 were identified on angiography and 41 at autopsy. In other studies, the distribution is very similar.
† Most aneurysms of the anterior cerebral artery are of the anterior communicating artery, rarely at other sites, such as the pericallosal artery.
‡ Most aneurysms of the internal carotid artery are at the origin of the posterior communicating artery, more rarely at other sites, such as the origin of the ophthalmic artery or the terminal bifurcation of the internal carotid artery into the middle and anterior cerebral arteries.
§ Aneurysms of the middle cerebral artery arise in 90% of cases from the point where the main stem of the artery divides into its main branches, although there is individual variation in whether this point is near to the temporal bone or more medially; in the remaining 10%, the aneurysm arises at the proximal segment of the middle cerebral artery, at the origin of lenticulostriate, fronto-orbital or early temporal branches (Hosoda *et al.*, 1995).
¶ Most aneurysms of the posterior circulation are at the tip of the basilar artery, less often they are at the origin of the posterior inferior cerebellar artery or at the junction between the posterior cerebral artery and the posterior communicating artery.

(Stehbens, 1989). Second, in experimental situations, the internal elastic lamina at the site of such gaps can withstand very high intraluminal pressure without breaking up or bulging out (Glynn, 1940). Finally, if an aneurysm has formed, any defect in the muscle layer is located not at the neck of the aneurysm but somewhere in the wall of the aneurysmal sac (Stehbens, 1989). Some investigators have postulated that the earliest change leading to the formation of aneurysms consists of local thickening of the intimal layer ('intimal pads'), which tend to develop distal and proximal to a branching site, perhaps as a result of haemodynamic strain (Walker & Allegre, 1954; Hassler, 1962). In younger people these pads consist mainly of smooth-muscle cells; in older people they are more fibrous (Hassler, 1962). It has been suggested that the formation of these pads, in which the intimal layer is inelastic, leads to increased strain in the more elastic portions of the vessel wall (Crompton, 1966). Occasionally, the aneurysm is found to consist of abnormally developed structures, such as primitive, myxoid connective tissue over the full thickness of the arterial wall (O'Boynick et al., 1994).

Despite aneurysms not being congenital in the strict sense, there is some degree of genetic predisposition for their formation, apart from the random factors of haemodynamics, and, in addition, some specific risk factors can be identified. It is well known that there are families in which three or more first- or second-degree relatives have had an SAH, and at a younger median age than the early 50s, which is the most common age at which sporadic aneurysms rupture (ter Berg et al., 1992; Alberts et al., 1995). Patients with a positive family history are younger and are more likely to have multiple aneurysms or aneurysms on the middle cerebral artery than patients with aneurysms and a negative family history (Norrgard et al., 1987; Ronkainen et al., 1995a). But, such families with at least three affected members form only a minute fraction of all SAHs, even though there must be many more than the published number of 50 families (Schievink et al., 1994c). Recently, a systematic search for fatal and non-fatal episodes of SAH amongst first-degree relatives of 163 so-called 'sporadic' cases with ruptured aneurysms showed a rate that was three to seven times higher than in second-degree relatives (Bromberg et al., 1995a). This increased risk for first-degree relatives was not statistically significant in another study of 149 incident cases with SAH and 298 external controls matched for age and sex (Wang et al., 1995), but in that study the criteria for the diagnosis of SAH through an interview were unspecified, medical records were not obtained for verification and the fate of almost 10% of first-degree relatives was unknown. In patients with at least one affected first-degree relative, the average outcome is worse than in truly isolated cases, a finding confirmed by a system-

atic review of patients with familial SAH reported in previous studies (Bromberg et al., 1995b).

> *In first-degree relatives of patients with subarachnoid haemorrhage the risk of subarachnoid haemorrhage is three to seven times higher than in second-degree relatives or in the general population.*

Risk factors

Some classical risk factors for stroke in general also apply to SAH. Hypertension and smoking have been identified as risk factors in prospectively studied cohorts of the population (Sacco et al., 1984; Shinton & Beevers, 1989; Knekt et al., 1991) and in a case–control study (Adamson et al., 1994). With regard to alcohol, prospective studies provide strong evidence to support the view that higher levels of alcohol intake are associated with an increased risk, at least of haemorrhagic stroke in general (van Gijn et al., 1993). For SAH alone, the numbers are small and the confidence intervals are therefore wide, but the findings are remarkably similar (Donahue et al., 1986; Stampfer et al., 1988). In contrast, studies differ about whether pregnancy is associated with an increased risk of aneurysmal SAH, with conclusions ranging from a fivefold increase in risk to no increase in risk at all (Fox et al., 1990; Simolke et al., 1991). A systematic overview of the studies reporting risk factors for SAH included eight longitudinal and 10 case–control studies that fulfilled predefined methodological criteria, such as the diagnosis of SAH being confirmed by CT, angiography or autopsy in at least 70% of patients (Teunissen et al., 1996). On aggregate, only smoking, hypertension and heavy drinking emerged as significant risk factors, with odds ratios in the order of 2 or 3. The risk was not significantly increased with the use of oral contraceptives, hormone replacement therapy or an increased level of plasma cholesterol. Seasonal variation does not seem to occur (Schievink et al., 1995a).

9.1.2 Non-aneurysmal perimesencephalic haemorrhage

In this radiologically distinct and strikingly harmless variety of SAH, the extravasated blood is confined to the cisterns around the midbrain, and the centre of the bleeding is immediately anterior to the midbrain or, in some cases, the only evidence of blood is found anterior to the pons (van Gijn et al., 1985b; Rinkel et al., 1991c). Here it is necessary to anticipate in some detail the radiological investigations discussed in Section 9.4.1 below, because in the acute phase this disease entity is defined only by the characteristic distribution of the extravasated blood on brain CT; in addition, the four-vessel angiogram should be normal, but this helps only to exclude other causes and not to identify the source, which is still unknown. There is no extension of the haemorrhage to the lateral Sylvian fissures or to the anterior part of the interhemispheric fissure. Some sedimentation of blood in the posterior horns of the lateral ventricles may occur, but frank intraventricular haemorrhage or extension of the haemorrhage into the brain parenchyma rules out this particular condition (Rinkel *et al.*, 1991c).

Perimesencephalic haemorrhage constitutes approximately 10% of all episodes of SAH and two-thirds of those with a normal angiogram (Rinkel *et al.*, 1991c; Farrés *et al.*, 1992; Ferbert *et al.*, 1992; Kitahara *et al.*, 1993; Pinto *et al.*, 1993). It can occur in any patient over the age of 20 years, but most patients are in their sixth decade, as with aneurysmal haemorrhage. A history of hypertension is not obtained more often than expected, and there is no history of 'sentinel headaches' (Rinkel *et al.*, 1991b). In one-third of the patients, strenuous activities immediately precede the onset of symptoms (Rinkel *et al.*, 1991b), a proportion similar to that found in aneurysmal haemorrhage (van Gijn *et al.*, 1985b).

> *There is a distinct and benign variety of subarachnoid haemorrhage, in which the distribution of extravasated blood on the brain CT scan is different from that with aneurysms, in the cisterns around the midbrain or ventral to the pons; the angiogram is completely normal; the long-term outcome is invariably excellent. This condition of perimesencephalic non-aneurysmal subarachnoid haemorrhage constitutes 10% of all subarachnoid haemorrhages and two-thirds of subarachnoid haemorrhages with a normal angiogram.*

The clinical features at onset may be milder than those in patients with aneurysmal rupture: the onset of the headache is gradual (minutes rather than seconds in 25% of the patients), loss of consciousness is exceptional and focal neurological abnormalities have not been observed so far. On admission, all patients are in fact in perfect clinical condition, apart from their headache (van Gijn *et al.*, 1985b; Rinkel *et al.*, 1991b). Typically, the early course is uneventful: rebleeds and delayed cerebral ischaemia simply do not occur. Although 20% of patients have acute hydrocephalus on their admission brain CT scan, only a few have symptoms from it, and even then an excellent outcome can be anticipated (Rinkel *et al.*, 1990a). The period of convalescence is short, and almost invariably patients are able to resume their previous work and other activities (Rinkel *et al.*, 1990b). Rebleeds after the hospital period have not been documented thus far, in a large series of 77 patients followed for an average of 4 years (Rinkel *et al.*, 1991a). This has

subsequently been confirmed by a study from Portugal, in which 36 patients were followed for 2 years (Canhao *et al.*, 1995).

For the time being, the definition of this mild variant of SAH remains a purely descriptive one, because postmortem studies have not been obtained and because there is no single test which allows separation from related conditions. Yet, the milder clinical features, the limited extension of the extravasated blood on brain CT and the normal angiograms in a large series of patients with this pattern of haemorrhage are all evidence against an aneurysm or in fact any arterial source of bleeding. Instead, rupture of a vein or a venous malformation in the prepontine or interpeduncular cistern seems a reasonable hypothesis. In two patients (one with a perimesencephalic pattern of haemorrhage), lacunar infarction developed in the vicinity of the haemorrhage and led to the conjecture that a small perforating artery had occluded and subsequently ruptured, but if this occurs at all it must surely be uncommon (Tatter *et al.*, 1995).

9.1.3 Arterial dissection (see also Section 7.1)

Dissection in general tends to be recognised more often in the carotid than in the vertebral artery, but SAH from a dissected artery is almost always found in the vertebral artery (Kaplan *et al.*, 1993; Rinkel *et al.*, 1993). Blunt rotational or hyperextension trauma, even if slight, is a common cause of vertebral artery dissection, particularly in the young; iatrogenic causes include not only osteopathic manipulation but also surgery for glioma (Nohjoh *et al.*, 1995). In middle-aged patients, dissection may occur more or less spontaneously (see Section 7.1). It is unknown what precise proportion of all SAHs arise from a dissected vertebral artery, but, after aneurysmal haemorrhages (85%) and perimesencephalic haemorrhages (10%), all other causes together account for only about 5%. In an autopsy study of fatal SAH, dissection was found in five of 110 patients (Sasaki *et al.*, 1991b). With vertebral artery dissection in general, the injury to the vessel occurs most often in its extracranial course; in about one in eight the intradural portion only is affected, and in a similar proportion the extracranial and intradural segment of the artery are both affected (Mokri *et al.*, 1988). If SAH occurs with a dissection starting in the extracranial portion, the plane of cleavage is subadventitial rather than subintimal, and extension into the intradural portion may result in rupture only there and not more proximally, because the outer wall of the artery is no longer protected by an external elastic lamina, whilst the muscle layer and the adventitial layer are thinner than in the extradural portion (Caplan *et al.*, 1988). It has been suggested that an extracranial pseudoaneurysm of the vertebral artery alone may give rise

Table 9.4 Clinical signs of vertebral artery dissection, as cause of SAH.

In a patient with SAH, suspect vertebral artery dissection if
1 Headache starts low in the neck and then moves up to the head (although this may also occur with ruptured aneurysms)
2 Palsies of the IXth or Xth cranial nerves occur (compression through subadventitial dissection)
3 Symptoms and signs occur that are attributable to dysfunction in the territory of supply of the posterior inferior cerebellar artery:

Lower part of cerebellar hemisphere
Vertigo
Inability to stand, or even sit
Dysarthria
VIIth nerve palsy (through secondary compression of pons)
Dysmetria (often absent)

Dorsolateral medulla oblongata
Horner's syndrome, ipsilateral
Rotatory nystagmus
Numbness of the face, ipsilateral
Numbness of the arm, trunk and leg, contralateral
Dysmetria, ipsilateral
Dysphagia
Hiccups

---

to SAH, but in that case one would have to assume that repeated haemorrhages lead to adhesions between the outer wall of the artery and the dural sleeve of a cervical root (Kaplan *et al.*, 1993). Sometimes dissection of the vertebral artery is associated with fenestration at the vertebrobasilar junction (Zhang *et al.*, 1994). Dissection with SAH may also affect the posterior inferior cerebellar artery (Fransen & De Tribolet, 1994).

Neurological deficits that may accompany SAH from vertebral artery dissection (Table 9.4) are palsies of the IXth and Xth cranial nerves, by subadventitial dissection (Senter & Sarwar, 1982), or of Wallenberg's syndrome, partial or complete, indicating subintimal dissection with impairment of blood flow in the territory of the posterior inferior cerebellar artery, resulting in ischaemia of the dorsolateral medulla (Caplan *et al.*, 1988). Rebleeds are common (30–70% in different series), after an interval of as short as a few hours or as long as a few weeks; recurrent events are fatal in approximately 50% of the patients (Caplan *et al.*, 1988; Aoki & Sakai, 1990; Yamaura *et al.*, 1990; Mizutani *et al.*, 1995).

Dissection of the intracranial portion of the internal carotid artery or one of its branches as a cause of SAH is extremely uncommon, much less common than dissection of the internal carotid artery in the neck, a condition encountered several times a year in most major neurology services (see Section 7.1). Reported cases have affected the terminal

portion of the internal carotid artery (Adams *et al.*, 1982; Massoud *et al.*, 1992), the middle cerebral artery (Kunze & Schiefer, 1971; Sasaki *et al.*, 1991a; Piepgras *et al.*, 1994) and the anterior cerebral artery (see Fig. 9.27; Guridi *et al.*, 1993).

9.1.4 Rare conditions causing subarachnoid haemorrhage (SAH)

Cerebral arteriovenous malformations (AVMs)

Cerebral AVMs were formerly believed to cause a substantial proportion of SAHs, but since the advent of CT it has become clear that haemorrhages from AVMs almost invariably involve the brain parenchyma (see Section 8.2.2). Subarachnoid bleeding at the convexity of the brain may occur from superficial AVMs, but only in less than 5% of all ruptured AVMs is there no intracerebral haematoma (Aoki, 1991). Exclusively intraventricular haemorrhage (see Section 9.1.5) may be associated with an AVM immediately under the ependymal surface (Darby *et al.*, 1988). A microangioma is conveniently and perhaps rightly implicated if angiography and magnetic resonance imaging (MRI) fail to show such an abnormality in cases of primary intraventricular haemorrhage. Saccular aneurysms form on feeding arteries of 10–20% of AVMs, presumably because of the greatly increased flow and the attendant strain on the arterial wall. If bleeding occurs in these cases, it is more often from the aneurysm than from the malformation, but the site of the aneurysms is different from the classical sites of saccular aneurysms on the circle of Willis, and again the haemorrhage is into the brain itself rather than into the subarachnoid space (Brown *et al.*, 1990; Marks *et al.*, 1992).

> *Very few arteriovenous malformations rupture only into the subarachnoid space. The vast majority form an intracerebral haematoma, with or without extension into the subarachnoid space.*

Dural arteriovenous malformations

Dural AVMs of the tentorium can give rise to a basal haemorrhage that is indistinguishable on CT from aneurysmal haemorrhage (see Section 8.2.7; Lasjaunias *et al.*, 1986). The anomaly is rare and can be found from adolescence to old age. Rebleeding may occur in patients with dural AVMs; in a series of five patients presenting with SAH, three had one or more rebleeds (Halbach *et al.*, 1987).

Spinal arteriovenous malformations

Spinal AVMs present with SAH in approximately 10%; in more than 50% of these patients, the first haemorrhage occurs before the age of 20 years (Kandel, 1980; Caroscio *et al.*, 1980). Symptoms may start with a sudden and excruciating pain in the lower part of the neck. Pain radiating from the neck to the shoulders or arms points to a cervical origin of the haemorrhage (Acciarri *et al.*, 1992). If such clues are absent, the true origin of the haemorrhage emerges only when spinal cord dysfunction develops, after a delay which may be as short as a few hours or as long as a few years (Kandel, 1980; Swann *et al.*, 1984). Rebleeds may occur, even repeatedly (Aminoff & Logue, 1974). Not only intradural malformations but also dural fistulas in the spinal axis may cause SAH (Willinsky *et al.*, 1990).

Saccular aneurysms of spinal arteries

Saccular aneurysms of spinal arteries are extremely rare, with approximately 12 patients on record (Handa *et al.*, 1992; Mohsenipour *et al.*, 1994). As with AVMs of the spinal cord, the clinical features of spinal SAH may be accompanied by those of a transverse lesion of the cord, partial or complete.

Trauma

Trauma and spontaneous SAH are sometimes difficult to disentangle. Patients may be found alone after having been beaten up in a brawl or hit by a drunken driver who made away, without external wounds to indicate an accident, with a decreased level of consciousness making it impossible to obtain a history and with neck stiffness causing the patient to be worked up for SAH. Conversely, patients who rupture an aneurysm whilst riding a bicycle or driving a car may cause an accident and even sustain a skull fracture, to make things really difficult, leading them to end up in hospital with a diagnosis of head injury (Sakas *et al.*, 1995). Meticulous reconstruction of traffic accidents may therefore be rewarding, especially in patients with disproportionate headache or neck stiffness.

> *Spontaneous subarachnoid haemorrhage may lead to head trauma, whilst head injury may cause superficial contusion with accumulation of blood in the subarachnoid space. If there is any doubt, it is vital to disentangle the course of events as accurately as possible.*

Fortunately, brain CT may help. If trauma is the cause of SAH, the blood is usually located in the superficial sulci at the convexity of the brain, adjacent to a fracture or to an

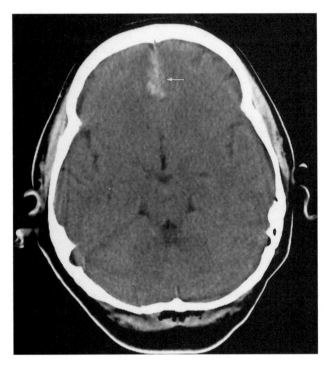

Figure 9.3 CT scan showing extravasated blood in the frontal interhemispheric fissure (arrow), as a result of trauma (34-year-old woman who had fallen from her horse).

intracerebral contusion, which findings dispel any lingering concern about the possibility of a ruptured aneurysm. In patients with basal–frontal contusions, however, the pattern of haemorrhage can resemble that of a ruptured anterior communicating artery aneurysm, and in patients with blood confined to the Sylvian fissure it may also be difficult to distinguish trauma from aneurysmal rupture by the pattern of haemorrhage alone (Fig. 9.3). In patients with direct trauma to the neck or with head injury associated with vigorous neck movement, the trauma can immediately be followed by massive basal haemorrhage resulting from a tear or even a complete rupture of one of the arteries of the posterior circulation, which is often rapidly fatal (Harland *et al.*, 1983; Dowling & Curry, 1988).

Mycotic aneurysms

Mycotic aneurysms as a cause of SAH are most frequently caused by infective endocarditis (see Section 6.4) or aspergillosis, but most strokes in the context of infective endocarditis are (haemorrhagic) infarcts or intracerebral haemorrhages from pyogenic arteritis (Hart *et al.*, 1990; Masuda *et al.*, 1992). Aneurysms associated with infective endocarditis are most often located on distal branches of the middle cerebral artery, but approximately 10% of the aneurysms develop at more proximal sites (see Fig. 6.10; Brust *et al.*, 1990). Therefore, rupture of a mycotic aneurysm causes an intracerebral haematoma in most patients, but some have a basal pattern of haemorrhage on CT that is very similar to that of a ruptured saccular aneurysm. CT-documented rebleeds have been reported (Steinberg *et al.*, 1992). Usually patients present with clinical features of infected heart valves before SAH occurs, but on rare occasions rupture of a mycotic aneurysm is the initial manifestation of infective endocarditis (Vincent *et al.*, 1980; Salgado *et al.*, 1987). Mycotic aneurysms may resolve after adequate antibiotic therapy (Brust *et al.*, 1990), but one patient is on record with late rupture after appropriate treatment (Bamford *et al.*, 1986). Mycotic aneurysms in patients with aspergillosis are usually located on the proximal part of the basilar or carotid artery (Lau *et al.*, 1991). Rupture of such an aneurysm causes a massive SAH in the basal cisterns, indistinguishable from that of a saccular aneurysm (Anonymous, 1988). Aspergillosis is difficult to diagnose but should particularly be suspected in patients undergoing long-term treatment with antibiotics or immunosuppressive agents. Most patients with haematogenous dissemination have pulmonary lesions, but X-ray films of the chest may be normal early in the course (Young *et al.*, 1970; Anonymous, 1988). Rupture of a mycotic aneurysm in patients with aspergillosis may be fatal (Lau *et al.*, 1991).

Cardiac myxoma

Cardiac myxoma is an extremely rare cause of aneurysm formation; the tumour may metastasise to an intracranial artery, infiltrate the wall and thus cause an aneurysm to develop, even more than 1 year after operation of the primary tumour (see Section 6.4; Furuya *et al.*, 1995).

Cocaine abuse

Cocaine abuse is associated with haemorrhagic as well as with ischaemic stroke (see Section 6.5.6). In patients with SAH related to the use of the alkaloid form of cocaine, 50% have no aneurysm on the angiogram (Levine *et al.*, 1990). The pattern of haemorrhage on brain CT may be comparable to that of a ruptured saccular aneurysm (Wojak & Flamm, 1987), and the diagnosis rests on a confirmatory history or on the results of toxicological tests. Rebleeds do occur, even in patients with a normal angiogram, and the outcome is often poor (Mangiardi *et al.*, 1988). The source of the haemorrhage in patients without an aneurysm is unknown. Although biopsy-proven vasculitis has been found (Krendel *et al.*, 1990), changes suggestive of vasculitis often fail to show up on angiograms, admittedly a very insensitive test (Mangiardi *et al.*, 1988; Levine *et al.*, 1990). Ingestion of *ephedrine* may also precipitate aneurysmal SAH (Bruno *et al.*, 1993).

Sickle cell disease

Sickle cell disease is commonly complicated by ischaemic stroke (see Section 7.6) and seldom by SAH (Overby & Rothman, 1985). Thirty per cent of patients with sickle cell disease and SAH are children (Carey *et al.*, 1990). CT scans in these children show blood in the superficial cortical sulci; angiograms reveal no aneurysm but often show multiple distal branch occlusions and a leptomeningeal collateral circulation. The SAH is attributed to rupture of these collaterals (Carey *et al.*, 1990). The outcome is poor: only three of 11 recently reviewed children recovered in a good functional state (Carey *et al.*, 1990). Most adult patients in whom sickle cell disease underlies SAH have a ruptured aneurysm at the base of the brain. The haemorrhage is located diffusely in the basal cisterns and the sickle cell disease may well be coincidental in these patients, but the management may include partial exchange transfusions (Love *et al.*, 1985).

Anticoagulation-related subarachnoid haemorrhage

Anticoagulation-related SAH seems rare. In a series of 116 patients on anticoagulant treatment and with intracranial extracerebral haemorrhage, seven had only SAH. In two of these seven patients the haemorrhage was associated with trauma, and in two other patients an aneurysm was found on angiography (Mattle *et al.*, 1989). Thus, in only about 3% of these patients was there no cause for the haemorrhage other than anticoagulation. Severe coagulopathy, other than by anticoagulant drugs, is also a rare cause of haemorrhage confined to the subarachnoid space, for example congenital deficiency of factor VII (Papa *et al.*, 1994). In a series of 13 patients with intracranial haemorrhage after liver transplantation, only three had an SAH on CT (Estol *et al.*, 1991). In all patients but one in this series, the intracranial haemorrhage was associated with systemic bleeding.

Pituitary apoplexy

Pituitary apoplexy has been proposed as one of the causes of SAH of unknown cause (Bjerre *et al.*, 1986). The precipitating event of arterial haemorrhage occurring in a pituitary tumour is thought to be tissue necrosis, involving one of the hypophyseal arteries. The initial features are a sudden and severe headache followed by nausea, vomiting, neck stiffness and sometimes a depressed level of consciousness (Reid *et al.*, 1985). The hallmark of pituitary apoplexy is that most patients suffer a sudden decrease in visual acuity: in one series of 15 patients, only two had normal visual acuity. The combination of sudden, severe headache and decreased vision (literally a 'blinding' headache) may also occur in patients in whom rupture of an aneurysm is complicated by subhyaloid haemorrhages, but in most patients with pituitary apoplexy eye movements are disturbed as well, because the haemorrhage compresses the oculomotor, trochlear and abducens nerves in the adjacent cavernous sinus (McFadzean *et al.*, 1991). Brain CT and MRI scanning indicate the pituitary fossa as the source of the haemorrhage and in most instances the adenoma itself is visible (Post *et al.*, 1980; McFadzean *et al.*, 1991).

Miscellaneous

Miscellaneous and exceedingly rare lesions that can give rise to SAH in the basal cisterns include cervical tumours, such as a meningioma or a cavernous angioma (Scotti *et al.*, 1987; Acciarri *et al.*, 1992); rupture of a small circumferential artery in the pontine cistern (Hochberg *et al.*, 1974); or isolated angiitis of the nervous system (see Section 7.2; Hankey, 1991). *Superficial siderosis of the central nervous system* may be a late complication of an episode of SAH from an aneurysm or AVM, or may be caused by chronic oozing of blood from a small meningeal or radicular vessel, with or without trauma or other known cause (Tomlinson & Walton, 1964; Bonito *et al.*, 1994; Fearnley *et al.*, 1995).

9.1.5 Spontaneous intraventricular haemorrhage

Intraventricular haemorrhage is usually associated with either SAH from a ruptured aneurysm (most often on the anterior communicating artery complex) or intracerebral haemorrhage. In both conditions, the outcome is worse with intraventricular rupture than without (Brott & Mandybur, 1986; Fogelholm *et al.*, 1992), and an intraventricular blood volume of more than 20 ml is invariably fatal (Young *et al.*, 1990; Roos *et al.*, 1995). In contrast, the outcome of 'primary' intraventricular haemorrhage, without detectable cause, is much better than if it is associated with SAH or intraparenchymal haemorrhage; patients may survive with intraventricular haemorrhages far exceeding 20 ml (Verma *et al.*, 1987; Roos *et al.*, 1995). The advent of CT proved that intraventricular haemorrhage is not the invariably lethal condition it was once thought, when the diagnosis was made only in those who died.

Idiopathic intraventricular haemorrhage is often specula-

Table 9.5 Causes of primary intraventricular haemorrhage.

Uncommon aneurysms
Posterior inferior cerebellar artery (Yeh *et al.*, 1985; Osenbach *et al.*, 1986; Ruelle *et al.*, 1988; Sadato *et al.*, 1991)
Anterior inferior cerebellar artery (Oana *et al.*, 1991)

AVMs
In the ependymal lining (Waga *et al.*, 1985; Darby *et al.*, 1988; Nakayama *et al.*, 1989; Donnet *et al.*, 1992)
Of the choroid plexus (Schmitt, 1983; van Rybroek & Moore, 1990)
Dural fistula of the superior sagittal sinus (Kataoka & Taneda, 1984)

Occlusive arterial disease
Moyamoya syndrome: idiopathic (Ruelle *et al.*, 1988), atherosclerotic (Masson *et al.*, 1986) or with associated aneurysm (Konishi *et al.*, 1985; Hamada *et al.*, 1994)
Lacunar infarction (Gates *et al.*, 1986)

Tumours
Pituitary tumour (Tsubota *et al.*, 1991)
Ependymoma (Poon & Solis, 1985)
Meningioma (Nachanakian *et al.*, 1983)

Infectious diseases
Brain abscess (Pascual *et al.*, 1987)
Parasitic granuloma (Wong & Ho, 1994)

Drugs
Cocaine (Levine *et al.*, 1990)
Amphetamine (Imanse & Vanneste, 1990)

tively attributed to occult AVMs in the ependymal wall, because sometimes they can actually be demonstrated (Waga *et al.*, 1985; Darby *et al.*, 1988; Nakayama *et al.*, 1989; Donnet *et al.*, 1992). Specific other causes may be found in exceptional cases, ranging from tumours, which are immediately obvious on CT scanning, to small aneurysms at uncommon sites, which only assiduous investigation can uncover (Table 9.5).

9.2 Clues from the history

The a priori probability of an aneurysm as the cause of SAH is so high that other conditions are worth considering only if there are very strong clues in the history (head trauma, infective endocarditis, sickle cell disease, pituitary adenoma) or in any antecedent events (violent head movements, cocaine ingestion), or if the first pain was felt in the neck rather than in the head (spinal SAH).

9.2.1 Medical history

In patients with a distant history of head injury, and particularly with a *skull fracture*, a *dural AVM* should be suspected, since healing of the fracture may be accompanied by the development of such a malformation (Chaudhary *et al.*, 1982). Even in patients not already known to suffer from a disorder of the heart valves, *mycotic aneurysms* may give rise to SAH, but such a presentation of infective endocarditis is exceptional, particularly compared with all other potential sources of bleeding (Vincent *et al.*, 1980; Salgado *et al.*, 1987). In practice, this possibility can be safely dismissed in a previously healthy patient in whom the haemorrhage is located at the base of the brain. A diagnosis of a ruptured mycotic aneurysm may well be entertained, however, with a history of malaise and a haemorrhage located at the convexity of the brain. Usually it will not be hard for the physician to get acquainted with the existence of *sickle cell disease*, a history of *cardiac myxoma*, the use of *anticoagulants* or the influence of other coagulation disorders.

Pituitary apoplexy may be difficult to diagnose if an adenoma was not known to exist and particularly if a decrease in the level of consciousness precludes a proper assessment of visual and oculomotor deficits. Usually, the underlying adenoma has insidiously manifested itself before the dramatic occurrence of the haemorrhage, such as by a dull retro-orbital pain, fatigue, a gradual decrease of visual acuity or a constriction of the temporal fields, but often these symptoms lead to the diagnosis only in retrospect and not before. There are many contributing conditions and factors that may precipitate haemorrhagic infarction of a pituitary tumour, such as pregnancy, raised intracranial pressure, the use of anticoagulants, cerebral angiography or the administration of gonadotrophin-releasing hormone (Reid *et al.*, 1985; Masson *et al.*, 1993).

9.2.2 Family history

A family history of SAH is an important clue in patients with sudden headache. It has been pointed out in Section 9.1.1 that rare families exist in which numerous relatives are struck down by ruptured aneurysms, but that even in cases of so-called sporadic SAH the risk in first-degree relatives is increased (Bromberg *et al.*, 1995a). Families in which aneurysm rupture has occurred in two or more first-degree relatives may have an underlying or associated disorder, such as Marfan's syndrome, Ehlers–Danlos syndrome type IV, pseudoxanthoma elasticum, hereditary haemorrhagic telangiectasia, polycystic kidney disease or coarctation of the aorta (see Table 9.2), but in most cases of familial aneurysms there is no such association.

9.2.3 Antecedent events

A history of even quite minor *neck trauma* or of *sudden, unusual head movements before the onset of headache* may provide a clue to the diagnosis of *vertebral artery dissection* as a cause of SAH. It has already been argued above that head trauma and primary SAH may be confused. Trauma should always be suspected in patients found unconscious in the street, even if there is marked neck stiffness and no superficial wound. Conversely, a traffic accident may sometimes be the result rather than the cause of SAH, and invaluable information may be obtained from the police or ambulance workers; in a patient known to have swerved from one side of the road to the other before crashing into someone else, the a priori probabilities are quite different from those in someone reported to have ignored a red traffic light.

Cocaine ingestion as a risk factor may not immediately be known in the case of an unconscious patient. Cocaine (or ephedrine) should be considered in young adults with SAH, particularly if the social background is unstable, although in some regions of the world the use of cocaine affects all social strata. Even if the family turns up in large numbers, one may find that not every relative is aware of illicit drugs being used or willing to volunteer this information even if they are.

9.2.4 Nature of the headache at onset

The key feature in diagnosing SAH from a *ruptured aneurysm* is the history of severe and unusual headache, classically in a *split second*. Such a history of 'a blow inside the head' is not specific for ruptured aneurysms or even for SAH in general. A similarly sudden headache may occur with some forms of benign vascular headache, migrainous or not, and with some forms of muscle contraction headache. Sexual activity may precipitate not only SAH, but also both of these types of innocuous headaches (Lance, 1976). Exceptional forms of common headaches may well outnumber common forms of a rare disease, such as a ruptured aneurysm (the incidence of aneurysmal haemorrhage being about eight per 100 000 population per year, so a family physician with a practice of 2000 people will, on average, see one such patient every 6 years or so). The actual proportion of SAH amongst all patients with 'thunderclap headache' in the population was unknown until recently. A survey amongst general practitioners in the Netherlands found that SAH was diagnosed in 37 of 148 patients with sudden headache (25%), in 12 of 103 patients (12%) in whom sudden headache was the *only* symptom and in 12 of 70 patients (17%) with headache alone who were referred to hospital (Linn *et al.*, 1994). There is no single clinical feature that distinguishes reliably and at an early stage between SAH and innocuous types of sudden headache (see Section 5.5.2). The discomfort and cost of referring the majority of patients for a brief consultation in hospital (which should include CT scanning and a delayed lumbar puncture if this is negative; see Section 5.3.3) is probably outweighed by the disaster of missing a ruptured aneurysm and being unpleasantly surprised by rebleeding or other secondary complications.

> *It is exceedingly rare for headache at the onset of aneurysmal haemorrhage in an awake patient to be mild or to last less than 2 hours, or for the symptoms to consist of non-specific 'dizziness'.*

A gradual onset of headache, in minutes rather than seconds, is recorded in about 25% of patients with non-aneurysmal perimesencephalic haemorrhage (Van Gijn *et al.*, 1985b; Rinkel *et al.*, 1991b), which again supports the notion of a non-arterial source of haemorrhage. But, the predictive value of this feature is low, as gradual onset of headache at onset also occurs in some 13% of patients with ruptured aneurysms (Van Gijn *et al.*, 1985b), whilst ruptured aneurysms are nine times as common as non-aneurysmal perimesencephalic haemorrhages (Rinkel *et al.*, 1993).

A biphasic headache may occur in patients with SAH from dissection of a vertebral artery: a severe occipital headache radiating from the back of the neck, followed after an interval of hours or days by a sudden exacerbation of a headache of a more diffuse type. The initial episode may represent the beginning of the dissection and not yet meningeal irritation; such occipital headaches are common also in patients with ischaemic deficits or lower cranial nerve palsies as a result of vertebral artery dissection, and headache may even be the only manifestation (Mokri *et al.*, 1988; Yamaura *et al.*, 1990). But, biphasic headache is not a necessary feature of SAH from dissection of a vertebral artery; the haemorrhage may well occur with the first symptoms (Aoki & Sakai, 1990).

A spinal AVM as the source of SAH may declare itself by the pain at onset being particularly severe in the lower part of the neck (upper neck pain is common also with ruptured intracranial aneurysms) or a sudden and stabbing pain between the shoulder-blades (*coup de poignard* or dagger thrust), with or without radiation to the arms. Even if there is severe headache initially, this may disappear before the backache or radicular pain.

> *Sudden pain in the lower neck or between the shoulder-blades is a pointer to spinal subarachnoid haemorrhage, particularly if the pain radiates to the shoulders or arms. Dissection of the thoracic aorta is another possibility.*

9.2.5 Loss of consciousness

Loss of consciousness occurred in approximately 50% of 479 patients with presumably aneurysmal haemorrhage who were well enough to be entered into a clinical trial of medical treatment (Vermeulen *et al.*, 1984). This means the overall proportion must be higher; in population-based studies 10–12% of patients died at home or during transportation (Linn *et al.*, 1994; Schievink *et al.*, 1995b), and in a large, unselected series of patients who reached hospital alive the case fatality within the first 24 hours was of the order of 23% (33/142) (Hijdra & van Gijn, 1982; see also Section 5.5.1). Therefore, patients entered into clinical trials constitute the surviving 80% of all patients initially affected, and in the entire cohort loss of consciousness must occur in at least 60%. Some patients complain of headache before they lose consciousness, and all patients have severe headache if they regain consciousness. Some patients may enter a confusional, agitated state (delirium), with or without preceding coma. Bizarre actions may include grimacing, spitting, making sucking or kissing sounds, spluttering, singing, whistling, yelling and screaming (Fisher, 1975). More than once, such behaviour has been misinterpreted as psychological in origin. Non-aneurysmal (perimesencephalic) SAH is typically associated with normal cognitive function; loss of consciousness or altered behaviour practically rules out this diagnosis. Head trauma should always be considered in patients who are found unconscious (see Section 9.2.3).

9.2.6 Epileptic seizures

Epileptic seizures occur in approximately 10% of patients with aneurysmal SAH (Sarner & Rose, 1967; Hart *et al.*, 1981; Hasan *et al.*, 1993; see also Section 5.5.1). Most of the seizures occur on the first day after the haemorrhage, but at the tail-end one-third of the patients have their first seizure after 6 months, and one-third of those after more than 1 year (Hart *et al.*, 1981). A large amount of cisternal blood on brain CT and the occurrence of rebleeding are the only independent predictors of epilepsy (Hart *et al.*, 1981). Seizures have not been documented in patients with perimesencephalic SAH, presumably of venous origin, but may well complicate haemorrhages from arterial sources other than aneurysms, such as dissection of the vertebral artery or an AVM.

Table 9.6 Focal neurological signs early after aneurysmal SAH, and their explanation.

Sign	Most common explanation
Hemiparesis	Large subarachnoid clot in Sylvian fissure (middle cerebral artery aneurysm)
Paraparesis	Aneurysm of anterior communicating artery
Cerebellar ataxia, Wallenberg's syndrome or both	Dissection of vertebral artery
IIIrd nerve palsy	Aneurysm of internal carotid artery, at the origin of posterior communicating artery; rarely aneurysm of basilar artery or superior cerebellar artery
VIth nerve palsy	Non-specific rise of cerebrospinal fluid pressure
IXth–XIIth nerve palsy	Dissection of vertebral artery

Note: intraparenchymal haematomas may give rise to other deficits, depending on their site.

9.3 Clues from the examination

9.3.1 Neck stiffness

This is a common sign in SAH of any cause but it takes some hours to develop and therefore can not be used to exclude the diagnosis if a patient is seen soon after the sudden-onset headache. Neck stiffness is also absent in deep coma. If present, the sign does not distinguish between different causes of SAH, and not even between haemorrhagic disorders and meningitis (see Section 5.5.1).

9.3.2 Focal neurological deficits

Classically, in the acute phase of aneurysmal SAH there are no signs other than those of meningeal irritation, but exceptions to this rule can provide useful information about the site or the extent of the haemorrhage (Table 9.6). In the second or third week after rupture, focal deficits are not uncommon; most often they represent secondary ischaemia (see Section 13.8).

Hemiparesis

Hemiparesis at onset occurs in approximately 15% of patients with a ruptured aneurysm, usually with aneurysms of the middle cerebral artery (Sarner & Rose, 1967). Because aneurysms vastly outnumber all other potential causes of

SAH, the presence or absence of hemiparesis does not contribute much to the diagnosis of rarer causes, in which hemiparesis is relatively common, for example with mycotic aneurysms, or uncommon, such as with intradural dissection of a vertebral artery. Deficits indicating lesions of the cerebellum or brainstem, such as dysmetria, scanning speech, rotatory nystagmus or Horner's syndrome, strongly suggest vertebral artery dissection.

Paraparesis

Paraparesis may complicate rupture of an aneurysm of the anterior communicating artery complex, as a manifestation of a bifrontal haematoma, if present initially, or of delayed ischaemia in the territory of both anterior cerebral arteries, if developing after an interval of several days (Greene et al., 1995).

IIIrd nerve palsy

IIIrd nerve palsy of variable degree is a well-recognised sign after rupture of aneurysms of the internal carotid artery at the origin of the posterior communicating artery (Hyland & Barnett, 1954). It can also occur with aneurysms of the basilar bifurcation or even of the superior cerebellar artery, but these are infrequent sites (Vincent & Zimmerman, 1980). IIIrd nerve palsy also occurs with unruptured aneurysms (Griffiths et al., 1994) or several days after the haemorrhage, presumably by expansion of the wall of the aneurysm without rupture. Most often the pupil is dilated and unreactive but in some patients the pupil is spared (Nadeau & Trobe, 1983; Kissel et al., 1983).

VIth nerve palsies

VIth nerve palsies, often bilateral in the acute stage, usually result from the sustained rise of cerebrospinal fluid (CSF) pressure, at the time of rupture or later, but occasionally aneurysms of the posterior circulation cause direct compression (Fisher, 1975).

Lower cranial nerve palsies

Lower cranial nerve palsies (IXth–XIIth nerve) may accompany dissection of the carotid artery in the neck, but, as mentioned above, this is an extremely uncommon cause of SAH (Sturzenegger & Huber, 1993). Subadventitial dissection of the vertebral artery may lead not only to SAH, but also to compression of the IXth or Xth nerve and to ischaemia in the territory of the posterior inferior cerebellar artery (see Table 9.4).

Rarely, the source of the haemorrhage is a giant aneurysm (Drake, 1979). This may have caused symptoms before the rupture, such as focal deficits via embolism (see Section 7.4), multiple cranial nerve palsies via mechanical distortion, or both.

9.3.3 Pyrexia

During the first 2–3 days after SAH, of aneurysmal or other origin, the body temperature rarely exceeds 38.5°C, but thereafter it may rise to over 39°C. This raises the possibility of an intercurrent infection, but an important distinction is that the pulse rate remains disproportionately low (see Section 5.5.1).

9.3.4 Hypertension

About 50% of the patients with aneurysmal SAH have a markedly raised blood pressure, although only 20–25% have a history of pre-existing hypertension (Artiola i Fortuny et al., 1980; Vermeulen et al., 1984). This probably also occurs with other sources of arterial haemorrhage, but less often with perimesencephalic non-aneurysmal SAH; however, it has not been systematically studied. In most patients the raised blood pressure is a reactive phenomenon, and the pressure returns to normal within a few days. It seems logical to assume that hypertension increases the risk of rebleeding, and indeed there is some evidence that this is so (Torner et al., 1981), although in that study the diagnosis of rebleeding was not always supported by CT scanning. On the other hand, antihypertensive therapy substantially increases the risk of delayed cerebral ischaemia (Wijdicks et al., 1990). The blood-pressure changes probably serve to counteract the decrease in cerebral perfusion resulting from increased CSF pressure and later vasospasm; at any rate, antihypertensive drugs are not indicated in a previously normotensive patient.

9.3.5 'Grading' patients with aneurysmal subarachnoid haemorrhage (SAH)

The neurological condition of the patient on admission, particularly the level of consciousness, is the most important clinical determinant of the eventual outcome (Hijdra et al., 1988). Several grading systems have been developed for this initial assessment, in most cases consisting of approximately five categories of severity, in hierarchical order. No single system has gained worldwide acceptance, but until recently the most widely used scales were those of Hunt and Hess (1968), and of Botterell, either in the original version (Botterell et al., 1956) or as modified by Nishioka (1966).

The constituent features of these grading systems are not only the level of consciousness, but also headache, neck stiffness and focal neurological deficit. Unfortunately, these more or less traditional systems are neither valid nor reliable.

Validity refers to whether a particular 'instrument' measures what it is supposed to measure, in this case prognosis. Headache and neck stiffness are very poor predictors of outcome in their own right, unless applied to patients from the pre-CT and pre-spectrophotometry era, which included non-aneurysmal haemorrhage or even patients with an innocuous but sudden headache followed by a traumatic lumbar puncture. Moreover, the construction of these grading scales attributes equal weight to the presence of an impaired level of consciousness, focal deficit or both, the actual grade depending on the severity. Finally, both these features are classified in vague terms.

The reliability of a scale refers to its reproducibility, particularly with different observers, and in view of the overlapping and equivocal terminology it is not surprising that a formal study of observer variability demonstrated formidable inconsistencies when the same patients were graded by different physicians, on either the Hunt and Hess scale or the Nishioka–Botterell scale (Lindsay et al., 1982). Up to four different grades were selected for the same patient! A similar inconsistency between observers was found with regard to the four clinical features on which the two scales are based (Lindsay et al., 1983).

Clearly, there is a need for a better grading system, which contains only relevant features for predicting prognosis (level of consciousness and the presence or absence of a focal deficit) and which defines and combines these in an unambiguous fashion. Classification into a few levels of the sum score of the Glasgow Coma Scale (GCS), which consists of eye-opening, motor response and verbal response (Teasdale & Jennett, 1974), proved more reliable than any of the previous systems used to classify the degree of wakefulness (see Section 4.2.2; Lindsay et al., 1983). Accordingly, a committee of the World Federation of Neurological Surgeons (WFNS) has proposed a new grading scale of five levels, essentially based on the GCS, with focal deficit making up one extra level for patients with a GCS score of 14 or 13 (Table 9.7). In other words, the WFNS Scale takes account of the fact that a focal neurological deficit in patients with SAH rarely occurs with a normal level of consciousness, and assumes that the presence or absence of such a deficit does not add much to the prognosis in patients with a GCS score of 12 or less (Drake et al., 1988). No formal studies of the validity and reliability of the WFNS Scale have yet been undertaken, but at least its core is made up by the GCS, which is extremely valid as a measure for outcome; the relia-

Table 9.7 Grading system for the initial classification of patients with SAH, according to the WFNS Scale. (From Drake *et al.*, 1988.)

WFNS grade	GCS	Focal deficit
I	15	Absent
II	14–13	Absent
III	14–13	Present
IV	12–7	Present or absent
V	6–3	Present or absent

bility of the GCS is also good (Teasdale & Jennett, 1974), although some have found this to apply only to experienced observers (Rowley & Fielding, 1991).

It is often tacitly assumed that the initial clinical condition is related only to the impact of the first haemorrhage. This is incorrect, as some complications can occur within hours of the original rupture: early rebleeding, cardiopulmonary dysfunction or acute hydrocephalus. Particularly, the presence of acute hydrocephalus may be sadly overlooked if the tell-tale history of increasing drowsiness in the first few hours after the bleed is not properly interpreted (van Gijn *et al.*, 1985a). It should therefore be emphasised that no grading scale, whatever its merits, should ever be used as the only guide to management; a patient without any deficit at all may, perhaps rightly, be regarded as a candidate for early surgery, but conversely a patient 'in a bad grade' should not be left alone to recover or aggressively treated according to a standard protocol (Bailes *et al.*, 1990), but should instead be investigated and treated according to the pathophysiological problem at hand.

> *'Grading' patients with subarachnoid haemorrhage is a misguided attempt to create a uniform baseline criterion. The patient's condition should be recorded in descriptive, not in codified terms: level of consciousness (Glasgow Coma Scale) and any focal neurological deficits. Specific causes of early neurological deficit should be identified: intracerebral haematoma, acute hydrocephalus or cardiorespiratory complications.*

9.4 Investigations

The following sections are devoted to investigations aimed at detecting and treating the underlying cause of SAH, but of course the investigations needed to assess a patient's general medical condition remain essential: full blood count, glucose, urea, electrolytes, chest X-ray and an electrocardiogram.

9.4.1 CT scanning

It was appreciated soon after the advent of CT scanning that the presence and distribution of subarachnoid blood from a ruptured aneurysm could be inferred from radiodense ('white') spots in the subarachnoid space at the base of the brain, which stood out against the much less dense ('black') background of normal CSF (Kendall *et al.*, 1976). In this section, we shall describe the patterns of bleeding in ruptured aneurysms, according to their site, and also the radiological characteristics of non-aneurysmal sources of haemorrhage.

Patterns of aneurysmal haemorrhage

The distribution of extravasated blood on brain CT (Table 9.8) is an invaluable guide in determining the presence and site of the offending aneurysm, and therefore also in planning the order and the extent of angiography, particularly in elderly patients, in whom surgical repair of unruptured aneurysms is not always indicated (see Chapter 13). Furthermore, identifying the source of haemorrhage from the scan is extremely helpful if more than one aneurysm is found (Lim & Sage, 1977), because there is a vast difference between the surgical management of a ruptured aneurysm (urgent) and an unruptured aneurysm (operation not urgent, if indicated at all). Even the uncommon event of two aneurysms rupturing at the same time can be correctly diagnosed by CT (Joslyn *et al.*, 1985).

Intracerebral haematomas give a good indication of the site of the ruptured aneurysm, whether they are truly parenchymal or only distend the subarachnoid space. In those cases, the prediction for the site of the ruptured aneurysm is correct in approximately 90% (Hillman, 1993). Haematomas from an aneurysm of the anterior cerebral artery usually arise near the anterior communicating artery (see Fig. 9.2). At least the most proximal part of the haematoma is located near the midline; the distal part may also be paramedian, in the gyrus rectus on one or both sides (Fig. 9.4), or it may split the frontal lobe more laterally (Fig. 9.5). A clot between the frontal horns is a particularly reli-

Table 9.8 Possible patterns of haemorrhage from a ruptured aneurysm on CT scanning (often in combinations).

Subarachnoid cisterns
Brain parenchyma
Ventricular system
Subdural space

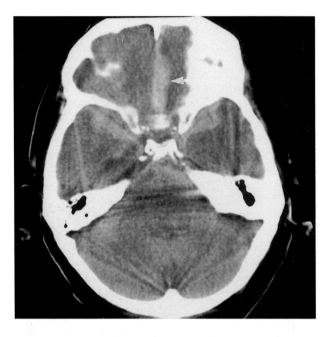

Figure 9.4 CT scan showing a haematoma from a ruptured aneurysm of the anterior communicating artery, in the gyrus rectus (arrow).

able indicator of a ruptured anterior communicating artery aneurysm (Jackson *et al.*, 1993), although it may be difficult to distinguish between a haematoma in the septum pellucidum (Fig. 9.6) and one in the subarachnoid space (Schulder *et al.*, 1987). A haematoma confined to the pericallosal cistern indicates that the aneurysm lies more distally on the anterior cerebral artery, usually at the origin of the pericallosal artery (Fig. 9.7).

Aneurysms arising from the internal carotid artery are most often situated at the origin of the posterior communicating artery, and intracerebral haematomas from rupture at this site are usually found in the medial part of the temporal lobe (Fig. 9.8). Very large haematomas at this location may also involve the frontal lobe. Haematomas from an aneurysm at the origin of the ophthalmic artery tend to involve the frontal lobe on one side and do not reach the midline, which distinguishes them from intracerebral bleeding from an aneurysm of the anterior communicating artery. If the aneurysm is located at the terminal bifurcation of the internal carotid artery (into the anterior and middle cerebral artery), the haematoma may extend into the head of the caudate nucleus (Hayward & O'Reilly, 1976). Middle cerebral

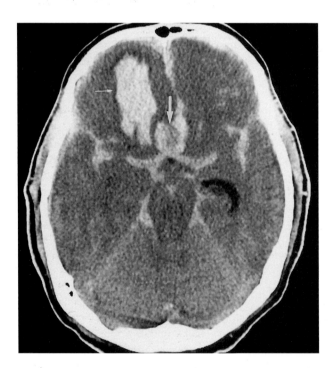

Figure 9.5 CT scan showing a haematoma (thin arrow) from a large ruptured aneurysm of the anterior communicating artery, in the middle of the right frontal lobe. The aneurysm is visible as a 'filling defect' (thick arrow) within the hyperdense subarachnoid blood.

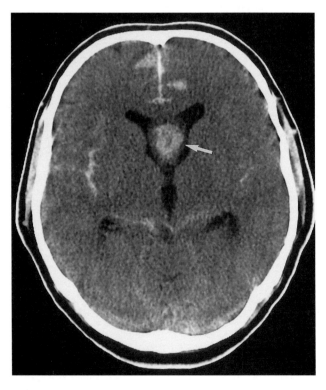

Figure 9.6 CT scan showing a haematoma in the cavum septum pellucidum (arrow), from a ruptured aneurysm of the anterior communicating artery.

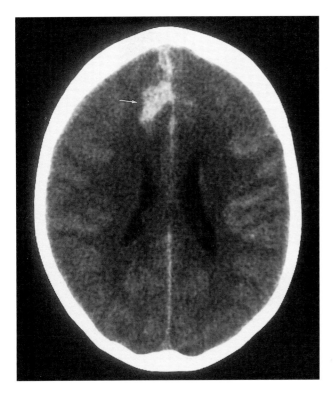

Figure 9.7 CT scan showing a haematoma in the right cingulate gyrus (arrow), from a ruptured aneurysm of the pericallosal artery.

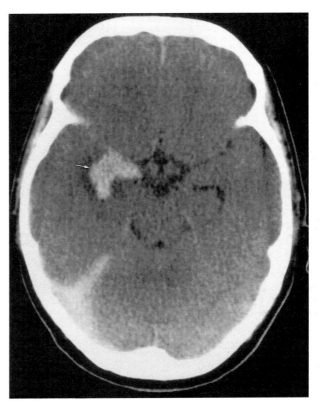

Figure 9.8 CT scan showing a haematoma in the medial part of the right temporal lobe (arrow), from a ruptured aneurysm of the posterior communicating artery, at its origin from the internal carotid artery.

artery aneurysms are located almost exclusively close to the temporal bone, where the trunk of the artery divides and turns superiorly and posteriorly to enter the lateral part of the Sylvian fissure. Haematomas from aneurysms of this type usually extend from this point posteriorly and superiorly, to follow the course of the lateral fissure (Fig. 9.9). Less often, the haemorrhage is directed medially, in which case it can be distinguished from a haematoma arising in the region of the basal ganglia, from rupture of a small perforating artery, by its lateral border being adjacent to the inner table of the skull (Fig. 9.10). Aneurysms arising from the posterior circulation rarely give rise to intraparenchymal haematomas.

The pattern of haemorrhage is less often specific for the site of the aneurysm if the extravasated blood is confined to the subarachnoid cisterns, especially if the haemorrhage is diffuse. Moreover, after an interval of 5 days 50% of patients no longer show cisternal blood (van Gijn & van Dongen, 1982) and in exceptional cases the abnormalities have all but disappeared within a single day (Fig. 9.11). The source of SAH can be inferred if the haemorrhage remains confined to or is most dense in a single cistern, near to an arterial branching site where aneurysms are known to arise (see Fig. 9.2). Sometimes the hyperdensity is very

subtle (Fig. 9.12), but with diffuse extravasation the source of haemorrhage may become clearer on a repeat scan. Aneurysms of the anterior cerebral artery near the anterior communicating artery are the most common site (see Table 9.2) and can be recognised from a region of hyperdensity in the most caudal part of the frontal interhemispheric fissure (Fig. 9.13). Haemorrhage involving the interhemispheric fissure at higher levels, particularly the supracallosal cistern (Fig. 9.14), implies an aneurysm at the origin of the pericallosal artery, although occasionally (two in 14 cases) haemorrhages from an aneurysm of the anterior communicating artery complex may extend this far (Jackson *et al.*, 1993). An asymmetrical distribution of subarachnoid blood in the region of the suprasellar cistern suggests an aneurysm of the internal carotid artery, usually at the origin of the posterior communicating artery, which site should be suspected when only one side of the suprasellar cisterns is filled with blood, perhaps with some extension to the basal part of the Sylvian fissure (Fig. 9.15). An aneurysm of the middle cerebral artery can be inferred from extravasation of blood at the junction of the basal and lateral parts of the Sylvian fissure (Fig. 9.16).

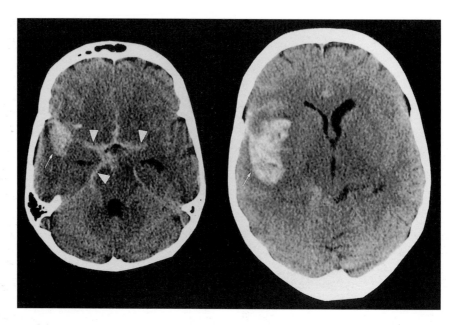

Figure 9.9 CT scan showing a haematoma in the lateral part of the right Sylvian fissure (arrows), from a ruptured aneurysm of the right middle cerebral artery, with diffuse subarachnoid blood also (arrowheads).

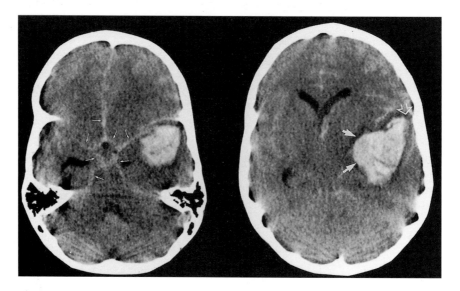

Figure 9.10 CT scan showing a haematoma from a ruptured aneurysm of the left middle cerebral artery; the haematoma has extended medially from the Sylvian fissure into the subinsular cortex and the putamen (thick arrows), thereby mimicking a primary intracerebral haemorrhage from a ruptured perforating artery in the basal ganglia. The characteristic features are the concomitant haemorrhage into the basal cisterns (left—thin arrows) and the extreme lateral extension of the haematoma, up to the inner table of the skull (open arrow).

The haemorrhage may further extend into the lateral fissure. Basilar artery aneurysms are almost invariably found at the terminal bifurcation; haemorrhages from this site are often directed forward and fill the suprasellar, interhemispheric and (basal) Sylvian cisterns (Fig. 9.17). The posterior inferior cerebellar artery is located near the base of the skull in the posterior fossa, a notoriously difficult region for CT; haemorrhages in this region are detected only when patients are examined within 3 days of onset (Kayama *et al.*, 1991). It is even more difficult if the aneurysm is extracranial (Alliez *et al.*, 1990). If subarachnoid blood is detected, its distribution is often non-specific (Fig. 9.18).

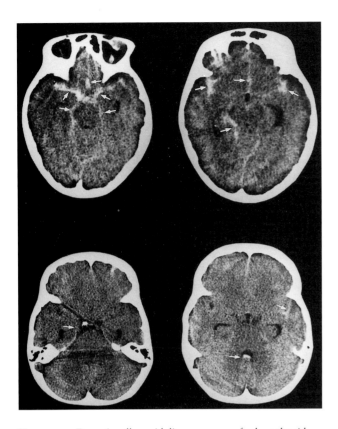

Figure 9.11 Exceptionally rapid disappearance of subarachnoid blood with CT scanning. Upper row: CT scan 4 hours after rupture of an aneurysm of the right posterior communicating artery, at its origin from the carotid artery. Abundant extravasation of blood, throughout the basal cisterns (arrows). Lower row: CT scan 24 hours after the haemorrhage; only a small amount of blood remains (arrows). (From van der Wee *et al.*, 1995; courtesy of the *Journal of Neurology, Neurosurgery and Psychiatry*.)

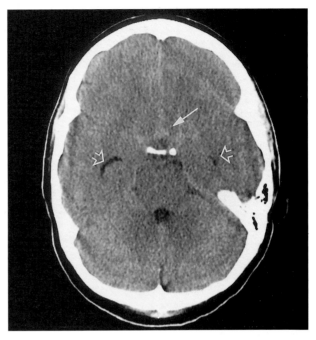

Figure 9.12 CT scan showing subtle amount of subarachnoid blood in anterior part of interhemispheric fissure (arrow), from ruptured aneurysm of the anterior communicating artery. There is also early hydrocephalus (open arrows point to the temporal horns of the lateral ventricles) and the basal cisterns are not as clearly seen as they should be (due to the presence of a small amount of diffuse subarachnoid blood).

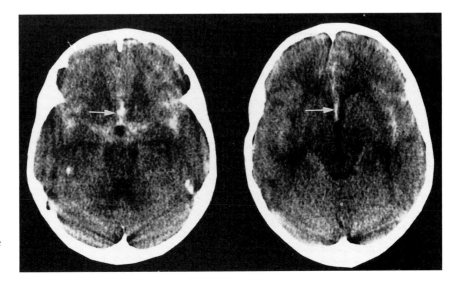

Figure 9.13 CT scan showing diffuse SAH from a ruptured aneurysm of the anterior communicating artery (the centre of the haemorrhage is in the frontal part of the interhemispheric fissure—arrows).

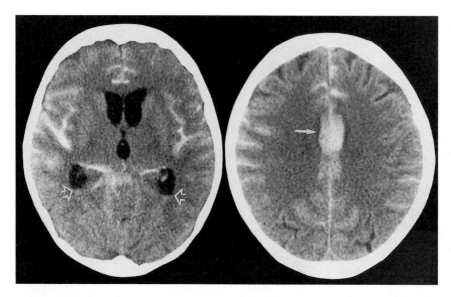

Figure 9.14 CT scan showing diffuse SAH, with most dense clot in the pericallosal cistern (arrow), from a ruptured aneurysm of a pericallosal artery. There is also hydrocephalus and a tiny amount of blood layering in the occipital horns of the lateral ventricles (open arrows).

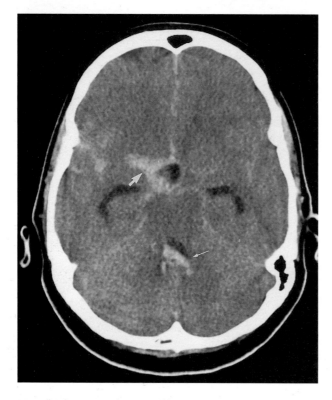

Figure 9.15 CT scan showing diffuse SAH, most dense in the right half of the suprasellar cistern (arrow) from a ruptured aneurysm of the posterior communicating artery, at its origin from the internal carotid artery. Note also the hydrocephalus and blood in the fourth ventricle (thin arrow).

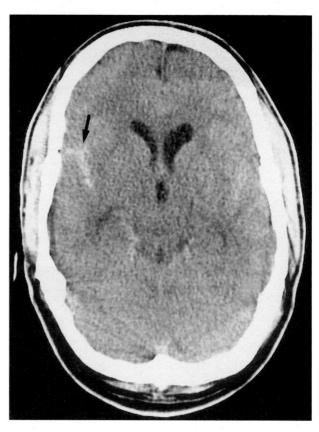

Figure 9.16 CT scan showing SAH, mainly in the lateral part of the right Sylvian fissure (arrow) from a ruptured aneurysm of the right middle cerebral artery.

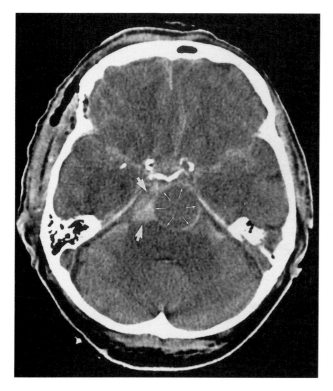

Figure 9.17 CT scan showing diffuse SAH, most dense in the prepontine cisterns (thick arrows) from a giant aneurysm of the basilar artery (thin arrows delineate the inner margins of the aneurysm).

Blood confined to the subarachnoid space may become undetectable on CT scanning within as little as 24 hours; at 5 days blood is undetectable in about 50% of all cases of subarachnoid haemorrhage.

Intraventricular haemorrhage

Intraventricular haemorrhage can occur with almost any type of intracranial haemorrhage (see Section 9.1.5), but most often with aneurysms. In fatal cases with massive intraventricular haemorrhage, transmission of pressure through the floor of the fourth ventricle can cause acute failure of pontine and medullary functions; this factor is responsible for 25–50% of early deaths after SAH (Hijdra & Van Gijn, 1982). Intraventricular haemorrhage occurs mostly with aneurysms of the anterior communicating artery, which can bleed through the lamina terminalis to fill the third and lateral ventricles (Little *et al.*, 1977; Weisberg *et al.*, 1991). Conversely, rupture of an aneurysm at the posterior inferior cerebellar artery may preferentially fill the fourth and third ventricles, from the back (Fig. 9.18).

Subdural haematomas

Subdural haematomas develop with aneurysmal rupture in 2–3% (Weir *et al.*, 1984; Kamiya *et al.*, 1991), most often associated with subarachnoid blood but sometimes as the only manifestation (Williams *et al.*, 1983; O'Leary &

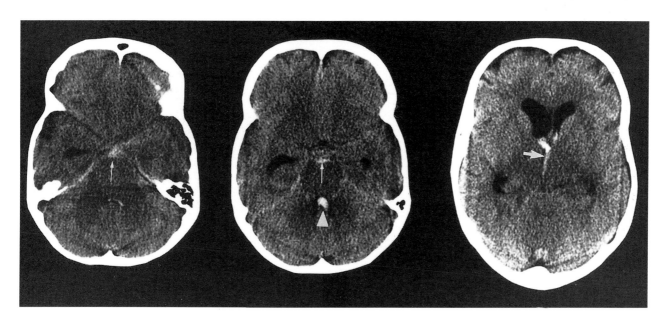

Figure 9.18 CT scan showing diffuse SAH, mostly in the posterior part of the suprasellar cistern (thin arrows), and with rupture into the fourth (arrowhead) and third (short arrow) ventricles from a ruptured aneurysm of the posterior inferior cerebellar artery.

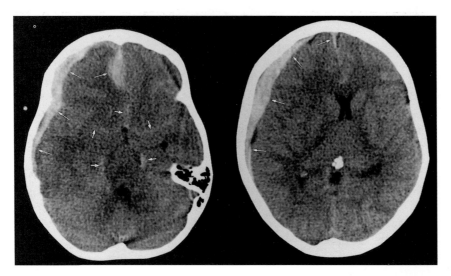

Figure 9.19 CT scan showing a subdural haematoma at the convexity of the right hemisphere and on the right side of the falx (thin arrows), in a 56-year-old woman with spontaneous SAH (site of aneurysm unknown). Diffuse blood is also visible throughout the basal cisterns (thick short arrows).

Sweeny, 1986; Kondziolka *et al.*, 1988; Ragland *et al.*, 1993). The most probable explanation is that the dome of the aneurysm sac adheres to the arachnoid membrane, usually as a result of a previous rupture, recognised or unrecognised (Clarke & Walton, 1953). The subdural collection is mostly found at the convexity of the brain, seldom in the interhemispheric fissure (Friedman & Brant Zawadzki, 1983). The ruptured aneurysm can be anywhere at the common sites (Weir *et al.*, 1984; Kamiya *et al.*, 1991). The distinction from subdural haematomas of traumatic origin can be made on the basis of any associated haemorrhage in the subarachnoid space, and also because the haematoma is more often unilateral, hyperdense and crescentic in shape than with trauma (Fig. 9.19) (Weir *et al.*, 1984).

Detection of aneurysms

The aneurysm itself is seldom seen on the unenhanced CT scan, and then only when it is very large or calcified or both (Figs 9.17 & 9.20) (van Gijn & van Dongen, 1980). High-resolution scanning, with a slice thickness of 1–5 mm, is more sensitive but not infallible (Schmid *et al.*, 1987). Scanning after injection of contrast and with reconstruction in multiple planes is a further refinement, and with this technique all 13 patients with aneurysms were detected in a series of 32 patients with oculomotor palsy (Teasdale *et al.*, 1990). Of course, these aneurysms were fairly large (7–15 mm), the oculomotor nerves having been involved, but in addition three smaller, unruptured aneurysms were detected, and the angiogram found no others. Spiral CT scanning is an improved technique that eliminates the problem of 'gaps' between slices, whilst so-called partial-volume phenomena ('dilution' of information within a slice) can be avoided by

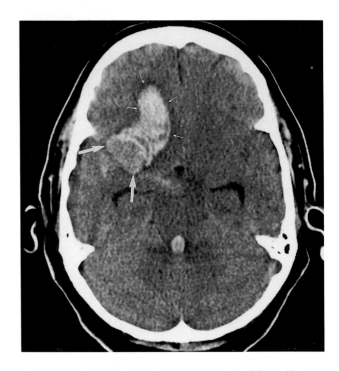

Figure 9.20 CT scan showing haematoma in the left frontal lobe (thin arrows), at a site not specific for any particular aneurysm, with large aneurysm visible (thick arrows) as a structure with density intermediate between densities of brain and blood. The aneurysm probably originates from the terminal bifurcation of the internal carotid artery, or from the middle cerebral artery.

data-processing techniques such as 'maximal intensity projection', which compress three-dimensional information in a single plane, from many different angles (Fig. 9.21). With these techniques, CT scanning is more sensitive than three-dimensional MRA (see Section 9.4.3) (Tsuchiya *et al.*, 1994)

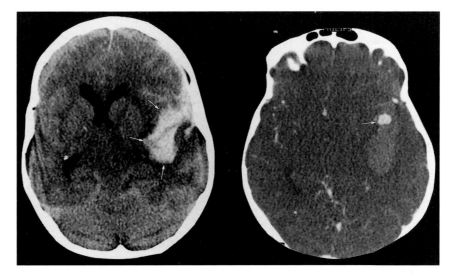

Figure 9.21 Visualisation of an aneurysm by CT scanning. Left: unenhanced CT scan showing haematoma in left Sylvian fissure (arrows). Right: aneurysm of left middle cerebral artery (arrow), visualised with spiral CT scanning after intravenous injection of contrast agent.

and sometimes even more sensitive than catheter angiography (Dorsch *et al.*, 1995). In general, however, aneurysms of less than 3 mm in size can not be identified by the three-dimensional tomographic technique, and catheter angiography is still superior (see Section 9.4.5) (Schwartz *et al.*, 1994). For the purpose of detecting aneurysms in asymptomatic patients, CT scanning, however sophisticated, is unlikely to gain an important role, because of the need for intravenous contrast and the small but inevitable risk of allergic reactions.

Non-aneurysmal (perimesencephalic) patterns of haemorrhage

Fifteen per cent of patients with SAH have a normal angiogram, and two-thirds of these show basal haemorrahges of a distinct kind: mainly or only in the perimesencephalic cisterns, a pattern of haemorrhage seen in only one of 92 patients with SAH and a demonstrable aneurysm (Van Gijn *et al.*, 1985b). On follow-up, no patients with perimesencephalic haemorrhage and a normal angiogram suffer from rebleeding, cerebral infarction or any other neurological cause of clinical deterioration, and all return to a normal life (see Section 9.1.2).

The distribution of cisternal blood in patients with a perimesencephalic type of haemorrhage (and a normal angiogram) has been studied in detail in a consecutive series of 52 patients (Rinkel *et al.*, 1991c). In all patients, the centre of the bleeding on CT was located immediately anterior to the midbrain or sometimes to the pons. Extension to the ambiens cisterns or to the basal parts of the Sylvian fissures was common, but the anterior interhemispheric fissure or the lateral Sylvian fissures were never completely filled with

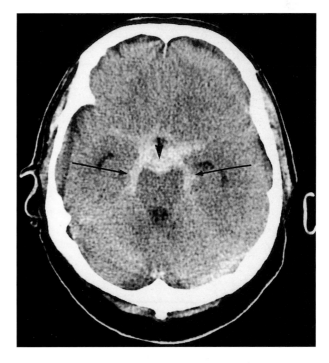

Figure 9.22 CT scan of non-aneurysmal perimesencephalic haemorrhage. The most dense clot is in the interpeduncular (thick arrow) and ambiens (long arrows) cisterns. The anterior part of the interhemispheric fissure and the lateral fissures are not filled, and there is no intraventricular haemorrhage. The angiogram showed no abnormality.

blood (Fig. 9.22). No intraventricular haemorrhage ever occurred, other than some sedimentation of blood in the posterior horns of the lateral ventricles, which may reflect an abnormal circulation of the CSF.

The possibility of distinguishing non-aneurysmal perimesencephalic haemorrhage from aneurysmal SAH on early CT scans has been studied in a consecutive series of 221 patients who subsequently underwent angiography (Rinkel *et al.*, 1991c). The scans were separately judged by two neuroradiologists. The predictive value of a perimesencephalic pattern of haemorrhage for a normal angiogram was determined conservatively, amongst only those CT scans (*n* = 37) with a predominance of extravasated blood in the posterior cisterns (15 with an aneurysm and 22 without). Prediction of a normal angiogram was correct in 95% and 94% for the two observers, with an excellent interobserver agreement (a kappa-value of 0.87, the maximum being 1.0). This shows that perimesencephalic non-aneurysmal haemorrhage can be reliably distinguished in the majority of patients. But, these results do not make angiography unnecessary. One patient with a basilar artery aneurysm on angiography (from a total of 15 such patients) was incorrectly classified as a non-aneurysmal pattern of perimesencephalic haemorrhage by both observers (Fig. 9.23). A study from another centre of perimesencephalic patterns of haemorrhage also found a single instance of a patient with a ruptured aneurysm, this time

amongst 38 patients (Pinto *et al.*, 1993). An estimate of the balance of risks leads to the conclusion that withholding surgical treatment in approximately 5% of patients with a perimesencephalic pattern of bleeding but an undetected basilar artery aneurysm is more unfavourable than the complications of 'unnecessary' angiography in the remaining 95%. Later studies have confirmed that a perimesencephalic pattern of bleeding occasionally arises from posterior circulation aneurysms, sometimes in unusual locations (Schievink *et al.*, 1994b). However, there is no need to repeat a normal angiogram in a patient with a perimesencephalic pattern of haemorrhage, whereas this is mandatory with aneurysmal patterns of haemorrhage on the CT scan (see Section 9.4.5).

> *Cerebral angiography is still required in patients with a perimesencephalic subarachnoid pattern of subarachnoid haemorrhage, even though the chance of finding an aneurysm is extremely small. However, repeating the angiogram after a negative initial angiogram is not required.*

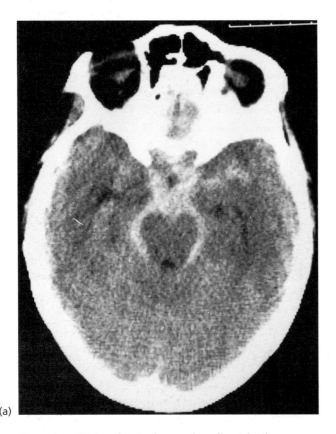

(a)

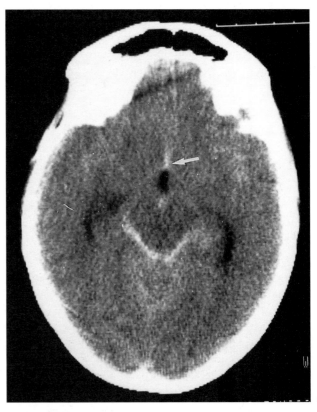

(b)

Figure 9.23 CT scan showing haemorrhage from a basilar artery aneurysm, mistaken by two neuroradiologists for a non-aneurysmal haemorrhage; in retrospect the speck of blood in front of the third ventricle (arrow) might have been a reason for suspecting aneurysmal haemorrhage. (From Rinkel *et al.*, 1991c; courtesy of the *American Journal of Neuroradiology*.)

Other sources of haemorrhage

Basal haemorrhages, indistinguishable on CT scanning from those associated with a ruptured aneurysm, may result from vertebral artery dissection, a dural fistula of the tentorium, an AVM in the neck region, cocaine abuse without an associated aneurysm or a mycotic aneurysm with aspergillosis.

Head trauma may result in SAH. If patients are found unconscious or were seen to have caused an unexplained traffic accident, the question may arise whether the trauma or the SAH was the primary event. With primary brain injury, usually the brain CT shows an adjacent contusion, different in shape and site from an aneurysmal haematoma. Only occasionally do basal contusions make the distinction more difficult. In some patients with shearing injury, pronounced accumulation of blood can be found in the posterior part of the ambiens cistern at the level of the tentorial margin (Takenaka *et al.*, 1990). The blood in the ambiens cistern may be part of more extensive intracranial haemorrhage, but it can be the only site of haemorrhage (Rinkel *et al.*, 1993). Blood confined to the ambiens cistern has also been reported in a patient on anticoagulants after the relatively mild trauma of a fall in the shower (Lavin & Troost, 1984). That site of the haemorrhage makes a ruptured saccular aneurysm as source of the haemorrhage very unlikely.

9.4.2 Magnetic resonance imaging (MRI)

In the acute stage of aneurysmal haemorrhage, particularly within the first 24 hours, subarachnoid blood can be detected by means of MRI as a region of hyperintensity on T2-weighted images (Fig. 9.24) (Satoh & Kadoya, 1988). According to the few studies available, all with, at best, incomplete blinding of observers and with a limited number of patients (20–30), MRI was slightly more sensitive than CT in the first few days after SAH (Jenkins *et al.*, 1988; Matsumura *et al.*, 1990; Ogawa *et al.*, 1993) or, in one case, than even angiography (Renowden *et al.*, 1994). Some studies specifically emphasise the advantages of MRI with aneurysms of the posterior inferior cerebellar artery (Stone *et al.*, 1988; Matsumura *et al.*, 1990). New echo techniques are continuously being developed; some, such as fluid-attenuated inversion recovery (FLAIR), seen especially suitable for detecting fresh subarachnoid blood (Noguchi *et al.*, 1994). On the other hand, other workers are more critical about the balance between sensitivity and specificity of MRI in the acute stage (Atlas, 1993). Moreover, the facilities for MRI are much less readily available than CT scans, and when conscious level is impaired the long scanning time increases the problem of movement artefacts.

After 4 days, T1-weighted images detect extravasated blood best, owing to the paramagnetic effect of the breakdown products of haemoglobin, i.e. oxyhaemoglobin and methaemoglobin (Fig. 9.25) (Di Chiro *et al.*, 1986; Spickler *et al.*, 1990). The hyperintensity of 'old' blood on T1-weighted images may last for at least 2 weeks (Matsumura *et al.*, 1990), but this mainly applies to intraparenchymal blood, which also disappears slowly on CT scans (Van Gijn & van Dongen, 1982). This makes MRI a unique method for identifying the site of the ruptured aneurysm in patients who are not referred until after 5–10 days, in whom brain CT often no longer shows evidence of subarachnoid blood (Barkovich & Atlas, 1988; Jenkins *et al.*, 1988).

Aneurysms can be identified by MRI in approximately

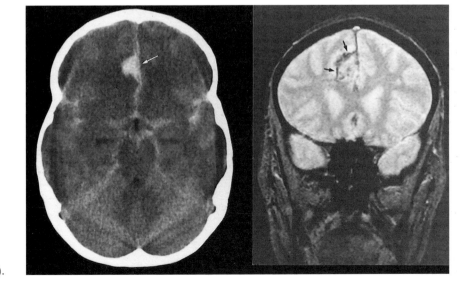

Figure 9.24 Left: axial CT scan after rupture of a pericallosal aneurysm, obtained within 24 hours, showing diffuse subarachnoid blood, with local haematoma in the frontal interhemispheric fissure (arrow). Right: coronal MRI (T2-weighted iamge) of aneurysmal SAH, on same day. The periphery of the haematoma is hypointense (methaemoglobin—arrows).

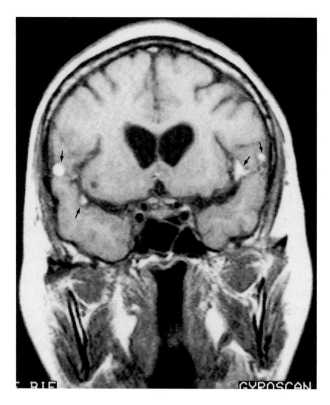

Figure 9.25 Coronal MRI scan (T1-weighted) of aneurysmal SAH, after 5 days. Remaining clots of subarachnoid blood in both Sylvian fissures are hyperintense (arrows).

50% of the cases, as a signal-void area, often associated with focal changes in the brain (Jenkins *et al.*, 1988; Matsumura *et al.*, 1990). This is most helpful if the angiogram has failed to show an expected aneurysm (Pertuiset *et al.*, 1989).

With arterial dissection, MRI (or CT) may detect a thrombus within the false lumen within the dissected wall of the artery (see Section 7.1) (Quint & Spickler, 1990; Schwaighofer *et al.*, 1990; Woimant & Spelle, 1995). In the case of chronic haemosiderosis, MRI scanning will show diffuse deposition of haemosiderin in the subpial layers of the brain and spinal cord (Bonito *et al.*, 1994; River *et al.*, 1994).

9.4.3 Magnetic resonance angiography (MRA)

The specialised technique of MRA is making rapid advances for the demonstration of saccular aneurysms (Ross *et al.*, 1990; Atlas *et al.*, 1994; Korogi *et al.*, 1994), but its main potential is for patients with unruptured aneurysms. The procedure is often not suitable in the acute phase after rupture of an aneurysm, because at present patients have to remain immobile for half an hour or so and artificial ventilation is not always possible in the vicinity of MRA equipment.

On the other hand, the complete safety of the procedure makes it an ideal instrument for screening subjects at risk, provided the sensitivity and specificity are acceptable.

At present MRA has a sensitivity in the order of 85% and a specificity of around 90% in comparison with conventional catheter angiography (Auffray *et al.*, 1994; Horikoshi *et al.*, 1994; Patrux *et al.*, 1994). With spiral CT scanning after contrast injection, the results are also slightly better than with MRA (Tsuchiya *et al.*, 1994). Particularly aneurysms of the carotid artery are more difficult to visualise with MRA or, conversely, are more often diagnosed but not confirmed by angiography than aneurysms at other sites (Horikoshi *et al.*, 1994; Patrux *et al.*, 1994). Aneurysms of the posterior circulation can be adequately detected, even if distal at the posterior inferior cerebellar artery (Price & Miller, 1994). The critical size of aneurysms is now 3 mm, below which they are usually missed by MRA (Futatsuya *et al.*, 1994; Houkin *et al.*, 1994; Huston *et al.*, 1994) and also by spiral CT (Schwartz *et al.*, 1994). Of course, there are exceptions on both sides, and occasionally a large aneurysm is missed by MRA (Turtz *et al.*, 1995). Three-dimensional projection techniques will surely improve on the results obtained so far, for example in allowing a better view of the neck of the aneurysm, information which is vital for the surgeon (Bontozoglou *et al.*, 1994). The time-of-flight technique of MRA results in a higher detection rate than the phase-contrast technique, in both cases wth three-dimensional reconstructions (Araki *et al.*, 1994; Huston *et al.*, 1994; Ikawa *et al.*, 1994).

On a few occasions, the technique has been actually applied in screening neurologically normal people, with a family history of SAH (Fig. 9.26) or with polycystic kidney disease (Ruggieri *et al.*, 1994; Ronkainen *et al.*, 1995b). So far, the high specificity suggested by studies of patients with ruptured aneurysms seems to be borne out, but a proper assessment of the value of screening for aneurysms should include follow-up of patients with negative studies and also a cost-effectiveness analysis, ideally including the psychological stress of a possibly abnormal test result in those being screened.

MRA is without risks and reasonably sensitive (90%), which makes it well suited as an instrument for screening people at risk of saccular aneurysms. However, such screening should not be introduced before the benefits and disadvantages have been properly assessed.

9.4.4 Ultrasound

The technique of transcranial Doppler can be combined with echo imaging (duplex technique) and with colour coding

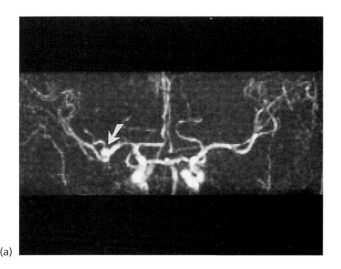
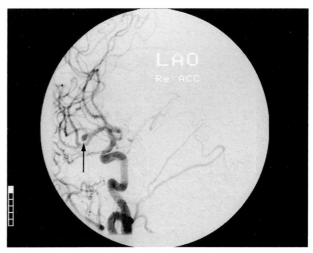

(a) (b)

Figure 9.26 (a) MRA of the circle of Willis viewed from the front. An aneurysm of the right middle cerebral artery (white arrow) is shown in an asymptomatic patient with affected relatives. (b) Confirmation by catheter angiography, in a reversed anterior oblique view (black arrow).

(transcranial colour-coded duplex sonography). A single study in which the investigator was blinded to the results of angiography (but not to those of CT or MRI) showed that this ultrasound technique detected 23 of 27 aneurysms, or 85% (Baumgartner *et al.*, 1994). Eventually MRA will probably turn out to be the most sensitive amongst the non-invasive techniques for the detection of aneurysms, as well as the most widely available. But, a feature unique to a dynamic technique such as ultrasound is the potential for assessing the degree to which aneurysms expand during each cardiac cycle (Wardlaw & Cannon, 1995), a characteristic which in asymptomatic aneurysms may be related to the risk of rupture.

9.4.5 Cerebral angiography

General consideration of risks and benefits

Catheter angiography is not an innocuous procedure. Only one prospective study has specifically addressed the complications of angiography in patients with recent SAH, with a risk of permanent stroke of 1% (Dion *et al.*, 1987), but the 95% confidence interval was wide (0–5%). Given an overall rate of 1% permanent neurological complications in patients with mild cerebrovascular disease (Hankey *et al.*, 1990), the true risk in patients with recent SAH is probably higher, if only because the aneurysm may rerupture during the procedure (Hayakawa *et al.*, 1978; Koenig *et al.*, 1979). In certain parts of the world, the aim of making as accurate a diagnosis as possible overrides pragmatic considerations, and an angiogram is felt to be justified in nearly every patient with SAH, but we feel that the potential benefit in terms of management decisions should outweigh the risks in an individual patient.

> *In general, angiography in patients with subarachnoid haemorrhage should be performed only with a view to surgery or, in exceptional cases, to establish a more firm prognosis.*

Timing and extent of angiography

In a patient with an aneurysmal pattern of haemorrhage on CT scanning, the timing of angiography is intricately linked with the timing of surgery. Many neurosurgeons advocate early clipping of the aneurysm, within 3 days of the initial bleed, in the belief that not only rebleeding but also ischaemia might be prevented, in the latter case by washing away extravasated blood (Mizukami *et al.*, 1982). However, comparative studies have not convincingly demonstrated the benefits of early surgery (see Section 13.5.2). This includes a randomised but relatively small study (Öhman & Heiskanen, 1989) and a study with many centres and large numbers but without random allocation (Kassell *et al.*, 1990). The latter study found the worst outcome in patients operated between days 7 and 10 after the initial haemorrhage. This is in accordance with the time course of cerebral ischaemia (Hijdra *et al.*, 1986) and that of cerebral vasospasm (Weir *et al.*, 1978), both phenomena being most common from days 4 to 12.

Angiography with a view to aneurysm-clipping should

therefore be performed at the earliest opportunity if the operation is planned within 3 days of SAH onset. If surgery is to be deferred until approximately day 12, the angiogram should be done either before day 4 or on day 10 or 11, to avoid the period of maximum risk for cerebral vasospasm. If the patient is in good condition, early angiography is to be preferred even with late surgery, because intervening complications can often be dealt with more promptly if the exact site of the offending aneurysm is known.

How extensive should angiography be if CT scanning gives a good indication of the site of the ruptured aneurysm, as is often the case? With aneurysms of the anterior communicating artery, studies of both carotid artery territories are necessary for identification of the artery bearing the aneurysm; with aneurysms of the carotid artery at the origin of the posterior communicating artery, the neurosurgeon often finds it useful to know whether the posterior cerebral artery is sufficiently filled via the basilar artery in the event that temporary clipping of the posterior communicating artery is required to control bleeding; but, with aneurysms of the middle cerebral artery, it is not usually necessary to have information about any other arterial territory. However, if the patient's age and clinical condition warrant treatment of any unruptured as well as the ruptured aneurysm (see Section 13.11), that is good reason for performing a four-vessel angiogram, i.e. to display all the branches of both carotid and vertebral arterial systems. An angiogram can not be termed 'negative' until both vertebral arteries have been visualised, preferably selectively; after all, aneurysms arising from the posterior inferior cerebellar artery or other proximal branches of the vertebral artery will be missed if the posterior circulation is investigated by injection of only a single vertebral artery.

Angiography has been used as a screening instrument for normal people with four or more affected siblings (Alberts *et al.*, 1995), but this has now been superseded by MRA (see Section 9.4.3).

Dissection of intracranial arteries

Here, the diagnosis rests on the angiographic demonstration of narrowing of the artery with signs of an intimal flap, a pseudoaneurysm or a double lumen (see Section 7.1). Angiography may be warranted if CT or MRI fails to confirm the clinical diagnosis of dissection, not with a view to treatment but for excluding other causes and for giving a prognosis. Timing of the study is difficult, because an early angiogram may be normal or show only non-specific arterial narrowing, whereas the abnormalities may have disappeared on a follow-up angiogram (Fig. 9.27) (Friedman & Drake, 1984).

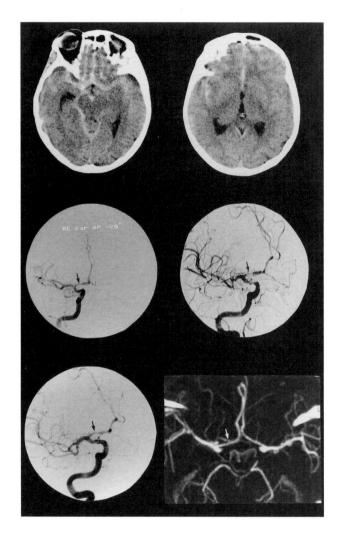

Figure 9.27 SAH from dissection of an intracranial artery. Top row: CT scan within hours of the haemorrhage, showing diffuse extravasation of blood in the basal cisterns, predominantly on the right side. Middle row, left: right carotid angiogram (anteroposterior view) after 1 day, showing a narrowed segment in the proximal part of the anterior cerebral artery (arrow). Middle row, right: second right carotid angiogram (oblique view) after 11 days, showing even more marked narrowing at the same site (arrow). Lower row, left: third right carotid angiogram (oblique view), 3 months after the haemorrhage; the affected segment has almost returned to a normal calibre (arrow). Bottom row, right: spiral CT scan after intravenous contrast, with maximal intensity projection, 9 months after the haemorrhage; the segment of the proximal right anterior cerebral artery is now completely normal (arrow).

In patients in whom CT scanning suggests that the haemorrhage originates near the tentorium, angiography should be directed at the detection of a dural AVM. In that case, it is important to visualise the external carotid artery, because branches of this artery can be the main or the sole feeders (Aminoff, 1973).

In the case of a spinal AVM, brain CT may show blood throughout the basal cisterns and ventricles, which may obscure the diagnosis (Acciarri *et al.*, 1992). Not only negative angiography of the cerebral circulation but also clinical clues such as sudden backache should form an indication for spinal angiography. However, this procedure is not always diagnostic (Kandel, 1980; Swann *et al.*, 1984). Also, angiography is impractical without localising signs or symptoms, because so many intercostal arteries have to be catheterised, and the procedure carries a risk of over 5% of a persisting neurological deficit (Logue, 1979). If a vascular malformation of the spinal cord is considered, MRI, particularly in the sagittal plane, is the first-line investigation for detecting the characterisic serpiginous structures, usually at the dorsal aspect of the cord, or at least for detecting an associated extradural or subdural haematoma (D'Angelo *et al.*, 1990; Mohsenipour *et al.*, 1994). There are no systematic studies available of the usefulness of spinal angiography after a negative MRI scan of the spinal cord.

Mycotic aneurysms were missed by angiography in 10% in older series, but even now they may be visible only on repeated studies. A policy of routine angiography in all patients with infective endocarditis is not justified by decision analysis, but after an intracranial haemorrhage surgical clipping and therefore angiography should be considered (van der Meulen *et al.*, 1992).

Aneurysmal patterns of haemorrhage but negative angiography

Although non-aneurysmal types of SAH were first distinguished 10 years ago (van Gijn *et al.*, 1985b), a steady stream of publications in which SAH patients with a normal angiogram were still treated as a single group has continued to clutter up the scientific literature. That they contribute so little knowledge is to some extent the result of the invariably retrospective design, but the most serious flaw is that they contain a mixed bag of patients (Rinkel *et al.*, 1993). The three most common subgroups are: (i) patients whose 'SAH' is not real but in whom the diagnosis results from a traumatic lumbar puncture (see Section 5.3.2); (ii) patients with non-aneurysmal types of haemorrhage; and (iii) patients with a pattern of haemorrhage that is entirely consistent with a ruptured aneurysm but who nevertheless have a normal angiogram. It is this last category of patients that we shall consider here.

Only two studies have been performed in which patients with an aneurysmal pattern of bleeding on CT were separately distinguished amongst a greater group with SAH and a negative angiogram. In the first, 36 such patients were identified (Rinkel *et al.*, 1991a). In the initial hospital period, rebleeding occurred in three (two of whom died), delayed cerebral ischaemia in one and symptomatic hydrocephalus in five patients. The patient who survived her rebleed underwent exploratory craniotomy at the suspected site of the aneurysm (on the middle cerebral artery) and the aneurysm was indeed found and clipped. On long-term follow-up, another patient rebled and died. One further patient suddenly developed an oculomotor palsy on the side where an aneurysm of the internal carotid artery had been suspected during the initial period of admission, but which had not been found on two angiographic studies. A third angiogram, at the time of the oculomotor palsy, finally showed the expected aneurysm, which was successfully clipped. Thus, not only had three of the 36 patients died, but another four remained incapacitated. Similarly, in the second study, 35 patients with a negative angiogram despite an aneurysmal pattern of haemorrhage on CT were followed for more than 2 years: three patients rebled (fatally in one case), two had delayed cerebral ischaemia and four had hydrocephalus (Canhao *et al.*, 1995). The occurrence of all these complications is in stark contrast to patients with a non-aneurysmal (perimesencephalic) pattern of haemorrhage, in whom death and disability from neurological causes do not occur.

The substantial rate of rebleeding in patients with an aneurysmal pattern of haemorrhage indicates that at least in some patients an aneurysm escapes radiological detection. Apart from technical reasons, such as insufficient use of oblique projections, this phenomenon may have several explanations. Narrowing of blood vessels by vasospasm has been invoked in some cases (Spetzler *et al.*, 1974; Bohmfalk & Story, 1980; Moritake *et al.*, 1981). Thrombosis of the neck of the aneurysm or of the entire sac is another possible reason (Edner *et al.*, 1978). Obliteration of the aneurysm by pressure of an adjacent haematoma may also occur, particularly with aneurysms of the anterior communicating artery (Di Lorenzo & Guidetti, 1988; Iwanaga *et al.*, 1990). Microaneurysms too small to be detected on angiography have also been implicated as a possible source of the haemorrhage but have rarely been demonstrated (Hayward, 1977; Spallone *et al.*, 1986).

Given the risk of a later rebleed, it is in patients with an aneurysmal pattern of haemorrhage on CT that repeat angiography seems most clearly indicated. The combined yield of a second angiogram in seven reported series was 22 aneurysms in 135 patients, or 16% (Ruelle *et al.*, 1985; Juul *et al.*, 1986; Spallone *et al.*, 1986; Suzuki *et al.*, 1987; Giombini *et al.*, 1988; Cioffi *et al.*, 1989; Iwanaga *et al.*, 1990). If it is taken into account that patients with perimesencephalic (non-aneurysmal) haemorrhage were not excluded from these series, the yield of repeat angiograms in patients with a diffuse or anteriorly located pattern of haemorrhage on CT scanning must be even higher. If a second angiogram also fails to demonstrate the suspected aneurysm, perhaps a third angiogram may be positive, after an interval of several months (Di Lorenzo & Guidetti, 1988; Rinkel *et al.*, 1991c). In a unique, consecutive series of 14 such patients subjected to a third angiogram, a single aneurysm was found (Suzuki *et al.*, 1987). MRI may in exceptional cases show the expected aneurysm, despite a normal angiogram (Pertuiset *et al.*, 1989; Renowden *et al.*, 1994). Spiral CT scanning with three-dimensional projection is an emerging technique, but its value in detecting 'occult' aneurysms has not yet transcended the stage of the case report (Dorsch *et al.*, 1995).

> *If angiography is completely negative (not only both internal carotid arteries but also both vertebral arteries having been injected) despite an aneurysmal pattern of haemorrhage on the CT scan, the search for a vascular lesion should be doggedly pursued (repeat angiography, spiral CT scanning, MRI).*

Few neurosurgeons perform exploratory craniotomy in patients with a suspected aneurysm despite repeatedly normal angiograms, but in those who do the rate of aneurysms found and obliterated seems satisfactory: five out of six in one report, the exception probably being a non-aneurysmal perimesencephalic haemorrhage (Jafar & Weiner, 1993). Such a course of action is especially indicated in patients with negative angiograms who nevertheless had, and survived, a rebleed.

Sudden headache with normal CT and normal CSF: should angiography be done?

If patients present within 1–2 weeks of an episode of sudden headache, the diagnostic value of a normal CT scan is very limited, but a lumbar puncture showing crystal-clear CSF will suffice to exclude SAH; at least with ruptured aneurysms, the CSF is invariably xanthochromic within this period (Vermeulen *et al.*, 1983, 1989). Nevertheless, the issue of distinguishing patients with non-haemorrhagic 'thunderclap headache' from those with ruptured aneurysms has been unnecessarily complicated by a few case reports of impressive but rare events. Ball (1975) found postmortem evidence of haemorrhage in the wall of an aneurysm, in a patient with a previous episode of headache. In addition, two patients with sudden headache and negative findings on CT as well as on lumbar puncture showed an aneurysm on cerebral angiography, accompanied by vasospasm; at operation no evidence of haemorrhage around the aneurysm was found, but it was claimed that the aneurysm had suddenly

enlarged, without rupturing (Day & Raskin, 1986; Clarke *et al.*, 1988). On the other hand, a follow-up study of 71 patients with non-haemorrhagic 'thunderclap headache', for an average period of 3.3 years, failed to produce a single episode of SAH; 12 patients had identical recurrences, but again without evidence of SAH, and 31 subsequently had regular episodes of tension headache or common migraine (Wijdicks *et al.*, 1988). It should be kept in mind that in the course of life a few per cent of all adults develop asymptomatic aneurysms (Chason & Hindman, 1958; Stehbens, 1963; McCormick & Nofzinger, 1965), and indiscriminate use of angiography is bound to uncover some of these. If it is assumed that the aneurysm was incidental in the two case reports cited above, migraine might explain both the headache and the development of vasospasm. Segmental and fully reversible vasospasm has been demonstrated in patients with severe headache but without an aneurysm (Call *et al.*, 1988). Haemorrhage confined to the wall of an aneurysm may indeed have occurred in an occasional patient but must be exceedingly rare amongst all patients with sudden headache. Cerebral angiography carries a permanent stroke rate of approxmately 1% (Hankey *et al.*, 1990). 'Thunderclap headache' does not warrant this potentially dangerous procedure if both the CT scan and the CSF are normal within 2 weeks of the event.

> *If a patient presents with a sudden severe headache and the CT scan and lumbar puncture are carried out in less than 2 weeks and are completely normal, with no evidence of intracranial haemorrhage, then cerebral angiography is not indicated.*

Late presentation with a history of sudden headache

A patient may present a few weeks or more after what sounds like a possible SAH (headache within a split second, lasting more than 2 hours). First of all, if the interval is between 2 and 6 weeks, a lumbar puncture may still show xanthochromia (Vermeulen *et al.*, 1989), but a normal CSF certainly does not exclude SAH. If there has been associated loss of consciousness, the probability of a ruptured aneurysm is considerable, and there is a good case for angiography or at least spiral CT scanning with intravenous contrast (see Section 9.4.1). If headache was the only symptom, the probability of SAH is approximately 10% (Linn *et al.*, 1994). In that case, we would opt for MRA with three-dimensional image projections (see Section 9.4.3). Given that the sensitivity of this technique is 80–90%, a normal MRA would leave a 1% risk of an undetected aneurysm, in someone whose chance of rebleeding, at that stage, is steadily decreasing towards an annual rate of 3%.

The disadvantages of catheter angiography probably outweigh the small residual risk of rebleeding after a normal MRA study.

References

Acciarri N, Padovani R, Pozzati E, Gaist G, Manetto V (1992). Spinal cavernous angioma: a rare cause of subarachnoid hemorrhage. *Surg Neurol* 37: 453–6.

Adams HP Jr, Aschenbrener CA, Kassell NF, Ansbacher L, Cornell SH (1982). Intracranial hemorrhage produced by spontaneous dissecting intracranial aneurysm. *Arch Neurol* 39: 773–6.

Adamson J, Humphries SE, Ostergaard JR, Voldby B, Richards P, Powell JT (1994). Are cerebral aneurysms atherosclerotic? *Stroke* 25: 963–6.

Alberts MJ, Quinones A, Graffagnino C, Friedman A, Roses AD (1995). Risk of intracranial aneurysms in families with subarachnoid hemorrhage. *Can J Neurol Sci* 22: 121–5.

Alliez B, Du Lac P, Trabulsi R (1990). [Extracranial aneurysm of the posterior inferior cerebellar artery: a case report] Anévrysme extra-cranien de l'artère cérébelleuse postéro-inférieure: une observation. *Neurochirurgie* 36: 137–40.

Aminoff MJ (1973). Vascular anomalies in the intracranial dura mater. *Brain* 96: 601–12.

Aminoff MJ, Logue V (1974). Clinical features of spinal vascular malformations. *Brain* 97: 197–210.

Anonymous (1988). Case records of the Massachusetts General Hospital. Weekly clinicopathological exercises. Case 7-1988: a 27-year-old man with acute myelomonocytic leukemia in remission and repeated intracranial hemorrhages. *N Engl J Med* 318: 427–40.

Aoki N (1991). Do intracranial arteriovenous malformations cause subarachnoid haemorrhage? Review of computed tomography features of ruptured arteriovenous malformations in the acute stage. *Acta Neurochir Wien* 112: 92–5.

Aoki N, Sakai T (1990). Rebleeding from intracranial dissecting aneurysm in the vertebral artery. *Stroke* 21: 1628–31.

Araki Y, Kohmura E, Tsukaguchi I (1994). A pitfall in detection of intracranial unruptured aneurysms on three-dimensional phase-contrast MR angiography. *Am J Neuroradiol* 15: 1618–23.

Artiola i Fortuny L, Adams CB, Briggs M (1980). Surgical mortality in an aneurysm population: effects of age, blood pressure and preoperative neurological state. *J Neurol Neurosurg Psychiatr* 43: 879–82.

Atlas SW (1993). MR imaging is highly sensitive for acute subarachnoid hemorrhage . . . not? *Radiology* 186: 319–22.

Atlas SW, Listerud J, Chung W, Flamm ES (1994). Intracranial aneurysms: depiction on MR angiograms with a multifeature-extraction, ray-tracing postprocessing algorithm. *Radiology* 192: 129–39.

Auffray E, de Kersaint Gilly A, Havet T *et al.* (1994). Contribution of MR-angiography to the diagnosis and the therapeutic indication and follow-up of intracranial aneurysms. *J Neuroradiol* 21: 17–29.

Bailes JE, Spetzler RF, Hadley MN, Baldwin HZ (1990). Management morbidity and mortality of poor-grade aneurysm patients. *J Neurosurg* 72: 559–66.

Ball MJ (1975). Pathogenesis of the 'sentinel headache' preceding berry aneurysm rupture. *Can Med Assoc J* 112: 78–9.

Bamford J, Hodges J, Warlow C (1986). Late rupture of a mycotic aneurysm after 'cure' of bacterial endocarditis. *J Neurol* 233: 51–3.

Bannerman RM, Ingall GB, Graf CJ (1970). The familial occurrence of intracranial aneurysms. *Neurology* 20: 283–92.

Barkovich AJ, Atlas SW (1988). Magnetic resonance imaging of intracranial hemorrhage. *Radiol Clin North Am* 26: 801–20.

Barth A, De Tribolet N (1994). Growth of small saccular aneurysms to giant aneurysms: presentation of three cases. *Surg Neurol* 41: 277–80.

Baumgartner RW, Mattle HP, Kothbauer K, Schroth G (1994). Transcranial color-coded duplex sonography in cerebral aneurysms. *Stroke* 25: 2429–34.

Bjerre P, Videbaek H, Lindholm J (1986). Subarachnoid hemorrhage with normal cerebral angiography: a prospective study on sellar abnormalities and pituitary function. *Neurosurgery* 19: 1012–15.

Bohmfalk GL, Story JL (1980). Intermittent appearance of a ruptured cerebral aneurysm on sequential angiograms: case report. *J Neurosurg* 52: 263–5.

Bonito V, Agostinis C, Ferraresi S, Defanti CA (1994). Superficial siderosis of the central nervous system after brachial plexus injury: case report. *J Neurosurg* 80: 931–4.

Bontozoglou N, Spanos H, Lasjaunias P, Zarifis G (1994). Three-dimensional display of the orifice of intracranial aneurysms: a new potential application for magnetic resonance angiography. *Neuroradiology* 36: 346–9.

Botterell EH, Lougheed WM, Scott JW, Vandewater SL (1956). Hypothermia, and interruption of carotid, or carotid and vertebral circulation, in the surgical management of intracranial aneurysms. *J Neurosurg* 13: 1–42.

Bromberg JEC, Rinkel GJE, Algra A *et al.* (1995a). Subarachnoid haemorrhage in first and second degree relatives of patients with subarachnoid haemorrhage. *Br Med J* 311: 288–9.

Bromberg JEC, Rinkel GJE, Algra A, Limburg M, Van Gijn J (1995b). Outcome in familial subarachnoid hemorrhage. *Stroke* 26: 961–3.

Brott T, Mandybur TI (1986). Case–control study of clinical outcome after aneurysmal subarachnoid hemorrhage. *Neurosurgery* 19: 891–5.

Brown RD Jr, Wiebers DO, Forbes GS (1990). Unruptured intracranial aneurysms and arteriovenous malformations: frequency of intracranial hemorrhage and relationship of lesions. *J Neurosurg* 73: 859–63.

Bruno A, Nolte KB, Chapin J (1993). Stroke associated with ephedrine use. *Neurology* 43: 1313–16.

Brust JC, Dickinson PC, Hughes JE, Holtzman RN (1990). The diagnosis and treatment of cerebral mycotic aneurysms. *Ann*

Neurol 27: 238–46.

Call GK, Fleming MC, Sealfon S, Levine H, Kistler JP, Fisher CM (1988). Reversible cerebral segmental vasoconstriction. *Stroke* 19: 1159–70.

Canhao P, Ferro JM, Pinto AM, Melo TP, Campos JG (1995). Perimesencephalic and nonperimesencephalic subarachnoid haemorrhages with negative angiograms. *Acta Neurochir Wien* 132: 14–19.

Caplan LR, Baquis GD, Pessin MS *et al.* (1988). Dissection of the intracranial vertebral artery. *Neurology* 38: 868–77.

Carey J, Numaguchi Y, Nadell J (1990). Subarachnoid hemorrhage in sickle cell disease. *Child Nerv Syst* 6: 47–50.

Caroscio JT, Brannan T, Budabin M, Huang YP, Yahr MD (1980). Subarachnoid hemorrhage secondary to spinal arteriovenous malformation and aneurysm: report of a case and review of the literature. *Arch Neurol* 37: 101–3.

Chapman AB, Rubinstein D, Hughes R *et al.* (1992). Intracranial aneurysms in autosomal dominant polycystic kidney disease. *N Engl J Med* 327: 916–20.

Chason JL, Hindman WM (1958). Berry aneurysms of the circle of Willis: results of a planned autopsy study. *Neurology* 8: 41–4.

Chaudhary MY, Sachdev VP, Cho SH, Weitzner I Jr, Puljic S, Huang YP (1982). Dural arteriovenous malformation of the major venous sinuses: an acquired lesion. *Am J Neuroradiol* 3: 13–19.

Cioffi F, Pasqualin A, Cavazzani P, Da Pian R (1989). Subarachnoid haemorrhage of unknown origin: clinical and tomographical aspects. *Acta Neurochir Wien* 97: 31–9.

Clarke CE, Shepherd DI, Chishti K, Victoratos G (1988). Thunderclap headache [letter]. *Lancet* ii: 625.

Clarke E, Walton JN (1953). Subdural haematoma complicating intracranial aneurysm and angioma. *Brain* 76: 378–404.

Crompton MR (1966). The pathogenesis of cerebral aneurysms. *Brain* 89: 797–814.

D'Angelo V, Bizzozero L, Talamonti G, Ferrara M, Colombo N (1990). Value of magnetic resonance imaging in spontaneous extradural spinal hematoma due to vascular malformation: case report. *Surg Neurol* 34: 343–4.

Darby DG, Donnan GA, Saling MA, Walsh KW, Bladin PF (1988). Primary intraventricular hemorrhage: clinical and neuropsychological findings in a prospective stroke series. *Neurology* 38: 68–75.

Day JW, Raskin NH (1986). Thunderclap headache: symptom of unruptured cerebral aneurysm. *Lancet* ii: 1247–8.

Di Chiro G, Brooks RA, Girton ME *et al.* (1986). Sequential MR studies of intracerebral hematomas in monkeys. *Am J Neuroradiol* 7: 193–9.

Di Lorenzo N, Guidetti G (1988). Anterior communicating aneurysm missed at angiography: report of two cases treated surgically. *Neurosurgery* 23: 494–9.

Dion JE, Gates PC, Fox AJ, Barnett HJM, Blom RJ (1987). Clinical events following neuroangiography: a prospective study. *Stroke* 18: 997–1004.

Donahue RP, Abbott RD, Reed DM, Yano K (1986). Alcohol and hemorrhagic stroke: the Honolulu Heart Program. *J Am Med Assoc* 255: 2311–14.

Donnet A, Balzamo M, Royere ML, Grisoli F, Ali Cherif A (1992). [Transient Korsakoff's syndrome after intraventricular hemorrhage] Syndrome de Korsakoff transitoire au decours d'une hémorragie intraventriculaire. *Neurochirurgie* 38: 102–4.

Dorsch NW, Young N, Kingston RJ, Compton JS (1995). Early experience with spiral CT in the diagnosis of intracranial aneurysms. *Neurosurgery* 36: 230–6.

Dowling G, Curry B (1988). Traumatic basal subarachnoid hemorrhage: report of six cases and review of the literature. *Am J Forensic Med Pathol* 9: 23–31.

Drake CG (1979). Giant intracranial aneurysms: experience with surgical treatment in 174 patients. *Clin Neurosurg* 26: 12–95.

Drake CG, Hunt WE, Sano K *et al.* (1988). Report of World Federation of Neurological Surgeons Committee on a Universal Subarachnoid Hemorrhage Grading Scale. *J Neurosurg* 68: 985–6.

Edner G, Forster DM, Steiner L, Bergvall U (1978). Spontaneous healing intracranial aneurysms after subarachnoid hemorrhage: case report. *J Neurosurg* 48: 450–4.

Estol CJ, Pessin MS, Martinez AJ (1991). Cerebrovascular complications after orthotopic liver transplantation: a clinicopathologic study. *Neurology* 41: 815–19.

Farrés MT, Ferraz Leite H, Schindler E, Mühlbauer M (1992). Spontaneous subarachnoid hemorrhage with negative angiography: CT findings. *J Comput Assist Tomogr* 16: 534–7.

Fearnley JM, Stevens JM, Rudge P (1995). Superficial siderosis of the central nervous system. *Brain* 118: 1051–66.

Ferbert A, Hubo I, Biniek R (1992). Non-traumatic subarachnoid hemorrhage with normal angiogram: long-term follow-up and CT predictors of complications. *J Neurol Sci* 107: 14–18.

Ferry PC, Kerber C, Peterson D, Gallo AA Jr (1974). Arteriectasis, subarachnoid hemorrhage in a three-month-old infant. *Neurology* 24: 494–500.

Finney LH, Roberts TS, Anderson RE (1976). Giant intracranial aneurysm associated with Marfan's syndrome: case report. *J Neurosurg* 45: 342–7.

Fisher CM (1975). Clinical syndromes in cerebral thrombosis, hypertensive hemorrhage, and ruptured saccular aneurysm. *Clin Neurosurg* 22: 117–47.

Fogelholm R, Nuutila M, Vuorela AL (1992). Primary intracerebral haemorrhage in the Jyvaskyla region, central Finland, 1985–89: incidence, case fatality rate, and functional outcome. *J Neurol Neurosurg Psychiatry* 55: 546–52.

Fox MW, Harms RW, Davis DH (1990). Selected neurologic complications of pregnancy. *Mayo Clin Proc* 65: 1595–618.

Fransen P, De Tribolet N (1994). Dissecting aneurysm of the posterior inferior cerebellar artery. *Br J Neurosurg* 8: 381–6.

Friedman AH, Drake CG (1984). Subarachnoid hemorrhage from intracranial dissecting aneurysm. *J Neurosurg* 60: 325–34.

Friedman MB, Brant Zawadzki M (1983). Interhemispheric subdural hematoma from ruptured aneurysm. *Comput Radiol* 7: 129–34.

Furuya K, Sasaki T, Yoshimoto Y, Okada Y, Fujimaki T, Kirino T (1995). Histologically verified cerebral aneurysm formation secondary to embolism from cardiac myxoma: case report. *J Neurosurg* 83: 170–3.

Futatsuya R, Seto H, Kamei T *et al.* (1994). Clinical utility of three-dimensional time-of-flight magnetic resonance angiography for the evaluation of intracranial aneurysms. *Clin Imaging* 18: 101–6.

Gates PC, Barnett HJM, Vinters HV, Simonsen RL, Siu K (1986). Primary intraventricular hemorrhage in adults. *Stroke* 17: 872–7.

Giombini S, Bruzzone MG, Pluchino F (1988). Subarachnoid hemorrhage of unexplained cause. *Neurosurgery* 22: 313–16.

Glynn LE (1940). Medial defects in the circle of Willis and their relation to aneurysm formation. *J Pathol Bacteriol* 51: 213–22.

Greene KA, Marciano FF, Dickman CA *et al.* (1995). Anterior communicating artery aneurysm paraparesis syndrome: clinical manifestations and pathologic correlates. *Neurology* 45: 45–50.

Griffiths PD, Gholkar A, Sengupta RP (1994). Oculomotor nerve palsy due to thrombosis of a posterior communicating artery aneurysm following diagnostic angiography. *Neuroradiology* 36: 614–15.

Guridi J, Gallego J, Monzon F, Aguilera F (1993). Intracerebral hemorrhage caused by transmural dissection of the anterior cerebral artery. *Stroke* 24: 1400–2.

Halbach VV, Higashida RT, Hieshima GB, Goto K, Norman D, Newton TH (1987). Dural fistulas involving the transverse and sigmoid sinuses: results of treatment in 28 patients. *Radiology* 163: 443–7.

Hamada J, Hashimoto N, Tsukahara T (1994). Moyamoya disease with repeated intraventricular hemorrhage due to aneurysm rupture: report of two cases. *J Neurosurg* 80: 328–31.

Handa T, Suzuki Y, Saito K, Sugita K, Patel SJ (1992). Isolated intramedullary spinal artery aneurysm presenting with quadriplegia: case report. *J Neurosurg* 77: 148–50.

Hankey GJ (1991). Isolated angiitis/angiopathy of the central nervous sytem. *Cerebrovasc Dis* 1: 2–15.

Hankey GJ, Warlow CP, Sellar RJ (1990). Cerebral angiographic risk in mild cerebrovascular disease. *Stroke* 21: 209–22.

Harland WA, Pitts JF, Watson AA (1983). Subarachnoid haemorrhage due to upper cervical trauma. *J Clin Pathol* 36: 1335–41.

Hart RG, Byer JA, Slaughter JR, Hewett JE, Easton JD (1981). Occurrence and implications of seizures in subarachnoid hemorrhage due to ruptured intracranial aneurysms. *Neurosurgery* 8: 417–21.

Hart RG, Foster JW, Luther MF, Kanter MC (1990). Stroke in infective endocarditis. *Stroke* 21: 695–700.

Hasan D, Schonck RS, Avezaat CJ, Tanghe HL, Van Gijn J, van der Lugt PJ (1993). Epileptic seizures after subarachnoid hemorrhage. *Ann Neurol* 33: 286–91.

Hassler OL (1962). Physiological intima cushions in the large cerebral arteries of young individuals. Part I. Morphological structure and possible significance for the circulation. *Acta Pathol Microbiol Scand* 55: 19–27.

Hayakawa I, Watanabe T, Tsuchida T, Sasaki A (1978). Perangiographic rupture of intracranial aneurysms. *Neuroradiology* 16: 293–5.

Hayward RD (1977). Subarachnoid haemorrhage of unknown aetiology: a clinical and radiological study of 51 cases. *J Neurol Neurosurg Psychiatr* 40: 926–31.

Hayward RD, O'Reilly GV (1976). Intracerebral haemorrhage: accuracy of computerised transverse axial scanning in predicting the underlying aetiology. *Lancet* i: 1–4.

Hijdra A, Van Gijn J (1982). Early death from rupture of an intracranial aneurysm. *J Neurosurg* 57: 765–8.

Hijdra A, Braakman R, Van Gijn J, Vermeulen M, van Crevel H (1987). Aneurysmal subarachnoid hemorrhage: complications and outcome in a hospital population. *Stroke* 18: 1061–7.

Hijdra A, Van Gijn J, Nagelkerke NJ, Vermeulen M, van Crevel H (1988). Prediction of delayed cerebral ischemia, rebleeding, and outcome after aneurysmal subarachnoid hemorrhage. *Stroke* 19: 1250–6.

Hijdra A, Van Gijn J, Stefanko S, van Dongen KJ, Vermeulen M, van Crevel H (1986). Delayed cerebral ischemia after aneurysmal subarachnoid hemorrhage: clinicoanatomic correlations. *Neurology* 36: 329–33.

Hillman J (1993). Selective angiography for early aneurysm detection in acute subarachnoid haemorrhage. *Acta Neurochir Wien* 121: 20–5.

Hochberg FH, Fisher CM, Roberson GH (1974). Subarachnoid hemorrhage caused by rupture of a small superficial artery. *Neurology* 24: 319–21.

Horikoshi T, Fukamachi A, Nishi H, Fukasawa I (1994). Detection of intracranial aneurysms by three-dimensional time-of-flight magnetic resonance angiography. *Neuroradiology* 36: 203–7.

Hosoda K, Fujita S, Kawaguchi T, Shose Y, Hamano S (1995). Saccular aneurysms of the proximal (M1) segment of the middle cerebral artery. *Neurosurgery* 36: 441–6.

Houkin K, Aoki T, Takahashi A, Abe H, Koiwa M, Kashiwaba T (1994). Magnetic resonance angiography (MRA) of ruptured cerebral aneurysm. *Acta Neurochir Wien* 128: 132–6.

Housepian EM, Pool JL (1958). Systematic analysis of intracranial aneurysms from the autopsy file of the Presbyterian Hospital 1914 to 1956. *J Neuropathol Exp Neurol* 17: 409–29.

Hunt WE, Hess RM (1968). Surgical risk as related to time of intervention in the repair of intracranial aneurysms. *J Neurosurg* 28: 14–20.

Huston J, Nichols DA, Luetmer PH *et al.* (1994). Blinded prospective evaluation of sensitivity of MR angiography to known intracranial aneurysms: importance of aneurysm size. *Am J Neuroradiol* 15: 1607–14.

Hyland HH, Barnett HJM (1954). The pathogenesis of cranial nerve palsies associated with intracranial aneurysms. *Proc Roy Soc Med* 47: 141–6.

Ikawa F, Sumida M, Uozumi T *et al.* (1994). Comparison of three-dimensional phase-contrast magnetic resonance angiography with three-dimensional time-of-flight magnetic resonance angiography in cerebral aneurysms. *Surg Neurol* 42: 287–92.

Imanse J, Vanneste J (1990). Intraventricular hemorrhage following amphetamine abuse. *Neurology* 40: 1318–19.

Iwanaga H, Wakai S, Ochiai C, Narita J, Inoh S, Nagai M (1990).

Ruptured cerebral aneurysms missed by initial angiographic study. *Neurosurgery* 27: 45–51.

Jackson A, Fitzgerald JB, Hartley RW, Leonard A, Yates J (1993). CT appearances of haematomas in the corpus callosum in patients with subarachnoid haemorrhage. *Neuroradiology* 35: 420–3.

Jafar JJ, Weiner HL (1993). Surgery for angiographically occult cerebral aneurysms. *J Neurosurg* 79: 674–9.

Jenkins A, Hadley DM, Teasdale GM, Condon B, Macpherson P, Patterson J (1988). Magnetic resonance imaging of acute subarachnoid hemorrhage. *J Neurosurg* 68: 731–6.

Joslyn JN, Williams JP, White JL, White RL (1985). Simultaneous rupture of two intracranial aneurysms: CT diagnosis. *Stroke* 16: 518–21.

Juul R, Fredriksen TA, Ringkjob R (1986). Prognosis in subarachnoid hemorrhage of unknown etiology. *J Neurosurg* 64: 359–62.

Kamiya K, Inagawa T, Yamaoto M, Monden S (1991). Subdural hematoma due to ruptured intracranial aneurysm. *Neurol Med Chir Tokyo* 31: 82–6.

Kandel EI (1980). Complete excision of arteriovenous malformations of the cervical cord. *Surg Neurol* 13: 135–9.

Kaplan SS, Ogilvy CS, Gonzalez R, Gress D, Pile Spellman J (1993). Extracranial vertebral artery pseudoaneurysm presenting as subarachnoid hemorrhage. *Stroke* 24: 1397–9.

Kassell NF, Torner JC, Jane JA, Haley EC Jr, Adams HP (1990). The International Cooperative Study on the Timing of Aneurysm Surgery. Part 2: surgical results. *J Neurosurg* 73: 37–47.

Kataoka K, Taneda M (1984). Angiographic disappearance of multiple dural arteriovenous malformations: case report. *J Neurosurg* 60: 1275–8.

Kayama T, Sugawara T, Sakurai Y, Ogawa A, Onuma T, Yoshimoto T (1991). Early CT features of ruptured cerebral aneurysms of the posterior cranial fossa. *Acta Neurochir Wien* 108: 34–9.

Kayembe KN, Sasahara M, Hazama F (1984). Cerebral aneurysms and variations in the circle of Willis. *Stroke* 15: 846–50.

Kendall BE, Lee BC, Claveria E (1976). Computerized tomography and angiography in subarachnoid haemorrhage. *Br J Radiol* 49: 483–501.

Kissel JT, Burde RM, Klingele TG, Zeiger HE (1983). Pupil-sparing oculomotor palsies with internal carotid-posterior communicating artery aneurysms. *Ann Neurol* 13: 149–54.

Kitahara T, Ohwada T, Tokiwa K *et al.* (1993). [Clinical study in patients with perimesencephalic subarachnoid hemorrhage of unknown etiology]. *No Shinkei Geka* 21: 903–8.

Knekt P, Reunanen A, Aho K *et al.* (1991). Risk factors for subarachnoid hemorrhage in a longitudinal population study. *J Clin Epidemiol* 44: 933–9.

Koenig GH, Marshall WH Jr, Poole GJ, Kramer RA (1979). Rupture of intracranial aneurysms during cerebral angiography: report of ten cases and review of the literature. *Neurosurgery* 5: 314–24.

Kondziolka D, Bernstein M, ter Brugge K, Schutz H (1988). Acute subdural hematoma from ruptured posterior communicating artery aneurysm. *Neurosurgery* 22: 151–4.

Konishi Y, Kadowaki C, Hara M, Takeuchi K (1985). Aneurysms associated with moyamoya disease. *Neurosurgery* 16: 484–91.

Korogi Y, Takahashi M, Mabuchi N *et al.* (1994). Intracranial aneurysms: diagnostic accuracy of three-dimensional. Fourier transform, time-of-flight MR angiography. *Radiology* 193: 181–6.

Krendel DA, Ditter SM, Frankel MR, Ross WK (1990). Biopsy-proven cerebral vasculitis associated with cocaine abuse. *Neurology* 40: 1092–4.

Kunze S, Schiefer W (1971). Angiographic demonstration of a dissecting aneurysm of the middle cerebral artery. *Neuroradiology* 2: 201–6.

Lance JW (1976). Headaches related to sexual activity. *J Neurol Neurosurg Psychiatr* 39: 1226–30.

Lasjaunias P, Chiu M, ter Brugge K, Tolia A, Hurth M, Bernstein M (1986). Neurological manifestations of intracranial dural arteriovenous malformations. *J Neurosurg* 64: 724–30.

Lau AHC, Takeshita M, Ishii M (1991). Mycotic (*Aspergillus*) arteriitis resulting in fatal subarachnoid hemorrhage: a case report. *Angiology* 42: 251–5.

Lavin PJ, Troost BT (1984). Traumatic fourth nerve palsy: clinicoanatomic correlations with computed tomographic scan. *Arch Neurol* 41: 679–80.

Levine SR, Brust JC, Futrell N *et al.* (1990). Cerebrovascular complications of the use of the 'crack' form of alkaloidal cocaine. *N Engl J Med* 323: 699–704.

Lim ST, Sage DJ (1977). Detection of subarachnoid blood clot and other thin, flat structures by computed tomography. *Radiology* 123: 79–84.

Lindsay KW, Teasdale GM, Knill Jones RP (1983). Observer variability in assessing the clinical features of subarachnoid hemorrhage. *J Neurosurg* 58: 57–62.

Lindsay KW, Teasdale G, Knill Jones RP, Murray L (1982). Observer variability in grading patients with subarachnoid hemorrahge. *J Neurosurg* 56: 628–33.

Linn FHH, Wijdicks EFM, van der Graaf Y, Weerdesteyn-van Vliet FA, Bartelds AI, Van Gijn J (1994). Prospective study of sentinel headache in aneurysmal subarachnoid haemorrhage. *Lancet* 344: 590–3.

Little JR, Blomquist GA Jr, Ethier R (1977). Intraventricular hemorrhage in adults. *Surg Neurol* 8: 143–9.

Logue V (1979). Angiomas of the spinal cord: review of the pathogenesis, clinical features, and results of surgery. *J Neurol Neurosurg Psychiatr* 42: 1–11.

Love LC, Mickle JP, Sypert GW (1985). Ruptured intracranial aneurysms in cases of sickle cell anemia. *Neurosurgery* 16: 808–12.

McCormick WF (1971). Problems and pathogenesis of intracranial arterial aneurysms. In: Toole JF, Mossy J, Janeway R, eds. *Cerebral Vascular Diseases*. New York: Grune & Stratton, 219–31

McCormick WF, Nofzinger JD (1965). Saccular intracranial aneurysms—an autopsy study. *J Neurosurg* 22: 155–9.

McFadzean RM, Doyle D, Rampling R, Teasdale E, Teasdale G (1991). Pituitary apoplexy and its effect on vision. *Neurosurgery* 29: 669–75.

Mangiardi JR, Daras M, Geller ME, Weitzner I, Tuchman AJ (1988). Cocaine-related intracranial hemorrhage: report of nine cases and review. *Acta Neurol Scand* 77: 177–80.

Marks MP, Lane B, Steinberg GK, Snipes GJ (1992). Intranidal aneurysms in cerebral arteriovenous malformations: evaluation and endovascular treatment. *Radiology* 183: 355–60.

Masson C, Martin N, Masson M, Cambier J (1986). [Intraventricular hemorrhage after carotid endarterectomy: role of moyamoya-type collateral circulation] Hémorrhagie intraventriculaire après endartériectomie carotidienne: rôle des suppléances de type moya moya. *Rev Neurol Paris* 142: 716–19.

Masson EA, Atkin SL, Diver M, White MC (1993). Pituitary apoplexy and sudden blindness following the administration of gonadotrophin releasing hormone. *Clin Endocrinol Oxf* 38: 109–10.

Massoud TF, Anslow P, Molyneux AJ (1992). Subarachnoid hemorrhage following spontaneous intracranial carotid artery dissection. *Neuroradiology* 34: 33–5.

Masuda J, Yutani C, Waki R, Ogata J, Kuriyama Y, Yamaguchi T (1992). Histopathological analysis of the mechanisms of intracranial hemorrhage complicating infective endocarditis. *Stroke* 23: 843–50.

Matsumura K, Matsuda M, Handa J, Todo G (1990). Magnetic resonance imaging with aneurysmal subarachnoid hemorrhage: comparison with computed tomography scan. *Surg Neurol* 34: 71–8.

Mattle H, Kohler S, Huber P, Rohner M, Steinsiepe KF (1989). Anticoagulation-related intracranial extracerebral haemorrhage. *J Neurol Neurosurg Psychiatr* 52: 829–37.

Mizukami M, Kawase T, Usami T, Tazawa T (1982). Prevention of vasospasm by early operation with removal of subarachnoid blood. *Neurosurgery* 10: 301–7.

Mizutani T, Aruga T, Kirino T, Miki Y, Saito I, Tsuchida T (1995). Recurrent subarachnoid hemorrhage from untreated ruptured vertebrobasilar dissecting aneurysms. *Neurosurgery* 36: 905–13.

Mohsenipour I, Ortler M, Twerdy K, Schmutzhard E, Attlmayr G, Aichner F (1994). Isolated aneurysm of a spinal radicular artery presenting as spinal subarachnoid haemorrhage [letter]. *J Neurol Neurosurg Psychiatr* 57: 767–8.

Mokri B, Houser OW, Sandok BA, Piepgras DG (1988). Spontaneous dissections of the vertebral arteries. *Neurology* 38: 880–5.

Moritake K, Handa H, Ohtsuka S, Hashimoto N (1981). Vanishing cerebral aneurysm in serial angiography. *Surg Neurol* 16: 36–40.

Muhonen MG, Godersky JC, VanGilder JC (1991). Cerebral aneurysms associated with neurofibromatosis. *Surg Neurol* 36: 470–5.

Munyer TP, Margulis AR (1981). Pseudoxanthoma elasticum with internal carotid artery aneurysm. *Am J Roentgenol* 136: 1023–4.

Nachanakian A, Gardeur D, Poisson M, Philippon J (1983). [Spontaneous intraventricular hemorrhage secondary to meningioma] Hémorrhagie intra-ventriculaire spontanée secondaire à un méningiome. *Neurochirurgie* 29: 47–9.

Nadeau SE, Trobe JD (1983). Pupil sparing in oculomotor palsy: a brief review. *Ann Neurol* 13: 143–8.

Nagamine Y, Takahashi S, Sonobe M (1981). Multiple intracranial aneurysms associated with moyamoya disease: case report. *J Neurosurg* 54: 673–6.

Nakagawa T, Hashi K (1994). The incidence and treatment of asymptomatic, unruptured cerebral aneurysms. *J Neurosurg* 80: 217–23.

Nakayama Y, Tanaka A, Yoshinaga S, Tomonaga M, Maehara F, Ohkawa M (1989). Multiple intracerebral arteriovenous malformations: report of two cases. *Neurosurgery* 25: 281–6.

Nishioka H (1966). Report on the cooperative study of intracranial aneurysms and subarachnoid hemorrhage. Section VII. I. Evaluation of the conservative management of ruptured intracranial aneurysms. *J Neurosurg* 25: 574–92.

Noguchi K, Ogawa T, Inugami A, Toyoshima H, Okudera T, Uemura K (1994). MR of acute subarachnoid hemorrhage: a preliminary report of fluid-attenuated inversion-recovery pulse sequences. *Am J Neuroradiol* 15: 1940–3.

Nohjoh T, Houkin K, Takahashi A, Abe H (1995). Ruptured dissecting vertebral artery aneurysm detected by repeated angiography: case report. *Neurosurgery* 36: 180–2.

Norrgard O, Angquist KA, Fodstad H, Forsell A, Lindberg M (1987). Intracranial aneurysms and heredity. *Neurosurgery* 20: 236–9.

Oana K, Murakami T, Beppu T, Yamaura A, Kanaya H (1991). Aneurysm of the distal anterior inferior cerebellar artery unrelated to the cerebellopontine angle: case report. *Neurosurgery* 28: 899–903.

O'Boynick P, Green KD, Batnitzky S, Kepes JJ, Pietak R (1994). Aneurysm of the left middle cerebral artery caused by myxoid degeneration of the vessel wall. *Stroke* 25: 2283–6.

Ogawa T, Inugami A, Shimosegawa E *et al.* (1993). Subarachnoid hemorrhage: evaluation with MR imaging. *Radiology* 186: 345–51.

Öhman J, Heiskanen O (1989). Timing of operation for ruptured supratentorial aneurysms: a prospective randomized study. *J Neurosurg* 70: 55–60.

Okamoto S, Handa H, Hashimoto N (1984). Location of intracranial aneurysms associated with cerebral arteriovenous malformation: statistical analysis. *Surg Neurol* 22: 335–40.

O'Leary PM, Sweeny PJ (1986). Ruptured intracerebral aneurysm resulting in a subdural hematoma. *Ann Emerg Med* 15: 944–6.

Osenbach RK, Blumenkopf B, McComb B, Huggins MJ (1986). Ocular bobbing with ruptured giant distal posterior inferior cerebellar artery aneurysm. *Surg Neurol* 25: 149–52.

Overby MC, Rothman AS (1985). Multiple intracranial aneurysms in sickle cell anemia: report of two cases. *J Neurosurg* 62: 430–4.

Papa ML, Schisano G, Franco A, Nina P (1994). Congenital deficiency of factor VII in subarachnoid hemorrhage. *Stroke* 25: 508–10.

Pascual J, Diez C, Carda JR, Vazquez Barquero A (1987).

355

Intraventricular haemorrhage complicating a brain abscess. *Postgrad Med J* 63: 785–7.

Patrux B, Laissy JP, Jouini S, Kawiecki W, Coty P, Thiebot J (1994). Magnetic resonance angiography (MRA) of the circle of Willis: a prospective comparison with conventional angiography in 54 subjects. *Neuroradiology* 36: 193–7.

Pertuiset B, Haisa T, Bordi L, Abou Ouf S, Eissa M (1989). Detection of a ruptured aneurysmal sac by MRI in a case of negative angiogram. Successful clipping of an anterior communicating artery aneurysm: case report. *Acta Neurochir Wien* 100: 84–6.

Piepgras DG, McGrail KM, Tazelaar HD (1994). Intracranial dissection of the distal middle cerebral artery as an uncommon cause of distal cerebral artery aneurysm: case report. *J Neurosurg* 80: 909–13.

Pinto AN, Ferro JM, Canhao P, Campos J (1993). How often is a perimesencephalic subarachnoid haemorrhage CT pattern caused by ruptured aneurysms? *Acta Neurochir Wien* 124: 79–81.

Poon TP, Solis OG (1985). Sudden death due to massive intraventricular hemorrhage into an unsuspected ependymoma. *Surg Neurol* 24: 63–6.

Post MJ, David NJ, Glaser JS, Safran A (1980). Pituitary apoplexy: diagnosis by computed tomography. *Radiology* 134: 665–70.

Price DB, Miller LJ (1994). MR angiography of peripheral posterior inferior cerebellar artery aneurysms. *J Comput Assist Tomogr* 18: 539–41.

Quint DJ, Spickler EM (1990). Magnetic resonance demonstration of vertebral artery dissection: report of two cases. *J Neurosurg* 72: 964–7.

Ragland RL, Gelber ND, Wilkinson HA, Knorr JR, Tran AA (1993). Anterior communicating artery aneurysm rupture: an unusual cause of acute subdural hemorrhage. *Surg Neurol* 40: 400–2.

Reid RL, Quigley ME, Yen SS (1985). Pituitary apoplexy: a review. *Arch Neurol* 42: 712–19.

Renowden SA, Molyneux AJ, Anslow P, Byrne JV (1994). The value of MRI in angiogram-negative intracranial haemorrhage. *Neuroradiology* 36: 422–5.

Riggs HE, Rupp C (1943). Miliary aneurysms: relation of anomalies of the circle of Willis to formation of aneurysms. *Arch Neurol Psych* 49: 615–16.

Rinkel GJE, Van Gijn J, Wijdicks EFM (1993). Subarachnoid hemorrhage wihout detectable aneurysm: a review of the causes. *Stroke* 24: 1403–9.

Rinkel GJE, Wijdicks EFM, Ramos LMP, Van Gijn J (1990a). Progressin in acute hydrocephalus in subarachnoid haemorrhage: a case report documented by serial CT scanning. *J Neurol Neurosurg Psychiatr* 53: 354–5.

Rinkel GJE, Wijdicks EFM, Vermeulen M, Hageman LM, Tans JT, Van Gijn J (1990b). Outcome in perimesencephalic (nonaneurysmal) subarachnoid hemorrhage: a follow-up study in 37 patients. *Neurology* 40: 1130–2.

Rinkel GJE, Wijdicks EFM, Vermeulen M, Hasan D, Brouwers PJAM, Van Gijn J (1991b). The clinical course of perimesencephalic nonaneurysmal subarachnoid hemorrhage.

Ann Neurol 29: 463–8.

Rinkel GJE, Wijdicks EFM, Hasan D *et al.* (1991a). Outcome in patients with subarachnoid haemorrhage and negative angiography according to pattern of haemorrhage on computed tomography. *Lancet* 338: 964–8.

Rinkel GJE, Wijdicks EFM, Vermeulen M *et al.* (1991c). Nonaneurysmal perimesencephalic subarachnoid hemorrhage: CT and MR patterns that differ from aneurysmal rupture. *Am J Neuroradiol* 12: 829–34.

River Y, Honigman S, Gomori JM, Reches A (1994). Superficial hemosiderosis of the central nervous system. *Move Disord* 9: 559–62.

Robinson RG (1967). Coarctation of the aorta and cerebral aneurysm: report of two cases. *J Neurosurg* 26: 527–31.

Román G, Fisher M, Perl DP, Poser CM (1978). Neurological manifestations of hereditary hemorrhagic teleangiectasis (Rendu–Osler–Weber disease): report of two cases and review of the literature. *Ann Neurol* 4: 130–44.

Ronkainen A, Hernesniemi J, Tromp G (1995a). Special features of familial intracranial aneurysms: report of 215 familial aneurysms. *Neurosurgery* 37: 43–7.

Ronkainen A, Puranen MI, Hernesniemi JA *et al.* (1995b). Intracranial aneurysms: MR angiographic screening in 400 asymptomatic individuals with increased familial risk. *Radiology* 195: 35–40.

Roos YBWEM, Hasan D, Vermeulen M (1995). Outcome in patients with large intraventricular haemorrhages: a volumetric study. *J Neurol Neurosurg Psychiatr* 58: 622–4.

Ross JS, Masaryk TJ, Modic MT, Ruggieri PM, Haacke EM, Selman WR (1990). Intracranial aneurysms: evaluation by MR angiography. *Am J Roentgenol* 155: 159–65.

Rowley G, Fielding K (1991). Reliability and accuracy of the Glasgow Coma Scale with experienced and inexperienced users. *Lancet* 337: 535–8.

Ruelle A, Lasio G, Boccardo M, Gottlieb A, Severi P (1985). Long-term prognosis of subarachnoid hemorrhages of unknown etiology. *J Neurol* 232: 277–9.

Ruelle A, Cavazzani P, Andrioli G (1988). Extracranial posterior inferior cerebellar artery aneurysm causing isolated intraventricular hemorrhage: a case report. *Neurosurgery* 23: 774–7.

Ruggieri PM, Poulos N, Masaryk TJ *et al.* (1994). Occult intracranial aneurysms in polycystic kidney disease: screening with MR angiography. *Radiology* 191: 33–9.

Sacco RL, Wolf PA, Bharucha NE *et al.* (1984). Subarachnoid and intracerebral hemorrhage: natural history, prognosis, and precursive factors in the Framingham Study. *Neurology* 34: 847–54.

Sadato N, Numaguchi Y, Rigamonti D, Salcman M, Gellad FE, Kishikawa T (1991). Bleeding patterns in ruptured posterior fossa aneurysms: a CT study. *J Comput Assist Tomogr* 15: 612–17.

Sakas DE, Dias LS, Beale D (1995). Subarachnoid haemorrhage presenting as head injury. *Br Med J* 301: 1186–7.

Salgado AV, Furlan AJ, Keys TF (1987). Mycotic aneurysm,

subarachnoid hemorrhage, and indications for cerebral angiography in infective endocarditis. *Stroke* 18: 1057–60.

Sarner M, Rose FC (1967). Clinical presentation of ruptured intracranial aneurysm. *J Neurol Neurosurg Psychiatr* 30: 67–70.

Sasaki O, Koike T, Tanaka R, Ogawa H (1991a). Subarachnoid hemorrhage from a dissecting aneurysm of the middle cerebral artery: case report. *J Neurosurg* 74: 504–7.

Sasaki O, Ogawa H, Koike T, Koizumi T, Tanaka R (1991b). A clinicopathological study of dissecting aneurysms of the intracranial vertebral artery. *J Neurosurg* 75: 874–82.

Satoh S, Kadoya S (1988). Magnetic resonance imaging of subarachnoid hemorrhage. *Neuroradiology* 30: 361–6.

Schievink WI, Prakash UB, Piepgras DG, Mokri B (1994a). Alpha 1-antitrypsin deficiency in intracranial aneurysms and cervical artery dissection. *Lancet* 343: 452–3.

Schievink WI, Limburg M, Oorthuys JW, Fleury P, Pope FM (1990). Cerebrovascular disease in Ehlers–Danlos syndrome type IV. *Stroke* 21: 626–32.

Schievink WI, Schaid DJ, Rogers HM, Piepgras DG, Michels VV (1994c). On the inheritance of intracranial aneurysms. *Stroke* 25: 2028–37.

Schievink WI, Wijdicks EFM, Parisi JE, Piepgras DG, Whisnant JP (1995b). Sudden death from aneurysmal subarachnoid hemorrhage. *Neurology* 45: 871–4.

Schievink WI, Wijdicks EFM, Piepgras DG, Nichols DA, Ebersold MJ (1994b). Perimesencephalic subarachnoid hemorrhage: additional perspectives from four cases. *Stroke* 25: 1507–11.

Schievink WI, Wijdicks EFM, Meyer FB, Piepgras DG, Fode NC, Whisnant JP (1995a). Seasons, snow, and subarachnoid hemorrhage: lack of association in Rochester, Minnesota. *J Neurosurg* 82: 912–13.

Schmid UD, Steiger HJ, Huber P (1987). Accuracy of high resolution computed tomography in direct diagnosis of cerebral aneurysms. *Neuroradiology* 29: 152–9.

Schmitt HP (1983). [Sports accident or natural death? Hematocephalus internus caused by rupture of a choroid plexus angioma] Sportunfall oder naturlicher Tod? Haematocephalus internus durch Rupture eines Plexus-choriodeus-Angioms. *Z Rechtsmed* 91: 129–33.

Schulder M, Hirano A, Elkin C (1987). 'Caval–septal' hematoma: does it exist? *Neurosurgery* 21: 239–41.

Schwaighofer BW, Klein MV, Lyden PD, Hesselink JR (1990). MR imaging of vertebrobasilar vascular disease. *J Comput Assist Tomogr* 14: 895–904.

Schwartz RB, Tice HM, Hooten SM, Hsu L, Stieg PE (1994). Evaluation of cerebral aneurysms with helical CT: correlation with conventional angiography and MR angiography. *Radiology* 192: 717–22.

Scotti G, Filizzolo F, Scialfa G, Tampieri D, Versari P (1987). Repeated subarachnoid hemorrhages from a cervical meningioma: case report. *J Neurosurg* 66: 779–81.

Senter HJ, Sarwar M (1982). Nontraumatic dissecting aneurysm of the vertebral artery. *J Neurosurg* 56: 128–30.

Shinton R, Beevers G (1989). Meta-analysis of relation between cigarette smoking and stroke. *Br Med J* 298: 789–94.

Simolke GA, Cox SM, Cunningham FG (1991). Cerebrovascular accidents complicating pregnancy and the puerperium. *Obstet Gynecol* 78: 37–42.

Spallone A, Ferrante L, Palatinsky E, Santoro A, Acqui M (1986). Subarachnoid haemorrhage of unknown origin. *Acta Neurochir Wien* 80: 12–17.

Spetzler RF, Winestock D, Newton HT, Boldrey EB (1974). Disappearance and reappearance of cerebral aneurysm in serial arteriograms: case report. *J Neurosurg* 41: 508–10.

Spickler E, Lufkin R, Teresi L *et al.* (1990). MR imaging of acute subarachnoid hemorrhage. *Comput Med Imaging Graph* 14: 67–77.

Stampfer MJ, Colditz GA, Willett WC, Speizer FE, Hennekens CH (1988). A prospective study of moderate alcohol consumption and the risk of coronary disease and stroke in women. *N Engl J Med* 319: 267–73.

Stehbens WE (1963). Aneurysms and anatomical variations of the circle of Willis. *Arch Pathol* 75: 45–64.

Stehbens WE (1982). Intracranial berry aneurysms in infancy. *Surg Neurol* 18: 58–60.

Stehbens WE (1989). Etiology of intracranial berry aneurysms. *J Neurosurg* 70: 823–31.

Steinberg GK, Guppy KH, Adler JR, Silverberg GD (1992). Stereotactic, angiography-guided clipping of a distal, mycotic intracranial aneurysm using the Cosman–Roberts–Wells system: technical note. *Neurosurgery* 30: 408–411.

Stone JL, Crowell RM, Gandhi YN, Jafar JJ (1988). Multiple intracranial aneurysms: magnetic resonance imaging for determination of the site of rupture. Report of a case. *Neurosurgery* 23: 97–100.

Sturzenegger M, Huber P (1993). Cranial nerve palsies in spontaneous carotid artery dissection. *J Neurol Neurosurg Psychiatr* 56: 1191–9.

Suzuki S, Kayama T, Sakurai Y, Ogawa A, Suzuki J (1987). Subarachnoid hemorrhage of unknown cause. *Neurosurgery* 21: 310–13.

Swann KW, Ropper AH, New PF, Poletti CE (1984). Spontaneous spinal subarachnoid hemorrhage and subdural hematoma: report of two cases. *J Neurosurg* 61: 975–80.

Takenaka N, Mine T, Suga S *et al.* (1990). Interpeduncular high-density spot in severe shearing injury. *Surg Neurol* 34: 30–8.

Tatter SB, Buonanno FS, Ogilvy CS (1995). Acute lacunar stroke in association with angiogram-negative subarachnoid hemorrhage: mechanistic implications of two cases. *Stroke* 26: 891–5.

Teasdale E, Statham P, Straiton J, Macpherson P (1990). Non-invasive radiological investigation for oculomotor palsy. *J Neurol Neurosurg Psychiatr* 53: 549–53.

Teasdale G, Jennett B (1974). Assessment of coma and impaired consciousness—a practical scale. *Lancet* ii: 81–4.

Ter Berg HW, Dippel DW, Limburg M, Schievink WI, Van Gijn J (1992). Familial intracranial aneurysms: a review. *Stroke* 23: 1024–30.

Teunissen LL, Rinkel GJE, Algra A, van Gijn J (1996). Risk factors for subarachnoid haemorrhage—a systematic review. *Stroke* 27: 544–9.

Tomlinson BE, Walton JN (1964). Superficial haemosiderosis of the central nervous system. *J Neurol Neurosurg Psychiatr* 27: 332–9.

Torner JC, Kassell NF, Wallace RB, Adams HP Jr (1981). Preoperative prognostic factors for rebleeding and survival in aneurysm patients receiving antifibrinolytic therapy: report of the Cooperative Aneurysm Study. *Neurosurgery* 9: 506–13.

Tsubota A, Shishiba Y, Shimizu T, Ozawa Y, Sawano S, Yamada S (1991). Masked Cushing's disease in an aged man associated with intraventricular hemorrhage and tuberculous peritonitis. *Jpn J Med* 30: 233–7.

Tsuchiya K, Makita K, Furui S (1994). 3D-CT angiography of cerebral aneurysms with spiral scanning: comparison with 3D-time-of-flight MR angiography. *Radiat Med* 12: 161–6.

Turtz A, Allen D, Koenigsberg R, Goldman HW (1995). Nonvisualization of a large cerebral aneurysm despite high-resolution magnetic resonance angiography: case report. *J Neurosurg* 82: 294–5.

Ujiie H, Sato K, Onda H *et al.* (1993). Clinical analysis of incidentally discovered unruptured aneurysms. *Stroke* 24: 1850–6.

van der Meulen JH, Weststrate W, Van Gijn J, Habbema JD (1992). Is cerebral angiography indicated in infective endocarditis? *Stroke* 23: 1662–7.

van der Wee N, Rinkel GJ, Hasan D, Van Gijn J (1995). Detection of subarachnoid haemorrhage on early CT: is lumbar puncture still needed after a negative scan? *J Neurol Neurosurg Psychiatr* 58: 357–9.

van Gijn J (1992). Subarachnoid haemorrhage. *Lancet* 339: 653–5.

van Gijn J, van Dongen KJ (1980). Computed tomography in the diagnosis of subarachnoid haemorrhage and ruptured aneurysm. *Clin Neurol Neurosurg* 82: 11–24.

van Gijn J, van Dongen KJ (1982). The time course of aneurysmal haemorrhage on computed tomograms. *Neuroradiology* 23: 153–6.

van Gijn J, Stampfer MJ, Wolfe CDA, Algra A (1993). The association between alcohol and stroke. In: Verschuren PM, ed. *Health Issues Related to Alcohol Consumption.* Washington: ILSI Press, 43–79.

van Gijn J, van Dongen KJ, Vermeulen M, Hijdra A (1985b). Perimesencephalic hemorrhage: a nonaneurysmal and benign form of subarachnoid hemorrhage. *Neurology* 35: 493–7.

van Gijn J, Hijdra A, Wijdicks EFM, Vermeulen M, van Crevel H (1985a). Acute hydrocephalus after aneurysmal subarachnoid hemorrhage. *J Neurosurg* 63: 355–62.

van Rybroek JJ, Moore SA (1990). Sudden death from choroid plexus vascular malformation hemorrhage: case report and review of the literature. *Clin Neuropathol* 9: 39–45.

Verma A, Maheshwari MC, Bhargava S (1987). Spontaneous intraventricular haemorrhage. *J Neurol* 234: 233–6.

Vermeulen M, Lindsay KW, Van Gijn J (1992). *Subarachnoid Haemorrhage.* London: WB Saunders.

Vermeulen M, Van Gijn J, Blijenberg BG (1983). Spectrophotometric analysis of CSF after subarachnoid

hemorrhage: limitations in the diagnosis of rebleeding. *Neurology* 33: 112–15.

Vermeulen M, Hasan D, Blijenberg BG, Hijdra A, Van Gijn J (1989). Xanthochromia after subarachnoid haemorrhage needs no revisitation. *J Neurol Neurosurg Psychiatr* 52: 826–8.

Vermeulen M, Lindsay KW, Murray GD *et al.* (1984). Antifibrinolytic treatment in subarachnoid hemorrhage. *N Engl J Med* 311: 432–7.

Vincent FM, Zimmerman JE (1980). Superior cerebellar artery aneurysm presenting as an oculomotor nerve palsy in a child. *Neurosurgery* 6: 661–4.

Vincent FM, Zimmerman JE, Auer TC, Martin DB (1980). Subarachnoid hemorrhage—the initial manifestation of bacterial endocarditis: report of a case with negative arteriography and computed tomography. *Neurosurgery* 7: 488–90.

Waga S, Shimosaka S, Kojima T (1985). Arteriovenous malformation of the lateral ventricle. *J Neurosurg* 63: 185–92.

Walker AE, Allegre GW (1954). The pathology and pathogenesis of cerebral aneurysms. *J Neuropathol Exp Neurol* 13: 248–59.

Wang PS, Longstreth WT Jr, Koepsell TD (1995). Subarachnoid hemorrhage and family history: a population-based case–control study. *Arch Neurol* 52: 202–4.

Wardlaw JM, Cannon J (1995). Intracranial aneurysms and their 'dynamics' demonstrated by TCD 'colour Doppler energy'. *Cerebrovasc Dis* 5: 228 (abstract).

Weir B, Grace M, Hansen J, Rothberg C (1978). Time course of vasospasm in man. *J Neurosurg* 48: 173–8.

Weir B, Myles T, Kahn M *et al.* (1984). Management of acute subdural hematomas from aneurysmal rupture. *Can J Neurol Sci* 11: 371–6.

Weisberg LA, Elliott D, Shamsnia M (1991). Intraventricular hemorrhage in adults: clinical–computed tomographic correlations. *Comput Med Imaging Graph* 15: 43–51.

Whisnant JP, Sacco SE, O'Fallon WM, Fode NC, Sundt TM Jr (1993). Referral bias in aneurysmal subarachnoid hemorrhage. *J Neurosurg* 78: 726–32.

Wijdicks EFM, Kerkhoff H, Van Gijn J (1988). Long-term follow-up of 71 patients with thunderclap headache mimicking subarachnoid haemorrhage. *Lancet* ii: 68–70.

Wijdicks EFM, Vermeulen M, Murray GD, Hijdra A, Van Gijn J (1990). The effects of treating hypertension following aneurysmal subarachnoid haemorrhage. *Clin Neurol Neurosurg* 92: 111–17.

Williams JP, Joslyn JN, White JL, Dean DF (1983). Subdural hematoma secondary to ruptured intracranial aneurysm: computed tomographic diagnosis. *J Comput Tomogr* 7: 142–53.

Willinsky R, Terbrugge K, Lasjaunias P, Montanera W (1990). The variable presentations of craniocervical and cervical dural arteriovenous malformations. *Surg Neurol* 34: 118–23.

Woimant F, Spelle L (1995). Spontaneous basilar artery dissection: contribution of magnetic resonance imaging to diagnosis. *J Neurol Neurosurg Psychiatr* 58: 540.

Wojak JC, Flamm ES (1987). Intracranial hemorrhage and cocaine use. *Stroke* 18: 712–15.

Wong CW, Ho YS (1994). Intraventricular haemorrhage and hydrocephalus caused by intraventricular parasitic granuloma suggesting cerebral sparganosis. *Acta Neurochir Wien* 129: 205–8.

Wright CJE (1949). Coarctation of the aorta with death from rupture of a cerebral aneurysm. *Arch Pathol* 48: 382–6.

Yamaura A, Watanabe Y, Saeki N (1990). Dissecting aneurysms of the intracranial vertebral artery. *J Neurosurg* 72: 183–8.

Yeh HS, Tomsick TA, Tew JM Jr (1985). Intraventricular hemorrhage due to aneurysms of the distal posterior inferior cerebellar artery: report of three cases. *J Neurosurg* 62: 772–5.

Young RC, Bennett JE, Vogel CL, Carbone PP, DeVita VT (1970). Aspergillosis: the spectrum of the disease in 98 patients. *Med Baltimore* 49: 147–73.

Young WB, Lee KP, Pessin MS, Kwan ES, Rand WM, Caplan LR (1990). Prognostic significance of ventricular blood in supratentorial hemorrhage: a volumetric study. *Neurology* 40: 616–19.

Zhang QJ, Kobayashi S, Gibo H, Hongo K (1994). Vertebrobasilar junction fenestration associated with dissecting aneurysm of intracranial vertebral artery. *Stroke* 25: 1273–5.

A practical approach to the management of stroke patients

This chapter will introduce the general principles of treating patients with stroke. Because treatment is aimed at improving the patient's outcome, the chapter includes a section on the prognosis of stroke and the factors which may help predict the progress of individual patients. It also introduces a model for treating patients that avoids the pitfalls of traditional thinking which splits treatment artificially into acute care, rehabilitation and continuing care.

IO.I   Aims of treatment

The aims of treatment can be summarised as: (i) optimising the patient's chance of surviving; and (ii) minimising the impact of the stroke on the patient and carers. In minimising the impact of the stroke one has to think not just about the short-term effects of the stroke on the patient's neurological impairments but also about its effect on their function (i.e. disability) and on their role in society (i.e. handicap). Therefore, it is useful to consider the results of a stroke in terms of the World Health Organization (WHO) International Classification of Disease (ICD) (WHO, 1980). This divides the consequences of disease into four levels.

I *Pathology*: the underlying pathology of the stroke, e.g. cerebral infarction due to embolic occlusion of a middle cerebral artery from thrombus in the left atrium, resulting from atrial fibrillation due to ischaemic heart disease. Specific medical and surgical treatments (e.g. thrombolytic or neuroprotective drugs) are directed at this level of the disease process.

2 *Impairments*: any loss or abnormality of specific psychological, physiological or anatomical structure or function (e.g. muscle weakness or spasticity, loss of sensation, dysphasia) caused by the stroke. Physical therapies, such as physiotherapy or electromyographic (EMG) biofeedback, are directed at this level.

3 *Disability*: any restriction or lack (resulting from an impairment) of ability to perform an activity in the manner or within the range considered normal for a human being (e.g. inability to walk, wash, feed, etc.) due to the stroke. Physical therapies are also used to try to reduce the disability related to impairments.

4 *Handicap*: the disadvantage for a given individual, resulting from an impairment or disability, that limits or prevents the fulfilment of a role (depending on age, sex, social and cultural factors) for that individual, e.g. inability to continue the same job. Although more difficult to define and measure than the other levels of disease, handicap is probably the level which best reflects the patient's and carer's perspective. Many aspects of treatment will impact on handicap but occupational therapy and social work are those most obviously aimed at influencing this level.

Although not included in the WHO ICD classification, *quality of life* is obviously an important aspect of a patient's outcome. However, there is no generally accepted definition of quality of life and therefore it is not surprising that it is difficult to measure it.

> The consequences of a stroke must be considered at five levels: pathology, impairment, disability, handicap and quality of life.

The most obvious effects of a stroke are physical, but in some situations these may not be as important as the cognitive, psychological, social and even financial consequences. Thus, treatment which aims to minimise the impact of the stroke on the patient and their carers must be directed at all of these types of problems.

10.1.1 Aspects of treatment

To optimise a patient's outcome with respect to their pathology, impairments, disability and handicap many aspects of treatment have to be considered. Because each patient has a unique blend of pathologies, impairments, disabilities and handicaps it follows that treatment must be preceded by a comprehensive assessment and should then be tailored to that individual patient. Traditionally, the discussion of the treatment of stroke is split into sections on: (i) general treatment in the acute phase; (ii) acute medical and surgical treatments; (iii) rehabilitation; and (iv) continuing care. However, this structure does not reflect the need for an integrated approach to the management of the patient. For example, patients may develop acute problems (e.g. pneumonia, pulmonary embolism or urinary tract infection) at any stage in their illness, quite often during what is commonly called rehabilitation (Dromerick & Reding, 1994; Kalra *et al.*, 1995). Conversely, certain aspects of rehabilitation, such as team work and early mobilisation, are just as important on the day of the stroke as they are later on.

The term rehabilitation seems to mean different things to different people. Unfortunately, to many physicians who are responsible for the care of stroke patients, the term is synonymous with physical therapy (e.g. physiotherapy, occupational therapy and speech and language therapy). Having referred the patient to one or more therapists, a physician then mistakenly believes that 'rehabilitation' has been organised. This is far too simplistic. Although there is no universally accepted definition of rehabilitation, most people would view it as a process aimed at minimising the functional effects of the stroke, minimising the impact of the stroke on the patient's and any carer's life, and maximising their autonomy. If we include in our definition *all* those components of care which have these aims, it is apparent that rehabilitation must embrace most aspects of care, ranging from the acute medical treatment through to making alterations to the patient's home prior to discharge and providing support later on. To achieve the best possible outcome for the patient requires a broad approach rather than one that just focuses on the primary pathology or just on the resulting impairments.

> Rehabilitation is not synonymous with physical therapies such as physiotherapy or occupational therapy; it is a far more complex process.

If thought of in this way it becomes artificial, and perhaps even harmful, to separate stroke management into acute care, rehabilitation and continuing care. There are aspects of what is traditionally thought of as rehabilitation which should start on the day of the stroke, and there are elements of acute care which may be important several months after the stroke. To compound the problem these separate components of care may even be provided by different staff in different institutions, which leads to a breakdown in communications and lack of continuity of care. Often, in this modular system of care, one encounters the patient who is 'waiting for rehabilitation', i.e. the patient in the department which normally deals with acute stroke patients for whom there is no immediate place in the rehabilitation facility and who is not progressing. Conversely, one comes across patients in 'a rehabilitation setting' who have developed acute medical problems (e.g. epilepsy or chest pain) and who are denied quick access to the necessary facilities or expertise to ensure their optimum management.

We have therefore abandoned the divisions of treatment into acute, rehabilitation, etc., and will present an integrated, problem- and goal-orientated approach which we believe overcomes the disadvantages of the traditional approach.

10.1.2 An integrated, problem- and goal-orientated approach

The patient's general management, as distinct from the specific treatment of their stroke pathology (see Chapters 11–14), is primarily aimed at preventing potential problems and solving existing ones which are identified at various stages of their illness. One can think of the management as many interwoven cycles or loops (Fig. 10.1). The assessment of a problem, or potential problem, includes not only its detection and perhaps measurement, but also consideration of its likely cause and prognosis. This assessment may often have to include the patient's or carer's expectations or wishes (see Section 10.3.4). Furthermore, we have to remember that assessment is not just a 'once only' activity, but one which should be repeated in different forms throughout the patient's illness so that their management is tailored to their changing needs.

For some problems this cycle can be completed in a few minutes (e.g. an obstructed airway is a short-loop problem), whilst for others the cycle might take weeks to complete (e.g. depression is a long-loop problem). Quite often a problem, e.g. dysphagia, will demand both an immediate intervention, e.g. stop oral fluids and give them by an alternative route, and longer term interventions, e.g. retraining to compensate for swallowing impairment. Thus, in reality the general management involves many such cycles layered on top of each other and cycling at different rates, with each having some influence on the others. This model of management applies equally well to acute general care, rehabilitation and continuing care.

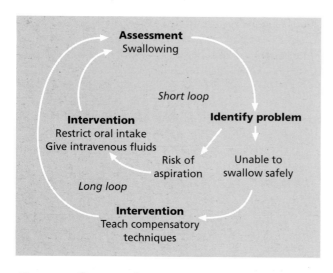

Figure 10.1 Illustrating 'short-' and 'long-loop' problems.

10.1.3 A guide to the following sections on management

We have tried to reflect our integrated approach in the structure of the following discussion on treatment, which is divided into several sections.

1 *What is this patient's prognosis?* Section 10.2 deals with the prognosis of stroke with respect to survival and function in groups of patients and in individual patients. After all, our efforts are aimed at improving the patient's prognosis.

2 *Delivering an integrated management plan.* Section 10.3 deals with general assessment of the patient, the role of the stroke team and its members, problem- and goal-orientated care.

3 *Some difficult ethical dilemmas.* In Section 10.4 we discuss some of the ethical dilemmas which arise in treating stroke patients.

4 *Specific medical and surgical treatments in the acute phase.* Chapters 11–14 deal with the pathophysiology of acute stroke and the drug and surgical treatments which aim to reduce the severity of brain injury.

5 *What are the patient's problems? A problem-orientated approach to management.* Chapter 15 deals with the problems which occur after stroke, and their assessment and interventions which may help to prevent or solve these problems.

6 *Preventing recurrent stroke and other serious vascular events.* Chapter 16 completes the description of the prognosis of stroke by focusing on the risks of further stroke and other vascular events before moving on to describe the various strategies to reduce these risks.

7 *Organising stroke services.* Chapter 17 focuses on the organisational issues which are important when trying to deliver the various aspects of treatment to large numbers of stroke patients as efficiently and equitably as possible.

10.2 What is this patient's prognosis?

10.2.1 Introduction

It is useful to predict the outcome of individual patients because this may enable one to do the following.

1 Have more informed discussions with the patient and/or their carers.

2 Set more accurate short- and long-term goals (see Section 10.3.3).

3 Weigh the potential risks and benefits of treatment options. For example, one might reserve a particularly hazardous but nevertheless effective treatment for patients in whom the prognosis is poor.

4 Plan treatment and make early decisions about later discharge and long-term placement to optimise the efficiency of the service.

5 Make rationing decisions where resources are limited. Thus, if a particular patient is very unlikely to make a good recovery, one could divert resources from that patient to another with a better prognosis who may gain more from the interventions available. It is also wasteful to consume resources on patients who will make a good recovery without any intervention at all. Of course, by adopting this approach, one must be wary of self-fulfilling prophecies, i.e. if one withdraws treatment from a patient they may do badly because of the lack of input.

Before considering how to predict an *individual's* prognosis we shall describe the prognosis of the 'average' patient, i.e. the outcome of an unselected cohort of stroke patients. Here, the prognosis with respect to survival and overall functional outcome is described since this is relevant to all aspects of treatment. The prognosis for particular individual impairments, disabilities and handicaps is dealt with in the appropriate sections of Chapter 15, whilst that related to the risk of late death, recurrent stroke and other vascular events is dealt with in Chapter 16. Subarachnoid haemorrhage will be dealt with in detail in Chapter 13.

10.2.2 Collecting reliable information about prognosis

If information concerning the prognosis of stroke is to be useful it must have been collected using sound methods which minimise bias and maximise precision, accuracy and generalisability (Table 10.1).

Prognosis or natural history?

It is important to distinguish these two aspects because they are not the same. Natural history refers to the *untreated* course of an illness from its onset, whilst prognosis refers to the probability of an outcome in an individual or group of patients over a defined period of time after the disease is first identified, and this is likely to be influenced by any treatment given. Usually, but not always, the prognosis with treatment is better than the natural history but it may be worse. This section describes the *prognosis* of stroke. No data on the natural history (strictly defined) are available because, even in developing countries, patients with stroke are usually given some treatment and in those places where minimal or no treatment is given, no studies of prognosis have been reported. The mere act of admission to hospital, even without any medical or physical therapy, could be regarded as 'treatment' and may influence outcome.

Table 10.1 Methodological features which are important in assessing a study of prognosis after stroke. (From Sackett *et al.*, 1991.)

---

1 *Were the patients identified at an early and uniform point in the course of their disease and were diagnostic criteria, disease severity, co-morbidity and demographic details for inclusion clearly specified?*

If they were, then this is called an 'inception cohort'

2 *Was the referral pattern described?*

Did the study avoid the following
(a) 'Referral filter bias' which occurs when an inception cohort is assembled on selected cases which are not representative of all cases occurring in the population. This is a particular problem with specialist centres which attract unusual cases (centripetal bias) or admit or track interesting cases (popularity bias)
(b) 'Diagnostic access bias' which occurs if cases are defined by technology (e.g. intracerebral haemorrhage by computerised tomography scanning), but the patient's access to the technology is influenced by factors such as their wealth which may affect their outcome

3 *Was complete follow-up achieved?*

Were all patients entered into the study accounted for in the results and was their clinical status known at final follow-up? Patients who are lost to follow-up may be systematically different from those who are not. For example, patients with a good recovery may be more mobile or at work and therefore more difficult to follow-up whilst patients may not be followed-up because they have died. Therefore, the effect of incomplete follow-up on perceived prognosis is difficult to predict

4 *Were objective outcome criteria developed and used and were the criteria reproducible and accurate?*

To make sense of prognostic data it is important to know what the authors meant by terms such as 'recurrent stroke' or 'independent' so that one can apply the data to one's own patients. It is also important that the criteria are applied consistently

5 *Was outcome assessment blind?*

In other words, were diagnostic suspicion bias and expectation bias avoided in the assessment of patient outcomes? If the observer has a preconceived view that a particular baseline factor is likely to be related to a particular outcome, knowledge of the presence or absence of that factor at the time of follow-up may bias that observer

6 *Was adjustment for extraneous prognostic factors carried out?*

Where authors relate certain baseline factors to the likelihood of specific outcomes it is important that they allow for other baseline factors. The most common example of this is age, which partly explains the observed relationships between other factors, e.g. atrial fibrillation and early death. Before applying predictive equations to one's own patients it is important that the equation has been tested on an independent test cohort other than the one in which it was developed

---

Sources of prognostic data

No published study of prognosis after stroke fulfils all the criteria summarised in Table 10.1. We have used data from the Oxfordshire Community Stroke Project (OCSP) because it meets, at least partly, most of these criteria (Bamford *et al.*, 1987, 1988, 1990a,b, 1991; Dennis *et al.*, 1993). Other methodologically sound studies come to broadly similar conclusions, although to compare them directly is difficult because of their different methods, their varying styles of reporting, and because much of the variation in prognosis can be accounted for by the play of chance as a result of relatively small sample sizes (Sacco *et al.*, 1982; Garraway *et al.*, 1983; Turney *et al.*, 1984; Kojima *et al.*, 1990; Anderson *et al.*, 1994).

10.2.3 Prognosis for death

The risk of dying within the first 7 and 30 days after a stroke is about 12% and 19%, respectively (Fig. 10.2). Surprisingly, the risk of death within 30 days of a recurrent stroke is not significantly greater, although because only small numbers of recurrent strokes occurred in the OCSP, real differences cannot be ruled out (Burn *et al.*, 1994). Patients with haemorrhagic stroke, either primary intracerebral or subarachnoid, have a much higher early risk of dying than those with ischaemic stroke, although patients with *major* ischaemic strokes, i.e. total anterior circulation infarc-

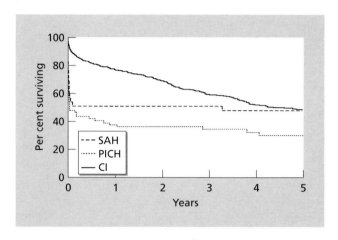

Figure 10.3 A Kaplan–Meier plot showing the proportion of patients surviving after a first-ever in a lifetime stroke due to cerebral infarction (CI; *n* = 545), primary intracerebral haemorrhage (PICH; *n* = 66) and subarachnoid haemorrhage (SAH; *n* = 33). (From Dennis *et al.*, 1993; reproduced with permission of the American Heart Association.)

Table 10.2 Death after different pathological types of first-ever in a lifetime stroke. Data from the OCSP.

Type of stroke	*n*	Case fatality (%)			
		7 days	30 days	6 months	1 year
All strokes	675	12	19	27	31
Subarachnoid haemorrhage	33	27	46	48	48
Primary intracerebral haemorrhage	66	40	50	58	62
All ischaemic stroke	545	5	10	18	23
Total anterior circulation infarction	92	17	39	57	60
Partial anterior circulation infarction	186	2	4	11	16
Lacunar infarction	138	2	2	7	11
Posterior circulation infarction	129	5	7	14	19

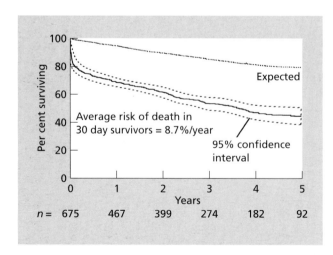

Figure 10.2 A Kaplan–Meier plot showing the proportion of patients surviving at increasing intervals after a first-ever in a lifetime stroke compared with the expected survival of people of the same age and sex who have not had a stroke. Data from the OCSP (Dennis *et al.*, 1993). The expected survival was derived from all-causes mortality rates for Oxfordshire (1985). (Reproduced with permission of the American Heart Association.)

tion (see Section 4.4.8), have a very high early risk of death (Fig. 10.3 & Table 10.2).

Causes of death

Knowing the causes of these early deaths is important if one is interested in treatments to avoid them (Fig. 10.4). In the

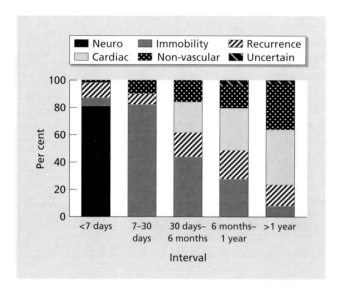

Figure 10.4 Histogram showing the proportion of patients dying from different causes at increasing intervals after a first-ever in a lifetime stroke. (From Bamford *et al.*, 1990b; Dennis *et al.*, 1993.)

first few days after stroke, most patients who die do so as a result of the direct effects of the brain damage (Bounds *et al.*, 1981; Silver *et al.*, 1984; Bamford *et al.*, 1990b). In brainstem strokes, the respiratory centre may be affected by the stroke itself, whilst in supratentorial cerebral infarction or haemorrhage, dysfunction of the brainstem results from displacement and herniation of oedematous supratentorial brain tissue (see Fig. 11.11). Deaths occurring within an hour or two of onset are unusual in cerebral infarction because it takes time for oedema to develop; almost all such very early deaths after stroke result from intracranial haemorrhage of some sort (Bamford *et al.*, 1990a).

> *Death within a few hours of stroke onset only occurs with intracerebral or subarachnoid haemorrhage, or rarely with massive brainstem infarction.*

Having survived the first few days, patients may then develop various potentially fatal complications of immobility, the most common being pneumonia (see Section 15.12) and pulmonary embolism (see Section 15.13). In addition, pressure sores (see Section 15.16), dehydration (see Section 15.18.1) with renal failure and urinary tract infection (see Section 15.12) may cause death where basic care is lacking. Because some strokes occur in the context of other serious conditions (e.g. myocardial infarction (see Section 7.7), cardiac failure (see Section 6.4) and cancer (see Section 7.9)), some early deaths can, at least in part, be attributed to these underlying problems. Also, because the risk of stroke recurrence is highest early after the first stroke, about 13%

in the first year (see Section 16.1), some patients will die from the direct or indirect effects of a recurrent stroke (Burn *et al.*, 1994). This is most common in patients with subarachnoid haemorrhage (see Section 13.5), especially if due to rupture of a saccular aneurysm where the recurrence or rebleed rate is about 30% (without intervention), accounting for perhaps 50% of deaths in the first 30 days (van Gijn, 1992). After subarachnoid haemorrhage, clinical worsening can also result from cerebral ischaemia related to vasospasm or to obstructive hydrocephalus (see Sections 13.6 and 13.9).

10.2.4 Prognosis for dependency

Stroke often leaves surviving patients with neurological impairments which prevent them performing everyday activities, so making them dependent on others. Figures 10.5 and 10.6 show the proportions of survivors who are independent and dependent in everyday activities at various times after a first-ever in a lifetime stroke and in strokes of different pathologies and clinical subtypes. Other studies have produced similar data (Dombovy *et al.*, 1987). It is likely that a greater proportion of patients will become dependent after recurrent strokes. Details of the prognosis with respect to particular impairments, disabilities and handicaps will be discussed in the specific sections dealing with their treatment (see Chapter 15), but it is relevant here to discuss the general pattern of recovery after stroke.

10.2.5 Patterns of recovery

Patients who survive an acute stroke almost always improve, to a greater or lesser extent. Improvement is reflected not just in a reduction in the neurological impairments but also in any resulting disability and handicap. Various mechanisms have been postulated to explain recovery. In the first few days after a stroke, neurones that were not irreversibly damaged during the primary event, may start to function because of improved blood supply, reversal of metabolic problems or resolution of cerebral oedema (see Section 11.1). Neuroplasticity, the process by which surviving neurones can take over some of the functions of those which have been irreversibly damaged, might explain some of the later improvement (Chollet *et al.*, 1991; Stephenson, 1993; Weiller *et al.*, 1993). However, much of the later recovery with respect to disability and handicap is probably due to adaptive changes, i.e. the patient learns techniques to compensate for their remaining impairments, and their environment is altered to maximise their autonomy. The overall 'pattern of recovery' will reflect all of these processes superimposed upon each other. Because it is so difficult to predict

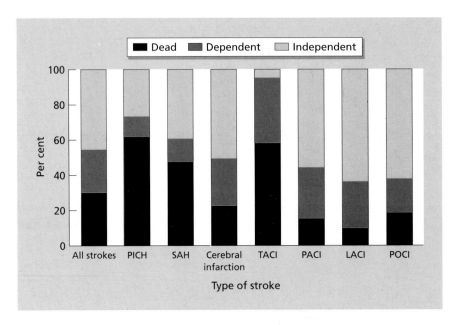

Figure 10.5 Histogram showing the proportion of patients with different outcomes (i.e. dead, dependent (Rankin 3, 4 or 5) or independent (Rankin 0, 1 or 2) in activities of daily living) 1 year after their first-ever in a lifetime stroke due to cerebral infarction (CI; *n* = 545) and its clinical subtypes (TACI, total anterior circulation infarction; PACI, partial anterior circulation infarction; LACI, lacunar infarction; POCI, posterior circulation infarction), primary intracerebral haemorrhage (PICH; *n* = 66) and subarachnoid haemorrhage (SAH; *n* = 33). (From Bamford *et al.*, 1990a, 1991.)

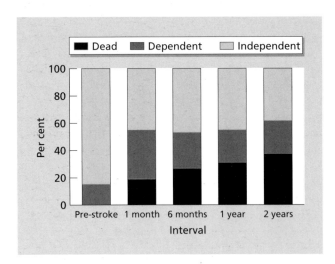

Figure 10.6 Histogram showing the proportion of patients with different outcomes (i.e. dead, dependent (Rankin 3, 4 or 5) or independent (Rankin 0, 1 or 2) in activities of daily living) at increasing intervals after their first-ever in a lifetime stroke. (From unpublished data from OCSP.)

an individual patient's functional outcome, the following general points can be made to patients and their relatives:

1 the rate of recovery is highest in the early period after the initial stroke;

2 improvement may continue for many months and in some patients for 1–2 years;

3 the rate and completeness of recovery varies from patient to patient and is relatively unpredictable, at least in the first few days and weeks after the stroke onset.

These generalisations are supported by our own experience and also data from studies where stroke patient's functional abilities have been repeatedly tested over a period of time (Skilbeck *et al.*, 1983; Wade *et al.*, 1983a, 1985; Wade & Langton Hewer, 1987; Gray *et al.*, 1990). Figure 10.7 shows two graphs which, on the face of it, support the idea that the 'pattern of recovery' follows an almost exponential trajectory. However, one needs to be careful in interpreting such data. These graphs show changes in groups of patients with respect to a particular function over time, which does not mean that all individual patients necessarily follow the same overall pattern. Also, the apparent plateau in recovery after a few months may simply reflect that the tools used to measure the function are often 'ordinal' rather than 'interval' scales (see Table 17.19), and also that there is a marked 'ceiling effect', i.e. the measure is not sensitive to improvements at the upper end of the range of performance (Wellwood *et al.*, 1995). Therefore, the apparent differences in patterns and duration of recovery for different impairments and disabilities may to some extent reflect the characteristics of the tools

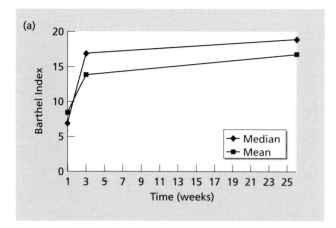
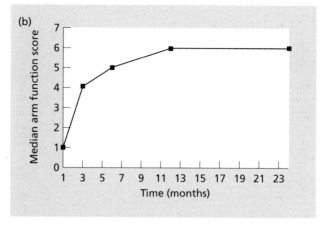

Figure 10.7 Patterns of recovery after stroke. (a) This graph shows the change in median and mean Barthel Index over 6 months in the survivors of 976 patients identified in a community-based study with a first-ever or recurrent stroke. (b) This graph shows the change in median arm function score amongst 84 patients (although not all patients were tested on each occasion) over a follow-up of about 2 years. Although the grouped data suggest an almost exponential recovery, this pattern was rarely observed in individual patients. (From Skilbeck *et al.*, 1983; Wade & Langton Hewer, 1987; reproduced with permission of the authors and the *Journal of Neurology, Neurosurgery and Psychiatry*.)

used to measure them. For example, it is often said that language function continues to improve for a very long time after a stroke, whilst recovery in arm function does not. This different perception may be due to patients being acutely aware of even small differences in fluency whilst they may only report an improvement in arm function if they can perform a new function with their hand. Certainly, there is scope for further research into the patterns of recovery after stroke taking these points into account.

The shape of so-called recovery curves may reflect the properties of the instrument used to measure function as much as the patient's rate of improvement.

10.2.6 Is this the prognosis of your patients?

The prognostic data presented in this section come mainly from the OCSP which, over a 4-year period, prospectively registered all patients from a well-defined population who had a first-ever in a lifetime stroke (Bamford *et al.*, 1988). After an assessment by a study neurologist as soon after the stroke as possible, patients were prospectively followed for up to 6 years (Dennis *et al.*, 1993). Patients were included whether referred to hospital or not and so this study provided prognostic data on an unselected community-based cohort of patients with a first-ever stroke. Studies of prognosis in other community-based series have provided broadly similar results (Sacco *et al.*, 1982; Garraway *et al.*, 1983; Turney *et al.*, 1984; Kojima *et al.*, 1990; Anderson *et al.*, 1994). However, the prognosis of

patients in one's own clinical practice may be different because of the following.

1 The stroke population is different from that in Oxfordshire; patients may be younger or older, of different racial or ethnic background, have more or less severe strokes, more or less co-morbidity, or a different pattern of stroke pathology. For example, there is evidence that a greater proportion of strokes in Japan are haemorrhagic (see Sections 5.2 and 17.2.1) and thus one might expect a higher early case-fatality rate (Table 10.2).

2 In any hospital the prognosis of patients will be affected by referral bias (see Table 10.1). In general, stroke patients referred to hospital can be expected to have a worse prognosis (i.e. a higher case fatality and worse functional outcome) because a greater proportion of milder cases are looked after by their family doctors at home (Bamford *et al.*, 1986). However, this is not always predictable since in some places younger patients, who have on average a better prognosis (Fig. 10.8), may be referred to hospital more often than older patients. Furthermore, some patients with very severe strokes which are likely to lead to death within a few hours, or who are already living in a nursing home, may not be admitted at all and so be under-represented in a hospitalised cohort. Differences in outcome between hospitals are probably more likely to reflect the differences in the proportions of patients with severe stroke rather than any differences in treatment given (see Section 17.6.3).

Hospital admission rates vary considerably from place to place, country to country and time to time. For example, in Oxfordshire only 55% of patients were admitted whilst in

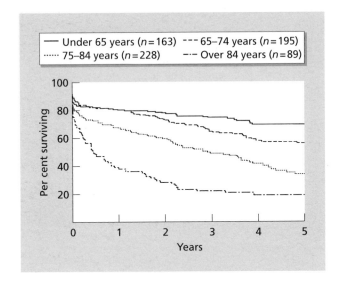

Figure 10.8 A Kaplan–Meier plot showing the proportion of patients of different ages surviving after a first-ever in a lifetime stroke. (From Dennis *et al.*, 1993; reproduced with permission of American Heart Association.)

Perugia, Italy 85% were admitted and in Umea, Sweden almost all stroke patients are admitted to hospital (Bamford *et al.*, 1986; Ricci *et al.*, 1991; Asplund *et al.*, 1995). The type of hospital (e.g. district general, university or tertiary referral hospital) and the specialities represented in it (e.g. neurosurgery, neurology, general medicine, care of the elderly, etc.), will have a major influence on case mix, so that clinicians working in different institutions will form, from their own experience, widely differing views of the prognosis of stroke patients (Horner *et al.*, 1995).

3 If patients are seen very early after stroke onset (e.g. because the hospital is in a city and has an accident and emergency unit), they are likely to have a worse prognosis than patients who are seen later (such as those referred to a distant tertiary referral centre) because they must survive long enough to be admitted (see Table 10.1).

4 Unless patients are followed-up using similar definitions of outcome and for the same time period as those in the published studies, their prognosis will be different (see Table 10.1). Also, the reasons why patients are lost to follow-up may be related to their outcome. For example, dead patients are sometimes lost to follow-up which biases the prognosis in a favourable direction, whilst patients who have made a good recovery and are mobile may be lost because they move away which biases the prognosis in the opposite direction (see Table 10.1). Furthermore, if all patients are not followed-up the perceived prognosis is likely to be overly influenced by the outcome of the last few patients who are remembered most vividly, or perhaps the patients who had particularly good or particularly bad outcomes.

5 If the estimate of the outcome is based on the follow-up of too few patients it may differ from that in published studies simply by chance alone ('the good or bad luck effect').

6 Patients may be managed more or less effectively than those in Oxfordshire and other published studies, and thus the outcomes may be better or worse. However, the likely impact of differences in treatment between centres is likely to be swamped by other factors which have a much greater influence on outcome (e.g. case mix; see Section 17.6.3).

10.2.7 Predicting outcome in individual patients

Unfortunately, it is difficult to predict an *individual* patient's outcome accurately enough to be of much value in clinical practice. It is also difficult to define the acceptable accuracy of any prediction because this depends on the consequences, or cost, of getting it wrong. Taking an extreme example, if one was sure that a patient with an apparently severe stroke, who was being supported on a ventilator, was not going to have an acceptable long-term quality of life, then one might withdraw ventilatory support. However, in this situation one would have to be very confident of one's prediction.

A broad range of factors have been shown to be associated with outcome including: (i) clinical features shortly after stroke onset; (ii) the results of both simple and complex investigations; and (iii) the patient's progress over the initial post-stroke period (Table 10.3). Many are inter-related, e.g. conscious level and lesion size on computerised tomography (CT), so multiple regression statistical techniques are needed to identify the factors which independently predict outcome. Most studies have focused on factors that are associated with death. However, a growing number also consider those factors which are related to a good or bad functional outcome and, in general, these are similar to those predicting death. Unfortunately, methodological problems have so far limited the usefulness of these studies (Table 10.4) (Jongbloed, 1990; Hier & Edelstein, 1991).

> *At present, it is impossible to predict an individual's outcome early after stroke onset with enough accuracy to be of much value in clinical practice.*

Predicting early death

Clinical features which alone or in combination indicate severe brainstem dysfunction, whether due to direct damage or as a result of raised intracranial pressure, are highly predictive of early death (Table 10.5). Unfortunately, many patients who die do not show these features and occasionally

Table 10.3 Some of the factors which have been associated with a high risk of death and poor functional outcome after stroke. (From Hier & Edelstein, 1991.)

DEMOGRAPHIC FEATURES
Increasing age

CLINICAL FEATURES

General
Atrial fibrillation
Cardiac failure
Ischaemic heart disease
Diabetes mellitus
Fever
Urinary incontinence
Previous stroke

Neurological
Reduced level of consciousness
Severe motor deficit
Impaired proprioception
Visuospatial dysfunction
Cognitive impairment
Total anterior circulation syndrome
Lower activities of daily living (ADL) score

SIMPLE LABORATORY TESTS
Hyperglycaemia
High haematocrit
Abnormal electrocardiogram

COMPLEX TESTS (CT or magnetic resonance imaging brain scan)
Large stroke lesion
Mass effect
Intraventricular blood (in primary intracerebral haemorrhage)
Hydrocephalus (in intracranial haemorrhage and cerebellar stroke)

patients with more than one of these features make an unexpectedly good recovery (fortunate for the patient, unfortunate for the predictor). Sometimes one sees patients with single predictive factors, e.g. just periodic respiration (see Section 15.2.2) and, in isolation, these factors can be associated with a good recovery; it is the combination of prognostic factors that is the more powerful predictor. Indeed, the poor inter-rater reliability of individual neurological signs, such as the plantar response, further limits the usefulness of isolated features.

Predicting longer term outcomes

It is even more difficult to predict longer term outcomes. Many of the factors that indicate a high early risk of death also indicate a high risk of long-term dependency if the patient survives (Table 10.5). In general, the predictive factors that have been identified reflect either the patient's pre-

stroke health status or the amount of brain damaged. In predicting longer term outcome one also has the problem that further events which may be related to the initial stroke (i.e. recurrent strokes and myocardial infarction) or may not (i.e. development of unrelated illness), can occur and have a major and often quite unpredictable effect on outcome. Attempts have been made to estimate an individual's risk of further vascular events, but this has proven even more difficult than prediction of early death and functional outcome (see Section 16.1).

Methods of prediction

A variety of different approaches have been taken in predicting outcome after stroke.

1 The simplest approach has been to identify a single factor, the presence or absence of which early after the stroke indicates the likelihood that the patient will have a good or bad outcome. The most widely used examples are reduced level of consciousness and urinary incontinence, which have both been related to a poor survival and functional outcome

Table 10.4 Methodological problems in studies of prediction of outcome after stroke.

Failure to describe adequately the group of patients in whom the work was done
Use of unrepresentative cohorts of patients, e.g. highly selected patients in rehabilitation settings
Many studies are retrospective which limit the range and perhaps the reliability of the baseline and outcome data
Failure to define adequately variables studied
Variation in the timing after stroke of the initial patient assessments
Failure to measure outcome at a relevant and uniform point after the stroke, i.e. 6 months post-stroke rather than at hospital discharge
Failure to use reliable and valid measures of outcome
Inadequate sample sizes
Failure to use appropriate statistical techniques to adjust for the effect of baseline variables
Failure to test the accuracy of any predictive model in an independent data set

Table 10.5 Neurological features that reflect brainstem dysfunction and which in combination are related to a very high risk of early death.

Decreased conscious level (Henon *et al.*, 1995)
Conjugate gaze palsy (tonic deviation of gaze) (Tijssen *et al.*, 1991)
Severe bilateral motor weakness
Abnormal respiratory pattern (e.g. periodic respiration)
Bilateral extensor plantar responses

(Wade & Langton Hewer, 1985; Gladman, 1992; Taub *et al.*, 1994). Measures of cognitive function at initial assessment have also been related to poor functional outcomes (Barer, 1990; Rose *et al.*, 1994; Taub *et al.*, 1994). Although such models are simple to use they are probably too inaccurate for clinical decision making (Gladman *et al.*, 1992). They have a more obvious use in stratifying patients who are being randomised in clinical trials.

> *Reduced conscious level and urinary incontinence in the first few days after stroke are both associated, in general, with a poor outcome. Unfortunately, this association is not reliable enough to be useful in managing individual patients.*

2 In general, it appears that the larger the volume of brain damaged the worse the clinical outcome, except for critically sited strokes, particularly in the brainstem, where even quite small lesions can be fatal. Most of the clinical indicators of poor prognosis relate quite closely to the size of the brain lesion. For example, the OCSP classification (see Section 4.4) reflects the volume of brain damage and so the prognosis of the different groups varies (see Fig. 10.5). Imaging techniques including CT, single-photon emission CT (SPECT) and magnetic resonance imaging (MRI) have so far added little to the accuracy of clinical predictors (Valdimarsson *et al.*, 1982; Allen, 1984a; Crisi *et al.*, 1984; Tuhrim *et al.*, 1991; Slattery & Hankey, 1992). None of this is at all surprising because the size of the stroke lesion on brain imaging can so often be predicted from the clinical findings. Moreover, a substantial proportion of patients have a normal or near normal CT scan early after even a major cerebral infarction, which weakens the predictive utility of any imaging (see Section 5.3.5).

> *In general, the larger the stroke lesion the worse the likely outcome, except for small critically sited lesions which may be associated with a poor outcome.*

3 Complex mathematical models based on regression analyses have been developed by several groups to predict both survival and functional outcome (Prescott *et al.*, 1982; Sheikh *et al.*, 1983; Wade *et al.*, 1983a; Allen, 1984b; Fullerton *et al.*, 1988; Anderson *et al.*, 1994; Fiorelli *et al.*, 1995). Although these are generally a little more accurate than models based on a single variable, any advantage may be offset by the practical difficulties in applying them (Weingarten *et al.*, 1990). Also, they have not been tested adequately in independent cohorts of sufficient size. Where they have been tested, as one would predict, they generally perform less well than in the cohort from which they were developed (Britton *et al.*, 1980; Tuhrim *et al.*, 1991; Gladman, 1992; Gompertz *et al.*, 1994). If such models are

to be used in routine clinical practice they need to be further refined, tested prospectively in large independent cohorts of patients, and made far more 'user friendly' so that they do not require the clinician to perform complex calculations. In selecting the factors which are included in these models more attention needs to be given to their inter-rater reliability so that predictions are repeatable.

4 Predictions based on measures of function early after a stroke (e.g. the Barthel Index) have been used to predict eventual functional outcome and may be particularly useful for those working in rehabilitation facilities (Granger *et al.*, 1989; Loewen & Anderson, 1990; Lincoln *et al.*, 1990).

5 Another approach to predict outcome is to observe the rate of change in some measure of the patient's condition early in the clinical course and from this predict the likely longer term outcome (Granger *et al.*, 1989). This might be likened to the growth curves used by paediatricians. Predictions for individuals would then depend on the pattern of recovery observed in large cohorts of patients.

6 Of course, the most widely used method of prediction is the informal judgement we make about patients during our daily work. Such informal predictions have rarely been evaluated but it will be important to ensure that any more formal predictive system is at least as accurate as our informal judgements before recommending it for widespread use.

The predictive systems developed up until now have been tested inadequately and are probably insufficiently accurate to influence important clinical decisions. However, they may be useful as a tool to guide less experienced clinicians in what to say to patients and carers, in who to randomise in trials of acute treatment, and in deciding which patient is likely to require an extended period of rehabilitation. Predictive systems may have more potential in adjusting outcome data from different *groups* of patients for differences in case mix so that their adjusted outcomes can be used as an indicator of the quality of care in clinical audit (see Section 17.6.3).

In the future we expect the fairly crude predictive models currently available to be replaced by more precise, better validated models. These might be used to predict not only survival and basic functional outcome but also the recovery of individual impairments, disabilities and handicaps which is so important in planning treatment. Such models may even be developed using neural networks in addition to the more conventional multiple regression analyses. One might combine several approaches to predicting a patient's outcome, so that one relies on the mathematical modelling in the early stages, but as more data become available from continued observation of the patient the 'recovery curve' can be plotted. One could imagine that these predictive systems be presented in several forms for clinical use: (i) wall charts;

(ii) clinical slide rules; (iii) on pocket calculators; or (iv) on personal computers or hospital-wide computer networks. Eventually, any such system, which will inevitably consume resources, will have to be tested to show that it improves the effectiveness and efficiency of stroke services.

10.3 Delivering an integrated management plan

10.3.1 Introduction

The term 'stroke' embraces a very wide spectrum of clinical presentations ranging from neurological deficits lasting just 1 day to those leading rapidly to death or causing lifelong disability. These deficits are layered on a complex mix of pre-existing pathology, personality, social and environmental factors. We have already seen the range of possible pathological types (see Chapter 5) and causes (see Chapters 6–9), but each patient requires a management plan tailored to his or her own individual needs. It is obvious that for a patient whose symptoms resolve completely within a few days, the emphasis should be on diagnosis and secondary prevention, whereas for a patient with a major disabling stroke the emphasis must be on treatment of the acute phase, prevention of complications and rehabilitation. The essential first step in formulating a management plan is a full and detailed assessment.

10.3.2 Assessment

The assessment should aim to answer the following questions.

1 Is it a vascular event (transient ischaemic attack (TIA) or stroke)? (see Chapter 3).
2 Where is the lesion? (see Chapter 4).
3 What sort of stroke lesion is it? (see Chapter 5).
4 What is the likely cause? (see Chapters 6–9).
5 What is this patient's prognosis? (see Section 10.2).
6 What are this patient's particular problems? (see Chapter 15).

The answers to these questions will determine the management of the patient and which therapeutic interventions are appropriate. The first five questions have been addressed in previous sections and before proceeding to discuss the assessment of specific problems to complete the diagnostic formulation (see Chapter 15), some general principles and the organisation of assessment must be considered.

In practice, the patient's first assessment is usually carried out by either a family practitioner in the patient's home, or by a hospital doctor in training. However, neither clinician may have had much training or experience in the assessment of patients with stroke. An average general practitioner in the UK is only likely to see about four new cases of stroke each year. Guidelines, a protocol or, in hospital, a clerking or admission form may be useful tools to ensure that each patient has a thorough and relevant assessment. We have demonstrated a significant improvement in the completeness of the assessment of stroke patients following the introduction of a stroke clerking or admission form (Davenport et al., 1995). The use of the form also makes it much easier to access the information subsequently and to identify relevant items which are missing.

> A clerking or admission form will improve the completeness and relevance of the initial assessment and will facilitate communication and audit.

Although a physician is often the first person to assess the patient it is important to emphasise that assessment should often involve other members of the multidisciplinary team (see Section 10.3.5). It is often very valuable, even on the day of the stroke, to involve the nurse, the physiotherapist and a speech and language therapist; advice on the patient's risk of pressure sores, lifting, handling and positioning and the patient's ability to swallow safely are all relevant to their care from the moment of hospital admission, or indeed from the moment of assessment at home. The components of the initial assessment and their use are summarised in Table 10.6. It is important to emphasise that assessment is not a 'once only' process but should continue throughout the course of the patient's recovery from stroke.

Health professionals involved in the initial assessment of stroke patients learn that, although the patient may be a

Table 10.6 Types of information which should be collected during the initial assessment of a stroke patient, and their potential value.

Type of information	Diagnosis	Cause	Prognosis	Problems	Secondary prevention
Demographics	×	×	×	×	
History of onset	×	×			
Risk factors	×	×	×	×	×
Co-existing disease		×	×	×	×
Medication		×		×	
Social details			×	×	
Pre-stroke function	×		×	×	×
General examination		×	×	×	×
Neurological examination	×	×	×	×	
Investigations	×	×	×	×	×

useful source of information, other people often provide more information which is essential to planning treatment. This is particularly important when the patient, for a variety of reasons, cannot communicate. It is often enormously valuable to spend a little time interviewing the family, neighbours, general practitioner, ambulance technicians or nursing staff even if this requires a telephone.

> *To complete an assessment it is often essential to talk to family or neighbours; essential information can often be collected by a telephone call to the appropriate person.*

Social environment is a very important factor in determining the overall effect that a stroke will have on an individual and their family. Accurate knowledge of social networks is, therefore, critical when setting longer term goals for rehabilitation and in planning discharge from hospital. Moreover, this allows one to build up a picture of the patient as a person rather than 'just another stroke' or 'that fibrillating hemiplegic in bed six'. It is so often difficult to see the person behind the facial weakness, severe dysarthria and dysphasia, hemiplegia and incontinence but that person is usually there and distressed by their predicament. Finding out about the patient's pre-stroke life might encourage members of the team who are caring for the patient to treat them with more understanding and sympathy. Also it is this background information which allows one to judge the likely effect that the individual's disabilities will have on their role in society, i.e. the likely handicap. This is important because one of the major aims of rehabilitation is to minimise handicap. For example, it may be more appropriate to put greater energy and resources into occupational therapy for a craftsman than a school teacher who might require relatively more speech therapy.

Although a lot of this background information can be collected over a longer period whilst the patient is recovering, it can be useful early on and may be more easily collected at the initial assessment. So often, the family, who may be the only source of this sort of information, melt away within a few hours of the admission and may then not reappear to be asked the relevant questions. Therefore, it is vital to seize the opportunity when a patient is first admitted, or at least in the next day or two, to obtain as much information from the family and friends as possible. Clearly, this may not be regarded as a medical priority but professionals other than doctors, in particular the nursing staff, are often equally well placed to collect it. It is important to remember that a complete picture of the patient's pre-stroke life may be useful when deciding how aggressively to manage a patient (e.g. neurosurgery for obstructive hydrocephalus). Because this background information is so important, but may not be available at the inital assessment, one needs some method to identify which items of data are missing so that they can be sought later on. The clerking or admission form, or a patient record which is shared by the different professions involved (the so-called 'combined' or 'single patient' record) should fulfil this role.

> *It is just as important to know the home and social circumstances of a stroke patient for early decision making (such as the desirability of emergency neurosurgery) as for later rehabilitation and discharge from hospital.*

By the end of the initial assessment one should have collected enough information to produce a diagnostic formulation including certainty of stroke diagnosis, site and size of the brain lesion, and the likely causes. This leads on to choices about the intensity of investigation required and enables the physician to talk to the patient and/or the family about the likely diagnosis, prognosis and management. At this stage it is valuable to consider, and even list, the particular problems the patient has, to ensure that they have all been identified and addressed. It may be useful to use a checklist of the most common ones which occur at this early stage (Table 10.7).

10.3.3 Identifying problems and setting goals

The patient's assessment, both initial and subsequently, should identify any major problems and it is these which determine the patient's management. Problems can occur at every level of the patient's illness, i.e. pathology, impairments, disabilities and handicap. For example, a problem at the pathological level might include 'diagnostic uncertainty' or 'raised erythrocyte sedimentation rate (ESR)' which

Table 10.7 Some important things to think about in the first day after a patient has had a severe stroke.

Maintenance of a clear airway
Co-existing or underlying disease
Swallowing ability
Hydration
Management of urinary incontinence
Prevention of
Deep venous thrombosis
Pressure sores
Aspiration
Trauma
Protection of a flaccid shoulder
Exclusion of fractures
Explanation for the patient and family

should lead on to further investigation if appropriate, whilst a problem at the level of handicap might be that the patient provided the only income for a large family who now have no money to feed themselves. Having identified a problem one can then formulate a plan to solve or at least alleviate that problem. Thus, a problem list can be turned into an action plan for the individual patient. Some problems can be dealt with very simply (e.g. antibiotics for a urinary tract infection). These are the 'short-loop problems'. The goal here is simply to remove the problem. Other problems such as immobility, which are more complex and which respond more slowly to therapy and may require several different types of intervention, are the 'long-loop problems' (see Section 10.1.2). With these it is useful to set a long-term goal of removing or alleviating the problem but it is also helpful to set intermediate shorter term goals which allow one to judge whether progress is being made towards the long-term goal.

Why a goal-orientated approach has several advantages

Setting goals allows forward planning. Intermediate goals allow members of the team to coordinate their work, assuming that goals are achieved on time, and so improve efficiency. For example, if a patient is to dress the lower half of their body, they must be able to stand. If the physiotherapist can estimate when the patient will stand independently, the occupational therapist can plan when to start working on dressing their lower half. Setting longer term goals can, for example, allow advanced planning of pre-discharge home visits and final discharges to the community, which can reduce the patient's length of stay in hospital by the number of days or weeks needed to plan a home visit or to make any necessary adaptations to the patient's home before discharge (e.g. stair rails).

If realistic goals are set they can be used to help motivate patients. Recovery from a stroke may be very slow, so slow that the patient and even the therapists are unable to discern any progress which is being made towards the long-term goal (e.g. to achieve independent mobility). If one sets and achieves intermediate goals (e.g. sitting balance), progress is more easily perceived and morale maintained. The management of patients with stroke in hospital is often allowed to drift without direction or leadership. The responsible clinician waves to the patient on a weekly ward round in the belief that the therapists are actively rehabilitating the patient. If the head of the multidisciplinary team maintains discipline, and encourages the setting of both short- and longer term goals, this drift can be avoided. This discipline benefits the patients, the team members and the service as a whole.

Describing goals

Where the goal is simply the removal of a problem, such as a urinary tract infection, it is fairly easy to describe it and then measure progress, e.g. relief of symptoms and sterile urine on a repeat culture. Similarly, long-term goals are often easy to describe but should take into account the patient's need for accommodation, physical and emotional support, how they might fill their time and what role they play in society (Wade, 1992). Judgements about whether these long-term goals have been achieved are relatively straightforward. For example, if the goal is to get a patient home to live with their family, or to return to work, one does not need any complex measures of outcome. In some areas, it is even fairly easy to set intermediate goals. For example, many patients with stroke have problems with mobility, but usually the patient will achieve certain physical milestones on the road to recovery (Fig. 10.9). Further improvement in mobility can be measured by recording the time it takes the patient to walk 10 m (Wade et al., 1987). Thus, it is a fairly simple process to set an intermediate goal, which the patient or carer can understand, in terms of the level of function and the date by which it should be achieved.

With other problems, e.g. language and activities of daily living (ADL), intermediate goals are less easily expressed and thus progress is less easily monitored. Although one could use a score on any one of the huge number of measures of language function or ADL as interim goals, these scores are not easily understood by patients and carers. For example, it is unlikely to mean much to a patient, or even the team members, to aim for a Barthel Index score of 12 out of a maximum of 20 in 2 weeks (see Section 17.6.3). Despite these difficulties, the team should attempt to identify problems, short-, intermediate and long-term goals and introduce some measures to determine whether progress is being made towards achieving them.

> In each stroke patient, long-term and intermediate goals should be agreed and described so that progress towards them can be measured. Moreover, everyone will feel a sense of achievement when the goals are met.

10.3.4 Goal setting: a diagnostic tool

Goals may also be useful in identifying new or previously unrecognised problems. If a patient is not achieving the goals which have been set this may be due to a number of causes which can be divided into team, patient and carer factors.

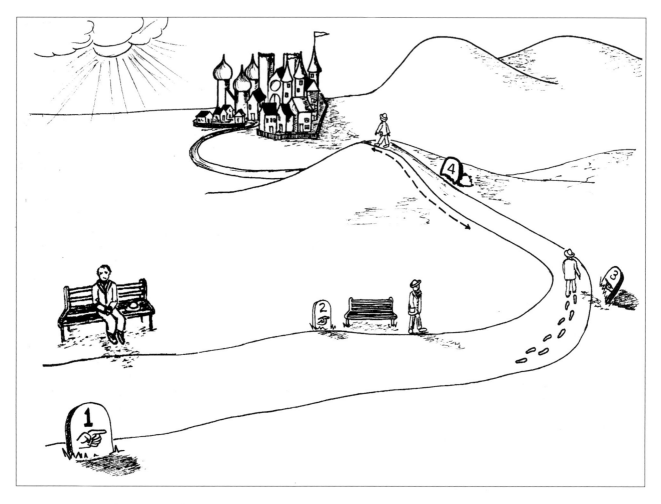

Figure 10.9 The 'road' to recovery after a hemiplegic stroke showing some mobility 'milestones'. 1, sitting balance for 1 minute; 2, standing for 10 seconds; 3, 10 steps unaided; 4, timed 10-m walk.

Team factors

If the goals are too ambitious because of inaccurate diagnosis, inadequate assessment or uncertainty about the prognosis, then patients will fail to achieve them, which will have a detrimental effect on the patient's and the team's morale. If goals are too easy, then progress may be slower than is possible. Also goal setting must be as realistic as possible if one is to use goal setting to coordinate care (see Section 10.3.3). To set realistic goals, which are more often achieved than not, requires an understanding of the prognosis and of the likely effectiveness of potential interventions. We have already seen that accurate predictions of progress and outcome are difficult in individual patients (see Section 10.2.7), but informal judgements made by the team may be more accurate because they are based on observation of the patient's progress over a period of time. Another reason why a patient

may not be achieving a goal might be lack of appropriate treatment. Thus, progress may be hampered by too little, or the wrong sort of therapy. However, since there is currently so little information about the optimum amount or the relative effectiveness of most interventions, it is difficult to sort this out. Team members will much more often have to modify their therapy based on their own experience rather than evidence from properly conducted randomised clinical trials.

Patient and carer factors

New, unrecognised medical or psychological problems (e.g. infection, recurrent stroke or depression) may not present overtly, especially in their early stages, but in a less specific way causing a patient's progress to slow, stop or reverse. One can draw a parallel with the concept of 'failure to thrive'

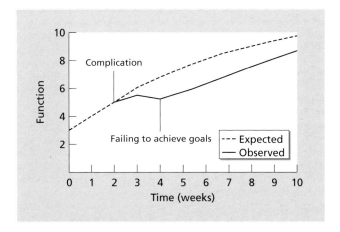

Figure 10.10 'Failure to thrive' after a stroke. Deviation from the expected recovery pattern might be due to any number of factors including recurrent stroke, infections, depression, etc.

in paediatric practice (Fig. 10.10). Where a patient is failing to achieve his or her goals (or milestones) then one needs to identify the cause.

> *Where a patient is failing to achieve his or her goals (or milestones) then one must identify the cause and, if possible, do something about it.*

Sometimes the patient or carer has different goals to those of the team looking after them. This is 'goal mismatch'. For example, a patient who does not want to live alone but would prefer to live with their daughter, may not achieve the level of independence expected. Therefore, when setting goals it is important to discuss them with the patient and carers, although they may be reticent to discuss such matters openly. It is also important to involve the patient, and perhaps the carer, in setting goals to ensure that the goals are really relevant to them. Many stroke patients are retired and thus leisure activities may be particularly important to their quality of life (see Section 15.33.3). The patient may be less interested in a goal aimed at self-care in dressing than being able to read or do the gardening. In hospital practice, where ADL function often determines length of stay, too much emphasis can be placed on ADL-related goals because of the pressures on the team to minimise costs by discharging the patient as early as possible.

10.3.5 The stroke team

Although a physician usually has overall responsibility for the management of the patient, other members of the multi-disciplinary team play an essential part. A systematic review of randomised trials has shown that compared with care on a general medical ward, well-organised care provided by a

multidisciplinary team is likely to reduce the mortality and need for institutionalisation in patients admitted to hospital with an acute stroke (Dennis & Langhorne, 1994; Stroke Unit Trialists' Collaboration, 1996). Because stroke patients have such a broad range of problems, their care demands input from several professions. In order that the professionals' input is coordinated, it is important that at least some of them work as a core team with regular meetings to discuss the patients' progress and problems (Table 10.8). Other professionals (Table 10.9), who may not be regular members of the team, should be available for consultation about individual patients. Although well established in rehabilitation settings, the team has an important role in all phases of treatment, even on the day of the stroke. Of course, the type and intensity of input from different members of the team will vary at different stages of the patient's illness.

By working closely together, and sharing information and skills, some blurring of the boundaries between the roles of the professions is possible and this can provide greater flexibility and efficiency. For example, if the nursing staff are trained by the speech and language therapist to carry out the more straightforward assessments of swallowing this will provide every patient with a simple and early screening assessment (even at weekends), enabling the speech and language therapist to focus on the patients with definite

Table 10.8 The core stroke team.

Physician
Nurses
Physiotherapist
Occupational therapist
Speech and language therapist
Social worker

Table 10.9 Other professionals who may be helpful in the management of particular stroke patients.

Others who may be consulted	Example of problem
Clinical psychologist	Antisocial behaviour
Psychiatrist	Severe depression
Neurosurgeon	Obstructive hydrocephalus
Vascular surgeon	Peripheral artery embolus
Radiologist	Unusual CT scan appearance
Rheumatologist	Painful shoulder
Orthopaedic surgeon	Fractured neck of femur
Ophthalmologist	Persistent diplopia
Dietician	Weight loss
Pharmacist	Formulations for dysphagia
Dentist	Ill-fitting dentures

swallowing or communication problems. Some have suggested that we should develop a hybrid therapist who could take on several roles, but this interesting idea has, not surprisingly, met with considerable opposition from the existing professions. This concept may have particular merits where, as in the community, it is difficult to coordinate the activities of a multidisciplinary team.

Figures 10.11 and 10.12 illustrate two models of how members of the stroke team can provide input to patients and their carers. They represent the extremes and it is likely that in the real world care would be provided in an intermediate way. Although the model represented in Fig. 10.12 realistically means that patients must be treated in a stroke rehabilitation unit, it has important advantages. Inevitably, because resources are limited, stroke patients receive relatively little time with the therapists. Where this input has been measured it may amount to less than 1 hour for each day spent in hospital (Garraway *et al.*, 1980). Training the nurses to practice with the patients the activities initiated by the therapists, should encourage consistency and increase the total amount of therapy received by patients. After all, the nurses are caring for patients on a ward throughout the 24-hour period. It is important that if, for example, the physiotherapists are teaching a patient how to transfer from bed to wheelchair that the patient continues to do this in the same way *between* physiotherapy sessions. Without this approach many of the skills the patient acquires during physiotherapy sessions may not be used during activities on the ward or, more importantly, at home. The same principles apply to input from other therapists. Whether therapy delivered by a non-specialist is as effective as therapy delivered by a highly trained specialist needs to be evaluated in ran-

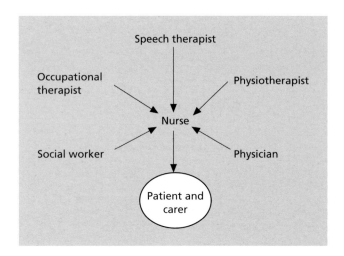

Figure 10.12 The model of care or rehabilitation which can be adopted on a geographically defined stroke unit where each member of the multidisciplinary team influences the nursing input to the patient and carer as well as having direct interaction with them.

domised trials. Studies have been performed to assess the relative effectiveness of speech and language therapists and volunteers in treating patients with aphasia (see Section 15.30). One of the important functions of the team meeting is to harmonise the activity of the therapists and the nurses who provide much of the daily input to the patients. This may be at least one of the reasons why stroke units seem to achieve better outcomes (see Section 17.4.2).

10.3.6 The roles of the team members

This section will outline the main functions of the core members of the team. In practice, and certainly where a team is functioning well, there will be some blurring of the roles of the team members with each performing the less specialised functions of the others.

Physician

Few doctors really understand the important role that they can play in the care of stroke patients beyond making the initial diagnosis, searching for a treatable cause, initiating secondary preventative measures and, perhaps in the future, giving acute medical therapies. The physician needs to be much more involved in the activities of the team for several reasons.

1 Usually, rightly or wrongly, political power in health services lies principally with doctors and, therefore, if stroke patients are to have access to adequate facilities the doctor must be involved.

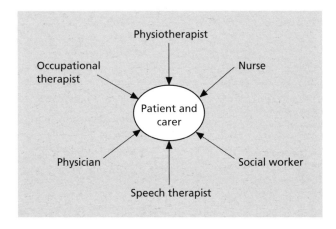

Figure 10.11 The traditional model of care or rehabilitation where each member of the multidisciplinary team interacts independently with the patient and/or carer.

2 The physician should be knowledgeable about the pathologies, both stroke and non-stroke, which underlie the patients' functional problems and thus understand the prognosis and likely effect of interventions. This is essential for predicting outcome and setting appropriate goals.

3 Stroke patients commonly have co-existing and complicating medical problems (e.g. diabetes, heart failure, deep venous thrombosis) which need to be identified and treated (Dromerick & Reding, 1994; Kalra *et al.*, 1995).

4 The physician will often have the broadest knowledge about stroke and is therefore in a good, although not necessarily unique, position to coordinate the team and to chair team meetings. This role is important because team meetings can become very time consuming and may lose direction without a strong chairperson. Overly long meetings are boring, demoralising and inefficient.

5 The final legal responsibility for the patient is the doctor's and therefore it is obvious that the doctor has to be involved at all stages of the patient's care.

Nursing staff

The nursing staff probably have the broadest role in the management of patients with stroke, which includes the following.

1 Daily assessment of the patient's problems, both existing and new, and of their abilities and disabilities. Every week our nurses assess the patients using the Barthel Index (see Table 17.18) which focuses their attention on important functional issues. Based on this assessment they evolve a care plan which aims to meet the individual's needs.

2 Provision of all the basic needs (e.g. feeding, washing, dressing, toileting, turning and transferring) of dependent patients after a stroke.

3 Provision of skilled nursing to prevent the development of complications such as pressures sores (see Section 15.16), painful shoulders (see Section 15.24), other injuries (see Section 15.26) and aspiration pneumonia (see Sections 15.12 and 15.17). This involves correctly positioning and handling the immobile patient (see Section 15.11). If one adopts a model of team working which approximates to that shown in Fig. 10.12, then the nurse's role will include many of the functions of other members of the team.

4 Supporting the patient and family. With increasing emphasis on improving easily measured clinical outcomes such as case fatality and disability, other aspects of caring for and about patients are easily forgotten but these are very important to patients and close family members (Pound et al., 1995); informing, reassuring, encouraging, advising, supporting and sympathising. The nurses usually have greatest contact with the patients and family and therefore have an important role in this area. Although in the UK, and many other developed countries, we have until now taken our nursing staff for granted, it should be remembered that in some other health care systems trained nurses are less available and much of the patient's day to day needs are met by relatives.

Physiotherapist

The physiotherapist has several important roles in caring for stroke patients, depending on their individual needs and the stage of their illness. Soon after a severe stroke the physiotherapist may be involved in the following.

1 Providing a detailed assessment of the motor and sensory problems of the patient to help estimate the patient's prognosis.

2 Assessing and treating chest problems, including pneumonia and retention of secretions. Speech and language therapists often find it useful to have a physiotherapist present at swallowing assessments to help position the patient and to deal promptly with any aspiration (see Section 15.17).

3 Advising nurses and other carers on the best way to position patients to prevent changes in tone which may lead ultimately to contractures and further limitation of function (see Section 15.20).

4 Training the nurses or informal carers the best way to handle the patient to avoid pain or injury to the patient or the carer. This will often involve teaching proper methods of transferring, lifting, standing and walking a patient.

5 Providing therapy to relieve the symptoms associated with painful shoulders or swollen limbs (see Sections 15.24 and 15.25).

6 Providing therapy to improve the patient's mobility and arm function (see Section 15.21).

7 Advising on walking aids and splints (see Section 15.32.1) which may sometimes improve a patient's function.

Occupational therapists

Occupational therapists fulfil several roles in the management of stroke patients. Their role is usually fairly limited in the very early period after a severe stroke but it becomes more important as the patient recovers and as self-care becomes more relevant. These roles include the following.

1 An early assessment of the patient to find out how each impairment is likely to restrict the patient's function. This requires an assessment of what the patient was able to do before the stroke and of what their home circumstances are, e.g. ease of access to the front door, bedroom, toilet or bathroom.

2 An assessment of the patient's visuospatial functioning. It is important to remember that many of the objective tests of these aspects of the stroke patient used an occupational therapist's assessment as the gold standard (see Section 15.29) (Stone *et al.*, 1991).

3 Training the patient and the carer to carry out everyday activities despite their impairments (see Section 15.32). This involves finding the best way of achieving a particular activity for that individual patient. Most input is spent on the activities of daily living (see Table 17.18), although in specialised units or those dealing with younger patients, therapy aimed at return to an occupation (see Section 15.33.2) or leisure activity (see Section 15.33.3) may be available.

4 Provision of aids and adaptations to allow patients to function better. In the UK this includes wheelchair provision, feeding and kitchen aids and bathroom aids, amongst many others (see Section 15.32).

5 Assessment of the patient's function in their own home. This is often done before discharge in patients who have been admitted to hospital and is an important element of discharge planning. It is important in identifying problems which are specific to the patient's home environment and which may be solved by further training or by provision of aids or adaptations.

Speech and language therapist

As the title suggests, the speech and language therapist has several roles in the care of stroke patients. These include the following.

1 Assessment of swallowing safety both initially and as the patient improves, so that their diet and fluid intake matches their swallowing abilities (see Section 15.17).

2 Teaching the patient, nurses or family who are involved with feeding, techniques that help overcome a swallowing impairment and to avoid aspiration.

3 Teaching the patients exercises that *may* increase the rate of recovery of swallowing problems.

4 Diagnosis and assessment of the patient's communication problems (see Section 15.30).

5 Informing carers, both formal and informal, of the nature of the patient's communication problems. Patients, their families and even the professionals caring for the patient often have great difficulty understanding what is wrong with a dysphasic patient. They may think the patient is 'confused', 'demented' or simply 'mad'. Because problems with communication so often lead to emotional distress, most therapists will take on a counselling role.

6 Teaching patients, carers or even volunteers strategies to allow the patient to communicate effectively using language (spoken or written), gesture or communication aids where appropriate.

7 Providing therapy which *may* enhance the recovery of communication difficulties (see Section 15.30).

Social worker

The role of the social worker is bound to vary in different societies. In the UK, Australia and the Netherlands the social worker is likely to be involved in the following.

1 Providing the patient and their family with practical advice and help at all stages of the patient's illness. For example, arranging subsidised transport for the family to visit the hospital, or extra home care for a dependent relative if the stroke patient had been their main carer before admission. Social workers often help with any financial problems which have arisen because the main 'bread winner' has had a stroke, e.g. by applying for allowances or grants.

2 Later in the illness, they have a major role in helping to plan the patient's discharge from hospital or change of accommodation. Social workers often spend a lot of time identifying the wishes and needs of the patient and family and then, with the rest of the team, trying to meet them. Where patients are unable to make decisions for themselves, and have no close family, the social worker may need to act as the patient's advocate and make arrangements for their financial affairs to be taken care of and perhaps even to arrange any change of accommodation (e.g. transfer to a nursing home).

3 A hospital-based social worker may, depending on local organisation, be responsible for following up the family after the patient's discharge from hospital to identify their changing need for support and to make adjustments to any care package.

4 Many social workers have counselling skills which can be helpful in allowing patients and families to come to terms with the change in circumstances brought about by the stroke. Some organise groups of patients, carers or both to help solve problems.

One function which should be shared by all members of the team is that of monitoring the patient's condition. Nurses and therapists, in particular, spend a lot of their time handling patients and observing the patient's performance, so they are often in an ideal position to notice the relatively minor changes that may be an early sign of a complication, which might benefit from early treatment.

> *All members of the team should be alert to changes in the patient's condition which may indicate the development of a complication.*

Are the interventions of the team members effective?

It is clear from a systematic review of randomised trials that compared with the traditional, disorganised pattern of care provided on general medical wards, care coordinated by a well-organised multidisciplinary team results in a better clinical outcome for stroke patients (Dennis & Langhorne, 1994; Stroke Unit Trialists' Collaboration, 1996). However, exactly which specific aspects of this model of care bring about these benefits is unclear (see Section 17.4.2). People often question the effectiveness of physiotherapy, occupational therapy, speech and language therapy and social work. They point to the lack of research evidence to support the effectiveness of these professionals or they emphasise particular studies which appear to demonstrate their ineffectiveness. Unfortunately, these 'negative' studies have, in general, asked the wrong questions, measured the wrong outcomes, been too small and have not evaluated the intervention in the context of a well-organised stroke team. This has possibly resulted in 'false-negative' studies with a resulting rejection of valuable team members. Failure to demonstrate a definite effect cannot be taken as proof of a lack of effect (Altman & Bland, 1995). Nobody who is closely involved in working with these team members could doubt their value and overall effectiveness. There may be uncertainty about the effectiveness, optimum dose and duration of some of the specific therapeutic manoeuvres they use but, as we have shown, this type of input forms only a small part of their contribution to the care of stroke patients. The evidence for the effectiveness of specific aspects of their work is discussed later (see Chapter 15).

10.3.7 Multidisciplinary team meetings

If the team is to work effectively it is important that it meets regularly. All the stroke units included in a recent systematic review of the randomised controlled trials held at least weekly meetings of the multidisciplinary team, separate from conventional ward rounds (Langhorne, 1995). These meetings have several important functions.

1 The entire team can be introduced to new patients and their problems.

2 Existing patients can be reviewed and if individual team members have noted a change in their condition, or a new problem, this can be communicated to the other members.

3 After reviewing each patient's progress, and the development of any problems, realistic goals can be set jointly and an appropriate course of action to meet those goals agreed (see Section 10.3.3).

4 Verbal reports of individual therapist's assessments, and in particular the results of pre-discharge home visits, can be discussed and detailed plans for discharge made.

5 Meetings have an educational role for the team members, students and visitors. For example, we often show the patient's brain CT, discuss the likely pathogenesis of the stroke and any rationale for treatment.

So that important details are not overlooked it may be useful to agree a formal structure to discussions. The structure we have adopted is discussed below. This is not rigidly adhered to but forms a framework for discussions about individual patients.

Structure of team discussion

The medical details of any new patients are presented by the physician including a brief account of the patient's symptoms and any relevant past history, including risk factors and the presumed cause of the stroke. The patient's social background is presented briefly by the clinician but other members of the team are often able to contribute extra details. The patient's neurological impairments are discussed and the therapists have often identified impairments which may not have been obvious to the physician. By the time of the meeting the nursing staff can report on the functional consequences of these impairments (i.e. disability) and, using the information about pre-stroke activities, some estimate of the stroke's likely effect on the patient's life after the stroke can be made (i.e. predicted handicap).

At each subsequent meeting we introduce the patient briefly with a resumé of their date of stroke, stroke pathology, clinical type and presumed cause. We then summarise the problems, goals and actions which were agreed at the last meeting. Each member of the team is then invited to update the rest of the team on the patient's progress, what problems and goals have been solved or achieved, what new goals they plan to set and how they plan to achieve them. Usually we do this in a set order which tends to reflect the way we think about patients, i.e. pathology, impairments, disabilities and handicaps. The physician starts by updating the team on any changes in the patient's medical condition or the results of any important investigations which may be relevant to other team members. The nurses then give an overall report on the patient's progress. The therapists follow: first the physiotherapist, then the speech therapist and lastly the occupational therapist. The first two tend to focus more on impairments and the patient's basic functions such as mobility, swallowing and communication, whilst the occupational therapist usually focuses on the broader range of disabilities and how these are likely to affect the patient's everyday life. Lastly, the social worker reports on any problems which close contact with the family may have revealed and any progress regarding discharge planning. This sequence also has the advantage that the occupational therapist and social worker can make use of the information from the others in formulating their own goals and actions.

The discussion is then opened up and longer term goals such as timing of home visits, discharges and case (family) conferences are set and we decide who will do what by the next meeting. This includes deciding who should communicate with the patient and family to ensure that they are involved with the goal setting process and that their views are taken into account.

Multidisciplinary teams may lack effectiveness if each member is not given an equal chance to contribute. Inevitably, teams will include some more assertive individuals and other less out-going members, the former tending to dominate discussions. It is important that the team leader, often the physician, ensures that individual members do not monopolise the discussions to the extent that others are not heard. The framework we have adopted lessens the likelihood of this arising, although of course not every member will have something useful to contribute in each case.

Involving patients and carers in team meetings

Neither the patient nor the family have been mentioned as having a direct input into the team meetings, although their input is obviously crucial in setting goals and planning discharge from hospital. We do not invite them to attend each meeting but we do try to find out their views on certain aspects of their care in advance of the meeting. We also try to ensure that the nature and conclusions of the discussion at the meeting are communicated back to the patient and/or family by the most appropriate team member, most often the nurse. Although it is sometimes vital to involve the patient and families in discussions we feel that their attendance at each weekly meeting would inhibit the discussion and might be distressing for them. It would also make meetings longer and more unwieldy.

We normally hold separate team meetings (case conferences or family meetings) which the patient, their family and any other people who are involved, such as district nurse and home care organiser, are invited to attend. These meetings are useful in planning hospital discharges in complex cases and in resolving differences of opinion between the team members and the patient or their family.

Team building

We have found it useful to have separate team meetings where patients are not discussed. On these occasions we discuss management issues, how the team is working, what the

problems are and any changes which might be made in the way we work. These sessions also allow individuals to tell the rest of the team about certain specialised aspects of their jobs. This, we believe, not only encourages some blurring of the distinctions between their functions but also aids team building. Each member can more fully appreciate the contribution made by other members.

Recording the work of the team

We have not yet found a very satisfactory method of recording the work of the team. Traditionally, each member has kept their own records so that they may refer to them, but this inevitably leads to much unnecessary duplication. However, a unified record has disadvantages, the main one being that different members of the team require information of varying detail. Thus, the physiotherapist's record will contain very detailed records of the patient's motor functioning which is irrelevant to the social worker. Also, the records may be needed simultaneously by the physiotherapist in the gym and the occupational therapist on a home visit. We have, therefore, kept individual records but encouraged the nurses to base their care plans on the discussions at the team meetings. This has been helped by their adoption of a problem-orientated approach so that the nurses regularly record the patients' problems, the goals and actions to attain the goals. A compromise where core details are collected once and shared, whilst more detailed records are kept by each team member, may provide the best and most efficient solution. In the future, increased use of information technology may facilitate a combined patient record which avoids some of these problems (Kalra & Fowle, 1994).

10.4 Some difficult ethical issues

Where patients are judged to be unlikely to have a reasonable quality of life if they survive, many clinicians would make a decision not to strive to ensure survival. This is an extremely difficult decision since, as we have already discussed (see Section 10.2.7), there are considerable difficulties in predicting outcome reliably. It is also an area where, until now, little research has been done (Alexandrov *et al.*, 1995; Grotta *et al.*, 1995).

The patient who has had a major stroke is often not in a position to make decisions about their treatment because they are, due to depressed conscious level, language or visuo-spatial problems, unable to understand or communicate. Under these circumstances, the family or potential carers should be included in the decision-making process. The family can often provide information which allow judgements about what the patient's likely wishes are. However, some relatives may have their own interests and not just those of the patient to consider. Younger relatives may gain financially from the death of an older relative and death removes the obligation to care for a severely disabled person.

One has to be careful in assessing the likely prognosis of an individual patient with an apparently severe stroke. A relatively minor stroke which is complicated by another medical problem (e.g. pneumonia) may be impossible to differentiate from a severe stroke (see Section 15.4). However, the complicating medical problem may, if identified, be treated easily to achieve a very satisfactory clinical outcome for the patient.

It is not always easy to distinguish between a patient who has had a catastrophic stroke and one who has had a less severe stroke which is complicated and worsened by infection, seizures or metabolic problems. The prognosis is much worse for the former than the latter patient.

Perhaps the most common dilemma is whether or not to give fluids to a patient with an 'apparently severe stroke' who is unable to swallow. Few would argue against giving parenteral fluids to a conscious patient on the basis of preventing dehydration, thirst and discomfort. However, if the patient is unconscious and thus probably unaware of discomfort, then there is more uncertainty about what to do for the best. Also, if the patient develops an infection very soon after the onset of the stroke, apart from the difficulties mentioned above in assessing the severity of stroke, the question arises as to how aggressively one should treat the patient. Are intravenous antibiotics, physiotherapy or even artificial ventilation and inotropic support appropriate?

There are some facts worth considering before making these difficult decisions. First, most patients who are unconscious after a stroke die in the first few days from the direct neurological effects of the stroke on brainstem function and not from dehydration or infection (see Section 10.2.3) (Bounds *et al.*, 1981; Silver *et al.*, 1984; Bamford *et al.*, 1990b). Therefore, by simply giving fluids, it is unlikely that the lives of many patients will be greatly prolonged but it may give more time to make an accurate assessment of prognosis.

If one elects to give a patient fluids, antibiotics or even naso-gastric nutritional support, this clearly does not have to be continued long term. However, in some countries there are laws which prevent clinicians from withdrawing treatment of this kind and many clinicians feel more uncomfortable about stopping a treatment which they have started than not starting it in the first place. Apart from worrying about medicolegal issues one has to consider the reaction of the family. However, in our experience, if the clinician has spent enough time informing the family of the patient's state and likely prognosis, and have involved them in the decisions, withdrawal of fluids, feeding or antibiotics is usually not a major problem. Unfortunately, there is a trend for such decisions, especially in severely brain-damaged children and patients in a persistent vegetative state, to be deferred to the legal profession.

We can not hope to have the answers to all these difficult problems but perhaps it is worth suggesting a general approach which we have found practicable.

1 *The first requirement is for prompt access to accurate and unbiased information about the patient's life prior to the stroke.* It is inadequate to base one's decisions on some measure of the severity of just the stroke since this may be difficult to estimate accurately (see Section 15.4) and other factors will influence prognosis (Alexandrov *et al.*, 1995). The patient's pre-stroke functional level and social activity are crucial in making these decisions. Unfortunately, this information is often not collected in sufficient detail during the acute phase because its relevance to acute care is not recognised. One might be less aggressive in treating a patient who was previously handicapped, miserable and in pain from severe arthritis and living in an institution than somebody with an equally severe stroke who was previously living at home independently with their family. Usually, the patient's pre-stroke handicap sets the ceiling on their potential post-stroke outcome so that these two patients have very different outlooks. It is still a difficult, some would say an impossible, judgement to say whether the first person's life is worth prolonging.

2 *Make a detailed assessment of the patient's condition* to make the best possible judgement about their prognosis.

3 *Formulate the alternative management plans which might be adopted.* These should include the most aggressive to the most conservative.

4 *Discuss all the options with other members of the team and any close family members.* The family needs to be given accurate information about the diagnosis, problems, likely outcomes and treatment possibilities. It is probably unfair to suggest that the decisions are theirs but any decision the clinician makes should ideally be compatible with their views. If one does not take the families' wishes in to account one is inviting trouble, complaints, and nowadays, litigation. It is worth making it clear to them that few decisions are irreversible (except perhaps for turning off a ventilator) since circumstances change. One is often in a much better position to make an accurate prognosis having observed the patient's progress over a few days than on the day of the stroke so that what appeared to be an appropriate intervention on day one may appear less appropriate after a few days. The development of better tools to help predict prognosis, and

studies that give a better understanding of the effect of our supportive interventions, should improve these difficult decisions in the future.

> *Involve other members of the team and the patient's family in any decisions about how aggressively one should strive to keep a patient alive.*

References

Alexandrov AV, Bladin CF, Meslin EM, Norris JW (1995). Do-not-resuscitate orders in acute stroke. *Neurology* 45: 634–40.

Allen CM (1984a). Predicting outcome after acute stroke: role of computerised tomography. *Lancet* 25 August: 464–5.

Allen CMC (1984b). Predicting the outcome of acute stroke: a prognostic score. *J Neurol Neurosurg Psychiatr* 47: 475–80.

Altman DG, Bland JM (1995). Absence of evidence is not evidence of absence. *Br Med J* 311: 485.

Anderson CS, Jamrozik KD, Broadhurst RJ, Stewart-Wynne EG (1994). Predicting survival for 1 year among different subtypes of stroke: results from the Perth Community Stroke Study. *Stroke* 25: 1935–44.

Asplund K, Bonita R, Kuulasmaa K *et al.* (1995). Multinational comparisons of stroke epidemiology: evaluation of case ascertainment in the WHO MONICA Stroke Study. *Stroke* 26: 355–60.

Bamford J, Sandercock PAG, Dennis MS, Warlow CP (1990a). A prospective study of acute cerebrovascular disease in the community: the Oxfordshire Community Stroke Project 1981–86. 2. Incidence, case fatality rates and overall outcome at one year of cerebral infarction, primary intracerebral and subarachnoid haemorrhage. *J Neurol Neurosurg Psychiatr* 53: 16–22.

Bamford J, Sandercock PAG, Jones L, Warlow CP (1987). The natural history of lacunar infarction: the Oxfordshire Community Stroke Project. *Stroke* 18: 545–51.

Bamford J, Sandercock P, Warlow C, Gray M (1986). Why are patients with acute stroke admitted to hospital? *Br Med J* 292: 1369–72.

Bamford J, Dennis MS, Sandercock P, Burn J, Warlow C (1990b). The frequency, cause and timing of death within 30 days of a first stroke: the Oxfordshire Community Stroke Project. *J Neurol Neurosurg Psychiatr* 53: 824–9.

Bamford J, Sandercock PAG, Dennis MS, Burn J, Warlow CP (1991). Classification and natural history of clinically identifiable subtypes of cerebral infarction. *Lancet* 337: 1521–6.

Bamford J, Sandercock P, Dennis M *et al.* (1988). A prospective study of acute cerebrovascular disease in the community: the Oxfordshire Community Stroke Project 1981–86. 1. Methodology, demography and incident cases of first-ever stroke. *J Neurol Neurosurg Psychiatr* 51: 1273–1380.

Barer DH (1990). The influence of visual and tactile inattention on predictions for recovery from acute stroke. *Quart J Med* 273: 21–32.

Bounds JV, Weibers DO, Whisnant JP, Okazaki H (1981). Mechanisms and timing of deaths from cerebral infarction. *Stroke* 12: 474–7.

Britton M, de Faire U, Helmers C, Miah K (1980). Prognostication in acute cerebrovascular disease. *Acta Med Scand* 207: 37–42.

Burn J, Dennis MS, Bamford J, Sandercock PAG, Wade D, Warlow CP (1994). Long-term risk of recurrent stroke after a first-ever stroke. The Oxfordshire Community Stroke Project. *Stroke* 25: 333–7.

Chollet F, DiPiero V, Wise RJS, Brooks DJ, Dolan RJ, Frackowiak RSJ (1991). The functional anatomy of motor recovery after stroke in humans: a study with positron emission tomography. *Ann Neurol* 29: 63–71.

Crisi G, Colombo A, de Santis M, Guerzoni MC, Calo M, Panzetti P (1984). CT and cerebral ischemic infarcts. Correlations between morphological and clinical prognostic findings. *Neuroradiology* 26: 101–5.

Davenport RJ, Dennis MS, Warlow CP (1995). Improving the recording of the clinical assessment of stroke patients using a clerking proforma. *Age Ageing* 24: 43–8.

Dennis MS, Langhorne P (1994). So stroke units save lives: where do we go from here? *Br Med J* 309: 1273–7.

Dennis MS, Burn JPS, Sandercock P, Bamford JM, Wade DT, Warlow CP (1993). Long term survival after first ever stroke: the Oxfordshire Community Stroke Project. *Stroke* 24: 796–800.

Dombovy ML, Basfird JR, Whisnant JP, Bergstalh EJ (1987). Disability and use of rehabilitation services following stroke in Rochester, Minnesota, 1975–1979. *Stroke* 18: 830–6.

Dromerick A, Reding M (1994). Medical and neurological complications during in-patient stroke rehabilitation. *Stroke* 25: 358–61.

Fiorelli M, Alperovitch A, Argentino C *et al.* (1995). Prediction of long-term outcome in the early hours following acute ischaemic stroke. *Arch Neurol* 52: 250–5.

Fullerton KJ, MacKenzie G, Stout RW (1988). Prognostic indices in stroke. *Quart J Med* 25: 147–62.

Garraway WM, Whisnant JP, Drury I (1983). The changing pattern of survival following stroke. *Stroke* 14: 699–703.

Garraway WM, Akhtar AJ, Prescott RJ, Hockey L (1980). Management of acute stroke in the elderly: preliminary results of a controlled trial. *Br Med J* 280: 1040–3.

Gladman JRF, Harwood DMJ, Barer DH (1992). Predicting the outcome of acute stroke: prospective evaluation of five multivariate models and comparison with simple methods. *J Neurol Neurosurg Psychiatr* 55: 347–51.

Gompertz P, Pound P, Ebrahim S (1994). Predicting stroke outcome: Guy's prognostic score in practice. *J Neurol Neurosurg Psychiatr* 57: 932–5.

Granger CV, Hamilton BB, Gresham GE, Kramer AA (1989). The stroke rehabilitation outcome study: part II. Relative merits of the total Barthel Index Score and a Four-Item subscore in predicting patient outcomes. *Arch Phys Med Rehab* 70: 100–3.

Gray CS, French JM, Bates D, Cartlidge NEF, James OFW, Venables G (1990). Motor recovery following acute stroke. *Age Ageing* 19: 179–84.

Grotta J, Pasteur W, Khwaja G, Hamel T, Fisher M, Ramirez A (1995). Elective intubation for neurologic deterioration after stroke. *Neurology* 45: 640–4.

Henon H, Godefroy O, Leys D *et al.* (1995). Early predictors of death and disability after acute cerebral ischaemic event. *Stroke* 26: 392–8.

Hier DB, Edelstein G (1991). Deriving clinical prediction rules from stroke outcome research. *Stroke* 22: 1431–6.

Horner RD, Matchar DB, Divine GW, Feussner JR (1995). Relationship between physician specialty and the selection and outcome of ischaemic stroke patients. *Health Serv Res* 30 (No 2): 275–88.

Jongbloed L (1990). Problems of methodological heterogeneity in studies predicting disability after stroke. *Stroke* 21 (Suppl. II): 32–4.

Kalra L, Fowle AJ (1994). An integrated system for multidisciplinary assessments in stroke rehabilitation. *Stroke* 24: 2210–14.

Kalra L, Yu G, Wilson K, Roots P (1995). Medical complications during stroke rehabilitation. *Stroke* 26: 990–4.

Kojima S, Omura T, Wakamatsu W *et al.* (1990). Prognosis and disability of stroke patients after 5 years in Akita, Japan. *Stroke* 21: 72–7.

Langhorne P (1995). What is a stroke unit? Survey of the randomised trials. *Cerebrovasc Dis* 5: 228 (abstract).

Lincoln NB, Jackson JM, Edmans JA *et al.* (1990). The accuracy of predictions about progress of patients on a stroke unit. *J Neurol Neurosurg Psychiatr* 53: 972–5.

Loewen SC, Anderson BA (1990). Predictors of stroke outcome using objective measurement scales. *Stroke* 21: 78–81.

Pound P, Bury M, Gompertz P, Ebrahim S (1995). Stroke patients' views of their admission to hospital. *Br Med J* 311: 18–22.

Prescott RJ, Garraway WM, Akhtar AJ (1982). Predicting functional outcome following acute stroke using a standard clinical examination. *Stroke* 13(5): 641–7.

Ricci S, Celani MG, La Rosa F *et al.* (1991). Sepivac: a community-based study of stroke incidence in Umbria, Italy. *J Neurol Neurosurg Psychiatr* 54: 695–8.

Rose L, Bakal DA, Fung TS, Farn P, Weaver LE (1994). Tactile extinction and functional status after stroke. A preliminary investigation. *Stroke* 25: 1973–6.

Sacco RL, Wolf PA, Kannel WB, McNamara PM (1982). Survival and recurrence following stroke. The Framingham Study. *Stroke* 13 (No 3): 290–5.

Sackett DL, Haynes RB, Guyatt GH, Tugwell MD (1991). *Clinical Epidemiology. A Basic Science for Clinical Medicine*, 2nd edn. Boston/Toronto/London: Little, Brown and Company, 173–85.

Sheikh K, Brennan PJ, Meade TW, Smith DS, Goldenberg E (1983). Predictors of mortality and disability in stroke. *J Epidemiol Commun Health* 37: 70–4.

Silver FL, Norris JW, Lewis AJ, Hachinski VC (1984). Early mortality following stroke: a prospective view. *Stroke* 15: 492–6.

Skilbeck CE, Wade DT, Langton Hewer R, Wood VA (1983). Recovery after stroke. *J Neurol Neurosurg Psychiatr* 46: 5–8.

Slattery JM, Hankey GJ (1992). Intracerebral haemorrhage: external validation and extension of a model for prediction of 30 day survival. *Ann Neurol* 32 (No 2): 225–6.

Stephenson R (1993). A review of neuroplasticity: some implications for physiotherapy in the treatment of lesions of the brain. *Physiotherapy* 79 (No 10): 699–704.

Stone SP, Wilson B, Wroot A *et al.* (1991). The assessment of visuo-spatial neglect after acute stroke. *J Neurol Neurosurg Psychiatr* 54: 345–50.

Stroke Unit Trialists' Collaboration (1996). A systematic review of specialist multidisciplinary team (stroke unit) care for stroke inpatients. In: Warlow C, van Gijn J, Sandercock P, eds. *Stroke Module of the Cochrane Database of Systematic Reviews, 1996* (updated 23 February 1996). Available in the Cochrane Library. London: BMJ Publishing Group.

Taub NA, Wolfe CDA, Richardson E, Burney PGJ (1994). Predicting the disability of first-time stroke sufferers at 1 year. 12 month follow up of a population based cohort in Southeast England. *Stroke* 25: 352–7.

Tijssen CC, Bento PM, Schulte MD, Anton CM, Leyten MD (1991). Prognostic significance of conjugate eye deviation in stroke patients. *Stroke* 22: 200–2.

Tuhrim S, Dambrosia JM, Price TR *et al.* (1991). Intracerebral haemorrhage: external validation and extension of a model for prediction of 30 day survival. *Ann Neurol* 29: 658–63.

Turney TM, Garraway M, Whisnant JP (1984). The natural history of hemispheric and brainstem infarction in Rochester, Minnesota. *Stroke* 15 (5): 790–4.

Valdimarsson E, Bergvall U, Samuelsson K (1982). Prognostic significance of cerebral computed tomography results in supratentorial infarction. *Acta Neurol Scand* 65: 133–45.

van Gijn J (1992). Subarachnoid haemorrhage. *Stroke Octet (Lancet)* 339: 653–5.

Wade DT (1992). Stroke: rehabilitation and long-term care. *Lancet Stroke Octet*: 38–40.

Wade T, Hewer RL (1985). Outlook after an acute stroke: urinary incontinence and loss of consciousness compared in 532 patients. *Quart J Med* 56: 601–8.

Wade DT, Langton Hewer R (1987). Functional abilities after stroke: measurement, natural history and prognosis. *J Neurol Neurosurg Psychiatr* 50: 177–82.

Wade DT, Skilbeck CE, Langton Hewer R (1983a). Predicting Barthel ADL score at 6 months after an acute stroke. *Arch Phys Med Rehab* 64: 24–8.

Wade DT, Wood VA, Hewer RL (1985). Recovery after stroke—the first 3 months. *J Neurol Neurosurg Psychiatr* 48: 7–13.

Wade DT, Langton Hewer R, Wood VA, Skilbeck CE, Ismail HM (1983b). The hemiplegic arm after stroke: measurement and recovery. *J Neurol Neurosurg Psychiatr* 46: 521–4.

Wade DT, Wood VA, Heller A, Maggs J, Langton Hewer R (1987). Walking after stroke. Measurement and recovery over the first 3 months. *Scand J Rehab Med* 19: 25–30.

Weiller C, Ramsay SC, Wise RJS, Friston KL, Frackowiak RSJ

(1993). Individual patterns of functional reorganisation in the human cerebral cortex after capsular infarction. *Ann Neurol* 33: 181–9.

Weingarten S, Bolus R, Riedinger MS, Maldonado L, Stein S, Ellrodt AG (1990). The principle of parsimony: Glasgow Coma Scale Score Predicts Mortality as well as the APACHE II score for stroke patients. *Stroke* 21: 1280–2.

Wellwood I, Dennis MS, Warlow CP (1995). A comparison of the Barthel Index and the OPCS disability instrument used to measure outcome after acute stroke. *Age Ageing* 24: 54–7.

WHO (1980). *International Classification of Impairments, Disabilities and Handicaps*. Conference papers. Geneva: World Health Organization.

Specific treatment of acute ischaemic stroke

The occlusion of a cerebral blood vessel initiates a series of events which can lead to irreversible neuronal damage and cell death (i.e. infarction) in a part of the brain. Several pathophysiological cascades run in sequence (and in parallel). In the vascular system, rapid changes in platelet and coagulation factors, the vessel wall (particularly the endothelium) and in the thrombus itself interact to produce a very dynamic state, not only at the site of the vessel occlusion, but also more remotely, in both the macro- and micro-circulation. In cerebral tissue, changes occur in neurones, glial cells and other structural components in differing degrees and at different times after the onset of ischaemia, which means that in humans cerebral infarction is a dynamic and highly unstable process, not a discrete event. In other words, infarction is *not* an 'all-or-nothing' episode which is instantaneous in onset, maximal in severity at the moment of onset and irreversibly complete within 6 hours. Specific treatments generally aim to affect one particular pathophysiological cascade at a certain point. This chapter therefore begins with a review of pathophysiology, particularly those aspects which relate to the specific types of treatment that are described in the rest of the chapter. As far as possible, we base the decision whether or not to use a particular treatment, not on its putative physiological effects, but on the evidence from randomised trials to demonstrate the balance of clinical risk and benefit associated with its use. In view of this, the section on each of the specific treatments aims to assess the strength of evidence available and, where possible, to base any recommendations on the results of a systematic review (or meta-analysis) of all the relevant randomised trials of that particular treatment.

11.1 Pathophysiology of acute ischaemic stroke

The pathophysiology of acute ischaemic stroke encompasses two sequential processes: (i) the vascular, haematological or cardiac events that cause the initial reduction (and subsequent change) in local cerebral blood flow; and (ii) then the alterations of cellular chemistry that are caused by ischaemia and which lead on to necrosis of neurones, glia and other brain cells. This section will discuss cerebral metabolism, regulation of cerebral blood flow (CBF), molecular consequences of cerebral ischaemia and how understanding these processes leads on to the development of various treatments for acute ischaemic stroke. The causes of cerebral ischaemia have been described in Chapters 6 and 7.

11.1.1 Cerebral metabolism

Energy demand

The human brain has a high metabolic demand for energy and, unlike other organs, uses glucose (about 75–100 mg/minute, or 125 g/day) as its sole substrate for energy metabolism. Glucose is metabolised in the brain entirely via the glycolytic sequence and the tricarboxylic acid cycle (Fig. 11.1). Each molecule of glucose is broken down in a series of enzymatic steps (glycolysis) to two molecules (2M) of pyruvate. During these reactions, the oxidised form of nicotinamide adenine dinucleotide (NAD$^+$) is reduced (to NADH) and 2M each of adenosine diphosphate (ADP) and intracellular phosphorus are converted to 2M of adenosine triphosphate (ATP). In the *presence* of oxygen, pyruvate is metabolised first by pyruvate dehydrogenase and then by a series of mitochondrial reactions to carbon dioxide (CO_2) and water (H_2O) with the formation of 36M of ATP. This is the maximum ATP yield. In the *absence* of oxygen, this sequence of events is blocked or retarded at the stage of pyruvate oxidation, leading to the reduction of pyruvate to lactate by NADH and lactic dehydrogenase. Anaerobic glycolysis, therefore, still leads to the formation of ATP, as well as lactate, but the energy yield is relatively small (2M rather than 36M of ATP from 1M of glucose). In addition, lactic acid accumulates within and outside cells (hence, the cell is acidified) and mitochondria lose their ability to sequester calcium, so any calcium entering or released within the cell will raise the intracellular calcium level (Siesjo, 1992a).

Figure 11.1 (*Opposite.*) The aerobic metabolism of glucose. The stages of the complete aerobic oxidation of glucose to CO_2 and H_2O and the conservation of free energy as ATP. For the glycolytic sequence to pyruvate we have the reaction: glucose + 2ADP + 2P$_i$ + 2NAD$^+$ → 2pyruvate + 2NADH + 2H$^+$ + 2ATP + 2H$_2$O, and for the tricarboxylic acid cycle: 2pyruvate + 5O$_2$ + 30ADP + 30P$_i$ → 6CO$_2$ + 30ATP + 34H$_2$O. To these are added the equation for the oxidation of two molecules of extra-mitochondrial NADH formed in the glycolytic conversion of glucose to pyruvate. Oxidation of extra-mitochondrial NADH may generate either two or three molecules of ATP per pair of electrons, depending on how the electrons from extra-mitochondrial NADH enter the mitochondria. If we assume that two molecules of ATP are formed in this process, we have 2NADH + 2H$^+$ + O$_2$ + 4ADP + 4P$_i$ → 2NAD$^+$ + 4ATP + 6H$_2$O. The sum of the above three equations is therefore: glucose + 6O$_2$ + 36ADP + 36P$_i$ → 6CO$_2$ + 36ATP + 42H$_2$O. The overall equation of anaerobic glycolysis is: glucose + 2ADP + 2P$_i$ → 2lactic acid + 2ATP + 2H$_2$O.

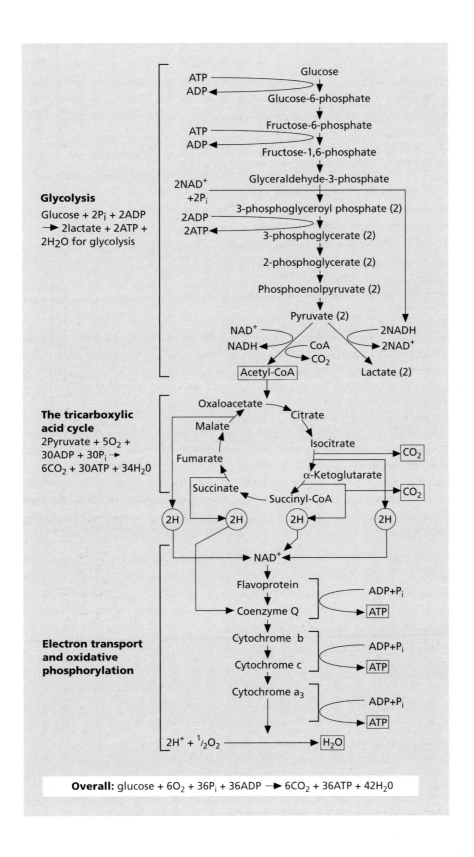

Glycolysis

Glucose + 2P$_i$ + 2ADP
→ 2lactate + 2ATP +
2H$_2$O for glycolysis

The tricarboxylic acid cycle

2Pyruvate + 5O$_2$ +
30ADP + 30P$_i$ →
6CO$_2$ + 30ATP + 34H$_2$0

Electron transport and oxidative phosphorylation

Overall: glucose + 6O$_2$ + 36P$_i$ + 36ADP → 6CO$_2$ + 36ATP + 42H$_2$0

> *The brain uses glucose as its only source of energy. During aerobic metabolism each molecule of glucose produces 36 molecules of adenosine triphosphate, but during anaerobic metabolism only two molecules of ATP are produced along with lactic acid.*

Neurones in the brain require a constant supply of ATP to maintain their integrity and to keep the major intracellular cation, potassium ions (K^+), within the cell and the major extracellular cations, sodium ions (Na^+) and calcium ions (Ca^{2+}), outside the cell. As the brain is unable to store energy, it requires a constant supply of oxygenated blood containing an adequate glucose concentration to maintain its function and structural integrity.

> *The resting brain consumes energy at the same rate as a 20-Watt light bulb.*

Global CBF reflecting both grey and white matter compartments, per unit of brain in a healthy young adult, is about 50–55 ml/100 g of brain per minute, with significantly higher values in those below 20 years of age and lower values in those over 60 years (Leenders *et al.*, 1990). For a brain of average weight (1300–1400 g in a 60–65-kg adult), which is only 2% of total adult body weight, the total CBF at rest is disproportionately large at about 800 ml/minute, which is 15–20% of the total cardiac output of blood (Kety, 1950). At this level of blood flow, whole brain oxygen consumption, usually measured as the cerebral metabolic rate of oxygen ($CMRO_2$), is about 3.3–3.5 ml/100 g of brain per minute, or 45 ml of oxygen per minute or 20% of the total oxygen consumption of the body at rest.

11.1.2 Cerebral blood flow (CBF) regulation

The fraction of oxygen extracted from the blood, the oxygen extraction fraction (OEF), is fairly constant throughout the brain because CBF, cerebral blood volume (CBV) and $CMRO_2$ as well as of glucose (CMRglu) are all coupled (Leenders *et al.*, 1990). In the normal resting brain, measurements of CBF are therefore a reliable reflection of cerebral metabolism ($CMRO_2$). If CBF falls, however (down to a level of 20–25 ml/100 g per minute), the OEF increases to maintain the $CMRO_2$ (see below). Over the past 50 years, methods of measuring CBF have become more accurate and reliable and have had a major impact on our understanding of the regulation of CBF and the pathogenesis of cerebral ischaemia (Kety & Schmidt, 1945; Baron, 1991; Pulsinelli, 1992). Positron emission tomography (PET) now enables CBF, $CMRO_2$, OEF and CMRglu to be measured in various regions of interest in the brain, both in normal people and after stroke (Baron, 1991).

Cerebral perfusion pressure (CPP)

Under normal conditions, blood flow through the brain is determined by the CPP at the base of the brain and by the cerebrovascular resistance (CVR) imposed by blood viscosity and the size of the intracranial arteries (i.e. flow = pressure/resistance). The CPP represents the difference between arterial pressure forcing blood into the cerebral circulation and the venous back pressure. The mean CPP is the mean systemic arterial pressure at the base of the brain when in the recumbent position which approximates to the diastolic blood pressure (about 80 mmHg) plus one-third of the pulse pressure (1/3 × about 40 mmHg) minus the intracranial venous pressure (about 10 mmHg), i.e. 80–85 mmHg.

Cerebrovascular resistance

Under normal conditions, when resting CPP is constant, any change in CBF must be caused by a change in CVR, usually as a result of alteration in the diameter of small intracranial arteries or arterioles. Under these circumstances, there is a direct correlation between CBF and the intravascular CBV. CBF and CBV will both increase as vessels dilate and both decrease as vessels constrict. The CBV:CBF ratio remains relatively constant over a wide range of CBF at normal CPP.

When an artery narrows causing CVR to increase, or when CBF increases, the blood-flow velocity in that segment of artery increases. Although it may seem paradoxical that a reduction in luminal diameter causes an increase in blood flow velocity, think of using a hose: putting one's finger over the nozzle generates a high-pressure jet of water. The narrower the lumen at the nozzle, the greater the pressure (and velocity of flow) in the stream of water until the lumen is nearly occluded, at which point velocity becomes substantially reduced and the water dribbles out of the hose. This is one of the principles governing the interpretation of blood flow velocities in the major basal arteries by transcranial Doppler ultrasound (see Section 6.6.4). Mean blood flow velocities within the intracranial arteries vary from 40 to 70 cm/second. As blood flow velocity (centimetres per second) is proportional to the second power of the vessel radius it cannot be equated linearly with volume blood flow (millilitres per second), which is proportional to the fourth power of the vessel radius (Kontos, 1989). If vessel calibre were constant, some assumptions could be made about volume flow from velocity measures but the calibre of large cerebral arteries varies with changes in blood pressure, arterial CO_2 partial pressure ($Paco_2$), intracranial pressure and age (Markwalder *et al.*, 1984).

Metabolic rate of cerebral tissue

In the resting brain with normal CPP, CBF is closely matched to the metabolic demands of the tissue. Therefore, grey matter (which has a high metabolic rate) has higher regional CBF than white matter, which has a relatively low metabolic rate. The ratio between CBF and metabolism is fairly uniform in all areas of the brain and, consequently, the OEF and functional extraction of glucose from the blood are much the same in different areas. Normally, regional OEF is about one-third and the regional glucose extraction fraction is about 10% (Powers, 1991). Similarly, local flow varies directly with local brain function by 10–20%, even though global CBF tends to be fairly stable under steady state conditions. For example, during voluntary hand movements, the metabolic activity of the contralateral motor cortex increases over a few seconds and is accompanied by rapid vasodilatation of the cerebral resistance vessels, leading to an increase in CBF and CBV, rather than any increase in the OEF or the glucose extraction fraction (Lassen et al., 1977). Conversely, low regional metabolic activity (as may occur in a cerebral infarct) is associated with reduced metabolic demand and low CBF. Therefore, low flow does not necessarily mean vessel occlusion but, in this case, non-functioning brain. Although this coupling of flow with metabolism and function has been suspected for over one century (Roy & Sherrington, 1890), the mechanism is unknown; it may be that the metabolically active areas of brain produce vasodilatory metabolites, or the resistance vessels may be under neural regulation or a combination of both (Lou et al., 1987).

> *In normal brain, blood flow is closely coupled with metabolic demand. However, if the brain is damaged, blood flow and metabolism become uncoupled and so normal flow no longer necessarily implies normal metabolism and function.*

Arterial carbon dioxide tension

$Paco_2$ has a potent effect on CBF; a 1-mmHg rise in $Paco_2$ within the range of 20–60 mmHg in normal individuals causes an immediate 3–5% increase in CBF due to dilatation of cerebral resistance vessels (Harper & Bell, 1963). In *chronic* respiratory failure however, causing CO_2 retention, CBF is normal (Fieschi & Lenzi, 1983). Changes in arterial oxygen tension (Pao_2) have a modest inverse effect on CBF, unless the Pao_2 falls below about 50 mmHg (6.7 kPa) (Brown et al., 1985), when the resultant decline in the oxygen saturation of the blood leads to a fall in CVR and an increase in CBF. Increasing the Pao_2 above the normal level has little effect on CBF.

Whole-blood viscosity

Normally, CBF is inversely related to whole-blood viscosity (Thomas, 1982). As the main determinant of whole-blood viscosity (at normal shear rates) is the haematocrit, it follows that CBF and the haematocrit are inversely related. But, this relationship is not because the high haematocrit raises viscosity and thereby slows flow (at least not in normal vessels); rather, the higher oxygen content of high haematocrit blood allows CBF to be lower and yet to maintain normal oxygen delivery to the tissues in accordance with metabolic demands (Brown & Marshall, 1985; Brown et al., 1985). A practical example is encountered in patients with leukaemia or paraproteinaemia who have very high blood viscosity but normal CBF (or even high CBF if anaemia co-exists), because CBF depends more on the oxygen content of the blood (which is normal or low) than the viscosity (which is high) (Brown et al., 1985). However, at very low shear rates, which might be found in ischaemic brain, for example, whole-blood viscosity depends more on plasma fibrinogen than haematocrit (Weaver et al., 1969). In addition, other local factors such as red cell aggregation, platelet aggregation and perhaps increasing red cell fragility as a result of anoxia, all of which increase blood viscosity, may come into play to reduce flow (Wood & Kee, 1985).

Autoregulation

Under normal conditions, CBF is maintained at a relatively constant level, irrespective of the systemic arterial blood pressure, as long as the mean blood pressure remains between about 60 and 160 mmHg (Fig. 11.2). This capacity to maintain a constant CBF is due to the phenomenon of autoregulation (Powers, 1991). Autoregulation is achieved primarily by varying pre-capillary resistance; compensatory vasodilatation of pial arterioles occurs when the blood pressure falls and compensatory vasoconstriction when the blood pressure rises. Whether myogenic, metabolic or neurogenic processes are responsible for this response is unknown. The autoregulatory curve is 'set' higher in patients with long-standing hypertension and, consequently, these patients develop symptoms of ischaemia at a relatively higher blood pressure (e.g. mean about 70 mmHg) than in non-hypertensive patients (e.g. mean 50 mmHg) (Fig. 11.2) (Strandgaard et al., 1973; Strandgaard, 1978; Barry et al., 1982). Autoregulation tends to become gradually less effective with increasing age so that elderly people are more likely to develop symptoms of cerebral ischaemia with a fall in blood pressure induced by, for example, postural change (Wollner et al., 1979). The reason is not clear but may be related to subclinical cerebral damage where the normal

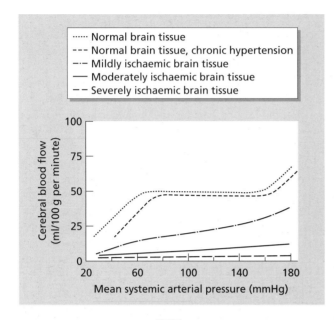

Figure 11.2 Autoregulation. Relationship between mean systemic arterial blood pressure and CBF in normal brain tissue and in focal cerebral ischaemia. Under normal conditions, CBF is maintained at a relatively constant level, independent of the systemic arterial blood pressure, as long as the mean pressure remains between about 60 and 160 mmHg. This capacity to maintain a constant CBF is due to the phenomenon of autoregulation. In chronic hypertension the curve is shifted to the right. During ischaemia, resting CBF decreases and autoregulation is impaired. This is particularly important during mild ischaemia when reductions in systemic arterial blood pressure can produce reductions in CBF from levels above 20 ml/100 g per minute, which is sufficient to sustain brain function, to lethal levels below 10 ml/100 g per minute. (From Strandgaard *et al.*, 1973; Dirnagl & Pulsinelli, 1990.)

mechanisms of cerebrovascular control may no longer operate. It is therefore not surprising that autoregulation is impaired in a variety of disease states such as head trauma, diffuse cerebral hypoxia, ischaemic stroke and vasospasm secondary to subarachnoid haemorrhage (Fig. 11.2) (Symon *et al.*, 1976; Fieschi & Lenzi, 1983; Strandgaard & Paulson 1984; Dearden, 1985). Autoregulation is also impaired if the $Paco_2$ is high, presumably because further vasodilatation cannot occur and so the perfusion reserve is exhausted (Aaslid *et al.*, 1989). In some patients who have had transient ischaemic attacks (TIAs) or mild ischaemic stroke, with subsequently normal angiograms, autoregulation and the cerebrovascular response to $Paco_2$ may be deranged for several weeks (Skinhoj *et al.*, 1970; Frackowiak, 1985). In all of these situations of impaired autoregulation, CBF varies directly with blood pressure, thus becoming 'pressure passive'.

> *Autoregulation is the ability of cerebral blood flow to remain constant in the face of changes in cerebral perfusion pressure.*

Despite recent reports that it may be possible to monitor autoregulation of CBF, or at least the lower limit of autoregulation, non-invasively with transcranial Doppler (TCD) ultrasound (Lagi *et al.*, 1994; Larsen *et al.*, 1994), it has hitherto been difficult to monitor cerebral autoregulation by non-invasive techniques (Aaslid *et al.*, 1991). Therefore, much of our knowledge in humans has been inferred from animal studies.

If mean arterial pressure falls below about 40–50 mmHg, compensatory vascular change and, therefore, cerebral perfusion reserve is exhausted, and CBF parallels the blood pressure (see Section 6.5.5) (Harper, 1966). Because oxygen delivery to the brain normally far exceeds demand, metabolic activity is maintained at a mean blood pressure of around 40–50 mmHg by increasing the oxygen extraction from the blood (Fig. 11.3). This state of increased OEF has been termed 'misery perfusion' (Baron *et al.*, 1981). However, when the OEF is maximal, a state of 'ischaemia' exists; flow is inadequate (< 20 ml/100 g brain per minute) to meet metabolic demands, cellular metabolism is impaired and $CMRO_2$ begins to fall (see below) (Powers *et al.*, 1984; Pulsinelli, 1992). As neuronal function ceases, the patient usually develops symptoms of neurological dysfunction (if the whole brain is ischaemic, non-focal symptoms such as faintness occur and if only part of the brain is ischaemic, focal symptoms such as hemiparesis occur).

If the CPP rises above the autoregulatory range where compensatory vasoconstriction is maximal (i.e. above about 160 mmHg in normal people), then hyperaemia occurs followed by vasogenic oedema, raised intracranial pressure and the clinical syndrome of hypertensive encephalopathy (see Section 3.5.6).

Cerebral perfusion reserve

The ratio of CBF:CBV (see above) is a measure of cerebral perfusion reserve. A CBF:CBV ratio below about 6.0 indicates maximal vasodilatation and CBV, and exhausted reserve, even if the CBF is still normal. If available, positron emission tomography (PET) scanning will show a rising OEF at this stage, to maintain $CMRO_2$ (Fig. 11.4) (Gibbs *et al.*, 1984). If PET is unavailable, the mean cerebral transit time (MCTT), which is the reciprocal of CBF:CBV, can be used instead (Merrick *et al.*, 1991; Naylor *et al.*, 1991).

In clinical practice, cerebral perfusion reserve is more commonly assessed indirectly by measuring CBF at baseline and then in response to a challenge with CO_2 inhalation

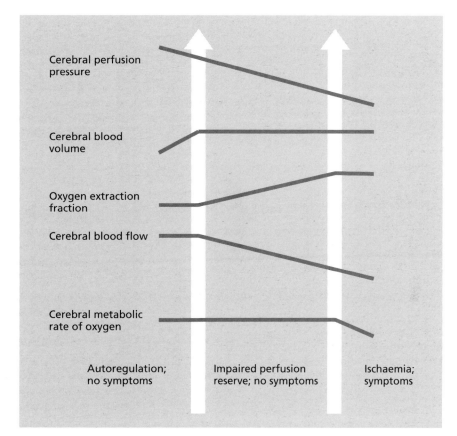

Figure 11.3 Schematic representation of the protective responses to a progressive fall in CPP. With falling CPP, intracranial arteries dilate to maintain CBF. This results in an increase in CBV. When vasodilatation (and CBV) is maximal, further falls in CPP result in a fall in CBF and, therefore, a fall in the CBF:CBV ratio, and an increase in the OEF to maintain tissue oxygenation. This represents a state of impaired cerebral perfusion reserve. When the OEF is maximal, further falls in CPP lead to reduction in $CMRO_2$ and the symptoms of cerebral ischaemia.

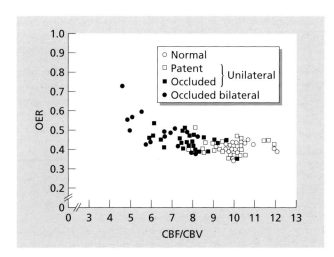

Figure 11.4 Relationship between OER and the CBF:CBV ratio in each of 82 middle cerebral artery regions from 32 patients with varying degrees of carotid artery stenosis and occlusion and nine normal subjects. (From Gibbs *et al.*, 1984; reproduced with permission of the *Lancet*.)

(Markwalder *et al.*, 1984; Herold *et al.*, 1988) or intravenous acetazolamide administration (Sullivan *et al.*, 1987), which increase CBF (unless the capacity for cerebral autoregulation is exhausted). The techniques for measuring CBF include the xenon-133 (^{133}Xe) inhalation system (Sullivan *et al.*, 1987); stable Xe CT (CT) (Yamashita *et al.*, 1992); single-photon emission computerised tomography (SPECT) with ^{133}Xe-, iodine-123 (^{123}I)-labelled isopropyliodoamphetamine or technetium-99m (^{99m}Tc)-labelled hexamethylpropyleneamine oxime (HMPAO) (Knop *et al.*, 1992; Masdeu *et al.*, 1994); and three-dimensional time-of-flight magnetic resonance angiography (Mandai *et al.*, 1994). TCD is also used to measure velocity flow in the middle cerebral artery as a surrogate for CBF (Markus & Harrison, 1992). Most users of TCD for assessing cerebrovascular reserve capacity prefer CO_2 stimulation to acetazolamide administration (Kleiser *et al.*, 1994).

It is important to recognise that these indirect methods of measuring perfusion reserve (i.e. SPECT, TCD, MCTT) are inaccurate when the normal relationships between CBF, CBV, OEF and vascular reactivity are distorted, as occurs in ischaemic and infarcted brain (Powers, 1991) (see also Section 6.6.4).

A common clinical scenario of impaired reserve is a patient with stenosis or occlusion of one or both internal carotid arteries, severe enough (at least 50% diameter stenosis) to produce a fall in CPP distally, and inadequate collateral CBF distally (Powers *et al.*, 1987; Schroeder, 1988; Powers, 1991). Under these circumstances, the brain is vulnerable to any further fall in CPP, as may occur when the patient stands up quickly, when undergoing anaesthesia (e.g. for coronary artery bypass surgery) or starts or increases antihypertensive medication or vasodilators (Widder *et al.*, 1994).

11.1.3 Pathophysiology of cerebral ischaemia

Thrombosis

Acute cerebral ischaemia begins with the occlusion of a cerebral blood vessel, usually by thrombus or embolus (Raichle, 1983). Modern ideas about the pathogenesis of vessel thrombosis began with Rudolph Virchow's dissertation in 1845 in which he enunciated his famous triad that thrombosis was due to changes in the vessel wall, changes in the pattern of blood flow and changes in the constituents of the blood. In fact, this concept had been already hinted at by John Hunter nearly 100 years earlier (Hunter, 1794).

It has since been established that vascular endothelial injury (i.e. as a result of rupture of an atheromatous plaque, due to haemorrhage into the plaque or ischaemic necrosis of the plaque) is the most critical event in the formation of a thrombus (see Section 6.2.2) (Ross, 1986). Exposure of subendothelial structures, particularly fibrillar collagen, to blood at high shear rates activates platelets and induces platelet adhesion (Fuster *et al.*, 1992). Activated platelets release ADP (which increases platelet aggregation) and arachidonic acid (which is metabolised by the enzyme cyclooxygenase to prostaglandin endoperoxides, which is converted by thromboxane synthetase to thromboxane A_2, a very potent vasoconstrictor and inducer of further platelet aggregation and secretion). The platelets also release other eicosanoids, such as prostaglandin F_{2alpha} and serotonin, which also induce vasoconstriction and platelet aggregation (Schror & Braun, 1990; Patrono *et al.*, 1990; D'Andrea *et al.*, 1994; van Kooten *et al.*, 1994). Vascular tone is modulated by peptides released from endothelial cells, which include the vasoconstrictor endothelin and the vasodilators prostacyclin and nitric oxide (endothelium-derived relaxing factor) (Yanagisawa *et al.*, 1988; Faraci & Brian, 1994; Levin, 1995; Loscalzo, 1995). In addition, platelet aggregation may activate leucocytes to induce an acute disturbance in endothelial-dependent relaxation that results in vasoconstriction (Akopov *et al.*, 1994). Endothelial injury also activates the coagulation cascade. The original cascade/waterfall hypothesis of blood coagulation is that there are two activating pathways: (i) the tissue factor or extrinsic pathway; and (ii) the contact or intrinsic pathway. A revised hypothesis of blood coagulation (Broze, 1992) is that there is a *single* coagulation pathway, triggered by vessel injury and tissue factor (TF) (the factor VIIa/TF complex). Activation of factor VIIa/TF leads to the activation of factor X and the generation of thrombin (IIa), which not only cleaves fibrinogen (producing a stable fibrin monomer) but also activates factor XI; factor XI activation occurs 'late' in the coagulation process, rather than being involved in the initiation of coagulation. Due to feedback inhibition of the factor VIIa/TF complex by TF pathway inhibitor (TFPI), factors VII, IX and XI are required for the production of additional factor Xa. As blood clot forms at the site of vessel injury, plasminogen, an inert circulating protein closely bound to the deposited fibrin, is slowly activated (by plasminogen activator which has been activated by kallikrein) to form plasmin, which digests the fibrin clot to give fibrin degradation products. The net result is that platelets and later fibrin accumulate at, and are limited to, the site of vascular injury. The rest of the vasculature remains free of platelet and fibrin deposits because, in circulating blood, the tendency of the coagulation mechanism to be activated is counterbalanced by inhibitory factors in the blood such as antithrombin III (which inactivates factors IX, X, XI and XII). However, at the point of vessel injury, the activation of the coagulation mechanism is so powerful that the inhibitors are overwhelmed. Also, endothelial cells normally promote a local non-thrombogenic state which is mediated by the release of certain membrane proteins. Thrombomodulin is one such protein which, in the presence of thrombin, binds protein C, converting it to an active form that re-enters the circulation and, in the presence of protein S, inactivates factors Va and VIIIa on the platelet surface (Rosenberg & Rosenberg, 1984).

> *Injured endothelium (e.g. as a result of atherosclerotic plaque) interacts with blood platelets to form nidi of loosely adherent platelets and fibrin that can break off and embolise distally, and also initiate the coagulation cascade that can lead to the formation of an occlusive thrombus.*

Pathologists recognise and describe three different types of thrombi (Deykin, 1967).

1 *Red thrombi* are composed mostly of red blood cells and fibrin. They form in areas of slowed blood flow and the vessel wall need not be obviously abnormal (e.g. deep venous thrombosis (DVT) in the leg veins).

2 *White thrombi* are made up of platelets and fibrin and

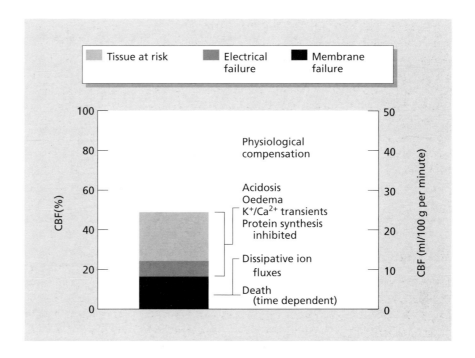

Figure 11.5 CBF thresholds for cell dysfunction and death. (From Siesjo, 1992a.)

have few red blood cells. They form in areas in which the endothelial surface or vessel wall is abnormal and blood flow is rapid (e.g. thrombosis complicating carotid atheroma).

3 *Disseminated fibrin deposition* occurs in small blood vessels.

When a major artery is suddenly occluded, arterial blood pressure and blood flow fall distal to the occlusion, and the region of brain supplied by that vessel is acutely deprived of blood supply and rendered ischaemic. The metabolic and clinical consequences of cerebral ischaemia depend not only on the cascade of events induced by thrombus formation (i.e. biosynthesis of thrombogenic and neurotoxic eicosanoids, breakdown of the blood–brain barrier, diffusion of these products into surrounding brain and reduced microvascular flow in the ischaemic penumbra around the initial focus), but also on the site, severity and duration of cerebral ischaemia and the availability of collateral blood flow (Heiss, 1992; Siesjo, 1992a) (Fig. 11.5).

Site of cerebral ischaemia

The brain cells which are most vulnerable to ischaemia are neurones, followed in decreasing sensitivity by oligodendroglia, astrocytes and endothelial cells. However, even within the population of neurones, there are many different types that also vary in sensitivity to ischaemia, and in some cases the vulnerability varies with the location of the cells. The most vulnerable neurones to mild ischaemia are the pyramidal neurones in the CA1 and CA4 zones of the hip-

pocampus, followed by neurones in the cerebellum, striatum and neocortex (Brierley, 1976; Heros, 1994).

Severity and duration of cerebral ischaemia

During moderate cerebral ischaemia (i.e. reduction of CBF to about 50% of normal), several compensatory mechanisms come into play which sacrifice electrophysiological activity (hence, the suppression of electroencephalogram (EEG) activity) in order to reduce energy use. This enables near-normal ATP concentrations and membrane ion gradients to be maintained and cell viability to be preserved, at least temporarily. If moderate ischaemia persists, however (i.e. for several hours), cell death occurs.

Critical flow thresholds

During moderate to severe cerebral ischaemia, autoregulation is impaired or lost and so CBF varies passively with the perfusion pressure (see Fig. 11.2 and Section 11.1.2) (Symon *et al.*, 1976). This has allowed investigators to reduce gradually CBF and assess the critical flow thresholds for certain functions. In experimental and human models of focal cerebral ischaemia, when blood flow falls below about 20 ml/100 g of brain per minute, the OEF becomes maximal, the $CMRO_2$ begins to fall (see Fig. 11.3) and normal neuronal function of the cerebral cortex is affected (Wise *et al.*, 1983; Powers *et al.*, 1984; Friberg & Olsen, 1991), electrical activity in cortical cells ceases (Heiss *et al.*, 1976) and evoked cerebral responses from the area of focal ischaemia decrease in amplitude (Heiss, 1992). This degree of ischaemia thus represents a threshold for *loss of neuronal electrical function* (i.e. electrical failure).

When blood flow falls to 15 ml/100 g of brain per minute, evoked potentials are lost and the EEG flattens. With further falls in flow, the EEG becomes isoelectric and the water and electrolyte content of ischaemic tissue changes due to cell pump failure (see below). The critical threshold for the beginning of irreversible cell damage is a CBF of about 10 ml/100 g of brain per minute (Siesjo, 1992a). For a short period, the neurones may remain viable and recover function if perfusion is restored. At this stage, lack of oxygen inhibits mitochondrial metabolism and activates the inefficient anaerobic metabolism of glucose, causing a local rise in lactate production and so a fall in pH, leading to intra- and extracellular acidosis (Fig. 11.5). The energy dependent functions of cell membranes to maintain ion homeostasis become progressively impaired; K^+ leaks out of cells into the extracellular space, Na^+ and water enter cells (cytotoxic oedema), and Ca^{2+} also moves into cells (where it causes mitochondrial failure and compromises the ability of intracellular membranes to control subsequent ion fluxes, leading to cytotoxicity) (Harris *et al.*, 1981; Cheung *et al.*, 1986; Siesjo, 1992a). Rapid efflux of K^+ and influx of Ca^{2+} represent a generalised collapse of membrane function. This degree of ischaemia represents a threshold for *loss of cellular ion homeostasis* (i.e. membrane failure) (Siesjo, 1992a).

This classic concept of the viability thresholds of ischaemia thus differentiates between two principal critical flow thresholds (loss of neuronal electrical function and then loss of cellular ion homeostasis), which are separated by an intermediate zone characterised by cessation of electrical activity of cells with preservation of their membrane potential (Siesjo, 1992a). These thresholds mark the upper and lower flow limits of the ischaemic penumbra (see below) which has hitherto been thought to suffer only functional but not structural injury. However, recent studies of functional and metabolic disturbances suggest a more complex pattern of thresholds. At declining flow rates, protein synthesis is inhibited first (at a threshold of about 55 ml/100 g brain per minute), followed by stimulation of anaerobic glycolysis (at 35 ml/100 g per minute), the release of neurotransmitters, disturbance of energy metabolism (at about 20 ml/100 g per minute) and finally anoxic depolarisation (<15 ml/g per minute) (Hossmann, 1994).

In addition to the *degree* of ischaemia, the *duration* of ischaemia also determines whether the thresholds are crossed (Fig. 11.6). With prolonged reductions in CBF below about 10 ml/100 g brain per minute, cellular transport mechanisms and neurotransmitter systems fail, potentially neuro-

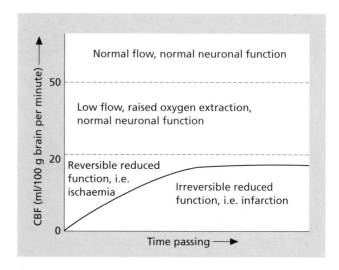

Figure 11.6 Combined effects of residual CBF and duration of ischaemia on reversibility of neuronal dysfunction during focal cerebral ischaemia. The solid line delineates the limits of severity and duration of ischaemia that allow survival of any neurones. (From Jones *et al.*, 1981; Heiss & Rosner, 1983.)

toxic transmitters are released (such as L-glutamate (Rothman & Olney, 1986)), free oxygen radicals and lipid peroxides are formed which damage cells further (McCord, 1985), and neurones release platelet activating factor which may be neurotoxic (Lindsberg *et al.*, 1991) (see below).

The concept of an ischaemic penumbra

The finding of two separate thresholds, one for cessation of electrical signals and the other for loss of ion homeostasis, has led to the concept of an ischaemic penumbra, i.e. of brain tissue (within and around a central core of dense ischaemic brain tissue) which is less densely ischaemic and which contains electrically inexcitable but essentially viable cells (Astrup *et al.*, 1981; Heiss, 1992; Siesjo, 1992a; Ginsburg & Pulsinelli, 1994; Heiss & Graf, 1994). These are areas of 'critical' or 'misery' perfusion where neuronal function is depressed because the metabolic demands of the tissue are not being met (blood flow is low and OEF is high), but the cells are still viable with maintained ion homeostasis. Because local perfusion reserve is exhausted, the neurones in the ischaemic penumbra are vulnerable to any further fall in perfusion pressure caused by, for example, hypovolaemia secondary to dehydration, medications that lower blood pressure and even by standing up quickly. The penumbral area can perhaps be prevented from becoming necrotic by avoiding these insults, by reperfusion and also by the use of neuroprotective drugs (see Section 11.13). The penumbra can therefore be defined as that part of an ischaemic area that is potentially salvageable. However, the ischaemic penumbra is not just a topographic locus, but rather it is a dynamic process, an evolving zone of bioenergetic upheaval (Ginsberg & Pulsinelli, 1994).

> As cerebral blood flow falls, a critical threshold is reached when the electrical activity of neurones is suppressed. As flow falls further, another threshold is reached when cellular integrity begins to breakdown. Cells falling in between these two thresholds make up the 'ischaemic penumbra'; they may not be functioning but they are still alive.

In any individual patient with acute cerebral infarction, it is not known how large the ischaemic penumbra is likely to be, how long it is likely to remain in this state, how important it is functionally and how much recovery is likely if flow is restored (Lassen et al., 1991). One of the reasons is that accurate information about the ischaemic penumbra can only be obtained from PET scanning. Despite the practical difficulties (Baron, 1991) there is now evidence from a small, but meticulous study using PET and CT, that there is prolonged persistence of substantial volumes of potentially viable brain tissue after ischaemic stroke (Marchal et al., 1996).

The time window for effective therapeutic intervention may be longer in humans than predicted from animal studies (Heiss & Graf, 1994) because it is unlikely to be absolute; ischaemia is probably a dynamic process of fluctuating severity over the first few hours and therefore it may not be possible to predict just how long the time window is to allow successful therapeutic intervention in any individual (Baron et al., 1995). We have learnt from randomised trials in acute myocardial infarction (MI) that thrombolysis is still effective in reducing case fatality even when given up to 24 hours after the onset of chest pain (White, 1992), despite the widely held belief prior to these studies, mainly based on animal models, that thrombolysis could not possibly be effective if given more than a few hours after acute MI (Fibrinolytic Therapy Trialists' (FTT) Collaborative Group, 1994). Recent PET studies in humans suggest the 'window' may be as long as 17 hours (Marchal et al., 1996). Therefore, we need to keep an open mind about the therapeutic time window and acknowledge that it may even vary for different interventions. For example, the time window for thrombolytics may be shorter than for neuroprotective agents than for antithrombotic agents; we do not know yet.

> In humans it is not clear how long ischaemic brain can survive and still be salvaged by reperfusion or measures to protect neurones from dying; in other words, the duration of the 'time window' for effective therapeutic intervention is unknown.

Reperfusion and brain damage

In the monkey, a middle cerebral artery occlusion that lasts for 30 minutes or longer often produces some tissue damage, and occlusion periods longer than 60 minutes frequently cause infarction. Nevertheless, animal experiments have shown that short-term recovery of electrical and metabolic functions is possible with reperfusion after ischaemic periods as long as 60 minutes, and that reperfusion within 4–8 hours can reduce the size of the lesion (Jones et al., 1981; Siesjo, 1992a). In addition, the demonstration of viable (penumbra) tissue by PET up to several hours after ischaemic stroke indicates that there is a therapeutic time window (of a few hours, perhaps even longer) during which the re-establishment of perfusion (spontaneously or by treatment) may be effective (Heiss & Graf, 1994).

However, although reperfusion within the revival times of ischaemic tissues may salvage cells and aid recovery, it may also be detrimental and lead to 'reperfusion damage' due to resupply of water and osmotic equivalents (exacerbating oedema) and of oxygen (which triggers production of injurious free radicals) (McCord, 1985). Frequently, reperfusion following 3–6 hours of arterial occlusion has been observed to be followed by massive tissue swelling (particularly the vasogenic component) with secondary compromise of circulation (see below) (Ito et al., 1979). It is unclear whether this is a problem in humans; there is some evidence that it is not (Wardlaw et al., 1993).

Availability of collateral blood flow

Occlusion of a cerebral artery reduces but seldom abolishes the delivery of oxygen and glucose to the relevant region of the brain because dense collateral channels partly maintain blood flow in the ischaemic territory. This incomplete ischaemia is responsible for the spatial and temporal dynamics of cerebral infarction (Pulsinelli, 1992). Some other areas of the brain, including the infarcted tissue, may show relative or absolute hyperaemia (called 'luxury perfusion') due to good collateral blood supply, recanalisation of the occluded artery, inflammation or vasodilatation in response to hypercapnia, i.e. flow is in excess of the metabolic demands and OEF is reduced.

11.1.4 Mediators of cell death

With prolonged reductions in CBF below about 10 ml/100 g brain per minute, infarction occurs and, even if flow is restored, function cannot recover. The mechanisms that give rise to ischaemic cell death have not been determined definitively but considerable evidence points to three major

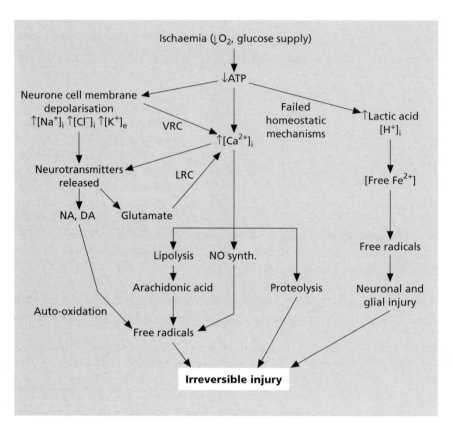

Figure 11.7 Potential mechanisms of ischaemic brain damage. This diagram illustrates the complexity of the process of ischaemic brain damage with multiple branching pathways and potential sites of interaction when the energy supply to the brain is depleted. $[Ca^{2+}]_i$, intracellular Ca^{2+} concentration; $[Cl^-]_i$, intracellular chloride ion concentration; DA, dopamine; Fe^{2+}, iron ions; $[H^+]_i$, intracellular hydrogen ion concentration; $[K^+]_e$, extracellular K^+ concentration; LRC, ligand-regulated Ca^{2+} channels; NA, noradrenaline; $[Na^+]_i$, intracellular Na^+ concentration; NO synth, nitric oxide synthase; VRC, voltage-regulated Ca^{2+} channels. (From Pulsinelli, 1992.)

mediators: unregulated increases in intracellular cytosolic Ca^{2+} concentration, acidosis and the production of free radicals (Fig. 11.7). The induction of immediate early genes and expression of heat shock proteins may modulate the process.

Increases in intracellular cytosolic Ca^{2+} concentration

Extracellular Ca^{2+} concentration is 10^4–10^5 times greater than its intracellular concentration and most of the mechanisms that maintain this gradient are either directly or indirectly energy dependent. Therefore, loss of ATP rapidly leads to a massive influx of Ca^{2+} into the cell as a result of impaired Ca^{2+} pump function (due to ATP depletion), an increase in membrane permeability to Ca^{2+}, release of Ca^{2+} from intracellular compartments and the release of endogenous excitatory amino acid neurotransmitters (such as glutamate) from depolarised nerve endings; glutamate activates several post-synaptic glutamate receptors/channel complexes causing Na^+ influx and depolarisation, followed by more

Ca^{2+} influx via ligand- and voltage-regulated ion channels (Fig. 11.8) (Lipton & Rosenberg, 1994).

There are five categories of glutamate receptor/channel complex, classified according to the agonist that most efficiently activates them: high- and low-affinity kainate; amino-3-hydroxy-5-methyl-4-isoxazole propionic acid (AMPA); N-methyl-D-aspartate (NMDA); and quisqualate receptors (Greenamyre & Porter, 1994; Muir & Lees, 1995). Glutamate itself is a mixed agonist; when released from presynaptic endings, it activates both AMPA and NMDA receptors. The AMPA receptor gates a channel that is permeable to monovalent cations (Na^+, K^+ and H^+); by allowing Na^+ to enter, the opening of this channel leads to depolarisation. The NMDA subtype of the glutamate receptor (Fig. 11.9) gates a channel permeable to both monovalent cations and Ca^{2+}. This channel is normally blocked by magnesium (Mg^{2+}) but, since this block is voltage dependent, it is relieved when the membrane depolarises. Therefore, activation of the AMPA receptor leads to Na^+ influx and depolari-

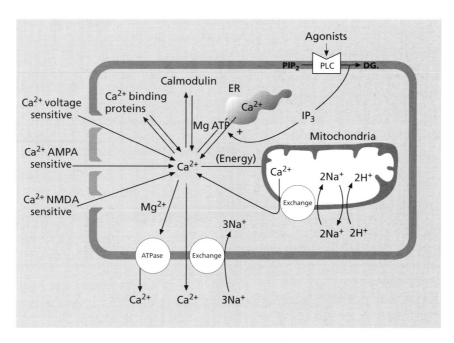

Figure 11.8 Ca^{2+} homeostasis in neurones. Ca^{2+} influx is regulated by voltage- and ligand (glutamate)-sensitive channels named for their most potent synthetic agonists (N-methyl-D-aspartate (NMDA) and amino-3-hydroxy-5-methyl-4-isoxazole propionic acid (AMPA)). DG, diacylglycerol; IP_3, inositol triphosphate; PIP_2, phosphatidyl inositol diphosphate; PLC, phospholipase C. Energy-dependent regulation of intracellular Ca^{2+} ($[Ca^{2+}]_i$) is via an ATP-dependent pump, translocation for Na^+ ions and uptake into endoplasmic reticulum (ER) and mitochondria. Energy-dependent Ca^{2+} homeostasis occurs via buffering of Ca^{2+} by calmodulin and other intracellular proteins (calbindin, parvalbumin). (From Pulsinelli, 1992; reproduced with permission of the *Lancet*.)

sation, thus relieving the block and allowing Ca^{2+} to enter via the NMDA channel. Depolarisation also allows Ca^{2+} to enter via voltage-sensitive Ca^{2+} channels of the L and T types. Inhibition is assumed to be mediated by activation of K^+ and chlorine (Cl^-) conductances (Siesjo, 1992a).

The consequence of a non-physiological unregulated rise in intracellular cytoplasmic Ca^{2+} is cell damage, believed to be caused by: activation of Ca^{2+} ATPase (which results in further consumption of cellular ATP); activation of Ca^{2+}-dependent phospholipases, proteases and nucleases; and alteration of protein phosphorylation, which secondarily affects protein synthesis and genome expression. Ca^{2+} activates phospholipases, which hydrolyse membrane-bound glycerophospholipids to free fatty acids and, in turn, facilitate free radical peroxidation of other membrane lipids; proteases which lyse structural proteins; and activates nitric oxide synthase which initiates free radical mechanisms.

Acidosis

Acidosis arises as a result of sustained tissue ischaemia and may contribute to tissue damage and prevent or retard recovery during reoxygenation by several mechanisms; these include oedema formation, inhibition of H^+ extrusion, inhi-

bition of lactate oxidation and inhibition of mitochondrial respiration (Siesjo, 1992b). Cellular acidosis may promote intracellular oedema formation by inducing Na^+ and Cl^- accumulation in the cell via coupled Na^+/H^+ and $Cl^-/$ hydrogen carbonate (HCO_3^-) exchange; acidosis activates the Na^+/H^+ exchange and H^+ leaks back into the cell via the Cl^-/HCO_3^- antiporter causing accumulation of Na^+ and Cl^- in the cell with osmotically obligated water. In other words, the cell tries to regulate intracellular pH at the expense of its own volume regulation (see also Section 11.1.5). Furthermore, extracellular acidosis may outcompete Na^+ at the external site of the Na^+/H^+ antiporter, thereby retarding or preventing H^+ extrusion from acidotic cells. Finally, acidosis may block the lactate oxidase form of the lactate dehydrogenase complex, retarding both oxidation of lactate accumulated during ischaemia and oxidative phosphorylation in isolated mitochondria, thus curtailing ATP production.

Production of free radicals

A free radical is any atom, group of atoms or molecule with an unpaired electron in its outer-most orbital (Halliwell, 1994). Since covalent chemical bonds usually consist of a

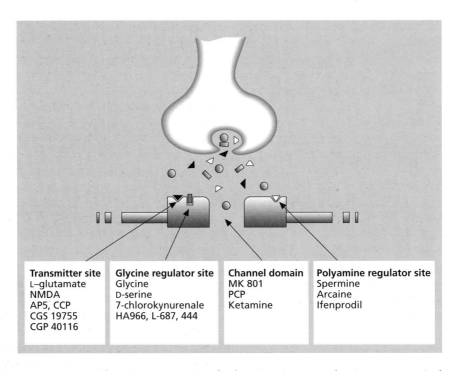

Transmitter site	Glycine regulator site	Channel domain	Polyamine regulator site
L–glutamate	Glycine	MK 801	Spermine
NMDA	D-serine	PCP	Arcaine
AP5, CCP	7-chlorokynurenale	Ketamine	Ifenprodil
CGS 19755	HA966, L-687, 444		
CGP 40116			

Figure 11.9 The glutaminergic synapse. Schematic representation of a glutaminergic synapse showing a presynaptic glutamatergic nerve terminal and an NMDA receptor in the cell membrane of a postsynaptic neurone. The NMDA receptor and channel complex possess a number of modulatory sites that can be pharmacologically manipulated to either enhance or attenuate glutamate-stimulated ionic fluxes. Interaction of glutamate or a glutamate-like agonist (e.g. NMDA) with the glutamate recognition (transmitter) site leads to activation of inward Ca^{2+} and Na^+ currents that can be damaging when in excess. The glycine and polyamine sites, when acted upon by selective agonists, serve to enhance the effects of glutamate receptor activation. Agents that block any of these sites will attenuate NMDA receptor-mediated ionic currents. Additionally, within the channel, there are non-competitive and Mg^{2+} binding sites that attenuate Ca^{2+} influx through the channel when pharmacologically blocked.

pair of electrons sharing an orbital, free radicals can be thought of as molecules with an 'open' or 'half' bond, and it is this which accounts for their extreme reactivity (Schmidley, 1990). Free radicals are produced in small quantities by normal cellular process in all aerobic cells; for example, 'leaks' in mitochondrial electron transport allow oxygen to accept single electrons, forming superoxide (O_2^-) (De Bono, 1994). However, they are inherently toxic; they can react with and damage proteins, nucleic acids, lipids and other classes of molecules such as the extracellular matrix glycosaminoglycans (e.g. hyaluronic acid). The sulphur-containing amino acids and the polyunsaturated fatty acids (found in high concentrations in the brain) are particularly vulnerable. Fortunately, cells possess appropriate defence mechanisms in the form of free radical scavengers (e.g. vitamins and their analogues such as alpha-tocopherol and ascorbic acid) and enzymes which metabolise free radicals or their precursors (e.g. superoxide dismutase, catalase and glutathione peroxidase) (De Bono, 1994).

During severe ischaemia, insufficient oxygen is available

to accept electrons passed along the mitochondrial electron transport chain, leading to eventual reduction ('electron saturation') of components of this system. In the presence of small amounts of oxygen, these molecules can then auto-oxidise. The residual oxygen molecules in severely ischaemic brain can not act as electron acceptors in the 'normal' fashion because oxidation–reduction ('redox') potential sufficient to favour stepwise electron transfer to them can not be generated by such low concentrations of molecular oxygen.

Free radicals may also be generated during cerebral ischaemia by the release of iron from ferritin stores within ischaemic brain cells (Davalos *et al.*, 1994). As the cerebrospinal fluid has a low concentration of ferritin-binding proteins, much of the iron released from damaged brain cells remains unbound and is therefore available to catalyse the generation of radical hydroxyl (OH·), the more malignant free radical species (see below), leading to iron-induced lipid peroxidation (a process that may be inhibited by lazaroids). This process is compounded by the fact that the central nervous system is relatively poorly endowed with superoxide dismutase, an enzyme which scavenges OH· and inhibits iron release from intracellular stores such as ferritin.

The free radical species of potential importance in cerebral ischaemia include O_2^- and OH·. Like other free radicals, they react with and damage proteins, nucleic acids and lipids, particularly the fatty acid component of membrane phospholipids, producing changes in the fluidity and permeability of the cellular membranes (lipid peroxidation) (Halliwell, 1994). These, and other mediators of inflammatory reactions such as platelet activating factor, contribute to ischaemic cell death by targeting the microvasculature and so causing microvascular dysfunction and disruption of the blood–brain barrier.

With reperfusion, reactive oxygen radicals may be generated as byproducts of the reactions of free arachidonic acid (released from membrane phospholipids during ischaemia) to produce prostaglandins and leukotrienes, and lead to reperfusion injury to the brain and its microvessels.

Altered gene expression

During early cerebral ischaemia, protein synthesis in virtually all cell types in the brain is generally suppressed. Protein synthesis recovers in regions where cells survive and remains decreased in cells or regions that go on to die. It is unknown whether the decrease in protein synthesis is simply secondary to ischaemic injury or whether it plays some causal role in mediating cell death. Depending on the severity of the ischaemia and the intrinsic nature of the neuronal populations, it is thought that a stress response and changes in gene expression are elicited by ischaemia, which may be vital to cell survival and repair. Specific genes are expressed and their corresponding proteins may be synthesised, such as immediate-early genes and their products (c-*fos*, c-*jun* and zinc finger gene), heat shock and other stress genes and proteins, growth factor/receptor genes and amyloid precursor protein. These genes seem likely to be involved in mediating ischaemic injury, or in protection or repair, because they are being selectively transcribed and translated in a cell environment where limited energy availability is suppressing the translation of the majority of genes. Molecular biological techniques are presently being applied to elucidate further the mechanisms of ischaemic neuronal death and repair and to see if it is possible to switch off or block injury-related genes, which programme cell death, and to facilitate protection or repair genes (Kogure & Kato, 1993; Sharp, 1994). One recent study shows that an (antisense) oligonucleotide, complementary to a piece of messenger ribonucleic acid (RNA), can disrupt or block expression of a gene, the c-*fos* proto-oncogene, that is induced in the intact brain by ischaemia (Liu *et al.*, 1994). Since the c-*fos* gene is a transcription factor believed to bind to the promoter of many target genes and regulate their expression, the results pave the way for understanding whether the target genes of the fos protein-mediated pathways help cells survive and regenerate, or mediate pathways that lead to cell death following ischaemic injury in brain. If it is shown that c-*fos* is 'bad' for the brain when it is induced in ischaemia, then the finding that ischaemic induction of fos protein can be markedly attenuated with the antisense oligonucleotide (Liu *et al.*, 1994) might have therapeutic implications. Other hypotheses of ischaemic neuronal death, based on a disturbance of mitochondrial gene expression, have also been proposed (Abe *et al.*, 1995).

11.1.5 Ischaemic cerebral oedema

Cerebral ischaemia not only causes loss of neuronal function but also cerebral oedema. Within minutes of onset of ischaemia, cytotoxic cerebral oedema occurs as a result of cell membrane damage allowing intracellular accumulation of water. The blood–brain barrier remains intact according to CT and isotope studies, and endothelial tight junctions are maintained (Bruce & Hurtig, 1979). The grey matter tends to be affected more than the white matter (Symon *et al.*, 1979) and the CT scan appearance of cytotoxic oedema is of well-circumscribed low density involving the cortex and subcortex. After several days of ischaemia, breakdown of the blood–brain barrier leads to vasogenic cerebral oedema as plasma constituents enter the brain extracellular space. The white matter tends to be more affected than the grey matter. The CT scan appearance of vasogenic oedema includes the characteristic finger-like projections of low density, which characteristically accompany cerebral tumours.

Animal studies and clinical observations suggest that cerebral oedema begins within hours of stroke onset and reaches a maximum volume at 2–4 days and then subsides over 1–2 weeks, but CT studies indicate that fluid volume after infarction peaks in 7–10 days and oedema remains detectable for 1 month (Bruce & Hurtig, 1979). Although the CT assessment of oedema may be unreliable (because of stroke-induced changes in blood volume and tissue density on CT), these findings do suggest that the peak frequency of herniation in the first week (see below) depends more on the rate of fluid accumulation than on the absolute volume of fluid accumulated.

In baboons, cerebral oedema can be exacerbated by reperfusion 2 hours after stroke onset but it is unknown whether this occurs in humans (see Section 11.1.3) (Bell *et al.*, 1985). Despite some evidence that early spontaneous reperfusion is not associated with a worsening of acute cerebral infarction and may lead to a better clinical outcome (von Kummer & Forsting, 1993; Wardlaw *et al.*, 1993), the recent thrombolytic trials (see Section 11.5) have reported that presumed reperfusion following thrombolytic therapy is associated with a higher rate of haemorrhagic transformation of the infarct and subsequent death and disability (see Section 11.5) (Donnan *et al.*, 1995; Hommel *et al.*, 1995; Kaste *et al.*, 1995). See Section 5.4 for a fuller discussion of haemorrhagic transformation of infarct.

Cerebral oedema correlates well with mass effect, midline shift, infarct size, neurological status and outcome. Correlation with infarct size perhaps explains why oedema does not seem to be so common or prominent in lacunar and small brainstem infarcts as it is in larger cortical/subcortical infarcts. Postmortem studies show microscopic cerebral oedema in almost all fatal strokes, whereas brain CT in life shows evidence of mass effect caused by oedema in less than 50% of acute (fatal and non-fatal) strokes (Bruce & Hurtig, 1979).

The effects of cerebral oedema are to compromise blood flow even further (by increasing pressure in the extravascular space, thus causing vascular congestion and sometimes haemorrhagic transformation) and to cause mass effect, brain shift and eventually brain herniation. The main danger of herniation is that it can initiate vascular and obstructive complications which aggravate the original expanding lesion, by compressing important vessels and tissues and causing cerebral ischaemia, congestion and oedema which, in turn, enhances the expanding process. In addition, the herniating brain can compress the aqueduct and subarachnoid spaces and so interfere with cerebrospinal fluid circulation, leading to hydrocephalus and elevated supratentorial cerebrospinal fluid pressure. There are three major patterns of supratentorial brain shift which can be identified by their end stages: (i) cingulate herniation; (ii) central transtentorial herniation; and (iii) uncal herniation (Plum & Posner, 1985).

Cingulate herniation

Cingulate herniation occurs when the expanding hemisphere shifts across the intracranial cavity, forcing the cingulate gyrus under the falx cerebri, compressing and displacing the internal cerebral vein and the ipsilateral anterior cerebral artery. This may lead to additional infarction in the territory of the anterior cerebral artery (Fig. 11.10).

Central transtentorial herniation

Central transtentorial herniation of the diencephalon is the end result of displacement of the hemispheres and basal

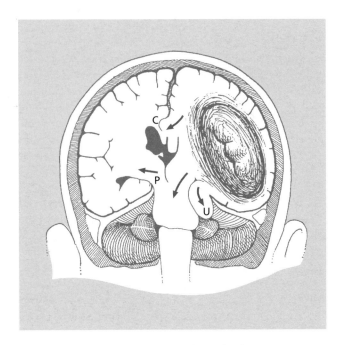

Figure 11.10 Uncal, transtentorial and cingulate herniation. A mass such as a cerebral haemorrhage, cerebral infarct or haemorrhagic infarct displaces the diencephalon and mesencephalon horizontally and caudally. The cingulate gyrus (C) on the side of the lesion herniates under the falx cerebri. The uncus (U) of the ipsilateral temporal lobe herniates under the tentorium cerebelli and becomes grooved and swollen and may compress the ipsilateral oculomotor (IIIrd cranial) nerve causing pupillary dilatation (Hutchinson's sign) (Hutchinson, 1867). The cerebral peduncle (P) opposite the supratentorial mass becomes compressed against the edge of the tentorium, leading to grooving (Kernohan's notch) and a paresis ipsilateral to the cerebral mass lesion (Kernohan & Woltman, 1929). Central downward displacement also occurs but is less marked than in Fig. 11.11. (From Plum & Posner, 1985.)

nuclei, compressing and eventually displacing the diencephalon and the adjoining midbrain rostrocaudally through the tentorial notch (Fig. 11.11). The great cerebral vein is compressed, which raises the hydrostatic pressure of the entire deep territory it drains. In addition, downward displacement of the midbrain and pons stretches the medial perforating branches of the basilar artery (the artery cannot shift downward because it is tethered to the circle of Willis), leading to paramedian brainstem ischaemia (and haemorrhage if perfusion continues).

Uncal herniation

Uncal herniation characteristically occurs when expanding lesions arising in the temporal fossa or temporal lobe shift the inner, basal edge of the uncus and hippocampal gyrus

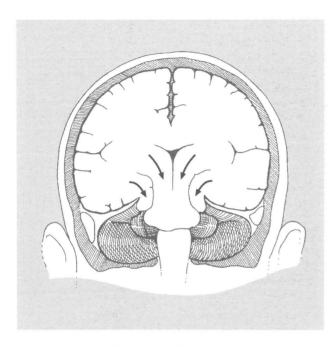

Figure 11.11 Central transtentorial herniation. Diffuse or multifocal swelling of the cerebral hemispheres (or bilateral subdural or extradural haematomas) compress and elongate the diencephalon from above. The mammillary bodies are displaced caudally. The cingulate gyrus is not herniated (From Plum & Posner, 1985.)

toward the midline so that they bulge over the incisural edge of the tentorium, and push the adjacent midbrain against the opposite incisural edge (see Fig. 11.10). At the same time the IIIrd cranial nerve and the posterior cerebral artery on the side of the expanding temporal lobe are often caught between the overhanging swollen uncus and the free edge of the tentorium or the petroclinoid ligament, leading to a IIIrd nerve palsy and occipital and medial temporal lobe infarction and swelling due to posterior cerebral artery territory ischaemia, which further compounds the problem.

Transtentorial herniation is the most common cause of death during the first week after acute stroke, accounting for about 80% of deaths in cerebral infarction and 90% in cerebral haemorrhage (Hachinski & Norris, 1985; Oppenheimer & Hachinski, 1992). The risk of death peaks within 24 hours for cerebral haemorrhage and at 4–5 days for cerebral infarction. Brainstem compression with subsequent haemorrhage and infarction accounts for the serious morbidity and mortality associated with herniation.

> *Transtentorial herniation is the most common cause of death within the first week of onset of both ischaemic stroke and primary intracerebral haemorrhage.*

11.1.6 Conclusion

Many different mediators have been implicated in brain cell survival and death in cerebral ischaemia. These include platelet activating factor, platelet adhesion and aggregation, eicosanoids, cytokines, leucocytes, coagulation and fibrinolysis, excitotoxins, Ca^{2+}, acidosis, free radicals, altered gene expression and cellular oedema. It has not been established whether these mediators act in a sequential, hierarchical fashion, or whether they are involved in a network of intricate relationships with overlapping effects. Efforts to treat ischaemic stroke successfully will require an integrated approach to understanding how the ischaemic process is initiated, and how the mediators interact and when.

11.2 General treatment considerations

The primary aim of most of the specific treatments is to reduce the volume of brain damaged by ischaemia, on the assumption that this will lead to less neurological impairment and so less disability and handicap in survivors. For patients with a large volume of brain damaged by infarction, reduction in infarct size may also reduce the risk of early death, particularly from ischaemic cerebral oedema and transtentorial herniation (see Section 11.1.5). As the pathophysiology of acute cerebral ischaemia is complex (see Section 11.1.3), many potential treatments have more than one mechanism or action and, for some, the precise mechanism is unknown.

11.2.1 Evaluating treatment for acute ischaemic stroke

Randomised trials

There is now little disagreement that the randomised controlled trial (RCT) is the best way to evaluate new (or old) treatments (Sackett *et al.*, 1991). Randomisation avoids the biases inherent in other research designs (e.g. case series without controls at all, series with retrospective controls, series with concurrent controls but non-random treatment allocation). However, RCTs often need to be surprisingly large to provide really reliable evidence on the balance of risk and benefit for a particular treatment, particularly if the measure of outcome is an uncommon, but serious, event such as death (Peto *et al.*, 1995). The effort of conducting large RCTs is substantial, and so many of the 'mega trials' have used a factorial design to assess two or three treatments at the same time without loss of statistical efficiency (Peto *et al.*, 1995). Our philosophy, both in this book and in our clinical practice, in deciding whether or not to adopt a particular treatment, is to place greatest emphasis on the evidence from randomised trials and from systematic reviews of randomised trials (see below). This style of practice is increasingly referred to as 'evidence-based medicine' and some of the general principles involved in translating results of trials (and of systematic reviews of trials) into clinical practice have been reviewed recently (Chalmers, 1995; Sackett, 1995). Unfortunately, the diffusion of these ideas into stroke medicine has been painfully slow.

> *We could answer many of the therapeutic questions posed in this book a great deal faster if a larger proportion of stroke patients were entered in to appropriate randomised trials.*

The need for adequate controls in evaluating treatments for stroke was realised as long ago as the 1950s because the assessment and prediction of the outcome in an individual patient was difficult, and it was even harder to assess, in a particular individual, whether or not treatment had been effective (see Section 10.2.7) (Dyken & White, 1956). Clinicians willing to admit uncertainty and undertake RCTs of different forms of treatment for acute stroke have been trying to overcome the methodological problems ever since. Dyken undertook the first quasi-randomised study of a medical treatment for acute stroke (Dyken & White, 1956). Thirty-six patients were alternately (but not randomly) assigned to cortisone or control. Thirteen of the cortisone patients died and 10 of the controls died; a trend against treatment. It is illuminating to read this 1956 article now and to realise that it has taken more than 30 years to make substantial progress with the clinical assessment of patients, the measurement of outcome and with achieving an adequate sample size in stroke trials.

The McMaster Group of Clinical Epidemiologists from Hamilton, Canada, have described the key features of a methodologically sound RCT. The report of a randomised trial should be evaluated critically to ensure the key features are present before clinicians decide whether or not to adopt that particular form of treatment in their own clinical practice (Sackett *et al.*, 1991). This book is strongly recommended reading. If the guidelines (Table 11.1) are applied to the trials in acute stroke, very few articles published before the 1990s emerge creditably. The weaknesses include: overcomplex eligibility criteria; inadequate sample size; inappropriate measures of outcome; poor standards of execution (i.e. poor trial discipline); and an unacceptably high proportion of patients 'lost' to follow-up. The reports of these studies often gave incomplete descriptions of the methods used (particularly the method of randomisation), failed to account for all patients randomised, used inappropriate

Table 11.1 Methodological criteria for the critical assessment of an article evaluating treatment. (From Sackett *et al.*, 1991.)

Was the assignment of patients to treatment really randomised?
Was the similarity between groups documented?
Was prognostic stratification used in treatment allocation?
Was foreknowledge of the randomly allocated treatment possible?

Were all clinically relevant outcomes reported?
Was case fatality as well as morbidity reported?
Were deaths from all causes reported?
Were quality of life assessments conducted?
Was outcome assessment blind to treatment allocation?

Were the study patients recognisably similar to your own?
Were reproducibly-defined exclusion criteria stated?
Was the setting primary, secondary or tertiary care?

Were both statistical and clinical significance considered?
If statistically significant, was the difference clinically important?
If not statistically significant, was the study big enough to show a
   clinically important difference if one really exists?

Is the therapeutic manoeuvre feasible in your practice?
Available, affordable, sensible?
Were contamination and co-intervention avoided?
Was the manoeuvre administered blind?
Was compliance measured?

*Were all patients who entered the study accounted for at its
   conclusion?*
(i.e. were drop-outs, withdrawals, non-compliers and those who
   crossed over handled appropriately in the analysis?)

---

statistical methods (often with inappropriate subgroup analysis) and provided conclusions that were not supported by the data presented. The picture is now changing and, in general, the design of stroke trials seems to be improving with larger sample sizes, better design and higher standards of execution and reporting. Measures of outcome after stroke are getting simpler, more reliable and valid; complex (and irrelevant) stroke scales to assess outcome (rather than initial stroke severity) may soon be a thing of the past (see Section 17.6.3) (van Gijn & Warlow, 1992).

> *The ideal would be that the evaluation of new treatments for stroke would be handled in the same way that, for example, new treatments for leukaemia are, i.e. it is normal practice that almost all patients with leukaemia in the UK are treated in the context of a randomised trial.*

The need for systematic reviews (or meta-analyses)

The biomedical literature is enormous. Clinicians are faced with a large amount of information to assimilate. For example, in 1995 over 800 references to reports of randomised controlled trials of different forms of stroke treatment, pre-

Table 11.2 Methodological criteria for the critical assessment of a review, an overview or a meta-analysis.

Were the question(s) and methods clearly stated?
Were the search methods used to locate relevant studies comprehensive?
Were explicit methods used to determine which articles to include in the review?
Was the methodological quality of the primary studies assessed?
Were the selection and assessment of the primary studies reproducible and free from bias?
Were differences in individual study results adequately explained?
Were the results of the primary studies combined appropriately?
Were the reviewers' conclusions supported by the data cited?

Note: this is a simple version for 'beginners' (Sackett *et al.*, 1991); a more up-to-date and detailed review is to be found in a recent paper (Cook *et al.*, 1995).

vention and rehabilitation had been identified with new studies being added at the rate of about five per week (Counsell *et al.*, 1995). To take just one example, 22 studies of Ca^{2+} antagonists in acute stroke were identified, of which 10 included fewer than 100 patients, only one study included more than 1000 patients; in total these studies included over 5000 patients (Counsell *et al.*, 1995). Of these 22 trials, 10 reported significant benefit from Ca^{2+} antagonists and 12 showed no effect or an adverse effect. Faced with such a confusing array of information, what can the busy clinician do? The temptation may be to focus on a selected few reports published in well-known English-language journals. Such selection will inevitably lead to a biased assessment of the effects of Ca^{2+} antagonists (or indeed of any treatment). The best way to minimise this bias is to review systematically all of the evidence from all of the RCTs (Sackett *et al.*, 1991; Counsell *et al.*, 1995). The criteria for a systematic review are outlined in Table 11.2. In fact, two recent systematic reviews of all the RCTs of one particular Ca^{2+} antagonist, nimodipine, independently confirmed that, based on the evidence available in 1994, treatment did not reduce death or the combined outcome of 'death or disability' (di Mascio *et al.*, 1994; Mohr *et al.*, 1994).

In a systematic review, the estimate of treatment effect is based on all of the data, which reduces the influence of random error. In other words, the confidence intervals for the estimate of treatment effect in the systematic reviews are narrower than for any one trial; the estimate is more precise and less prone to the play of chance. Subgroup analysis is popular with clinical trialists and people who like to generate hypotheses to explain the 'negative' or 'positive' results of particular trials. It is a dangerous sport, since often even surprisingly large effects observed in subgroups are due to the play of chance and not to the treatment itself (Antiplatelet

Trialists' Collaboration, 1994a; Counsell *et al.*, 1994). Claims for benefits of treatment based on a subgroup analysis of a single trial, or of a meta-analysis, need to be viewed with caution; the suggestion that nimodipine is effective when given within 12 hours, but hazardous if given more than 24 hours after stroke onset, may well not be real but due to the play of chance (Counsell *et al.*, 1994; Mohr *et al.*, 1994). It is interesting to assess the impact of this large amount of information on clinical practice; some clinicians will be aware of some of the 'positive' reports, some aware of the 'negative' studies and a few will be aware of the systematic reviews. It is perhaps not surprising that the use of Ca^{2+} antagonists varies enormously (see Section 11.2.2). There is, therefore, a great need for a series of systematic reviews of all the different forms of treatment for acute stroke, which are periodically updated as new evidence becomes available (Counsell *et al.*, 1995). A number of recent publications have given useful guidelines for systematic reviews and how to translate the results into clinical practice (Chalmers, 1995; Rothwell, 1995; Sackett, 1995; Cook *et al.*, 1995).

Meta-analysis is not statistical trickery; it is simply the best way to obtain the least biased and most precise estimate of a treatment effect from a group of approximately similar trials of the same intervention.

In response to this need, the Cochrane Collaborative Stroke Review Group is now coordinating a series of systematic reviews of different forms of health care for the treatment and prevention of stroke (Counsell *et al.*, 1995; The Cochrane Collaboration, 1996). Where a Cochrane systematic review of a particular intervention has been performed, it will be referred to in the text. For almost all trials an analysis of the effect of treatment on death has been possible, although even for this most fundamental outcome event some trials did not provide adequate detail. For some interventions such as heparin therapy, it has been possible to assess the effect of treatment on some of the common complications of stroke such as DVT and pulmonary embolism, but even in these trials, reliable analyses of the effect of treatment on disability and rare but important side effects, such as haemorrhagic transformation of the infarct, are not possible (Sandercock *et al.*, 1993; Counsell & Sandercock, 1996b). In the vast majority of trials, effects on disability have either not been reported at all or reported in a way that did not permit a systematic review. Thus, the effect on disability and handicap remains unclear for many treatments.

11.2.2 Treatments currently in use worldwide

There are enormous variations in the use of specific treatments for acute stroke both between and within different

	Number of patients randomised	Glycerol (%)	Corticosteroids (%)	Ca²⁺ antagonists (%)	Haemodilution (%)
Argentina	149	0	19	8	1
Australia	390	0	1	6	0
Austria	173	0	1	18	58
Belgium	145	1	4	7	0
Canada	87	0	0	9	7
Chile	51	0	0	25	0
Czech Republic	284	3	11	50	37
Denmark	18	0	6	0	0
Eire	41	0	12	2	0
Finland	49	0	2	12	0
Greece	110	2	1	1	2
Hungary	82	12	0	13	10
India	33	0	6	6	0
Israel	83	0	2	0	0
Italy	2 248	50	7	21	1
The Netherlands	585	0	1	2	0
New Zealand	345	0	1	6	0
Norway	381	0	1	2	0
Poland	382	26	3	12	9
Portugal	265	9	11	17	0
Slovak Republic	63	0	2	32	0
Slovenia	29	0	0	52	10
South Africa	48	0	2	42	0
Spain	320	1	2	8	1
Sri Lanka	5	0	0	20	0
Sweden	503	0	1	5	0
Switzerland	1 107	0	3	16	5
Turkey	175	1	28	21	1
UK	4 048	0	2	5	0
US	74	0	0	8	0
All countries	12 273	10	4	11	3

Table 11.3 Use of glycerol, corticosteroids, Ca²⁺ antagonists and haemodilution amongst 12 273 patients randomised in the IST (by 25/8/95). (From Ricci, 1995.)

countries. Over 30 countries are participating in the International Stroke Trial (IST) and substantial variation in the use of ancillary treatments has been reported (Table 11.3); glycerol treatment was used in 50% of patients treated in Italian centres, and 26% of patients treated in Polish centres, yet was hardly used at all in the remaining countries. Half the patients treated in centres in the Czech Republic and Slovenia received Ca²⁺ antagonists, more than 20% of patients received this treatment in Chile, Italy, the Slovak Republic, South Africa and Turkey; this is remarkable but sadly rather typical for a treatment which has not been proven beyond all reasonable doubt to be effective. Similarly, there were substantial between-country variations in the use of haemodilution and corticosteroids. In the US, a survey of neurologists reported that, in the treatment of acute ischaemic stroke, some clinicians used intravenous heparin in virtually all their patients, whereas others used it

in none (Marsh et al., 1989). A survey of consultant opinion in the UK suggested that, in the treatment of their patients with acute ischaemic stroke, about 10% of physicians used low-dose subcutaneous heparin routinely and less than 1% used intravenous heparin routinely (Lindley et al., 1995). In contrast, in Germany, the use of low-dose heparin is considered to be a mandatory standard therapy and so participation in the IST (in which 50% of the patients are allocated to avoid heparin; see Section 11.3.2) was considered unethical. Our knowledge of clinical practice in China and Asia is less well defined, but a recent survey in China suggested that the use of medically active herbal therapy was very common (yet the benefits had not been established by randomised trials) and that treatments used in the West (aspirin, heparin, thrombolytic and antioedema therapy) were used, but very variably in different centres (Chen et al., 1995). This world-wide therapeutic chaos must in part reflect the lack of really reliable evidence from appropriately large RCTs and the lack of widely disseminated systematic reviews of existing trial evidence.

> *Many agents are used routinely, in the mistaken belief that they are effective and safe, to treat patients with acute stroke, yet there is no clear evidence to support the use of any of them. We do not currently use any of the agents mentioned in this chapter routinely.*

11.2.3 Treatment of any specific underlying cause

Although the majority of ischaemic strokes are in one way or another related to atheroma and its thromboembolic complications (see Section 6.2), intracranial small vessel disease (see Section 6.3) and mostly embolism from the heart (see Section 6.4), a small proportion are due to other conditions which are mostly discussed in detail in Chapter 7. The more commonly encountered conditions, for which there is at least some evidence about the balance of risk and benefit from a specific treatment, are mentioned individually under the section dealing with that treatment; the remainder are dealt with briefly.

- Trauma and arterial dissection (see Section 11.3.3).
- Inflammatory vascular disorders (see Section 11.9).
- Congenital arterial anomalies (see Section 11.16).
- Embolism from arterial aneurysms (see Section 11.16).
- Migraine (see Section 11.16).
- Stroke in association with acute MI (see Section 11.3.3).
- Infections (see Section 11.16).
- Cancer (see Section 11.16).
- Malignant angioendotheliosis (see Section 11.16).
- Female sex hormones (see Sections 11.16 and 16.6).
- Pregnancy (see Section 11.16).
- Moyamoya syndrome (see Section 11.16).
- Mitochondrial cytopathy (see Section 11.16).
- Cholesterol embolisation syndrome (see Section 11.16).

It is important to emphasise that, although conditions like arteritis may be infrequent, failure to recognise and treat them may lead to a poor outcome or even death. A systematic approach to history taking, examination and investigation will minimise the risk of failing to identify a potentially treatable condition (see Chapters 5–7).

11.3 Anticoagulants

11.3.1 Rationale

The rationale for using anticoagulants applies to both the arterial and venous circulations (Hirsh, 1991). In large arter-

ies and in the single perforating arteries involved in lacunar infarction, the aim of treatment is to prevent local propagation of the occluding thrombus, to tip the balance in favour of spontaneous lysis of the occluding thrombus and to prevent early re-embolisation from any proximal arterial or cardiac sources. In small arteries and the microvessels, anticoagulation might also prevent sludging which may contribute to ischaemia in the penumbra zone around the infarct core. In the venous circulation, prevention of DVT and pulmonary embolism, common complications of immobility after stroke, is clearly important (see Section 15.13). However, anticoagulants could theoretically increase the risk of symptomatic intracranial haemorrhage arising *de novo* (as intracerebral, subarachnoid or subdural bleeding) or as symptomatic haemorrhagic transformation of cerebral infarction (HTI). Of course, HTI can occur spontaneously, as part of the natural evolution of an initially bland infarct, even in patients not receiving any antithrombotic treatment (see Section 5.4) (Wardlaw & Warlow, 1992). A systematic review of the literature suggests that asymptomatic petechial HTI occurs in about 10–50% of patients, and that symptomatic HTI (usually associated with the formation of a haematoma) occurs in about 5% of untreated patients. It is more likely to occur in patients with a major neurological defect or a large infarct on CT/magnetic resonance imaging (MRI) (Hart *et al.*, 1995). If a policy of immediate anticoagulation of patients with acute ischaemic stroke does, even modestly, increase the risk of symptomatic HTI, this could offset any of the potential benefits mentioned earlier. Randomised trials provide the best means to assess this balance of risk and benefit.

11.3.2 Evidence

By mid-1995, 14 RCTs in patients with acute presumed ischaemic stroke had been completed and were available for review (Counsell & Sandercock, 1996b). In nine trials all (or virtually all) patients had a CT scan to exclude intracerebral haemorrhage before treatment was started, generally within 48 hours of stroke onset and continued for 2 weeks. Six trials tested standard unfractionated heparin, six tested some other form of heparin (low-molecular-weight heparin or heparinoid) and two tested heparin given for just 24 hours followed by oral anticoagulation. The trials included 1470 patients of whom 261 died. There was a consistent trend across all trials towards an excess of early deaths (i.e. during the treatment period) with a 33% *increase* in the odds of early death (95% confidence interval (CI): 13% reduction to a 105% increase). By the end of the scheduled follow-up, the observed difference between treatment and control reverted to a non-significant 7% reduction in the odds of death (95%

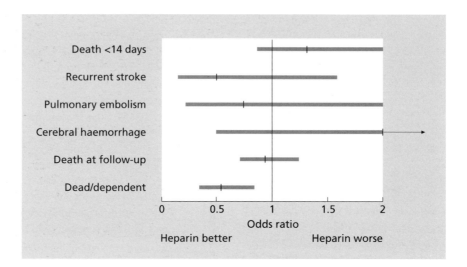

Figure 11.12 Results of a systematic review of the 14 randomised trials comparing heparin with control in patients with acute ischaemic stroke; relative effects on different outcomes. The estimate of treatment effect is expressed as an odds ratio (short vertical line) and its 95% confidence interval (horizontal error bar). An odds ratio of 1 corresponds to a treatment effect of zero, an odds ratio less than 1 suggests treatment is better than control and an odds ratio greater than 1 suggests treatment is worse than control. (From Counsell *et al.*, 1996a.)

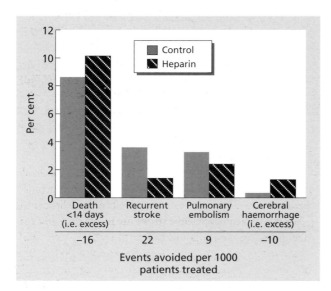

Figure 11.13 Results of a systematic review of the 14 randomised trials comparing heparin with control in acute ischaemic stroke: absolute risks of events in hospital (generally within the first 14 days of randomisation). None of the differences was statistically significant. (From Counsell *et al.*, 1996a.)

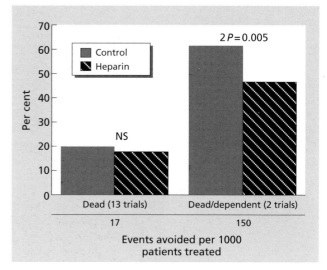

Figure 11.14 Results of a systematic review of the 14 randomised trials comparing heparin with control: absolute risks of different outcomes at final follow-up. Data on deaths at final follow-up were available for 13 trials, and on the numbers of patients dead or dependent at final follow-up for two trials. (From Counsell *et al.*, 1996a.)

CI: 29% reduction to 23% increase in the odds of death) (Figs 11.12–11.14). Only two trials reported data on functional outcome at final follow-up: the odds of being dead or dependent at final follow-up were reduced by 43% amongst heparin-allocated patients. The odds of DVT were reduced by 81% with anticoagulants, which was highly statistically significant, but the trials did not have sufficient statistical

power to provide reliable evidence on whether or not the observed reductions in pulmonary embolism and early recurrence of stroke were real or just due to the play of chance. Similarly, the trials lacked power to determine whether or not the excess of symptomatic intracranial haemorrhage (four of 296 heparin treated versus one out of 269 control patients) was real or not. Therefore, although there was clear evidence of protection against DVT and a promising effect on functional outcome, the trials included in the overview did not provide reliable evidence on the overall balance of risk and benefit of early anticoagulation, particularly for major events such as death, heamorrhagic transformation of the infarct, early recurrence of stroke and survival free of dependency. An up-to-date list of completed trials (and trials in progress) is in Counsell and Sandercock (1996b). The largest is the IST, a multicentre RCT evaluating the safety and efficacy of antithrombotic treatment, started within 48 hours of stroke onset and continued for 14 days. Patients with acute stroke are eligible provided there are no clear indications for, or clear contraindications to, immediate treatment with aspirin, heparin or the combination. The trial uses a 3 × 2 factorial design which enables each regimen to be tested separately and in combination. The regimens tested are: aspirin 300 mg daily versus 'avoid aspirin' and subcutaneous heparin 12 500 U twice daily versus subcutaneous heparin 5000 U twice daily versus 'avoid heparin'. The two main analyses will be of, in each treatment group, the proportion of patients who: die from any cause within 14 days, and who are dead or dependent in everyday activities at 6 months (International Stroke Trial Pilot Study Collaborative Group, 1996). The study began in 1993 and should have recruited its target of about 20 000 patients in 1996. Until the IST results are available, routine heparin therapy for treatment of ischaemic stroke cannot be recommended.

> *There should be no double standards for randomised trials and clinical practice, yet patients given treatments in routine practice are often not given any explanation or information. Many patients refused randomisation in the International Stroke Trial when they were told that aspirin and heparin might cause intracranial bleeding. Given clear information, patients can often make appropriate choices, yet how many tens of thousands of patients with acute stroke have been given these two drugs (before the current trials began) without a word of explanation of the potential risks?*

11.3.3 Who to treat

Patients at high risk of deep venous thrombosis

Patients with hemiplegia or immobility have a very high absolute risk of DVT and thereby the most to gain from heparin prophylaxis. In some European countries (Germany and France) such patients are *routinely* given low-dose subcutaneous heparin. A recent guideline issued by the American Heart Association also recommended routine use of heparin for DVT prophylaxis in stroke patients (Adams *et al.*, 1994), which rather conflicts with advice given elsewhere in the same guideline *not* to use heparin as a treatment for the cerebral lesion of acute ischaemic stroke. We would *not* recommend routine use of even low-dose heparin for DVT prophylaxis after stroke because of worries about the increased risk of intracranial bleeding and of death during the treatment period (see Section 11.3.2), but would rather recommend graded compression stockings, since they reduce the risk of DVT, at least in postoperative patients where they have been mostly tested, without causing cerebral haemorrhage (see Section 15.13) (Wells *et al.*, 1994).

Suspected cardioembolic ischaemic stroke: patient not already on anticoagulants

In the US, intravenous heparin is widely used for emergency anticoagulant therapy in patients with a suspected cardioembolic stroke (Marsh *et al.*, 1989). However, there has only been one RCT specifically targeted on this problem, which included a mere 45 patients (Hakim *et al.*, 1983). The more recent European Atrial Fibrillation Trial assessed the value of anticoagulants (and aspirin) in long-term secondary prevention after an ischaemic stroke or TIA (see Section 16.5.2): it did not specifically address the use of anticoagulants during the acute phase to prevent very early re-embolisation (European Atrial Fibrillation Trial Study Group, 1993). There is therefore no reliable evidence from large RCTs on the balance of risk and benefit from immediate anticoagulation in patients with suspected acute cardioembolic ischaemic stroke.

We agree with the Special Writing Group for the Stroke Council of the American Heart Association who concluded: 'Because data about the safety and efficacy of heparin in patients with acute ischaemic stroke are insufficient and conflicting, no recommendation can be offered' (Adams *et al.*, 1994). Table 11.4 lists categories of patients who are most and least likely to gain from early anticoagulation. All patients with suspected cardioembolic stroke should have a CT scan, since about 5–10% turn out to have primary intracerebral haemorrhage (Sandercock *et al.*, 1992). Patients with atrial fibrillation (AF) who have had a stroke or TIA are likely to benefit from long-term oral anticoagulant therapy as secondary prevention, provided there are no contraindications (see Section 16.5 for further details on the selection of patients with AF most likely to benefit from long-term oral anticoagulants). About 3600 of the 20 000 patients in the IST will have AF, so more substantial data on the balance of risk and benefit from *immediate* antithrombotic treatment in suspected cardioembolic stroke will be available by 1997 (Koudstaal, 1995).

Table 11.4 Which patients with acute ischaemic stroke of suspected cardioembolic origin should be considered for immediate anticoagulation and which should have anticoagulants deferred (or avoided completely)?

ANTICOAGULANTS NOT WORTHWHILE

Low risk of recurrent cardioembolic stroke without anticoagulants
Low-risk cardiac lesion (mitral valve prolapse, mitral annulus calcification, patent foramen ovale with no evidence of DVT, atrial septal aneurysm, aortic sclerosis)
Other, non-cardiac lesion more likely cause of cerebral infarct
  (a) severe ipsilateral carotid stenosis
  (b) likely disease of intracranial small vessels (i.e. lacunar infarct)

Little to gain from long-term anticoagulation
Suspected cholesterol embolisation syndrome (i.e. ischaemic stroke during cardiac catheterisation, after cerebral angiography or other vascular procedure)
Already severely disabled before the stroke
Moribund or predicted to be severely disabled in the long term

High risk of cerebral haemorrhage on anticoagulants
Infective endocarditis
Large cerebral infarct with midline shift and/or evidence of major haemorrhagic transformation (HTI) on brain CT
Likely to comply poorly with anticoagulation therapy and its monitoring after discharge
Severe, uncontrolled hypertension

Absolute contraindication to anticoagulants
Primary intracerebral haemorrhage (controversial; see Section 15.13)
History of bleeding disorder (e.g. haemophilia)

IMMEDIATE ANTICOAGULANTS PROBABLY WORTHWHILE

Best time to start anticoagulants unclear
Acute myocardial infarction within past few weeks and confirmed ischaemic stroke or TIA
Disabling ischaemic stroke and atrial fibrillation

IMMEDIATE ANTICOAGULANTS VERY LIKELY TO BE WORTHWHILE

Start as soon as possible
TIA or ischaemic stroke with complete recovery with 1–2 days + atrial fibrillation

Best time to start unclear
Non-disabling ischaemic stroke, no HTI, and atrial fibrillation

---

In a patient with acute ischaemic stroke and atrial fibrillation, the risk of stroke recurrence within the first 14 days is low in absolute terms, so we would not generally use anticoagulants within that period when the risk of haemorrhagic transformation of the infarct is probably highest.

Acute stroke in patients with acute myocardial infarction (see also Section 7.7)

The first step in management is to determine if the stroke was due to primary intracerebral haemorrhage, either spontaneous or iatrogenic caused by thrombolytic or anticoagulant treatment given for the MI (see Section 12.2.4 for the management of such intracerebral haematomas). Other patients may have iatrogenic ischaemic strokes due to particulate emboli reaching the brain as a complication of some invasive cardiological procedure such as coronary angiography or angioplasty. The value of anticoagulants in the latter patients is not clear, as the embolic material is often atheromatous debris from the large arteries rather than fresh thrombus or platelet aggregates (see Cholesterol embolisation syndrome, Section 11.16). Patients with full-thickness (Q wave) anterior MI have a higher than average risk of developing left ventricular (LV) thrombus (see Section 7.7). Although two small trials (SCATI Group, 1989; Turpie *et al.*, 1989) showed that medium-dose subcutaneous heparin (12 500 U twice daily) reduced the frequency of LV thrombus, an overview of the two megatrials, ISIS-3 and GISSI-2, showed that routine use of this regimen did not reduce early death or prevent stroke in patients with acute MI (Peto *et al.*, 1995). The value of anticoagulants in a patient with MI complicated by acute ischaemic stroke with a likely source of embolism (such as proven LV thrombus) is unclear. Anticoagulants, given to stroke-free MI survivors for several months, probably reduce the risk of having a stroke in the longer term, but the optimal intensity and timing of the start of treatment have not been defined (Vaitkus *et al.*, 1992). We would seriously consider giving anticoagulants for 6 months to a patient whose MI was complicated by acute ischaemic stroke likely due to embolism from the left ventricle.

'Progressing hemispheric stroke' and 'progressive basilar thrombosis'

The first step is to find out why the stroke is 'progressing'. There are numerous causes for a worsening neurological deficit besides propagating cerebral arterial thrombosis (see Section 15.5). Many textbooks and reviews recommend immediate intravenous heparin; some even recommend thrombolytic treatment (Hacke *et al.*, 1995). There have been two small trials of intravenous heparin in patients with non-progressing stroke and treatment was associated with a non-significant doubling of the risk of death (Counsell *et al.*, 1996b). These data are not encouraging. We would not use anticoagulants routinely in such patients, but might do so on rare occasions as a last resort. Further trials of anticoagulants in such patients are clearly needed.

Carotid or vertebral artery dissection

Patients with dissection of the extracranial carotid or vertebral arteries can deteriorate because of artery-to-artery embolisation arising from thrombus formed at the site of dissection (see Section 7.1). On the evidence derived from uncontrolled series of small numbers of patients, many clinicians are inclined to use anticoagulants. However, anticoagulants could both increase bleeding into the dissected arterial wall, and therefore worsen the situation, and possibly accentuate any HTI. However, there have been no RCTs, although one is said to be in the planning stage. In a patient with a confirmed dissection, we would generally avoid anticoagulation if the patient was clinically stable or improving. We would consider anticoagulation if the patient was deteriorating and other, more plausible, causes for deterioration such as cerebral herniation or pneumonia had been excluded. After the acute phase, re-endothelialisation occurs at the site of the dissection. Remodelling and healing may, within a few months, lead to an arterial lumen which appears virtually normal (Mokri *et al.*, 1986; Sturzenegger *et al.*, 1995). In other cases, the artery remains occluded, but because the thrombus has been covered with endothelium, there is probably little risk of further thromboembolism. Some clinicians find it helpful to re-image vessels non-invasively with ultrasound or MR angiography a few months after the dissection and, if the vessel has returned to normal, consider stopping any antithrombotic therapy. For those few patients with dissection whom we do anticoagulate we do not routinely re-image the vessel before stopping treatment.

The balance of risk (haemorrhage) and benefit (less venous thromboembolism and possibly less handicap) of heparin for immediate treatment in acute ischaemic stroke is unknown. We only use this treatment outside clinical trials in some patients with progressing stroke likely to be due to progressing thromboembolism. If we are going to use oral anticoagulation for long-term secondary prevention we tend to start the treatment a week or two after stroke onset.

11.3.4 Who not to treat

Any patient with acute stroke who is being considered for *full-dose* anticoagulants should not start on treatment until brain CT has excluded intracranial haemorrhage. But, can *less intensive* anticoagulant regimens be started before a CT scan? The issue is controversial, but the IST should provide evidence on the balance of risk and benefit of the policy of 'start antithrombotic therapy in patients considered clinically unlikely to have intracranial haemor-

Table 11.5 Contraindications to and cautions with full-dose anticoagulants (these depend on individual circumstances and are seldom absolute). (From Scottish Intercollegiate Guidelines Network, 1996.)

Uncorrected major bleeding disorder
    Thrombocytopenia
    Haemophilia
    Liver failure
    Renal failure
Uncontrolled severe hypertension
    Systolic pressure over 200 mmHg
    Diastolic pressure over 120 mmHg
Potential bleeding lesions
    Active peptic ulcer
    Oesophageal varices
    Intracranial aneurysm
    Proliferative retinopathy
    Recent organ biopsy
    Recent trauma or surgery to head, orbit, spine
    Recent stroke, but patient not had brain CT scan or MRI
    Confirmed intracranial or intraspinal bleeding
History of heparin-induced thrombocytopenia or thrombosis
    (if heparin planned)
If warfarin planned
    Homozygous protein C deficiency (risk of skin necrosis)
    History of warfarin-related skin necrosis
    Uncooperative/or unreliable patients (long-term therapy)
    Risk of falling
    Unable to monitor INR

rhage whilst CT scanning is being arranged' (International Stroke Trial Pilot Study Collaborative Group, 1996). Other relative contraindications and cautions are given in Table 11.5.

11.3.5 When to start

Although we do not use anticoagulants routinely ourselves for the acute treatment of stroke and, in general, only use them within the context of a RCT (i.e. IST), there are circumstances where we may feel compelled to use them (see Section 11.3.3). In those few patients where we do use anticoagulants (whether given as prophylaxis for venous thromboembolism or as a treatment for the cerebral lesion itself during the acute phase of ischaemic stroke), on theoretical grounds one should start treatment as soon as possible after stroke onset. There may be a 'therapeutic window' for heparin, so that the therapeutic effect declines with increasing delay between symptom onset and start of treatment. Equally, the risk of intracerebral bleeding may alter with time (a 'hazard window'?). If the aim is to prevent early recurrent ischaemic stroke, there is no clear guidance from

RCTs of the optimum time for starting treatment. However, the risk of early recurrence of ischaemic stroke is relatively low both for patients in AF and in sinus rhythm (Sandercock *et al.*, 1992; Koudstaal, 1995), and so we think that one should not feel compelled to use immediate anticoagulant therapy for this reason alone. The risk of spontaneous HTI is highest during the first 2 weeks and occurs most commonly in large infarcts (Wardlaw & Warlow, 1992; Hart *et al.*, 1995). Patients who are drowsy or who have uncontrolled hypertension seem at highest risk of HTI (Hart *et al.*, 1995). The IST will provide further evidence on the optimum starting time for anticoagulants: in other words, whether it is better to start treatment immediately or to delay starting for a week or two. The risk of HTI is probably negligible in patients with TIA or with an ischaemic stroke which resolves within 1 day or so; if such a patient has a clear indication for the use of anticoagulants we would start treatment immediately.

11.3.6 Agent/dose/route/adverse effects

Agent

Oral anticoagulants do not act sufficiently fast to have a major role within the first few hours of onset of an ischaemic stroke. Anticoagulants must be given by injection if they are to achieve a rapid effect. The majority of the evidence on heparin in acute stroke relates to trials which used low-dose unfractionated heparin (5000 U subcutaneously two or three times daily) (Sandercock *et al.*, 1993; Counsell & Sandercock, 1996b). What little direct randomised evidence there is in patients with acute stroke suggests that more intensive heparin regimens (either with higher dose unfractionated heparin or with low-molecular-weight heparin or with heparinoid) may provide greater protection against DVT (Kay *et al.*, 1995; Counsell & Sandercock, 1996a,b). Unfortunately, these greater benefits may be offset by a higher risk of HTI and of early death (Sandercock *et al.*, 1993; Counsell & Sandercock, 1996a,b). Warfarin should not be used during pregnancy (see Sections 11.16 and 16.5).

Dose and route

An overview of the two trials testing intravenous heparin showed that in the acute phase of stroke there was a doubling of the risk of death, although this was not statistically significant; further trials are clearly required (Counsell & Sandercock, 1996b). Again, the IST should provide reliable evidence on the relative merits of different intensities of anticoagulation in the acute phase of stroke, i.e. low-dose (5000 U twice daily) and medium-dose (12 500 U twice

daily) subcutaneous unfractionated heparin. For clinicians who wish to use some form of heparin now, evidence from an overview of six randomised trials in non-stroke patients with established DVT, which compared subcutaneous with intravenous heparin, suggested that the subcutaneous route was more effective and possibly safer than the intravenous route (Hommes *et al.*, 1992). Subcutaneous administration of heparin is cheaper and avoids the inevitable restricted mobility of being attached to an intravenous infusion pump (Robinson *et al.*, 1993). Details of heparin and warfarin administration are given in Section 16.5.

Adverse effects

Tables 11.6 and 11.7 list the most important adverse effects of, and cautions with, the use of heparin. The most life-threatening risks are of massive non-cerebral haemorrhage

Table 11.6 Adverse effects of heparin.

LOCAL MINOR COMPLICATIONS OF SUBCUTANEOUS HEPARIN AT INJECTION SITE
Discomfort
Bruising

LOCAL COMPLICATIONS OF INTRAVENOUS HEPARIN AT CANNULA SITE (OR ELSEWHERE)
Pain at cannula site
Infection at cannula (sometimes with severe systemic infection)
Reduced patient mobility because of infusion lines and pump

MAJOR SYSTEMIC COMPLICATIONS

Intracranial bleeding
Haemorrhagic transformation of cerebral infarct (potentially disabling or fatal)
Intracerebral haematoma
Subarachnoid haemorrhage
Subdural haematoma

Extracranial haemorrhages
Subcutaneous (can be massive)
Visceral (haematemesis, melaena, haematuria)

Thrombocytopenia
Type I: dose and duration related, reversible, mild, usually asymptomatic, not serious and often resolves spontaneously
Type II: idiosyncratic, allergic, severe (may be complicated by arterial and venous thrombosis). Affects 3–11% of patients treated with intravenous heparin and less than 1% of patients treated with subcutaneous heparin (Hirsh, 1991; Schmitt & Adelman, 1993; Aster, 1995; Warkentin *et al.*, 1995)

Osteoporosis

Skin necrosis

Alopecia

---

and intracranial haemorrhage. Management of severe non-cerebral bleeding consists of stopping any heparin administration; estimation of the clotting time; and reversal with intravenous protamine sulphate in a dose of 1 mg for every

100 IU of heparin infused in the previous hour (Scottish Intercollegiate Guidelines Network, 1996). Protamine should be given slowly over 10 minutes and the patient monitored for hypotension and bradycardia. Not more than 40 mg of protamine should be administered in any one injection. Patients on oral anticoagulants who suffer a head injury or develop any of the neurological symptoms listed in Table 11.7 or who require a diagnostic lumbar puncture should be investigated and treated as described in Tables 11.7–11.9 (Scottish Intercollegiate Guidelines Network, 1996). Reversal of warfarin therapy requires consultation with the local haematology specialist (see Table 11.8).

Table 11.7 Cautions in patients on anticoagulants who have a head injury, develop headaches, neurological symptoms or require a lumbar puncture. (From Scottish Intercollegiate Guidelines Network, 1996.)

Intracranial bleeding
Head injury, headache, drowsiness, confusion or focal neurological symptoms or signs in patients on anticoagulant drugs

Any patient on anticoagulants who sustains a significant head injury (i.e. any loss of consciousness or amnesia or the presence of a scalp laceration) *must* undergo brain CT to exclude intracranial haemorrhage

Headache (especially of recent onset, or increasing in severity), impaired consciousness, confusion, or focal neurological symptoms or signs must *always* arouse the suspicion of intracranial or subdural haemorrhage, and brain CT *must* be performed (see Section 3.5.2)

Intraspinal bleeding
Lumbar puncture, myelography, epidural or spinal anaesthesia, transhepatic percutaneous shunting. All of these procedures carry a risk of spinal haemorrhage and paraplegia and should not be performed in any patients on anticoagulants until the anticoagulation has been reversed. The need for lumbar puncture or myelography should be discussed with a neurologist or neurosurgeon before anticoagulants are reversed, since reversal carries a risk of thromboembolism and alternative investigation (e.g. MRI scanning) may be preferable

Table 11.8 Strategy for reversal of oral anticoagulation. (From Scottish Intercollegiate Guidelines Network, 1996.)

Life-threatening haemorrhage (intracranial or major gastrointestinal bleeding)
Intravenous vitamin K_1 0.5 mg, repeated if necessary
and
50 IU factor IX complex concentrate/kg (also contains factors II and X) along with 50 IU factor VII concentrate (if available)/kg
or, less effectively
Fresh frozen plasma, approximately 1 L for adult

Less severe haemorrhage (e.g. haematuria, epistaxis)
Stop warfarin for 1–2 days
Give vitamin K_1 0.5 mg intravenously or 2 mg orally

High INR but no haemorrhage
Stop warfarin for several days and review
Consider giving vitamin K_1 0.5 mg intravenously or 2 mg orally

---

Table 11.9 Options for reversal of warfarin therapy. (From Scottish Intercollegiate Guidelines Network, 1996.)

Method	Dose	Advantage	Disadvantage
Stop warfarin		Simple	May take several days for prothrombin time to normalise, particularly with liver disease
Vitamin K_1	0.5 mg intravenously	Safe if given slowly	2–6 hours to take effect
Factor IX complex concentrate (also contains factors II and X)	50 IU factor IX/kg	Acts immediately. Small volume can be given quickly	Exposes patients to pooled blood product which rarely may transmit hepatitis B (but safe from hepatitis C and HIV). Effect is temporary (8–24 hours) and should be combined with vitamin K_1
Factor VII concentrate	50 IU factor VII/kg	Should be given with factor IX complex concentrate	As for factor IX complex
Fresh frozen plasma	1 L for adult	Acts immediately	Large intravenous volume load. Allergic reactions. Not virally inactivated. Not as efficacious as factor IX complex concentrate. Difficult to give repeat infusions because of large volume

Acute stroke in a patient already receiving anticoagulants

The first step is, as ever, to do a brain CT; if this shows intracranial haemorrhage then anticoagulants should be stopped and urgently reversed, with vitamin K and administration of clotting factors (with the advice of the local haematology specialist) (Hart *et al.*, 1995) (see Tables 11.7–11.9, and Section 12.2.4). Patients with mechanical heart valves are at risk of valve thrombosis and re-embolisation if anticoagulants are withdrawn, so the management of such patients requires careful communication between the stroke physician, the haematologist and the cardiologist. If the scan shows an infarct with a slight degree of HTI, anticoagulants do not necessarily need to be stopped. If the CT is normal or shows bland infarction, the reason for the infarction must be sought. Often, the cause is inadequate warfarin dose, but infective endocarditis must be ruled out; if it has, more careful supervision to maintain the international normalised ratio (INR) above 2.0 should minimise the risk of further ischaemic strokes (European Atrial Fibrillation Trial Study Group, 1995). However, recurrent ischaemic stroke despite an adequate INR may necessitate the addition of low-dose aspirin (see Section 16.5.4) (Turpie *et al.*, 1993).

11.4   Antiplatelet therapy

11.4.1   Rationale

On the arterial side, aspirin may prevent distal and proximal propagation of arterial thrombus as well as re-embolisation and, in the microcirculation, prevent platelet aggregation (and release of thromboxane and other neurotoxic eicosanoids) (see Section 11.1.3) (Antiplatelet Trialists' Collaboration, 1994b). In the venous circulation, antiplatelet therapy reduces DVT and pulmonary embolism: in patients at high risk as a result of general surgery, antiplatelet therapy reduced DVT by 39% and pulmonary embolism by 64% (Antiplatelet Trialists' Collaboration, 1994c). However, antiplatelet agents do have significant antihaemostatic effects. In the overview of the RCTs, antiplatelet therapy was consistently associated with a small but definite excess of intracranial and other non-cerebral haemorrhages (Antiplatelet Trialists' Collaboration, 1994a). The effects of antiplatelet agents, given in the acute phase of ischaemic stroke, have not been investigated extensively. Clarke *et al.* (1991) studied the effect of aspirin, heparin and recombinant tissue plasminogen activator (rTPA) on cerebral bleeding in a rabbit model of acute embolic ischaemic stroke. Aspirin, and to a lesser extent heparin and rTPA, was associated with

an excess of intracerebral haemorrhage. The animals that developed intracerebral haemorrhage all died. It is therefore possible that, in humans, the balance of risk and benefit of antiplatelet therapy could be completely different (and even hazardous) when used in the treatment of acute ischaemic stroke in contrast to the clear net benefits observed when used for the prevention of stroke (see Section 16.4).

11.4.2   Evidence

The first RCT of antiplatelet therapy in the prevention of stroke was reported in 1969 (Acheson *et al.*, 1969). Many further studies with somewhat conflicting results then followed. However, proof beyond reasonable doubt of the benefits of antiplatelet therapy in high-risk individuals in the long-term prevention of stroke, MI and vascular death did not emerge until 1988 when a systematic review of all of the trials then available was published (Antiplatelet Trialists' Collaboration, 1988). Aspirin was established as an effective treatment for patients with acute MI in the same year (ISIS-2 Collaborative Group, 1988).

A more extensive review of the worldwide literature in 1994 identified 174 randomised trials involving over 100 000 patients, and yet antiplatelet therapy had been hardly assessed at all as a treatment for the acute phase of stroke (Antiplatelet Trialists' Collaboration, 1994a). The five completed trials included a mere 500 patients and showed that antiplatelet therapy was associated with non-significant reductions in pulmonary embolism, early recurrent stroke, death and in the proportion of patients 'dead or dependent' at final follow-up (Counsell & Sandercock, 1996c) (Figs 11.15 & 11.16). These data are inadequate to guide clinical practice. Of course, if aspirin was proven to be effective and safe when started within the first few hours of symptom onset as a treatment for acute ischaemic stroke, it could be very widely used. Perhaps ten million patients with acute ischaemic stroke in Europe and the US might be suitable for treatment over the next decade. However, if aspirin is to be used on such a scale, then particularly reliable evidence of its effects — both good and bad — will be required.

> *At present there is no indication for routine use of aspirin or any other antiplatelet drug in the early treatment of acute stroke.*

Potential hazards of antiplatelet therapy in acute ischaemic stroke

In the five completed trials, there was a non-significant excess of intracranial haemorrhages amongst antiplatelet-

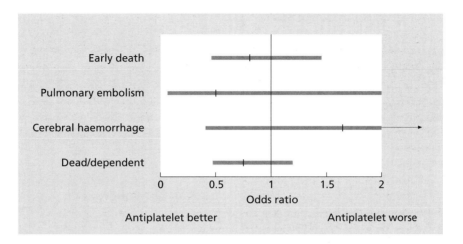

Figure 11.15 Results of a systematic review of the five randomised trials of antiplatelet therapy in acute stroke. Relative effects on different outcomes. The estimate of treatment effect is expressed as an odds ratio (short vertical line) and its 95% confidence interval (horizontal error bar). An odds ratio of 1 corresponds to a treatment effect of zero, an odds ratio less than 1 suggests treatment is better than control and an odds ratio greater than 1 suggests treatment is worse than control. There was no statistically significant difference between the treated and control groups for any of the outcomes. (From Counsell *et al.*, 1996c.)

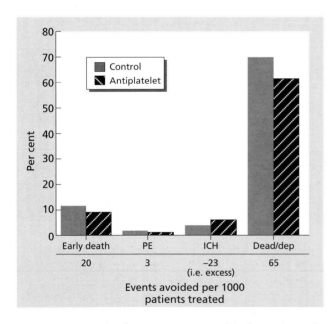

Figure 11.16 Results of a systematic review of the five randomised trials comparing antiplatelet therapy with control in acute ischaemic stroke: absolute differences. Dead/dep, percentage dead or dependent at final follow-up; ICH, intracranial haemorrhage; PE, pulmonary embolism. There was no statistically significant difference between the treated and control groups for any of the outcomes. (From Counsell *et al.*, 1996c.)

allocated patients (Counsell & Sandercock, 1996c). The excess, equivalent to about 20 fatal or disabling intracerebral haemorrhages per 1000 patients treated, if confirmed by a larger study, would be highly significant to patients and doctors (and might outweigh any reductions in less important events such as DVT).

Current studies

Two large trials are in progress, the first IST and the Chinese Acute Stroke Trial (CAST). Both plan to recruit about 20 000 patients. In the IST, patients are allocated, in an open factorial design, to treatment policies of: aspirin, heparin, the combination or to 'avoid both aspirin and heparin' for 14 days. In CAST, patients are allocated, in a double-blind design, to 1 month of aspirin or matching placebo. Aspirin alone is a highly effective antithrombotic therapy in the acute phase of MI, and evidence from a recent systematic review suggested that the addition of heparin to aspirin did not confer any extra benefit but did increase the risk of major haemorrhage by about 50% (R. Collins, personal communication, 1996). The factorial design in IST will clarify whether or not the addition of heparin to aspirin in patients with acute ischaemic stroke adds net clinical benefit or merely increases the risk of fatal or disabling intracranial haemorrhage. Both IST and CAST are expected to report results in late 1996/1997. An updated systematic review of all of the randomised trials should be available soon after both of these trials have been completed. Since the available data are inadequate to guide clinical practice, we would not recommend antiplatelet therapy for *routine* use in acute ischaemic stroke. However, some points about our own practice are worth mentioning (see Sections 11.4.3 and 11.4.4).

11.4.3 Who to treat

Transient ischaemic attack or minor stroke that has almost completely recovered within the first few hours

It is often difficult, when assessing a patient within the first few hours of symptom onset, to know whether or not the deficit will recover completely (or almost completely) within 24 hours. If we were reasonably confident that the patient was recovering very rapidly, within just a few hours of symptom onset, and the final diagnosis was likely to be a TIA or minor ischaemic stroke, we would routinely start antiplatelet therapy for secondary prevention (see Section 16.4).

Patients already on antiplatelet therapy

The priority is to perform a brain CT or an MRI scan to determine whether the stroke is haemorrhagic or ischaemic; if haemorrhagic, antiplatelet therapy should be stopped. If the stroke is ischaemic we are uncertain whether it is better to stop, because the treatment has 'failed' to prevent the stroke (and because we need to minimise the risk of intracranial haemorrhage), or to continue. The IST should provide some, albeit limited, guidance on this issue, since about 20% of patients are already on aspirin at randomisation. By the end of the trial about 4000 patients on aspirin at entry will have been randomised between stopping and continuing their treatment. The question of what to do for long-term secondary prevention in patients who have a stroke whilst already on antiplatelet therapy is discussed later (see Section 16.5.2).

11.4.4 Who not to treat

It should go without saying that a patient with proven intracranial haemorrhage should not be treated with antiplatelet agents. However, there have been a few small inconclusive trials in patients with aneurysmal subarachnoid haemorrhage in which the primary aim was to prevent ischaemic deficits *after* a ruptured aneurysm had been clipped; further trials are being planned (Antiplatelet Trialists' Collaboration, 1994a; J. van Gijn, personal communication).

11.4.5 Agent/dose/route/adverse effects

These issues are discussed in detail in relation to secondary prevention (see Section 16.4.4). For the few patients with acute ischaemic stroke in whom we do give immediate treatment with antiplatelet therapy, we would use aspirin at a dose of at least 150 mg daily. The initial dose has to be high (and certainly higher than is required for long-term secondary prevention), in order to inhibit thromboxane biosynthesis as quickly and completely as possible (Patrono *et al.*, 1990; Patrono, 1994). For patients who can swallow safely (see Section 15.17), aspirin can be given by mouth; for the remainder, it can be given rectally by suppository or by intravenous injection (as 100 mg of the lysine salt, infused over 10 minutes).

11.5 Thrombolysis

11.5.1 Rationale

Restoration of blood flow, to reperfuse the ischaemic brain as soon as possible after the cerebral vessel has been occluded, may lead to reduction in the volume of brain damaged by ischaemia volume on brain CT, less likelihood of major cerebral oedema and a better clinical outcome (see Section 11.1.3). Therefore, therapeutic attempts to hasten reperfusion with thrombolytic drugs ought to be helpful, provided any benefit is not negated by early hazard.

11.5.2 Evidence

Non-randomised and early randomised evidence

An exhaustive review of the world literature up to 1992 showed that thrombolytic treatment had been used in patients with acute stroke for over 40 years in at least 2500 patients (with its use in many more probably not reported) (Wardlaw & Warlow, 1992). However, only 700 of those patients had been studied in the context of RCTs. A review of the non-randomised trials yielded some useful information, suggesting that treatment did seem to increase the proportion of patients with early arterial recanalisation (Wardlaw & Warlow, 1992). A systematic review of the trials which used CT scanning to exclude intracranial haemorrhage before randomisation showed a non-significant trend towards reduced mortality and a significant reduction by about 50% in the odds of 'death or deterioration' (Wardlaw & Warlow, 1992). Some clinicians feel that these data provide sufficiently conclusive evidence to support thrombolytic treatment in selected patients. The 'target' population is any patient with major cerebral vessel occlusion (e.g. occlusion of the main stem of the middle cerebral artery or basilar trunk) who presents within a few hours of symptom onset (Hacke *et al.*, 1995). However, we and many others believe that further randomised evidence is needed, so a number of larger RCTs were set up. The results from that group of

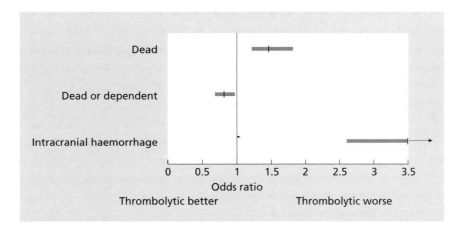

Figure 11.17 Results of a systematic review of the 11 randomised trials of thrombolytic treatment in acute CT-confirmed ischaemic stroke: relative effects on major outcome events. The estimate of treatment effect is expressed as an odds ratio (short vertical line) and its 95% confidence interval (horizontal error bar). An odds ratio of 1 corresponds to a treatment effect of zero, an odds ratio less than 1 suggests treatment is better than control and an odds ratio greater than 1 suggests treatment is worse than control. There were significant differences ($P < 0.01$) in outcomes of treatment versus control. (From Wardlaw *et al.*, 1996.)

'second-generation' thrombolytic trials became available during 1995 and 1996.

By 1996, 11 randomised trials, which included about 2800 patients, had reported at least interim data (Wardlaw *et al.*, 1996). A further study, the National Institute of Health (NIH) study, completed its target for recruitment of over 600 patients by 1995 and the results have recently become available (National Institute of Neurological Disorders and Stroke rt-PA Stroke Study Group, 1995). This is still a relatively small body of data in comparison to that available from the RCTs in acute MI, where over 50 000 patients had been randomised before clinicians generally accepted the evidence that thrombolysis saved lives (Fibrinolytic Therapy Trialists' (FTT) Collaborative Group, 1994; Peto *et al.*, 1995). Furthermore, it required a systematic review of the data from those trials to establish which patients with acute MI were most likely to benefit from treatment (Fibrinolytic Therapy Trialists' (FTT) Collaborative Group, 1994). The updated Cochrane Database of Systematic Reviews (CDSR) review of the trials of thrombolytic treatment in acute stroke (based on 11 trials reporting mortality data) showed a significant excess of deaths from all causes by the end of scheduled follow-up: 23.1% of thrombolytic-allocated patients compared with 18.8% of control-allocated patients; i.e. a significant 44% increase in the odds of death (95% CI: 19–75%) (Wardlaw *et al.*, 1996). Much of this hazard was related to an excess of *early* deaths and a significant 3.5-fold excess of symptomatic intracranial haemorrhages (10.3% amongst fibrinolytic-allocated patients compared with 3.0% amongst control-

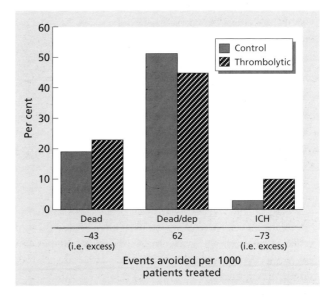

Figure 11.18 Results of a systematic review of the 11 trials of thrombolytic treatment for acute ischaemic stroke: absolute differences. Dead/dep, percentage dead or dependent at final follow-up; ICH, intracranial haemorrhage. All the differences between treatment and control were significant ($P < 0.01$). (From Wardlaw *et al.*, 1996.)

allocated patients). However, an analysis of the composite outcome measure 'death or disability' showed at least the possibility of worthwhile net long-term benefit: at final follow-up, 51% of controls were dead or disabled compared with 45% of thrombolytic-allocated patients; a marginally significant 20% reduction in the odds of a poor outcome (95% CI: 5–33%) (Fig. 11.17). The relative benefit may seem modest, but the level of absolute benefit is not small: about 60 stroke patients may avoid having a bad outcome for every 1000 treated with thrombolytic therapy (i.e. one needs to treat 16 patients to prevent one poor outcome) (Fig. 11.18). A separate more detailed review of the recent trials is being prepared in parallel with the Cochrane review by the Thrombolysis in Acute Stroke Pooling Project (TAS-PP). The analysis for the TAS-PP review will be based on collation of individual patient data from each trial, which may take some time; an expected publication date has not yet been set (J.P. Boissel, personal communication, 1996). TAS-PP will, however, allow exploratory analyses to examine factors which predict the early hazard, particularly of intracranial haemorrhage. Concomitant aspirin therapy (Multicentre Acute Stroke Trial (MAST-I) Group, 1995), delay of more than 3 hours from symptom onset (Donnan *et al.*, 1995) and the presence of visible infarction on pre-randomisation brain CT (Hacke *et al.*, 1995) have all been identified as possible adverse factors. Similarly, TAS-PP aims to identify predictors of a good outcome.

> *There is no doubt that thrombolytic treatment of acute ischaemic stroke carries a significant early risk of intracranial haemorrhage. However, there is a possibility that there may be a reduction in disability in survivors of the acute phase. At present, the balance between early hazard and possible long-term benefit is unclear.*

Implications for practice

For many neurologists and stroke physicians these results will confirm their view that thrombolytic treatment is, at best, not beneficial and, at worst, harmful. The early hazard will rightly deter many clinicians, but some stroke patients might view the situation differently, especially if they would prefer to die from the stroke than to survive in a disabled state (Solomon *et al.*, 1994). If further evidence, from trials and systematic reviews of trials, confirms that patients with acute ischaemic stroke who survive thrombolytic treatment are less disabled, then many patients might accept the short-term risk for longer term benefit. Indeed, many patients already accept this kind of trade-off; for example, patients at risk of stroke do seem to be prepared to accept the 5–6% risk of stroke and/or death complicating carotid surgery in order to reap the long-term benefits (see Section 16.7). But, for now, there is not enough evidence to support routine use of thrombolysis in acute ischaemic stroke.

Implications for research

The systematic reviews need to be continually brought up to date, published and widely debated to clarify whether there is worthwhile net benefit to: identify which patients are most likely to suffer early hazard; which patients will gain the greatest long-term benefit; and to help design appropriately large simple trials to test any hypotheses generated by the reviews (Bath, 1995; Peto *et al.*, 1995). The trials will need to include several thousand patients to clarify these issues. Large trials are *essential*; we must ensure that we do not abandon this treatment prematurely. If large trials are to be practicable, the way we care for stroke patients will need to alter radically. The whole health system will need a new *modus operandi* with a much greater sense of urgency to ensure that stroke patients are admitted, have a CT scan to exclude intracerebral haemorrhage and are randomised within a few hours of stroke onset (Bath, 1995).

11.5.3 Who to treat

Thrombolysis cannot be recommended as routine treatment for any category of patient with acute ischaemic stroke, and we do not use it in our patients. However, some comment is needed for specific categories of patients.

Acute occlusion of the basilar artery or the main stem of the middle cerebral artery

There have been two small RCTs in which most, if not all, of the patients had occlusion of the relevant cerebral vessel confirmed angiographically before randomisation (Mori *et al.*, 1992; Yamaguchi *et al.*, 1993). At least two additional trials in patients with arteriographically confirmed vessel occlusion, comparing intra-arterial thrombolysis with control, are under way (G. del Zoppo & G. Donnan, personal communications, 1996). None of these trials, either separately or combined in a systematic review, showed clear evidence of benefit (Wardlaw *et al.*, 1996). There have been no randomised trials restricted to patients with acute occlusion of the basilar artery. Despite the lack of randomised evidence, some clinicians still advocate the use of thrombolysis for such patients (Hacke *et al.*, 1994). We do not.

Suspected cardioembolic stroke

A small trial comparing rTPA with control in 98 patients with suspected cardioembolic ischaemic stroke showed a non-significant trend towards benefit with thrombolysis (Yamaguchi *et al.*, 1993). There is some suggestion that occlusion of a cerebral artery may be more susceptible to lysis if it is due to embolism from a cardiac source than from an arterial lesion in the extracranial arteries (Chimowitz *et al.*, 1994). We would not use thrombolytic therapy in a patient with acute, suspected cardioembolic stroke.

Ischaemic stroke following angiography or interventional radiology

There are many possible causes of stroke (both ischaemic and haemorrhagic) after such procedures (see Sections 6.6.4 and 13.5.4). If brain CT has excluded intracranial haemorrhage, and if the intra-arterial catheter is still in place, the radiologist may inject contrast material to see if an occlusive lesion can be visualised. Unfortunately, it may be difficult to ascertain whether the vessel has occluded because of local thrombosis, intimal dissection, arterial spasm or emboli dislodged by the catheter from proximal arterial sites. Even if the vessel is occluded by emboli, it may not be possible to determine whether the emboli consist of atheromatous debris or fresh thrombus. Nonetheless, interventional radiologists like to intervene, and there are several anecdotal reports of the use of thrombolysis to clear the obstruction. A single report of an uncontrolled study in 11 patients who had acute ischaemic strokes during interventional neuroradiological procedures (10 of 11 were having coils or balloons inserted into inoperable intracranial aneurysms), suggested that thrombolysis within 4 hours of symptom onset with an unspecified intra-arterial dose of urokinase was not catastrophic, but then a similar clinical outcome might have been observed without any treatment (Berenstein *et al.*, 1994).

11.5.4 Agent/dose/adverse effects

Agent

The debate about which agent is most effective and safe for patients with acute MI rages almost as fiercely now as it did in 1992 with the suggestion from ISIS-3 that streptokinase and rTPA had similar effects on death, but that the hazard of intracranial bleeding was higher with rTPA than with streptokinase (ISIS-3 Collaborative Group, 1992). A careful systematic review of all the trials directly randomising between the two agents is badly needed to quell the debate and one is planned for late 1996 (Fibrinolytic Therapy Trialists' Collaborative Group, personal communication, 1996). There are no studies which have directly randomised sufficiently large numbers of patients with acute ischaemic stroke between streptokinase, rTPA and urokinase to allow reliable comparison of the safety and efficacy of these agents. Only

indirect comparisons are available and these are not the most reliable way to compare treatment effects; nonetheless, they did not show major differences in efficacy between the three agents so no firm recommendation on the 'best' agent can be made (Wardlaw *et al.*, 1996).

Dose

There is a suggestion that low-dose urokinase and low-dose rTPA are associated with a lower risk of symptomatic intracranial haemorrhage, but the comparisons are confounded by a number of factors, such as baseline severity of stroke, race and time to randomisation, so no firm recommendation on the 'best' dose can be given (Wardlaw *et al.*, 1996).

Adverse effects

Intracranial haemorrhage is the most feared adverse effect of thrombolytic treatment, and it has been discussed extensively already. Streptokinase infusions can cause hypotension and this was a problem in the Australian Streptokinase (ASK) study (Donnan *et al.*, 1995). In MAST-I there was a major interaction of streptokinase with aspirin; the risk of symptomatic intracranial haemorrhage was significantly higher for the combination of aspirin and streptokinase than for either drug separately (Multicentre Acute Stroke Trial (MAST-I) Group, 1995). In all of the other trials, aspirin was not randomly allocated, so it was very difficult to determine whether any differences between trials in the frequency of symptomatic intracranial haemorrhage were due to concomitant aspirin treatment or to other factors (such as thrombolytic agent, dose, delay, etc.).

11.6   Defibrination

There are several defibrinating agents. Ancrod, a purified fraction of venom from the Malayan pit viper, has a number of effects: rapid defibrination, reduction in blood viscosity and some degree of anticoagulation (Hossmann *et al.*, 1983; Pollak *et al.*, 1990). Other agents are less well characterised (Cerebrovascular Research Group, 1982; Hao, 1984). Therefore, defibrination might have net beneficial effects in patients with acute ischaemic stroke, provided that its use is not associated with a substantial excess of major bleeds.

There have been at least three small RCTs of Ancrod, which have included a total of 202 patients (Hossmann *et al.*, 1983; Pollak *et al.*, 1990; Ancrod Stroke Study Investigators, 1994) and possibly additional studies of other

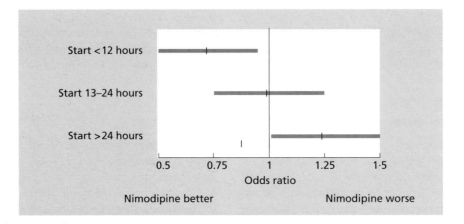

Figure 11.19 Results of a systematic review of the trials of nimodipine in patients with acute ischaemic stroke; subgroup analyses. The estimate of treatment effect is expressed as an odds ratio (short vertical line) and its 95% confidence interval (horizontal error bar). An odds ratio of 1 corresponds to a treatment effect of zero, an odds ratio less than 1 suggests treatment is better than control and an odds ratio greater than 1 suggests treatment is worse than control. Comparisons for less than 12-hours and greater than 24-hour subgroups are marginally significant ($P < 0.05$). (Redrawn from Mohr *et al.*, 1994.)

agents (C. Counsell, personal communication). The largest study with 132 patients showed a non-significant trend towards a reduction in death and 'death or dependency' (Ancrod Study Investigators, 1994). The frequency of intracranial haemorrhage was similar in treated patients and controls, but the study had inadequate power to exclude a moderate to substantial hazard of treatment. Two further trials are under way: a study in the US which plans to recruit 460 patients, and a study in Europe which will recruit 618 patients; results are not expected before 1997/1998.

11.7 Calcium (Ca^{2+}) antagonists

Influx of Ca^{2+} through voltage-sensitive channels may have a major role in neuronal death from ischaemia; this influx can be inhibited with a number of agents, so-called Ca^{2+} channel blockers or antagonists (see Section 11.1.4).

There have been over 20 RCTs of different classes of Ca^{2+} antagonists given as immediate treatment for patients with acute ischaemic stroke. Twelve of the trials testing only nimodipine have recently been reviewed and these included 3518 patients of whom 670 died (Di Mascio *et al.*, 1994). The observed relative reduction in the number of deaths was only 2% (95% CI, 18% reduction to an 18% excess). On the basis of this evidence, routine use of Ca^{2+} antagonists in acute ischaemic stroke cannot be recommended. A selective meta-analysis of nine trials of 120 mg oral nimodipine (trials testing a higher dose were excluded because of adverse effects) showed, in a subgroup analysis, that patients treated within 12 hours of onset had a favourable outcome (Mohr *et al.*, 1994) (Fig. 11.19). However, it is hazardous to undertake a selective subgroup analysis in a trial or meta-analysis which has an overall negative result, because the outcome in one particular subgroup may well, by chance alone, be better than average. An analysis of treatment effects in all other patients will then inevitably show that treatment is associated with a worse than average outcome (Counsell *et al.*, 1994). This was seen in the overview of Ca^{2+} antagonists, since patients treated more than 24 hours after onset of symptoms with nimodipine had a significantly increased risk of a poor outcome (Fig. 11.19). Thus, the apparent benefits of early nimodipine (and the apparent hazards of late nimodipine) could have been due to the play of chance and not to a real treatment benefit or hazard. A recent trial of intravenous nimodipine in acute ischaemic stroke showed that treatment was associated with higher early mortality, larger infarct volume and worse long-term outcome (Wahlgren *et al.*, 1994). An additional trial of oral nimodipine showed a higher proportion of patients with poor functional outcome amongst nimodipine-allocated patients (Kaste *et al.*, 1994). A further RCT of very early oral nimodipine in acute stroke (the Very Early Nimodipine Use in Stroke (VENUS) study) is underway in the Netherlands; this study is based in general practice and patients are randomised before transfer to hospital to maximise the opportunity for early therapy (M. Limburg, personal communication). A further systematic review of all trials of all Ca^{2+} antagonists in acute ischaemic stroke is planned as part of the Cochrane review process.

> *There is no evidence to support the routine use of Ca²⁺ antagonists in acute ischaemic stroke.*

Since the balance of benefits and risk remains unclear, we do not use Ca^{2+} antagonists routinely in acute ischaemic stroke patients.

11.8 Naftidrofuryl

The mechanism of action of this agent is not entirely clear but it is said to be, broadly speaking, protective to ischaemic neurones (Steiner & Clifford Rose, 1986). There have been three small trials, none of which provided convincing evidence of benefit (Admani, 1978; Steiner & Clifford Rose, 1986; Gray *et al.*, 1990). A further trial of intravenous Naftidrofuryl (the Praxilene in Stroke Treatment in Northern Europe (PRISTINE) study) is due to report its results in 1996 (T.J. Steiner, personal communication, 1996). For the time being this treatment can not be recommended for routine use in patients with acute ischaemic stroke.

11.9 Corticosteroids

Corticosteroids (such as dexamethasone) reduce vasogenic cerebral oedema, which tends to develop about 24–48 hours or more after stroke onset, particularly in and around large infarcts (see Section 11.1.5). There have been at least 14 apparently randomised trials in acute stroke (Qizilbash & Murphy, 1993). A systematic review of the 10 methodologically sound studies (including 619 patients) showed that treatment was associated with a non-significant 4% increase in the odds of death (95% CI: 28% reduction to 50% increase) (Qizilbash & Murphy, 1993). Inclusion of the four less well-designed studies (an additional 100 patients) suggested that treatment increased the odds of death by 20% (95% CI: 15% reduction to 68% increase). These data were inadequate to confirm or refute moderate benefit (or moderate hazard). Indirect evidence from studies of corticosteroids in patients with primary intracerebral haemorrhage showed no clear reduction in mortality, but a significant excess of adverse effects, such as infections, amongst corticosteroid-treated patients (Poungvarin *et al.*, 1987).

Corticosteroids are used haphazardly in different countries (see Table 11.3). We do not use them as a routine treatment for unselected patients with ischaemic stroke, nor do we use them in patients who have massive cerebral oedema complicated by transtentorial herniation. Our only indication is in patients with inflammatory vascular disorders (e.g. giant cell arteritis, polyarteritis nodosa, systemic lupus erythematosus; see Section 7.2). If we suspect the diagnosis and if the patient is acutely ill or is at high risk of complications without corticosteroids (such as a high risk of blindness in patients with untreated giant cell arteritis), then we start with 60–80 mg oral prednisolone daily, whilst arranging a biopsy of the relevant artery: temporal artery for giant cell arteritis or meningeal and brain biopsy for granulomatous angiitis of the nervous system. If granulomatous angiitis is confirmed histologically, cyclophosphamide should probably be added to corticosteroids (Hankey, 1991).

11.10 Glycerol, mannitol and other treatments to reduce intracranial pressure

Glycerol is a hyperosmolar agent which is said to reduce cerebral oedema and possibly increase CBF (Rogvi-Hansen & Boysen, 1995), mannitol is an osmotically active agent and hemispherectomy is a surgical procedure to remove necrotic brain (Kalia & Yonas, 1993). All these treatments aim to reduce intracranial pressure and thereby improve CPP. Surgical decompression of massive cerebellar infarcts may improve CPP and also relieve obstructive hydrocephalus, but requires further study (Muffelmann *et al.*, 1995).

There have been 10 RCTs of glycerol in acute stroke, involving 593 patients (Rogvi Hansen & Boysen, 1995). A systematic review of the evidence from these trials showed that glycerol was associated with a marginally significant 42% reduction in the odds of early death (95% CI: 6–64% reduction in the odds of death). However, at final follow-up, early glycerol treatment was associated with only a non-significant 18% reduction in the odds of death (95% CI: 46% reduction to 23% increase). An analysis of the effects of treatment on functional outcome was not possible. A further trial of glycerol is underway in Italy (Azzinibdu *et al.*, 1994). Mannitol and decompressive surgery have not been evaluated by adequately designed RCTs.

We do not use glycerol at all in our own clinical practice, although it is often used in Italy; about 50% of patients entered by the 60 Italian centres participating in the IST received glycerol (see Table 11.3). Until the current trial of glycerol is completed, and the systematic review updated, glycerol cannot be recommended for routine use. The use of mannitol is also not recommended. Hemispherectomy is unproven. The selection of patients with cerebellar infarction for decompressive surgery and/or shunting remains controversial (MacDonnell *et al.*, 1987; Mathew *et al.*, 1995).

11.11   Haemodilution

Haemodilution is generally achieved by giving an infusion of dextran, hydroxyethyl starch or albumin (Asplund, 1995). Such infusions increase blood volume (hypervolaemic haemodilution). In patients with acute stroke in whom an increase in total blood volume may be undesirable, haemodilution can be achieved isovolaemically by simultaneously removing several hundred millilitres of blood. This treatment leads to reduced whole blood viscosity, and if the optimum haematocrit is achieved, an increase in cerebral oxygen delivery. This increase in cerebral oxygen delivery, if achieved in practice, might be neuroprotective and so reduce infarct volume.

Fifteen RCTs including 2268 patients have been reviewed systematically (Asplund, 1995). No overall effect on survival was seen. In survivors, neurological outcome was similar in the haemodilution and control groups. The proportion of patients independent in daily activities on final follow-up did not differ between the groups. No subgroup could be identified in which treatment was clearly beneficial. DVT and pulmonary embolism were possibly reduced in the treatment group. This benefit was partly offset by a trend towards an increase in 'other circulatory events' in the treated group.

Given this information, we can see no reason to use this treatment in routine clinical practice, although it is used quite widely in Austria and in some parts of Eastern Europe (see Table 11.3).

11.12   Blood pressure reduction

The observational data relating blood pressure soon after stroke onset with subsequent outcome do not give a clear picture and a systematic review of all the available studies is required (see Section 15.7). At least one study has suggested that higher initial blood pressure is associated with a favourable outcome (Allen, 1984), whereas others have suggested that an increasing level of baseline blood pressure in patients with impaired consciousness is associated with a progressively higher probability of a poor outcome (Phillips, 1994). The data from the first 8000 patients randomised in the IST suggested a U-shaped relationship with early death and poor long-term outcome being more frequent in patients with blood pressures in the highest and lowest quartiles of systolic blood pressure (Fig. 11.20) (Phillips *et al.*, 1995). Of course, any relationship between blood pressure and outcome is likely to be confounded by stroke severity and by co-morbid conditions (which may raise or lower blood

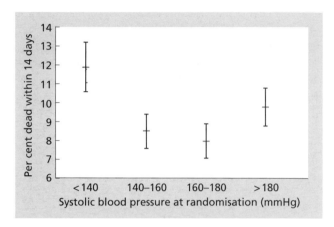

Figure 11.20 U-shaped relationship between 14-day case fatality and systolic blood pressure at randomisation amongst 8000 patients randomised in the IST by 1995. Horizontal lines indicate the 14-day case fatality rate (%). The vertical error bars show the 95% confidence interval. (From Phillips *et al.*, 1995.)

pressure). These data are all compatible with the hypothesis that adjusting the level of blood pressure to a notional 'optimum' may lead to a better outcome, but do not give a clear rationale to underpin a trial evaluating interventions to alter blood pressure in acute stroke (i.e. is it better to have blood pressure high, and risk breaking through the upper limit of autoregulation if this has not already been impaired by the stroke and so cause cerebral oedema, or low and risk worsening cerebral ischaemia?).

There has been only one small trial which specifically aimed to compare blood pressure reduction with control in patients with acute ischaemic stroke (Lisk *et al.*, 1993). However, there have been several additional trials in patients with acute stroke, in which the intervention definitely or probably affected blood pressure: intravenous nimodipine (Wahlgren *et al.*, 1994), oral nimodipine (Mohr *et al.*, 1994) and beta-blockers (Barer *et al.*, 1988) to name but a few. A systematic review of these trials is planned, but the precipitate fall in blood pressure associated with intravenous nimodipine did *increase* the risk of early death and of a poor long-term outcome, probably by increasing cerebral infarct volume.

There is no clear indication to reduce blood pressure routinely in all patients, so any guidelines are based on observational data and are therefore unreliable. In our own practice, we do not routinely reduce blood pressure within the first few days, unless there is clear evidence from fundoscopy (or other clinical evidence) of organ damage by accelerated hypertension. Patients who have persistently high blood pressures at 7–14 days after stroke are likely to benefit from long-term antihypertensive drug therapy for secondary prevention (see Section 16.3.1). There is no reliable evidence on the optimal timing of the start of treatment, but it is more convenient to start treatment for patients with sustained hypertension, not previously detected, in long-term secondary prevention about 1–2 weeks after stroke onset, before the patient is discharged from hospital.

> *What to do about the blood pressure in acute stroke is unclear: raise it, lower it or leave it alone. We tend to leave it alone unless there is evidence of hypertensive encephalopathy. We normally start treatment for persisting hypertension about 1–2 weeks after stroke onset.*

11.13 Neuroprotective agents

There are many points in the pathophysiological cascade between vessel occlusion and irreversible cell death where pharmacological intervention might be beneficial (see Sections 11.1.3 and 11.1.4), and the pharmaceutical industry has been able to develop a very large number of compounds for clinical development and testing (Muir & Lees, 1995; Dorman *et al.*, 1996). There is no doubt that, in animal models, many neuroprotective agents reduce the volume of brain damaged by cerebral infarction when given either after or before the ischaemic insult (Touzani *et al.*, 1994).

However, really reliable evidence about the balance of risk and benefit from these agents in humans will only emerge if some appropriately large simple trials are undertaken (Dorman & Sandercock, 1996). The methodological considerations which have been mentioned in relation to other interventions apply equally to neuroprotective agents, but two specific points are worth making.

1 The trials should have sufficient power to detect moderate treatment effects (since the effects of these drugs will surely be less striking in humans than they are in experimental animals).

2 These agents should be tested in both ischaemic and haemorrhagic stroke (Dorman & Sandercock, 1996).

The situation is changing very rapidly, and it is possible that one of the neuroprotective compounds currently undergoing trials may gain a licence for use in acute ischaemic stroke by 1996. The agents that are currently available for testing in clinical trials are listed in Table 11.10.

> *It is probable that the extremely large reductions in cerebral infarct volumes achieved with neuroprotective agents in experimental animal models will translate into only moderate reductions in disability when used in human acute stroke; neuroprotective therapy is unlikely to prove a panacea for acute stroke.*

In 1995, none of the agents in Table 11.10 had a product licence for use in acute stroke, and there is therefore no indication to use any of them routinely in clinical practice. Some agents may prove to be effective in patients with primary intracerebral haemorrhage as well as in cerebral infarction (in which case, treatment could be started immediately, whilst brain CT is awaited, or even started before admission to hospital). Some agents are relatively simple to administer, with a short intravenous infusion lasting only a few hours, whereas others may require infusions to be maintained for several days or require careful electrocardiographic (ECG) monitoring to detect prolongation of the QT_c interval, which may herald serious cardiac arrhythmias. The

Table 11.10. Neuroprotective agents and their presumed mode of action (1995). (From Dorman *et al.*, 1996.)

Presynaptic	NMDA receptor modulators	Postsynaptic	Ca²⁺ channel antagonists	Metabolic activator	Antileucocyte	Free radical scavengers	Anti-oedema agents	Neurotrophic	Other
619C89	Cerestat	Gangliosides	Destrorphan	Glycerol	Anti-ICAM-1	Corticosteroids	Corticosteroids	Citicholine	Cerestat
Barbiturates	CGS 19755	Lubeluzole	Dextromethorphan	Magnesium		Glycerol	Glycerol	Gangliosides	CGS 19755
GABA agonists	Dextromethorphan		Eliprodril	Naftidrofuryl		Mannitol	Mannitol		Dextromethorphan
			Flunarizine	Protirelin		Tirilazad	Neurotropin		Dextrorphan
Chlormethiazole	Dextrophan		Isradipine				Propentofylline		Eliprodril
Lubeluzole	Eliprodril		Lubeluzole						Flunarizine
Propentofylline	Magnesium		Magnesium						Gangliosides
RS-87476	Remacemide		Nicardipine						Iradipine
			Nimodipine						Magnesium
			Propentofylline						Nicardipine
			PY 108 068						Nimodipine
			Remacemide						Opiate antagonists
			RS 87476						Propentofylline
									PY 108 068
									Remacemide
									RS 87476

GABA, gamma-aminobutyric acid; ICAM-1, intracellular cell adhesion molecule 1.

Table 11.11 Miscellaneous treatments for acute ischaemic stroke which have been tested in RCTs.

Acupuncture	Phosphocreatine
Arnica (homeopathic)	Piracetam
Beta-blocker	Prostacyclin
Choline precursor	Spironolactone
Heparin-induced extracorporeal	Theophylline
low-density lipoprotein	Thromboxane A_2 antagonists
precipitation	Veinoglobulin
Hydergine	Ventilation therapy
Intravenous magnesium	Vincamine
Ornithine alpha-ketoglutarate	
Opiate antagonists (naloxone)	

current trials are small and therefore unlikely to define the 'time window' for effective intervention very clearly, and a few 'megatrials' with several tens of thousands of patients may be required to determine, in humans, whether the 'window' is just a few hours or perhaps as long as 24 or even 48 hours. Such megatrials will also help to define which categories of patient are most likely to gain from treatment and which are the most likely to suffer adverse effects (confusion, hallucinations and agitation have been common in the early trials).

11.14   Other specific agents

A bewildering variety of agents have been suggested as effective in acute stroke. Those which have been tested in RCTs are listed in Table 11.11. None is clearly beneficial. A comprehensive bibliography of RCTs, the Controlled Clinical Trial Register, is available in the Cochrane Library (which also includes the Cochrane Database of Systematic reviews). The 1997 edition should include the bibliography of trials relevant to stroke assembled by the stroke module of the Cochrane Collaboration (The Cochrane Library, 1996).

11.15   Immediate carotid endarterectomy and interventional radiology

For patients with severe carotid stenosis and an ischaemic stroke in the ipsilateral hemisphere, early restoration of normal vascular anatomy and so flow in the internal carotid artery might improve outcome. There are undoubtedly a few patients in whom the predominant cerebral problem is low flow in the ipsilateral hemisphere and it is this group that is theoretically most likely to benefit from urgent surgical restoration of flow. For others, the problem is artery-to-artery embolisation and, in them, the rationale is removal of

the embolic source before a recurrent disabling ischaemic stroke occurs. Some surgeons are prepared to consider surgical removal of an occluding thrombus, but this is likely to be incomplete since thrombus which has propagated distally into the carotid syphon cannot be removed surgically.

There have been no RCTs comparing immediate with deferred carotid surgery (or immediate versus deferred angioplasty) in patients with acute ischaemic stroke. Arguments based on non-randomised clinical series of patients do nothing but confuse the issue. Those in favour of surgery (mostly surgeons) cite series showing an apparently low surgical morbidity from operations performed within the first day or two of the onset of stroke, whereas other more conservative people (generally physicians and neurologists) cite surgical series with prohibitively high morbidity and case fatality. Similarly, enthusiastic proponents of interventional radiology claim that it can be used safely in acute stroke to deal with severe carotid stenosis (Higashida *et al.*, 1995).

In theory, it should be straightforward to identify patients with a mild neurological deficit that is either fluctuating or worsening in association with a very severe stenosis of the relevant carotid artery. In practice, such patients are only rarely encountered. We would only advocate the use of any surgical or interventional radiology procedure during the acute phase of ischaemic stroke within the context of a RCT.

11.16   Specific treatments for miscellaneous rare causes of ischaemic stroke

Congenital arterial anomalies and unruptured aneurysms

Kinks, loop and coils of the carotid or vertebral arteries should be managed conservatively (see Section 7.3). If one suspects embolisation from an unruptured intracerebral aneurysm (see Section 7.4) the options are to clip the aneurysm surgically, to treat it by endovascular coiling, to give antiplatelet agents or to do nothing. The balance of risks and benefits for each of these approaches is completely unknown.

Migraine

The pathophysiological relationship between migraine and acute ischaemic stroke is not clear (see Section 7.5) and there is no sensible clear rationale for using any particular treatment. Treatment of suspected acute migrainous cerebral infarction should follow the same principles as for nonmigrainous infarction.

Infections

Infective endocarditis (see Section 6.4), if confirmed by blood culture, requires standard treatment with intravenous antibiotics. The choice of antibiotic and duration of treatment should be made in conjunction with the microbiologists, and the management of any cardiac complications will require cardiological advice. Other specific infections causing stroke (e.g. syphilis, Lyme disease and human immunodeficiency virus (HIV)) should be treated according to the usual protocols.

Cancer (see Section 7.9)

If the malignant lesion happens to be an atrial myxoma, then surgical excision is required. Marantic endocarditis (see Section 6.4) complicating malignancy, even if it can be diagnosed reliably, is not treatable.

Malignant angioendotheliosis (see Section 7.6)

This requires specific oncological treatment with radiotherapy and/or chemotherapy.

Sex hormones

Young women who have an ischaemic stroke whilst taking the oral contraceptive should probably stop it and use an alternative form of contraception (see Section 7.10). Elderly women on hormone replacement therapy who have a stroke can probably continue safely but many may choose to stop after the stroke (see Section 7.10).

Pregnancy (see Section 7.11)

If there is a need for anticoagulation during pregnancy, heparin and not warfarin should be used during the first trimester since warfarin may cause fetal abnormalities (Scottish Intercollegiate Guidelines Network, 1996). Prolonged heparin therapy can cause osteoporosis in the mother (see Section 16.5.4 and Table 11.6).

Moyamoya syndrome (see Section 7.13)

No specific treatments are available to treat or prevent this disorder, the precise cause of which is unknown.

Mitochondrial cytopathy (see Section 7.15)

No specific treatments are available, although corticosteroids and co-factor therapy may be helpful sometimes (Di

Mauro & Moraes 1993; Fox & Dunne, 1993; Hammans & Morgan-Hughes, 1994).

Cholesterol embolisation syndrome (see Section 7.16)

This condition may be exacerbated by thrombolytic or anticoagulant therapy. If severe, renal failure may develop, requiring haemodialysis (Fine et al., 1987; Hyman et al., 1987; Anonymous, 1991).

References

Aaslid R, Lindegaard KF, Sorteberg W, Nornes H (1989). Cerebral autoregulation dynamics in humans. Stroke 20: 45–52.

Aaslid R, Newell DW, Stooss R, Sorteberg W, Lindegaard KF (1991). Assessment of cerebral autoregulation from simultaneous arterial and venous transcranial doppler recordings in humans. Stroke 22: 1148–54.

Abe K, Aoki M, Kawagoe J (1995). Ischaemic delayed neuronal death. A mitochondrial hypothesis. Stroke 26: 1478–89.

Acheson J, Danta G, Hutchinson EC (1969). Controlled trial of dipyridamole in cerebral vascular disease. Br Med J 1: 614–15.

Adams HP, Brott TG, Crowell RM et al. (1994). Guidelines for the management of patients with acute ischaemic stroke. A Statement for Healthcare Professionals from a Special Writing Group of the Stroke Council, American Heart Association. Circulation 90(3): 1588–1601.

Admani AK (1978). New approach to treatment of recent stroke. Br Med J 2: 1678–9.

Akopov SE, Sercombe R, Seylaz J (1994). Leucocyte-induced acute endothelial dysfunction in middle cerebral artery in rabbits. Stroke 25: 2246–52.

Allen CM (1984). Predicting the outcome of acute stroke: a prognostic score. J Neurol Neurosurg Psychiatr 47: 475–80.

Ancrod Stroke Study Investigators (1994). Ancrod for the treatment of acute ischaemic brain infarction. Stroke 25: 1755–9.

Anonymous (1991). Cholesterol embolism. Lancet 338: 1365–6.

Antiplatelet Trialists' Collaboration (1988). Secondary prevention of vascular disease by prolonged antiplatelet treatment. Br Med J 296: 320–31.

Antiplatelet Trialists' Collaboration (1994a). Collaborative overview of randomised trials of antiplatelet therapy. I. Prevention of death, myocardial infarction, and stroke by prolonged antiplatelet therapy in various categories of patients. Br Med J 308: 81–106.

Antiplatelet Trialists' Collaboration (1994b). Collaborative overview of randomised trials of antiplatelet therapy. II. Maintenance of vascular graft or arterial patency by antiplatelet therapy. Br Med J 308: 159–68.

Antiplatelet Trialists' Collaboration (1994c). Collaborative overview of randomised trials of antiplatelet therapy. III. Reduction in venous thrombosis and pulmonary embolism by antiplatelet prophylaxis among surgical and medical patients. *Br Med J* 308: 235–46.

Asplund K (1995). Haemodilution in acute stroke. In: Warlow C, van Gijn J, Sandercock P, eds. *Stroke Module of Cochrane Collaboration Database of Systematic Reviews*. London: BMJ Publishing.

Aster RH (1995). Heparin-induced thrombocytopenia and thrombosis. *N Engl J Med* 332(20): 1374–6.

Astrup J, Siesjo BK, Symon L (1981). Thresholds in cerebral ischaemia—the ischaemic penumbra. *Stroke* 12: 723–5.

Azzinibdu G, Casmiro M, D'Alessandro R, Fiorani L, Nonino F (1994). Italian trial on glycerol in ischaemic stroke (Trial Italiano sul Glicerolo nell'Ictus: TIGI). *Stroke* 25: 2113 (abstract).

Barer DH, Cruickshank JM, Ebrahim SB, Mitchell JR (1988). Low dose beta blockade in acute stroke ('BEST' trial): an evaluation. *Br Med J* 296: 737–41.

Baron JC (1991). Pathophysiology of acute cerebral ischaemia: PET studies in humans. *Cerebrovasc Dis* 1 (Suppl. 1): 22–31.

Baron JC, von Kummer, del Zoppo G (1995). Treatment of acute ischaemic stroke: challenging the concept of a rigid time window. *Stroke* 26: 2219–21.

Baron JC, Bousser MG, Rey A, Guillard A, Comar D, Castaigne P (1981). Reversal of focal 'misery-perfusion syndrome' by extra-intracranial arterial bypass in haemodynamic cerebral ischaemia: a case study with 15O positron emission tomography. *Stroke* 12: 454–9.

Barry DI, Strandgaard S, Graham DI (1982). Cerebral blood flow in rats with renal and spontaneous hypertension: resetting of the lower limit of autoregulation. *J Cereb Blood Flow Metab* 2: 347.

Bath PMW (1995). Treating acute ischaemic stroke. Still no effective drug treatment available. *Br Med J* 311: 139–40.

Bell BA, Symon L, Branston NM (1985). CBF and time thresholds for the formation of ischaemic cerebral oedema and effect of reperfusion in baboons. *J Neurosurg* 62: 31–41.

Berenstein A, Siller KA, Setton A, Nelson PK, Levin DN, Kupersmith M (1994). Intra arterial urokinase for acute ischaemic stroke during interventional neuroradiological procedures. *Neurology* 44 (Suppl. 2): A356 (abstract).

Brierley J (1976). Cerebral hypoxia. In: Blackwood W, Corsellis J, eds. *Greenfield's Neuropathology*. London: Arnold, E., 43–85.

Brown MM, Marshall J (1985). Regulation of cerebral blood flow in response to changes in blood viscosity. *Lancet* i: 604–9.

Brown MM, Wade JPH, Marshall J (1985). Fundamental importance of arterial oxygen content in the regulation of cerebral blood flow in man. *Brain* 108: 81–93.

Broze GJ Jnr (1992). The role of tissue factor pathway inhibitor in a revised coagulation cascade. *Semin Haematol* 29(3): 159–69.

Bruce DA, Hurtig HI (1979). Incidence, course, and significance of cerebral oedema associated with cerebral infarction. In: Price TR, Nelson E, eds. *Cerebrovascular Diseases*. New York: Raven, 191–8.

Cerebrovascular Research Group (1982). China made defibrase in the treatment of cerebral thrombosis: a clinical controlled study. *Bull Human Med Coll* 7(2): 163–7.

Chalmers I (1995). Applying overviews and meta analyses at the bedside—discussion. *J Clin Epidemiol* 45(1): 67–70.

Chen ZM, Zie JX, Collins R, Peto R, Liu LS (1995). Survey of hospital care of patients with acute stroke in China. *Cerebrovasc Dis* 5(4): 228 (abstract).

Cheung JY, Bonventre JV, Malis CD, Leaf A (1986). Calcium and ischaemic injury. *N Engl J Med* 314: 1670–6.

Chimowitz M, Arbor A, Pessin M, Furlan A, Wolpert S, del Zoppo G (1994). The effect of source of cerebral embolus on susceptibility to thrombolysis. *Neurology* 44 (Suppl. 2): A356 (abstract).

Clark WM, Madden KP, Lyden PD, Zivin JA (1991). Cerebral haemorrhage risk of aspirin or heparin therapy with thrombolytic treatment in rabbits. *Stroke* 22: 872–6.

Cook DJ, Sackett DL, Spitzer WO (1995). Methodologic guidelines for systematic reviews of randomised control trials in health care from the Potsdam consultation on meta-analysis. *J Clin Epidemiol* 48(1): 167–71.

Counsell C, Sandercock P (1996a). The use of low molecular weight heparins or heparinoids compared to standard unfractionated heparin in acute ischaemic stroke: a systematic review of the randomised trials. In: Warlow C, van Gijn J, Sandercock P, eds. *Stroke Module of Cochrane Database of Systematic Reviews*. (Database on disk and CD-ROM.) *The Cochrane Collaboration Issue 3*, Oxford: Update Software. London: BMJ Publishing.

Counsell C, Sandercock P (1996b). Efficacy and safety of anticoagulant therapy in patients with acute presumed ischaemic stroke: a systematic review of the randomised trials comparing anticoagulants with control. In: Warlow C, van Gijn J, Sandercock P, eds. *Stroke Module of Cochrane Database of Systematic Reviews*. (Database on disk and CD-ROM.) *The Cochrane Collaboration Issue 3*, Oxford: Update Software. London: BMJ Publishing.

Counsell C, Sandercock P (1996c). Efficacy and safety of antiplatelet therapy in patients with acute presumed ischaemic stroke: a systematic review of the randomised trials comparing immediate antiplatelet therapy with control. In: Warlow C, van Gijn J, Sandercock P, eds. *Stroke Module of Cochrane Database of Systematic Reviews*. (Database on disk and CD-ROM.) *The Cochrane Collaboration Issue 3*, Oxford: Update Software. London: BMJ Publishing.

Counsell C, Clarke MJ, Slattery J, Sandercock P (1994). The miracle of DICE therapy for acute stroke: fact or fictional product of subgroup analysis? *Br Med J* 309: 1677–81.

Counsell C, Warlow C, Sandercock P, Fraser H, van Gijn J (1995). The Cochrane Collaboration Stroke Review Group. Meeting the need for systematic reviews in stroke care. *Stroke* 26: 498–502.

D'Andrea G, Cananzi AR, Perini F (1994). Platelet function in acute ischaemic stroke: relevance of granule secretion. *Cerebrovasc Dis* 4: 163–9.

Davalos A, Fernandez-Real JM, Ricart W (1994). Iron-related damage in acute ischaemic stroke. *Stroke* 24: 1543–6.

Dearden NM (1985). Ischaemic brain. *Lancet* ii: 255–9.

De Bono DP (1994). Free radicals and antioxidants in vascular biology: the roles of reaction kinetics, environment and substrate turnover. *Quatern J Med* 87: 445–53.

Deykin D (1967). Thrombogenesis. *N Engl J Med* 276: 622–8.

Di Mascio R, Marchioli R, Tognoni G (1994). From pharmacological promises to controlled clinical trials to meta-analysis and back: the case of nimodipine in cerebrovascular disorders. *Clin Trials Meta-anal* 29: 57–79.

DiMauro S, Moraes CT (1993). Mitochondrial encephalomyopathies. *Arch Neurol* 50: 1197–1208.

Dirnagl U, Pulsinelli W (1990). Autoregulation of cerebral blood flow in experimental focal brain ischaemia. *J Cereb Blood Flow Metab* 10: 327–36.

Donnan GA, Davis SM, Chambers BR *et al.* (1995). Trials of streptokinase in severe acute ischaemic stroke. *Lancet* 345: 578–9.

Dorman P, Sandercock P (1996). Design considerations in trials of neuroprotective therapy. *Stroke* (submitted).

Dorman P, Counsell C, Sandercock P (1996). Systematic review of clinical trials of neuroprotective therapy for acute stroke. *CNS Drugs* (in press).

Dyken ML, White P (1956). Evaluation of cortisone in the treatment of cerebral infarction. *J Am Med Assoc* 162: 1531–4.

European Atrial Fibrillation Trial Study Group (1993). Secondary prevention in non-rheumatic atrial fibrillation after transient ischaemic attack or minor stroke. *Lancet* 342: 1255–62.

European Atrial Fibrillation Trial Study Group (1995). Optimal oral anticoagulant therapy in patients with nonrheumatic atrial fibrillation and recent cerebral ischaemia. *N Engl J Med* 333(1): 5–10.

Faraci FM, Brian JE (1994). Nitric oxide and the cerebral circulation. *Stroke* 25: 692–703.

Fibrinolytic Therapy Trialists' (FTT) Collaborative Group (1994). Indications for fibrinolytic therapy in suspected acute myocardial infarction: collaborative overview of early mortality and major morbidity results from all randomised trials of more than 1000 patients. *Lancet* 343: 311–22.

Fieschi C, Lenzi GL (1983). Cerebral blood flow and metabolism in stroke. In: Ross Russell RW, ed. *Vascular Disease of the Central Nervous System*. Edinburgh: Churchill Livingstone, 101–27.

Fine MJ, Kapoor W, Falanga V (1987). Cholesterol crystal embolisation: a review of 221 cases in the English literature. *Angiology* 38: 769–84.

Fox C, Dunne J (1993). Corticosteroid responsive mitochondrial encephalomyopathy. *Aust N Z J Med* 23: 522.

Frackowiak RSJ (1985). The pathophysiology of human cerebral ischaemia: a new perspective obtained with positron. *Quatern J Med* 57: 713–27.

Friberg L, Olsen TS (1991). Cerebrovascular instability in a subset of patients with stroke and transient ischaemic attack. *Arch Neurol* 48: 1026–31.

Fuster V, Badimon L, Badimon JJ, Chesebro JH (1992). The pathogenesis of coronary artery disease and the acute coronary syndromes. *N Engl J Med* 326: 310–18.

Gibbs JM, Wise RJS, Leenders KL, Jones T (1984). Evaluation of cerebral perfusion reserve in patients with carotid artery occlusion. *Lancet* i: 310–14.

Ginsberg MD, Pulsinelli WA (1994). The ischaemic penumbra, injury thresholds and the therapeutic window of acute stroke. *Ann Neurol* 36: 553–4.

Gray CS, French JM, Venables GS, Cartlidge NE, James OF, Bates D (1990). A randomised double blind controlled trial of naftidrofuryl in acute stroke. *Age Ageing* 19: 356–63.

Greenamyre JT, Porter RHP (1994). Anatomy and physiology of glutamate in the CNS. *Neurology* 44 (Suppl. 8): S7–S13.

Hachinksi VC, Norris JW (1985). *The Acute Stroke*. Philadelphia: David FA Company.

Hacke W, Schwab S, De Georgia M (1994). Intensive care of acute ischaemic stroke. *Cerebrovasc Dis* 4: 385–92.

Hacke W, Kaste M, Fieschi C *et al.* (1995). The European Cooperative Acute Stroke Study (ECASS). Intravenous thrombolysis with recombinant tissue plasminogen activator in the treatment of acute hemispheric stroke. *J Am Med Assoc* 274: 1017–25.

Hakim AM, Furlan AJ, Hart RG (1983). Immediate anticoagulation of embolic stroke: a randomised trial. *Stroke* 14: 668–76.

Halliwell B (1994). Free radicals, antioxidants, and human disease: curiosity, cause or consequence? *Lancet* 344: 721–4.

Hammans SR, Morgan-Hughes JA (1994). Mitochondrial myeopathies: clinical features, investigation, treatment and genetic counselling. In: Schapira AHV, DiMauro S, eds. *Mitochondrial Disorders in Neurology*. Oxford: Butterworth-Heinemann, 49–74.

Hankey GJ (1991). Isolated angitis/angiopathy of the central nervous system. *Cerebrovasc Dis* 1: 2–15.

Hao WX (1984). Effect of antithrombotic enzyme of Agkistrodon halys venom in the treatment of cerebral thrombosis. Report of 322 cases. *Chung Hua Shen Ching Ching Shen Ko Tsa Chih* 17(4): 223–5.

Harper AM (1966). Autoregulation of cerebral blood flow: influence of the arterial blood pressure on the blood flow through the cerebral cortex. *J Neurol Neurosurg Psychiatr* 29: 398–403.

Harper AM, Bell RA (1963). The effect of metabolic acidosis and alkalosis on the blood flow through the cerebral cortex. *J Neurol Neurosurg Psychiatr* 26: 341–4.

Harris RJ, Symon L, Branston NM (1981). Changes in extracellular calcium activity in cerebral ischaemia. *J Cereb Blood Flow Metab* 1: 203–9.

Hart RG, Boop BS, Anderson DC (1995). Oral anticoagulants and intracranial haemorrhage. Facts and hypotheses. *Stroke* 26: 1471–7.

Heiss WD (1992). Experimental evidence of ischaemic thresholds and functional recovery. *Stroke* 23: 1668–72.

Heiss WD, Graf R (1994). The ischaemic penumbra. *Curr Opin Neurol* 7: 11–19.

Heiss WD, Rosner G (1983). Functional recovery of cortical neurones as related to degree and duration of ischaemia. *Ann Neurol* 14: 294–301.

Heiss WD, Hayakawa T, Waltz AG (1976). Cortical neuronal

function during ischaemia. Effects of occlusion of one middle cerebral artery on single unit activity in cats. *Arch Neurol* 33: 813–20.

Herold S, Brown MM, Frackowiak RSJ, Mansfield AO, Thomas DJ, Marshall J (1988). Assessment of cerebral haemodynamic reserve: correlation between PET parameters and CO_2 reactivity measured by intravenous 133 xenon injection technique. *J Neurol Neurosurg Psychiatr* 51: 1045–50.

Heros RC (1994). Stroke: early pathophysiology and treatment. *Stroke* 25: 1877–81.

Higashida RT, Isai FY, Halbach VV, Barnwell SL, Dourd CF, Hieshima GB (1995). Interventional neurovascular techniques—state of the art therapy. *J Intern Med* 237: 105–15.

Hirsh J (1991). Heparin. *N Engl J Med* 324(22): 1565–74.

Hommel M, Boissal JP, Cornu C *et al.* (1995). Termination of trial of streptokinase in severe acute ischaemic stroke. *Lancet* 345: 57.

Hommes DW, Bura A, Mazzolai L, Buller HR, ten Cate JW (1992). Subcutaneous heparin compared with continuous intravenous heparin administration in the initial treatment of deep vein thrombosis. *Arch Intern Med* 116: 279–84.

Hossmann Ka (1994). Availability thresholds and the penumbra of focal ischaemia. *Ann Neurol* 36: 557–65.

Hossmann V, Heiss WD, Bewermeyer H, Wiedemann G (1983). Controlled trial of ancrod in ischaemic stroke. *Arch Neurol* 40: 803–8.

Hunter J (1794). A treatise on the blood, inflammation and gunshot wounds. In: Palmer JF, ed. *The Work of John Hunter* (1937) London: Longman.

Hutchinson J (1867). Four lectures on compression of the brain. *Clin Lect Reps Lond Hosp* 4: 10–55.

Hyman BT, Landas SK, Ashman RF, Schelper RL, Robinson RA (1987). Warfarin-related purple toes syndrome and cholesterol microembolisation. *Am J Med* 82: 1233–7.

International Stroke Trial Pilot Study Collaborative Group (1996). International Stroke Trial (IST) Pilot Study: design, baseline data and outcome in 984 randomised patients. *J Neurol Neurosurg Psychiatr* 60: 371–6.

ISIS-2 Collaborative Group (1988). Randomised trial of intravenous streptokinase, oral aspirin, both or neither among 17 187 cases of suspected acute myocardial infarction: ISIS-2. *Lancet* 2: 349–60.

ISIS-3. Third International Study of Infarct Survival Collaborative Group (1992). ISIS-3: a randomised comparison of streptokinase versus tissue plasminogen activator versus anistreplase and of aspirin plus heparin versus aspirin alone among 41 299 cases of suspected acute myocardial infarction. *Lancet* 339(8796): 753–70.

Ito U, Ohno K, Nakamura R (1979). Brain oedema during ischaemia and after restoration of blood flow. Measurement of water, sodium, potassium content and plasma protein permeability. *Stroke* 10: 542–7.

Jones TH, Morawetz RB, Crowell RM (1981). Thresholds of focal cerebral ischaemia in awake monkeys. *J Neurosurg* 54: 773–82.

Kalia KK, Yonas H (1993). An aggressive approach to massive middle cerebral artery infarction. *Arch Neurol* 50: 1293–7.

Kaste M, Fogelholm R, Erila T (1994). A randomised double blind placebo controlled trial of nimodipine in acute ischaemic hemispheric stroke. *Stroke* 25: 1348–53.

Kaste M, Hacke W, Fieschi C (1995). Results of the European Co-operative Acute Stroke Study (ECASS). *Cerebrovasc Dis* 5: 255.

Kay R, Wong SK, Yu LY *et al.* (1995). Low molecular weight heparin for the treatment of acute ischemic stroke. *N Engl J Med* 333: 1588–93.

Kernohan JW, Woltman HW (1929). Incisura of the crus due to contralateral brain tumour. *Arch Neurol Psych* 21: 274–87.

Kety SS (1950). Circulation and metabolism of the human brain in health and disease. *Am J Med* 8: 205–17.

Kety SS, Schmidt CF (1945). The determination of cerebral blood flow in man by the use of nitrous oxide in low concentrations. *Am J Physiol* 143: 53–66.

Kleiser B, Scholl D, Widder B (1994). Assessment of cerebrovascular reactivity by Doppler CO_2 and Diamox testing: which is the appropriate method. *Cerebrovasc Dis* 4: 134–8.

Knop J, Thie A, Fuchs C, Siepmann G, Zeumer H (1992). 99MTC–HMPAO–SPECT with acetazolamide challenge to detect haemodynamic compromise in occlusive cerebrovascular disease. *Stroke* 23: 1733–42.

Kogure K, Kato H (1993). Altered gene expression in cerebral ischaemia. *Stroke* 24: 2121–7.

Kontos HA (1989). Validity of cerebral arterial blood flow calculations from velocity measurements. *Stroke* 20: 1–3.

Koudstaal PJ (1995). Effect of atrial fibrillation on early deaths and recurrent strokes in the International Stroke Trial. *Cerebrovasc Dis* 5(4): 232–44 (abstract).

Lagi A, Bacalli S, Cencetti S, Paggetti C, Colzi L (1994). Cerebral autoregulation in orthostatic hypotension. A transcranial Doppler study. *Stroke* 25: 1771–5.

Larsen FS, Olsen KS, Hansen BA, Paulson OB, Knudsen GM (1994). Transcranial Doppler is valid for determination of the lower limit of cerebral blood flow regulation. *Stroke* 25: 1985–8.

Lassen NA, Fieschi C, Lenzi GL (1991). Ischaemic penumbra and neuronal death: comments on the therapeutic window in acute stroke with particular reference to thrombolytic therapy. *Cerebrovasc Dis* 1 (Suppl.): 32–5.

Lassen NA, Roland PE, Larsen B, Melamed E, Soh K (1977). Mapping of human cerebral functions: a study of the regional cerebral blood flow pattern during rest, its reproducibility and the activations seen during basic sensory and motor functions. *Acta Neurol Scand* 64 (Suppl.): 262–3.

Leenders KL, Perani D, Lammertsma AA (1990). Cerebral blood flow, blood volume and oxygen utilisation. Normal values and effect of age. *Brain* 113: 27–47.

Levin ER (1995). Endothelins. *N Engl J Med* 333: 356–61.

Lindley RI, Amayo EO, Marshall J, Sandercock P, Warlow C (1995). Acute stroke treatment in the UK hospitals: the Stroke Association Survey of Consultant Opinion. *J Roy Coll Phys* 29: 479–84.

Lindsberg PJ, Hallenbeck JM, Feuerstein G (1991). Platelet-activating factor in stroke and brain injury. *Ann Neurol* 30: 117–29.

Lipton SA, Rosenberg PA (1994). Excitatory amino acids as a final common pathway for neurologic disorders. *N Engl J Med* 330: 613–22.

Lisk DR, Grotta JC, Lamki LM (1993). Should hypertension be treated after acute stroke? A randomised controlled trial using single photon emission computed tomography. *Arch Neurol* 50: 855–62.

Liu PK, Salminen A, He YY (1994). Suppression of ischaemia-induced Fos expression and AP-1 activity by an antisense oligonucleotide to c-fos mRNA. *Ann Neurol* 36: 566–76.

Loscalzo J (1995). Nitric oxide and vascular disease. *N Engl J Med* 333: 251–3.

Lou HC, Edvinsson L, MacKenzie ET (1987). The concept of coupling blood flow to brain function: revision required? *Ann Neurol* 22: 289–97.

McCord JM (1985). Oxygen-derived free radicals in post-ischaemic tissue injury. *N Engl J Med* 312: 159–63.

MacDonell RAL, Kalnins RM, Donnan GA (1987). Cerebellar infarction: natural history, prognosis and pathology. *Stroke* 18: 849–55.

Mandai K, Sueyoshi K, Fukunaga R (1994). Evaluation of cerebral vasoreactivity by three-dimensional time of flight magnetic resonance angiography. *Stroke* 25: 1807–11.

Marchal G, Beaudoin V, Rioux P et al. (1996). Prolonged persistence of substantial volumes of potentially viable brain tissue after stroke: a correlative PET–CT study with voxel-based data analysis. *Stroke* 27: 599–606.

Markus HS, Harrison MJG (1992). Estimation of cerebrovascular reactivity using transcranial Doppler, include the use of breath-holding as the vasodilatory stimulus. *Stroke* 23: 668–73.

Markwalder TM, Grolimund P, Seiler RW, Roth F, Aaslid R (1984). Dependency of blood flow velocity in the middle cerebral artery on end-tidal carbon dioxide partial pressure—A transcranial ultrasound Doppler study. *J Cereb Blood Flow Metab* 4: 368–72.

Marsh EE, Adams HP, Biller J et al. (1989). Use of antithrombotic drugs in the treatment of acute ischaemic stroke. A survey of neurologists in practice in the United States. *Neurology* 29: 1631–4.

Masdeu JC, Brass LM, Holman L, Kushner MJ (1994). Brain single-photon emission computed tomography. *Neurology* 44: 1970–7.

Mathew P, Teasdale G, Bannan A, Oluoch-Olunya D (1995). Neurosurgical management of cerebellar haematoma and infarct. *J Neurol Neurosurg Psychiatr* 59: 287–92.

Merrick MV, Ferrington CM, Cowen SJ (1991). Parametric imaging of cerebral vascular reserves. 1. Theory, validation and normal values. *Eur J Med* 18: 171–7.

Mohr JP, Orgogozo JM, Hennerici M (1994). Meta-analysis of oral nimodipine trials in acute ischaemic stroke. *Cerebrovasc Dis* 4: 197–203.

Mokri B, Sundt TM, Houser W, Piepgras DG (1986). Spontaneous dissection of the cervical internal carotid artery. *Ann Neurol* 19: 126–38.

Mori E, Yoneda Y, Tabuchi M (1992). Intravenous recombinant tissue plasminogen activator in acute carotid artery territory stroke. *Neurology* 42: 976–82.

Muffelmann B, Busse O, Jaub M, Hornig C, Tettenborn B, Krieger D (1995) GASCIS—multicentre trial about space occupying cerebellar strokes. *Cerebrovasc Dis* 594: 240 (abstract).

Muir KW, Lees KR (1995). Clinical experience with excitatory amino acid antagonist drugs. *Stroke* 26(3): 503–13.

Multicentre Acute Stroke Trial (MAST-I) Group (1995). Are thrombolytic and antithrombotic agents safe and useful in acute ischaemic stroke? A randomised controlled trial with streptokinase, aspirin and combination of both treatments. *Lancet* 346: 1509–14.

National Institute of Neurological Disorders and Stroke rt-PA Stroke Study Group (1995). Tissue plasminogen activator for acute ischemic stroke. *N Engl J Med* 333: 1581–7.

Naylor AR, Merrick MV, Slattery JM, Notghi A, Fennington CM, Miller JD (1991). Parametric imaging of cerebral vascular reserve. 2. Reproducibility, response to CO_2 and comparison with middle cerebral artery velocities. *Eur J Nucl Med* 18: 259–64.

Oppenheimer S, Hachinski V (1992). Complications of acute stroke. *Lancet* 339: 721–4.

Patrono C (1994). Aspirin as an antiplatelet drug. *N Engl J Med* 330: 1287–94.

Patrono C, Ciabattoni G, Davi G (1990). Thromboxane biosynthesis in cardiovascular diseases. *Stroke* 21 (Suppl. IV): IV130–3.

Peto R, Collins R, Gray R (1995). Large-scale randomised evidence: large, simple trials and overviews of trials. *J Clin Epidemiol* 48(1): 23–40.

Phillips SJ (1994). Pathophysiology and management of hypertension in acute ischaemic stroke. *Hypertension* 23(1): 131–6.

Phillips SJ, Sandercock P, Slattery J (1995). U-shaped relationship between systolic blood pressure and early death after acute ischaemic stroke. *Can J Neurol Sci* 22(1): S44 (abstract).

Plum F, Posner JB (1985). *The Diagnosis of Stupor and Coma.* Philadelphia: Davis FA Company, 96–100.

Pollak Ve, Glas-Greenwalt P, Olinger CP, Wadhwa NK, Myre SA (1990). Ancrod causes rapid thrombolysis in patients with acute stroke. *Am J Med Sci* 299: 319–25.

Poungvarin N, Bhoopat W, Viriyavejakul A (1987). Effects of dexamethasone in primary supratentorial intracerebral haemorrhage. *N Engl J Med* 316: 1229–33.

Powers WJ (1991). Cerebral haemodynamics in ischaemic cerebrovascular disease. *Ann Neurol* 29: 231–40.

Powers WJ, Grabb RL Jnr, Raichel ME (1984). Physiological responses to focal cerebral ischaemia in humans. *Ann Neurol* 16: 546–52.

Powers WJ, Press GA, Grabb RL Jnr, Gado M, Raichle ME (1987). The effect of haemodynamically significant carotid artery disease on the haemodynamic status of the cerebral circulation. *Ann*

Intern Med 106: 27–35.

Pulsinelli W (1992). Pathophysiology of acute ischaemic stroke. *Lancet* 339: 533–6.

Qizilbash N, Murphy M (1993). Meta analysis of trials of corticosteroids in acute stroke. *Age Ageing* 22 (Suppl. 2): 4 (abstract).

Raichle M (1983). The pathophysiology of brain ischaemia. *Ann Neurol* 13: 2–10.

Ricci S (1995). Between country variations in the use of medical treatments for acute stroke. *Cerebrovasc Dis* 5(4): 272 (abstract).

Robinson AM, McLean KA, Greaves M, Channer KS (1993). Subcutaneous versus intravenous administration of heparin in the treatment of deep vein thrombosis: which do patients prefer? A randomised cross-over study. *Postgrad Med J* 69: 115–16.

Rogvi-Hansen B, Boysen G (1995). IV glycerol treatment in acute ischaemic stroke. In: Warlow C, van Gijn J, Sandercock P, eds. *Stroke Module of Cochrane Database of Systematic Reviews.* (Database on disk and CD-ROM.) *The Cochrane Collaboration Issue 3*, Oxford: Update Software. London: BMJ Publishing.

Rosenberg RD, Rosenberg JS (1984). Natural antocoagulant mechanisms. *J Clin Invest* 74(1): 1–6.

Ross R (1986). The pathogenesis of atherosclerosis—an update. *N Engl J Med* 314: 488–500.

Rothman SM, Olney JW (1986). Glutamate and the pathophysiology of hypoxic–ischaemic brain damage. *Ann Neurol* 19: 105–11.

Rothwell PM (1995). Can overall results of clinical trials be applied to all patients? *Lancet* 345: 1616–19.

Roy CS, Sherrington CS (1890). On the regulation of the blood supply of the brain. *J Physiol* 11: 85–108.

Sackett DL (1995). Applying overviews and meta-analyses at the bedside. *J Clin Epidemiol* 48(1): 61–6.

Sackett DL, Haynes RB, Guyatt GH, Tugwell P (1991). *Clinical Epidemiology. A Basic Science for Clinical Medicine.* Toronto: Little, Brown and Company, 173–85.

Sandercock P, van den Belt AGM, Lindley RI, Slattery J (1993). Antithrombotic therapy in acute ischaemic stroke: an overview of the completed randomised trials. *J Neurol Neurosurg Psychiatr* 56: 17–25.

Sandercock P, Bamford J, Dennis M *et al.* (1992). Atrial fibrillation and stroke: prevalence in different types of stroke and influence on early and long term prognosis (Oxfordshire Community Stroke Project). *Br Med J* 305: 1460–5.

SCATI Group (1989). Randomised controlled trial of subcutaneous calcium–heparin in acute myocardial infarction. The SCATI (Studio sulla Calciparina nell'Angina e nella Trombosi Ventricolare nell'Infarto) Group. *Lancet* 2: 182–6.

Schmidley JW (1990). Free radicals in central nervous system ischaemia. *Stroke* 21: 1086–90.

Schmitt BP, Adelman B (1993). Heparin-associated thrombocytopenia: a critical review and pooled analysis. *Am J Med Sci* 305(4): 208–15.

Schroeder T (1988). Haemodynamic significance of internal carotid artery disease. *Acta Neurol Scand* 77: 353–72.

Schror K, Braun M (1990). Platelets as a source of vasoactive mediators. *Stroke* 21 (Suppl. IV): IV32–5.

Scottish Intercollegiate Guidelines Network (1996). *Antithrombotic Therapy. A National Clinical Guideline Recommended for use in Scotland by the Scottish Intercollegiate Guidelines Network.* HMSO, Edinburgh (in press).

Sharp FR (1994). The sense of antisense fos oligonucleotides. *Ann Neurol* 36: 555–6.

Siesjo BK (1992a). Pathophysiology and treatment of focal cerebral ischaemia Part I: pathophysiology. *J Neurosurg* 77: 169–84.

Siesjo BK (1992b). Pathophysiology and treatment of focal cerebral ischaemia Part II: mechanisms of damage and treatment. *J Neurosurg* 77: 337–54.

Skinhoj E, Hoedt-Rasmussen K, Paulson OB, Lassen NA (1970). Regional cerebral blood flow and its autoregulation in patients with transient focal cerebral ischaemic attacks. *Neurology* 20: 485–93.

Solomon NA, Glick HA, Russo CJ, Lee J, Schulman KA (1994). Patient preferences for stroke outcomes. *Stroke* 25: 1721–5.

Steiner TJ, Clifford Rose F (1986). Randomised double blind placebo controlled clinical trial of naftidrofuryl in hemiparetic CT-proven acute cerebral hemisphere infarction. In: Clifford Rose F, ed. *Stroke: Epidemiological, Therapeutic and Socio-economic Aspects.* Royal Society of Medicine Services International Congress and Symposium Series No 99. London: Royal Society of Medicine Services Limited, 85–98.

Strandgaard S (1978). Autoregulation of cerebral circulation in hypertension. *Acta Neurol Scand* 57 (Suppl. 66): 1–82.

Strandgaard S, Paulson OB (1984). Cerebral autoregulation. *Stroke* 15: 413–41.

Strandgaard S, Olesen J, Skinhoj E, Lassen NA (1973). Autoregulation of brain circulation in severe arterial hypertension. *Br Med J* I: 507–10.

Sturzenegger M, Mattle HP, Rivoir A, Baumgartner RW (1995). Ultrasound findings in carotid artery dissection: analysis of 43 patients. *Neurology* 45: 691–8.

Sullivan HG, Kingsbury TB, Morgan ME (1987). The rCBF response to Diamox in normal subjects and cerebrovascular disease patients. *J Neurosurg* 67: 525–34.

Symon L, Branston NM, Chikovani O (1979). Systemic brain oedema following middle cerebral artery occlusion in baboons: relationship between regional cerebral water content and blood flow at 1 to 2 hours. *Stroke* 2: 184–91.

Symon L, Branston NM, Strong AJ (1976). Autoregulation in acute focal ischaemia. An experimental study. *Stroke* 7: 547–54.

The Cochrane Collaboration (1996). *The Cochrane Collaboration Issue 1*, Oxford: Update Software. Updated quarterly. London: BMJ Publishing Group.

Thomas DJ (1982). Whole blood viscosity and cerebral blood flow. *Stroke* 13: 285–7.

Touzani O, Young AR, MacKenzie ET (1994). The window of therapeutic opportunity following focal cerebral ischaemia. In: Krieglstein J, Oberpichler-Schwenk H, eds. *Pharmacology of Cerebral Ischaemia.* Stuttgart: Medpharm, 575–88.

Turpie AGG, Robinson JG, Doyle DJ (1989). Comparison of high-dose with low-dose subcutaneous heparin to prevent left ventricular mural thrombosis in patients with acute transmural anterior myocardial infarction. *N Engl J Med* 320: 353–7.

Turpie AGG, Gent M, Laupacis A, Latour Y, Gunnstensen J, Basile F (1993). A comparison of aspirin with placebo in patients treatment with warfarin after heart valve replacement. *N Engl J Med* 329: 524–9.

Vaitkus PT, Berllin JA, Schwartz JS, Barnathan ES (1992). Stroke complicating acute myocardial infarction. A meta-analysis of risk modification by anticoagulation and thrombolytic therapy. *Arch Intern Med* 152: 2020–4.

van Gijn J, Warlow C (1992). Down with stroke scales. *Cerebrovasc Dis* 2: 239–47.

van Kooten F, Ciabattoni G, Patrono C, Schmitz PIM, van Gijn J, Koudstaal PJ (1994). Evidence for episodic platelet activation in acute ischaemic stroke. *Stroke* 25: 278–81.

von Kummer R, Forsting M (1993). Effects of recanalisation and collateral blood supply on infarct extent and brain oedema after middle cerebral artery occlusion. *Cerebrovasc Dis* 3: 252–5.

Wahlgren NG, MacMahon DG, de Keyser J, Indredavik B, Ryman T (1994). Intravenous Nimodipine West European Stroke Trial (INWEST) of nimodipine in the treatment of acute ischaemic stroke. *Cerebrovasc Dis* 4: 204–10.

Wardlaw J, Yamaguchi T, del Zoppo G, Hacke W (1996). Thrombolysis in acute ischaemic stroke. In: Warlow C, van Gijn J, Sandercock P, eds. *Stroke Module, Cochrane Database of Systematic Reviews.* (Database on disk and CD-ROM.) *The Cochrane Collaboration Issue 3*, Oxford: Update Software. London: BMJ Publishing.

Wardlaw JM, Warlow C (1992). Thrombolysis in acute ischaemic stroke: does it work? *Stroke* 23: 1826–39.

Wardlaw JM, Dennis M, Lindley RI, Warlow C, Sandercock P, Sellar R (1993). Does early reperfusion of a cerebral infarct influence cerebral infarct swelling in the acute stage or the final clinical outcome? *Cerebrovasc Dis* 3: 86–93.

Warkentin TE, Levine MN, Hirsh J *et al.* (1995). Heparin-induced thrombocytopenia in patients treated with low molecular weight heparin or unfractionated heparin. *N Engl J Med* 332(20): 1330–5.

Weaver JPA, Evans A, Walder DN (1969). The effect of increased fibrinogen content on the viscosity of blood. *Clin Sci* 36: 1–10.

Wells PS, Lensing AWA, Hirsh J (1994). Graduated compression stockings in the prevention of postoperative venous thromboembolism: a meta analysis. *Arch Intern Med* 154: 67–72.

White HO (1992). Thrombolytic therapy for patients with myocardial infarction presenting after six hours. *Lancet* 340: 221–2.

Widder B, Kleiser B, Krapf H (1994). Course of cerebrovascular reactivity in patients with carotid artery occlusion. *Stroke* 25: 1963–7.

Wise RJS, Bernadi S, Frackowiak RJS, Legg NJ, Jones T (1983). Serial observations on the pathophysiology of acute stroke. The transition from ischaemia to infarction as reflected in regional oxygen extraction. *Brain* 106: 197–222.

Wollner L, McCarthy ST, Soper NDW, Macy DJ (1979). Failure of cerebral autoregulation as a cause of brain dysfunction in the elderly. *Br Med J* I: 1117–18.

Wood JH, Kee DB (1985). Haemorrheology of the cerebral circulation in stroke. *Stroke* 16: 765–72.

Yamaguchi T, Hayakawa T, Kiuchi H (1993). Intravenous tissue plasminogen activator ameliorates the outcome of hyperacute embolic stroke. *Cerebrovasc Dis* 3: 269–72.

Yamashita T, Hayashi M, Kashiwagi S (1992). Cerebrovascular reserve capacity in ischaemia due to occlusion of a major arterial trunk: studies by Xe-CT and the acetazolamide test. *J Comput Assist Tomogr* 16: 750–5.

Yanagisawa M, Kurihara H, Kimura S (1988). A novel potent vasoconstrictor peptide produced by vascular endothelial cells. *Nature* 332: 411–15.

Specific treatment of
primary intracerebral haemorrhage

12

12.1 Pathophysiology

The pathophysiology of primary intracerebral haemorrhage (PICH) is surprisingly complex (see Section 8.2.1). Rupture of a blood vessel inevitably leads to disruption of white matter tracts and some irreversible damage to neurones in the deep nuclei or the cortex. The protective encasement of the skull may become a disadvantage with sudden increases in volume within the intracranial cavity, as is the case with intracerebral haemorrhage. Apart from the brain tissue destroyed by the haemorrhage itself, the attendant increase in intracranial pressure may threaten the other parts of the brain, particularly — but not exclusively — when the intracranial pressure reaches levels of the same order of magnitude as the arterial pressure. Direct mechanical compression of the brain tissue surrounding the haematoma and, to some extent, vasoconstrictor substances in extravasated blood lead to impaired blood supply (Mendelow, 1993). Cellular ischaemia leads to further swelling from oedema, which is initially cytotoxic and later vasogenic (see Section 11.1.5). Hydrocephalus may be an additional space-occupying factor, especially with cerebellar haematomas, but a large haematoma in the region of the basal ganglia may also cause enlargement of the opposite lateral ventricle, through midline shift and obstruction of the third ventricle, whilst the ipsilateral ventricle is compressed (Ropper, 1986). The zone of ischaemia around the haematoma may be exacerbated by systemic factors such as hypotension or hypoxia. There may also be loss of cerebral autoregulation in the vasculature supplying the region of the haematoma. Some perifocal ischaemic damage occurs at the time of bleeding and cannot be prevented, but the question to be considered here is whether the vicious cycle of ongoing ischaemia causing steadily increasing pressure can be detected in its early stages and interrupted.

12.2 Management

12.2.1 Initial management

Once the diagnosis of PICH has been confirmed by computerised tomography (CT) scanning or magnetic resonance imaging (MRI), the next step is to identify the cause before treatment is initiated (see Chapter 8). For example, if surgical evacuation of a life-threatening haematoma is considered, medical measures may have to be taken first (such as substitution of clotting factors in patients with liver failure or on anticoagulant treatment). The surgeon should think twice if amyloid angiopathy is a likely cause, because the operation may provoke new haemorrhages at distant sites (Waga *et al.*, 1983).

Repeated CT scanning is indicated in case of clinical deterioration, which may be caused by rebleeding at the same or sometimes at a distant site, hydrocephalus or there are no changes, in which case the search for systemic disorders should be intensified (see Section 15.5).

It is important to know when intervention is useless, because the outlook is either very good or very bad; in both cases, only supportive care is called for. Predictive models include level of consciousness, age, pulse pressure, haematoma volume and intraventricular extension of the haemorrhage as the most important factors (Lisk *et al.*, 1994; Tuhrim *et al.*, 1995). A fatal outcome can be anticipated when there is no motor or other response to pain, and all brainstem reflexes (including the gag reflex) have been lost for at least a few hours, as a result of infratentorial haemorrhage or transtentorial herniation. As these patients are invariably ventilated it is important to exclude an effect of sedative drugs and neuromuscular blocking agents. Volumetric analysis alone may also guide prognosis: with supratentorial haemorrhages the prognosis is poor when the volume of the haematoma exceeds 50 ml (Franke *et al.*, 1990; Fogelholm *et al.*, 1992), or if the volume of intraventricular haemorrhage exceeds 20 ml (Young *et al.*, 1990).

Factors determining the prognosis of patients with primary intracerebral haemorrhage are: level of consciousness (Glasgow Coma Scale); age; volume of haematoma (poor prognosis if supratentorial haematoma >50 ml); and intraventricular extension of haemorrhage (poor prognosis if volume >20 ml).

12.2.2 Reduction of intracranial pressure

In patients with intracerebral haemorrhage, there are often factors other than the local effects of the haematoma itself that contribute to raised intracranial pressure. Frequently, these can be treated more directly than the intracerebral lesion, so it is important to be aware of them. They include fever, hypoxia, hypertension, seizures and elevations of intrathoracic pressure (Ropper, 1993). A vexing and unsolved question is whether it is useful to measure the actual intracranial pressure by the introduction of an intraventricular catheter or other device, at least in patients with a decreased level of consciousness. Such regimens can certainly be rationalised (Ropper & King, 1984), but any invasive procedure can give rise to complications and the presumed advantages in terms of outcome have not been subjected to controlled studies. Therefore, we prefer to err on the side of caution and base management on clinical and radiological measures.

Hyperventilation

Undoubtedly, hyperventilation decreases intracranial pressure, but the cure may be at least as bad as the disease. The intracranial pressure goes down because hypocapnia (usually down to values of the order of 4 kPa) causes vasoconstriction; in other words, ischaemia by compression is exchanged for ischaemia by vasoconstriction. Moreover, experimental evidence suggests that the effect on the vessel diameter is short lived, of the order of 6 hours; in patients with head injury, hypocapnia affects mainly normal brain vasculature, with a paradoxical increase of blood flow in the injured parts, which may be followed by increased oedema (Darby *et al.*, 1988). A randomised controlled trial of prolonged hyperventilation in head-injured patients showed a worse outcome in the treatment group, although the numbers were small (Muizelaar *et al.*, 1991). For patients with intracerebral haematomas no controlled trials of hyperventilation have been performed, but the experience with head trauma is not encouraging. Provisionally it seems best to reserve this treatment for bridging a few hours in patients for whom surgical evacuation is planned (see Sections 12.2.5 and 12.2.6).

Osmotic agents

Osmotic agents include mannitol, urea and glycerol, in doses between 0.5 and 2 g/kg; iodide-containing contrast agents for angiography may have the same effect, although used for a different purpose. Osmotic agents extract water from the extracellular into the intravascular compartment of the brain, provided the blood–brain barrier between these two compartments is still intact. Shrinking of the brain therefore occurs especially in oedematous, but otherwise intact regions that surround a lesion with profoundly damaged tissue and the magnitude of the reduction in intracranial pressure parallels the proportion of brain regions with preserved autoregulation (Muizelaar *et al.*, 1984; Bell *et al.*, 1987). The interval between the infusion and the decrease of intracranial pressure is usually less than 1 hour, but the effect of a single dose lasts not more than 4–6 hours because the concentration of the solute becomes equilibrated between the intravascular and extracellular compartments. Potential dangers of this treatment include hypotension, hypokalaemia, renal failure from hyperosmolality, haemolysis and congestive heart failure (Yu *et al.*, 1992; Ropper, 1993).

Small controlled trials of intravenous glycerol have claimed benefit for patients with acute stroke, in general, presumably mostly ischaemic (see Section 11.10) (Bayer *et al.*, 1987). A somewhat larger trial (more than 100 patients in each group) specifically included patients with intracerebral haemorrhage, and showed no benefits (Yu *et al.*, 1992).

Despite the lack of evidence from controlled studies, mannitol (20–25% solution) has become the mainstay of osmotic therapy in many centres. The ideal dose cannot be predicted, but a safe regimen is to give 0.75–1 g/kg initially, then 0.25–0.5 kg every 3–5 hours, depending on clinical findings and osmolality (the aim being 295–305 mosm/L initially; if needed, 310–320 mosm/L) (Ropper, 1993). With such regimens at least the central venous pressure should be monitored.

Corticosteroids

Corticosteroids reduce peritumoural oedema and at first sight it seems rational to expect a similar effect on oedematous brain tissue around an intracerebral haemorrhage. There have been two small trials, the first undertaken in the early 1970s, before the advent of CT (Tellez & Bauer, 1973), and a more recent study in Thailand (Poungvarin *et al.*, 1987). Neither trial showed a difference in case fatality between the treated and control groups. The pooled odds ratio for the effect of steroids within the first 2–3 weeks was 1.0 (95% confidence interval (CI): 0.5–2.1). As in acute ischaemic stroke, there was no clear evidence that steroids reduced case fatality, and the confidence interval included the possibilities that steroids could equally have substantially reduced case fatality or substantially increased it. Only the trial by Poungvarin *et al.* (1987) reported on the proportion of patients making a complete recovery by the 21st day, and although there was a non-significant trend in favour of treatment (odds ratio 0.7, 95% CI: 0.2–2.4), any modest benefits in terms of functional improvement were, in this trial at least, outweighed by the medical complications of steroid treatment. Almost 50% of the steroid-treated group developed some complication (such as infection, diabetes or bleeding) compared with 13% amongst controls; this difference was highly significant. The trial included patients with all levels of consciousness, in a stratified design; it might be argued on the basis of a subgroup analysis that corticosteroids may yet do some good in patients with a Glasgow Coma Scale score of 8 or more, but—quite apart from the pitfalls of data-dependent subgroup analyses in general—an advantage emerged only for the case fatality on day 7, and was lost on subsequent days. Thus, any benefit in terms of neurological function is only likely to be moderate, whereas the adverse effects are clearly substantial.

> *Mannitol is widely used in patients with primary intracerebral haemorrhage and a depressed level of consciousness, to decrease intracranial pressure and alleviate the space-occupying effect of the haematoma, although this custom is not backed up by randomised trials with clinical outcome rather than pressure as the outcome variable. With corticosteroids the benefits have so far not been proved to outweigh the disadvantages.*

12.2.3 Prevention of deep venous thrombosis and pulmonary embolism

Patients suffering from PICH have a substantial risk of deep venous thrombosis (between 30 and 70%, depending on the severity of the stroke and the degree of immobilisation) and a risk of pulmonary embolism which is perhaps 1–5%, or possibly higher (Dickmann *et al.*, 1988). Yet, physicians are intuitively cautious in using antithrombotic drugs in patients with intracerebral haematomas. On the other hand, drug regimens that prevent clotting subsequent to venous stasis do not necessarily increase the risk that a small artery in the brain ruptures a second time. The definitive answer should of course come from clinical trials, not from theoretical considerations.

Subcutaneous heparin

Subcutaneous heparin, usually given as three doses of 5000 U daily, reduces the frequency of deep venous thrombosis by 68%, at least after general, orthopaedic and urologic surgery (see Section 11.3) (Collins *et al.*, 1988). In a small, but so far unique, clinical trial in 46 patients with PICH this regimen was applied 4 days after the haemorrhage in the active treatment group and 10 days after the haemorrhage in the control group (Dickmann *et al.*, 1988). Forty per cent (nine out of 23) of the control group developed some evidence of pulmonary embolism (as detected by perfusion scintigraphy of the lungs) against 22% (five out of 22) in the control group. The number of deaths was far too small to exclude the possibility that routine heparin prophylaxis for such patients could substantially increase the risk of fatal intracerebral rebleeding. In a subsequent non-randomised study, in 68 patients with PICH, treatment was started on day 2, 4 or 10 after the haemorrhage (Boeer *et al.*, 1991). For what it is worth, the rate of pulmonary embolism was significantly less in the group with treatment started on day 2 than in the other two groups, without a concomitant increase in rebleeding. As the group with early treatment was studied after the two control groups, the results may well have been influenced by factors other than the interval until the initiation of treatment.

Aspirin

Aspirin is also effective in preventing deep venous thrombosis (approximately 39% risk reduction) as well as pulmonary embolism in an overview of all trials in the perioperative period and in medical patients at increased risk (see Section 11.4.1) (Antiplatelet Trialists' Collaboration, 1994). Its safety in patients with intracerebral haemorrhage has not been studied, but it is improbable that the risk of rebleeding with aspirin is greater than with subcutaneous heparin.

Compression stockings

These are of course the safest method of prophylaxis in patients with PICH, although occasionally pressure sores may be induced (see Section 15.13). The efficacy of this measure was studied in 12 methodologically sound clinical trials, mostly in patients with moderate risk (abdominal, gynaecological and neurosurgery), the collective evidence pointing towards a risk reduction in deep venous thrombosis of the order of 70% (Wells *et al.*, 1994). The occurrence of pulmonary embolism was not included in the analysis. Thus, unless the disadvantages of heparin are proved to be merely theoretical, application of graduated compression stockings seems to offer the greatest protection and the smallest risk, although the method is fairly labour intensive and the stockings can be uncomfortable after a time.

> *Subcutaneous heparin and the application of graduated compression stockings both decrease the occurrence of deep venous thrombosis in bedridden patients by approximately 70% and aspirin by approximately 39%, as judged from clinical trials in a variety of postoperative conditions. Because the safety of heparin and aspirin is largely unknown in patients with primary intracerebral haemorrhage, compression stockings are the preferred method of prophylaxis, despite being labour intensive.*

12.2.4 Iatrogenic intracerebral haemorrhage

Anticoagulant drugs

Anticoagulant drugs are associated with an increased rate of intracerebral haemorrhages, although it is difficult to estimate the actual risk because the underlying condition for which the treatment was given also contributes to the risk (confounding by indication; see Section 8.4.1). It seems rational to reverse the deficiency of clotting factors as quickly as possible, especially in view of the frequent progression of clinical deficits that occurs in these patients, but the validity of this reasoning has never been put to the test in a clinical trial (Kase *et al.*, 1985). The first step is intravenous injection of 10–20 mg of vitamin K, at not more than 5 mg/minute, followed by infusion of a concentrate of the coagulation factors II, VII, IX and X or fresh frozen plasma. Infusion of the factors alone restores the coagulation system more rapidly than whole plasma, and is safer from the point of view of transmission of virus particles (see Section 11.3.6) (Anonymous, 1990; Fredriksson *et al.*, 1992).

Fibrinolytic drugs

Fibrinolytic drugs used after myocardial infarction are complicated by PICH in only a small proportion (see Section 8.4.3), but the case fatality is high. This grim prognosis warrants attempts at intervention, even without the benefits of controlled clinical trials (Eleff *et al.*, 1990). These measures include control of any hypertension and infusion of cryoprecipitate; the use of antifibrinolytic drugs is controversial even from a theoretical point of view. Life-threatening arrhythmias may occur, often before the onset of the neurological symptoms, and these should be promptly treated (Sloan *et al.*, 1995).

Aspirin

Aspirin treatment is associated with a small risk of PICH (see Section 8.4.2). It is reasonable to stop the drug once the diagnosis is made, although no disasters have been documented in instances in which aspirin treatment was continued, or even instituted (in most trials of aspirin for the secondary prevention of cerebral ischaemia a handful of patients with small intracerebral haemorrhages have been erroneously included, before CT scanning established the true diagnosis).

12.2.5 Surgery for supratentorial haemorrhage

The frequency of surgical intervention for PICH varies from practically nil, even in developed countries, to 20% of all patients in a metropolitan community (Greater Cincinnati) (Broderick *et al.*, 1994). This variation must reflect clinical uncertainty, which itself must be based on the lack of appropriate evidence from randomised controlled trials. There are four possible surgical procedures to treat PICH: simple aspiration, craniotomy with open surgery, endoscopic evacuation and stereotactic aspiration (Kaufman, 1993). Four controlled clinical trials have been performed in this area; these have been subjected to critical review (Prasad, 1993), the results of which we shall include in the following sections.

Simple aspiration

Simple aspiration was attempted mainly in the 1950s but was abandoned because only small amounts of clot could be obtained, and because the procedure could precipitate 'blind' rebleeding (McKissock *et al.*, 1959; Mitsuno *et al.*, 1966).

Open surgery

Open surgery has been the method for removing haematomas in three trials (McKissock *et al.*, 1961; Juvela *et al.*, 1989; Batjer *et al.*, 1990). The combined results of the three studies (Fig. 12.1) show that craniotomy is definitely harmful, because it increases the proportion of patients who are dead or dependent by 13% (95% CI: 3–23%) (Prasad, 1993). The largest trial was reported in 1961, so it is conceivable that the results would have been better with current neuroradiological and microsurgical techniques, but this remains to be proved.

Endoscopic evacuation

Endoscopic evacuation by stereotactic methods was studied in a randomised controlled trial involving two groups of 50 patients (Auer *et al.*, 1989). The interpretation of the authors was that surgery had no effect in putaminal and thalamic haemorrhage, but that it was beneficial in subcortical haematomas, provided the patients are aged 60 years or less and are alert or somnolent. The problem with this analysis is not only that it concerns subgroups, but also that no overall analysis was reported and that some outcome categories were not reported at all. Recalculation of the results for all patients according to the proportion who were dead or dependent showed that surgery reduced this proportion by 18%, which just missed being statistically significant (95% CI: 0–36%). The effect appears stronger in patients under 60 years and with haematoma volumes exceeding 50 ml.

Contrary to the authors' own conclusion, the effect of the intervention was uniform across subgroups of patients with haematomas at various sites, and possibly with different levels of consciousness (Prasad, 1993). Stereotactic endoscopic evacuation is a promising technique, but its benefits and specific indications remain to be confirmed by further well-conducted and large clinical trials.

Stereotactic aspiration

Stereotactic aspiration without endoscopy, usually combined with instillation of fibrinolytic agents, has been reported in more than 400 patients with supratentorial haemorrhage, either intraparenchymal (Matsumoto & Hondo, 1984; Niizuma *et al.*, 1989; Mohadjer *et al.*, 1992; Miller *et al.*, 1993) or intraventricular (Rohde *et al.*, 1995). The time has now come for controlled trials of this technique before it is adopted into routine clinical practice.

12.2.6 Surgery for infratentorial haemorrhage

Cerebellar haematomas

Cerebellar haematomas have fairly characteristic clinical features (see Section 8.8.2), with the exception of massive haemorrhages, which are clinically indistinguishable from brainstem strokes (Gerritsen van der Hoop *et al.*, 1988; Ogata *et al.*, 1988), and very small haemorrhages, which may simulate a peripheral disorder of the vestibular system (Dunne *et al.*, 1987; Gerritsen van der Hoop *et al.*, 1988).

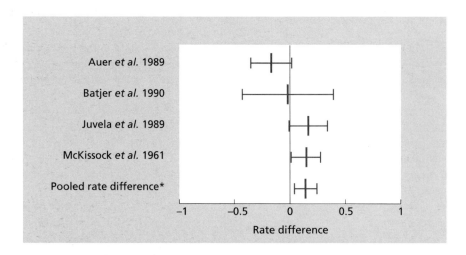

Figure 12.1 The results of a systematic review of four randomised trials which examined the effect of surgery for supratentorial haematoma. Auer *et al.* (1989) evaluated stereotactic surgery so their results were not included in the pooled analysis. The vertical lines show the difference in the proportion of patients who were dead or dependent at final follow-up. The horizontal error bars indicate the 95% confidence intervals. A rate difference of greater than 1 indicates that more patients were dead or disabled in the surgically treated group. *Excluding Auer *et al.* (1989). (From Prasad, 1993; reproduced with the author's permission.)

For decades there has been a strong impression that surgical evacuation saves lives in patients with cerebellar haematomas who have clinical evidence of progressive compression of the brainstem (Fisher *et al.*, 1965). So strong is this impression that a clinical trial in this category of patients is as unlikely to be mounted as it would be in acute appendicitis. This is not to say there are no areas of controversy. First, there is no doubt that some patients can be managed conservatively, but there is uncertainty about the selection criteria (Ott *et al.*, 1974). In general, an impaired level of consciousness seems a good indication for surgery, provided the brainstem reflexes have not been lost for hours, in which case the outcome is invariably fatal (Gerritsen van der Hoop *et al.*, 1988). Some neurosurgeons advocate surgery with large haematomas (>3 cm in diameter), even in alert patients, based on the experience that delayed deterioration of consciousness may be so rapid that the patient cannot be salvaged at this later stage (Brillman, 1979; Lui *et al.*, 1985). On the other hand, patients with cerebellar haematomas larger than 3 cm in size may retain a nearly normal level of consciousness (drowsy, disorientated or both) and subsequently survive without operation (Bogousslavsky *et al.*, 1984; Gerritsen van der Hoop *et al.*, 1988). Second, some neurosurgeons argue that the main problem is not direct compression of the brainstem but obstructive hydrocephalus, and that ventriculostomy is a sufficient measure to prevent a fatal outcome (Shenkin & Zavala, 1982). Such an approach may be justified in some patients, with progressive obtundation and hydrocephalus without clinical signs of brainstem compression, but against generalisation of this point of view is the rapid disappearance of pupillary, corneal and oculocephalic reflexes in other patients, something not seen with acute hydrocephalus from different causes (van Gijn *et al.*, 1985), and also the failure of ventricular shunting to prevent death, despite initial improvement (Gerritsen van der Hoop *et al.*, 1988).

> *Surgical evacuation of cerebellar haematomas can be life saving, often with surprisingly few neurological sequelae. Sound indications for evacuation are the combination of a depressed level of consciousness with signs of progressive brainstem compression (unless all brainstem reflexes have been lost for more than a few hours, in which case a fatal outcome is unavoidable), or haematoma greater than 3 cm. If the patient has a depressed level of consciousness and hydrocephalus, without signs of brainstem compression and with a haematoma less than 3 cm, ventriculostomy can be carried out as an initial (and perhaps only) procedure.*

As with supratentorial haemorrhage, some patients with cerebellar haemorrhage have been successfully treated by

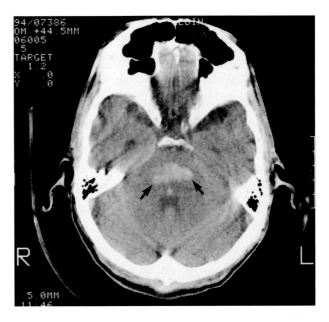

Figure 12.2 CT brain scan showing a pontine haematoma (arrows) in a patient who walked, unsteadily, into (and out of) the outpatient clinic.

stereotactic aspiration, with or without instillation of fibrinolytic drugs (Niizuma & Suzuki, 1987). Any advantage of these techniques over the conventional approach with suboccipital craniotomy remains to be proved.

Pontine haemorrhages

Pontine haemorrhages are not as invariably fatal as when the diagnosis could only be made at postmortem (Fig. 12.2), but the case fatality is still about 60% (see Section 8.8.2) (Kushner & Bressman, 1985; Masiyama *et al.*, 1985). The management of these patients is usually conservative, but some case reports have documented successful stereotactic aspiration (Beatty & Zervas, 1973; Bosch & Beute, 1985; Niizuma & Suzuki, 1987). The natural history may or may not have been influenced by these interventions, and surgical failures in similar cases may have received less publicity.

References

Anonymous (1990). Guidelines on oral anticoagulation: second edition. British Society for Haematology. British Committee for Standards in Haematology. Haemostasis and Thrombosis Task Force. *J Clin Pathol* 43: 177–83.

Antiplatelet Trialists' Collaboration (1994). Collaborative overview of randomised trials of antiplatelet therapy—III:

reduction in venous thrombosis and pulmonary embolism by antiplatelet prophylaxis among surgical and medical patients. *Br Med J* 308: 235–46.

Auer LM, Deinsberger W, Niederkorn K *et al.* (1989). Endoscopic surgery versus medical treatment for spontaneous intracerebral hematoma: a randomized study. *J Neurosurg* 70: 530–5.

Batjer HH, Reisch JS, Allen BC, Plaizier LJ, Su CJ (1990). Failure of surgery to improve outcome in hypertensive putaminal hemorrhage. A prospective randomized trial. *Arch Neurol* 47: 1103–6.

Bayer AJ, Pathy MS, Newcombe R (1987). Double-blind randomised trial of intravenous glycerol in acute stroke. *Lancet* i: 405–8.

Beatty RM, Zervas NT (1973). Stereotactic aspiration of a brain stem hematoma. *Neurosurgery* 13: 204–7.

Bell BA, Smith MA, Kean DM *et al.* (1987). Brain water measured by magnetic resonance imaging. Correlation with direct estimation and changes after mannitol and dexamethasone. *Lancet* i: 66–9.

Boeer A, Voth E, Henze T, Prange HW (1991). Early heparin therapy in patients with spontaneous intracerebral haemorrhage. *J Neurol Neurosurg Psychiatr* 54: 466–7.

Bogousslavsky J, Regli F, Jeanrenaud X (1984). Benign outcome in unoperated large cerebellar haemorrhage. Report of 2 cases. *Acta Neurochir Wien* 73: 59–65.

Bosch DA, Beute GN (1985). Successful stereotaxic evacuation of an acute pontomedullary hematoma. Case report. *J Neurosurg* 62: 153–6.

Brillman J (1979). Acute hydrocephalus and death one month after non-surgical treatment for acute cerebellar hemorrhage—case report. *J Neurosurg* 50: 374–6.

Broderick J, Brott T, Tomsick T, Tew J, Duldner J, Huster G (1994). Management of intracerebral hemorrhage in a large metropolitan population. *Neurosurgery* 34: 882–7.

Collins R, Scrimgeour A, Yusuf S, Peto R (1988). Reduction in fatal pulmonary embolism and venous thrombosis by perioperative administration of subcutaneous heparin. Overview of results of randomized trials in general, orthopedic, and urologic surgery. *N Engl J Med* 318: 1162–73.

Darby JM, Yonas H, Marion DW, Latchaw RE (1988). Local 'inverse steal' induced by hyperventilation in head injury. *Neurosurgery* 23: 84–8.

Dickmann U, Voth E, Schicha H, Henze T, Prange H, Emrich D (1988). Heparin therapy, deep-vein thrombosis and pulmonary embolism after intracerebral hemorrhage. *Klin Wochenschr* 66: 1182–3.

Dunne JW, Chakera T, Kermode S (1987). Cerebellar haemorrhage —diagnosis and treatment: a study of 75 consecutive cases. *Quatern J Med* 64: 739–54.

Eleff SM, Borel C, Bell WR, Long DM (1990). Acute management of intracranial hemorrhage in patients receiving thrombolytic therapy: case reports. *Neurosurgery* 26: 867–9.

Fisher CM, Picard EH, Polak A, Dalal P, Ojemann R (1965). Acute hypertensive cerebellar haemorrhage. *J Nerv Ment Dis* 140: 38–57.

Fogelholm R, Nuutila M, Vuorela AL (1992). Primary intracerebral haemorrhage in the Jyvaskyla region, central Finland, 1985–89: incidence, case fatality rate, and functional outcome. *J Neurol Neurosurg Psychiatr* 55: 546–52.

Franke CL, de Jonge J, van Swieten JC, Op de Coul AAW, Van Gijn J (1990). Intracerebral hematomas during anticoagulant treatment. *Stroke* 21: 726–30.

Fredriksson K, Norrving B, Stromblad LG (1992). Emergency reversal of anticoagulation after intracerebral hemorrhage. *Stroke* 23: 972–7.

Gerritsen van der Hoop R, Vermeulen M, Van Gijn J (1988). Cerebellar hemorrhage: diagnosis and treatment. *Surg Neurol* 29: 6–10.

Juvela S, Heiskanen O, Poranen A *et al.* (1989). The treatment of spontaneous intracerebral hemorrhage. A prospective randomized trial of surgical and conservative treatment. *J Neurosurg* 70: 755–8.

Kase CS, Robinson RK, Stein RW *et al.* (1985). Anticoagulant-related intracerebral hemorrhage. *Neurology* 35: 943–8.

Kaufman HH (1993). Treatment of deep spontaneous intracerebral hematomas. A review. *Stroke* 24: 1101–6.

Kushner MJ, Bressman SB (1985). The clinical manifestations of pontine hemorrhage. *Neurology* 35: 637–43.

Lisk DR, Pasteur W, Rhoades H, Putnam RD, Grotta JC (1994). Early presentation of hemispheric intracerebral hemorrhage: prediction of outcome and guidelines for treatment allocation. *Neurology* 44: 133–9.

Lui TN, Fairholm DJ, Shu TF, Chang CN, Lee ST, Chen HR (1985). Surgical treatment of spontaneous cerebellar hemorrhage. *Surg Neurol* 23: 555–8.

McKissock W, Richardson A, Walsh L (1959). Primary intracerebral haematoma: results of surgical treatment in 244 consecutive cases. *Lancet* ii: 683–6.

McKissock W, Richardson A, Taylor J (1961). Primary intracerebral haemorrhage: a controlled trial of surgical and conservative treatment in 180 unselected cases. *Lancet* ii: 221–6.

Masiyama S, Niizuma H, Suzuki J (1985). Pontine haemorrhage: a clinical analysis of 26 cases. *J Neurol Neurosurg Psychiatr* 48: 658–62.

Matsumoto K, Hondo H (1984). CT-guided stereotaxic evacuation of hypertensive intracerebral hematomas. *J Neurosurg* 61: 440–8.

Mendelow AD (1993). Mechanisms of ischemic brain damage with intracerebral hemorrhage. *Stroke* 24 (Suppl. I): 115–17.

Miller DW, Barnett GH, Kormos DW, Steiner CP (1993). Stereotactically guided thrombolysis of deep cerebral hemorrhage: preliminary results. *Cleve Clin J Med* 60: 321–4.

Mitsuno T, Kanaya H, Shirakata S, Ohsawa K, Ishikawa Y (1966). Surgical treatment of hypertensive intracerebral hemorrhage. *J Neurosurg* 24: 70–6.

Mohadjer M, Braus DF, Myers A, Scheremet R, Krauss JK (1992). CT-stereotactic fibrinolysis of spontaneous intracerebral hematomas. *Neurosurg Rev* 15: 105–10.

Muizelaar JP, Lutz HA 3rd, Becker DP (1984). Effect of mannitol on ICP and CBF and correlation with pressure autoregulation in severely head-injured patients. *J Neurosurg* 61: 700–6.

Muizelaar JP, Marmarou A, Ward JD *et al.* (1991). Adverse effects of prolonged hyperventilation in patients with severe head injury: a randomized clinical trial. *J Neurosurg* 75: 731–9.

Niizuma H, Suzuki J (1987). Computed tomography-guided stereotactic aspiration of posterior fossa hematomas: a supine lateral retromastoid approach. *Neurosurgery* 21: 422–7.

Niizuma H, Shimizu Y, Yonemitsu T, Nakasato N, Suzuki J (1989). Results of stereotactic aspiration in 175 cases of putaminal hemorrhage. *Neurosurgery* 24: 814–19.

Ogata J, Imakita M, Yutani C, Miyamoto S, Kikuchi H (1988). Primary brainstem death: a clinico-pathological study. *J Neurol Neurosurg Psychiatr* 51: 646–50.

Ott KH, Kase CS, Ojemann RG, Mohr JP (1974). Cerebellar hemorrhage: diagnosis and treatment. A review of 56 cases. *Arch Neurol* 31: 160–7.

Poungvarin N, Bhoopat W, Viriyavejakul A *et al.* (1987). Effects of dexamethasone in primary supratentorial intracerebral hemorrhage. *N Engl J Med* 316: 1229–33.

Prasad K (1993). *A randomised controlled trial of stereotactic aspiration surgery in primary supratentorial intracerebral haemorrhage.* MSc thesis, McMaster University, 1–148.

Rohde V, Schaller C, Hassler WE (1995). Intraventricular recombinant tissue plasminogen activator for lysis of intraventricular haemorrhage. *J Neurol Neurosurg Psychiatr* 58: 447–51.

Ropper AH (1986). Lateral displacement of the brain and level of consciousness in patients with an acute hemispheral mass. *N Engl J Med* 314: 953–8.

Ropper AH (1993). Treatment of intracranial hypertension. In: Ropper AH, ed. *Neurological and Neurosurgical Intensive Care*, 3rd edn. New York: Raven Press, 29–52.

Ropper AH, King RB (1984). Intracranial pressure monitoring in

comatose patients with cerebral hemorrhage. *Arch Neurol* 41: 725–8.

Shenkin HA, Zavala H (1982). Cerebellar strokes: mortality, surgical indications, and results of ventricular drainage. *Lancet* ii: 429–31.

Sloan MA, Price TR, Petito CK *et al.* (1995). Clinical features and pathogenesis of intracerebral hemorrhage after rt-PA and heparin therapy for acute myocardial infarction: the Thrombolysis in Myocardial Infarction (TIMI) II pilot and randomized clinical trial combined experience. *Neurology* 45: 649–58.

Tellez H, Bauer RB (1973). Dexamethasone as treatment in cerebrovascular disease. 1. A controlled study in intracerebral hemorrhage. *Stroke* 4: 541–6.

Tuhrim S, Horowitz DR, Sacher M, Godbold JH (1995). Validation and comparison of models predicting survival following intracerebral hemorrhage. *Crit Care Med* 23: 950–4.

Van Gijn J, Hijdra A, Wijdicks EFM, Vermeulen M, van Crevel H (1985). Acute hydrocephalus after aneurysmal subarachnoid hemorrhage. *J Neurosurg* 63: 355–62.

Waga S, Shimosaka S, Sakakura M (1983). Intracerebral hemorrhage remote from the site of the initial neurosurgical procedure. *Neurosurgery* 13: 662–5.

Wells PS, Lensing AWA, Hirsh J (1994). Graduated compression stockings in the prevention of postoperative venous thromboembolism. A meta-analysis. *Arch Intern Med* 154: 67–72.

Young WB, Lee KP, Pessin MS, Kwan ES, Rand WM, Caplan LR (1990). Prognostic significance of ventricular blood in supratentorial hemorrhage: a volumetric study. *Neurology* 40: 616–19.

Yu YL, Kumana CR, Lauder IJ *et al.* (1992). Treatment of acute cerebral hemorrhage with intravenous glycerol. A double-blind, placebo-controlled, randomized trial. *Stroke* 23: 967–71.

Specific treatment of aneurysmal subarachnoid haemorrhage

13

13.1   General principles

This chapter deals only with the treatment of patients with aneurysms. The management of non-aneurysmal causes of subarachnoid haemorrhage (SAH) depends on the underlying condition (see Section 9.1). The most common non-aneurysmal form of SAH is idiopathic perimesencephalic haemorrhage, probably from a venous source (see Section

438

9.1.2); these patients can be mobilised as their headache wears off and can look forward to a long and happy life, at least as far as the blood vessels of their brain are concerned. There are numerous other causes, all extremely rare, and the management is equally diverse (Rinkel *et al.*, 1993). An example is endovascular balloon occlusion of the extracranial part of the vertebral artery after dissection of this artery with SAH (Tsukahara *et al.*, 1995).

The essence of managing patients with aneurysmal SAH is deceptively simple: make the diagnosis, locate the aneurysm and put a clip on it. Yet, 50% of the patients still die, at least in secondary referral centres, and 50% of the survivors remain severely disabled (Hijdra *et al.*, 1987a). The reason is that the course of the disease is beset by complications, of which the most important are rebleeding, delayed cerebral ischaemia, hydrocephalus and a variety of systemic disorders. Distinguishing the different causes of secondary deterioration has many pitfalls (van Crevel, 1980). Precise observations and definitions are therefore necessary for the management of individual patients, as well as for the exchange of scientific information.

The precision of these definitions was the subject of a survey of 184 articles about SAH published in nine neurosurgical or neurological journals in the period 1985–1992, and the results were disappointing (van Gijn *et al.*, 1994). The specific outcome events, i.e. rebleeding, ischaemia and hydrocephalus, were sufficiently defined in only 31%, incompletely in 22% and not at all in 47%. The proportion of acceptable definitions was similar when the articles were analysed according to the type of complication or to the year of publication. The four exclusively neurosurgical journals provided adequate definitions for any of the three outcome events in only 20% (of 209 instances), whereas the five mainly neurological journals published fewer articles on the subject (74 instances of outcome events), but more often with precise criteria (65%). Different research groups may not always agree on the precise formulation of criteria for the complications of SAH, but the least one can ask from authors is an attempt at some kind of definition. The criteria we propose for distinguishing the different complications after SAH will be discussed in the sections about the management of each complication, but it should be emphasised at the outset the vital role of repeat computerised tomography (CT).

> *Articles reporting the frequency of specific complications of subarachnoid haemorrhage are only worth reading if an adequate definition of those complications is given.*

Surgical repair of the ruptured aneurysm is the main aim of treatment in most (although not all) patients with this condition, but the contribution of the neurologist in the non-surgical management can be considerable.

1 The neurologist is trained in assessing subtle changes in the neurological condition, and — not being tied up in the operating theatre — can be quickly on the spot to investigate any changes that the nursing staff have detected during the continuous observation that is so vital in these patients.

2 Important systemic complications may occur after aneurysmal haemorrhage, and the neurologist is in an ideal position to investigate these and, if necessary, to liaise quickly with general physicians, anaesthetists and other specialists.

It is only in close collaboration with neurosurgeons and radiologists, however, that the neurologist can adequately fulfil this role. Ideally, the investigation and treatment of patients with aneurysmal SAH should be planned on at least a day-to-day mutual consultation amongst these disciplines, with adaptation to any changes in the neurological condition that occurs. At any rate, patients should not be cared for in general medical or neurological wards that have no immediate access to neurosurgical expertise and modern neuroradiological facilities. The threshold for admission to an intensive care unit should be low, as close observation can not be guaranteed on general wards. The need for expert referral applies even to patients 'in a poor grade': these may be the very patients that need urgent intervention because of, for example, a haematoma, hydrocephalus or hypovolaemia (Wijdicks, 1995). In this chapter we shall first discuss general outcome and then follow the clinical course of a patient with SAH, especially the prevention and management of the possible complications.

13.2 Prognosis

Meaningful interpretation of patient outcome in any reported series requires an accurate description of the state of the patient on admission, the most relevant features of which will be discussed below, and on the length of time the patient has already survived the bleed (Alvord *et al.*, 1972). The state of the patient will, in turn, depend heavily on the selection criteria for admission (Maurice-Williams & Marsh, 1985). The average outcome will be much poorer in centres admitting patients regardless of their clinical condition than in, for example, a neurosurgical centre, where the policy is to operate on all patients within the first 3 days, with the result that moribund patients will usually be referred elsewhere, often as much by preselection on the part of the referring physicians as by discouragement from the centre in question (see Fig. 9.1). For the same reason, reports dealing with only operated patients are meaningless, almost by definition.

Even comprehensive series reflecting the overall management of patients with SAH can not serve as a basis for comparison, unless one can be reasonably certain that the entire community has been included (Phillips *et al.*, 1980).

13.2.1 Methods of outcome assessment

Most studies attempt not only to tabulate case fatality but also to define morbidity. Before the 1980s, surviving patients were usually categorised into 'good', 'fair' or 'poor', but with widely varying definitions of each. Fortunately, the Glasgow Outcome Scale (Table 13.1) is now widely used (van Gijn *et al.*, 1994). This scale was originally proposed for assessing patients with head injury, but its general terminology allows its use as a measure of outcome for any brain disease (Jennett & Bond, 1975). The World Federation of Neurological Surgeons has recommended its future use in patients with SAH (Drake *et al.*, 1988). It is a simple hybrid of a disability and handicap scale, very similar to the Rankin or Oxford Handicap Scale that is often used in assessing outcome after ischaemic stroke (see Section 17.6.3). As with the Rankin Scale, there is little variation between observers who use the Glasgow Outcome Scale (Maas *et al.*, 1983). The main difference between the two scales is that the Glasgow Outcome Scale does not allow a distinction within the stratum of patients who are independent with some impairment, i.e. between those who do or do not need some help every day; whether this is a disadvantage in terms of sensitivity in comparisons between groups has not been investigated.

> *At the very least, any study of the outcome after subarachnoid haemorrhage should report the case fatality at about 1 month and the morbidity at about 6 months using the Glasgow Outcome Scale or the Rankin Scale.*

Table 13.1 The Glasgow Outcome Scale. (From Jennett & Bond, 1975.)

Grade	Description	Definition
1	Good recovery	Patient can lead an independent life, with or without minimal neurological deficit
2	Moderately disabled	Patient has neurological or intellectual impairment but is independent
3	Severely disabled	Patient conscious but totally dependent on others to get through daily activities
4	Vegetative survival	
5	Dead	

13.2.2 Natural history

Only studies up to the mid-1960s can illustrate the results of conservative treatment alone, although it should be kept in mind that at that time not only the methods of treatment but also the methods of diagnosis differed from current practice, and that these series necessarily included varieties of non-aneurysmal haemorrhage that CT scanning would now exclude. With this qualification, Pakarinen's population-based study from Finland can be regarded as the standard of management results before the era of aneurysm surgery; the total case fatality was 62%, most of which occurred in the first 6 weeks (Pakarinen, 1967).

Death outside hospital occurs in 8–17% of all patients (Crawford & Sarner, 1965; Phillips *et al.*, 1980; Ljunggren *et al.*, 1985; Inagawa *et al.*, 1995; Schievink *et al.*, 1995a). This proportion is unlikely to have changed over the years, and it may be nearly impossible to change it ever. Of those patients who do reach hospital alive, a further 10–12% die within 24 hours of the first bleed (Locksley, 1966; Hijdra & van Gijn 1982; Broderick *et al.*, 1994). In the most recent of these two series, serial CT scanning identified rebleeding in 50% (16 of 31) of the patients who died within the first day, a proportion perhaps still underestimated because deterioration may well occur before the first CT scan is done (see Section 13.5.1).

Keeping in mind that some 25% of all patients die within 24 hours of the onset of symptoms, outside or just inside hospital, and that these deaths are almost unavoidable, it is the subsequent case fatality and morbidity that is the realistic target for our medical and surgical interventions. In a large hospital series (not a population series) reported in the 1980s, another 35% of those surviving the first day died within the subsequent 3 months, approximately equal parts being contributed by a poor condition from the initial haemorrhage, rebleeding and delayed cerebral ischaemia (Hijdra *et al.*, 1987a). If comparisons between series were in order—which they are not—we might be tempted to comment that not much seems to have been achieved in 20 years, since Pakarinen's time. Since then, however, a number of definite or highly probable advances have been made: the operating microscope, liberal administration of fluids, avoidance of antihypertensive drugs, and nimodipine for prevention of delayed cerebral ischaemia. But, given the overpowering influence of the effects of early haemorrhage (or haemorrhages) on the overall death rate, the only potential benefits of intervention relate to the 24% of all deaths that are caused by late rebleeding and delayed cerebral ischaemia (hydrocephalus rarely causes death by itself). So, whatever the future developments in the management of patients with

SAH, the effect on *overall* death rate is likely to remain modest.

For patients who survive SAH and do not have their ruptured aneurysm clipped, the risk of rebleeding is a substantial 3%/year (Jane *et al.*, 1985) (see Section 13.5.1).

13.2.3 Factors related to outcome

Outcome after SAH depends on a variety of factors, many of which are inter-related. A multivariate analysis by means of proportional hazards regression has been performed on two different series of patients: the multicentre American Cooperative Study, based on 3521 patients (Kassell *et al.*, 1990a), and the 479 patients from the Dutch–Scottish trial of tranexamic acid (TEA) (D.W.J. Dippel, unpublished observations). The most important determinants were selected from the data sets of both studies (Table 13.2): first, the level of consciousness on admission (four categories in the American study, not strictly defined, and in the European study according to the Glasgow Coma Scale); and second, the amount of subarachnoid blood (maximal thickness of the clot in the American study (Fisher *et al.*, 1980) versus a sum score for each of 10 cisterns in the European series (Hijdra *et al.*, 1990)). Of course, the amount of blood may merely reflect the damage that occurred at the time of the haemorrhage, as is the case for the level of consciousness, and the prognostic importance of this factor by no means implies that removal of subarachnoid blood will improve outcome. Not surprisingly, age was an adverse factor in both studies; in another study dedicated to the age factor, the excess case fatality in patients over 65 years resulted mostly from intracranial complications, whereas the proportion of medical complications was not markedly different (Muizelaar *et al.*, 1988).

Table 13.2 Factors with independent prognostic value for poor outcome after SAH.

Prognostic factor	Kassell *et al.* (1990a)	D.W.J. Dippel (unpublished observations)
Decreased level of consciousness on admission*	+++	+++
Loss of consciousness at onset	−	+
Increasing age	++	+
Large amount of blood on CT scan*	++	++
High blood pressure on admission	+	−
Pre-existing medical condition	+	−
Aneurysm in posterior circulation*	+	−

* For definitions and further discussion, see text.

−, +, ++, +++, prognostic value, in increasing order.

The site of the aneurysm emerged as a predictive factor only in the larger, American data set. In univariate analysis case fatality was lowest for internal carotid and middle cerebral artery aneurysms, and highest for anterior cerebral and vertebrobasilar aneurysms, but in the multivariate analysis only aneurysms of the posterior circulation were independently (and unfavourably) associated with outcome. This was confirmed in a smaller series from the Mayo Clinic (Schievink *et al.*, 1995b).

> *The main adverse factors for outcome after subarachnoid haemorrhage are level of consciousness, amount of blood in the subarachnoid space, increasing age and an aneurysm in the posterior rather than the anterior circulation.*

13.3 Indications for immediate operation

13.3.1 Intracerebral haematomas

Intraparenchymal haematomas occur in 30% of patients with ruptured aneurysms (van Gijn & van Dongen, 1982). Not surprisingly, the average outcome is worse than in patients with purely subarachnoid blood (Hauerberg *et al.*, 1994). When large haematomas are associated with gradual deterioration in the level of consciousness in the first 2 days (Fig. 13.1), immediate evacuation of the haematoma should be considered seriously, even without preceding angiography. The impression is that operation is not only life saving in patients with impending transtentorial herniation, particularly with temporal haematomas, but may even result in independent survival (Brandt *et al.*, 1987). Fortunately, this impression has been backed up by a randomised study, although a small one, in which 11 of 15 patients in the operated group survived, against three of 15 in the conservatively treated group (Heiskanen *et al.*, 1988).

> *If patients with large haematomas, likely to be caused by a ruptured aneurysm, become increasingly drowsy in the first few hours after subarachnoid haemorrhage, they are candidates for immediate surgical evacuation of the haematoma, even without preceding angiography.*

13.3.2 Symptomatic hydrocephalus

Gradual obtundation within 24 hours of haemorrhage, sometimes accompanied by slow pupillary responses to light and downward deviation of the eyes, is fairly characteristic for acute hydrocephalus (van Gijn *et al.*, 1985). If the diagnosis is confirmed by CT this can be a reason for early

441

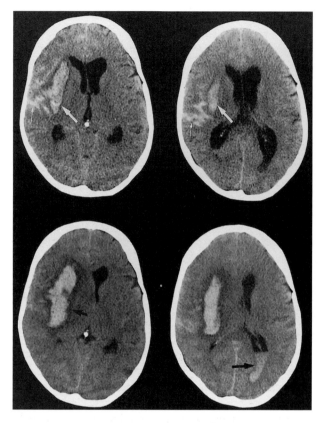

Figure 13.1 'Enlarging haematoma'. Top: CT scan on day of SAH from a ruptured aneurysm of the right middle cerebral artery, in a 51-year-old man on anticoagulant treatment because of myocardial infarction with mitral valve insufficiency. Haematoma in the right Sylvian fissure (thin arrow) and in the subinsular cortex (thick arrow); at the time of the scan anticoagulation had already been reversed by infusion of a concentrate of coagulation factors. Bottom: CT scan 5 days after the haemorrhage, showing a marked increase of the space-occupying effect, with compression of the right lateral ventricle and the third ventricle. The increased mass effect results not only from a newly formed rim of oedema around the haematoma (short arrow), but also from an increase in size of the haematoma itself. There had been no new neurological signs or other clinical features indicating rebleeding. The newly formed collection of blood in the posterior horn of the left lateral ventricle (long arrow) is often seen in the absence of rebleeding (sedimentation effect).

ventricular drainage, although some patients do improve spontaneously in the first 24 hours; the management priorities of acute hydrocephalus are discussed more fully below in the section on secondary deterioration (see Section 13.9).

13.3.3 Early death without possibilities for surgical intervention

Not all patients who arrive moribund can be salvaged. In one consecutive series of 31 patients who died on the first day, 17 showed dysfunction of the brainstem, associated with massive intraventricular haemorrhage on CT, including distension of the fourth ventricle with blood (in nine cases, together with an intracerebral haematoma). In six patients neither a supratentorial haematoma nor intraventricular haemorrhage could explain the progressive dysfunction of the brainstem and the fatal outcome, the CT scan showing no abnormality other than subarachnoid blood (Hijdra & van Gijn, 1982). The most likely explanation is a prolonged period of global cerebral ischaemia at the time of haemorrhage, as a result of the pressure in the cerebrospinal fluid spaces being elevated to the level of that in the arteries, for as long as a few minutes. Such a potentially lethal arrest of the circulation to the brain is indeed suggested by autopsy evidence, and by the recording of intracranial pressure or transcranial Doppler sonography at the time of recurrent aneurysmal haemorrhage (Smith, 1963; Grote & Hassler, 1988).

Ventricular fibrillation may occur but is probably a relatively rare cause of sudden death in patients with ruptured aneurysm (see Section 13.10.2). The only prospective study of this problem concerned 43 consecutive episodes of cardiorespiratory complications in patients with aneurysmal haemorrhage (first or recurrent, but mostly the latter). Thirty-seven episodes consisted of primary respiratory arrest; in one case followed within minutes by ventricular fibrillation. Only two patients had ventricular fibrillation at onset, and in four patients the course of events was uncertain because they died suddenly, without vital signs having been recorded (Hijdra *et al.*, 1984).

13.4 General care

13.4.1 Blood pressure

Management of hypertension (blood pressure above about 200/110 mmHg) is a difficult issue in patients with SAH. Following intracranial haemorrhage, the upper and lower limits of the autoregulation of cerebral blood flow become closer, which makes the perfusion of brain more dependent on arterial blood pressure (Kaneko *et al.*, 1983). Consequently, there is a very real risk of ischaemia in areas with loss of autoregulation when surges of blood pressure are aggressively treated. Many neurologists and physicians therefore advise against treating hypertension following aneurysmal rupture (Calhoun & Oparil, 1990). The empirical evidence from clinical trials is sparse, but does not support the use of antihypertensive drugs. In the American Cooperative Study (1963–70) (Torner *et al.*, 1981b), 1005 patients with ruptured aneurysms were randomised between four treatment modalities, two of which were drug-induced lowering of the blood pressure and bed rest alone (the other two were carotid ligation and intracranial surgery). In the unbiased intention-to-treat analysis, blood pressure reduction failed to reduce either mortality or the rate of rebleeding within the first 6 months after the initial event; on-treatment analysis suggested that induced hypotension decreased the rate of rebleeding in comparison with bed rest, but not the case fatality rate (Torner et al., 1981b). It should be kept in mind that the diagnosis of rebleeding had to be made in the pre-CT era and was therefore probably inaccurate (see Section 13.7.1). The same caveat applies to the finding from the same study that the rate of rebleeding was not dependent on the degree of blood pressure reduction (Nibbelink et al., 1981). A retrospective review of a series of patients, documented by means of serial CT scanning, in whom hypertension had been treated, showed less frequent rebleeding but a higher rate of cerebral infarction than in untreated patients, despite the blood pressures being, on average, still higher than in the controls (Wijdicks et al., 1990). This suggests that hypertension after SAH is a compensatory reaction, at least to some extent, and one that should not be interfered with. In keeping with this a further study from the same centre suggested that the combined regimen of avoiding antihypertensive medication and increasing fluid intake may decrease the risk of cerebral infarction (Hasan et al., 1989c).

It seems best only to use antihypertensive therapy in patients with extreme elevations of blood pressure as well as evidence of rapidly progressive end organ deterioration, diagnosed from either clinical signs (e.g. new retinopathy, heart failure, etc.) or laboratory evidence (e.g. signs of left ventricular failure on chest X-ray, proteinuria or oliguria with a rapid rise of creatinine levels). Effective treatments are diazoxide (50–150 mg by intravenous bolus, repeated after 5–10 minutes, or 15–30 mg/minute by intravenous infusion, up to 600 mg) or labetalol hydrochloride (20–80 mg by intravenous bolus every 10 minutes, or 2 mg/minute by intravenous infusion, up to 300 mg) (Calhoun & Oparil, 1990; Gifford, 1991). Labetalol, however, may be ineffective in patients previously treated with beta-blockers and is contraindicated in heart failure and asthma. Nitroprusside (intravenously) has also been advocated in hypertensive crises, but is probably not a first-line drug in this situation because animal studies have shown that it increases intracranial pressure (Candia et al., 1978). It is reasonable to aim at a 25% decrease in mean arterial pressure below the initial baseline. For monitoring the blood pressure an arterial line is almost mandatory. In practice, however, there is rarely any need for antihypertensive therapy. In many patients surges of high blood pressure can be attenuated by adequate pain management or sedation, for example when the patient is resisting the ventilator.

> *Hypertension in the acute phase of subarachnoid haemorrhage can be left untreated unless there are signs of organ damage. Existing antihypertensive drugs can be continued.*

13.4.2 Fluids and electrolytes

Fluid management in SAH is critical to prevent a reduction in plasma volume, which may contribute to the development of cerebral ischaemia. However, the arguments for an aggressive regimen are indirect. Approximately one-third of the patients decrease their plasma volume by more than 10% within the preoperative period, which is significantly associated with a negative sodium balance; in other words, there is loss of sodium as well as of water (Wijdicks et al., 1985b; Hasan et al., 1990). Moreover, fluid restriction in patients with hyponatraemia is associated with an increased risk of cerebral ischaemia (Wijdicks et al., 1985a); this was done in the past because hyponatraemia was erroneously attributed to water retention (via inappropriate secretion of antidiuretic hormone). Finally, a non-randomised study with historical controls suggested that a daily intake of at least 3 L of saline (against 1.5–2.0 L in the past) was associated with a decrease in total case fatality and risk of cerebral ischaemia, whilst rebleeding and acute hydrocephalus were equally frequent in the two periods (Hasan et al., 1989c). The interpretation of this study is difficult not only because the design was less than optimal, but also because the liberal administration of saline in the second period was confounded by avoidance of antihypertensive drugs. Despite the incomplete evidence, it seems reasonable to prevent hypovolaemia. We favour 2.5–3.5 L/day of normal saline, unless contraindicated by signs of impending cardiac failure (see below). The amount of intravenous saline should be reduced if the patient is also receiving nutritional solution via the enteral route; most commercially prepared enteral solutions deliver 1–2 cal/ml (4–8 J/ml). Nevertheless, it appears that many patients need a daily fluid intake of 4–6 L to balance the production of urine plus estimated insensible losses (via perspiration and expired air). Central venous pressure (directly measured value kept above 8 mmHg) or pulmonary wedge pressures (kept above 7 mmHg) may guide fluid requirements, but daily calculation of fluid balance is the main measure for estimating how much fluid should be given. It is advisable to measure central venous pressure, via a catheter in the subclavian or internal jugular vein, in patients who develop hyponatraemia or a negative fluid balance; pulmonary artery balloon catheters are used in patients with a history of cardiopulmonary disease.

A high fluid intake is essential in patients with aneurysmal subarachnoid haemorrhage, to compensate for 'cerebral salt wasting' and to prevent hypovolaemia, because this predisposes to cerebral ischaemia. The minimum is 2.5–3.5 L of normal saline, or more, to balance the volume of urine, or in case of fever.

Fluid intake should be increased gradually in patients with fever, which is a common result of SAH. In the first few days an infectious origin is unlikely, even more so if the pulse rate is normal (Rousseaux *et al.*, 1980).

13.4.3 Analgesics and general nursing care

During the preoperative period the patient should be kept on complete bed rest, traditionally in dimmed light, on the assumption that any form of excitement increases the risk of rebleeding. Patients with a normal angiogram can usually be allowed to sit up as soon as the headache subsides, but in patients with an aneurysmal pattern of haemorrhage on the CT scan it is rational to keep them under the close supervision of the nursing staff until the repeat angiogram has been done (see Section 9.4.5). Continuous assessment of the level of consciousness is essential, preferably by means of the Glasgow Coma Scale (see Section 4.2.2) (Teasdale & Jennett, 1974), remembering that with inexperienced observers errors of more than one point may occur (Rowley & Fielding, 1991). Any change in consciousness may signify early cerebral ischaemia, rebleeding, enlargement of the ventricles or a systemic medical complication. The nurses should be familiar with the peak times of occurrence of rebleeding and cerebral ischaemia, and they should be able to detect the early signs of delirium, which is seldom caused by SAH per se but more often by the combined effects of isolation, sleep deprivation, narcotic drugs or alcohol withdrawal.

Headache can sometimes be managed with mild analgesics such as paracetamol with or without dextropropoxyphene; salicylates should be avoided until the aneurysm has been clipped because of their inhibitory effect on haemostasis. However, usually the pain is so severe that codeine needs to be added, and this will not mask neurological signs. Sometimes, pain can be alleviated with anxiolytic drugs such as midazolam (5 mg intramuscularly or via an infusion pump). Even a synthetic opiate such as piritramide may be needed to obtain relief. As a last resort, severe headache can be treated with morphine given intravenously in small increments of 1–2 mg; many patients benefit from the euphoriant effect. A potential adverse effect of morphine is hypotension because it is a potent vasodilator. The blood pressure should be checked frequently until the pain has subsided. Constipation is a common disadvantage of morphine

and codeine. Coughing and straining must be rigorously prevented because of the attendant overshoots in arterial blood pressure. Stool softeners should be prescribed routinely. Enemas are contraindicated because they markedly increase intra-abdominal pressure and secondarily intracranial pressure. A bladder catheter is needed in patients who cannot void voluntarily, a proper control of the fluid balance requiring that the volume of urine is precisely measured; condom devices leak or slip off too often to be of any use in these critically ill patients. Intermittent catheterisation may substantially decrease the risk of urinary infections but the procedure is too stressful for patients with SAH.

Headache is a typical and distressing problem in awake patients with subarachnoid haemorrhage. The 'analgesic staircase' consists of frequent doses (every 3–4 hours) of paracetamol 500 mg orally; add codeine 20 mg orally; piritramide 20 mg subcutaneously; morphine 2 mg intravenously, with 1–2-mg increments.

If they are pulling at equipment, confused patients should be restrained by means of girdles and velcro wristbands that can be attached to the side of the bed. Of course, specific causes of confusion should be excluded, such as hypoxia, alcohol withdrawal, infection or a blocked urinary catheter. Self-extubation is a potentially life-threatening event and sedation, restraint or proximity of nursing personnel do not necessarily decrease the risk (Coppolo & May, 1990).

A reliable intravenous route should be maintained for emergency administration of plasma expanders or anticonvulsants. Oral administration of antacids is said to be sufficient to protect against stress bleeding; H_2 receptor antagonists are expensive and should be considered only in mechanically ventilated patients or patients with a previous history of ulcers.

Deep venous thrombosis (DVT) is not as common after SAH as in patients with ischaemic stroke, presumably because the patients are restless rather than immobile and on the whole younger; in a large and prospective series the diagnosis was clinically apparent in only 4% (Vermeulen *et al.*, 1984a). In general, DVT can be prevented by subcutaneous low-dose heparin or heparinoids (see Section 15.13), but the obvious concern is that anticoagulation will not be confined to the venous system and the risk of rebleeding will be increased; no systematic studies have disproved this hypothesis, but many physicians prefer to err on the side of caution and do not give heparin. Graduated compression stockings are of confirmed benefit in preventing DVT in patients undergoing general surgical or orthopaedic procedures (Wells *et al.*, 1994). Because these stockings must be individually fitted to be efficacious, some favour pneumatic devices that apply intermittent venous compression to the legs, but these can be successfully employed only if backed up by a repair service that keeps them running (Clarke Pearson *et al.*, 1984). The devices are well tolerated by patients and can be managed easily by the nursing staff. It has been argued that impedance plethysmography or duplex Doppler sonography should be performed to exclude clinically occult thrombosis before any kind of compression is applied to the calves, but no systematic studies have addressed the question whether the danger of dislodging emboli to the lungs is imaginary or not.

The prophylactic use of antiepileptic medication is controversial. Seizures in the first few weeks after aneurysmal rupture occur in about 10% of the patients and may be easily confused with rebleeding (Rose & Sarner, 1965; Hart *et al.*, 1981; Hasan *et al.*, 1993). The majority occur soon after the initial haemorrhage. Predictive factors for epileptic seizures have not been consistently identified. Intracranial haematomas and intracranial surgery probably increase the risk, but a randomised trial of antiepileptic drugs after supratentorial craniotomy for benign lesions (not only aneurysms) failed to show benefits in terms of seizure rate or case fatality, although the confidence intervals were wide (Foy *et al.*, 1992). Currently, we think that the possible disadvantage of a serious drug reaction outweighs the benefits. If phenytoin is given, absorption by the oral route is severely impaired when patients receive continuous nasogastric tube feedings (Bauer, 1982). Absorption will improve if the continuous feeding is stopped 2 hours before the dose is given, the suspension or crushed tablets are flushed down the nasogastric tube with 60 ml of water and 2 additional hours are allowed to elapse before feeding is resumed, but larger than usual doses will still be required.

Our recommendations for the general management of patients with SAH are summarised in Table 13.3. Before discussing the diagnosis and prevention of all the possible complications we would like to address the *prevention* of the two most common ones: rebleeding and cerebral ischaemia.

Table 13.3 Recommendations for nursing and general management of patients with SAH.

NURSING
Continuous observation (Glasgow Coma Scale, pupils, any focal deficits)

NUTRITION
Oral route
Only with intact cough and swallowing reflexes
Keep stools soft by adequate fluid intake and by restriction of milk content; if necessary add laxatives

Nasogastric tube
Deflate endotracheal cuff (if present) on insertion
Confirm proper placement by X-ray
Begin with small test feeds of 5% dextrose
Prevent aspiration by feeding in sitting position and by checking gastric residue every hour
Tablets should be crushed and flushed down (phenytoin levels will not be adequate in conventional doses)

Total parenteral nutrition should be used only as a last resort

BLOOD PRESSURE
Do not treat hypertension unless there is clinical or laboratory evidence of progressive organ damage

FLUIDS AND ELECTROLYTES
Give at least 3 L/day (normal saline)
Insert an indwelling bladder catheter if voiding is involuntary
Compensate for a negative fluid balance and for fever

PAIN
Start with paracetamol and/or dextropropoxyphene; avoid aspirin
Midazolam can be used if pain is accompanied by anxiety (5 mg intramuscularly or infusion pump)
For severe pain, use codeine or, as a last resort, morphine

PREVENTION OF DVT AND PULMONARY EMBOLISM
Apply compression stockings or intermittent compression by pneumatic devices

13.5 Prevention of rebleeding

13.5.1 Risk of rebleeding

In the first few hours after the initial haemorrhage, up to 15% of patients experience a sudden episode of clinical deterioration that suggests rebleeding (Kassell & Torner, 1983; Hijdra *et al.*, 1987b). As this often occurs before the first CT scan, or even before admission to hospital, a definite diagnosis is difficult and the true frequency of rebleeding on the first day is invariably underestimated. A study from Japan, in which 150 patients were investigated after an amazingly short delay of 6 hours or less from symptom onset, found that of the 33 patients who rebled, 29 did so on the first day, and 23 within the first 6 hours (Inagawa *et al.*, 1987). In patients who survive the first day, the risk of rebleeding is rather evenly distributed over the next 4 weeks, and amounts to 32% in patients not treated with antifibrinolytic agents but with placebo (Hijdra *et al.*, 1987b). Given that one-third of the patients in this latter series had undergone aneurysm clipping around day 12, the risk of rebleeding without medical or surgical intervention in the 4 weeks after the first day can be estimated at 35–40%. A more precise estimate is difficult to obtain because, currently, patients in good condition have their operation much sooner, within 3 days. In previous studies, before the advent of CT, the occurrence of rebleeding was probably overestimated (Vermeulen *et al.*, 1984b). Between 4 weeks and 6 months after the haemorrhage the risk of rebleeding gradually decreases, from the initial level of 1–2%/day to a constant level of about 3%/year (Winn *et al.*, 1977).

> *The risk of rebleeding after rupture of an intracranial aneurysm, without medical or surgical intervention is: in all patients about 20% on the first day; in survivors of the first day about 40% in the first month; and the cumulative risk for all patients in the first month is about 50%.*

The case fatality of rebleeding is high: around 50%, compared with the 35% overall case fatality within 3 months for patients with SAH who survive the first day, which proportion includes the fatal rebleeds (see Section 13.2.2) (Hijdra *et al.*, 1987b). Unfortunately, there are few prognostic factors that predict an increased risk of rebleeding. Some studies suggest that rebleeding occurs more often in patients with a decreased level of consciousness (Torner *et al.*, 1981a; Aoyagi & Hayakawa, 1984), but this could not be confirmed when the diagnosis of rebleeding was rigorous, based on serial CT scanning (Hijdra *et al.*, 1987b). In a single series of patients studied with serial CT scanning, a statistically significant but small excess risk of rebleeding was found for patients who had lost consciousness at the initial haemorrhage and for those with direct intraventricular haemorrhage (D.W.J. Dippel, unpublished observations). Even if the difference between subgroups was substantial, therapeutic measures for the prevention of rebleeding cannot be restricted to only high-risk groups because of the prevention paradox (Rose, 1992); treatment would then be denied to most patients eventually going on to suffer the event in question, in this case rebleeding (see also Section 18.4).

> *Rebleeding of a ruptured aneurysm can not be predicted reliably.*

13.5.2 The timing of surgery

The classical study from Atkinson Morley's Hospital, London, was the first to establish in a randomised controlled trial that operation (at that time mainly carotid ligation) was preferable to conservative management for patients who had recovered from the immediate effects of rupture of a posterior communicating artery aneurysm (McKissock *et al.*, 1960). A subsequent study showed no difference between surgical and conservative treatment of aneurysms of the anterior communicating artery complex, but surgical treatment of intracranial aneurysms continued without further controlled trials being done (McKissock *et al.*, 1965). In those days the aneurysm was usually clipped after at least 12 days had elapsed. The second week was notorious for its ischaemic complications, even without operation, and attempts at very early intervention were disappointing.

Improvements in anaesthetic technique, and especially the introduction of the operating microscope, have radically changed this. Nowadays, many neurosurgeons adhere to a policy of early clipping of the aneurysm, i.e. within 3 days of the initial bleed. Of course, the main rationale for early surgery is optimal prevention of rebleeding, but some also believe that ischaemia might be prevented by early operation because the clots that surround blood vessels in the subarachnoid space can be washed away and no longer contribute to the development of vasospasm (Mizukami *et al.*, 1982). On the other hand, a clinical trial of intraoperative thrombolysis with tissue plasminogen activator (tPA) failed to show a convincing benefit (Findlay *et al.*, 1995), and in an uncontrolled and small study there was no difference in outcome according to the dose of tPA that was used (Öhman *et al.*, 1991). Another theoretical advantage of early aneurysm clipping is that if cerebral ischaemia does still develop there is an opportunity for hypertensive and hypervolaemic treatment without fear of rebleeding.

The advantages of early surgery have not yet been proven by systematic studies. A remarkable study was done in Finland and, to date, it is the only randomised trial of the timing of operation. The 216 patients were allocated to surgery within 3 days, after 7 days or in the intermediate period (Öhman & Heiskanen, 1989). The outcome tended to be better after early than after intermediate or late surgery, but as the difference was not statistically significant a disadvantage of early surgery could not be excluded. No difference in the outcome after early or late operation was found in a study with a completely different design, with many centres and large numbers but without random allocation (Kassell *et al.*, 1990b). That study found the worst outcome in patients operated on between day 7 and 10 after the initial haemorrhage. This disadvantageous period for performing the operation in the second week after SAH coincides with the peak time of cerebral ischaemia (Hijdra *et al.*, 1986), and of cerebral vasospasm (Weir *et al.*, 1978), both of which are most common from day 4 to 12.

> *Although early aneurysm surgery in patients in good clinical condition is now the usual practice, this policy is vulnerable to challenge and reversal because it has not been supported by any randomised controlled trial.*

13.5.3 Antifibrinolytic drugs

The purpose of treatment with antifibrinolytic drugs is to reduce the risk of rebleeding before definitive surgical intervention is possible. Its rationale is the notion that rebleeding is caused by lysis of the blood clot that seals the aneurysm at the site of the initial rupture. The first report on antifibrinolytic treatment in SAH was published in 1967. Almost 30-years later, this mode of treatment has remained controversial (Adams, 1987; Weir, 1987). The two most commonly used antifibrinolytic drugs are TEA (usual dose 1 g intravenously or 1.5 g orally, four to six times daily), or epsilon-aminocaproic acid (EACA; 3–4.5 g 3-hourly intravenously or orally). Both agents are structurally similar to lysine and so block the lysine binding sites by which the plasminogen molecules bind to complementary sites on fibrin. In this way these drugs prevent fibrinolysis in general, and lysis of the clot on the recently ruptured aneurysm in particular. TEA has indeed been shown to enter the clot adherent to the aneurysm and to cross the barrier between the blood and the cerebrospinal fluid (Fodstad et al., 1981). It is assumed that it takes 36 hours to achieve complete inhibition of fibrinolysis in the cerebrospinal fluid.

Before the mid-1980s, about 30 papers had addressed the efficacy of these drugs (Vermeulen & Muizelaar, 1980; Ramirez-Lassepas, 1981). Only 10 studies were controlled, seven had a randomised treatment allocation and in only three was assessment blind. These three studies showed no advantage of antifibrinolytic treatment over placebo, but the number of patients included was so small that clinically important effects might easily have been missed. An additional problem with many studies was that the analysis included rebleeding alone, without the overall outcome being taken into account, and that even then the diagnosis of rebleeding was not usually confirmed by brain CT.

The importance of relevant outcome criteria and other methodological issues became only too clear in 1984 from the results of a large randomized double-blind, placebo-controlled trial (479 patients), conducted in the Netherlands and Scotland. The rate of rebleeding was reduced from 24% in the control group to 9% in the TEA-treated group, but the overall outcome in terms of disability in the two groups was strikingly similar. This could be explained by a concomitant increase in the rate of ischaemic complications: 15% in the control group and 24% in the TEA group (Vermeulen et al., 1984a). From a pragmatic point of view patients had been included with a diagnosis of SAH that was *presumably* aneurysmal in origin, before angiography had been carried out; the results were similar, however, if the analysis was restricted to patients in whom the presence of an aneurysm was subsequently confirmed. The statistical power of the study was large enough for the 95% confidence interval of the difference in case fatality rate for the two groups to be as narrow as −6 to +11%. In the same year the participants in the Cooperative Aneurysm Study reported a similar trade-off between medical prevention of rebleeding and an increase in the risk of delayed cerebral infarction, but from a non-randomised comparison, between 467 patients who were treated with antifibrinolytic drugs and 205 who were not (Kassell et al., 1984). A meta-analysis of all randomised studies with antifibrinolytic trials, including one small trial performed later, showed no significant advantage over placebo (Roos et al., to be published as part of the Cochrane Collaboration).

Antifibrinolytic drugs prevent rebleeding after aneurysmal rupture, but because they increase the risk of cerebral ischaemia there is no useful effect on overall outcome.

So far, antifibrinolytic drugs have been shown to work, but not to help. This does not necessarily mean the end of their application in patients with SAH if the attendant ischaemia could be prevented. How this treatment precipitates cerebral ischaemia is still unclear; possible explanations include increased blood viscosity, the development of microthrombi, delayed clearance of blood clots around the arteries at the base of the brain and the development of hydrocephalus through delayed resorption of blood. In the Dutch–Scottish trial of TEA, it was after day 6 that the rate of cerebral infarction in patients on the active drug started to exceed that in the placebo group, which then raised the possibility that a shorter period of treatment might still inhibit rebleeding yet avoid the ischaemic complications (Vermeulen et al., 1984a). After all, the rationale for giving the drug for up to 4 weeks (or until operation) was the notion that the continuing presence of fibrin/fibrinogen degradation products in the cerebrospinal fluid, up to the fifth week, indicates ongoing fibrinolytic activity; but, this idea was subsequently proved wrong (Vermeulen et al., 1985). Disappointingly, however, a pilot study in which TEA was given for only a 4-day period produced the reverse of the desired result: the rate of rebleeding was as high as one would expect in untreated patients, and cerebral ischaemia was as frequent as in previous patients on long-term treatment (Wijdicks et al., 1989).

Since the 'negative' result of the Dutch–Scottish trial, it has emerged that several measures are effective in the prevention of ischaemic complications: (i) maintenance of an adequate intake of water and sodium; (ii) the avoidance of antihypertensive treatment; (iii) the use of calcium antagonists; and (iv) if necessary, expansion of the plasma volume (see Section 13.6). It is not unduly optimistic to expect that antifibrinolytic drugs might prevent rebleeds and yet improve overall outcome if they were combined with these measures to prevent cerebral ischaemia. A preliminary study in which antifibrinolytic drugs and calcium antagonists were combined showed promising results (Beck *et al.*, 1988). A new clinical trial is underway in the Netherlands, in which all patients are maximally protected against ischaemia and 50% are randomized to additional treatment with antifibrinolytic drugs; it is expected to end in 1998. Until the results of this or similar new trials are available, routine administration of antifibrinolytic drugs is not indicated.

13.5.4 Endovascular occlusion

For giant aneurysms of the posterior circulation, or of the carotid siphon, the endovascular approach is used to insert an inflatable balloon. Very few centres have experience with the endovascular application of coils that can be mechanically or electrically detached within aneurysms. The purpose is to entirely pack the aneurysm with coils; the remaining lumen should then become occluded by a process of reactive thrombosis. Yet, in two patients studied postmortem there were no signs of organisation of thrombi, endothelialisation of the neck of the aneurysm or a decrease in size of the aneurysm (Molyneux *et al.*, 1995). Up to the present time the indication for such treatment has often been limited to aneurysms of the posterior circulation that are difficult to access surgically (Guglielmi *et al.*, 1992). Complete thrombosis of the aneurysm after introduction of a coil seems most likely to succeed if the neck of the aneurysm is smaller than 4 mm (Fernandez Zubillaga *et al.*, 1994). Nevertheless, this approach has also been used to treat giant aneurysms (Casasco *et al.*, 1992; Nakahara *et al.*, 1992; Numaguchi *et al.*, 1992). It is conceivable that this technique will also gain ground in the treatment of surgically accessible aneurysms. No controlled trials have yet been reported in which the procedure has been compared with craniotomy and clipping, but one is being launched from Oxford, by Molyneux and collaborators.

13.6   Prevention of delayed cerebral ischaemia

13.6.1 Pathogenesis and risk factors

Unlike stroke occurring as a result of disease of the extra- or intracerebral arteries, cerebral ischaemia or infarction after SAH is not confined to the territory of a single cerebral artery or one of its branches (Fig. 13.2) (Hijdra *et al.*, 1986). Vasospasm is often implicated, because its peak frequency from day 5 to 14 coincides with that of delayed ischaemia

(Weir *et al.*, 1978), and also because it is often generalised, in keeping with the multifocal or diffuse nature of the clinical manifestations and of the ischaemic lesions found on CT and at autopsy (Heros *et al.*, 1983; Kistler *et al.*, 1983). Nevertheless, it is incorrect to use the term 'vasospasm' as being synonymous with delayed cerebral ischaemia, for four reasons.

1 Arterial narrowing does not necessarily signify contraction of smooth muscle in the arterial wall, but may represent necrosis and secondary oedema (Conway & McDonald, 1972; Hughes & Schianchi, 1978; Smith *et al.*, 1983; Findlay *et al.*, 1989). Intimal proliferation is another possibility, a process shown to underlie restenosis in coronary arteries after balloon angioplasty (Post *et al.*, 1994).

2 Arterial narrowing can be asymptomatic even if severe (Millikan, 1975; Fisher *et al.*, 1977).

3 The interpretation of angiographic appearances relating to the severity or even the presence of arterial narrowing is subject to variation between observers (Eskesen *et al.*, 1987).

4 Vasospasm is certainly not the only factor in the pathogenesis of cerebral infarction in patients with ruptured aneurysms (Table 13.4).

Many of the risk factors for delayed cerebral ischaemia factors are dependent on each other or on intermediate factors in complex interactions, which are poorly understood. These include the development of hyponatraemia and hypovolaemia (see Section 13.10.1). Some have postulated a close relationship between the location of subarachnoid blood and the occurrence of vasospasm and delayed cerebral ischaemia, but based on a series of only 41 patients (Kistler *et al.*, 1983). Although there is little doubt that the overall amount of subarachnoid blood as determined on CT scan is the most powerful predictor of delayed ischaemia, larger series have failed to show any relationship between the anatomical distribution or even the side of infarction and the site of the extravasated blood in the subarachnoid space (Hijdra *et al.*, 1986; Brouwers *et al.*, 1992). In addition, delayed cerebral ischaemia does not occur in perimesencephalic non-aneurysmal SAH, even after matching for the

Table 13.4 Determinants of delayed cerebral ischaemia after SAH.

Arterial narrowing (Kistler *et al.*, 1983)
Depressed level of consciousness after the onset (Brouwers *et al.*, 1992)
Amount of subarachnoid blood on early CT scanning (Hijdra *et al.*, 1988; Öhman *et al.*, 1991; Brouwers *et al.*, 1992)
Hyponatraemia and hypovolaemia (Wijdicks *et al.*, 1985a,b; Hasan *et al.*, 1990)
Treatment with antihypertensive drugs (Wijdicks *et al.*, 1990)
Treatment with antifibrinolytic drugs (Vermeulen *et al.*, 1984a)

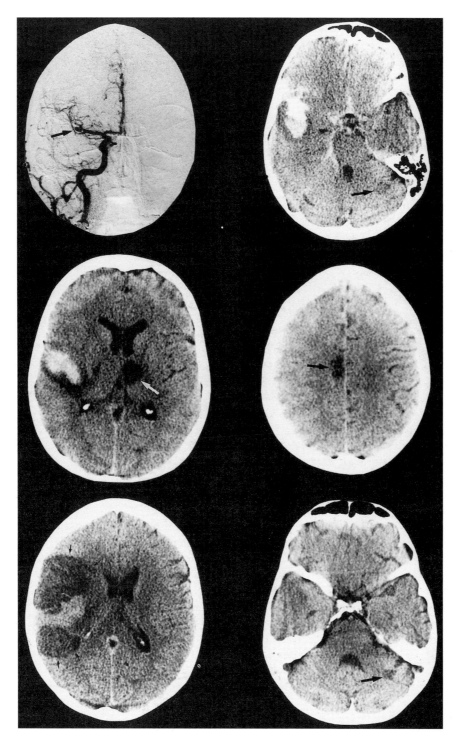

Figure 13.2 Delayed cerebral ischaemia after SAH, with scattered lesions. Cerebral angiography and CT scans of a 43-year-old woman with SAH. Angiography on the day of the haemorrhage (upper row, left) showed an aneurysm of the right middle cerebral artery (arrow), consistent with the initial CT scan (not shown). On the second day after she had a gradual decline in the level of consciousness a repeat CT scan (upper row, right) showed unchanged blood in the basal cisterns, with an intracranial haematoma at the site of the aneurysm, and a newly developed focal hypodensity in the left cerebellar hemisphere (arrow). On the fifth day after the haemorrhage, she developed a hemiparesis on the left, with a further decline in the level of consciousness. CT now showed infarcts in the left thalamus (middle row, left—white arrow), and in the distal territory of the right anterior cerebral artery (middle row, right—black arrow). Ten days after the haemorrhage, the haematoma had resolved, leaving a large area of ischaemia (bottom row, left—arrows). One month after the haemorrhage, the left cerebellar infarct is still clearly visible (bottom row, right—arrow). (Courtesy of J.W. Hop.)

449

amount of extravasated blood; thus, damage to the wall of an artery seems to be one necessary factor for the development of delayed ischaemia (Rinkel *et al.*, 1991).

> *The occurrence of cerebral ischaemia after subarachnoid haemorrhage is strongly related to the total amount of subarachnoid blood, but much less to the distribution of the extravasated blood, and occurs only if the source is a ruptured aneurysm.*

In summary, any causal relationship between the amount of extravasated blood and the development of delayed cerebral ischaemia is not explained sufficiently by the production of some toxic substances that might be released from clots around the large arteries at the base of the brain. As loss of consciousness at the time of the haemorrhage is an important predictive factor for delayed cerebral ischaemia, it is possible that global ischaemia during this brief period of massive increase in intracranial pressure may sensitise neurones to marginal perfusion, associated with later complications such as diffuse vasospasm or hypovolaemia.

Practical measures that can help to prevent ischaemia are avoidance of antihypertensive drugs, an adequate intake of fluid and sodium, routine administration of calcium antagonists and limitation of sodium loss by means of fludrocortisone acetate. The first two measures are backed by indirect rather than direct evidence (see Section 13.4.2).

13.6.2 Calcium antagonists

Calcium entry blocking drugs have been used because they inhibit the contractile properties of smooth muscle cells, particularly those in cerebral arteries, and also because they may, to some extent, protect neurones against the deleterious effect of calcium influx after ischaemic damage (see Section 11.7) (Greenberg, 1987). Nimodipine was first tested only in small randomised trials, in which the drug was administered orally (Allen *et al.*, 1983; Philippon *et al.*, 1986; Neil Dwyer *et al.*, 1987) or intravenously (Öhman & Heiskanen, 1988; Jan *et al.*, 1988). In some of these studies the number of ischaemic complications was less in patients treated according to protocol, but the differences were not statistically significant when the overall outcome after 3 months in all randomised patients was taken into account. A multicentre study in Canada included only patients with clinical deficits and found a significantly better outcome in patients allocated to (oral) nimodipine, but not all randomised patients were included in the analysis (Petruk *et al.*, 1988).

The most authoritative study of nimodipine to date is from the UK, in which 554 patients were randomised between placebo or nimodipine, given orally every 4 hours for 21 days (Pickard *et al.*, 1989). If the patient was unable to swallow, the tablets were crushed and washed down a nasogastric tube with normal saline. This regimen resulted in a significant reduction of poor outcomes (as defined on the Glasgow Outcome Scale: death, vegetative state or severe disability) from 33 to 20% (i.e. a relative reduction of 40%; 95% confidence interval (CI): 20–55%). The rate of cerebral infarction was reduced by 34% (95% CI: 13–50%). The authors kept strictly to the rules of a pragmatic study by including all randomised patients in the analysis; they even refrained from separately analysing the treatment results in the subgroup of patients with an angiographically demonstrated aneurysm. It should be emphasised that these results do not necessarily apply to nimodipine if administered intravenously because this route may lead to a decrease in blood pressure, particularly in hypertensive patients. Nevertheless, a meta-analysis of all seven randomised controlled trials (including the UK trial) gave an overall reduction of poor outcome from delayed cerebral ischaemia that was very similar to that of the large British trial alone: odds ratio 0.47, 95% CI: 0.36–0.62 (Di Mascio *et al.*, 1993).

> *Oral nimodipine about halves the risk of a poor outcome after subarachnoid haemorrhage.*

Interestingly, several studies with nimodipine found there was no difference between treated patients and controls with regard to the frequency of arterial narrowing on a repeat angiogram (Philippon *et al.*, 1986; Petruk *et al.*, 1988; Pickard *et al.*, 1989). Therefore, at least with this particular calcium antagonist, the protective effect on neurones seems to be more important than any amelioration of vasospasm.

Nicardipine, a different calcium antagonist administered by the intravenous route, has been tested in a multicentre clinical trial in the US, involving 906 patients. The overall outcome after 3 months was no different in the treated and control groups, despite a statistically significant decrease in the occurrence of episodes of delayed ischaemia, and a similar decrease in the rate of vasospasm as assessed by means of angiography or transcranial Doppler ultrasound, in selected patients (Haley *et al.*, 1993a,b). A confounding factor was an excess of hypervolaemic/hypertensive treatment in the control group. A subsequent study tested the effect of halving the dose of nicardipine (0.075 instead of 0.15 mg/kg per hour), in a randomised design; the rate of ischaemic episodes and the overall outcome were identical in the two groups (Haley *et al.*, 1994). The disappointing results with nicardipine could perhaps be attributed to lowering blood pressure with intravenous administration, as is the case with intravenous nimodipine. The collective evidence leaves no other conclusion than that the intravenous administration of calcium entry blockers in patients with SAH is ineffective.

13.6.3 Fludrocortisone acetate

Because of its mineralocorticoid activity (reabsorption of sodium in the distal tubules of the kidney) fludrocortisone might, in theory, prevent a negative sodium balance, hypovolaemia and ischaemic complications (Wijdicks *et al.*, 1988b). A randomised study in which patients with SAH were entered soon after admission showed that fludrocortisone acetate significantly reduced natriuresis in the first 6 days after the haemorrhage. Reductions in the occurrence of plasma volume depletion and of ischaemic complications were not statistically significant, but these beneficial effects may have been masked because patients in the control group were often treated with plasma expanders after they had developed clinical signs of ischaemia (Hasan *et al.*, 1989a). These results are insufficiently conclusive to warrant routine administration of fludrocortisone to all patients with SAH, but they do support its use in patients developing hyponatraemia (see Section 13.10.1).

13.6.4 Free radical scavengers

Tirilazad mesylate, a 21-aminosteroid free radical scavenger, has been shown to reduce infarct size in animal models of SAH. The safety of varying doses of this new drug has been confirmed in a randomised phase II trial (Haley *et al.*, 1995) and two efficacy studies with reportedly positive results in males have just been completed but not yet published.

13.6.5 Aspirin

A retrospective analysis of 242 patients who had survived the first 4 days after SAH showed that patients who had used salicylates before their haemorrhage (as detected by history and urine screening) had a significantly decreased risk of delayed cerebral ischaemia, with or without permanent deficits (relative risk 0.40, 95% CI: 0.18–0.93) (Juvela, 1995). This interesting observation warrants a prospective and randomised study of salicylates or other antiplatelet drugs as a preventive measure against delayed cerebral ischaemia, preferably after clipping of the aneurysm to avoid rebleeding being precipitated by the antiplatelet and so antihaemostatic action.

13.7 Management of rebleeding

13.7.1 Diagnosis

In a consecutive series of 39 patients with a CT-proven rebleed, of whom 36 were awake at the time, 35 lost consciousness (preceded by headache in one-third); in the remaining patient a sudden increase in headache was the only symptom, and serial CT scanning failed to detect 'silent' rebleeding in any awake patient (Hijdra *et al.*, 1987b). In patients with a first episode of SAH, loss of consciousness occurs in slightly less than 50% (Vermeulen *et al.*, 1984a). This difference in the rate of unconsciousness at onset already indicates that rebleeding has a more severe impact on the brain than the first bleed (Fig. 13.3), which is confirmed by the higher case fatality rate (50%). Most patients with fatal rebleeds immediately lose consciousness, with loss of brainstem reflexes but without initial apnoea (Hijdra *et al.*, 1987b).

It should not be assumed, however, that a sudden deterioration of consciousness in a patient with a ruptured aneurysm is sufficient evidence for the diagnosis of rebleeding. Other causes underlie about one-third of all episodes of sudden deterioration (Table 13.5) (Vermeulen *et al.*, 1984a), and the frequency of rebleeding is overestimated to an even greater degree if the mode of onset is not precisely known (Maurice-Williams, 1982). Once the respiratory and circulatory state of the patient has stabilized sufficiently, it is mandatory to confirm the diagnosis of rebleeding by repeat brain CT, which may show successive layers of fresh blood in the brain parenchyma or the ventricular system, each corresponding to an episode of clinical deterioration (Vermeulen *et al.*, 1984b). Lumbar puncture, apart from its dangers, is unreliable for the diagnosis of rebleeding (Vermeulen *et al.*, 1983).

13.7.2 To resuscitate or not?

The question whether patients with a rebleed should be resuscitated and artificially ventilated if respiratory arrest

Table 13.5 Causes of sudden deterioration in patients with aneurysmal SAH. (From Vermeulen *et al.*, 1984.)

Rebleeding (two-thirds) (see Section 13.7)
Epileptic seizure (see Section 13.4.3)
Delayed cerebral ischaemia, with atypical, sudden onset
  (see Section 13.8)
Ventricular fibrillation (see Section 13.10.2)
Undetermined

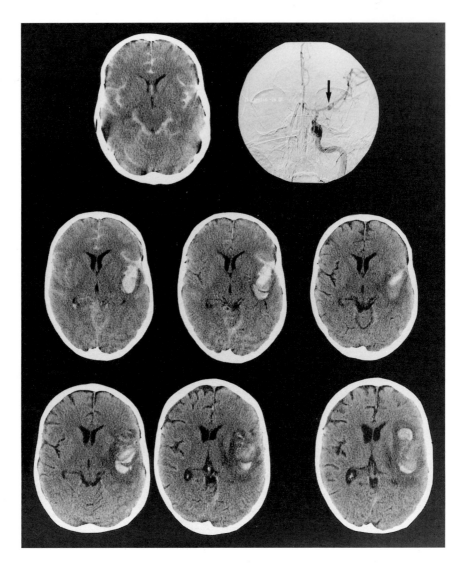

Figure 13.3 Serial CT scans with multiple episodes of rebleeding. Top, left: diffuse haemorrhage throughout all subarachnoid spaces, in a 45-year-old man (day 0). Middle row, left: CT scan showing a haematoma in the left Sylvian fissure, after a sudden episode of clinical deterioration (day 1). Top, right: angiogram, made on day 3, after substantial improvement in the level of consciousness; aneurysm of the left middle cerebral artery (arrow). Middle row, centre: CT scan made after angiography (day 3), following a second episode of sudden deterioration. New compartment of blood at posterior end of previous haematoma (arrow). Middle row, right: resorption of haematoma (day 12). Bottom row, left and centre: CT scan showing fresh blood, after third episode of clinical deterioration (day 15). Bottom, right: CT scan showing fresh haematoma at site of aneurysm, following a fourth episode with sudden decrease in the level of consciousness (day 24). Eventually, the patient was successfully operated on day 53.

occurs is not academic: in the previously mentioned series of 39 patients with a CT-confirmed rebleed, 14 had initial respiratory abnormalities that called for assisted ventilation. Spontaneous respiration returned within 1 hour in eight of these 14 patients, and in three more between 1 and 24 hours (Hijdra *et al.*, 1987b).

In a study of episodes of respiratory arrest in which first bleeds were also included, the answer to the question whether the patient would or would not regain spontaneous respiration could not be predicted from the anatomical site of haemorrhage on CT, the initial presence or absence of brainstem reflexes or the type of respiratory disorder (Hijdra *et al.*, 1984). Many patients with initial apnoea who were successfully resuscitated, nevertheless died from subsequent complications, but the message to be stressed here is that survival without brain damage is possible even after respiratory arrest. This is another important reason why patients with a recently ruptured aneurysm should be under close and continuous observation. After resuscitation, it will usually become clear within a matter of hours whether the patient will indeed survive the episode or whether dysfunction of the brainstem will persist; there are no grounds for the fear that the intervention will only result in prolongation of a vegetative state.

> *Sudden apnoea in a patient with subarachnoid haemorrhage usually signifies rebleeding. With full resuscitative measures spontaneous respiration will rapidly return in approximately 50% of the cases, followed within hours by return of brainstem reflexes and consciousness, if these functions had been lost at the same time. If it does not, then organ donation should be considered.*

In those patients who progress to brain death from a devastating rebleed, usually with massive hydrocephalus and large intraventricular clots, the resuscitation procedure has at least allowed organ donation to be considered, with some benefits to others.

13.7.3 Emergency clipping of the aneurysm

A large haematoma that causes brain shift without being associated with gross intraventricular haemorrhage is an infrequent finding after rebleeding, occurring in around 10% (Hijdra *et al.*, 1987b). In these rare cases, evacuation of the haematoma may be indicated. A more frequent consideration after rebleeding is that amongst the survivors, 50–75% suffer a further rebleed (Hijdra *et al.*, 1987b; Inagawa *et al.*, 1987). This implies that emergency clipping of the aneurysm should be seriously considered in patients who regain consciousness after rebleeding. Of course, the risk of the operation is increased after a rebleed but the risks of a wait-and-see policy at that stage seem even more intimidating. The management of rebleeding is summarised in Table 13.6.

13.8 Management of cerebral ischaemia

13.8.1 Diagnosis

The clinical manifestations of delayed cerebral ischaemia evolve gradually, over several hours, and usually between day 4 and 12 after the haemorrhage. In 25% of the patients ischaemia causes hemispheric focal deficits, in another 25% a decrease in the level of consciousness, and in the remaining 50% these two features evolve together (Hijdra *et al.*, 1986). The diagnosis of cerebral ischaemia should be based not only on this clinical picture, but also on the results of a repeat

Table 13.6 Management of rebleeding.

In case of respiratory arrest, resuscitate and ventilate; within hours either spontaneous respiration will return or all other brainstem functions will be lost

Repeat CT scan

Consider emergency clipping of aneurysm after recovery, as the majority will rebleed again, with a high case fatality; any intracerebral haematoma can be removed at the same time

---

Table 13.7 Causes of subacute clinical deterioration after SAH.

Cerebral ischaemia (see Section 13.8.1)
Hydrocephalus (see Section 13.9.1)
Unsuspected rebleeding (see Section 13.7.1)
Systemic complication (see Section 13.10)

---

brain CT (see Fig. 13.1). The scan serves to exclude other causes of subacute deterioration, such as oedema surrounding an intracerebral haematoma, dilatation of the ventricular system or unsuspected rebleeding (Table 13.7). Positive evidence of ischaemia is shown by CT in about 80% of patients after exclusion of these other causes, at least after a few days (Hijdra *et al.*, 1986). Magnetic resonance imaging (MRI) is probably more sensitive in detecting early changes in the water content of the brain parenchyma, but MRI facilities are not readily available in most centres; in addition, the acquisition time needed to obtain good images is often too long for ill and restless patients. Single photon emission CT (SPECT) scanning may be helpful (Davis *et al.*, 1990), but hypoperfusion may also result from oedema around a resolving haematoma or, if it occurs in the basal parts of the brain, from hydrocephalus (Hasan *et al.*, 1991b). Transcranial Doppler sonography is very specific, but only moderately sensitive, in suggesting cerebral ischaemia by means of the increased blood flow velocity from arterial narrowing in the middle cerebral artery or in the posterior circulation, because vasospasm may have occurred in more distal vessels (Sloan *et al.*, 1989, 1994). Of course, demonstration of arterial narrowing is no proof in itself that clinical deterioration has been caused by ischaemia. Factors such as intracranial pressure, arterial blood pressure and respiration may all influence the form of the velocity wave, but completely normal blood velocities would at least lower the probability of ischaemia as the cause of any clinical deterioration.

13.8.2 Induced hypertension and volume expansion

Since the 1960s, induced hypertension has been used to combat ischaemic deficits in patients with SAH (Farhat & Schneider, 1967). Later, induced hypertension was often combined with volume expansion. Particularly remarkable was the case of a 50-year-old woman with a ruptured middle cerebral artery aneurysm who developed aphasia and a right-sided hemiparesis postoperatively. Her deficits cleared when she was treated with noradrenaline and blood transfusion, by which her blood pressure was raised from 120/70 to 180/110 mmHg. Numerous attempts, in the next few days, to allow the blood pressure to fall to normal ranges were each time met by worsening of the neurological condition. This treatment regimen was also successful in five of six other patients (Kosnik & Hunt, 1976). Kassell *et al.* (1982) reported the effect of induced hypertension and volume expansion in a larger series of 58 patients with progressive neurological deterioration and angiographically confirmed vasospasm. They were able to reverse the deficits in 47 cases, and permanently in 43. In 16 patients who had responded to this treatment, the neurological deficits recurred when the blood pressure transiently dropped, but again resolved when the pressure increased. Similar results have been obtained by Awad *et al.* (1987), although the degree of improvement was rather vaguely described. The most plausible explanation for these phenomena is a defect of cerebral autoregulation that makes the perfusion of the brain passively dependent on the systemic blood pressure.

The risks of deliberately increasing the arterial pressure and plasma volume include rebleeding of an unclipped aneurysm, increased cerebral oedema or haemorrhagic transformation in areas of infarction, congestive heart failure and myocardial infarction. Therefore, the circulatory system should be closely monitored with an arterial line and either a central venous or pulmonary artery catheter. These monitoring procedures carry their own risks (infection, pneumothorax, haemothorax, ventricular arrhythmia and pulmonary infarction). Some have found that the development of neurological deficits was more closely related to the pulmonary capillary wedge pressure than to the blood pressure, or to a measure of cardiac output (Finn *et al.*, 1986). A currently recommended regimen (Table 13.8), although not supported by rigorously controlled trials, is to start with plasma volume expansion with 5% albumin, 250 mg four to six times a day; others use a plasma protein fraction or Hetastarch. The aim is to raise the central venous filling pressure to approximately 8–12 mmHg, or the pulmonary capillary wedge pressure to about 14–18 mmHg. The haematocrit is kept around 40%. If no clinical improvement is obtained with these measures, one might consider raising

Table 13.8 Management of cerebral ischaemia.

Stop nimodipine
Immediately administer 500 ml albumin 5% or 20%
Repeat brain CT to rule out other causes of deterioration
Insert external jugular vein catheter or pulmonary arterial balloon catheter; maintain central venous pressure between 8–10 mmHg, or pulmonary wedge pressure between 14–18 mmHg
Keep arterial pressure 20–40 mmHg above baseline values
Maintain fluid intake with at least 3 L of normal saline per 24 hours
Correct hyponatraemia (see Table 13.10)

the blood pressure with dopamine or dobutamine to a level of 20–40 mmHg above pretreatment values (Biller *et al.*, 1988). These procedures should only be carried out in an intensive care unit with facilities for specialised care and close monitoring.

13.8.3 Transluminal angioplasty

The endovascular approach is being used in the treatment of several vascular diseases. In the treatment of symptomatic vasospasm after SAH, dilatation with a balloon catheter is rather novel. Very few centres have any experience with this application of transluminal angioplasty (Higashida *et al.*, 1989; Newell *et al.*, 1989; Nichols *et al.*, 1994). These centres have reported sustained improvement in nine of 13 and eight of 10 cases, respectively. Rebleeding may be precipitated by this procedure, even after the aneurysm has been clipped (Newell *et al.*, 1989; Linskey *et al.*, 1991). Postmortem study in two patients showed that the procedure had resulted in stretching and disruption of a degenerated muscular layer as well as of proliferated collagen tissue (Honma *et al.*, 1995). In view of the risks, the high costs and the lack of controlled trials, transluminal angioplasty should presently be regarded as a strictly experimental procedure. The same applies to anecdotal reports of intra-arterial infusion of papaverine, following super-selective catheterisation (Kaku *et al.*, 1992).

13.8.4 Pharmacological intervention

Calcitonin gene-related peptide (CGRP) is a potent vasodilator in the carotid vascular bed, but a randomised, multicentre, single-blind clinical trial in 62 patients failed to bear out any benefits in terms of overall outcome: the relative risk of a poor outcome in CGRP-treated patients was 0.88 (95% CI: 0.60–1.28) (Anonymous, 1992).

13.9   Management of acute hydrocephalus

13.9.1   Diagnosis

In several series of patients admitted within 3 days of SAH and who were not selected for aneurysm surgery, the frequency of acute hydrocephalus (defined as a bicaudate index above the 95th percentile for age; Fig. 13.4) was consistently around 20% (van Gijn et al., 1985; Milhorat, 1987; Hasan et al., 1989b, 1991a). Of those, only 10–28% had a normal level of consciousness, but approximately one-third of the patients in this group deteriorated in the next few days (Hasan et al., 1989b).

The classical presentation of acute hydrocephalus is that of a patient who is alert immediately after the initial haemorrhage, but who in the next few hours becomes increasingly drowsy, to the point that the patient only moans and localises to pain. But, only 50% of all patients with acute hydrocephalus present in this way (Van Gijn et al., 1985). In the other 50%, consciousness is impaired from the onset, or the course is unknown because the patient was alone at the time of haemorrhage. If the patient is admitted very early and secondary deterioration occurs because of hydrocephalus, serial investigation by CT may show that the level of consciousness correlates more or less inversely with the width of the lateral ventricles (Fig. 13.5) (Rinkel et al., 1990). When different patients are compared within one series, however, the relationship between the level of consciousness and the degree of ventricular dilatation is rather erratic (van Gijn et al., 1985;

Hasan et al., 1989b). Ocular signs do not always accompany obtundation as a result of acute hydrocephalus; they help to corroborate but not to exclude the diagnosis. In a prospective study in which 30 of 34 patients with acute hydrocephalus had an impaired level of consciousness, nine of these 30 had small, non-reactive pupils, and four of these nine also showed persistent downward deviation of the eyes, with otherwise intact brainstem reflexes (van Gijn et al., 1985). These eye signs reflect dilatation of the proximal part of the aqueduct, which causes dysfunction of the pretectal area (Swash, 1974). All nine patients with non-reactive pupils had a relative ventricular size of more than 1.20 and were in coma, i.e. they did not open their eyes, did not obey commands and did not utter words (Glasgow Coma Scale score of 7 or less with the maximum at 14, i.e. without distinction between purposive withdrawal and abnormal flexion for the motor response of the arm).

> *Repeat CT scanning is required to diagnose or exclude hydrocephalus in a patient with subarachnoid haemorrhage who deteriorates within hours or days of the initial event, with or without eye signs of hydrocephalus (small, unreactive pupils and downward deviation of gaze). Patients with intraventricular blood or with extensive haemorrhage in the perimesencephalic cisterns are predisposed to developing acute hydrocephalus.*

Intraventricular blood was found to be associated with acute hydrocephalus in all studies that addressed this question, at least if there was enough to suggest direct intraven-

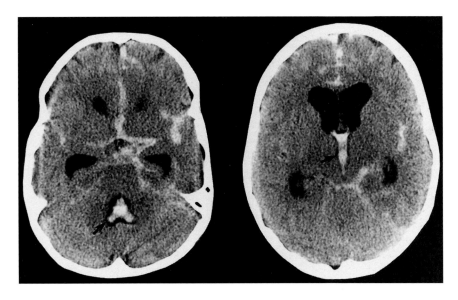

Figure 13.4 Acute hydrocephalus after SAH, through obstruction of cerebrospinal fluid flow: the third (right—arrow) and fourth (left—arrow) ventricles are both filled with blood (day 0); the patient was a 24-year-old woman, who probably had suffered an earlier episode 7-days before (not investigated). The site of the aneurysm was not identified.

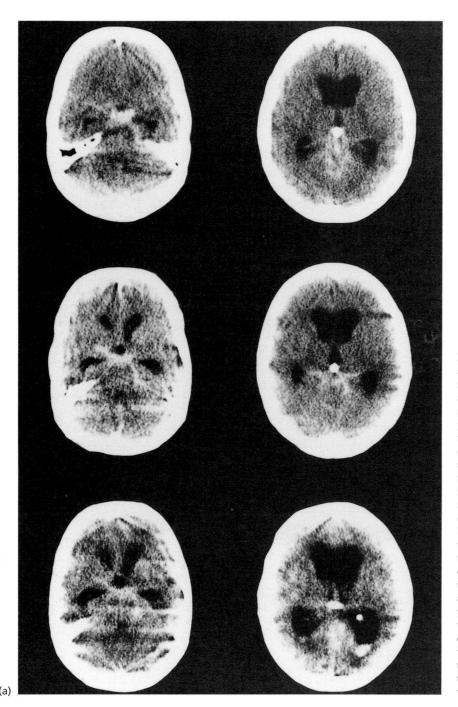

(a)

Figure 13.5 (a) Non-contrast CT scans in a patient with SAH (incidentally, this was not from a ruptured aneurysm, but from an unidentified source, presumably a ruptured vein (see Section 9.1.2)), in the perimesencephalic cisterns. In this case, the site at which the cerebrospinal fluid is obstructed is not so much the ventricular system itself but the tentorial hiatus, through which the outflow from the fourth ventricle has to pass in order to reach the arachnoid villi at the convexity of the brain. Left: slice at the level of the basal cisterns. Right: slice at the level of the pineal gland. Upper row (4 hours after the ictus): haemorrhage in the basal cisterns, with most of the blood located in the interpeduncular fossa and the left ambiens cistern; relative size of lateral ventricles 1.4. Middle row (9 hours after the ictus): amount of blood in the basal cistern unchanged; relative size of lateral ventricles 1.4. Bottom row (28 hours after the ictus): some sedimentation of blood in the posterior horns; relative size of lateral ventricles 1.8.

tricular haemorrhage rather than just sedimentation in the posterior horns reflecting diffusion of red blood cells throughout the cerebrospinal fluid spaces (van Gijn *et al.*, 1985; Graff-Radford *et al.*, 1989; Hasan *et al.*, 1991a). On the other hand, not all patients with acute hydrocephalus have intraventricular blood (the proportions varied between 35 and 65% in these studies), and it is an erroneous notion that acute hydrocephalus is, by definition, the result of intraventricular obstruction. In some patients, it is probable that clots obstructing the tentorial hiatus are partly or wholly responsible for the development of hydrocephalus (Hasan & Tanghe, 1992; Rinkel *et al.*, 1992).

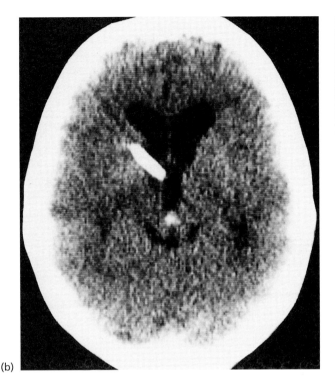

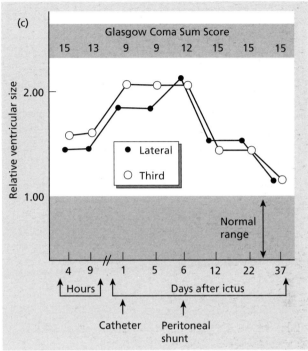

Figure 13.5 *Continued.* (b) CT scan 5 weeks after the haemorrhage, and 4 weeks after insertion of a ventricular catheter; relative size of lateral ventricles 1.2. (c) Serial measurements of the relative size of the lateral and third ventricles, and total scores on the Glasgow Coma Scale. (From Rinkel *et al.*, 1990; reproduced with permission of the authors and of the *Journal of Neurology, Neurosurgery and Psychiatry*.)

13.9.2 Possible interventions (Table 13.9)

Wait-and-see

A policy of wait-and-see for 24 hours is eminently justified in patients with dilated ventricles who are alert, because only about one-third of these patients will become symptomatic in the next few days (Hasan *et al.*, 1989b). Waiting for 1 day can be rewarding even if the level of consciousness is decreased. The reason is that spontaneous improvement within this period has been documented in approximately 50% of the patients (seven of 13) with acute hydrocephalus who were only drowsy (Glasgow Coma Score of 13, 14 being the maximum), and also in almost 50% of the patients (19 of 43) who had a Glasgow Coma Score of 12 or worse but no massive intraventricular haemorrhage (Hasan *et al.*, 1989b). On the other hand, it is not always easy to make a definitive decision on the need for surgical measures even after 1 day has elapsed, because patients may temporarily improve to some extent but then reach a plateau phase or again deteriorate; such fluctuations were encountered in about one-third of the cases (Hasan *et al.*, 1989b). Any

Table 13.9 Management of acute hydrocephalus.

Consider diagnosis if level of consciousness gradually deteriorates, particularly on the first day after the bleed

Repeat the CT scan and compare the bicaudate index with that on any previous scan

Spontaneous improvement occurs within 24 hours in 50% of the patients (except those with massive intraventricular haemorrhage); take action if patient further deteriorates or fails to improve within 24 hours

Lumbar punctures are reasonably safe if there is no brain shift, and effective in about 50% of the patients who have no intraventricular obstruction

External drainage of the ventricles is very effective in restoring the level of consciousness, but carries a high risk of rebleeding (consider emergency clipping at the same time), and of infection (this may to some degree be prevented by prophylactic antibiotics or subcutaneous tunnelling)

deterioration in the level of consciousness warrants active intervention.

Lumbar puncture

Lumbar puncture has been suggested as a therapeutic measure (Kolluri & Sengupta, 1984) but not formally studied until recently (Hasan *et al.*, 1991a). In a prospective but uncontrolled study, the authors treated 17 patients in this way; they had acute hydrocephalus with neither a haematoma nor gross intraventricular haemorrhage, i.e. less than complete filling of the third or fourth ventricle. Between one and seven spinal taps per patient were performed in the first 10 days, the number depending on the rate of improvement; each time a maximum of 20 ml of cerebrospinal fluid was removed, the aim being a closing pressure of 15 cmH$_2$O. Five of the 17 patients had a decreased level of consciousness on admission, and in them the lumbar punctures were started immediately; in 11 of the remaining 12 patients deterioration occurred a few days after admission, and the last patient had a fluctuating level of consciousness. Of the total of 17 patients, 12 showed initial improvement: six fully recovered, two showed incomplete improvement but fully recovered after insertion of an internal shunt and four patients died of other complications several days after the lumbar punctures had been started. Of the five remaining patients in whom lumbar puncture had no effect, two recovered after an internal shunt and three died of other complications. The rate of rebleeding (two of the 17 patients) was similar to what might have been expected, but of course the numbers were small (Hasan *et al.*, 1991a). Until controlled trials are available, and we think these are still needed and ethically justifiable, the tentative conclusion is that lumbar puncture seems a safe and reasonably effective way of treating those forms of acute hydrocephalus that are not obviously caused by intraventricular obstruction.

> *In patients deteriorating from acute hydrocephalus after subarachnoid haemorrhage it is worth trying lumbar punctures if spontaneous improvement does not occur within 24 hours, and if the probable site of obstruction is in the subarachnoid space, not in the ventricular system.*

External drainage

External drainage of the cerebral ventricles by a catheter inserted through a burr hole is, in many centres, the most common method of treating acute hydrocephalus. Internal drainage is rarely considered in the first few days because the blood in the cerebrospinal fluid will almost inevitably block the shunt system. After insertion of an external catheter, the improvement is usually rapid and sometimes dramatic (van Gijn *et al.*, 1985; Hasan *et al.*, 1989b). But, other problems

tend to intervene soon, particularly rebleeding and ventriculitis.

Rebleeding after insertion of an external drain occurs significantly more often than in patients with acute hydrocephalus who are not shunted or in patients without hydrocephalus (Raimondi & Torres, 1973; Papo *et al.*, 1984; van Gijn *et al.*, 1985; Hasan *et al.*, 1989b). None of these studies had a randomised design for assessing the effect of shunt insertion, but as the occurrence of rebleeding, in general, is not known to be associated with any determinant except loss of consciousness at the time of haemorrhage (weak factor; see Section 13.5.1) or the administration of TEA (strong factor; see Section 13.5.3), it is hard to see how the development of hydrocephalus or the selection for external drainage could be confounding factors that explain the excess of rebleeding after placement of a ventricular catheter. It is more plausible that the sudden decrease in intracranial pressure (particularly cerebrospinal fluid pressure), which is much more rapid than with lumbar puncture, disrupts the subtle forces that seal the clot at the site of the previous rupture. It has been suggested that an excess of rebleeding can be prevented by keeping the pressure of the cerebrospinal fluid not only below 25 mmHg but also above 15 mmHg (Pickard, 1984), but this has not been borne out by subsequent experience (Hasan *et al.*, 1989b). Milhorat (1987) advocated capitalisation on the expected improvement after external drainage by performing early aneurysm surgery at the same time. His results sound impressive: of 42 patients with acute hydrocephalus, 35 underwent external drainage and 29 survived. This is clearly yet another area where a randomised controlled trial is needed to settle the issue.

Ventriculitis is a frequent complication after external drainage, especially if drainage is continued for more than 3 days; of 31 patients treated with external drainage, 17 had died after 3 months and infection contributed to the death of five (Hasan *et al.*, 1989b). The use of prophylactic antibiotics or a long subcutaneous tunnel has been advocated but these measures have not been subjected to a controlled study.

13.10 Management of systemic complications

Neurologists and neurosurgeons are regularly confronted by non-neurological complications in patients with aneurysmal SAH which need intensive therapeutic intervention. Hyponatraemia is the most common of these but several other systemic disorders may cause secondary deterioration. Clinical detection of these metabolic derangements requires a high index of suspicion.

13.10.1 Hyponatraemia

In general, the causes of hyponatraemia vary according to the patient's volume status. In most, but not all cases, the total body sodium has remained constant but the water content of the extracellular volume is at fault, and hyponatraemia can be best classified according to the extracellular volume status. After the syndrome of inappropriate secretion of antidiuretic hormone (SIADH) was initially described in the 1950s (Bartter & Schwarz, 1967), hyponatraemia in SAH has often been incorrectly attributed to this syndrome. In SIADH there is a continuing secretion of ADH, not appropriate to changes of plasma volume and osmolality. The extracellular volume increases and by the expansion of the intravascular component of this volume a *dilutional hyponatraemia* ensues. Natriuresis takes place because the volume expansion increases the glomerular filtration rate and inhibits the secretion of aldosterone. Balance studies have shown that the degree of natriuresis is relatively small and approximately equals intake. The high concentration of urinary sodium in SIADH can be simply explained by the fact that the sodium intake must be excreted in a small volume of urine.

Hyponatraemia, with or without intravascular volume change, is the most common electrolyte disturbance following aneurysmal rupture. In one series of 290 patients with SAH only 10% developed hyponatraemia (Dóczi et al., 1981), but in other studies the frequency was higher. In a recent series of 244 prospectively studied patients admitted within 72 hours after the initial bleed, 34% developed hyponatraemia, defined as a sodium level of 134 mmol or less on at least two consecutive days (Hasan et al., 1989c).

The clinical manifestations of hyponatraemia include an impaired level of consciousness, asterixis, hemiparesis, seizures and coma (Arieff et al., 1976). These usually do not occur until the plasma sodium is less than 125 mmol/L, but irritability, restlessness and confusion can result from a rapid decline of sodium, particularly if the downward trend continues over a few days. Sodium levels below 100 mmol/L almost always give rise to seizures and, rarely, ventricular tachycardia or fibrillation (Arieff, 1986).

Hyponatraemia after SAH develops most commonly between the second and 10th day (Wijdicks et al., 1985a). Its cause is still uncertain. A prospective study of 21 patients demonstrated that the plasma volume decreased in most patients who developed hyponatraemia, and that this was preceded by a negative sodium balance in all instances. Serum vasopressin levels were increased or normal on admission, but had decreased by the time hyponatraemia occurred. An additional finding was that plasma volume considerably decreased, even in some patients with normal sodium levels,

usually as a result of excessive natriuresis (Wijdicks et al., 1985b). These findings supported the notion of *cerebral salt wasting* rather than the syndrome of inappropriate ADH secretion as the cause of hyponatraemia after SAH. It is clear that the volume status in these patients is extremely important.

A possible contributing factor in the development of hyponatraemia may be hydrocephalus, particularly enlargement of the third ventricle (van Gijn et al., 1985; Wijdicks et al., 1988a). This relationship is independent of the amount of cisternal blood or the location of the ruptured aneurysm but is partly dependent on the amount of intraventricular blood. Mechanical pressure on the hypothalamus can perhaps disturb sodium and water homeostasis. Two substances have been identified as being related to natriuresis and possibly acting as intermediary factors: a digoxin-like substance (Wijdicks et al., 1985b) and atrial natriuretic factor (Diringer et al., 1988; Rosenfeld et al., 1989; Wijdicks et al., 1991).

Correction of hyponatraemia in SAH is truly a problem of correcting volume depletion (Table 13.10). Acute symptomatic hyponatraemia is rare and requires urgent treatment with 3% saline. But, myelinolysis in the pons and the white matter of the hemispheres may complicate over-rapid infusion of sodium; a retrospective survey suggests the maximal rate of correction should be by 12 mmol/L per day (Sterns et al., 1986), but others maintain that more rapid correction is safe as long as the sodium level does not exceed 126 mmol/L during the first 24 hours (Ayus et al., 1987). A mild degree of hyponatraemia (125–134 mmol/L) is usually well tolerated, self-limiting and needs not to be treated in itself. Hyponatraemia in patients with evidence of a negative fluid balance or excessive natriuresis is corrected with isotonic saline (sodium concentration: 154 mmol/L) or with a mixture of glucose and saline (sodium concentration: 130 mmol/L). A central venous pressure between 8 and 10 mmHg or a pulmonary capillary wedge pressure of

Table 13.10 Management of hyponatraemia.

Almost invariably caused by sodium *depletion*, not by sodium dilution (SIADH)

Associated hypovolaemia increases risk of delayed cerebral ischaemia

Give isotonic saline (with or without albumin to expand plasma volume) or a mixture of glucose and saline; no free water

If necessary, add fludrocortisone acetate, 400 μg/day in two doses, orally or intravenously

Keep central venous pressure between 8 and 10 mmHg, or pulmonary capillary wedge pressure between 8 and 12 mmHg

8–12 mmHg indicates adequate filling of the intravascular compartment. Alternatively, albumin in a 5% solution in isotonic saline can be given to expand the intravascular volume. If necessary, up to 6 or even 9 L should be infused per 24 hours, and only rarely is it impossible to maintain a steady state in fluid balance with these measures. In resistant cases fludrocortisone acetate can be added (400 µg/day in two doses, intravenously or orally). In the only randomized study fludrocortisone acetate reduced the occurrence of a negative sodium balance (Hasan *et al.*, 1989a). There were no relevant side effects associated with overt hypervolaemia, such as marked hypertension or pulmonary oedema.

> *Hyponatraemia after subarachnoid haemorrhage usually reflects cerebral salt wasting (sodium depletion) and not secretion of antidiuretic hormone (sodium dilution). Hypovolaemia being the underlying cause of the hyponatraemia, it should be vigorously treated to prevent cerebral ischaemia.*

13.10.2 Disorders of heart rhythm

Aneurysmal rupture is commonly associated with cardiac arrhythmias and electrocardiographic (ECG) abnormalities. A commonly accepted explanation is sustained sympathetic stimulation, sometimes resulting in structural damage to the myocardium, which is often evident on echocardiograms (Pollick *et al.*, 1988). The histological features of myocardial damage are contraction bands, focal myocardial necrosis and subendocardial ischaemia. A more unconventional theo-

ry is the existence of an arrhythmogenic centre in the insular cortex (Svigelj *et al.*, 1994).

The most common ECG abnormalities in SAH (Fig. 13.6) are ST- and T-segment changes, prominent U waves, QT prolongation and sinus arrhythmias (Marion *et al.*, 1986; Stober *et al.*, 1988; Brouwers *et al.*, 1989). Life-threatening arrhythmias such as ventricular fibrillation or 'torsade de pointe' may be seen on 24-hour monitoring, but are extremely rare (Carruth & Silverman, 1980; Hijdra *et al.*, 1984; Andreoli *et al.*, 1987). A striking finding in a large and recent series of patients investigated by serial ECGs was that every patient had at least one abnormal ECG (Brouwers *et al.*, 1989). Virtually all ECG abnormalities changed to other abnormalities, without any consistent order, and then disappeared during the observation period of 10 days. Some patients had ECG changes that closely resembled those in acute myocardial infarction and these spontaneously disappeared the following day without any change in neurological or cardiac condition. Potentially dangerous arrhythmias or actual death from cardiac failure did not occur in this limited series. In contrast, others found runs of ventricular tachycardia in 20% of those monitored, and prolonged QT intervals in 60% (Estanol *et al.*, 1979). Prolonged QT intervals often represent delayed ventricular repolarisation and predispose to ventricular arrhythmias. The prognostic value of these ECG changes is not known, but in patients with SAH they are more important as indicators of intracranial disease than as predictors of potentially serious cardiac complications (Brouwers *et al.*, 1989; Manninen *et al.*, 1995).

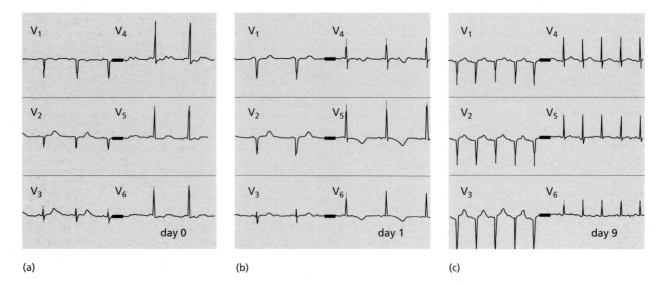

Figure 13.6 ECG abnormalities in a 74-year-old woman with SAH. (a) Day 1: ischaemic ST segment, prominent U wave and prolonged QT$_c$ interval. (b) Day 1: sinus bradycardia, ischaemic ST segment, ischaemic T wave, prolonged QT$_c$ interval and signs of left ventricular hypertrophy. (c) Day 9: sinus tachycardia, transient pathological Q wave and ischaemic ST segment.

Abnormalities of heart rhythm after subarachnoid haemorrhage represent 'smoke' rather than 'fire' and rarely need to be treated.

Generally, severe ventricular arrhythmias are of short duration. Beta-blockade has been proposed as preventive treatment aiming at lowering the sympathetic tone. In patients with head injury a double-blind, randomised study found that beta-blockers reduced catecholamine-induced cardiac necrosis, but not in-hospital case fatality (Cruickshank *et al.*, 1987). In patients with SAH, routine administration of beta-blockers is not warranted until there is evidence of improved overall outcome; the net benefits may be disappointing because beta-blockers also lower blood pressure. Clearly, controlled clinical trials are needed in patients with SAH.

13.10.3 Neurogenic pulmonary oedema

Neurogenic pulmonary oedema is a dramatic and dangerous complication. Usually, it has an extremely rapid onset, although a delayed course has been reported (Fisher & Aboul Nasr, 1979). What triggers pulmonary oedema is unclear. Elevated intracranial pressure can lead to a massive sympathetic discharge mediated by the anterior hypothalamus. Systemic hypertension often co-exists, but pulmonary oedema may present or even worsen during the lowering of systemic or pulmonary pressures. It has also been suggested that increased sympathetic activity leads to generalised vasoconstriction, including the pulmonary vasculature, and that direct damage to endothelial cells may result in increased permeability (Theodore & Robin, 1976).

Fortunately, this complication is rare. Its occurrence corresponds with the magnitude of aneurysmal haemorrhage and so it is rarely seen in patients with a normal level of consciousness (Weir, 1978). The typical clinical picture consists of unexpected dyspnoea, cyanosis and production of pink and frothy sputum. Many patients are pale, sweat excessively and are hypertensive. A chest X-ray usually demonstrates impressive pulmonary oedema (Fig. 13.7) which may disappear in a matter of hours following positive end-expiratory pressure ventilation (Wauchob *et al.*, 1984). Diuretics are often used as standard therapy and it has been claimed that labetalol or chlorpromazine are also beneficial (Wohns *et al.*, 1985; Harrier, 1988).

Neurogenic pulmonary oedema may be complicated by reversible decompensation of the left ventricle, clinically manifested by sudden hypotension following initially elevated blood pressures, transient lactic acidosis, mild elevation of the creatine kinase MB fraction and varied ECG changes during the first day, followed by widespread and persistent

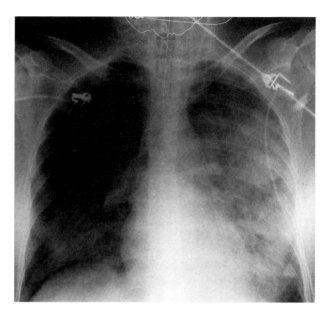

Figure 13.7 Chest X-ray with neurogenic pulmonary oedema (same patient as in Fig. 13.4).

T-wave inversions (Mayer *et al.*, 1994). In these cases of pulmonary oedema with secondary cardiac injury, treatment with pressor agents may be indicated.

13.10.4 Vitreous haemorrhages

Preretinal haemorrhages associated with SAH (see Sections 3.2.6 and 5.5.1) may break into the vitreous cavity (Terson's syndrome). This occurs in one or in both eyes, usually at the time of the initial haemorrhage, but sometimes several days later, and then mostly in association with rebleeding or sometimes arteriography. It may, however, take days or weeks before the patient is sufficiently alert to complain about blurred vision. In most cases, the vitreous haemorrhage clears spontaneously in a matter of weeks to months. In patients with bilateral severe haemorrhages, vitrectomy may be indicated to improve vision during the period of neurological recovery (Weingeist *et al.*, 1986; Huber *et al.*, 1988).

13.11 Management of unruptured aneurysms

Most aneurysms never rupture. On the assumption that 5% of the population eventually develop at least one aneurysm (see Section 9.1.1), and that the annual incidence of aneurysmal SAH is approximately six per 100 000, which corresponds with a lifetime risk of 0.5%, only about one in 10 cerebral aneurysms ever rupture. An intact aneurysm may be detected during angiography in patients who have already had a SAH from another aneurysm, or in patients without a history of intracranial haemorrhage who have angiography for a different reason. There is a possibility, but no conclusive evidence, that the risk of rupture is greater in patients with previous bleeds. In yet other patients, an aneurysm may be detected in the course of a screening programme (with brain CT or MR angiography) for a familial disorder, e.g. in families with autosomal dominant polycystic kidney disease (Chapman *et al.*, 1992), in families with SAH in three or more relatives (ter Berg *et al.*, 1992), and even in people with a single first-degree relative suffering from SAH (Bromberg *et al.*, 1995). In all these situations the practical dilemma is whether the operative risk associated with preventive clipping of the aneurysm is outweighed by the morbidity from eventual rupture of unoperated aneurysms. 'Intuition' fails in such a balance between short-term risks and long-term risks, although it was found some years ago that many neurosurgeons had adopted an approach either of 'never operate' or of 'always operate' (van Crevel *et al.*, 1986). It is especially in such situations that the technique of decision analysis is helpful. The most important factors can be estimated: (i) the annual risk of rupture (about 1% overall); (ii) the case fatality and morbidity after rupture; (iii) the risk of surgery (for the aneurysm in question *and* for the neurosurgeon in question); (iv) the life expectancy; and (v) the disutility of being handicapped, which is generally perceived as a greater disadvantage, even per year, in the immediate than in the more distant future (van Crevel *et al.*, 1986).

> *An unruptured aneurysm is not necessarily a 'time bomb', because only one in 10 ever ruptures. Whether surgery is warranted depends on the patient's age, the size of the aneurysm and the family history.*

The size of the aneurysm is probably an important factor. In the largest follow-up study of unruptured aneurysms, 15 of 51 aneurysms that were more than 10 mm in diameter ruptured in a mean follow-up period of 8 years, against none of 102 aneurysms that were less than 10 mm (Wiebers *et al.*, 1987). The growth rate of asymptomatic aneurysms may be an important determinant of the risk of rupture, a factor about which very little is known at present (Obuchowski *et al.*, 1995). A study from Finland found a relatively rapid enlargement in asymptomatic aneurysms that eventually ruptured, although many did so before growing to 10 mm, the median size before rupture being 4 mm (Juvela *et al.*, 1993). This last series consisted almost entirely of patients who had first come to attention because of a ruptured aneurysm and who had one or more unruptured aneurysms as well; because of this ascertainment bias, the relatively

small size at rupture does not necessarily apply to patients with a single incidental aneurysm. In general, the 'size principle' seems to go against the experience of neurosurgeons that most ruptured aneurysms measure less than 10 mm (Jane *et al.*, 1985). The most likely explanation is that the vast majority of aneurysms are of small size, and that even a minute fraction of those rupturing will still outnumber a greater proportion of the smaller number of larger aneurysms that rupture. The corollary of this finding is the 'prevention paradox' formulated by Rose (1992): screening the population for people at high risk (large aneurysms) will do little to change the burden of the disease because most patients who actually have a SAH are at low risk from smaller aneurysms (see Section 18.4).

In individual patients with incidentally discovered aneurysms of 10–25 mm, these are associated with an annual risk of rupture of the order of 3–4%, and surgical treatment seems warranted for the time being, with an upper age limit of around 69 years for men and 75 years for women (Auger & Wiebers, 1991); the risk of death or disabling deficits from surgery with these middle-sized aneurysms is around 5% (Solomon *et al.*, 1994). Of course, one is justified in adjusting the life expectancy according to the 'biological age' of a given patient. Smaller aneurysms, with an annual risk of rupture that is 0.5% or less, should best be left unoperated, even at the age of 45 years (van Crevel *et al.*, 1986), and even though the risk of operation is also very small (Solomon *et al.*, 1994). In 1996 refinements of this advice may evolve from a collaborative project involving 3500 patients, coordinated by Dr Wiebers at the Mayo Clinic (the International Study of Unruptured Intracranial Aneurysms).

What about the need for screening patients not known to have an aneurysm but who have first-degree relatives with SAH? Even in families with three or more first-degree relatives definitely affected, where any coincidence can be discounted, the risks of catheter angiography by means of iodinated contrast agents, intravenous or intra-arterial, are only marginally outweighed by the net benefits of surgery if an aneurysm is detected, according to the results of decision analysis. However, the recent advent of MR angiography, without any attendant risk (see Section 9.4.3), has now considerably lowered the threshold for screening in such families; a first study from Finland reporting a yield of 10% (Ronkainen *et al.*, 1994). It is not yet clear how often a negative study should be repeated. Another unanswered question is whether MR angiography is now indicated in first-degree relatives of patients with 'sporadic' SAH. Studies suggesting an increased risk for family members, in general, suffer from a number of problems: (i) incomplete ascertainment of all living relatives; (ii) failure to separate different degrees of kinship; and (iii) no allowance for expected incidence (Norrgård *et al.*, 1987). A study in which these disadvantages were avoided found an odds ratio for first- against second-degree relatives of 6.5 for definite or probable episodes of SAH (95% CI: 2.0–21); if possible episodes were also included, the odds ratio dropped to 2.8 (95% CI: 1.4–5.7). The frequency in second-degree relatives was of the same order of magnitude as for the general population (Bromberg *et al.*, 1995). These results certainly warrant a pilot study of screening amongst first-degree relatives of patients with 'sporadic' SAH in which not only the number of aneurysms detected and operated is entered into the equation, but also the costs and the delicate balance between reassurance and new worries in the subjects under study.

References

Adams HP Jr (1987). Antifibrinolytics in aneurysmal subarachnoid hemorrhage. Do they have a role? Maybe. *Arch Neurol* 44: 114–15.

Allen GS, Ahn HS, Preziosi TJ *et al.* (1983). Cerebral arterial spasm—a controlled trial of nimodipine in patients with subarachnoid hemorrhage. *N Engl J Med* 308: 619–24.

Alvord EC, Loeser JD, Bailey WL, Copass MK (1972). Subarachnoid hemorrhage due to ruptured aneurysms—a simple method of estimating prognosis. *Arch Neurol* 27: 273–84.

Andreoli A, di Pasquale G, Pinelli G, Grazi P, Tognetti F, Testa C (1987). Subarachnoid hemorrhage: frequency and severity of cardiac arrhythmias. A survey of 70 cases studied in the acute phase. *Stroke* 18: 558–64.

Anonymous (1992). Effect of calcitonin-gene-related peptide in patients with delayed postoperative cerebral ischaemia after aneurysmal subarachnoid haemorrhage. European CGRP in Subarachnoid Haemorrhage Study Group. *Lancet* 339: 831–4.

Aoyagi N, Hayakawa I (1984). Analysis of 223 ruptured intracranial aneurysms with special reference to rerupture. *Surg Neurol* 21: 445–52.

Arieff AI (1986). Hyponatremia, convulsions, respiratory arrest and permanent brain damage after elective surgery in healthy women. *N Engl J Med* 314: 1529–35.

Arieff AI, Llach F, Massry SG (1976). Neurological manifestations and morbidity of hyponatremia: correlation with brain water and electrolytes. *Medicine (Baltimore)* 55: 121–9.

Auger RG, Wiebers DO (1991). Management of unruptured intracranial aneurysms: a decision analysis. *J Stroke Cerebrovasc Dis* 1: 174–81.

Awad IA, Carter LP, Spetzler RF, Medina M, Williams FC Jr (1987). Clinical vasospasm after subarachnoid hemorrhage: response to hypervolemic hemodilution and arterial hypertension. *Stroke* 18: 365–72.

Ayus JC, Krothapalli RK, Arieff AI (1987). Treatment of symptomatic hyponatremia and its relation to brain damage. A prospective study. *N Engl J Med* 317: 1190–5.

Bartter FC, Schwarz WB (1967). The syndrome of inappropriate secretion of antdiuretic hormone. *Am J Med* 42: 790–806.

Bauer LA (1982). Interference of oral phenytoin absorption by continuous nasogastric feedings. *Neurology* 32: 570–2.

Beck DW, Adams HP, Flamm ES, Godersky JC, Loftus CM (1988). Combination of aminocaproic acid and nicardipine in treatment of aneurysmal subarachnoid hemorrhage. *Stroke* 19: 63–7.

Biller J, Godersky JC, Adams HP Jr (1988). Management of aneurysmal subarachnoid hemorrhage. *Stroke* 19: 1300–5.

Brandt L, Sonesson B, Ljunggren B, Såveland H (1987). Ruptured middle cerebral artery aneurysm with intracerebral hemorrhage in younger patients appearing moribund: emergency operation? *Neurosurgery* 20: 925–9.

Broderick JP, Brott TG, Duldner JE, Tomsick T, Leach A (1994). Initial and recurrent bleeding are the major causes of death following subarachnoid hemorrhage. *Stroke* 25: 1342–7.

Bromberg JEC, Rinkel GJE, Algra A *et al.* (1995). Subarachnoid haemorrhage in first and second degree relatives of patients with subarachnoid haemorrhage. *Br Med J* 311: 288–9.

Brouwers PJAM, Wijdicks EFM, Van Gijn J (1992). Infarction after aneurysm rupture does not depend on distribution or clearance rate of blood. *Stroke* 23: 374–9.

Brouwers PJAM, Wijdicks EFM, Hasan D *et al.* (1989). Serial electrocardiographic recording in aneurysmal subarachnoid hemorrhage. *Stroke* 20: 1162–7.

Calhoun DA, Oparil S (1990). Treatment of hypertensive crisis. *N Engl J Med* 323: 1177–83.

Candia GJ, Heros RC, Lavyne MH, Zervas NT, Nelson CN (1978). Effect of intravenous sodium nitroprusside on cerebral blood flow and intracranial pressure. *Neurosurgery* 3: 50–3.

Carruth JE, Silverman ME (1980). Torsade de pointe atypical ventricular tachycardia complicating subarachnoid hemorrhage. *Chest* 78: 886–8.

Casasco A, Arnaud O, Gobin P *et al.* (1992). [Giant intracranial aneurysm. Elective endovascular treatment using metallic coils.] Anevrysmes geants intracraniens. Traitement endovasculaire electif par des spires metalliques. *Neurochirurgie* 38: 18–26.

Chapman AB, Rubinstein D, Hughes R *et al.* (1992). Intracranial aneurysms in autosomal dominant polycystic kidney disease. *N Engl J Med* 327: 916–20.

Clarke Pearson DL, Synan IS, Hinshaw WM, Coleman RE, Creasman WT (1984). Prevention of postoperative venous thromboembolism by external pneumatic calf compression in patients with gynecologic malignancy. *Obstet Gynecol* 63: 92–8.

Conway LW, McDonald LW (1972). Structural changes of the intradural arteries following subarachnoid hemorrhage. *J Neurosurg* 37: 715–23.

Coppolo DP, May JJ (1990). Self-extubations. A 12-month experience. *Chest* 98: 165–9.

Crawford MD, Sarner M (1965). Ruptured intracranial aneurysm —a community study. *Lancet* ii: 1254–7.

Cruickshank JM, Neil Dwyer G, Degaute JP *et al.* (1987). Reduction of stress/catecholamine-induced cardiac necrosis by beta 1-selective blockade. *Lancet* 2: 585–9.

Davis S, Andrews J, Lichtenstein M *et al.* (1990). A single-photon emission computed tomography study of hypoperfusion after subarachnoid hemorrhage. *Stroke* 21: 252–9.

Di Mascio R, Marchioli R, Tognoni G (1993). From pharmacological promises to controlled clinical trials to meta-analysis and back: the case of nimodipine in cerebrovascular disorders. *Clin Trials Meta-anal* 29: 57–79.

Diringer M, Ladenson PW, Stern BJ, Schleimer J, Hanley DF (1988). Plasma atrial natriuretic factor and subarachnoid hemorrhage. *Stroke* 19: 1119–24.

Dóczi T, Bende J, Huszka E, Kiss J (1981). Syndrome of inappropriate secretion of antidiuretic hormone after subarachnoid hemorrhage. *Neurosurgery* 9: 394–7.

Drake CG, Hunt WE, Sano K *et al.* (1988). Report of World Federation of Neurological Surgeons Committee on a Universal Subarachnoid Hemorrhage Grading Scale. *J Neurosurg* 68: 985–6.

Eskesen V, Karle A, Kruse A, Kruse Larsen C, Praestholm J, Schmidt K (1987). Observer variability in assessment of angiographic vasospasm after aneurysmal subarachnoid haemorrhage. *Acta Neurochir Wien* 87: 54–7.

Estanol BV, Dergal EB, Cesarman E *et al.* (1979). Cardiac arrhythmias associated with subarachnoid hemorrhage: prospective study. *Neurosurgery* 5: 675–9.

Farhat SM, Schneider RC (1967). Observations on the effect of systemic blood pressure on intracranial circulation in patients with cerebrovascular insufficiency. *J Neurosurg* 27: 441–5.

Fernandez Zubillaga A, Guglielmi G, Vinuela F, Duckwiler GR (1994). Endovascular occlusion of intracranial aneurysms with electrically detachable coils: correlation of aneurysm neck size and treatment results. *Am J Neuroradiol* 15: 815–20.

Findlay JM, Weir BK, Kanamaru K, Espinosa F (1989). Arterial wall changes in cerebral vasospasm. *Neurosurgery* 25: 736–45.

Findlay JM, Kassell NF, Weir BKA *et al.* (1995). A randomized trial of intraoperative, intracisternal tissue plasminogen activator for the prevention of vasospasm. *Neurosurgery* 37: 168–78.

Finn SS, Stephensen SA, Miller CA, Drobnich L, Hunt WE (1986). Observations on the perioperative management of aneurysmal subarachnoid hemorrhage. *J Neurosurg* 65: 48–62.

Fisher A, Aboul Nasr HT (1979). Delayed nonfatal pulmonary edema following subarachnoid hemorrhage. Case report. *J Neurosurg* 51: 856–9.

Fisher CM, Kistler JP, Davis JM (1980). Relation of cerebral vasospasm to subarachnoid hemorrhage visualized by computerized tomographic scanning. *Neurosurgery* 6: 1–9.

Fisher CM, Roberson GH, Ojemann RG (1977). Cerebral vasospasm with ruptured saccular aneurysm—the clinical manifestations. *Neurosurgery* 1: 245–8.

Fodstad H, Pilbrant A, Schannong M, Strömberg S (1981). Determination of tranexamic acid and fibrin/fibrinogen degradation products in cerebrospinal fluid after aneurysmal subarachnoid haemorrhage. *Acta Neurochir Wien* 58: 1–13.

Foy PM, Chadwick DW, Rajgopalan N, Johnson AL, Shaw MD (1992). Do prophylactic anticonvulsant drugs alter the pattern of seizures after craniotomy? *J Neurol Neurosurg Psychiatr* 55: 753–7.

Gifford RW Jr (1991). Management of hypertensive crises. *J Am Med Assoc* 266: 829–35.

Graff-Radford NR, Torner J, Adams HP Jr, Kassell NF (1989). Factors associated with hydrocephalus after subarachnoid hemorrhage. A report of the Cooperative Aneurysm Study. *Arch Neurol* 46: 744–52.

Greenberg DA (1987). Calcium channels and calcium channel antagonists. *Ann Neurol* 21: 317–30.

Grote E, Hassler W (1988). The critical first minutes after subarachnoid hemorrhage. *Neurosurgery* 22: 654–61.

Guglielmi G, Vinuela F, Duckwiler G *et al.* (1992). Endovascular treatment of posterior circulation aneurysms by electrothrombosis using electrically detachable coils. *J Neurosurg* 77: 515–24.

Haley EC Jr, Kassell NF, Torner JC (1993a). A randomized controlled trial of high-dose intravenous nicardipine in aneurysmal subarachnoid hemorrhage. A report of the Cooperative Aneurysm Study. *J Neurosurg* 78: 537–47.

Haley EC Jr, Kassell NF, Torner JC (1993b). A randomized trial of nicardipine in subarachnoid hemorrhage: angiographic and transcranial Doppler ultrasound results. A report of the Cooperative Aneurysm Study. *J Neurosurg* 78: 548–53.

Haley EC Jr, Kassell NF, Alves WM, Weir BKA, Hansen CA (1995). Phase II trial of tirilazad in aneurysmal subarachnoid hemorrhage. A report of the Cooperative Aneurysm Study. *J Neurosurg* 82: 786–90.

Haley EC Jr, Kassell NF, Torner JC, Truskowski LL, Germanson TP (1994). A randomized trial of two doses of nicardipine in aneurysmal subarachnoid hemorrhage. A report of the Cooperative Aneurysm Study. *J Neurosurg* 80: 788–96.

Harrier HD (1988). Use of labetalol in trauma. *Crit Care Med* 16: 1159–60.

Hart RG, Byer JA, Slaughter JR, Hewett JE, Easton JD (1981). Occurrence and implications of seizures in subarachnoid hemorrhage due to ruptured intracranial aneurysms. *Neurosurgery* 8: 417–21.

Hasan D, Tanghe HL (1992). Distribution of cisternal blood in patients with acute hydrocephalus after subarachnoid hemorrhage. *Ann Neurol* 31: 374–8.

Hasan D, Lindsay KW, Vermeulen M (1991a). Treatment of acute hydrocephalus after subarachnoid hemorrhage with serial lumbar puncture. *Stroke* 22: 190–4.

Hasan D, Wijdicks EFM, Vermeulen M (1990). Hyponatremia is associated with cerebral ischemia in patients with aneurysmal subarachnoid hemorrhage. *Ann Neurol* 27: 106–8.

Hasan D, van Peski J, Loeve I, Krenning EP, Vermeulen M (1991b). Single photon emission computed tomography in patients with acute hydrocephalus or with cerebral ischaemia after subarachnoid haemorrhage. *J Neurol Neurosurg Psychiatr* 54: 490–3.

Hasan D, Vermeulen M, Wijdicks EFM, Hijdra A, Van Gijn J (1989b). Effect of fluid intake and antihypertensive treatment on cerebral ischemia after subarachnoid hemorrhage. *Stroke* 20: 1511–15.

Hasan D, Vermeulen M, Wijdicks EFM, Hijdra A, Van Gijn J

(1989c). Management problems in acute hydrocephalus after subarachnoid hemorrhage. *Stroke* 20: 747–53.

Hasan D, Schonck RS, Avezaat CJ, Tanghe HL, Van Gijn J, van der Lugt PJ (1993). Epileptic seizures after subarachnoid hemorrhage. *Ann Neurol* 33: 286–91.

Hasan D, Lindsay KW, Wijdicks EFM *et al.* (1989a). Effect of fludrocortisone acetate in patients with subarachnoid hemorrhage. *Stroke* 20: 1156–61.

Hauerberg J, Eskesen V, Rosenorn J (1994). The prognostic significance of intracerebral haematoma as shown on CT scanning after aneurysmal subarachnoid haemorrhage. *Br J Neurosurg* 8: 333–9.

Heiskanen O, Poranen A, Kuurne T, Valtonen S, Kaste M (1988). Acute surgery for intracerebral haematomas caused by rupture of an intracranial arterial aneurysm. A prospective randomized study. *Acta Neurochir Wien* 90: 81–3.

Heros RC, Zervas NT, Varsos V (1983). Cerebral vasospasm after subarachnoid hemorrhage: an update. *Ann Neurol* 14: 599–608.

Higashida RT, Halbach VV, Cahan LD *et al.* (1989) Transluminal angioplasty for treatment of intracranial arterial vasospasm. *J Neurosurg* 71: 648–53.

Hijdra A, Van Gijn J (1982). Early death from rupture of an intracranial aneurysm. *J Neurosurg* 57: 765–8.

Hijdra A, Brouwers PJ, Vermeulen M, Van Gijn J (1990). Grading the amount of blood on computed tomograms after subarachnoid hemorrhage. *Stroke* 21: 1156–61.

Hijdra A, Vermeulen M, Van Gijn J, van Crevel H (1987b). Reruptature of intracranial aneurysms: a clinicoanatomic study. *J Neurosurg* 67: 29–33.

Hijdra A, Vermeulen M, Van Gijn J, van Crevel H (1984). Respiratory arrest in subarachnoid hemorrhage. *Neurology* 34: 1501–3.

Hijdra A, Braakman R, Van Gijn J, Vermeulen M, van Crevel H (1987a). Aneurysmal subarachnoid hemorrhage. Complications and outcome in a hospital population. *Stroke* 18: 1061–7.

Hijdra A, van Gijn J, Nagelkerke NJJ, Vermeulen M, van Crevel H (1988). Prediction of delayed cerebral ischaemia, rebleeding and outcome after aneurysmal subarachnoid hemorrhage. *Stroke* 19: 1250–6.

Hijdra A, Van Gijn J, Stefanko S, van Dongen KJ, Vermeulen M, van Crevel H (1986). Delayed cerebral ischemia after aneurysmal subarachnoid hemorrhage: clinicoanatomic correlations. *Neurology* 36: 329–33.

Honma Y, Fujiwara T, Irie K, Ohkawa M, Nagao S (1995). Morphological changes in human cerebral arteries after percutaneous transluminal angioplasty for vasospasm caused by subarachnoid hemorrhage. *Neurosurgery* 36: 1073–81.

Huber A, Klöti R, Landolt E (1988). Terson's syndrome. *Neuro-ophthalmology* 8: 223–33.

Hughes JT, Schianchi PM (1978). Cerebral artery spasm—a histological study at necropsy of the blood vessels in cases of subarachnoid hemorrhage. *J Neurosurg* 48: 515–25.

Inagawa T, Kamiya K, Ogasawara H, Yano T (1987). Rebleeding of ruptured intracranial aneurysms in the acute stage. *Surg Neurol* 28: 93–9.

Inagawa T, Tokuda Y, Ohbayashi N, Takaya M, Moritake K (1995). Study of aneurysmal subarachnoid hemorrhage in Izumo City, Japan. *Stroke* 26: 761–6.

Jan M, Buchheit F, Tremoulet M (1988). Therapeutic trial of intravenous nimodipine in patients with established cerebral vasospasm after rupture of intracranial aneurysms. *Neurosurgery* 23: 154–7.

Jane JA, Kassell NF, Torner JC, Winn HR (1985). The natural history of aneurysms and arteriovenous malformations. *J Neurosurg* 62: 321–3.

Jennett B, Bond M (1975). Assessment of outcome after severe brain damage: a practical scale. *Lancet* i: 480–4.

Juvela S (1995). Aspirin and delayed cerebral ischemia after aneurysmal subarachnoid hemorrhage. *J Neurosurg* 82: 945–52.

Juvela S, Porras M, Heiskanen O (1993). Natural history of unruptured intracranial aneurysms: a long-term follow-up study. *J Neurosurg* 79: 174–82.

Kaku Y, Yonekawa Y, Tsukahara T, Kazekawa K (1992). Superselective intra-arterial infusion of papaverine for the treatment of cerebral vasospasm after subarachnoid hemorrhage. *J Neurosurg* 77: 842–7.

Kaneko T, Sawada T, Niimi T (1983). Lower limit of blood pressure in treatment of acute hypertensive intracranial hemorrhage (AHCH). *J Cereb Blood Flow Metab* 3 (Suppl. 1): S51–2.

Kassell NF, Torner JC (1983). Aneurysmal rebleeding: a preliminary report from the Cooperative Aneurysm Study. *Neurosurgery* 13: 479–81.

Kassell NF, Torner JC, Adams HP Jr (1984). Antifibrinolytic therapy in the acute period following aneurysmal subarachnoid hemorrhage. Preliminary observations from the Cooperative Aneurysm Study. *J Neurosurg* 61: 225–30.

Kassell NF, Torner JC, Jane JA, Haley EC Jr, Adams HP (1990b). The International Cooperative Study on the Timing of Aneurysm Surgery. Part 2: surgical results. *J Neurosurg* 73: 37–47.

Kassell NF, Peerless SJ, Durward QJ, Beck DW, Drake CG, Adams HP (1982). Treatment of ischemic deficits from vasospasm with intravascular volume expansion and induced arterial hypertension. *Neurosurgery* 11: 337–43.

Kassell NF, Torner JC, Haley EC Jr, Jane JA, Adams HP, Kongable GL (1990a). The International Cooperative Study on the Timing of Aneurysm Surgery. Part 1: overall management results. *J Neurosurg* 73: 18–36.

Kistler JP, Crowell RM, Davis KR *et al.* (1983). The relation of cerebral vasospasm to the extent and location of subarachnoid blood visualized by CT scan: a prospective study. *Neurology* 33: 424–36.

Kolluri VR, Sengupta RP (1984). Symptomatic hydrocephalus following aneurysmal subarachnoid hemorrhage. *Surg Neurol* 21: 402–4.

Kosnik EJ, Hunt WE (1976). Postoperative hypertension in the management of patients with intracranial arterial aneurysms. *J Neurosurg* 45: 148–54.

Linskey ME, Horton JA, Rao GR, Yonas H (1991). Fatal rupture of the intracranial carotid artery during transluminal angioplasty for vasospasm induced by subarachnoid hemorrhage. Case report. *J Neurosurg* 74: 985–90.

Ljunggren B, Saveland H, Brandt L, Zygmunt S (1985). Early operation and overall outcome in aneurysmal subarachnoid hemorrhage. *J Neurosurg* 62: 547–51.

Locksley HB (1966). Report of the Cooperative Study on intracranial aneurysms and subarachnoid hemorrhage. Section V, part II. Natural history of subarachnoid hemorrhage, intracranial aneurysms, and arteriovenous malformations. *J Neurosurg* 25: 321–68.

Maas AI, Braakman R, Schouten HJ, Minderhoud JM, van Zomeren AH (1983). Agreement between physicians on assessment of outcome following severe head injury. *J Neurosurg* 58: 321–5.

McKissock W, Richardson A, Walsh L (1960). 'Posterior-communicating aneurysms'. A controlled trial of conservative and surgical treatment of ruptured aneurysms of the internal carotid artery at or near the point of origin of the posterior communicating artery. *Lancet* i: 1203–6.

McKissock W, Richardson A, Walsh L (1965). Anterior communicating aneurysms. A trial of conservative and surgical treatment. *Lancet* i: 873–6.

Manninen PH, Ayra B, Gelb AW, Pelz D (1995). Association between electrocardiographic abnormalities and intracranial blood in patients following acute subarachnoid hemorrhage. *J Neurosurg Anesthesiol* 7: 12–16.

Marion DW, Segal R, Thompson ME (1986). Subarachnoid hemorrhage and the heart. *Neurosurgery* 18: 101–6.

Maurice-Williams RS (1982). Ruptured intracranial aneurysms: has the incidence of early rebleeding been over-estimated? *J Neurol Neurosurg Psychiatr* 45: 774–9.

Maurice-Williams RS, Marsh H (1985). Ruptured intracranial aneurysms: the overall effect of treatment and the influence of patient selection and data presentation on the reported outcome. *J Neurol Neurosurg Psychiatr* 48: 1208–12.

Mayer SA, Fink ME, Homma S *et al.* (1994). Cardiac injury associated with neurogenic pulmonary edema following subarachnoid hemorrhage. *Neurology* 44: 815–20.

Milhorat TH (1987). Acute hydrocephalus after aneurysmal subarachnoid hemorrhage. *Neurosurgery* 20: 15–20.

Millikan CH (1975). Cerebral vasospasm and ruptured intracranial aneurysm. *Arch Neurol* 32: 433–49.

Mizukami M, Kawase T, Usami T, Tazawa T (1982). Prevention of vasospasm by early operation with removal of subarachnoid blood. *Neurosurgery* 10: 301–7.

Molyneux AJ, Ellison DW, Morris J, Byrne JV (1995). Histological findings in giant aneurysms treated with Guglielmi detachable coils. Report of two cases with autopsy correlation. *J Neurosurg* 83: 129–32.

Muizelaar JP, Vermeulen M, van Crevel H *et al.* (1988). Outcome of aneurysmal subarachnoid hemorrhage in patients 66 years of age and older. *Clin Neurol Neurosurg* 90: 203–7.

Nakahara I, Handa H, Nishikawa M *et al.* (1992). Endovascular coil embolization of a recurrent giant internal carotid artery aneurysm via the posterior communicating artery after cervical carotid ligation: case report. *Surg Neurol* 38: 57–62.

Neil Dwyer G, Mee E, Dorrance D, Lowe D (1987). Early intervention with nimodipine in subarachnoid haemorrhage. *Eur Heart J* 8 (Suppl. K): 41–7.

Newell DW, Eskridge JM, Mayberg MR, Grady MS, Winn HR (1989). Angioplasty for the treatment of symptomatic vasospasm following subarachnoid hemorrhage. *J Neurosurg* 71: 654–60.

Nibbelink DW, Torner JC, Henderson WG (1981). Randomised treatment study—drug-induced hypotension. In: Sahs AL, Nibbelink DW, Torner JC, eds. *Aneurysmal Subarachnoid Hemorrhage—Report of the Cooperative Study*. Baltimore: Urban & Schwartzenberg, 77–106.

Nichols DA, Meyer FB, Piepgras DG, Smith PL (1994). Endovascular treatment of intracranial aneurysms. *Mayo Clin Proc* 69: 272–85.

Norrgård O, Ångquist KA, Fodstad H, Forsell A, Lindberg M (1987). Intracranial aneurysms and heredity. *Neurosurgery* 20: 236–9.

Numaguchi Y, Pevsner PH, Rigamonti D, Ragheb J (1992). Platinum coil treatment of complex aneurysms of the vertebrobasilar circulation. *Neuroradiology* 34: 252–5.

Obuchowski NA, Modic MT, Magdinec M (1995). Current implications for the efficacy of noninvasive screening for occult intracranial aneurysms in patients with a family history of aneurysms. *J Neurosurg* 83: 42–9.

Öhman J, Heiskanen O (1988). Effect of nimodipine on the outcome of patients after aneurysmal subarachnoid hemorrhage and surgery. *J Neurosurg* 69: 683–6.

Öhman J, Heiskanen O (1989). Timing of operation for ruptured supratentorial aneurysms: a prospective randomized study. *J Neurosurg* 70: 55–60.

Öhman J, Servo A, Heiskanen O (1991). Effect of intrathecal fibrinolytic therapy on clot lysis and vasospasm in patients with aneurysmal subarachnoid hemorrhage. *J Neurosurg* 75: 197–201.

Pakarinen S (1967). Incidence, aetiology and prognosis of primary subarachnoid haemorrhage. *Acta Neurol Scand* 43 (Suppl. 29): 1–128.

Papo I, Bodosi M, Merei TF, Luongo A (1984). [Hydrocephalus following subarachnoid hemorrhage] L'hydrocephalie aprés hemorragie sous-arachnoidienne. *Neurochirurgie* 30: 159–64.

Petruk KC, West M, Mohr G *et al.* (1988). Nimodipine treatment in poor-grade aneurysm patients. Results of a multicenter double-blind placebo-controlled trial. *J Neurosurg* 68: 505–17.

Philippon J, Grob R, Dagreou F, Guggiari M, Rivierez M, Viars P (1986). Prevention of vasospasm in subarachnoid haemorrhage. A controlled study with nimodipine. *Acta Neurochir Wien* 82: 110–14.

Phillips LH, Whisnant JP, O'Fallon WM, Sundt TM (1980). The unchanging pattern of subarachnoid hemorrhage in a community. *Neurology* 30: 1034–40.

Pickard JD (1984). Early posthaemorrhagic hydrocephalus [editorial]. *Br Med J* 289: 569–70.

Pickard JD, Murray GD, Illingworth R *et al.* (1989). Effect of oral nimodipine on cerebral infarction and outcome after subarachnoid haemorrhage: British aneurysm nimodipine trial. *Br Med J* 298: 636–42.

Pollick C, Cujec B, Parker S, Tator C (1988). Left ventricular wall motion abnormalities in subarachnoid hemorrhage: an echocardiographic study. *J Am Coll Cardiol* 12: 600–5.

Post MJ, Borst C, Kuntz RE (1994). The relative importance of arterial remodeling compared with intimal hyperplasia in lumen renarrowing after balloon angioplasty. A study in the normal rabbit and the hypercholesterolemic Yucatan micropig. *Circulation* 89: 2816–21.

Raimondi AJ, Torres H (1973). Acute hydrocephalus as a complication of subarachnoid hemorrhage. *Surg Neurol* 1: 23–6.

Ramirez-Lassepas M (1981). Antifibrinolytic therapy in subarachnoid hemorrhage caused by ruptured intracranial aneurysm. *Neurology* 31: 316–22.

Rinkel GJE, Van Gijn J, Wijdicks EFM (1993). Subarachnoid hemorrhage without detectable aneurysm. A review of the causes. *Stroke* 24: 1403–9.

Rinkel GJE, Wijdicks EFM, Ramos LMP, Van Gijn J (1990). Progression of acute hydrocephalus in subarachnoid haemorrhage: a case report documented by serial CT scanning. *J Neurol Neurosurg Psychiatr* 53: 354–5.

Rinkel GJE, Wijdicks EFM, Vermeulen M, Hasan D, Brouwers PJAM, Van Gijn J (1991). The clinical course of perimesencephalic nonaneurysmal subarachnoid hemorrhage. *Ann Neurol* 29: 463–8.

Rinkel GJE, Wijdicks EFM, Vermeulen M, Tans JTJ, Hasan D, Van Gijn J (1992). Acute hydrocephalus in nonaneurysmal perimesencephalic hemorrhage: evidence of CSF block at the tentorial hiatus. *Neurology* 42: 1805–7.

Ronkainen A, Hernesniemi J, Ryynanen M, Puranen M, Kuivaniemi H (1994). A ten percent prevalence of asymptomatic familial intracranial aneurysms: preliminary report on 110 magnetic resonance angiography studies in members of 21 Finnish familial intracranial aneurysm families. *Neurosurgery* 35: 208–12.

Rose FC, Sarner M (1965). Epilepsy after ruptured intracranial aneurysm. *Br Med J* 1: 18–21.

Rose G (1992). *The Strategy of Preventive Medicine*. Oxford: Oxford Medical Publications.

Rosenfeld JV, Barnett GH, Sila CA, Little JR, Bravo EL, Beck GJ (1989). The effect of subarachnoid hemorrhage on blood and CSF atrial natriuretic factor. *J Neurosurg* 71: 32–7.

Rousseaux P, Scherpereel R, Bernard MH, Graftieaux JP, Guyot JF (1980). Fever and cerebral vasospasm in intracranial aneurysms. *Surg Neurol* 14: 459–65.

Rowley G, Fielding K (1991). Reliability and accuracy of the Glasgow Coma Scale with experienced and inexperienced users. *Lancet* 337: 535–8.

Schievink WI, Wijdicks EFM, Parisi JE, Piepgras DG, Whisnant JP (1995a). Sudden death from aneurysmal subarachnoid hemorrhage. *Neurology* 45: 871–4.

Schievink WI, Wijdicks EFM, Piepgras DG, Chu CP, O'Fallon WM, Whisnant JP (1995b). The poor prognosis of ruptured

intracranial aneurysms of the posterior circulation. *J Neurosurg* 82: 791–5.

Sloan MA, Burch CM, Wozniak MA et al. (1994). Transcranial Doppler detection of vertebrobasilar vasospasm following subarachnoid hemorrhage. *Stroke* 25: 2187–97.

Sloan MA, Haley EC Jr, Kassell NF et al. (1989). Sensitivity and specificity of transcranial Doppler ultrasonography in the diagnosis of vasospasm following subarachnoid hemorrhage. *Neurology* 39: 1514–18.

Smith B (1963). Cerebral pathology in subarachnoid haemorrhage. *J Neurol Neurosurg Psychiatr* 26: 67–70.

Smith RR, Clower BR, Peeler DF Jr, Yoshioka J (1983). The angiopathy of subarachnoid hemorrhage: angiographic and morphologic correlates. *Stroke* 14: 240–5.

Solomon RA, Fink ME, Pile Spellman J (1994). Surgical management of unruptured intracranial aneurysms. *J Neurosurg* 80: 440–6.

Sterns RH, Riggs JE, Schochet SS Jr (1986). Osmotic demyelination syndrome following correction of hyponatremia. *N Engl J Med* 314: 1535–42.

Stober T, Anstatt T, Sen S, Schimrigk K, Jager H (1988). Cardiac arrhythmias in subarachnoid haemorrhage. *Acta Neurochir Wien* 93: 37–44.

Svigelj V, Grad A, Tekavcic I, Kiauta T (1994). Cardiac arrhythmia associated with reversible damage to insula in a patient with subarachnoid hemorrhage. *Stroke* 25: 1053–5.

Swash M (1974). Periaqueductal dysfunction (the Sylvian aqueduct syndrome): a sign of hydrocephalus? *J Neurol Neurosurg Psychiatr* 37: 21–6.

Teasdale G, Jennett B (1974). Assessment of coma and impaired consciousness—a practical scale. *Lancet* ii: 81–4.

ter Berg HW, Dippel DW, Limburg M, Schievink WI, Van Gijn J (1992). Familial intracranial aneurysms. A review. *Stroke* 23: 1024–30.

Theodore J, Robin ED (1976). Speculations on neurogenic pulmonary edema (NPE). *Am Rev Respir Dis* 113: 405–11.

Torner JC, Nibbelink DW, Burmeister LF (1981b). Statistical comparisons of end results of a randomised treatment study. In: Sahs AL, Nibbelink DW, Torner JC, eds. *Aneurysmal Subarachnoid Hemorrhage—Report of the Cooperative Study*. Baltimore: Urban & Schwartzenberg, 249–75.

Torner JC, Kassell NF, Wallace RB, Adams HP Jr (1981a). Preoperative prognostic factors for rebleeding and survival in aneurysm patients receiving antifibrinolytic therapy: report of the Cooperative Aneurysm Study. *Neurosurgery* 9: 506–13.

Tsukahara T, Wada H, Satake K, Yaoita H, Takahashi A (1995). Proximal balloon occlusion for dissecting vertebral aneurysms accompanied by subarachnoid hemorrhage. *Neurosurgery* 36: 914–20.

van Crevel H (1980). Pitfalls in the diagnosis of rebleeding from intracranial aneurysm. *Clin Neurol Neurosurg* 82: 1–9.

van Crevel H, Habbema JD, Braakman R (1986). Decision analysis of the management of incidental intracranial saccular aneurysms. *Neurology* 36: 1335–9.

van Gijn J, van Dongen KJ (1982). The time course of aneurysmal haemorrhage on computed tomograms. *Neuroradiology* 23: 153–6.

van Gijn J, Bromberg JE, Lindsay KW, Hasan D, Vermeulen M (1994). Definition of initial grading, specific events, and overall outcome in patients with aneurysmal subarachnoid hemorrhage. A survey. *Stroke* 25: 1623–7.

van Gijn J, Hijdra A, Wijdicks EFM, Vermeulen M, van Crevel H (1985). Acute hydrocephalus after aneurysmal subarachnoid hemorrhage. *J Neurosurg* 63: 355–62.

Vermeulen M, Muizelaar JP (1980). Do antifibrinolytic agents prevent rebleeding after rupture of a cerebral aneurysm? A review. *Clin Neurol Neurosurg* 82: 25–30.

Vermeulen M, Van Gijn J, Blijenberg BG (1983). Spectrophotometric analysis of CSF after subarachnoid hemorrhage: limitations in the diagnosis of rebleeding. *Neurology* 33: 112–15.

Vermeulen M, Van Gijn J, Hijdra A, van Crevel H (1984b). Causes of acute deterioration in patients with a ruptured intracranial aneurysm. A prospective study with serial CT scanning. *J Neurosurg* 60: 935–9.

Vermeulen M, van Vliet HH, Lindsay KW, Hijdra A, Van Gijn J (1985). Source of fibrin/fibrinogen degradation products in the CSF after subarachnoid hemorrhage. *J Neurosurg* 63: 573–7.

Vermeulen M, Lindsay KW, Murray GD *et al.* (1984a). Antifibrinolytic treatment in subarachnoid hemorrhage. *N Engl J Med* 311: 432–7.

Wauchob TD, Brooks RJ, Harrison KM (1984). Neurogenic pulmonary oedema. *Anaesthesia* 39: 529–34.

Weingeist TA, Goldman EJ, Folk JC, Packer AJ, Ossoinig KC (1986). Terson's syndrome. Clinicopathologic correlations. *Ophthalmology* 93: 1435–42.

Weir B (1987). Antifibrinolytics in subarachnoid hemorrhage. Do they have a role? No. *Arch Neurol* 44: 116–18.

Weir B, Grace M, Hansen J, Rothberg C (1978). Time course of vasospasm in man. *J Neurosurg* 48: 173–8.

Weir BK (1978). Pulmonary edema following fatal aneurysm rupture. *J Neurosurg* 49: 502–7.

Wells PS, Lensing AWA, Hirsh J (1994). Graduated compression stockings in the prevention of postoperative venous thromboembolism. A meta-analysis. *Arch Intern Med* 154: 67–72.

Wiebers DO, Whisnant JP, Sundt TM Jr, O'Fallon WM (1987). The significance of unruptured intracranial saccular aneurysms. *J Neurosurg* 66: 23–9.

Wijdicks EFM (1995). Worst-case scenario: management in poor-grade aneurysmal subarachnoid hemorrhage. *Cerebrovasc Dis* 5: 163–9.

Wijdicks EFM, Vermeulen M, Hijdra A, Van Gijn J (1985a). Hyponatremia and cerebral infarction in patients with ruptured intracranial aneurysms: is fluid restriction harmful? *Ann Neurol* 17: 137–40.

Wijdicks EFM, Vermeulen M, van Brummelen P, Van Gijn J (1988b). The effect of fludrocortisone acetate on plasma volume and natriuresis in patients with aneurysmal subarachnoid hemorrhage. *Clin Neurol Neurosurg* 90: 209–14.

Wijdicks EFM, Ropper AH, Hunnicutt EJ, Richardson GS, Nathanson JA (1991). Atrial natriuretic factor and salt wasting after aneurysmal subarachnoid hemorrhage. *Stroke* 22: 1519–24.

Wijdicks EFM, van Dongen KJ, Van Gijn J, Hijdra A, Vermeulen M (1988a). Enlargement of the third ventricle and hyponatremia in aneurysmal subarachnoid haemorrhage. *J Neurol Neurosurg Psychiatr* 51: 516–20.

Wijdicks EFM, Vermeulen M, Murray GD, Hijdra A, Van Gijn J (1990). The effects of treating hypertension following aneurysmal subarachnoid hemorrhage. *Clin Neurol Neurosurg* 92: 111–7.

Wijdicks EFM, Vermeulen M, ten Haaf JA, Hijdra A, Bakker WH, Van Gijn J (1985b). Volume depletion and natriuresis in patients with a ruptured intracranial aneurysm. *Ann Neurol* 18: 211–16.

Wijdicks EFM, Hasan D, Lindsay KW *et al.* (1989). Short-term tranexamic acid treatment in aneurysmal subarachnoid hemorrhage. *Stroke* 20: 1674–9.

Winn HR, Richardson AE, Jane JA (1977). The long-term prognosis in untreated cerebral aneurysms: I. The incidence of late hemorrhage in cerebral aneurysm: a 10-year evaluation of 364 patients. *Ann Neurol* 1: 358–70.

Wohns RN, Tamas L, Pierce KR, Howe JF (1985). Chlorpromazine treatment for neurogenic pulmonary edema. *Crit Care Med* 13: 210–11.

Specific treatment of arteriovenous malformations

I4

14.1 Introduction

This chapter will deal only with arteriovenous malformations (AVMs) in the strict sense of the term, and not with the variety of microangiomas (cavernous angiomas, venous angiomas and telangiectasias; see Section 8.2.6) for which intervention is rarely indicated unless the lesion presents with haemorrhage; in those cases, craniotomy is often combined with stereotactic techniques and intraoperative ultrasound for accurate localisation (Davis & Kelly, 1990). A general point to be made about the management of AVMs in the brain is that there is no hurry. Even if the malformation has presented with haemorrhage, the risk of early rebleeding is low. It is extremely unusual for recurrent haemorrhages to supervene whilst the attendant physicians and surgeons are still in the process of balancing the risks and benefits of the various treatment options.

> *Recurrent haemorrhage from arteriovenous malformations may occur, but the interval is commonly counted in months or years, and not in days or weeks, as with ruptured aneurysms. This leaves time for ample consultation between neurologists, neurosurgeons and neuroradiologists on whether intervention is feasible and desirable.*

The delay is necessary not only for thinking. If a haemorrhage has been the presenting feature and has resulted in neurological deficits, one needs to take the degree of recovery into consideration; at the very least, a few weeks are required for the eventual disability to be estimated with any confidence. These considerations also imply that if a first angiogram has not shown the expected AVM it is safe to wait a few weeks before repeating the study, in case the AVM had been compressed by the mass effect of the haematoma (Willinsky *et al.*, 1993; Halpin *et al.*, 1994).

14.1.1 Heterogeneity of arteriovenous malformations (AVMs)

An important point to consider is that no two patients with AVMs are the same or have the same prognosis, which makes it difficult to outline a general management strategy, much more so than, for example, for ruptured aneurysms at the base of the brain. This is not only because the clinical manifestations are diverse: haemorrhage, epilepsy, progressive neurological deterioration, benign intracranial hypertension or migrainous headaches. The most important determinants of the therapeutic management are the size, location and venous drainage of the malformation. For example, a small and superficial AVM in one occipital lobe is much more easily accessible to surgical treatment than an anomaly involving almost an entire hemisphere, with feeders from all major arteries and with extensive drainage into the deep venous system. For this reason, Spetzler and Martin (1986) have proposed a grading system for AVMs that takes account of these three key features. This grading system

Table 14.1 Grading system for AVMs, according to Spetzler and Martin (1986).

Graded feature	Points assigned
Size of AVM	
Small (<3 cm)	1
Medium (3–6 cm)	2
Large (>6 cm)	3
Eloquence of adjacent brain	
Non-eloquent	0
Eloquent	1
Pattern of venous drainage	
Superficial only	0
Deep	1

Grade = [size] + [eloquence] + [venous drainage], i.e. [1, 2 or 3] + [0 or 1] + [0 or 1].

(Table 14.1, Figs 14.1–14.3) bears mainly on the feasibility of surgical treatment and not so much on the risk of haemorrhage. Of course, it is more useful to describe the three features separately than to rely on the sum score alone, in which important information gets lost.

In addition, a cautionary note is appropriate about the dangers of making too facile a distinction between 'eloquent' and so-called 'silent' areas of the brain. Because surgery in specialised areas of the cerebral cortex results in easily recognisable deficits such as hemiparesis, aphasia or a visual field defect does not imply that less specialised areas of the brain are functionally unimportant. Surgical excision of, say, the right temporal lobe will not result in impairments that are obvious when the patient is making a brief visit to a hospital clinic. But, a conversation with the patient's life partner will drastically cure any previous belief on the part of the physician that 'silent' areas of the brain can be excised without consequences for the patient's mood or character. To illustrate this point with a comparison: if the function of the intact brain is symbolised by a beautiful painting, lesions in 'eloquent' brain areas can be compared with holes or blots in the picture, whereas lesions in 'silent' areas correspond with darkening of the varnish and fading of the colours.

The term 'silent area of the brain' should be interpreted as an area with a general rather than a specific function (such as language or movements), not as an area that is redundant.

14.1.2 Clinical presentations other than haemorrhage

Intracranial haemorrhage is the initial manifestation of AVMs in at least 50% of cases, although the exact proportion depends to some extent on whether the series has been collected in a neurological or neurosurgical centre (Svien & McRae, 1965; Crawford *et al.*, 1986). The clinical features are similar in children and adults, except that in neonates high-volume intracranial shunts may cause congestive heart failure or hydrocephalus (Kelly *et al.*, 1978).

Clinical presentations of arteriovenous malformations are haemorrhage (50%), epilepsy (35%), ischaemia (10%), benign intracranial hypertension or migrainous headaches (rare).

Epilepsy, usually with partial seizures, is the initial manifestation in about one-third of the cases, and progressive neurological deterioration in about 10%. Insidiously developing neurological deficits can be focal or more general, in the form of problems with memory or cognition; in both cases the explanation is that shunting through a low-resistance AVM results in underperfusion of the surrounding normal brain tissue, a phenomenon called vascular 'steal' (Brown *et al.*, 1988; Leblanc & Little, 1990). Some argue against this, because in such patients the blood flow velocity in feeding arteries, as measured with transcranial Doppler techniques, is not higher than in patients with AVMs without haemorrhagic focal deficits, and the pathophysiology of AVMs is probably more complex than can be explained by velocity alone (Mast *et al.*, 1995). The syndrome of benign intracranial hypertension, with headache or visual symptoms, may result if the malformation drains into the superior sagittal sinus, which leads to increased cerebrospinal fluid pressure (Chimowitz *et al.*, 1990). Finally, migrainous headaches may, in a tiny minority, be associated with AVMs in the occipital region (Bruyn, 1984). There is little to distinguish these patients from ordinary migraineurs, except that the hemianopic deficit is always on the same side, and that hemianopia may follow rather than precede the headache. However, in view of the dilemmas with regard to invasive treatment of AVMs it is far from certain that a patient with migraine benefits from the knowledge that there is an underlying AVM, quite apart from the cost, discomfort and risk of all the negative investigations in the vast majority of atypical migraineurs.

14.1.3 Can the natural history be improved upon?

Even if the presentation and the future risks of patients with AVMs were less heterogeneous, balancing the pros and cons of the available treatment options would be difficult, for several reasons. First, the natural history of AVMs in general is known only vaguely, because all the series have been retrospectively collected, usually with a limited period of follow-

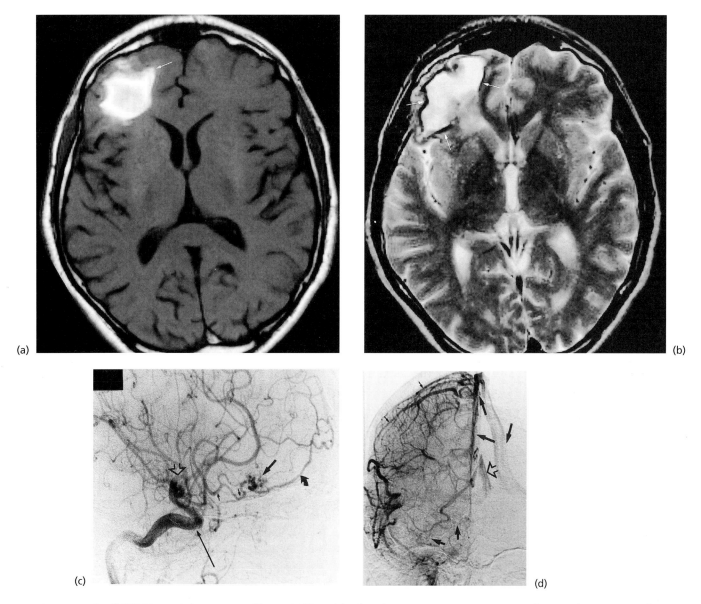

Figure 14.1 Small AVM (<3 cm), in a 59-year-old man. (a) T1-weighted axial magnetic resonance (MRI) scan showing a haematoma in the right frontal lobe (arrow). (b) T2-weighted MR scan, showing a rim of haemosiderin (low signal) around the haematoma (arrow). (c) Right carotid angiogram, arterial phase, oblique lateral view: small AVM in frontal lobe (thick solid arrow), fed by a branch of the anterior cerebral artery (short thin arrows). An early draining vein is visible (curved arrow). The middle cerebral artery (viewed mainly end on because of the projection—open arrow) and internal carotid artery (long thin arrow) are also seen. (d) Right carotid angiogram, venous phase, antero-posterior view: drainage via veins on the cortical surface (short arrows). Note the veins draining the AVM (short thick arrow) have virtually emptied as they fill earlier than the normal cortical veins (small arrows). The superior sagittal sinus (thick solid arrows), straight sinus (open arrow) and normal cortical veins (thin arrows) are also shown.

up, and because easily operable lesions are almost never included, causing a bias towards AVMs that are large or deep or situated in 'eloquent' areas of the brain. Despite these shortcomings, a reasonable estimate is an annual risk of bleeding of 2–3%, with little difference for patients with or without a previous haemorrhage (Aminoff, 1987; Heros & Tu, 1987; Brown *et al.*, 1988; Ondra *et al.*, 1990). The case fatality rate for a first bleed is about 10%, considerably lower than for ruptured aneurysms, where approximately 50% of first episodes are fatal in hospital series (see Section

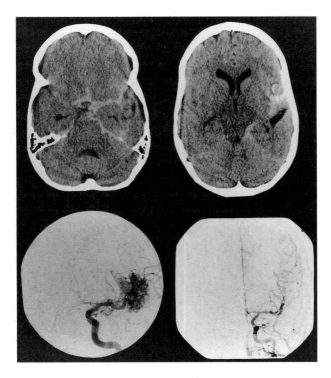

Figure 14.2 Medium-sized AVM (3–6 cm), in a 31-year-old woman. Top: CT scan, showing subarachnoid haemorrhage, predominantly in the left Sylvian fissure. Bottom, left: left carotid angiogram, antero-posterior view, shows AVM in the left temporal lobe supplied by branches of the left middle cerebral artery. Bottom, right: repeat angiogram after excision of the AVM.

13.2.2). The risk of future bleeding is greater in patients over 60 years (Crawford *et al.*, 1986), if there is an associated saccular aneurysm, in which case the risk is about 7%/year (Brown *et al.*, 1988), if there is only a single draining vein, or

if venous drainage is impaired or confined to the deep venous system (Miyasaka *et al.*, 1992).

> *The average risk of haemorrhage from an arteriovenous malformation is 2–3% per annum. Unfavourable factors (with higher risk) are an associated saccular aneurysm, age over 60 years and venous drainage via the deep venous system or via a single vein.*

A second problem is that the benefits and risks of any treatment can be measured only over many years, particularly if the lesion has not been completely obliterated and if the side effects of treatment do not emerge until years later, as with radiosurgery. Nevertheless, decision analyses have been attempted, especially with a view to surgical treatment (Iansek *et al.*, 1983; Aminoff, 1987). A third factor that is difficult to quantify in decision analyses is the patient's psychological attitude to living with an unoperated lesion in the brain that may unexpectedly bleed. Some patients show admirable *sang-froid* in coping with this knowledge, but in others their life may turn out to be so much dominated by the perceived danger that they insist on intervention even when the balance of risks would seem to argue against such a course of action. Finally, the balance between benefits and risks for any form of treatment (surgical excision, endovascular embolisation and radiosurgery) has never been assessed in randomised controlled trials. Despite the heterogeneity of lesions, such trials, necessarily in the form of a multicentre effort, are the only possible way of therapeutic advancement in this area, unless in the improbable circumstance that some form of intervention is completely harmless. The available options for treatment are: medical treatment; surgical excision; endovascular embolisation; radiosurgery; and some combination of these treatment modalities.

(a)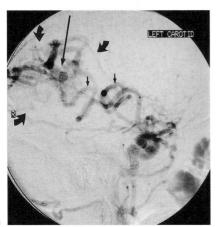

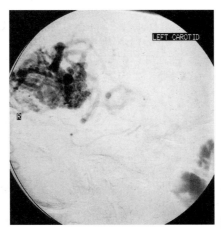 (b)

Figure 14.3 (a) Cerebral angiogram (left common carotid injection, lateral projection) of a large parieto-occipital AVM (> 6 cm), fed by dilated branches of the middle cerebral artery (short arrows). The nidus is beginning to fill (long arrow). The full extent is indicated by the curved arrows. (b) Film from later in the sequence showing the nidus more clearly.

14.2 Medical treatment

In all patients with AVMs, antithrombotic drugs should probably be avoided, including aspirin and other non-steroidal anti-inflammatory drugs that interfere with cyclo-oxygenase and thereby with platelet aggregation. Hypertension, if present, should be controlled. In patients with symptomatic epilepsy, anticonvulsants are usually indicated. At this time there is no evidence in favour of anticonvulsant treatment in patients with AVMs who have never had seizures, even in patients with neurological sequelae after a haemorrhage.

Pregnant patients with unoperated AVMs should be managed in the same way as other patients, until childbirth. It is controversial whether anticonvulsant medication should be changed to a supposedly 'safe' drug such as carbamazepine: (i) because there are no adequately controlled studies; and (ii) because organogenesis is often completed by the time a woman discovers she is pregnant (Donaldson, 1989). During delivery the risk of rupture with bearing down and its attendant overshoots of arterial pressure is usually thought to be high enough to justify an elective Caesarian section at 38-weeks gestation (Donaldson, 1989).

14.3 Surgical excision

Excision of an AVM is the most definitive treatment and, therefore, this approach is preferred if the operation is technically feasible and if the risks of neurological sequelae seem acceptable. Deep-seated lesions in the thalamus or basal ganglia can also be resected, but with higher risk (Tew et al., 1995). Ligation of feeding arteries alone is now considered out of date, as invariably new feeding vessels will emerge, being subject to the draining forces resulting from the low resistance of dilated veins that can be accessed without a capillary network; in the few cases where this does not occur, the brain tissue in the involved area may become irreversibly ischaemic.

Details of operative technique can be found elsewhere (Stein, 1992). Here, only the general principles will be outlined. A superselective angiogram is essential for accurate localisation during the operation; particularly of the superficial veins which can usually be recognised on the angiogram by their shape. From here, the feeding arteries at the margin of the malformation are uncovered by microdissection, although these are often hidden in the depths of the sulci. Often, there is a well-defined layer of glial tissue between the AVM and the normal brain, in which plane the dissection can be carried out. Small arteries are occluded by cautery, bipolar cautery having the great advantage that the vessel does not stick to the forceps with the danger of bleeding when the forceps are retracted. Metallic clips are used for larger feeding arteries, but care is necessary to ensure that feeders supplying both brain tissue and the AVM are left alone and that only the branches to the malformation itself are ligated. In this fashion surgeons slowly work their way around the malformation, a meticulous process that takes hours and sometimes even the greater part of a day. During this process, it is often possible to decrease the size of draining veins by gentle cauterisation.

The deepest part of the AVM is often found near the ventricular system, with numerous small arteries that are often related to the anterior or posterior choroidal arteries, or both, and that have subependymal draining veins. Some surgeons prefer to use hypotension in this phase of the operation. One large draining vein, superficial or deep, should be left intact until the very end of the procedure.

After the operation, close monitoring is needed for the first 24 hours, in view of the danger of haemorrhage or brain swelling. These complications are most common in AVMs 6 cm or more in diameter, particularly if preoperative single photon emission computerised tomography (SPECT) scanning has shown hypoperfusion of the parenchyma distal to the AVM nidus, and in AVMs arising directly off proximal cerebral arteries or, conversely, in a distal or border zone location (Awad et al., 1994). Haemorrhages may originate not only in the field of operation, e.g. from small remaining portions of the AVM, but also from small vessels at some distance from the lesion, because these cannot withstand the pressure of the large volume of blood that has been redirected; the so-called breakthrough phenomenon (Spetzler et al., 1978). Brain swelling may result from a redistribution of blood flow, or more specifically from occlusion of venous outflow (al Rodhan et al., 1993). The risk of postoperative seizures can perhaps be decreased by prophylactic anticonvulsants if the patient is not already on such medication; the benefits are estimated to exceed the risks, although no evidence from controlled clinical trials is available, but at any rate the drugs should be stopped after a few months if no fits have occurred. If ischaemic deficits are found to have occurred as a result of the operation, clinical improvement is still possible in the long term, by adaptive phenomena or because not all the damage to neurones has been irreversible (Heros et al., 1990). Even in carefully selected patients the net rate of serious permanent morbidity is of the order of 8% (Heros et al., 1990).

14.4 Endovascular embolisation

The development of microcatheters has allowed the delivery

of foreign material into AVMs, with the aim of occluding the anomalous vessels and thereby reducing the risk of subsequent haemorrhage and other complications (Luessenhop & Presper, 1984). The substances that were used initially consisted of particulate matter, such as ceramic pellets, silastic pellets, gelfoam and isopropyl alcohol fragments. At present, rapidly polymerising liquid glues are often preferred, of which bucrylate is the most commonly used (Vinuela *et al.*, 1983). With time it has become clear that total obliteration of the AVM by means of embolisation is difficult to achieve. In many centres the rationale of the procedure is mainly that of an adjunct to surgery, especially with deep AVMs; preoperative embolisation can often successfully decrease the size of the malformation to such a degree that subsequent surgery is probably safer and more complete than it would have been otherwise (Stein & Wolpert, 1980; Luessenhop & Rosa, 1984; Fournier *et al.*, 1991; Deruty *et al.*, 1995; Lawton *et al.*, 1995). Not only the technical difficulties of the operation are reduced but also the haemodynamic changes are more gradual, which decreases the risk of the breakthrough phenomenon mentioned above. Some surgeons inject embolising material at the time of operation into cannulated blood vessels, but the course of the material is more difficult to control under such circumstances than when the vascular bed downstream from the catheter can be visualised with soluble contrast (Deruty *et al.*, 1985).

Complications of endovascular embolisation in the immediate phase include: (i) cerebral infarction by inadvertent obliteration of an artery to normal brain; (ii) haemorrhage associated with manipulation of the catheter or with distension of the microballoon even before injection of embolising material; (iii) haemorrhage as a result of haemodynamic changes leading to rupture of a feeding artery, a draining vein or dilated capillaries (Kvam *et al.*, 1980; Luessenhop & Presper, 1984; Vinuela *et al.*, 1986); and (iv) pulmonary infarction after passage of the embolic material through the malformation. Rarely, delayed haemorrhage occurs, which may be explained by toxic effects of bucrylate on the vessel wall, with angionecrosis and extravasation of bucrylate (Deruty *et al.*, 1985; Vinters *et al.*, 1986). Although complications of embolisation are few in the series reported by the world experts cited above, these results cannot necessarily be generalised. In a series of 53 consecutive patients treated in the Netherlands by a dedicated neuroradiologist to whom patients were referred from all parts of the country, five patients died and 17 had permanent deficits, four of which were no longer able to lead an independent life (J. de Jonge, unpublished observations).

14.5 Radiosurgery

Focused radiation is an important option in the management of AVMs that are considered inaccessible to surgical treatment, i.e. lesions in the deep regions of a cerebral hemisphere, in the brainstem or in important primary projection areas such as for language or for motor control of the dominant hand. With these techniques collimated bundles of high-energy radiation are directed from many different angles at the lesion, resulting in a steep dosage gradient between the target and the normal brain tissue surrounding it; lesions of more than 3.5 cm in size cannot be treated in this fashion, because otherwise the dose to normal tissues would be excessive. The rationale for this treatment is that radiation damages and eventually occludes the blood vessels constituting the AVM (Ogilvy, 1990). This takes place in the long term, after months to years, and consists of proliferation of endothelial cells, deposition of collagen in the subendothelial region and thickening of the muscle layer; these alterations occur more extensively in arteries than in veins, particularly in small arteries. Two different techniques have been developed: the 'gamma-knife' and the linear accelerator, on the one hand, delivering photons, and the proton beam technique on the other (Heros & Korosue, 1990). Both methods use a stereotactic device for the delivery of radiation and require an extensive infrastructure of physical instruments that restricts the application of these techniques to only a few centres in the world.

The *gamma-knife*, developed by the Swedish neurosurgeon. Leksell, is a system that uses a cobalt source for generating highly collimated gamma-rays that converge at a focal point in the brain. A summary of the results in three groups of patients treated with the gamma-knife has shown that between 79 and 84% of the patients had complete angiographic obliteration of the AVM after 2 years (Lindquist & Steiner, 1988). Two groups using the related technique with a *linear accelerator*, which can deliver radiation to a defined volume of tissue, have reported similar results, with complete obliteration after 2 years in approximately 70% (Betti *et al.*, 1989; Colombo *et al.*, 1989). The rate of symptomatic radiation necrosis with either the gamma-knife or the linear accelerator was of the order of 3%. It should be kept in mind that as a rule, these two techniques were applied only in patients with AVMs measuring less than 3.5 cm in diameter.

The other method, the *proton beam* technique, uses the so-called Bragg peak of the proton beam generated at the Harvard University cyclotron (Kjellberg *et al.*, 1983b). The proton beam is designed to reach its peak in a defined volume of tissue. The reported rate of complete obliteration was only of the order of 22% (Kjellberg *et al.*, 1983a,b), but this series was associated with less than 2% of serious complications, and involved a high proportion of larger lesions and a lower dose of radiation (Heros & Korosue, 1990). Yet, the risk of haemorrhage from any AVM is not reduced or may even be increased until complete obliteration has been achieved (Ogilvy, 1990). For smaller lesions, measuring less than 3.5 cm in diameter, a group in Stanford used helium-ion Bragg-peak radiation and found an obliteration rate of 39% after 1 year, 84% after 2 years and 97% after 3 years (Steinberg *et al.*, 1990). Even 70% of larger lesions were no longer detectable on angiography after 3 years. On the other hand, the rate of disabling neurological complications as a result of treatment was 9%. Little is known at this time about possible side effects in the long term, particularly tumour formation.

In summary, if any intervention at all is needed, the technique of focused radiation is not much safer and is probably less effective than surgical resection, certainly in the short term. This approach should be reserved for AVMs that are completely inaccessible to surgery or embolisation, i.e. small and deep lesions, fed by small blood vessels (Stein, 1992).

> *The techniques for removal of arteriovenous malformations have not been properly compared with the natural history. Provisionally, it seems that* open surgery *is best for superficial arteriovenous malformations,* endovascular embolisation *is preferable for deep and large (> 3.5 cm) lesions, often in combination with open surgery, and* radiosurgery *is reserved for small, deep arteriovenous malformations.*

References

al Rodhan NR, Sundt TM Jr, Piepgras DG, Nichols DA, Rufenacht D, Stevens LN (1993). Occlusive hyperemia: a theory for the hemodynamic complications following resection of intracerebral arteriovenous malformations. *J Neurosurg* 78: 167–75.

Aminoff MJ (1987). Treatment of unruptured cerebral arteriovenous malformations. *Neurology* 37: 815–19.

Awad IA, Magdinec M, Schubert A (1994). Intracranial hypertension after resection of cerebral arteriovenous malformations. Predisposing factors and management strategy. *Stroke* 25: 611–20.

Betti OO, Munari C, Rosler R (1989). Stereotactic radiosurgery with the linear accelerator: treatment of arteriovenous malformations. *Neurosurgery* 24: 311–21.

Brown RD Jr, Wiebers DO, Forbes G *et al.* (1988). The natural history of unruptured intracranial arteriovenous malformations. *J Neurosurg* 68: 352–7.

Bruyn GW (1984). Intracranial arteriovenous malformation and migraine. *Cephalalgia* 4: 191–207.

Chimowitz MI, Little JR, Awad IA, Sila CA, Kosmorsky G, Furlan AJ (1990). Intracranial hypertension associated with unruptured cerebral arteriovenous malformations. *Ann Neurol* 27: 474–9.

Colombo F, Benedetti A, Pozza F, Marchetti C, Chierego G (1989). Linear accelerator radiosurgery of cerebral arteriovenous malformations. *Neurosurgery* 24: 833–40.

Crawford PM, West CR, Chadwick DW, Shaw MD (1986). Arteriovenous malformations of the brain: natural history in unoperated patients. *J Neurol Neurosurg Psychiatr* 49: 1–10.

Davis DH, Kelly PJ (1990). Stereotactic resection of occult vascular malformations. *J Neurosurg* 72: 698–702.

Deruty R, Lapras C, Pierluca P *et al.* (1985). Embolisation peropératoire des malformations arterio-veineuses cérébrales par le butyl-cyanoacrylate (18 cas). *Neurochirurgie* 31: 21–9.

Deruty R, Pelissou-Guyotat I, Amat D *et al.* (1995). Multidisciplinary treatment of cerebral arteriovenous malformations. *Neurol Res* 17: 169–77.

Donaldson JO (1989). *The Neurology of Pregnancy*, 2nd edn. London: W.B. Saunders.

Fournier D, TerBrugge KG, Willinsky R, Lasjaunias P, Montanera W (1991). Endovascular treatment of intracerebral arteriovenous malformations: experience in 49 cases. *J Neurosurg* 75: 228–33.

Halpin SF, Britton JA, Byrne JV, Clifton A, Hart G, Moore A (1994). Prospective evaluation of cerebral angiography and computed tomography in cerebral haematoma. *J Neurol Neurosurg Psychiatr* 57: 1180–6.

Heros RC, Korosue K (1990). Radiation treatment of cerebral arteriovenous malformations [editorial comment]. *N Engl J Med* 323: 127–9.

Heros RC, Tu YK (1987). Is surgical therapy needed for unruptured arteriovenous malformations? *Neurology* 37: 279–86.

Heros RC, Korosue K, Diebold PM (1990). Surgical excision of cerebral arteriovenous malformations: late results. *Neurosurgery* 26: 570–7.

Iansek R, Elstein AS, Balla JI (1983). Application of decision analysis to management of cerebral arteriovenous malformation. *Lancet* 1: 1132–5.

Kelly JJ, Mellinger JF, Sundt TM (1978). Intracranial arteriovenous malformations in childhood. *Ann Neurol* 3: 338–43.

Kjellberg RN, Davis KR, Lyons S, Butler W, Adams RD (1983a). Bragg peak proton beam therapy for arteriovenous malformation of the brain. *Clin Neurosurg* 31: 248–90.

Kjellberg RN, Hanamura T, Davis KR, Lyons SL, Adams RD (1983b). Bragg-peak proton-beam therapy for arteriovenous malformations of the brain. *N Engl J Med* 309: 269–74.

Kvam DA, Michelsen WJ, Quest DO (1980). Intracerebral hemorrhage as a complication of artificial embolization. *Neurosurgery* 7: 491–4.

Lawton MT, Hamilton MG, Spetzler RF (1995). Multimodality treatment of deep arteriovenous malformations: thalamus, basal ganglia, and brain stem. *Neurosurgery* 37: 29–36.

Leblanc R, Little JR (1990). Hemodynamics of arteriovenous malformations. *Clin Neurosurg* 36: 299–317.

Lindquist C, Steiner L (1988). Stereotactic radiosurgical treatment of arteriovenous malformations. In: Lunsford LD, ed. *Modern Stereotactic Neurosurgery*. Boston: Martinus Nijhoff, 491–505.

Luessenhop AJ, Presper JH (1984). Surgical embolization of cerebral arteriovenous malformations through internal carotid and vertebral arteries: long term results. *J Neurosurg* 60: 14–22.

Luessenhop AJ, Rosa L (1984). Cerebral arteriovenous malformations. Indications for and results of surgery, and the role of intravascular techniques. *J Neurosurg* 60: 14–22.

Mast H, Mohr JP, Osipov A *et al.* (1995). 'Steal' is an unestablished mechanism for the clinical presentation of cerebral arteriovenous malformations. *Stroke* 26: 1215–20.

Miyasaka Y, Yada K, Ohwada T, Kitahara T, Kurata A, Irikura K (1992). An analysis of the venous drainage system as a factor in hemorrhage from arteriovenous malformations. *J Neurosurg* 76: 239–43.

Ogilvy CS (1990). Radiation therapy for arteriovenous malformations: a review. *Neurosurgery* 26: 725–35.

Ondra SL, Troupp H, George ED, Schwab K (1990). The natural history of symptomatic arteriovenous malformations of the brain: a 24-year follow-up assessment. *J Neurosurg* 73: 387–91.

Spetzler RF, Martin NA (1986). A proposed grading system for arteriovenous malformations. *J Neurosurg* 65: 476–83.

Spetzler RF, Wilson CB, Weinstein P, Mehdorn M, Townsend J, Telles D (1978). Normal perfusion pressure breakthrough phenomenon. *Clin Neurosurg* 25: 651–72.

Stein BM (1992). Surgical decisions in vascular malformations of the brain. In: Barnett HJM, Mohr JP, Stein BM, Yatsu FM, eds. *Stroke: Pathophysiology, Diagnosis and Management*, 2nd edn. New York: Churchill Livingstone, 1093–133.

Stein BM, Wolpert SM (1980). Arteriovenous malformations of the brain. II. Current concepts and treatment. *Arch Neurol* 37: 69–75.

Steinberg GK, Fabrikant JI, Marks MP *et al.* (1990). Stereotactic heavy-charged-particle Bragg-peak radiation for intracranial arteriovenous malformations. *N Engl J Med* 323: 96–101.

Svien J, McRae JA (1965). Arteriovenous anomalies of the brain. *J Neurosurg* 23: 23–8.

Tew JM Jr, Lewis AI, Reichert KW (1995). Management strategies and surgical techniques for deep-seated supratentorial arteriovenous malformations. *Neurosurgery* 36: 1065–72.

Vinters HV, Lundie MJ, Kaufmann JC (1986). Long-term pathological follow-up of cerebral arteriovenous malformations treated by embolization with bucrylate. *N Engl J Med* 314: 477–83.

Vinuela F, Fox AJ, Pelz D, Debrun G (1986). Angiographic follow-up of large cerebral AVMs incompletely embolized with isobutyl-2-cyanoacrylate. *Am J Neuroradiol* 7: 919–25.

Vinuela FV, Debrun GM, Fox AJ, Girvin JP, Peerless SJ (1983). Dominant-hemisphere arteriovenous malformations: therapeutic embolization with isobutyl-2-cyanoacrylate. *Am J Neuroradiol* 4: 959–66.

Willinsky RA, Fitzgerald M, Terbrugge K, Montanera W, Wallace M (1993). Delayed angiography in the investigation of intracerebral hematomas caused by small arteriovenous malformations. *Neuroradiology* 35: 307–11.

What are this person's problems?
A problem-based approach to the general management of stroke

15

··

15.1 Introduction

The patient's general management, as distinct from the specific treatment of their stroke pathology (see Chapters 11–14), is primarily aimed at identifying and solving existing problems, as well as preventing potential problems, at different stages of their illness. This chapter will cover the common problems which occur in patients who have had a stroke. Each section is loosely structured as follows.

1 *General description of each problem* which will include a definition, its frequency, causes and clinical significance.

2 *Assessment* including methods of detection, simple clinical assessments and measures which may be appropriate for use in goal setting, audit or research.

3 *Prognosis and treatment* including what is known about recovery and those interventions which may hasten recovery.

Unfortunately, relatively little research has focused on these aspects of stroke. In particular, there have been, almost without exception, no large randomised controlled trials or systematic reviews to guide our management. Indeed, there are major methodological difficulties in performing such studies (Table 15.1). Therefore, the content of this chapter will reflect more our own clinical experience rather than high-quality evidence which, at present, is simply unavailable. Many of the topics are not specific to stroke medicine but might be included in any textbook of internal medicine. We have not attempted to provide comprehensive reviews, but instead have concentrated on those aspects of assessment and management which are particularly relevant to stroke patients.

15.2 Airway, breathing and circulation

Inadequate airway, breathing or circulation are life threatening and immediate resuscitative measures must be taken. Even if not an immediate threat to survival, it seems sensible

Table 15.1 Problems in performing randomised trials and systematic reviews of therapy interventions.

Ethical problems of performing randomised controlled trials

Difficulty in getting patients, and therapists, to accept the possibility of 'no treatment'

Therapists' certainty about the effectiveness of their therapy in individual patients

Difficulty in blinding patients to treatment allocation

Difficulties in defining a therapy which has to be tailored to the individual patient

Moderate treatment effects mean that large numbers of patients need to be randomised

The need to randomise large numbers of patients may necessitate multicentre trials but these raise difficulties in standardising and monitoring treatment

Therapy is very labour intensive and therefore expensive so that bodies which fund research may not be willing to fund the therapy

Difficulties agreeing suitable measures of outcome which are sensitive both to the things which therapists expect to influence, and which are relevant to the patient and family

Heterogeneity of reported outcome measures which hinders systematic review of trials

Problems due to complex interactions with other therapies given simultaneously to optimise the delivery of oxygen and glucose to the brain to minimise brain damage and so achieve the best possible outcome for the patient (see Section 11.1.3).

15.2.1 Maintenance of a clear airway

Patients who have a decreased level of consciousness, impaired bulbar function or who have aspirated may have an obstructed, or partially obstructed airway. Central cyanosis, noisy airflow with grunting, snoring or gurgling, an irregular breathing pattern and indrawing of the suprasternal area and intercostal muscles may all indicate an obstructed airway. It is important that apnoeic spells due to an obstructed airway are not mistakenly attributed to peri-

odic respiration (e.g. Cheyne–Stokes) (see Section 15.2.2). If an obstructed airway is suspected, the oropharynx should be cleared of any foreign matter with a sweep of a gloved finger, the patient's jaw pulled forward and the neck extended to stop the tongue falling back to obstruct the airway (Fig. 15.1). Positioning the patient in the coma or recovery position (Fig. 15.2) may be enough to keep the airway clear, although in some situations an oropharyngeal airway or even endotracheal intubation may be required.

> Do not mistakenly attribute apnoeic spells due to intermittent airway obstruction to periodic or Cheyne–Stokes respiration.

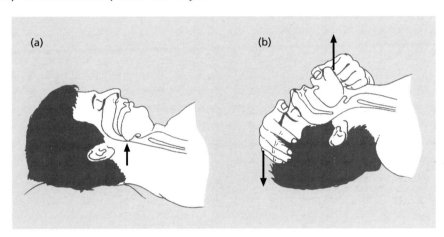

Figure 15.1 It is obviously essential to maintain a patent airway in a patient with a decreased level of consciousness. (a) In a comatose patient with their head in a resting or flexed position the tongue falls backwards to obstruct the hypopharnyx (arrow) and the epiglottis obstructs the larnyx. (b) Tilting the head back by lifting the chin stretches the anterior neck structures which opens the airway.

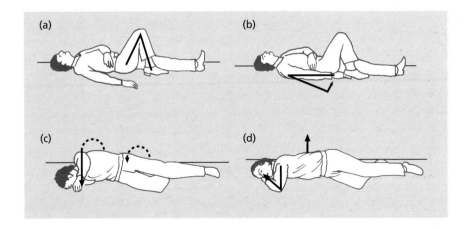

Figure 15.2 If the patient has a decreased level of consciousness and is not maintaining their airway (but does not require resuscitation) one can help maintain an open airway by putting the patient in the recovery position. (a) Flex the patient's leg closest to you. (b) Put their hand closest to you under their buttock. (c) Gently roll the patient towards you. (d) Tilt their head backwards and put their upper hand under their lower cheek to prevent the patient rolling onto their face. Their head should be kept low to encourage secretions to drain away.

15.2.2 Inadequate breathing

Strokes may directly, or more often indirectly, impair the function of the respiratory centre in the medulla which results in various disordered patterns of breathing.

Periodic respiration (Cheyne–Stokes), where there are regular alternating phases of hyperventilation and hypoventilation, is probably the most common abnormality. Other neurological functions, e.g. wakefulness, often vary in phase with the cycle as well. Periodic respiration, although originally described in left ventricular failure, has been observed in normal wakeful and sleeping subjects, patients with central sleep apnoea and those with acute and chronic neurological damage (Cheyne, 1818; Sprecht & Fruhmann, 1972; Webb, 1974; North & Jennett, 1974; O'Sullivan *et al.*, 1984). In 121 (12%) of 991 patients hospitalised with acute stroke, periodic respiration was recorded in the medical notes but this is likely to be an underestimate because the patients were not continuously monitored (Turney *et al.*, 1984). Another study of 32 conscious patients with ischaemic stroke demonstrated periodic respiration in 17 (53%) using non-invasive monitoring techniques (Nachtmann *et al.*, 1995). The mechanisms of periodic respiration are still debated but it probably reflects a change in the sensitivity of the brainstem respiratory centre to the arterial pressure of carbon dioxide ($Paco_2$) and slowed central circulation with a resultant delay in the feedback loop controlling respiration (Brown & Plum, 1961; Karp *et al.*, 1961). Whilst periodic respiration may, in an unconscious or drowsy patient, be associated with a poor chance of survival, it is seen quite frequently in patients who are alert and who subsequently make a reasonable recovery (Rout *et al.*, 1971; Nachtmann *et al.*, 1995).

> *Periodic respiration (Cheyne–Stokes) does not necessarily imply a hopeless prognosis.*

Other patterns of breathing associated with brainstem dysfunction include hyperventilation ('forced respiration'), irregular breathing, 'sighing' respiration and, ultimately, complete apnoea (North & Jennett, 1974). 'Central' sleep apnoea has been described in a patient with lateral medullary infarction (Askenasy & Goldhammer, 1988).

Associated with these abnormalities of breathing pattern one can observe changes in blood gas tension, pH and middle cerebral artery blood velocities which might exacerbate cerebral ischaemia, but their relevance has not been researched adequately (Rout *et al.*, 1971; Askenasy & Goldhammer, 1988; Wardlaw, 1993; Nachtmann *et al.*, 1995).

Co-existing cardiopulmonary disease is probably a more frequent cause of inadequate ventilation than the abnormal breathing patterns due to the stroke itself.

The adequacy of ventilation should be assessed clinically by checking for central cyanosis and examining the chest and, where there is doubt, by measuring the arterial blood gases. Pulse oximetry may be useful in monitoring patients' progress. If the patient is hypoxic the inspired oxygen should be increased, but with care if the patient has chronic lung disease and a tendency to hypercapnoea, in which case 24% oxygen should be used initially with careful monitoring of the patient's respiration, neurological function (see Section 15.5) and arterial blood gases. Sitting the patient up may help to improve oxygenation, as well as reduce the intracranial pressure, but may cause other problems (see Section 15.11) (Elizabeth *et al.*, 1993). Treatment for any co-existing lung or cardiac disease should be given and occasionally it may be necessary to intubate and artificially ventilate the patient. Often, however, such aggressive management is considered inappropriate because of the patient's small probability of regaining a good quality of life (see Section 10.4). Sedative drugs, given to promote sleep, to facilitate imaging or to control seizures may precipitate periodic respiration or respiratory failure and should be avoided if possible. Although theophylline has been used successfully to reverse periodic respiration, the indications for its use are unclear (Nachtmann *et al.*, 1995).

15.2.3 Poor circulation

Both severe brainstem dysfunction and massive subarachnoid haemorrhage can cause major circulatory problems such as neurogenic pulmonary oedema, cardiac arrhythmias and erratic blood pressure with severe hyper- or hypotension (see Section 13.10). More frequently, circulatory failure, with or without hypotension or hypoxia related to pulmonary oedema, is due to co-existent heart disease (e.g. congestive cardiac failure, myocardial infarction, atrial fibrillation), hypovolaemia (e.g. dehydration, bleeding) or severe infection.

Cardiac arrhythmias

Cardiac arrhythmias are quite common after an acute stroke, although they rarely cause significant problems (Reinstein *et al.*, 1972; Lavy *et al.*, 1974; Norris *et al.*, 1978; Britton *et al.*, 1979; Mikolich *et al.*, 1981; Rem *et al.*, 1985). The most clinically important, in terms of frequency and effect on management, is atrial fibrillation which occurs in about 17% of patients with stroke, 18% of those with cerebral infarction and 11% of those with primary intracerebral haemorrhage (Sandercock *et al.*, 1992). In the majority of cases, atrial fibrillation precedes the stroke and in some it is presumably the cause of the stroke (see Section 6.4). Of course, a small proportion of ischaemic strokes (5% in the Oxfordshire Community Stroke Project) occur in the context of a recent (within 6 weeks) myocardial infarction (see Section 7.7) (Sandercock *et al.*, 1989). *Routine* monitoring of the patient's cardiac rhythm is probably not necessary unless there is a clinical problem (e.g. palpitations, syncope or unexplained breathlessness).

> *Cardiac arrhythmias are quite common after an acute stroke, but seldom seem to be a problem unless they are due not to the stroke itself but to a recent or complicating myocardial infarction.*

Myocardial injury

It is important to identify the presence and likely cause of any circulatory failure based on clinical assessment of the cardiovascular system backed up with relevant investigations (e.g. cardiac enzymes, electrocardiogram (ECG) or echocardiography). However, the interpretation of a raised plasma creatine kinase (CK) may be difficult where the patient has fallen, been injured, lain on a hard floor or had a generalised seizure which may all increase the CK level. Measurement of more cardiac specific isoenzymes (i.e. muscle–brain (MB) fraction) may only partially resolve the difficulties (Norris *et al.*, 1979). Transient rises in cardiac enzymes have been attributed to focal regions of myocardial necrosis (i.e. myocytolysis) which have been identified at autopsy, but the clinical importance of these findings is uncertain (Dimant & Grob, 1977; Norris *et al.*, 1979).

Patients with circulatory failure, atrial fibrillation and recent myocardial infarction have a poor prognosis for survival after stroke (Sandercock *et al.*, 1992). In addition, there is some evidence that patients with symptomatic coronary disease achieve less good functional recovery (Roth *et al.*, 1988). Active treatment of these problems is likely to improve the patients' outcome but a detailed account is beyond the scope of this book.

Gastrointestinal haemorrhage

Although so-called 'stress ulceration' with associated bleeding is well described in critically ill patients, including those with head injury, little has been written about gastrointestinal haemorrhage after stroke (Schuster *et al.*, 1984; Gottlieb *et al.*, 1986; Metz *et al.*, 1993). Wijdicks *et al.* (1994) reported a frequency of only 0.1% in patients admitted to the Mayo Clinic, but their study relied on routinely coded data and may well have underestimated the real frequency.

In one of our hospitals, 18 (3%) of 607 patients admitted with a stroke had a documented upper gastrointestinal bleed, 50% of which were associated with systemic hypotension (systolic blood pressure < 100 mmHg) or a fall of at least 2 g/dl in haemoglobin concentration (Davenport *et al.*, 1996a). Bleeds were more common in elderly patients and those with severe strokes and, perhaps for this reason, few patients were thoroughly investigated to establish the source of bleeding. Clearly, hypotension and anaemia might both exacerbate cerebral ischaemia and worsen the neurological outcome. Indeed, 10 (56%) of our 18 patients died and only five of the eight survivors eventually got home. Although there is little evidence to support routine prophylaxis with acid-inhibiting drugs after stroke, one should obviously be aware of these patients' bleeding potential when prescribing antithrombotic and anti-inflammatory medication (Messer *et al.*, 1983; Somerville *et al.*, 1986; Machfoed *et al.*, 1993; Roderick *et al.*, 1993; Ben-Menachem *et al.*, 1994; Cook *et al.*, 1994).

15.3 Reduced level of consciousness

About 15% of stroke patients in the Oxfordshire Community Stroke Project had a reduced level of consciousness (Table 15.2) during the first few days after the stroke, whilst 420 (42%) of 991 patients admitted to the Mayo Clinic were recorded as having a reduced level of consciousness (Turney *et al.*, 1984). Clearly, the higher proportion in the hospital-based study is likely to have been due to referral bias, i.e. severe strokes were over-represented. Drowsiness or unconsciousness usually arise from direct (e.g. haemorrhage or infarction) or more commonly indirect damage (from raised intracranial pressure) to the brainstem. Occasionally, patients with large, apparently unilateral, cerebral infarcts become drowsy very early, before one would expect enough oedema to have developed to raise intracranial pressure significantly (Melo *et al.*, 1992). The mechanism of this drowsiness is unclear (Plum & Posner, 1980). Level of consciousness is an important indicator of the severity of the stroke and a valuable prognostic variable (see Section 10.2.7). The patient's level of consciousness is frequently used to guide the need for intervention, and those who are drowsy or unconscious are at greater risk of developing secondary complications, e.g. aspiration, pressure sores, etc.

The most commonly used measure of level of consciousness is the Glasgow Coma Scale (GCS) (see Table 4.3), which documents the patient's spontaneous actions as well as those in response to verbal and painful stimuli. Although useful, this scale, which was originally designed for patients with

Table 15.2 The frequency of various clinical features amongst 675 patients with a first-ever in a lifetime stroke at their initial assessment by a study neurologist. (From the Oxfordshire Community Stroke Project, unpublished data.)

Clinical feature	Number (%)	Not assessable (%)
Glasgow Coma Scale (motor <6)	86 (13)	15 (2)
Glasgow Coma Scale (eyes <4)	98 (15)	16 (2)
Glasgow Coma Scale (eyes + motor <10)	111 (16)	16 (2)
High blood pressure (systolic >160 mmHg)	311 (46)	19 (3)
Very high blood pressure (systolic >200 mmHg)	90 (13)	19 (3)
High blood pressure (diastolic >100 mmHg)	131 (19)	22 (3)
Very high blood pressure (diastolic >120 mmHg)	23 (3)	22 (3)
Epileptic seizures within 24 hours	14 (2)	0 (0)
Facial weakness	256 (38)	40 (6)
Arm or hand weakness	344 (51)	32 (5)
Leg weakness	307 (45)	34 (5)
Hemiparesis (at least two of face, arm and leg)	331 (49)	0 (0)
Sensory loss (proprioception)	101 (15)	168 (25)
Sensory loss (spinothalamic)	196 (29)	140 (21)
Homonymous visual field defect	113 (18)	134 (20)
Gaze palsy	50 (7)	36 (5)
Mental test score <8/10	85 (13)	135 (20)
Visuospatial dysfunction	81 (12)	179 (27)
Dysphasia	122 (19)	111 (16)
Dysarthria	135 (20)	27 (19)

Table 15.3 The Reaction Level Scale. The patient's reaction level is assessed on an eight-point scale according to whether they are mentally responsive (points 1–3) or not (points 4–8). Mental responsiveness is judged on whether the patient does any of the following: respond verbally, make eye contact or fix, obey commands or ward off pain in response to 'light' (by verbal command or touch) or 'strong' stimulation (by repeated loud verbal command, shaking or painful stimulation). Painful stimuli include retromandibular pressure or pressure on the nailbed.

Level	Description
Mentally responsive	
1	Alert. No delay of response
2	Drowsy or confused. Responsive to 'light' stimulation but drowsy or disorientated in time, place or person
3	Very drowsy or confused. Responsive only to 'strong' stimulation
Mentally unresponsive (unconscious)	
4	Unconscious but localises pain (moves hand to site of painful stimulus) but does not ward off pain
5	Unconscious but withdraws from painful stimulus
6	Unconscious but produces stereotyped flexion movements to painful stimulus
7	Unconscious but produces only stereotyped extension movements to painful stimulus
8	Unconscious with no response to painful stimulus

Full guidelines have been published by Starmark *et al.* (1988).

Table 15.4 Common complications in patients with a depressed level of consciousness after a stroke.

Complication	Section
Urinary incontinence	15.14
Faecal incontinence or constipation	15.15
Airway obstruction	15.2.1
Fever and infection	15.12
Aspiration	15.17
Dehydration	15.18.1
Malnutrition	15.19
Pressure sores	15.16

head injury, has a number of problems when applied to stroke. The most important is that many patients with stroke are dysphasic and, therefore, have a reduced score on the verbal response scale. Thus, a patient may have a reduced total score on the GCS but a normal level of consciousness. Also, inexperienced users may apply the motor scale to the affected side in a patient with a hemiparesis and obtain a reduced motor response rather than the 'best' response. However, as long as the score is not summed across the response levels, the GCS provides valuable information. The Reaction Level Scale, a unidimensional scale, although less widely used than the GCS, is an alternative tool for monitoring level of consciousness and may be more easily interpreted in aphasic patients (Table 15.3) (Johnstone *et al.*, 1993).

Patients who have a reduced level of consciousness are at greater risk of developing certain complications (Table 15.4), so that expert nursing care is needed to minimise these risks. Also, a falling level of consciousness may alert one to

an important and potentially reversible condition (Table 15.5). Therefore, patients with severe strokes, and in whom active treatment would be considered, should be monitored using the GCS for the first few days, especially where staff change, to avoid delays in initiating investigation and treatment of any worsening. The investigation and treatment of patients with a falling level of consciousness is the same as for those with other indicators of worsening (see Section 15.5).

Table 15.5 Remediable causes of a reduced level of consciousness after stroke.

Causes	Section
General	
Hypoxia	15.2.2
Hypotension	15.2.3
Severe infection	15.12
Electrolyte imbalance	15.18
Drugs, e.g. benzodiazepines, opiate analgesics	
Neurological	
Epileptic seizures	15.8
Raised intracranial pressure	11.10, 12.2.2
Obstructive hydrocephalus	12.2.6

Table 15.6 Causes of apparently severe strokes.

Non-neurological	
Infection	Respiratory
	Urinary
	Septicaemia
Metabolic	Dehydration
	Electrolyte disturbance
	Hypoglycaemia
Drugs	Major and minor tranquillisers
	Baclofen
	Lithium toxicity
	Anticonvulsant toxicity
Hypoxia	Pulmonary embolism
	Chronic respiratory disease
	Pulmonary oedema
Hypercapnoea	Chronic respiratory disease
Others	Limb or bowel ischaemia in patients with a cardiac or aortic arch source of embolism
Neurological	
Obstructive hydrocephalus in patients with stroke in the posterior fossa	
Epileptic seizures	

15.4 Severe stroke versus apparently severe stroke

Occasionally, a patient will present with the clinical features of severe stroke (e.g. reduced level of consciousness) which indicate a poor outcome. However, one must always be aware that severe concurrent illnesses or the presence of stroke complications (Table 15.6) may make a patient's stroke appear much worse than it really is. For example, a patient with a pure motor stroke (lacunar syndrome) (see Section 4.4.6) and a severe chest or urinary infection may be

drowsy or confused. It is then difficult to differentiate this clinical picture from that due to a major middle cerebral artery territory infarction (total anterior circulation infarction). Of course, an infection is more easily treated than a large volume of necrotic brain, so with appropriate therapy the prognosis of the two patients will be quite different. General signs such as fever, confusion and agitation along with more specific signs such as increased respiratory rate, tender abdomen or purulent urine, usually indicate co-existing disorders. Simple investigations such as a white cell count, erythrocyte sedimentation rate, urea and electrolytes, urine microscopy and culture, chest X-ray, ECG and blood cultures are useful, not only to identify the cause of the stroke (see Sections 6.6.1 and 6.6.2), but also to alert one to serious co-existing non-stroke pathology. Seizures that have occurred since stroke onset make the assessment of stroke severity particularly difficult so that treatment may need to be given to prevent further seizures (see Section 15.8). The treatment of apparently severe strokes will depend on the specific problem identified or suspected.

A 70-year-old man was found unconscious at home and admitted to hospital. In the receiving unit he had a partial seizure with secondary generalisation. Subsequent neurological examination revealed a reduced conscious level (Glasgow Coma Scale: eye 2, motor 4, verbal 1), deviated gaze and a flaccid paralysis of the right side. The brain computerised tomography scan on the day of admission was normal. A diagnosis of a severe ischaemic stroke was made and the decision not to resuscitate was recorded in the notes. He was given intravenous fluids but no regular anticonvulsants. He was later reviewed by the stroke physician who reversed the decision not to resuscitate and started regular anticonvulsants after an initial loading dose. The patient improved and was discharged from hospital without residual neurological deficits 4-days later. Therefore, do not write off people with apparently severe strokes and recent seizures.

15.5 Worsening after a stroke

Although stroke onset is usually abrupt, the patient's neurological condition may worsen hours, days or, rarely, weeks after the initial assessment. Patients may exhibit a reducing level of consciousness, worsening of existing neurological deficits or new deficits indicating dysfunction in another part of the brain. A large number of terms including 'stroke in evolution', 'stroke in progression' and 'progressing stroke' have been applied to this situation, which probably reflects the considerable level of interest in the problem (Gautier,

1985; Asplund, 1992). After all, here is a situation where one might be able to intervene to prevent a major stroke. Unfortunately, definitions vary and the literature (as well as the clinicians) is confused. Clearly, if we accept that the neurological deficit commonly increases over minutes or hours, then the earlier in the course of the stroke we first see the patient, the more likely we are to observe subsequent worsening. Indeed, it is likely that as we attempt to introduce acute treatments for stroke, we will become much more aware of the 'normal' worsening over the first few hours and days after stroke onset. We will probably see patients earlier in the development of their stroke and monitor them more closely because they will be in clinical trials or given a specific treatment for acute stroke.

Worsening may have a number of causes, some reversible, and so it is important to detect and treat them early. The literature has tended to emphasise the neurological causes (probably because it is mainly written by neurologists), but it is important not to miss the non-neurological ones (Table 15.7). There is, not surprisingly, considerable overlap with the causes of 'apparently severe stroke' (see Table 15.6).

To ensure that clinical worsening is identified as early as possible, i.e. when the potential for reversal is usually greatest, it is important to monitor the patient's condition. Regular measurement of the indices in Table 15.8 will usually alert one to any problem. However, experienced nursing staff who have regular close contact with the patient will often detect a problem at an early stage before it becomes obvious to other members of the team. Family members who often spend long periods with ill patients may also detect subtle but important changes in the patient's condition. It is important that the physician caring for the patient encourages free communication so that this sort of information is made known to those directing the patient's care.

Although there is a long list of the causes of worsening it is important to consider first those that are most readily reversible (see Table 15.7). The majority can be diagnosed by a clinical assessment supplemented by simple laboratory investigations. An urgent repeat brain computerised tomography (CT) scan is advisable in some situations, e.g. deterioration in conscious level in a patient with a posterior fossa stroke or subarachnoid haemorrhage who may be developing obstructive hydrocephalus, which may be amenable to neurosurgical intervention. The detection of haemorrhagic transformation of infarction in a patient receiving antithrombotic drugs may influence the decision to continue the medication or not, although there is no evidence about the best policy in this situation (see Sections 5.4, 11.3.2 and 11.4.2). A brain CT which shows that the deterioration was due to an early recurrent ischaemic stroke, especially one in a different arterial territory to the initial stroke, may

Table 15.7 Causes of worsening after stroke.

Neurological
Progression/completion of the stroke
Extension/early recurrence
Haemorrhagic transformation of an infarct (see Section 5.4)
Development of oedema around the infarct or haemorrhage* (see Section 11.1.5)
Obstructive hydrocephalus in patients with stroke in the posterior fossa or after subarachnoid haemorrhage* (see Sections 12.2.6 and 13.9)
Epileptic seizures* (see Section 15.8)
Vasospasm* (in subarachnoid haemorrhage; see Sections 13.6 and 13.8)
Incorrect diagnosis
    Cerebral tumour
    Cerebral abscess*
    Encephalitis*
    Chronic subdural haematoma*

*Non-neurological**
See Table 15.6

---

* Remediable causes of worsening.

Table 15.8 Indices to monitor and detect worsening.

Conscious level, i.e. Glasgow Coma Scale
Pupillary responses
Limb movement
Temperature
Pulse rate
Blood pressure
Fluid balance

---

encourage the clinician to investigate further for a proximal arterial or cardiac source of embolism. Clearly, any treatment will depend on the reason for the worsening (see relevant sections).

15.6 Co-existing medical problems

Co-existing medical problems are common in stroke patients because they are usually elderly and have associated vascular disease (Table 15.9). Although we have already mentioned the importance of cardiorespiratory diseases in the immediate management of the patient (see Section 15.2), these and other conditions can be important for many other reasons, not least that they may require treatment in their own right. Severe non-stroke illness can make a mild stroke *appear* severe and thus lead to an inaccurate prognosis and possibly

Table 15.9 Frequency of co-existing pathology amongst 675 patients with a first-ever in a lifetime stroke. (From the Oxfordshire Community Stroke Project, unpublished data.)

	n	(%)
Previous angina	106	(16)
Previous myocardial infarction	112	(17)
Cardiac failure	52	(8)
Intermittent claudication	112	(17)
Diabetes mellitus	63	(9)
Previous epileptic seizures	19	(3)
Previous malignancy	74	(11)
Dependent before stroke (Rankin >2)	103	(15)

No data were available on respiratory or musculoskeletal problems.

inappropriate treatment (see Section 15.4). Co-existent cardiorespiratory diseases (e.g. angina, cardiac failure, chronic airway disease) and those of the musculoskeletal system (e.g. arthritis, back pain, amputation) often compound stroke-related disability. So, for example, one might, after several months rehabilitation, have taught a patient with a severe hemiparesis to walk again, but if they also have chronic airway disease the added effort of walking with a hemiplegic gait over that with a normal gait may mean that the patient can not walk any useful distance. It is important to be aware of the limitations on rehabilitation imposed by pre-existing pathology before spending months trying to make a patient walk. It may be more realistic to teach the patient to be independent in a wheelchair. Even if one cannot estimate the impact of non-stroke pathology on recovery, knowledge of its existence may explain why a patient is not achieving their rehabilitation goals (see Section 10.3.4).

Although most patients who survive a stroke improve over weeks or months, many of the co-existing problems, which contribute to disability, progress. Thus, a patient may reach their optimal functional recovery some months after a stroke and then deteriorate due to progression of a co-morbid condition. If this kind of deterioration can be anticipated it may allow for a more flexible package of care to cope with such fluctuations. There can be few things more disappointing than to strive to discharge a patient into one form of accommodation and then hear that within a few months their condition has deteriorated to such an extent that the accommodation is no longer suitable. This can shatter the morale of the patient and their carer.

> *Functional deterioration months after a stroke is unlikely to be due to the initial stroke and much more likely to be caused by the progression of some co-morbid condition such as angina, arthritis or intermittent claudication.*

A thorough history and examination at the time of admission, perhaps with a reassessment when the patient is more active, should identify the main co-existing medical problems. An assessment of the patient's pre-stroke functional status (i.e. what could and could not they do?) is invaluable but is rarely recorded in medical records unless specifically prompted (Davenport *et al.*, 1995). One approach might be to estimate routinely a pre-stroke Barthel Index (see Table 17.18) since this covers most of the important activities of daily living (ADL). This sort of ADL checklist is also often of value in making a prognosis and in setting rehabilitation goals since, depending on the cause and duration, the pre-stroke functional impairment will determine the best achievable post-stroke functional status. If a patient who has, as a result of arthritis, been immobile for 10 years before the stroke it is ridiculous to try to get the patient to walk after the stroke. Unfortunately, this is often attempted simply because nobody has obtained an accurate picture of the patient's pre-stroke function. This is more likely to happen where the patient has difficulties with communication and no carer is available.

An assessment of the patient's pre-stroke function may also be very important in making decisions within the first few hours after the stroke. Although it may be impossible for anyone to judge a person's quality of life other than that person themselves, one may deduce something from the patient's function. This may be important where, for example, one is considering antibiotics for a severe infection, or neurosurgery for acute obstructive hydrocephalus in a patient with a cerebellar stroke. It may not be appropriate to submit a previously very disabled or demented patient, who will almost certainly have a poor long-term outcome, to uncomfortable procedures (see Section 10.4).

Clearly, one should aim to minimise the effect of co-morbidity by giving as effective a treatment as possible. Where it is not possible to influence the disease directly it is important to take account of co-morbidity in one's overall approach to the patient. One's short- and long-term goals have to take it into account.

15.7 High blood pressure after stroke

High blood pressure is often noted on admission to hospital after a stroke but it then falls over the next few days to a greater extent than in patients admitted for reasons other than stroke (Wallace & Levy, 1981; Britton *et al.*, 1986; Carlsson & Britton, 1993). Although the raised blood pressure may, in part, reflect the physical and mental stress of hospital admission, or the 'white coat' effect, some of the rise seems to be due to the acute stroke itself (Wallace & Levy

1981; Britton *et al.*, 1986; Fotherby *et al.*, 1993). Raised blood pressure detected during the initial assessment may also indicate chronic hypertension since about 50% of stroke patients are hypertensive before the onset of the stroke (i.e. at least two readings of >160/90 mmHg; Sandercock *et al.*, 1989). These patients will tend to have higher blood pressures than those without previous hypertension and are more likely to show evidence of end organ damage, e.g. hypertensive retinopathy, impaired renal function and left ventricular hypertrophy. Blood pressure in the acute phase is generally higher in patients with intracerebral haemorrhage than with ischaemic stroke (Allen, 1983; Carlberg *et al.*, 1991).

The blood pressure should be measured in the standard way with a sphygmomanometer and an appropriately sized cuff kept at the level of the patient's heart. Recent studies suggest, contrary to previous belief, that there is no consistent difference between the blood pressure measured in the plegic and unaffected arm, although there is often a difference between arms which is unrelated to the side of the stroke and probably reflects occlusive vascular disease affecting one arm (Panayiotou *et al.*, 1993). Therefore, the blood pressure should be checked in both arms on at least one occasion and monitored consistently in the arm giving the highest reading to avoid a spurious label of labile blood pressure. If the blood pressure is raised on admission it should be monitored to establish whether or not it falls spontaneously. If the blood pressure is high it is advisable to look for evidence of end organ damage including: hypertensive retinopathy; left ventricular hypertrophy on clinical assessment, ECG or echocardiography; and renal dysfunction with proteinuria or renal failure. The presence of end organ damage suggests that the high blood pressure is not simply a response to the acute stroke.

There is considerable uncertainty about the relative risks and benefits of lowering the blood pressure in a patient with acute stroke. Treatment may theoretically reduce the likelihood of rebleeding in intracerebral and subarachnoid haemorrhage and of brain oedema and haemorrhagic transformation in cerebral infarction. However, lowering the blood pressure may reduce cerebral perfusion where cerebral autoregulation is impaired and thus further increase ischaemic damage (see Section 11.12) (Powers, 1993; Phillips, 1994). There have been no large randomised trials specifically aimed at establishing the balance of risk and benefit. However, three small randomised-controlled trials of calcium channel blockers (intravenous nimodipine, oral nimodipine and intravenous nicardipine) in acute stroke demonstrated that the functional status and early survival may be worse in the treated group, probably because the hypotension increased infarct

Table 15.10 Circumstances in which immediate blood pressure lowering treatment is indicated after an acute stroke.

Papilloedema or retinal haemorrhages and exudates
Marked renal failure with microscopic haematuria and proteinuria
Left ventricular failure
Features of hypertensive encephalopathy, e.g. seizures, reduced conscious level
Aortic dissection

Note: even these features may be misleading in acute stroke because left heart failure may frequently be related to co-existent ischaemic heart disease, and seizures and drowsiness may occur due to the stroke itself.

volume (Lisk *et al.*, 1993; Kaste *et al.*, 1994; Wahlgren *et al.*, 1994).

Until randomised trials have been completed which answer this question directly we offer the following advice. If the blood pressure remains elevated (i.e. >160/90 mmHg after a couple of weeks) or where there is evidence of end organ damage, we would give the patient general advice (i.e. salt restriction, weight loss and moderation of alcohol intake) and start an antihypertensive drug, accepting that this timing is arbitrary. The rationale for delayed treatment of hypertension is discussed in Section 16.3. Our management is similar whatever the pathological type of stroke. Where the patient is already on antihypertensive treatment it seems reasonable to continue it as long as the patient has not become hypovolaemic, which may increase its effect and lead to marked and potentially damaging hypotension. If the blood pressure is very high (i.e. >220/>120 mmHg) there may be certain circumstances which prompt earlier initiation of blood-pressure-lowering drugs (Table 15.10). The aim of therapy should be a moderate reduction in blood pressure over a day or so rather than minutes. An oral beta-blocker (in the absence of heart failure or other contraindication) is a reasonable first choice but some authorities advise intravenous nitroprusside or labetalol, with very careful intra-arterial monitoring of blood pressure for resistant cases (Phillips, 1993). The former drug has the advantage of a very short half-life so that turning off the infusion quickly reverses the hypotensive effect.

Do not aggressively lower the blood pressure in the first few days after a stroke unless there is evidence of accelerated hypertension.

15.8 Epileptic seizures

About 2% of stroke patients have a seizure on the day of their stroke (i.e. onset seizure) and about 50% of these are generalised (Kilpatrick *et al.*, 1990; Oxfordshire Community Stroke Project, unpublished data) (see Section 6.5.6 and Table 15.2). This may be an underestimate since not all onset seizures are witnessed. In the Oxfordshire Community Stroke Project the risk of having a first seizure, excluding onset seizures, was about 5% in the first year after a stroke and about 1–2%/year thereafter (Oxfordshire Community Stroke Project, unpublished data). Hospital-based studies tend to overestimate the risks because of patient selection. Seizures may recur in about 50% of the patients, but are rarely troublesome if accurately diagnosed and appropriately treated. Patients with onset seizures, haemorrhagic strokes and cerebral infarcts involving the cerebral cortex (i.e. total anterior circulation infarction) have the highest overall risk of seizures (Olsen *et al.*, 1987; Kilpatrick *et al.*, 1992; Oxfordshire Community Stroke Project, unpublished data). Patients who are functionally independent have a very low risk of post-stroke seizures so that a theoretical risk of seizures is not a reason to stop a return to normal driving (Oxfordshire Community Stroke Project, unpublished data).

> *The risk of having an epileptic seizure after a first-ever in a lifetime stroke is about 5% in the first year and 1–2%/year thereafter.*

The diagnosis of seizures should, as usual, be based on a detailed description of the attack from the patient and/or witness and may very occasionally be confirmed by electroencephalography during a seizure. If patients have seizures in the first few days after the stroke, and especially if they are partial, one should generally investigate them further. Other cerebral and non-cerebral pathologies complicated by post-seizure impairments (e.g. Todd's paresis) may mimic strokes (see Section 3.5.1). Because the neurological deficits and conscious level may be temporarily much worse immediately after a seizure, 'onset seizures' can make the assessment of stroke severity unreliable (see Section 15.4). We have also seen occasional patients who have had non-convulsive status epilepticus, who may, for example, be severely dysphasic, and who have improved dramatically with anticonvulsant treatment. Also, seizures should not automatically be attributed to the stroke since many other causes may be present coincidentally, or as a consequence of the stroke (Table 15.11). Appropriate investigations should be performed to exclude these.

Any precipitating cause should be treated. Status epilepticus should be managed in the normal way. Usually, an isolated seizure does not require anticonvulsants but if seizures recur or, depending on the patient's wishes and their activities (particularly driving), treatment after the first seizure may be warranted since the risk of further seizures is about 50%. Patients who have had a seizure should be advised not

Table 15.11 Causes of epileptic seizures after 'stroke'.

General
Alcohol withdrawal
Anticonvulsant withdrawal
Hypoglycaemia (see Section 15.18.4)
Hyperglycaemia (see Section 15.18.3)
Hyper/hyponatraemia (see Sections 15.18.1 and 15.18.2)
Drugs
    Baclofen given for spasticity
    Antibiotics for infections, e.g. ciprofloxacin
    Antidepressants given for emotionalism or depression
    Phenothiazines given for agitation or hiccups
    Antiarrhythmics for associated atrial fibrillation

Neurological
Due to the primary stroke lesion
Haemorrhagic transformation of infarction (see Section 5.4)
Underlying pathology
    Arteriovenous malformation (see Section 8.2.2)
    Intracranial venous thrombosis (see Section 8.2.5)
    Mitochondrial cytopathy (see Section 7.15)
    Hypertensive encephalopathy (see Section 3.5.6)

Wrong diagnosis (see Section 3.5)
Herpes simplex encephalitis
Cerebral abscess
Cerebral tumour
Subdural empyema

to drive and, depending on the national regulations, may have to inform the authorities. However, many patients who have seizures are too disabled to drive anyway (see Section 15.32.2).

15.9 Headache

Headache is quite a common symptom in stroke and may provide clues to the type and cause (see Sections 3.2.3 and 6.5.6). Although it may be severe initially it is not usually very persistent. Having established that there is no sinister underlying cause, most patients simply require reassurance that the pain will settle, adequate analgesia and antiemetics for any associated nausea.

15.10 Hiccups (singultus)

Hiccups are due to involuntary diaphragmatic contractions with closure of the glottis. The precise mechanism is unclear. They may be persistent and troublesome in patients with strokes affecting the medulla. If they persist, other causes should be considered and excluded by appropriate investigations (e.g. uraemia, diaphragmatic irritation). Numerous folk cures, e.g. sudden frights and drugs (Table 15.12) have been suggested as effective treatments; the latter may occasionally be worth trying where hiccups are persistent and distressing to the patient but most have significant adverse effects. The management of hiccups has recently been thoroughly reviewed (Kolodzik & Eilers, 1991; Launois *et al.*, 1993).

15.11 Immobility and positioning

Immobility is a major consequence of: impaired conscious level; severe motor deficits including weakness, ataxia and apraxia; and less commonly of sensory (i.e. proprioceptive) and visuospatial deficits. Immobility makes the patient vulnerable to a number of complications such as infections (see Section 15.12), deep venous thrombosis (DVT) and pulmonary embolism (see Section 15.13), pressure sores (see Section 15.16), contractures (see Section 15.20) and falls and the resulting injuries (see Section 15.26). Immobile patients are unable to position themselves to maintain comfort, facilitate activities such as drinking and passing urine or to relieve pressure over bony prominences. They are in the ignominious situation of always having to ask others to position them appropriately.

Little formal research has been done in the area of positioning after stroke. For example, after a stroke should the patient be nursed sitting or lying, and if lying, on which side? The answers to these questions may be important in a number of respects.

1 *Maintenance of a clear airway.* In unconscious patients correct positioning is vital to maintain a clear airway and to reduce the risk of aspiration (see Section 15.2.1).

2 *Oxygenation.* When patients with acute stroke are sat up their blood oxygen saturation is significantly higher than when nursed lying flat (Elizabeth *et al.*, 1993) (see Section 15.2.2).

3 *Cerebral perfusion.* Patients who are hypovolaemic may have reduced systemic blood pressure when nursed sitting which may reduce cerebral perfusion and possibly increase cerebral ischaemia. However, if intracranial pressure falls on sitting, this may increase the cerebral perfusion pressure.

4 *Cerebral oedema.* Intracranial pressure is highly dependent on posture, being higher in patients nursed flat and lower when sitting up (Feldman *et al.*, 1992).

The relationships between oxygenation, cerebral perfusion, intracranial pressure and cerebral blood flow are so complex that it is difficult to predict the optimum position for nursing an individual patient (Fig. 15.3). Whether our own anecdotal observation that some patients with severe strokes are more alert when sitting up than when lying is explained by reduced intracranial pressure, reduced cerebral oedema, or improved oxygenation and increased stimulation is not at all clear.

Table 15.12 Some of the common drugs used to treat hiccups. (From Launois *et al.*, 1993.)

Chlorpromazine
Haloperidol
Metoclopramide
Sodium valproate
Phenytoin
Carbamazepine
Nifedipine
Amitriptyline
Baclofen

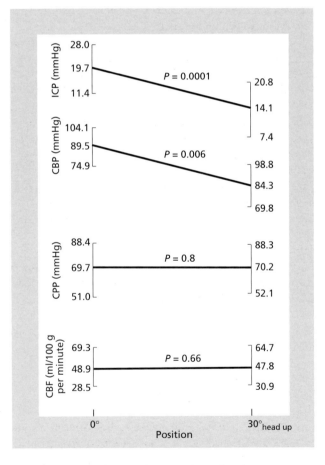

Figure 15.3 Graph showing the inter-relationships between intracranial pressure (ICP), carotid blood pressure (CBP), cerebral perfusion pressure (CPP) and cerebral blood flow (CBF) with changes in posture in patients with head injury. (Data from Feldmann *et al.*, 1992.)

5 *Tone*. The position of a patient influences the tone in their trunk and limbs (see Section 15.20). Positioning of the patient is used by physiotherapists and nurses to promote higher or lower tone, whichever seems most appropriate for that particular patient. Spasticity and the tendency to develop contractures may be reduced by careful positioning to reduce tone (see Section 15.20), whilst patients who have low tone in their truncal muscles may benefit from positioning which promotes increased tone and leads to better truncal control. The positioning charts which are so often strategically placed by the patient's bed to guide nursing care give the impression that we know what we are doing. However, although there is some agreement about the optimum positioning of patients with hemiplegia (e.g. fingers extended, spine straight), there are many areas of uncertainty (e.g. optimum position of the head, foot and unaffected limbs) (Carr & Kenney, 1992). There is clearly a need for further research into this area.

6 *Swallowing* is easier and safer with the patient sitting up with their neck flexed (see Section 15.17).

7 *Pressure area care*. For immobile patients who cannot shift their own weight, their position must be changed sufficiently frequently to avoid developing ischaemia of the skin and subcutaneous tissues over the points of weight bearing (see Section 15.16).

8 *Limb oedema*. The ankles, and in hemiplegia the paralysed arm, frequently become oedematous and painful, which may raise muscle tone and reduce function (see Section 15.25).

9 *Stimulation*. It is difficult for patients to see what is going on around them when lying flat. This lack of sensory stimulation and contact with daily events will encourage sleep and may lead to boredom, reduced morale and sometimes exacerbate confusion.

The team should assess each patient and decide which of these potential problems are most important in that individual. For example, is the patient hypoxic or dysphagic or at particular risk of pressure sores? Depending on this assessment a positioning regimen which sets out the best positions and the frequency of re-positioning should be agreed.

15.12 Fever and infection

Fever is quite common after stroke and is associated with a worse outcome (Hindfelt, 1976; Castillo *et al.*, 1994; Azzimondi *et al.*, 1995; Reith *et al.*, 1996). It is unclear whether this is because fever is: simply a marker of a severe stroke (i.e. due to loss of central temperature control or resorption of subarachnoid blood); an indication of an infective complication (e.g. pneumonia or urinary infection); and,

Table 15.13 Causes of fever after a stroke.

Causes	Section
Urinary infection	15.14
Pneumonia	
Coincidental upper respiratory tract infection	
DVT	15.13
Pulmonary embolism	15.13
Pressure sores	15.16
Vascular problems, e.g. infarction of myocardium, bowel or limb	
Infective endocarditis	6.4, 7.8
Infected intravenous access site	
Drug allergy	

whether fever itself increases cerebral damage. The last is an attractive, although unproven concept, since it is consistent with research in animal models which has shown that hyperthermia increases and hypothermia decreases ischaemic cerebral damage (Busto *et al.*, 1987, 1989; Chen *et al.*, 1991; Moyer *et al.*, 1992). Table 15.13 lists some of the potential causes of fever after stroke, of which infections are probably the most common (Przelomski *et al.*, 1986).

Immobile stroke patients are prone to infections, the most common sites being the chest and urinary tract (Dromerick & Reding, 1994; Kalra *et al.*, 1995; Davenport *et al.*, 1996b). Chest infections are much more common in the acute stage, occurring in as many as 20% of patients, whilst urinary infections occur throughout the period of recovery (Davenport *et al.*, 1996b). Chest infections may be due to aspiration, failure to clear secretions, immobility or reduced chest wall movement on the side of a hemiparesis. In one autopsy study, pneumonia was usually bilateral and where it was unilateral there was no excess on the side of the hemiparesis (Mulley, 1981). However, others have found more clinical signs of pneumonia on the side of the hemiparesis (Kaldor & Berlin, 1981).

Studies, based on retrospective reviews of case notes, have shown that between 25 and 44% of patients developed urinary tract infections whilst receiving in-patient rehabilitation for an acute stroke (Dromerick & Reding, 1994; Kalra *et al.*, 1995). Infections are an important cause of mortality and morbidity after stroke and often interrupt rehabilitation (Bounds *et al.*, 1981).

Chest infections may be minimised by careful positioning of the patient, physiotherapy and suction to avoid the accumulation of secretions, and care to avoid aspiration (see Section 15.17). Urinary infections can be avoided by maintaining adequate hydration and thus urine output, and by avoiding unnecessary bladder catheterisation (see Section

489

15.14). There is little evidence to support the use of prophylactic antibiotics to reduce the overall risk of infections after stroke. Ensuring that the patient receives adequate nutrition may also be important because malnutrition is known to lead to immune paresis (see Section 15.19).

The patient's temperature should be monitored at least 6-hourly during the first few days after the stroke and thereafter if there are any other signs of infection or functional deterioration. However, fever may not accompany infection, especially in elderly and immunocompromised patients. Any functional deterioration or failure to attain a rehabilitation goal should prompt a search for occult infection. Obviously, the cause of fever should be identified using clinical assessment supplemented with appropriate investigations (e.g. neutrophil count, cultures of urine, sputum or blood, chest X-ray, C reactive protein). The treatment of fever will depend on the cause but it seems reasonable, given the possibility that fever itself may be harmful, to prescribe antipyretic medication such as paracetamol. Obviously, appropriate antibiotics and supportive treatment (e.g. physiotherapy, oxygen) should be given in established infection.

15.13 Venous thromboembolism

Clinically apparent DVT is relatively uncommon in stroke, occurring in less than 5%. However, more sensitive diagnostic techniques such as iodine-125 (^{125}I) fibrinogen leg scanning show that around 50% of patients with hemiplegia develop a DVT during the first 10 days after stroke, almost always in the paretic leg (Warlow *et al.*, 1976; Sandercock *et al.*, 1993; Kalra *et al.*, 1995; Davenport *et al.*, 1996b). Others have shown that DVT commonly develops over the first few months in patients who remain immobile (Cope *et al.*, 1973; Oczkowski *et al.*, 1992). Pulmonary embolism is an important cause of death after stroke and is probably under-recognised (Bounds *et al.*, 1981). Difficulty breathing or tachypnoea may be wrongly attributed to pulmonary infection or cardiac failure rather than pulmonary embolism. The frequency of pulmonary embolism, which depends on patient selection and the criteria for diagnosis, has been reported in 6–16% of patients with acute stroke, and in up to 50% of those undergoing autopsy (Warlow *et al.*, 1976; McCarthy & Turner, 1986; Sandercock *et al.*, 1993).

DVT should be suspected if a patient's leg becomes swollen, hot or painful or if the patient develops a fever. Where the patient develops a clinical DVT or pulmonary embolism, confirmatory investigations should probably only be carried out if treatment with anticoagulants is being considered. We would normally use venography to confirm the presence of a DVT, although ultrasound and plethysmography are reasonably accurate alternatives to confirm thrombosis in the proximal leg veins but will not reliably detect thrombi confined to the calf (Weinmann & Salzman, 1994). A ventilation/perfusion isotope lung scan may be helpful in determining the likelihood that respiratory symptoms are due to pulmonary embolism.

Unfortunately, the clinical diagnosis of DVT can be difficult because many paretic legs become swollen due to dependency and lack of movement. If a paretic leg swells whilst a patient is still being nursed in bed, DVT is a likely cause, but where a patient's leg is dependent for part of the day the clinical diagnosis of DVT is much less certain. Non-stroke patients who develop a DVT will often complain of discomfort or swelling, but stroke patients who have communication difficulties, sensory loss or neglect may not complain, so that clinical detection will depend on the vigilance of members of the multidisciplinary team.

> *The clinical diagnosis of deep venous thrombosis in stroke patients is particularly difficult because, on the one hand, a swollen leg may be due to paralysis and dependency whilst, on the other hand, a patient may not complain about pain and swelling because of language and perceptual problems.*

Manoeuvres which may reduce the risk of DVT and pulmonary embolism include the following.

1 *Early mobilisation* of the patient and avoidance of prolonged bed rest, although the effectiveness of this regimen has not been tested in randomised trials.

2 Routine use of *full-length graduated compression stockings*. A systematic review of randomised trials of graduated compression stockings in patients undergoing *surgery* showed a 68% (95% confidence interval (CI): 53–73%) reduction in the odds of developing DVT (Wells *et al.*, 1994). There are not enough data to tell us whether below-knee stockings are just as effective. It seems reasonable to generalise these results to immobile stroke patients, although stroke patients may have particular problems. For example, great care should be taken in patients with diabetes or symptoms or signs of peripheral vascular disease in whom stockings may produce ischaemic skin damage over bony prominences (Fig. 15.4). Many patients find the stockings uncomfortable if worn for long periods, especially in hot weather, and full-length stockings may be difficult to keep dry in patients who are incontinent of urine. The stockings should be removed daily to check for problems with the skin.

3 *Heparin* has been shown to reduce the risk of DVT in patients with ischaemic stroke but we are still uncertain whether this benefit outweighs the potential risks of heparin,

If a patient with a confirmed ischaemic stroke has a proven DVT or pulmonary embolism, the conventional treatment is adjusted dose heparin, either given subcutaneously or intravenously, followed by oral anticoagulants for perhaps 6 months, although this duration might depend on the patient's mobility and there is little evidence to guide us in this. However, one has to balance the potential risks of such treatment in ischaemic stroke where haemorrhagic transformation may be increased, and in patients with established intracranial haemorrhage. We do not believe that intracranial haemorrhage is an absolute contraindication to anticoagulation since, if a patient has a life-threatening pulmonary embolus, the risk of anticoagulation may be worth taking. We have occasionally anticoagulated patients using adjusted dose intravenous heparin within 1 week of an intracerebral haemorrhage without obvious ill effects. There are few studies which help us make this difficult decision but anticoagulation may be less hazardous than one might expect (Dickmann *et al.*, 1988; Boeer *et al.*, 1991).

15.14 Urinary problems

Between one- and two-thirds of patients admitted to hospital are *incontinent of urine* in the first few days after an acute stroke (Brocklehurst *et al.*, 1985; Borrie *et al.*, 1986; Barer, 1989a; Benbow *et al.*, 1991). Urinary incontinence is more common in severe strokes (i.e. those with a poor outcome; see Section 10.2.7). Urinary incontinence may be due to the stroke itself but perhaps 20% of patients have been incontinent prior to the stroke (Borrie *et al.*, 1986; Benbow *et al.*, 1991). Although detrusor instability is the most common single cause of urinary incontinence after the first 4 weeks, many other factors may contribute in the acute stage (Table 15.14). Urinary incontinence is an important cause of distress to patients and carers, increases the risk of pressure sores, often interferes with rehabilitation (e.g. by interrupting physiotherapy sessions) and influences the patient's requirements for ongoing nursing care.

To identify patients with urinary incontinence one simply has to ask the carer or nursing staff. These are the people most aware of urinary problems since they have to deal with the consequences. It is important to ask, since many people consider incontinence an inevitable consequence of stroke and thus not worthy of mention. It is often useful, but frequently overlooked, to ask the patients themselves what they think is causing their incontinence. More detailed information, including urinary volumes, frequency and times of voiding, which can be collected using a micturition chart, may be useful in identifying the causes of incontinence (e.g. diuretics, communication difficulties) and in formulating a

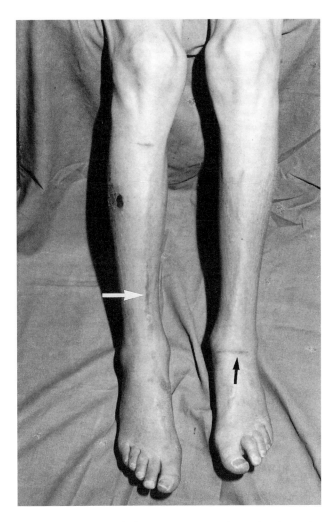

Figure 15.4 Photograph showing a patient with peripheral vascular disease and diabetes mellitus who was fitted with graduated compression stockings. Note the necrotic skin over the anterior border of the tibia (white arrow) and where the stockings were creased at the ankle (black arrow). There were also necrotic areas over both heels which failed to heal and led to a right above-knee amputation following an unsuccessful revascularisation procedure.

e.g. haemorrhagic transformation of cerebral infarction and in patients with primary intracerebral haemorrhage (see Section 11.3) (Dickmann *et al.*, 1988; Sandercock *et al.*, 1993; Counsell & Sandercock, 1995). Routine heparin for DVT prophylaxis can not be recommended in stroke patients at present. It seems likely that other antithrombotic drugs (e.g. aspirin) might reduce the incidence of venous thromboembolism but the balance of risk and benefit in acute stroke is unclear (see Section 11.4).

4 *Other methods* of prophylaxis, e.g. external pneumatic compression and functional electrical stimulation, have been suggested but have not been evaluated adequately (Prasad *et al.*, 1982; Desmukh *et al.*, 1991).

Table 15.14 Factors which may contribute to urinary incontinence.

Reduced conscious level
Immobility (can not get to the toilet in time)
Communication problems (can not indicate need to go to the toilet)
Impaired upper limb function (can not manipulate clothes or the urinal)
Loss of inhibition of bladder contraction (detrusor instability)
Urinary infection (often without other symptoms)
Urinary overflow due to outflow obstruction (e.g. prostatism)
Faecal impaction
Excess urinary flow due to high fluid intake, diuretics and poorly controlled diabetes
Too few carers/nurses (can not attend to patients in time)
Importance of maintaining continence underestimated by carers/nurses

Table 15.15 Drugs used to inhibit bladder contractility and their adverse effects.

Tricyclic antidepressants
Imipramine
Amitriptyline
Nortriptyline

Others
Flavoxate hydrochloride
Oxybutynin hydrochloride
Propantheline bromide

Common adverse effects
Dry mouth
Blurred vision
Nausea/vomiting
Constipation/diarrhoea
Confusion in the elderly
Retention where there is bladder neck obstruction
Precipitation of acute glaucoma

management plan.

Where the cause of urinary incontinence is unclear and if it persists for more than a few days, the patient should be investigated. Urine microscopy should identify infection. Measurement of post-micturition bladder volumes (by bladder ultrasound or catheterisation) may be useful in assessing bladder contractility and outflow. We reserve formal urodynamic studies for the few patients with unexplained, troublesome incontinence which persists for weeks after the stroke.

Some of those who are incontinent soon after stroke will die, but in many survivors urinary incontinence resolves spontaneously over the first week or two (Wade & Langton Hewer, 1985; Brocklehurst *et al.*, 1985; Borrie *et al.*, 1986). Between 20% and one-third of surviving patients are still incontinent a few months after the stroke (Brocklehurst *et al.*, 1985; Borrie *et al.*, 1986). Often, the patients with persisting problems were incontinent before their stroke, immobile or confused (Borrie *et al.*, 1986). If a patient is incontinent, but able to understand, then a careful explanation of the cause and likely prognosis should be given to allay their fears. Carers often benefit from such information too. Because urgency of micturition is such a common cause of incontinence, simple steps such as regular toiletting, offering dysphasic patients some means to alert the nurses to their needs, improving their mobility or providing a commode by the bed can all be effective (Gelber *et al.*, 1993). Obviously, one should strive to treat the underlying cause (e.g. infection, outflow obstruction) and where possible remove exacerbating factors (e.g. excessive fluids, uncontrolled hyperglycaemia or diuretics). Urodynamic studies are helpful in distinguishing patients who are incontinent due to detrusor hyper- and hyporeflexia. Such patients may respond to anticholinergic or cholinergic drugs, respectively (Table 15.15),

although 'bladder retraining' may be more effective and has fewer adverse effects (Gelber *et al.*, 1993).

An indwelling catheter should be avoided if possible because this makes resolution of urinary incontinence impossible to detect and may lead to a number of complications (Table 15.16). Other aids and appliances may be useful (Table 15.17) in avoiding unnecessary catheterisation. However, when patients are at high risk of pressure sores (see Section 15.16), and other means have failed to keep them dry, a catheter may be the best option. Catheterisation may also be required to relieve urinary retention (see below) until any cause or precipitating factor can be removed, e.g. enlarged prostate, urinary infection, severe constipation, anticholinergic drugs.

Occasionally, if urinary incontinence is a bar to discharge into the community, long-term catheterisation may be the preferred option. This issue should be discussed with the patient and, where appropriate, their carer. Continence advisors, nurses with specialist training in the management of incontinence and access to information, aids and appliances, can often provide help to other professionals, patients and their carers. In many parts of Britain, laundry services run by health authorities or social services provide invaluable assistance to families having to cope with incontinence.

Urinary retention, which may be acute or chronic, is quite common in stroke patients, more so in men. The main cause is pre-existing bladder outflow obstruction which may be precipitated by constipation, immobility and drugs such as tricyclic antidepressants which have antimuscarinic effects. Urinary retention may present with dribbling incontinence, agitation or confusion and is easily missed in patients with a reduced conscious level, communication difficulties or other

Table 15.16 Problems (and solutions) of indwelling urinary catheters. (From Belfield, 1989.)

Problem	Solution
Pain on insertion	Explain to the patient what is going to happen Use plenty of anaesthetic gel
Paraphimosis	Ensure foreskin is not left retracted after insertion
Poor self-esteem	Explain why catheter is needed, how it works and how long it will be in place Provide a discreet drainage bag
Immobility because of drainage bag	Use well-supported leg bag for mobile patients
Leakage	Use appropriate size of catheter Inhibit any involuntary bladder contraction causing bypassing with an antimuscarinic drug Change catheter if blocked
Blockage	Ensure adequate urine flow Remove encrusted catheter
Infection	Avoid unnecessary catheterisation since no proven method of preventing infection
Catheter fell out due to urethral dilatation or pelvic floor laxity	Ensure balloon inflated to correct volume or use larger volume balloon
Catheter rejection due to bladder contraction	Avoid large volume balloon Inhibit with antimuscarinic drug
Catheter pulled out by patient	Manage without a catheter to avoid further trauma
Pain on catheter removal	Avoid routine changes Explain procedure to patient Allow adequate time for balloon deflation
Failure of balloon deflation	Introduce ureteric catheter stylet along inflation channel

cognitive problems. It is important to palpate the patient's abdomen on admission and, later, if urinary problems or agitation develop, to exclude a distended bladder.

15.15 Faecal incontinence and constipation

Constipation is common after stroke and may lead to faecal smearing or incontinence. Immobility, poor fluid and food intake and constipating analgesics are common causative factors. Faecal incontinence occurs in about 25% of stroke patients admitted to hospital, usually those with severe strokes who have a depressed conscious level, are immobile or unable to communicate (Brocklehurst *et al.*, 1985).

Table 15.17 Aids and appliances which may be useful in patients with urinary incontinence. (From Smith, 1989.)

Absorbent pads and pants
These vary in the volume of urine they can absorb, their shape and method of holding them in position

Urinals
Useful for men who are immobile or have urgency which gives them insufficient time to reach the toilet. They can be fitted with a non-spill valve for patients who have poor manual dexterity (Fig. 15.5)

Bedside commode
Useful where urgency is associated with poor mobility so the patient has insufficient time to get to the toilet (see Fig. 15.20)

Penile sheath
Often viewed as an alternative to an indwelling catheter in men without bladder outflow obstruction, but they easily fall off and are therefore unsuitable for agitated or confused patients. Other problems include skin erosions due to urinary stasis or the adhesive strip and twisting of the sheath and penile retraction during voiding which causes leakage

Achieving continence of faeces is often a crucial step in discharging a patient home since incontinence is so practically and socially difficult to cope with and is invariably a cause of considerable strain for the carer.

The frequency of bowel movements should be monitored. Simple monitoring will detect constipation and diarrhoea and may help to establish the pattern of any faecal incontinence. Occasionally, it may be useful to culture the stool or to X-ray the abdomen to exclude infection or high faecal impaction, respectively, if the patient has faecal incontinence associated with diarrhoea. More detailed investigation is usually not required unless there are persistent unexplained problems.

> *Faecal incontinence which is not associated with severe cognitive problems is almost always remediable by dealing with constipation or diarrhoea.*

Avoidance of constipation by ensuring an adequate intake of fluid and fibre is the best approach, but laxatives, suppositories and, occasionally, enemas are sometimes required. However, laxatives may cause incontinence in immobile patients.

15.16 Pressure sores

Pressure sores occur when local pressure on skin and subcutaneous tissues exceeds the capillary opening pressure for long enough to cause ischaemia. In addition, friction may cause blistering and tears in the skin. Pressure sores usually

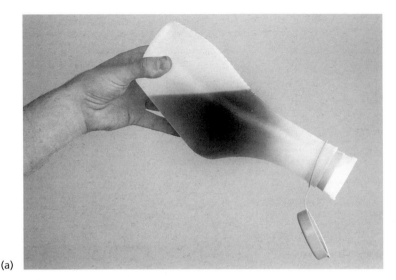

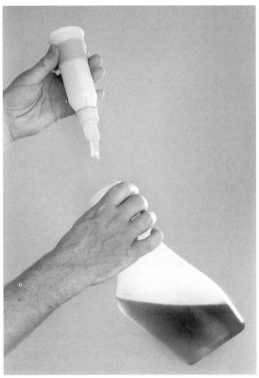

Figure 15.5 Some patients have difficulty manipulating a urinal which leads to spills and, effectively, incontinence. (a) This urinal can be inverted without leaking. (b) A simple one-way valve inserted in the neck of the urinal prevents the contents spilling.

(a)

(b)

occur over weight-bearing bony prominences (Fig. 15.6). Sores occur in patients who are immobile and unable to redistribute their own weight when lying or sitting. The reported frequency of pressure sores in hospitalised stroke patients is about 3%, but this is bound to vary depending on the population studied and the diagnostic criteria (Kalra *et al.*, 1995). One might expect the frequency to be less in the sorts of institutions which publish their results. Pressure sores are more common in patients who are malnourished, infected, incontinent or have serious underlying disease. They cause pain, increase spasticity, slow the recovery process and may even lead to death. They prolong length of stay in hospital, often require intensive treatment and can

therefore be extremely expensive to health services (Scales *et al.*, 1982; Clough, 1994). They can and should be prevented, although they may develop in the interval between the onset of the stroke and admission to hospital.

Pressure sores can be prevented by good nursing. Immobile patients should be examined regularly to identify early signs of pressure damage, i.e. skin erythema. It is important that patients who are at particular risk of developing pressure sores are identified as early as possible so that preventative measures can be taken. The Norton Scale (Table 15.18) was the first of many clinical scoring systems to be developed to indicate an individual patient's risk of pressure sores. Most scales include some measure of mobil-

Domain	Score				
	4	3	2	1	
Physical condition	Good	Fair	Poor	Very bad	
Mental state	Alert	Apathetic	Confused	Stuporous	
Activity	Ambulant	Walks with help	Chairbound	Bedbound	
Mobility	Full	Slightly limited	Very limited	Immobile	
Incontinence	None	Occasional	Usually urine	Double	
Total score					

Table 15.18 The Norton Scale. A score of less than 15 indicates a vulnerability to pressure sores, whilst a score of less than 12 indicates the patient is at high risk.

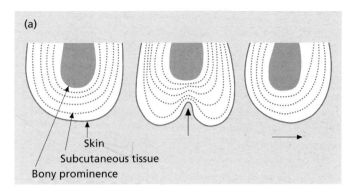

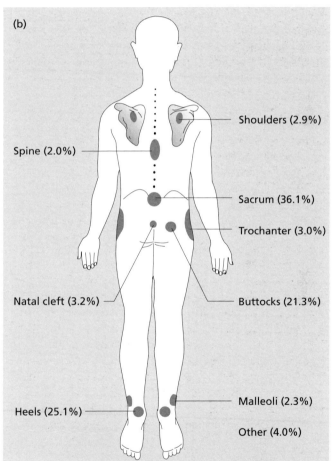

Figure 15.6 Showing (a) the distortions of tissues over a bony prominence due to compression or shear which may lead to pressure sores and (b) the anatomical distribution of established pressure sores based on data from a cross-sectional survey in the UK of pressure sores in patients being nursed on the Pegasus Airwave System. Patients with cerebrovascular disease were the largest group in this sample but only comprised 14.1% of patients. (From St Clair, 1992.)

ity, continence, cognitive function and nutritional status and none, based on less than ideal evaluations, is clearly superior to the others (Barratt, 1988; Cullum *et al.*, 1995).

The clinician should be alert to behaviour which, in patients with communication and cognitive problems, may indicate a painful pressure area. Such patients may repeatedly move themselves out of a desired position. For example, patients, colloquially known as 'thrusters', with a painful

sacrum may force themselves out of chairs by extending their bodies at the waist. This may become a major problem for nursing staff.

If patients develop pressure sores it is useful to have some objective measure of their severity so that healing or lack of healing can be monitored. Photographs incorporating a centimetre scale are a convenient and reliable method to demonstrate change, but where this facility is not available, tracing the limits of the sore or simply measuring it in several planes is useful (Allman *et al.*, 1987). Several grading scales have been developed for use in research but because they are less objective than say a photograph their inter-rater reliability is inferior (Shea, 1975). Patients who are at risk of sores, or who have established pressure sores, should be investigated to exclude malnutrition, hypoalbuminaemia, anaemia and occult infection, all of which can slow healing (Allman *et al.*, 1987).

The most important step in preventing or healing pressure sores is to relieve the pressure on the tissues for long enough and at frequent enough intervals to allow the tissues to receive an adequate blood supply. This can usually be achieved by regular turning of patients (1 or 2-hourly depending on the assessment of risk) but this takes up a lot of skilled nursing resources. Although the introduction of a variety of special mattresses and cushions (Table 15.19) may reduce the need for regular turning, most patients still need to be turned. Some beds are designed to turn the patient automatically (e.g. the net suspension bed).

Pressure-relieving mattresses and cushions can be divided into 'passive' and 'active' systems (Fig. 15.7). The 'passive' systems distribute the patient's weight through a larger area and make it easier for patients to re-position themselves (Kemp *et al.*, 1993; Hofman *et al.*, 1994). 'Active' systems usually work by inflating and deflating air cells to relieve pressure on each point at regular intervals. Although the 'active' systems are probably more effective than the 'passive' systems (Bliss *et al.*, 1967; Exton-Smith *et al.*, 1982; Bliss, 1995) they are expensive and can make certain nursing tasks more difficult, e.g. positioning a patient to reduce the risk of contractures, to help breathing or to facilitate swallowing, because they offer a less firm base. The ultimate

Table 15.19 Specialised mattresses and cushions.

Passive systems

Sheepskin fleeces and bootees which reduce skin shear and moisture. The natural fleeces are better than man-made ones. They are made ineffective by poor cleaning and being covered by sheets

Padded mattresses containing polyester fibres, e.g. Spenco

Polystyrene bead system

Foam mattresses (e.g. Vaperm) vary in their pressure-relieving properties

Gel pads can be used under heels and sacrum

Roho cushions are effective but very expensive (see Fig. 15.7)

Active systems

Ripple mattresses and airwave systems provide alternating pressure. The larger the cells the better but they tend to break down and leak

Low air loss systems (e.g. Mediscus) providing constant low pressure although effective tend to be noisy, expensive and complex needing regular maintenance and training (see Fig. 15.7)

Floatation beds, deep water beds, are difficult to nurse patients on, are very heavy and some patients get motion sickness

Dry floatation providing constant low pressure produced by glass microspheres blown by air. Air can be turned off when the patient needs to be repositioned. Effective but bulky and expensive

Mechanical beds turn the patient, e.g. net suspension bed. Effectiveness uncertain. Patients may not like being suspended (on view). Useful to turn patients who are in pain

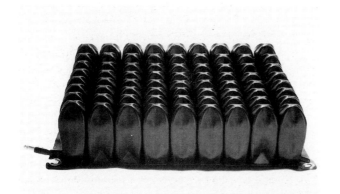

(a)

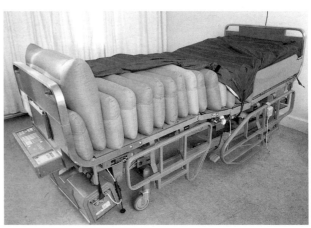

(b)

Figure 15.7 Pressure-relieving cushion and bed. (a) A Roho cushion. (b) A low air loss bed.

choice of preventative method will depend on an assessment of the individual patient's risk of pressure sore, the availability of nurses, the patient's other needs, e.g. positioning, and available resources. Further research is required to identify the most cost-effective strategy for preventing pressure sores. Studies will have to take into account patients' absolute risk of developing sores, the reduction in risk with each intervention and the cost of the intervention, as well as the cost of treating any pressure sores which develop. However, we believe that, whatever technology is employed, adequate numbers of skilled nursing staff will still be essential if pressure sores are to be prevented.

For patients with established pressure sores the relief of pressure probably remains the most important factor in promoting healing. 'Active' pressure-relieving systems are probably more effective than 'passive' ones in treatment as well as prevention (Ferrell et al., 1993). In addition, it is important to optimise the patient's general condition by providing a good diet with adequate protein intake and by treating concurrent illness aggressively (e.g. infections, cardiac failure). The pain associated with pressures sores may increase tone and lead to contractures which may hinder rehabilitation (Allman et al., 1987; Hofman et al., 1994). The discomfort may affect the patient's morale and further worsen their outcome. Adequate analgesia should be given to patients and opiates may sometimes be required, especially prior to renewal of dressings. Antibiotics may be required if there is local or systemic infection (spreading cellulitis, osteomyelitis). Debridement to remove necrotic tissue and skin grafting to achieve skin coverage may sometimes be necessary. A bewildering variety of local dressings and treatments (e.g. vitamin C, ultrasound, ultraviolet light) which aim to promote healing and reduce infection are available but most have not been evaluated adequately in randomised trials (Taylor et al., 1974; Wills et al., 1983; ter Riet et al., 1992, 1995). For a more detailed account the reader is referred to a recent systematic review of the management of pressure sores (Cullum et al., 1995).

15.17 Swallowing problems

Up to 45% of patients admitted to hospital with an acute stroke have some evidence of aspiration when asked to drink a small volume of water (Gordon et al., 1987). However, estimates of the frequency of swallowing difficulties vary because of differences in definitions, timing and methods of detecting dysphagia and in selecting patients for study. Swallowing difficulties have been associated with a high case fatality and poor functional outcome and certainly put patients at risk of aspiration, pneumonia, dehydration

and malnutrition (Gordon et al., 1987; Barer, 1989b; Holas et al., 1994). However, much of the excess mortality and morbidity is probably due to the severity of the stroke rather than the swallowing difficulties themselves.

15.17.1 Mechanisms of dysphagia

A number of mechanisms of dysphagia after stroke have been identified using videofluoroscopy (Veis & Logemann, 1985).

1 Poor oral control (oral preparatory phase) and delayed triggering of the swallow 'reflex', leading most often to aspiration before the swallow, i.e. liquid trickles over the back of the tongue before the swallow has been started. In addition, patients with weakness or incoordination of the face or tongue often have difficulty keeping fluids in their mouth, and in chewing and manipulation of the food to produce a well-formed food bolus.

2 Failure of laryngeal adduction which leads to aspiration during the swallow itself.

3 Reduced pharyngeal 'peristalsis' or cricopharyngeal dysfunction may allow food to collect in the pharynx and spill over, past the vocal cords and into the trachea. Thus, aspiration will occur after the swallow.

Delayed triggering of the swallow reflex is the most common mechanism but in most patients more than one abnormality can be identified. Veis and Logemann's study included few patients within days of their stroke so that their findings may not apply to the majority of patients who have difficulties with swallowing for just the first few days (Veis & Logemann, 1985; Barer, 1989b).

15.17.2 Detection of dysphagia

Despite their frequency, and the serious consequences of failing to detect them, swallowing problems are often not sought systematically in patients admitted to hospital with an acute stroke (Davenport et al., 1995). There is also no agreement about the best method of screening for dysphagia. Although videofluoroscopy (Fig. 15.8) is usually considered the 'gold standard' test, it has a number of limitations, including its lack of practicality in acute stroke (Table 15.20).

Because of the limitations of videofluoroscopy, several groups have developed clinical tests which can be performed at the bedside (DePippo et al., 1992; Horner et al., 1993; Kidd et al., 1993; Stanners et al., 1993). Unfortunately, none (Table 15.21) detects all patients who aspirate, which may be important since silent aspirators may be at greatest risk of complications (Holas et al., 1994). Clinicians often use the gag reflex to indicate swallowing safety but this has been

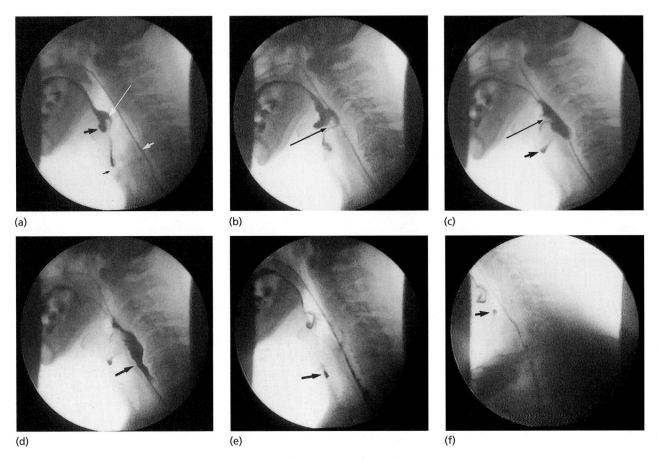

(a)   (b)   (c)

(d)   (e)   (f)

Figure 15.8 A series of six frames taken from a videofluoroscopy examination in a stroke patient with swallowing difficulties. We have shown only the lateral view. (a) The food bolus containing radiodense material has been propelled into the pharynx by the tongue and has filled the vallecular space (large black arrow). Food is spilling over from the vallecular space, past the epiglottis (long white arrow) and is heading for the vocal cords (small black arrow). Note the nasogastric tube (short white arrow). The pharyngeal swallow has not yet been triggered. (b) The pharyngeal swallow has triggered (at last) with elevation and inversion of the epiglottis (arrow). (c) The epiglottis is fully inverted (long arrow). No further laryngeal penetration has occurred, indicating effective (but rather belated) laryngeal closure. However, some of the food bolus has passed the vocal cords (short arrow). (d) The food bolus is passing through the cricopharyngeal sphincter (arrow). (e) The swallow is complete but part of the food bolus remains below the vocal cords (arrow). The patient has not coughed indicating that sensation is impaired, i.e. this patient has silent aspiration. (f) The patient has been asked to cough and this voluntary cough is effective in clearing the aspirated food back into the pharynx (arrow). (Videofluoroscopy provided by Diane Fraser.)

Table 15.20 Limitations of videofluoroscopy.

Lack of general availability, especially in the acute situation

Lack of evidence that aspiration detected by this method is
  clinically important since studies have shown that normal people
  aspirate under some circumstances

Patients are tested under unfamiliar and artificial conditions which
  may influence their swallowing performance and limit the
  generalisability of the results

Exposure of patients to radiation

Use of radiological contrast which may cause lung damage
  if inhaled

---

shown to be innaccurate and unreliable (kappa = 0.3) (Ellul & Barer, 1993; Smithard *et al.*, 1993; Stanners *et al.*, 1993). Until further studies have demonstrated which method of assessment most reliably detects clinically important swallowing problems, i.e. those which worsen the outcome, we suggest the following approach to screening for dysphagia.

The gag reflex is not a useful indicator of a stroke patient's swallowing ability.

1 Identify those patients who are *likely* to have problems swallowing, i.e. those with severe hemispheric or brainstem strokes, or impaired consciousness. Table 15.22 lists those

Table 15.21 The performance of bedside swallowing assessments in the detection of aspiration defined by videofluoroscopy as the 'gold standard'.

Study	Test	Sensitivity (%)	Specificity (%)	Aspiration (%)
Smithard *et al.* (1993)	Doctors	30	69	25
	Informal speech therapist	10	95	
Splaingard *et al.* (1988)	Formal testing by speech and language therapists	42	91	40
DePippo *et al.* (1992)	80 ml water swallow	80	54	45
Kidd *et al.* (1993)	50 ml water swallow	80	86	41
Horner *et al.* (1993)	Weak/absent cough	84	56	49
	Dysphonia	97	29	49
	Reduced gag reflex	67	70	49
Stanners *et al.* (1993)	Weak/absent cough	70	78	24
	Dysphonia	60	45	24
	Reduced gag reflex	60	45	24

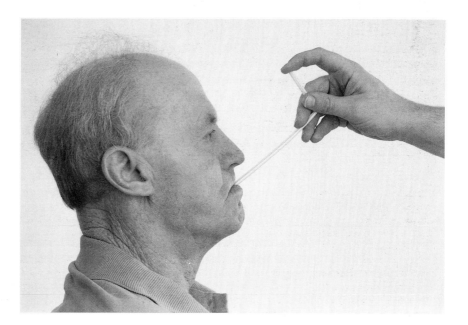

Figure 15.9 One can control the volume of liquid a patient receives during a swallowing assessment with a drinking straw used as a pipette.

Table 15.22 Features that indicate a likelihood of swallowing problems.

Severe stroke
    Decreased level of consciousness
    Severe weakness and loss of truncal control
    Dysphasia, neglect or hemianopia
Old age
Confusion
Facial weakness
Poor or absent voluntary cough
Moist or bubbling voice
Evidence of chest infection
Reduced pharyngeal sensation

features that should alert one to a high risk of swallowing difficulty.

2 For patients without these features, or where access to a speech and language therapist with an interest in swallowing difficulties is limited, a doctor or nurse can usefully assess swallowing. Ask the patient to swallow a total of perhaps 50 ml of water, initially in 5-ml aliquots, whilst sitting supported in the upright position, with neck flexed and the head tilted to the unaffected side. Suction equipment should be available. The volume and speed of delivery of the water can be controlled using a drinking straw as a pipette (Fig. 15.9). Patients may, if simply handed a cup to drink from, attempt to drink the whole quantity and aspirate large volumes.

After each swallow, wait for an involuntary cough and ask the patient to speak; a cough or a change in the patient's voice (i.e. wet voice) may indicate aspiration. This crude test has been shown to identify most patients who aspirate (Kidd *et al.*, 1993). One should be particularly careful in assessing patients with existing respiratory disease who may be compromised by even minor degrees of aspiration.

3 If swallowing difficulties are likely or are demonstrated on simple bedside testing, put the patient on 'nil by mouth' and hydrate them via an alternative route until a more detailed assessment can be made. Fluids may be given intravenously, subcutaneously or via a nasogastric tube; each route has its advantages and disadvantages and practice varies which reflects the lack of evidence about whether or not one route is superior to another (Challiner *et al.*, 1992). The patient's mouth should be kept moist and clean with regular care.

15.17.3 Prognosis and management

Most patients with swallowing difficulties immediately after their stroke either die or the dysphagia improves within 1–2 weeks so that persisting dysphagia is relatively uncommon. In one study only one patient of 357 had dysphagia 6 months after stroke onset (Barer, 1989b). However, ongoing assessment of patients' swallowing abilities by a speech and language therapist is valuable in guiding their fluid and feeding regimen, so that patients are not unnecessarily deprived of nutrition or put at risk of aspiration. Speech and language therapists may not be any more accurate in detecting swallowing problems than nurses or doctors, but they will usually perform a more detailed assessment including: feeding the patient in various positions (e.g. leaning to one side or the other); with different food textures (e.g. liquid, thickened fluids, purée or solids); with increasing bolus size; with different methods of delivery; and with different verbal cues or instructions (Smithard *et al.*, 1993). They may also advise videofluoroscopy if a patient has swallowing difficulties which persist for more than 1–2 weeks, perhaps where percutaneous endoscopic gastrostomy (PEG) is being considered (see Section 15.19) or where silent aspiration is suspected in a patient with repeated chest infections.

Based on their swallowing assessment, which may or may not include videofluoroscopy, speech and language therapists may be able to teach the patient and carers methods of compensating for their problems until recovery occurs (DePippo *et al.*, 1994). Simple interventions which might allow a patient to swallow safely include the following.

1 Teaching the patient manoeuvres such as the 'chin tuck' or 'head turn' which make aspiration less likely.

2 Tailoring the consistency of fluids and food to the patient's swallowing abilities. For instance, thickened fluids are usually more easily swallowed than water because they move less rapidly through the oropharynx and so give more time for the initiation of the swallow.

3 Choosing an appropriate type of drinking vessel. If the patient has not got a severe facial weakness and can suck, a drinking straw is often helpful. Beakers with spouts tend to encourage the patient to drink with an extended neck which opens the airway and encourages aspiration (Fig. 15.10).

Unfortunately, there has been little formal evaluation of these techniques and there is no evidence to suggest that therapy actually speeds the return of a normal swallow (DePippo *et al.*, 1994).

15.18 Metabolic disturbances

Metabolic disturbances, which may occasionally mimic stroke (see Section 3.5.3), occur commonly in patients with

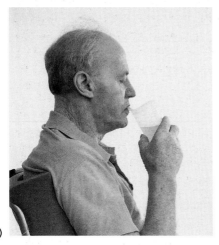 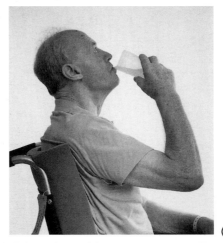

(a) (b)

Figure 15.10 Although beakers with a spout may prevent spills they have unfortunate associations with childhood which can make them unpopular with some patients. Also, they encourage patients to extend their neck when drinking which may lead to aspiration. The way *not* to do it: (a) bring the spout to the lips; (b) throw back the head, *open* the airway and inhale!

severe strokes (Berkovic *et al.*, 1984). They are important because they may cause 'worsening' (see Section 15.5) but are often easily reversed.

15.18.1 Dehydration

Patients with stroke are vulnerable to dehydration because of the following.

1 Swallowing difficulties are common after acute stroke (see Section 15.17).

2 Immobility often means patients are dependent on others to provide them with drinks (see Section 15.11). They may even have been lying on the floor for several hours before being found.

3 They may have communication problems (see Section 15.30) so they cannot ask for drinks.

4 They may have visual neglect (see Section 15.29) so may not see the jug of water beside them.

5 They are often elderly and therefore may have reduced sensitivity to thirst (O'Neill & McLean, 1992).

6 They may have a fever, chest infection (see Section 15.12), hyperglycaemia (see Section 15.18.3) or be taking diuretic therapy which increase their fluid losses.

Clinical signs (Table 15.23) are helpful in identifying dehydration, but are not so reliable in older patients (Gross *et al.*, 1992). Tachycardia, poor peripheral perfusion and a low jugular venous pressure are useful in severe cases but it is often impractical to test for orthostatic hypotension. Investigations, including the haematocrit, urea and electrolytes are probably more reliable and where a patient is unwell with hypotension or renal failure, cannulation of a

Table 15.23 Clinical indicators of dehydration.

General signs
Thirst
Reduced skin turgor
Dry mucous membranes
Sunken eyes

Cardiovascular
Cool peripheries
Collapsed peripheral veins
Postural hypotension
Low jugular venous pulse or central venous pressure
Low urine output

Investigations
Raised haemoglobin concentration
Raised packed cell volume
Raised serum sodium (evidence of water depletion)
Raised urea (out of proportion to the serum creatinine)

---

central vein to measure the right atrial pressure directly and to monitor fluid replacement may be valuable. In hospital, charting of patients' fluid intake and output can be helpful but fluid charts are often innaccurate, not least because it is more difficult, although not impossible, to monitor output when patients are incontinent (see Section 15.14).

Hypernatraemia is usually due to water depletion without concomitant sodium depletion and often occurs if patients do not drink adequate amounts. It is only diagnosed by measuring the serum sodium since it is difficult to detect clinically. Very occasionally, hypernatraemia indicates a diabetic hyperosmolar state.

Patients who are unable or unwilling to take adequate oral fluids to prevent or reverse dehydration should be offered fluid replacement by another route, i.e. intravenously, subcutaneously or by nasogastric tube. There is very little evidence to suggest that any one route is better than another (Challiner *et al.*, 1992). If patients are willing and able to take fluids orally they should be given adequate access to fluids (i.e. the cup and jug should be placed within their reach and not on the side of their neglect) and, importantly, regular encouragement to drink. Where the patient is hypernatraemic adequate isotonic fluid replacement will usually normalise the serum sodium.

Always ensure that patients, or at least those who can swallow safely, have ready access to fluids.

15.18.2 Hyponatraemia

Hyponatraemia appears to be a relatively unusual problem after ischaemic stroke and primary intracerebral haemorrhage compared with subarachnoid haemorrhage (see Section 13.4.2). One study suggested that hyponatraemia was more common in patients with haemorrhagic than ischaemic stroke, but this remains to be confirmed (Kusuda *et al.*, 1989). It may be due to excess salt loss, e.g. diuretics, or may be dilutional (reflecting inappropriate secretion of antidiuretic hormone) in response to the brain injury or medical complications. Dilution is the normal explanation for hyponatraemia after ischaemic stroke or intracerebral haemorrhage, but after subarachnoid haemorrhage, hyponatraemia has been attributed to excessive renal salt loss (see Section 13.4.2). Joynt *et al.* (1981) demonstrated higher levels of antidiuretic hormone in stroke patients than controls but none of their patients had hyponatraemia. Hyponatraemia may occasionally cause patients to deteriorate neurologically, so it is important to detect since it is usually reversible.

We would advise measuring the urea and electrolytes in patients with severe stroke and those with swallowing problems. A low serum sodium should prompt a search for the cause. This will include a review of the medication, a clinical assessment of hydration (Table 15.23) and fluid balance and, depending on the circumstances, some investigations (e.g. blood sugar, creatinine, plasma osmolality, urine osmolality and sodium concentration and, where available, antidiuretic hormone level). The serum sodium should be monitored if the initial sodium level was abnormal in patients who are not taking a normal diet and fluids, or if the patient deteriorates (see Section 15.5).

The treatment of hyponatraemia will obviously depend on the cause, e.g. stopping diuretics, fluid restriction in dilutional hyponatraemia and cautious administration of intravenous saline where salt wasting is confirmed (see Sections 13.4.2 and 13.10.1). It is usually recommended that hyponatraemia is corrected slowly to reduce the risk of central pontine myelinolysis (Burcar *et al.*, 1977; Harris *et al.*, 1993).

15.18.3 Hyperglycaemia

Hyperglycaemia (defined as a random plasma glucose of >8.0 mmol/L or a fasting level of >6.7 mmol/L) occurs in up to 43% of patients with acute stroke (van Kooten *et al.*, 1993). Of these, about 25% are known to have diabetes mellitus already and another 25% have a raised HbA1c which suggests that they had raised blood glucose for some period before the stroke, referred to as 'latent diabetes' (van Kooten *et al.*, 1993). However, 50% of the patients with hyperglycaemia have a normal HbA1c suggesting that the hyperglycaemia was very recent and may be due to the stroke itself. Whether the hyperglycaemia is due to release of catecholamines and corticosteroids as part of the stress response is controversial (Myers *et al.*, 1981; Candelise *et al.*, 1985; Oppenheimer *et al.*, 1985; O'Neill *et al.*, 1991; van Kooten *et al.*, 1993).

Hyperglycaemia after a stroke appears to be related to a poor outcome (Candelise *et al.*, 1985). This could be explained by more severe strokes producing a greater stress response and, thus, hyperglycaemia so that hyperglycaemia is simply a marker of severe stroke. However, some animal work suggests that hyperglycaemia can, depending on the blood flow, exacerbate ischaemic neuronal damage. Much of the excess morbidity and mortality associated with hyperglycaemia may in fact result from the micro- and macrovascular complications of known or latent diabetes.

A random blood glucose should be measured in all patients with stroke. In those with hyperglycaemia an HbA1c will help distinguish those with latent diabetes from those with hyperglycaemia due to the stroke itself. A glucose tolerance test after the acute stage of the illness (i.e. when the patient is medically stable) may be helpful in sorting out which patients have diabetes or impaired glucose tolerance and which simply had hyperglycaemia related to the acute stroke. Patients with established diabetes and latent diabetes should be assessed to exclude vascular (both micro and macro) and neurological complications.

There have been no randomised trials designed to determine whether rigorous control of blood glucose after stroke influences outcome. However, it seems sensible, until this question has been answered, to maintain reasonable control of blood sugar after an acute stroke, although hypoglycaemia must be avoided. This may require an insulin infusion and intravenous fluids. Treatment may, if nothing else, prevent dehydration and incontinence due to polyuria resulting from an osmotic diuresis.

15.18.4 Hypoglycaemia

Hypoglycaemia may mimic stroke or transient ischaemic attack (TIA) (see Sections 3.3.2 and 3.5.3), but also occur after stroke because patients' food intake and any requirement for hypoglycaemic agents may be less. Since hypoglycaemia may, if severe or undetected, cause worsening of the neurological deficit, the blood sugar should be monitored particularly carefully in diabetic patients on hypoglycaemic medication.

15.19 Nutrition

Several studies have shown that malnutrition is quite common in elderly patients admitted to hospital (Albiin *et al.*, 1982; Sandstrom *et al.*, 1985; Cederholm & Hellstrom, 1992). Malnutrition decreases immune competence, predisposes to pressure sores (see Section 15.16) and is associated with an increased length of stay and higher mortality (Davalos *et al.*, 1994). There have been few formal studies of nutrition in patients after stroke; their estimates of its frequency vary depending on, as usual in these matters, the methods of patient selection and the definitions of malnutrition. Smithard *et al.* (1993) showed that 29% of men and 52% of women admitted to their unit had triceps skinfold thickness below the normal reference value; Axelsson *et al.* (1988) found that 23% of patients admitted with acute stroke had a low serum albumen and 16% were judged to be poorly nourished on a range of anthropometric and serum protein measurements; Davalos *et al.* (1994) found that 12% had protein-energy malnutrition, whilst Unosson *et al.* (1994) found only 8% to be protein-energy malnourished using a more rigorous definition of malnutrition where patients had to have abnormalities of anthropometric measurements, serum proteins and antigen skin testing.

Published studies do not appear to have investigated other aspects, such as vitamin status, after stroke. Nutritional status may worsen in the weeks after admission to hospital with acute stroke but does not only occur in patients dependent in feeding (Axelsson *et al.*, 1988; Smithard *et al.*, 1993; Unosson *et al.*, 1994). It seems likely that patients who cannot swallow or feed themselves, have ill-fitting dentures, increased nutritional needs because of infection or a tendency to depression or apathy, will be at particular risk of becoming malnourished unless positive measures are taken.

Although malnutrition is a concern, obesity can also be a problem during recovery from stroke. Where patients have restricted mobility, especially where they rely on others for help with transfers, obesity can be a crucial factor in how long they remain in hospital and how much support they require. It is also a problem in the long term in achieving adequate control of vascular risk factors such as hypertension (see Section 16.3.1) and diabetes. Patients quite often gain weight after stroke presumably because of decreased energy expenditure and excessive calorie intake.

The published studies of nutritional status have used a variety of indicators but many of these techniques are not appropriate for routine clinical practice. However, it would seem sensible to at least measure the patients' weight, height, serum albumen and full blood count to give some measure of nutritional status. There may be practical problems in weighing patients accurately when they can neither sit nor stand independently but these might be overcome using a weighing bed. Where patients remain dependent, have problems with feeding or appear obese, their weight should be monitored regularly.

It is useful to involve the speech and language therapist and dietician in the assessment and care of patients who have swallowing problems or in whom nutritional intake may be inadequate for other reasons, e.g. confusion. Patients often eat very slowly after stroke and need supervision to ensure safe swallowing. Simple measures such as providing appetising food of an appropriate consistency (see Section 15.17), placing the patient's meal in their intact visual field and ensuring that the patient has well-fitting dentures should not be overlooked. Staff shortages may mean that patients receive insufficient food which will eventually cause malnutrition or have food forced into them hurriedly by unthinking staff, which is very demeaning and adversely affects morale. Where trained staff are unable to cope, the patient's family or even volunteers can be trained to help with feeding.

If the patient cannot swallow enough food, supplements of liquid feeds given via a large or small bore nasogastric tube or via PEG may be needed. In surgical patients, randomised trials have indicated that supplementary feeding may reduce the length of hospital stay and improve outcomes (Bastow *et al.*, 1983). Uncontrolled studies in stroke patients indicate a possible association between early initiation of enteral nutrition and shorter length of stay in hospital, but clearly this needs to be confirmed or refuted by randomised trials (Nyswonger & Helmchen, 1992). The timing and method of enteral feeding varies considerably between centres, which probably reflects the paucity of evidence that any one regimen is superior. The results of one trial, which randomised only 30 acute stroke patients with dysphagia to feeding via PEG or nasogastric tube, suggested that PEG feeding is associated with fewer treatment failures, better nutritional status and a rather implausible 80% reduction in the relative risk of dying (Norton *et al.*, 1996). These apparent effects may have been due to differences in patients at baseline and need to be confirmed in larger trials. Some of the advantages and disadvantages of the two approaches are listed in Table 15.24.

Patients who are obese, in particular if this causes problems with mobility or control of diabetes or blood pressure, should be encouraged to lose weight and be offered dietary advice.

Eating not only fulfils our nutritional requirements but plays an important role in our social lives and is a source of pleasure. Eating with other people during the recovery phase encourages communication and social interaction. Patients who are concerned by their appearance after a stroke (e.g. due to facial weakness) may gain confidence from this opportunity to socialise. On the other hand, dribbling whilst eating may distress the patient and inhibit social interaction.

Table 15.24 Advantages and disadvantages of nasogastric (NG) and PEG feeding. (From Finucane *et al.*, 1991; Pender *et al.*, 1993; Raha & Woodhouse, 1994.)

	Advantages	Disadvantages
NG tube	Widely available Cheap	Often pulled out Unsightly Uncomfortable May lead to aspiration Nasal irritation/ulcer Interference with swallow
PEG	Rarely displaced Cosmetically acceptable Long-term use practical	Limited availability Expensive Aspiration when sedated Wound infections Bleeding Peritonitis

15.20 Spasticity and contractures

Immediately after a stroke the muscular tone in the limbs may be lower, the same as, or higher than normal (Gray *et al.*, 1990). The reasons for this variation and subsequent changes are unclear. In patients with a hemiparesis the tone in the arm is usually greater in the flexors than extensors, whilst in the leg it is said to be greater in the extensors than the flexors (i.e. spasticity). This is consistent with the typical hemiplegic posture (i.e. arm flexed and internally rotated whilst the leg is extended at the hip and knee and the foot is plantar flexed and inverted). Tone in the truncal muscles may also be abnormally high or low. Tone may increase in any muscle group so much that it restricts the active movement which the residual muscle strength can produce. Imbalance in muscle tone can eventually result in shortening of muscles and permanent deformity and restriction of the full range of movement, i.e. contractures. Closely allied to spasticity are 'associated reactions' which are involuntary movements of the affected side (most typically flexion of the arm) elicited by a variety of stimuli including the use of unaffected limbs (e.g. self-propelling a wheelchair; yawning or coughing) and the upright posture (Mulley, 1982; Cornall, 1991). Associated reactions become more obvious with increases in tone. Spasticity and contractures may cause pain, deformity, disability and, if severe, secondary complications such as pressure sores at points of contact between soft tissues (e.g. on the inner aspect of the knees in a patient with contractures of the adductors of the thighs).

Physicians are trained to assess the tone in a limb by asking the patient to relax and then moving the limb through its range of movement at each joint at different speeds and noting the resistance to these movements. Unfortunately, many physicians do not appreciate how much the tone is influenced by factors such as the patient's posture and mental state. Tone may change from minute to minute. This makes it difficult to assess objectively with good inter-rater reliability. Physiotherapists, who spend far more time handling patients than physicians, are more aware of changes in tone and try to use these changes in their therapy. Formal measurement of tone can be attempted using clinical scales (e.g. the modified Ashworth scale; Table 15.25) or technology such as electrogoniometry. Unfortunately, the inter-rater reliability of the clinical scales is poor and the technological solutions are not widely available or practical in routine clinical practice (Bohannon & Smith, 1987).

Contractures are easier to assess than spasticity because, by definition, the deformity is fixed. Thus, one can objectively measure the range of movement around a joint and repeat the measure to determine whether or not an intervention has improved the range.

Table 15.25 The modified Ashworth scale for the clinical assessment of muscle tone. (From Ashworth, 1964.)

Score	Description
0	No increase in muscle tone
1	Slight increase in muscle tone, manifested by a catch and release, or by a minimal resistance at the end of the range of motion when the affected part(s) is moved in flexion or extension
1+	Slight increase in muscle tone, manifested by a catch, followed by minimal resistance throughout the remainder (less than half) of the range of movement
2	More marked increase in muscle tone through most of the range of movement but affected parts easily moved
3	Considerable increase in muscle tone, passive movement difficult
4	Affected parts rigid in flexion or extension

Physiotherapists aim to modulate changes in tone to the patient's advantage. For instance, they may try to increase the tone in a flaccid leg to provide the patient with a more secure base on which to walk or reduce tone in the arm to facilitate more active movement. Therapists modulate tone by careful positioning, by exercises and by avoiding factors that promote spasticity such as anxiety and pain. Patients with a hemiparesis may attempt to 'overuse' their sound side to achieve mobility but, as a consequence, the tone may increase in the affected side. If not controlled, this can lead to loss of function and contractures. Using the unaffected leg to self-propel a wheelchair is said to lead to increased spasticity in the affected arm and leg (Ashburn & Lynch, 1988; Cornall, 1991). The aim of many of the facilitation and inhibition techniques used by therapists is to use basic reflexes and postural changes in tone to promote function. These techniques, although widely accepted and used by therapists, have not been evaluated adequately in randomised trials (see Section 15.21).

Unwanted changes in tone, which might eventually lead to contractures, may be avoided by correctly positioning the patient. Unfortunately, there appears to be quite a lot of uncertainty about the optimum positions for patients with hemiplegia (Carr & Kenney, 1992). There are also practical difficulties in keeping patients in the required position, i.e. the patients tend to move. Carers should be taught to move patients' limbs passively even in the very acute stages to maintain a good range of movement. Factors which might increase tone excessively (such as pain from pressure sores, a painful shoulder or anxiety) should be controlled as far as possible. Where spasticity

Table 15.26 Adverse effects of antispasticity drugs.

Adverse effect	Baclofen	Diazepam	Dantrolene
Sedation/central nervous system depression	++	+++	+
Confusion	+	+	
Hypotonia/weakness	+	+	++
Unsteadiness/ataxia	+	++	+
Exacerbation of epileptic seizures	++		
Psychosis/hallucinations	++		
Headache	+	+	
Urinary retention	+	+	+
Hypotension	+	+	
Nausea/vomiting	+	+	
Diarrhoea/constipation	+	+	+
Abnormal liver function	+	+	+++
Hyperglycaemia	+		
Visual disturbance	+	+	
Skin rashes	+	+	+
Pericarditis/pleural effusions			+
Blood dyscrasia		+	
Withdrawal symptoms	+	++	
Drug interactions	++	+	+

+, reported occasionally; ++, quite frequent; +++, potentially fatal.

is not adequately controlled by these techniques, or where the patient is suffering from painful muscle spasms, certain drugs have been advocated. These include diazepam, baclofen and dantrolene. Although some small randomised trials have shown benefits in patients with established spasticity, others have not confirmed their effectiveness in acute stroke and in our experience they rarely make much difference and have a number of unwanted adverse effects (Table 15.26) (Burt & Currie, 1978; Ketel & Kolb, 1984; Katrak *et al.*, 1992). Adverse effects are much more common in older patients but can be minimised by starting with low doses and increasing the dose slowly until the desired effect is achieved, or adverse effects necessitate withdrawal.

Botulinum toxin has been used in patients with troublesome spasticity with some apparent short-term improvement both in spasticity and function, although no controlled evaluation of this expensive technique is available (Hesse *et al.*, 1994; Bhakta *et al.*, 1996). Very rarely, surgical procedures are used to reduce deformities due to contractures. Anecdotally, the prevalence of severe contractures appears to have declined dramatically over the last 30 years which is probably a result of improvements in the standards of general care.

15.21 Limb weakness, poor truncal control and unsteady gait

These aspects of the patient's condition are impossible to separate and will therefore be discussed together. Weakness of an arm, leg or both, sometimes with unilateral facial weakness, are probably the most common and widely recognised impairments related to stroke. However, there are often associated but less obvious problems with the axial muscles which impair truncal control and walking.

Facial weakness, which affects about 40% of patients (see Table 15.2), apart from its cosmetic effects, may contribute to dysarthria (see Section 15.30) and cause problems with the oral preparatory phase of swallowing (see Section 15.17). Weakness of the upper limb, which affects about 50% of patients (see Table 15.2), along with changes in tone, can lead to a painful shoulder (see Section 15.24) and swelling of the hand (see Section 15.25). Poor arm function is a major cause of dependency in activities of daily living. Weakness of the leg, which affects about 45% of patients (see Table 15.2), may be severe enough to immobilise the patient and thus predispose to the complications of immobility (see Section 15.11). Leg weakness, making it difficult to stand, transfer or walk independently, is one of the most important factors prolonging hospital stay in stroke patients. In patients with hemiparesis, which affects about 55% of patients, the arm is usually weaker than the leg (see Table 15.2).

Physiotherapists generally feel (and rightly so in our opinion) that physicians place too much emphasis on the assessment of muscle power because the associated abnormalities of tone, truncal control and patterns of movement account for many of the functional consequences of stroke. In assessing a patient with stroke it may be more useful to observe the range and control of voluntary movements of the limbs. For instance, does the patient have only coarse movement around the hip or shoulder or have they retained movement at the more distal joints? In stroke patients, distal movements are usually more severely impaired than proximal ones. The assessment of motor function and truncal control has already been described (see Section 4.2.3).

Recovery from a hemiplegic stroke has been likened to early infant development, in that the recovery of truncal control follows the same general pattern as that of a growing child. Head control develops first, followed by rolling over, sitting balance and then standing balance, and lastly the patient can walk with increasing steadiness and speed (see Fig. 10.7). After a stroke it is useful to know where the patient is on this 'developmental ladder' when assessing prognosis and setting goals for rehabilitation. It is important to assess truncal control and gait since truncal ataxia can occur without limb incoordination in patients with midline cerebellar lesions. It is not unknown for patients to undergo full gastrointestinal and metabolic investigation to elucidate the cause of vomiting before their truncal ataxia is noted and a cerebellar stroke diagnosed. It also seems absurd that, although immobility is the main reason for a stroke patient needing to stay in hospital for rehabilitation, mobility and balance are often not assessed properly by doctors admitting stroke patients (Davenport *et al.*, 1995). Having stressed the importance of testing truncal control and gait, it is important that in doing so neither the patient nor the doctor are put at risk of injury. Poor handling and lifting technique may dislocate a patient's flaccid shoulder, result in a fracture from a fall and may even injure the doctor's back! Physiotherapists should ideally provide appropriate training to *all* staff who are involved in handling patients to avoid these problems.

The severity of weakness of individual muscle groups is often graded using the Medical Research Council (MRC) Scale (Table 15.27) (Medical Research Council, 1982). However, this was originally designed to assess motor weakness arising from injuries to single peripheral nerves, not stroke. Unfortunately, although widely used, the MRC scale is often misused and the optional expansion to include extra grades (e.g. 4+, 5−) makes it even less reliable in the routine recording of motor weakness. The Motricity Index, a modification of the MRC Scale (Table 15.27) for use in patients with stroke, allows the observer to grade the severity of the hemiparesis rather than each separate muscle group (Demeurisse *et al.*, 1980). This can be useful in charting patients' progress for research purposes but is of limited value in routine clinical practice because it is difficult to remember the weights applied to individual movements and it requires a small block to assess grip strength. There are several tools available for objectively measuring and recording motor function (Table 15.28).

Spontaneous recovery of motor function is highly variable. The more severe the initial impairment, the less likely is full recovery. The pattern of recovery of motor function parallels that of other stroke-related deficits, with the most rapid recovery occurring in the first few weeks and then the pace of improvement slowing over subsequent months (see Section 10.2.5). In patients with hemiparesis it is generally thought that motor function in the leg usually improves more than that in the arm, although this has been questioned recently (Duncan *et al.*, 1994). Also, unless the patient has some return of grip within 1 month of the stroke, useful return of function is unlikely although not impossible (Sunderland *et al.*, 1989).

Physiotherapy is the main therapeutic option in hemiparesis although several other physical agents (e.g. acupuncture,

electrical stimulation) have been used. Techniques vary, but the two broad approaches most commonly employed are the 'facilitation and inhibition' techniques and the 'functional' approach. The facilitation and inhibition techniques are based on the premise that posture and sensory stimuli can modify basic reflex patterns which emerge after cerebral damage. If one observes a hemiplegic patient one might notice that the erect posture exaggerates the typical hemiplegic posture. Similarly, turning the head towards the affected side decreases the flexor tone in the arm, whilst turning the head away from the affected arm increases the tone. Several workers have developed different treatments based on facilitation and inhibition, the best known being those of Bobath (1978) and Brunnstrom (1970). Although these techniques differ, certain features have been identified as common to all (Table 15.29). These techniques aim to achieve as

Table 15.27 The MRC Scale of weakness and the Motricity Index which was developed from the MRC Scale for use in stroke patients.

MRC SCALE

0	No contraction
1	Flicker or trace of contraction
2	Active movement with gravity eliminated
3	Active movement against gravity
4	Active movement against resistance
5	Full strength

THE MOTRICITY INDEX

Arm

Pinch grip	—
Elbow flexion (from 90°)	—
Shoulder abduction (from chest)	—
Total arm score	—

Leg

Ankle dorsi-flexion (from plantar flexed)	—
Knee extension (from 90°)	—
Hip flexion	—
Total leg score	—

Scoring system for pinch grip

0	Pinch grip, no movement
11	Beginnings of prehension
19	Grips block (not against gravity)
22	Grips block against gravity
26	Against pull but weak
33	Normal

Scoring system for movements other than pinch grip

0	No movement
9	Palpable contraction only
14	Movement but not against gravity/limited range
19	Movement against gravity/full range
25	Weaker than other side
33	Normal

Table 15.28 Measurements of motor function. (From Wade, 1992.)

IMPAIRMENTS
MRC Scale (see Table 15.27)
Motricity Index (see Table 15.27)
Trunk control test
Motor club assessment
Rivermead motor assessment
Dynamometry

DISABILITY

Arm
Nine-hole peg test
Frenchay arm test/battery
Action Research arm test

Truncal control/mobility
Standing balance
Functional ambulation category
Timed 10-m walk
Truncal control
Rivermead mobility index (see Table 15.44)
Subsection of OPCS scale (Martin *et al.*, 1988)

OPCS, Office of Population Censuses and Surveys.

Table 15.29 Common features of facilitation/inhibition-based therapy. (From Flanagan, 1967.)

Recognition of the intimate relationship between sensation and movement
Recognition of the importance of basic reflex activity
Use of sensory input and different postures to facilitate or inhibit reflex activity and movement
Motor relearning based on repetition of activity and frequency of stimulation
Treatment of the body as an integrated unit rather than focusing on one part
Close personal interaction between the therapist and patient

---

normal a posture and pattern of movement on the affected side as possible. On the other hand, the functional approach simply aims, through training and strengthening of the unaffected side, to compensate for the impairment to achieve maximum function. For example, patients may be encouraged to transfer and walk as soon as possible after the stroke. Supporters of the facilitation and inhibition approach claim that although the functional approach might achieve earlier independence, it results in more abnormal patterns of movement which in the long term may lead to contractures and loss of function. Undoubtedly, there is a place for both approaches in clinical practice. Quite often, where a patient has not achieved useful independent mobility despite a prolonged period of physiotherapy (using the facilitation and

inhibition approach), we will opt to switch to a functional approach to maximise the patient's autonomy. For example, we will train patients to transfer independently and self-propel a wheelchair.

Although physiotherapists appreciate the complex nature of the motor problems in hemiparesis, including the subtle problems which affect the contralateral limbs, this focus on the motor impairments may distract attention from the associated sensory, cognitive and visuospatial problems which may often be more important in limiting the patient's functional recovery.

There has been very little formal evaluation of the physiotherapy techniques. Although several small randomised trials have been reported, no definite conclusions about the relative merits of different approaches can be drawn (Stern *et al.*, 1970; Inaba *et al.*, 1973; Dickstein *et al.*, 1986; Jongbloed *et al.*, 1989; Wagenaar *et al.*, 1990; Gelber *et al.*, 1993). In any case, comparisons of different techniques may have limited relevance to current clinical practice as many therapists adopt an eclectic approach, using selected aspects of each technique for appropriate individual patients.

We doubt whether anybody involved in stroke rehabilitation would seriously question whether physiotherapists are effective (see Section 10.3.6). Nonetheless, there are some important questions about physiotherapy after stroke which need to be addressed in properly designed randomised controlled trials.

1 When should physiotherapy start?
2 How long should it continue?
3 What is the optimum intensity of physiotherapy?
4 Is therapy provided by relatively unskilled therapists as effective as that provided by skilled therapists?
5 Which patients gain most from physiotherapy and can we prospectively identify them?
6 Which specific therapeutic interventions are the *most* effective?

Certainly, the results of randomised trials support the hypothesis that physiotherapy does have an effect on function and that the size of the effect is probably influenced by the intensity of treatment (Smith *et al.*, 1981; Sunderland *et al.*, 1992, 1994; Wade *et al.*, 1992). Systematic reviews of existing trials should help guide treatment and future research. There are many methodological problems in performing randomised trials of physiotherapy techniques (as well as those used by other therapists) and in applying their results and so progress will be slow (see Table 15.1).

Other interventions

The effectiveness of a number of physical techniques including, electromyographic (EMG) biofeedback, functional electrical stimulation, sensory stimulation, and acupuncture have been tested in small randomised trials (Han-Hwa *et al.*, 1993; Magnusson *et al.*, 1994). Although some have provided encouraging results there is insufficient evidence to recommend their widespread use. Indeed, two meta-analyses of published trials of EMG biofeedback came to differing conclusions regarding whether there was evidence of significant benefit or not (Schleenbaker & Mainous, 1993; Glanz *et al.*, 1995).

In this section we have dealt with interventions that aim to decrease disability by improving impairments. The complementary strategy involving the appropriate provision of mobility aids, e.g. walking sticks, splints and wheelchairs is dealt with elsewhere (see Section 15.32.1).

15.22   Sensory impairments

About one-third of patients, in whom it can be reliably assessed, have impairment of at least one sensory modality, but in about 20% it may be impossible to assess sensation adequately because of reduced conscious level, confusion or communication problems (see Table 15.2). Sensory problems are more easily identified in patients with right rather than left hemisphere stroke, probably because of the communication difficulties associated with left hemisphere strokes. Severe sensory loss may be as disabling as paralysis, especially when it affects proprioception. Loss of pain and temperature sensation in a limb, or sensory loss with neglect, may put a patient at risk of injury from heat, etc. Disordered sensation with numbness or paraesthesia, even without functional difficulties may, if persistent, be as distressing to some patients as central post-stroke pain (see Section 15.23). We have discussed some of the difficulties in assessing sensory function earlier (see Section 4.2.4).

> *Patients often complain bitterly about what appears to the doctor to be a minor change in sensation. Do not underestimate the effect which facial numbness or tingling in a hand can have on the morale of a patient.*

Little is known specifically about the recovery of sensation after stroke, although it probably follows the pattern of recovery seen in most other impairments (see Section 10.2.5). Although patients may be given sensory stimulation as part of their therapy nothing is known about the effect this or any other intervention has on sensation (Yekutiel & Guttman, 1993).

Where patients have lost temperature or pain sensation in a limb, especially if there is associated neglect, it is important to counsel them about commonsense strategies to reduce the risk of injury to the limb.

15.23   Pain

Pain is a common complaint amongst stroke patients. There are many potential sources, some of which are coincidental and others of which are in some way due to the stroke (Table 15.30). Usually, the cause becomes obvious after one has asked the patient about the distribution, nature and onset of the pain and has examined the relevant area. However, some pains (e.g. due to spasticity, axial arthritis and central post-stroke pain) may be difficult for patients to describe and localise. Although central post-stroke pain is typically described as a superficial burning, lacerating or pricking sensation triggered by touch or cold, patients' descriptions vary considerably (Leijon *et al.*, 1989). It is usually associated with some abnormality of sensation and may start immediately after the stroke or after a delay of weeks or months. Fortunately, central post-stroke pain is relatively uncommon (although we are not aware of any methodologically sound incidence studies) because it is often very distressing and resistant to treatment.

The treatment of pain depends on the likely cause. Simple analgesics along with some reassurance that the pain does not indicate any serious problem may be all that is needed. Pain due to spasticity should initially be treated by carefully positioning the patient to reduce tone (see Section 15.20). Antispasticity drugs are occasionally required, seldom work and have significant adverse effects (see Table 15.26). Musculoskeletal pain can be treated with simple analgesics and, if these are ineffective, a non-steroidal anti-inflammatory drug. If a joint becomes acutely painful it may be necessary to rest it and investigate to exclude more serious

Table 15.30 Causes of pain after stroke.

Headache due to vascular pathology (see Sections 3.2.3 and 15.9)
Painful shoulder (see Section 15.24)
DVT (see Section 15.13)
Pressure sores (see Section 15.16)
Limb spasticity (see Section 15.20)
Fractures (see Section 15.26)
Arterial occlusion with ischaemia of limb, bowel or myocardium
Co-existing arthritis exacerbated by immobility or therapy
Instrumentation, e.g. catheter, intravenous cannulae, nasogastric tube
Central post-stroke pain (thalamic pain/Dejerine–Roussy syndrome)

causes, e.g. septic arthritis, fracture or gout exacerbated by diuretics or aspirin.

Central post-stroke pain is a particularly difficult problem which is often resistant to therapy. Antidepressants (e.g. amitryptiline), anticonvulsants (e.g. carbamazepine, phenytoin, valproate, clonazepam) and antiarrhythmic drugs (e.g. mexiletine) have all been advocated; indeed, amitryptiline was shown to be significantly more effective than placebo in one small randomised trial (Leijon & Boivie, 1989). Another small randomised trial failed to demonstrate any effect using naloxone (Bainton *et al.*, 1992). Physical methods such as acupuncture and transcutaneous electrical nerve stimulation (TENS) may have some place in difficult cases. Stereotactic mesencephalic tractotomy may relieve symptoms in severe cases which are resistant to other treatment modalities but carries significant morbidity and mortality (Shieff & Nashold, 1987).

15.24   Painful shoulder

Shoulder pain is a common problem in stroke patients with arm weakness. Although the literature concerning painful shoulder is extensive, it is generally unenlightening (Roy, 1988; Van Langenberghe *et al.*, 1988). However, in a recent community-based study which overcame many of the methodological problems of earlier studies, approximately one-third of patients reported painful shoulders, usually on the hemiparetic side (R. Bonita, personal communication, 1994). About 8% of patients had a painful shoulder before the stroke onset. Painful shoulder was uncommon in patients without hemiparesis and its frequency was not influenced by age. Two-thirds of patients who were destined to suffer a painful shoulder in the first year developed symptoms in the first week after the stroke.

Although many factors (Table 15.31) have been associated with painful shoulders their role in aetiology is unclear. A small proportion of patients who complain of a painful shoulder after a stroke have the other clinical features which comprise the syndrome of reflex sympathetic dystrophy or shoulder–hand syndrome (Table 15.32). Although our understanding of the epidemiology and causes of painful shoulder is incomplete, no-one involved in stroke rehabilitation can doubt its importance. It causes patients great discomfort, it may seriously affect morale and can inhibit recovery. In some patients it persists for months and even years.

It is difficult to make firm recommendations regarding prevention and treatment when our understanding of the cause is so incomplete. Treatment of an established painful shoulder is often ineffective so that any measures which

Table 15.31 Factors associated with painful shoulder after stroke.

Associated features
Low tone allowing shoulder glenohumeral
    subluxation/malalignment
Spasticity
Severe weakness of the arm
Sensory loss
Neglect
Visual field deficits

Neurological mechanisms
Reflex sympathetic dystrophy (shoulder–hand syndrome)
Central post-stroke pain
Brachial plexus injury

Orthopaedic problems
Adhesive capsulitis (frozen shoulder)
Rotator cuff tears due to improper handling or positioning
Acromioclavicular arthritis
Glenohumeral arthritis
Bicipital tendinitis
Subdeltoid tendinitis

Table 15.32 Features of reflex sympathetic dystrophy.

Pain and tenderness in humeral abduction, flexion and external
    rotation
Pain and swelling over the carpal bones
Swelling of metacarpophalangeal and proximal interphalangeal
    joints
Changes in temperature, colour and dryness of the skin
Loss of dorsal skin creases and nail changes
Osteoporosis

Note: there is probably considerable overlap between reflex sympathetic dystrophy and the cold arms described by Wanklyn *et al.* (1994) (see Section 15.25).

might prevent its development are important. It is probably useful to introduce general measures on the stroke unit or ward which have been said to decrease the frequency of the problem in non-randomised studies (Table 15.33). It may also be useful to identify individuals who are at particularly high risk (based on the factors in Table 15.31) and make all staff aware of the potential problem.

More specific interventions including slings and cuffs to support the flaccid arm and prevent subluxation are used (Figs 15.11 & 15.12). Some designs may reduce subluxation whilst others do not, but their effect on the frequency of painful shoulder is unproven (Brooke *et al.*, 1991). Many therapists worry that the use of such appliances will inhibit recovery of the arm because they hold the arm in a position which promotes spasticity. Functional electrical stimulation has been shown in one small randomised trial to

Table 15.33 General measures which may reduce the frequency of painful shoulder after stroke.

Instruct *all* staff and carers to

1 Support the flaccid arm to reduce subluxation

Teach patients not to allow the affected arm to hang unsupported when sitting or standing. Whilst sitting they might use one of several arm supports which attach to the chair or wheelchair. All are more effective than a pillow which spends most of the time on the floor. Shoulder/arm orthoses may, depending on their design, prevent subluxation but have not been shown to reduce the frequency of painful shoulder (see Fig. 15.12)

2 Avoid pulling on the affected arm when handling the patient

Staff and carers should be trained in methods of handling and lifting patients to avoid traction injuries

3 Avoid any activity which causes shoulder discomfort

Therapy sessions sometimes do more harm than good

4 Maintain range of passive shoulder movements

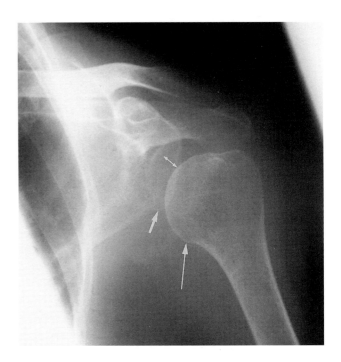

Figure 15.11 X-ray of shoulder showing glenohumeral subluxation, a common finding in stroke patients, but does it matter? Note the widened joint space (double-headed arrow) and the increased distance between the lower border of the glenoid cavity (short arrow) and the lower border of the humeral head (long arrow). (Photograph provided by Dr Allan Stephenson.)

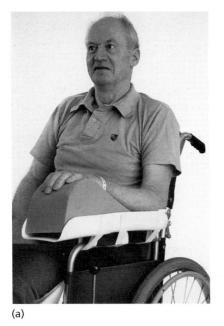
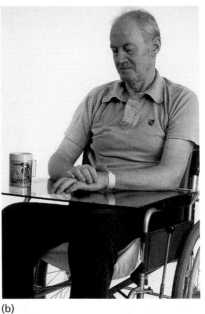
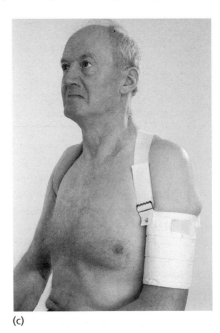

(a) (b) (c)

Figure 15.12 By supporting the weight of the arm, glenohumeral subluxation can be reduced. This may be achieved when the patient is sitting using an arm support (a) which attaches to the chair or wheelchair or, alternatively, a perspex tray (b) which, because it is transparent, allows the patient to check on the position of their feet. Both are better than pillows which invariably end up on the floor. Several designs of sling (c) are available to reduce subluxation when patients are upright.

Table 15.34 Treatments used for painful shoulders.

PHYSIOTHERAPY
Positioning and mobilisation
Exercises
Heat or cold (Partridge *et al.*, 1990)

SUPPORT
Shoulder/arm orthoses (see Fig. 15.12)
Bobath sling
Rood support
Arm supports for bed or chairs
Lapboard (see Fig. 15.12)
Forearm support
Wheelchair outrigger (see Fig. 15.12)

MEDICATION

Systemic
Analgesics
Non-steroidal anti-inflammatory drugs
Corticosteroids (Braus *et al.*, 1994)
Antispastic drugs (see Table 15.25)
Phenoxybenzamine
Antidepressants

Local
Corticosteroid injection of shoulder
Local anaesthetic
Stellate ganglion block

OTHER PHYSICAL
Ultrasound (Inaba & Piorkowski, 1972)
Acupuncture
Biofeedback
TENS (Leandri *et al.*, 1990)

SURGERY
Sympathectomy
Humeral head suspension
Relief of contractures

reduce subluxation and prevent painful shoulder (Faghri *et al.*, 1994).

When a patient complains of shoulder pain it is important to exclude a dislocation, fracture or specific shoulder syndromes, e.g. painful arc (supraspinatus tendinitis) which may respond better to specific measures (e.g. local steroid injection). In established painful shoulder many treatments have been suggested, some have been evaluated in small randomised trials, but further studies are needed to define the best treatments (Table 15.34) (Inaba & Piorkowski, 1972; Leandri *et al.*, 1990; Partridge *et al.*, 1990; Braus *et al.*, 1994). Some interventions are probably harmless and if they produce even short-term relief they are worth trying. Others have potentially important adverse effects and costs and

therefore need to be evaluated further before being adopted into routine clinical practice.

Shoulder pain after stroke is common, ill understood, difficult to prevent and none of the suggested treatments is supported by reliable evidence.

15.25 Swollen and cold limbs

Swelling with pitting oedema, and sometimes pain, quite often occurs in the paralysed or neglected hand, arm or leg, usually within the first few weeks. The swelling may limit the movement of the affected part and the pain does not only restrict movement but also exacerbates spasticity and associated reactions (see Section 15.20). Some patients complain of coldness of the limb, more often of the arm than the leg (Wanklyn *et al.*, 1994). Swelling often occurs in the legs of patients who sit for prolonged periods (see Section 15.13) and in a paralysed arm. Gravity and lack of muscle contraction, which reduces venous and lymphatic return, presumably play a part. There are a number of other causes which need to be considered (Table 15.35). People with fractures or acute ischaemia of the limb usually complain of severe pain, but stroke patients with sensory loss, visuospatial dysfunction or communication difficulties may not, which can lead to these diagnoses being overlooked.

The other causes of a swollen limb should be excluded by clinical examination and appropriate investigation before attributing the swelling simply to immobility or dependency. Investigation is not usually necessary but venography to exclude DVT of the leg, simple X-ray of a swollen wrist or ankle to exclude a fracture, and a serum albumen may be useful. One can monitor the effect of any intervention by simply measuring the circumference of the limb.

The treatment obviously depends on the cause. Where the swelling appears to be due to immobility we recommend the following.

Table 15.35 Causes of swollen limb after stroke.

Gravity in a dependent limb
Lack of muscle contraction
DVT (see Section 15.13)
Compression of veins or lymphatics by tumour, etc.
Cardiac failure
Hypoalbuminaemia (see Section 15.19)
Occult injury (see Section 15.26)
Acute ischaemia
Reflex sympathetic dystrophy (see Table 15.32)

1 Elevation of the affected limb when at rest.

2 Encourage active movement (this may be impossible with severe weakness but is important if neglect is the main cause).

3 Consider using a graduated compression stocking on the leg or a bandage on the arm, although the latter may worsen swelling of the hand.

4 Intermittent compression of the limb, e.g. Flowtron boot. In addition, where the limb is painful, simple analgesia may ameliorate the secondary effects of pain on tone which lead to spasticity and contractures. Diuretics should be avoided unless there is evidence of heart failure, since immobile stroke patients have a tendency to become dehydrated (see Section 15.18.1) and incontinent (see Section 15.14).

15.26   Falls and fractures

Falls are common after stroke. Between 25 and 39% have been reported as falling during in-patient rehabilitation, the higher figure coming from a prospective study in a unit dealing mainly with elderly patients (Dromerick & Reding, 1994; Nyberg & Gustafson, 1995). Falls are also frequent amongst stroke patients who are dependent in ADL following discharge from hospital; in one study, 79% of such patients fell in the first 6 months at home and the majority fell more than once (Forster & Young, 1995). Many factors contribute to this tendency to fall (Table 15.36).

A small proportion of falls occurring in hospital ($<5\%$), or in the first few months at home (about 1%), result in serious injury, most often fractures of the hip, pelvis or wrist, but other injuries (e.g. head and soft tissue), fear and loss of confidence are very common consequences (Nyberg & Gustafson, 1995; Forster & Young, 1995). Most hip fractures affect the hemiparetic side probably because the patients tend to fall to that side, but the osteoporosis which develops on the side of the weakness may be a contributory factor (Chiu *et al.*, 1992; Hamdy *et al.*, 1993). Stroke patients presumably have an increased long-term risk of fractures but we are not aware of any controlled studies which confirm this.

> *Stroke patients with communication problems, sensory loss or neglect may not report injury or pain so it is important to look for signs of fracture, i.e. deformity, swelling, bruising, on admission and after any accident. One should have a low threshold for X-raying suspected fractures.*

One could avoid falls and thus fractures by keeping the patient in bed, but this is clearly not a solution during reha-

Table 15.36 Factors likely to contribute to falls after stroke.

The patient
Muscle weakness (especially of quadriceps)
Sensory loss (especially visual impairments)
Impaired balance, righting reflexes and ataxia
Confusion
Visuospatial neglect, e.g. denial of hemiparesis
Deformity, e.g. plantar flexion causing toe catching
Epileptic seizures
Postural hypotension due to drugs or dehydration

The environment
Inappropriate footwear, e.g. slippers
Slippery floors, deep pile carpets and loose rugs
Excess furniture
Poorly placed rails and inappropriate aids
Lack of supervision
Fire doors (these may close automatically and hit slow-moving
    stroke patients)
Drugs
    Sedatives and hypnotics
    Hypotensive drugs
    Antispastic drugs
    Anticonvulsants

bilitation. The risk of falls and injuries may be minimised by the physiotherapist, nursing staff and carer working closely together to ensure that patients are mobilising with adequate supervision and support. It is also useful to identify patients who are at particular risk of falling. These include the elderly with mobility and balance problems, and particularly those with cognitive difficulties who forget to ask for help. Avoidance of any relevant environmental causes should also help reduce the risk of falls (Table 15.36). Whether drugs such as the bisphosphonates will be shown to prevent osteoporosis and thus reduce the risk of fractures after stroke remains to be seen.

15.27   Visual problems

Many stroke patients have pre-existing visual problems due to refractive errors, cataracts, glaucoma, diabetic retinopathy and senile macular degeneration. Although it is beyond the scope of this book to deal with their specific management, it is important that the clinician is aware of them and their cause because they may have an important influence on the patient's function.

> *Simple measures such as ensuring that the patient's glasses are clean, available and on their nose are obvious but easily overlooked.*

15.27.1 Visual field defects

About 20% of stroke patients have a demonstrable field defect (see Table 15.2) (Turney *et al.*, 1984). However, a similar proportion are not assessable because of reduced conscious level or communication difficulties. The prevalence in hospital patients will obviously depend on patient selection and the methods used to detect defects. Apart from their value in localising the stroke lesion (see Section 4.2.6), visual field defects have some predictive value. A homonymous visual field defect in association with motor and cognitive deficits is usually due to a large stroke lesion and is associated with a relatively poor prognosis (see Section 10.2.7). Some patients who are mobile but unaware of their field loss may be at greater risk of injury. Many patients with field defects find reading and watching television difficult, although some of their difficulty may be due to associated problems with cognition and concentration. Homonymous field defects have important implications for patients (and sometimes unfortunate pedestrians and cyclists!) who wish to drive (see Section 15.32.2). Some of the difficulties in detecting field defects in stroke patients have already been discussed in Section 4.2.6.

There have been very few studies of the recovery of visual field defects after stroke. Gray *et al.* (1989) found that only 14 (17%) of 81 patients with an acute hemispheric stroke and complete homonymous hemianopia (>50% of the hemifield was lost) had normal visual fields 1 month after their stroke. Most of any recovery occurred within the first 10 days. Thirteen (72%) patients with only an incomplete hemianopia initially (<50% of the hemifield was lost) recovered over the same period. This study supports our clinical impression that usually, although there are exceptions, visual field defects persist unless they resolve early.

No treatment is known to enhance the recovery of visual field defects so that interventions which aim to reduce the resulting disability and handicap are most important. In the acute stage it is sensible to avoid putting patients with a homonymous field defect in a bed next to the wall so that they can not see anything going on around them. One can imagine that this 'sensory deprivation' might be bad for morale. It may be possible to teach the patient to compensate for a field defect by head turning, etc. Hemianopia, even without associated neglect, makes reading difficult. Loss of the right visual field means that the patient has to track the words into a blind field, especially where they have no macular sparing. Loss of the left visual field makes it difficult to find the start of each line and patients lose their place easily. This can sometimes be helped by using a ruler to underline each line and by putting their hand or a bright coloured object at the left-hand margin to train them to look at this before starting a new line. Large print will make reading easier. Fresnel's lenses, which shift images in the hemianopic field into the intact one, have been advocated by some workers, particularly where there is associated visual neglect. So far, only very small randomised trials testing their effectiveness have been reported so no definite recommendations regarding their use can be made (Bainbridge & Reding, 1994). Patients with field defects spend a lot of money on new glasses within a few months of their stroke because they mistakenly believe that the problem is with their eyes. It is therefore important that the nature of the problem is explained to the patient and any carer and that new glasses are only prescribed where there is an uncorrected refractive error.

> *Explain to patients the nature and cause of their visual problems so they do not waste their money on inappropriate new glasses.*

15.27.2 Disordered eye movements, diplopia and oscillopsia

Strokes may lead to palsies of conjugate gaze so the patient is unable to look in particular direction(s). Most commonly, this is a problem with lateral gaze because of damage to the contralateral cerebral hemisphere or ipsilateral pons. If the stroke affects the rostral dorsal midbrain, vertical gaze is impaired. Palsies of conjugate gaze were present in about 8% in the Oxfordshire Community Stroke Project (see Table 15.2) but are more common in hospital-based series (Turney *et al.*, 1984; Stone *et al.*, 1993). Strokes involving the brainstem, and in particular the oculomotor nuclei or nerves or the medial longitudinal fasciculus, may cause disconjugate eye movements.

Eye movements after stroke help to localise the stroke lesion but, in addition, the presence of a palsy of conjugate gaze in a supratentorial stroke is associated with a poor outcome (see Table 10.5). Gaze palsies rarely cause disability or handicap. Double vision, which may result from disconjugate eye movements, and oscillopsia associated with nystagmus, are much more troublesome and can make patients even more unsteady than otherwise and prevent them from reading or watching television. The practical difficulties in assessing eye movements after stroke have been discussed earlier (see Section 4.2.7).

The most effective way of relieving patients of double vision in the early stages is a patch over one eye (it probably does not matter which, although alternation is traditionally recommended). Diplopia often resolves in a few weeks of the stroke but if it remains a problem it can be helped by using glasses fitted with prism lenses. However, prisms are no use where diplopia is associated with a variable degree of divergence. Of course, patients should be warned not to spend a lot of money on new glasses until they have reached a stable state. Oscillopsia rarely seems to persist which is fortunate since there are no effective remedies.

15.27.3 Visual hallucinations

Occasionally, patients report vivid visual hallucinations after strokes (see Section 3.2.2). Usually, these resolve but if persistent it may be worth considering investigations to exclude epileptic seizures. Visual hallucinations, sometimes associated with confusion, are frequently seen after administering neuroprotective drugs (see Section 11.13), so if these drugs are shown to improve the outcome of stroke this problem may become much more common. Usually, patients simply require explanation and reassurance, although if hallucinations are associated with marked agitation a major tranquilliser may be needed.

15.28 Cognitive dysfunction

The majority of patients with stroke are elderly and so pre-existing cognitive problems are common. In the Oxfordshire Community Stroke Project about 15% of patients had a Hodkinson Abbreviated Mental Test Score of less than 8/10, indicating significant cognitive dysfunction, in addition to those who were not assessable because of decreased conscious level or communication problems (see Table 15.2). In one hospital-based series disorientation (< 8/10 on the Mini Mental State Examination orientation subtest) affected at least 40% within the first 10 days and persisted for 3 months in 50% of these (Desmond *et al.*, 1994). Disorientation is more common in large hemispheric strokes but complicating infections and other illnesses are often contributory factors (Table 15.37). Confusion with disorientation, poor memory and disruptive behaviour are distressing to other patients and carers and severely hamper rehabilitation. Dementia in stroke patients is associated with a worse long-term survival (Tatemichi *et al.*, 1994).

Cognitive impairments are often overlooked in elderly patients admitted to hospital (Arden *et al.*, 1993). Unstructured assessments have been shown to have poor inter-rater reliability (kappa = 0.2–0.4) (see Table 4.5). It is important to obtain an estimate of the patient's pre-stroke cognitive function by talking to relatives so that acute confusion can be differentiated from longer standing confusion, which is less likely to be reversible. Where the patient can communicate it is useful to use one of the many short mental test scores, e.g. Hodkinson Abbreviated Mental Test Score

Table 15.37 Causes of confusion or dementia after stroke.

Coincidental
Alzheimer's disease

Common aetiology
Large hemispheric lesions
Vascular dementia
Amyloid angiopathy (see Section 8.2.3)
Giant cell arteritis (see Section 7.2)
Isolated angiitis of the central nervous system (see Section 7.2)
Infective endocarditis (see Sections 6.4 and 8.2.8)

Complications
Infections (see Section 15.12)
Hypoxia, hypotension, etc. (see Section 15.2)
Metabolic abnormalities (see Section 15.18)
Depression (see Section 15.31)
Hydrocephalus (see Section 12.2.6)
Drugs

Conditions mimicking stroke (see Section 3.5)
Herpes encephalitis (see Section 3.5.5)
Chronic subdural haematoma (see Section 3.5.2)
Cerebral abscess (see Section 3.5.5)
Cerebral tumour (see Section 3.5.2)
Creutzfeldt–Jakob disease (see Section 3.5.8)

Table 15.38 Hodkinson Abbreviated Mental Test. (From Hodkinson, 1972.)

Patient's age
Time (estimated to nearest hour)
Mr John Brown, 42 West St, Gasteshead (should be repeated to ensure that the patient has heard it correctly and then recalled at end of test)
Name of hospital/place
Current year
Recognition of two people (e.g. doctor, nurse)
Patient's date of birth
Dates of World War I*
Present monarch†
Count down from 20 to 1

* It may now be more appropriate to ask for dates of World War II.
† Clearly in some countries it would be more relevant to ask who the president is.

(Table 15.38) or even a longer one such as the Mini Mental State Examination (Folstein *et al.*, 1975; Grace *et al.*, 1995). Having such a measure at the baseline assessment allows subsequent changes to be identified and the cause sought. Where the patient is unable to communicate one usually has to rely on a history from others and observation of the patient's behaviour. The diagnosis, management and prognosis of the stroke may all be affected by the duration, severity and cause of cognitive impairment.

Depending on the assessment one may identify a cause for the cognitive problems, e.g. acute infection for which specific treatment can be given. Having excluded treatable causes, one might conclude that if the cognitive problem was not present before the stroke, then the stroke itself accounts for the problem (assuming that the diagnosis is secure). In this situation one can expect some spontaneous recovery over the next few weeks or months although problems frequently persist (Desmond *et al.*, 1994). Where the cognitive problems are long standing and pre-date the stroke, and treatable causes such as hypothyroidism or depression have been excluded, the process is likely to progress. This has important implications for planning the patient's further management. We know that patients with persisting cognitive dysfunction are more likely to remain dependent. If patients are disorientated or have memory problems the 'carry over' between therapy sessions is often poor, leading to slow progress with rehabilitation. Also, cognitive problems will have a strong influence on the amount of support and the type of accommodation the patient will need at the end of their rehabilitation.

> *Look systematically for irreversible cognitive problems at an early stage and get on with planning long-term placement and a suitable package of care.*

15.29   Visuospatial dysfunction

Visuospatial dysfunction includes visual and sensory neglect, visual and sensory inattention or extinction, constructional dyspraxias and agnosias (see Table 4.10). Unfortunately, the nomenclature is complex and confused by different people using different terms for the same phenomena.

The frequency of visuospatial dysfunction amongst stroke patients varies widely in the published literature because of patient selection, the timing of assessments and the use of different definitions and assessments. Visual neglect has been reported in 33–85% of patients with right hemisphere strokes and 0–24% of those with left hemisphere strokes (Stone *et al.*, 1993). More sensitive tests will naturally increase the apparent frequency of the problem. Stone *et al.*, (1993) reported a high frequency of visuospatial dysfunction amongst 171 consecutive admissions to two hospitals in London, examined within 2–3 days of an acute hemispheric stroke using the Behavioural Inattention Test (Table 15.39). This battery contains various tests which aim to assess both

Table 15.39 Frequency of visuospatial problems amongst hospitalised patients within 3 days of a hemispheric first stroke (Stone *et al.*, 1993). The differences in frequency between left and right were statistically significant for all but non-belonging, gaze paresis and visual field defects. The relatively high frequency of these phenomena in this series (cf. Table 15.2) probably reflects the severity of the strokes in this hospital-referred series and the sensitivity of the test battery used.

| | Per cent with phenomena | | Per cent not assessable | |
	Right hemisphere (*n* = 69)	Left hemisphere (*n* = 102)	Right	Left
Visual neglect	82	65	11	27
Hemi-inattention	70	49	9	15
Tactile extinction	65	35	25	58
Allaesthesia	57	11	15	55
Visual extinction	23	2	13	21
Anosognosia	28	5	13	45
Anosodiaphoria	27	2	13	48
Non-belonging	36	29	20	53
Gaze paresis	29	25	0	3
Visual field defect	36	46	11	9

Table 15.40 Components of the Behavioural Inattention Battery. (From Wilson *et al.*, 1987.)

Full version	Modified version
Line crossing	Pointing to objects in ward
Letter cancellation	Food on the plate
Star cancellation (see Fig. 4.13)	Reading a menu
Figure and shape drawing	Reading a newspaper article
Line bisection	Line cancellation
Representational drawing	Star cancellation (see Fig. 4.13)
Picture scanning	Coin selection
Telephone dialling	Figure copying
Menu reading	
Article reading	
Telling and setting time	
Coin sorting	
Address and sentence copying	
Map navigation	
Card sorting	

sensory neglect (patient's perception of incoming stimuli) and motor neglect (the patient's willingness to explore external space) (Table 15.40). Visuospatial dysfunction is associated by many with stroke in the non-dominant hemisphere, although Stone *et al.* (1993) found a surprisingly high frequency in patients with left hemisphere strokes. These may be underestimated in clinical practice because of the practical difficulties in assessing patients with a paralysed dominant hand or problems with language (see Section 4.2.5). Using unstructured and non-standardised testing of visuospatial dysfunction (usually including bilateral simultaneous stimulation for sensory and visual inattention, clock drawing and simple figure copying) we identified only 16% of assessable patients (25% were not assessable because of reduced level of consciousness, language problems or paralysis) in the Oxfordshire Community Stroke Project as having visuospatial dysfunction (see Table 15.2). Visuospatial problems are major causes of disability and handicap, impede functional recovery and have been associated with a poor outcome (Denes *et al.*, 1982; Kinsella & Ford, 1985; Barer, 1989).

Testing visuospatial function is one of the most difficult aspects of the examination and therefore frequently omitted in routine practice (Davenport *et al.*, 1995). It is not surprising that the inter-rater reliability of unstructured testing is relatively poor (kappa = 0.4) (see Table 4.5). We have already described some simple bedside assessments which are useful in detecting impairments of functional importance as well as in helping to localise the stroke lesion (see Table 4.9).

Recovery of visuospatial function, as with most other stroke-related impairments, is most rapid in the first week or two and then slows (see Section 10.2.5). Between 10 and 20% of patients with visual neglect in the acute stage have persisting problems 3-months later and recovery after this time is usually slow (Stone *et al.*, 1992). However, this study used a sensitive instrument to detect even mild cases so that in routine clinical practice where only more marked impairments are detected the prognosis may be worse. Stone *et al.* (1992) also showed that if visual neglect was severe and associated with anosognosia it was less likely to resolve. Visual neglect associated with right hemisphere lesions may continue to improve, albeit slowly, for longer than that associated with left hemisphere lesions. These findings need to be confirmed but they may be useful in identifying patients who would be suitable for randomisation in trials comparing treatments for visual neglect.

Visuospatial dysfunction poses major problems to those involved in rehabilitation. For instance, it is difficult to persuade patients with anosognosia or denial to become involved in therapy. There have been very few randomised trials of interventions aimed at improving visuospatial function after stroke and they have all suffered from the difficulties outlined previously (see Table 15.1). The few small randomised trials which have been reported suggest that specific interventions may improve patients' performance on test batteries but this does not generalise to improved functioning in ADL (Weinberg *et al.*, 1979; Gordon *et al.*, 1985; Lincoln *et al.*, 1985; Robertson *et al.*, 1990; Rossi

et al., 1990; Gray *et al.*, 1992; Hajek *et al.*, 1993; Robertson, 1993). In other words, any benefit of therapy appears to benefit performance on selected tasks but not on general visuospatial abilities.

We therefore have to adopt strategies which do not necessarily influence the severity of the underlying impairment but may reduce the resulting disability and handicap and help carers to cope. Carers are often bemused, frustrated or angered by the behavioural consequences of visuospatial dysfunction and it is very important to spend time explaining the unusual nature of the deficit. If this is not done, then carers may wrongly conclude that the patient is dementing, wilfully obstructive or even deliberately ignoring them.

Patients with unilateral neglect are often positioned so that they have their intact side facing a wall to encourage them to respond to stimuli on the affected side. However, since there is little evidence that this strategy influences outcome, we generally aim to position the patient in the middle of the ward so they receive stimulation from both sides on the basis that their morale might suffer if they are not stimulated (Loverro & Reding, 1988).

In our experience, patients with unilateral neglect and hemiparesis can be taught to walk, but often this is of limited functional use because they are so prone to falls. Unless supervised when walking, the patient's attention may become drawn to the unaffected side, which appears to inhibit activity on the affected side which leads to the fall. It can be difficult to persuade a patient who is unaware of their hemiparesis that they should only try to walk when supervised and that unsupervised walking carries a risk of falls and fractures (see Section 15.26).

Patients with neglect are at risk in other situations, e.g. the kitchen, because they are unaware of dangers to their affected side so that measures have to be taken to reduce this risk, e.g. use a microwave rather than a conventional cooker.

15.30 Communication difficulties

The most common problems with communication after stroke are dysphasia and dysarthria, which both affect about 20% of assessable patients (see Table 15.2). Dysphasia is almost invariably associated with dysgraphia and sometimes also dyslexia. Patients occasionally talk very quietly after a stroke (i.e. dysphonia), which sometimes appears to be due to difficulties in coordinating speech and breathing. Other abnormalities include aprosody which occurs with non-dominant hemisphere lesions. However, problems with language usually reflect dysfunction of the dominant hemisphere, although it is often difficult to localise the lesion more definitely because lesions in various locations have been associated with dysphasia (see Section 4.2.5). Dysarthria often results from unilateral hemispheric strokes as well as from those affecting the brainstem and cerebellum and is not particularly helpful in lesion localisation. It is important to assess the patient's ability to communicate for several reasons.

1 To identify the clinical syndrome and thus the likely underlying cause (see Sections 4.4.5 and 6.5).

2 To find a way for the patient to express his or her feelings and make their needs known to the carers and so avoid unnecessary distress caused by, e.g. urinary incontinence (see Section 15.14).

3 To find out how much the patient is capable of understanding so that one can tailor information-giving to their level of understanding. Also, therapists need to find a way of asking the patient to follow quite complex instructions, although many are masters of non-verbal communication.

4 To assess the patient's prognosis and in setting reasonable rehabilitation goals.

5 To protect the patient from losing control of their affairs. We have seen lawyers, oblivious to a patient's severe dysphasia and dyslexia, explaining complex documents and asking for their signature.

Although communication problems may be obvious, it is not always easy, as we have already discussed (see Section 4.2.5) to distinguish dysphasia from dysarthria. Table 4.8 outlines a simple assessment of language function. It is important not to overlook pre-existing impairments such as deafness, ill-fitting dentures and poor vision which can adversely affect a patient's ability to communicate. Before testing comprehension the patient must be wearing their hearing aid which should be turned on and functioning properly.

It is quite common for language function to vary with factors such as fatigue, anxiety and intercurrent illness. However, different members of the rehabilitation team may judge the severity of an individual patient's problems differently. In our experience, nurses often overestimate the patient's ability to understand language in part because, in dealing with the patient, they use a lot of non-verbal cuing which is of course of immense value.

More formal testing of language function using one of the standardised instruments (e.g. Western Aphasia Test, Aachen Aphasia Score, Porch Index of Communication Ability, Boston Diagnostic Aphasia Examination) is sometimes useful where there is doubt about the diagnosis or in research projects, but these are usually administered by a speech and language therapist. The Frenchay Aphasia Screening Test (FAST) has been developed for use in routine clinical practice by non-experts and has reasonable reliability and validity (Enderby et al., 1986; O'Neill et al., 1990).

Dysarthria after a stroke usually improves spontaneously and rarely causes major long-term problems. This is fortunate since, although speech and language therapists give patients exercises aimed at improving the clarity of speech, there has been little formal evaluation of these techniques. Dysphasia often improves markedly after a stroke but is more often a source of long-term disability and handicap than dysarthria. One study found that about 10% of survivors were still dysphasic 6 months after a stroke (Matsumoto et al., 1973). Persisting problems appear to be more likely where the initial dysphasia is severe, in particular if understanding is poor, the patient produces jargon speech, or if there is associated oral or speech dyspraxia.

> *Having established that the patient has a communication problem one should ensure that all the simple measures to optimise a patient's ability to communicate are taken, e.g. correct false teeth, hearing aid and spectacles are being used. These simple things are easily overlooked but can make a great difference to the patient.*

There is considerable controversy about the effectiveness of speech and language therapy in dysphasia. The results of the randomised trials which have attempted to test the effectiveness of therapy have been disappointing, mainly because of methodological weaknesses, as outlined in Table 15.1 (Whurr et al., 1992). But, other criticisms include the use of weak or low-intensity interventions, inappropriate control therapies, unblinded assessments of outcome and large numbers of patients lost to follow-up or not complying with treatment. Although some studies have shown that intensive treatment may be effective (Hagen, 1973; Wertz et al., 1986), others have shown no clear evidence of benefit from the low-intensity treatment which is routinely available in the UK (Lincoln et al., 1984). Several small randomised trials have shown that, at least for selected patients, similar outcomes can be achieved from input of volunteers working with guidance from a speech and language therapist and regular therapy from trained therapists (Meikle et al., 1979; David et al., 1982; Wertz et al., 1986; Hartman & Landau, 1987; Marshall et al., 1989). However, many (especially language therapists) dispute the validity of these trials because they tested heterogeneous and insufficiently intensive courses of treatment and used relatively crude outcome measures. They point to single case studies which provide some evidence for the effectiveness of therapy, although many others do not accept this type of experimental design as a reliable indicator of effectiveness. A systematic review of the research to date, and more randomised trials, are required to identify specific, reproducible interventions which may be

effects but it is important not to use subtherapeutic doses in the mistaken belief that depression after a stroke is somehow more drug sensitive. There is no clear evidence that any one drug is more effective than another in this setting, although the frequency and type of adverse effects associated with each group of antidepressants often determines the choice of medication (Song *et al.*, 1993; Lauritzen *et al.*, 1994). In elderly patients with a past history of depression who have previously relapsed when treatment has stopped, one should probably continue treatment indefinitely to prevent a relapse which may have serious functional consequences. Even where there is some doubt about the diagnosis of depression after stroke, perhaps because of communication difficulties, a trial of antidepressants may be worthwhile. Some drugs which are started after a stroke (e.g. beta-blockers, methyldopa to treat newly discovered hypertension) can cause depression so that it is important to review the drug chart before starting antidepressants. Electroconvulsive therapy may occasionally be required and has been used after stroke without complications (Murray *et al.*, 1986).

> *Start with a small dose of antidepressant and gradually increase the dose to minimise adverse effects. It is important not to use subtherapeutic doses in the mistaken belief that depression after a stroke is somehow more drug sensitive.*

15.31.2 Emotionalism

About 15% of patients have difficulty controlling the expression of emotion following stroke (House *et al.*, 1989b; Anderson *et al.*, 1995). This problem has been described using a variety of overlapping terms including emotionalism, pathological emotionalism, emotional lability, emotional incontinence, pathological crying/laughing and pseudobulbar affect. The patient abruptly starts to weep, or less commonly to laugh uncontrollably, perhaps with no obvious precipitant. More often, episodes are triggered by a kind word (e.g. how are you feeling?) or a thought with emotional overtones (e.g. thinking of grandchildren), but the emotional response is out of proportion to the degree of 'internal sadness' (or mirth). Usually, the episodes are short lived but may occur frequently enough to disrupt completely a conversation, therapy session or social event. Such outbursts cause considerable distress to the patient and their carer and may be a major obstacle to rehabilitation and social integration. Although classically described as a characteristic of pseudobulbar palsy (i.e. as with bilateral strokes) emotionalism usually occurs after a single, unilateral stroke. It is most common early on although may not be noticed in the first

few days because of everything else that is going on. Usually, episodes of emotionalism become less severe and less frequent with time (House *et al.*, 1989b). Patients with emotionalism have more psychological symptoms and tend to have worse cognitive function than unaffected patients so it is important not to overlook these additional sources of distress (House *et al.*, 1989b).

> *Emotionalism after stroke can occur with single or multiple lesions in more or less any part of the brain. It is usually triggered by some sort of emotion (such as seeing grandchildren), but the response is completely out of proportion to the stimulus.*

Emotionalism should be suspected if the patient is more tearful or cries more easily than before the stroke. Ask the patient, carer or staff whether the crying is of sudden onset and whether the patient can control it. Patients may describe similar problems controlling laughter, but this is less common. Having established that crying is a problem, one needs to assess whether this is solely due to emotionalism or whether it reflects frustration or depression. Crying which always occurs when the patient is trying, with difficulty, to perform a task (e.g. an aphasic patient trying to speak) suggests that the emotional outburst is due to frustration, although this does not mean that there are no other psychological problems as well. One needs to talk to the patient, the carers and staff to assess whether or not the patient is depressed (see Section 15.31.1). It can be useful to ask the patient to keep a diary to document the frequency and severity of emotional outbursts, especially if one is planning to instigate treatment.

Patients and carers are often confused and distressed by emotionalism. Therefore, it is important to explain that the problem is due to the stroke, that it is relatively common and that it usually becomes less severe with time. Do not walk away when the patient bursts into tears, but take the opportunity to explain the nature of the problem to them. If it is a persistent problem and is either causing major distress to the patient and family or disrupting therapy sessions, antidepressants can be effective. Symptoms are usually improved within the first few days of initiating the treatment, unlike the symptoms of depression which rarely respond in less than a few weeks. Small doses are often effective. It is best to start with 25 mg of amitryptyline in the first instance, taken at bedtime (Schiffer *et al.*, 1985; Robinson *et al.*, 1993). If the symptoms are not better in 1 week increase the dose slowly until the patient responds or begins to have dose-related adverse effects. If the patient does not respond, fluoxetine can be tried, or one of the other 5-hydroxytryptamine (5-HT) re-uptake inhibitors, since they also appear to be effective and there are anecdotal reports of success where a tricyclic has been ineffective (Sloan *et al.*, 1992; Andersen *et al.*, 1993).

15.31.3 Boredom

Patients who remain in hospital for a long period of rehabilitation often complain of boredom, not surprisingly because much of their time is spent doing nothing (Lincoln *et al.*, 1989). Boredom is a particular problem during weekends and evenings when the patients are not receiving therapy, or at least not receiving it from the therapists. It may also be a problem for patients after discharge home if they are housebound, socially isolated or unable to resume their normal leisure or work activities. Boredom leads to reduced motivation, low morale and can ultimately affect the patient's recovery. The team should remain alert to the problem and ask patients about it. There are a number of ways to alleviate boredom in hospitalised patients, which include the following.

1 Be as flexible as possible about visiting hours to maximise social contact with family and friends.

2 Provide patients with a variety of leisure activities on the unit. Some units even employ leisure activity coordinators!

3 Encourage families to take patients out of the hospital wherever this is practical, e.g. walks in the grounds, trips to the pub, trips home for a meal.

4 Introduce volunteers on the unit to work with the patients and develop group activities at weekends.

5 Encourage patients to keep their own timetable so they can plan their free time.

6 Provide individual televisions with remote controls, videos and even computer games.

These interventions may be integrated with the rehabilitation programme and incorporated in goal setting, and so benefit the patient in other ways. Unfortunately, even in specialised stroke units, patients spend far too much of their time staring into space. For patients at home there are often clubs, day centres and voluntary organisations which can help to get them out of the house to meet other people and to get involved in leisure activities.

15.32 Dependency in activities of daily living (ADL)

In previous sections we have discussed many of the impairments which result from a stroke. In this section we will concentrate on the resulting disabilities and the measures which can be taken to limit them. The frequency in stroke survivors is shown in Table 15.43.

Table 15.43 Frequency of dependency in ADL (based on the Barthel Index) amongst 246 consecutive patients surviving 1 year after their first-ever in a lifetime stroke in the Oxfordshire Community Stroke Project (M.S. Dennis, unpublished data).

Function	Dependent (%)	Independent (%)
Bowel function	23 (9)	223 (91)
Grooming	26 (11)	220 (89)
Toileting	30 (12)	216 (88)
Transfers	33 (13)	213 (87)
Walking inside	36 (15)	210 (85)
Bladder function	41 (17)	205 (83)
Feeding	44 (18)	202 (82)
Dressing	53 (22)	193 (78)
Stairs	64 (26)	182 (74)
Walking outside	76 (31)	171 (69)
Bathing	80 (33)	166 (67)

15.32.1 Mobility

Sections 15.11 and 15.21 addressed the immediate problems of immobility and the interventions described were those aimed at preventing complications and reducing the impairment. This section will deal with the disability and handicap as a consequence of reduced mobility. Many patients have mobility problems 1 year after their stroke (Table 15.43). Although the neurological consequences of the stroke account for the majority of these problems, other pathologies, in particular arthritis and hip fractures, add to the burden of walking disability (Collen & Wade, 1991).

Simple history taking is surprisingly informative; self-reported ability to turn over in bed, sit up, transfer (i.e. bed to chair and sitting to standing), walk (and use of walking aids, furniture) and climb stairs (up, down or both, with or without rails) will give a fairly clear picture of the patient's residual problems. It is useful to know whether the patient can (and does) walk outside, their range and whether physical or verbal support from another person is needed. It is also important to establish the reason for any problems, i.e. is it due to painful joints or feet, breathlessness, angina, intermittent claudication, loss of confidence, environmental factors such as big steps, lack of handrails or even the neighbour's aggressive dog? It is useful to observe the patient and the carer carrying out the various manoeuvres in their own home since environmental factors so often determine the level of handicap associated with impaired mobility. Several scales are available for measuring the mobility of patients (Table 15.44). The timed 10-m walk is particularly useful because it is simple, objective and requires no more equipment than a stopwatch.

Where the patient has residual problems, a physiotherapist or occupational therapist can improve mobility (Wade *et*

Table 15.44 Rivermead Mobility Index. (From Collen *et al.*, 1991.)

1 *Turning over in bed*
   Do you turn over from your back to your side without help?
2 *Lying from sitting*
   From lying in bed, do you get up to sit on the edge of the bed on your own?
3 *Sitting balance*
   Do you sit on the edge of the bed without holding on for 10 seconds?
4 *Sitting to standing*
   Do you stand up (from any chair) in less than 15 seconds, and stand there for 15 seconds (using hands, and with an aid if necessary)?
5 *Standing unsupported*
   Observe standing for 10 seconds without any aid or support.
6 *Transfer*
   Do you manage to move, e.g. from bed to chair and back without any help?
7 *Walking inside, with an aid if needed*
   Do you walk 10 m, with an aid or furniture if necessary, but with no stand-by help?
8 *Stairs*
   Do you manage a flight of stairs without help?
9 *Walking outside (even ground)*
   Do you walk around outside, on pavements without help?
10 *Walking inside (with no aid)*
   Do you walk 10 m inside with no calliper, splint, aid or use of furniture, and no stand-by help?
11 *Picking off floor*
   If you drop something on the floor do you manage to walk 5 m, pick it up and then walk back?
12 *Walking outside (uneven ground)*
   Do you walk over uneven ground (grass, gravel, dirt, snow, ice, etc.) without help?
13 *Bathing*
   Do you get in and out of a bath or shower unsupervised and wash yourself?
14 *Up and down four steps*
   Do you manage to go up and down four steps with no rail and without help, but using an aid if necessary?
15 *Running*
   Do you run 10 m without limping in 4 seconds (fast walk is acceptable)?

Note: only question 5 depends on direct observation. The index forms a hierarchy so that one does not have to ask all the questions. However, the authors point out that by asking all the questions, and finding out why patients can not manage certain actions, useful information is obtained to guide management.

al., 1992). Therapy in the patient's own home may be more helpful than in a hospital out-patient department since the therapist can then address the everyday problems that the patient is experiencing 'in the wild'. For example, patients can be taught to climb their *own* stairs and to overcome the particular problems associated with the layout of their *own*

Table 15.45 Walking aids. (From Mulley, 1991.)

Shoes
Should be comfortable, supportive and have non-slip soles
Occasionally, a smooth sole facilitates a smooth swing phase in patients with foot drop when walking on carpets

Walking sticks
Tailored to the patient (i.e. length, handle shape, weight and appearance). A long stick can be used to encourage patients to put weight through their affected leg (see Fig. 15.13d)
Replace worn rubber ferrule
Should be held in the unaffected hand in patients with hemiparesis but this means the patient's functioning hand is no longer available for other tasks
Other uses include extending the patient's reach and 'self-defence'

Tripods and quadrapods
Provide a broader base of support than a walking stick
Their weight may cause associated reactions (see Section 15.20)
Not useful on uneven ground

Walking frames (see Fig. 15.13)
Available in many sizes and shapes with or without wheels
Useful where balance is poor, especially if the patient tends to lean backwards
Often give patients confidence
Needs good upper limb function and, of course, prevents patient from using hands or carrying things; many patients attach a basket or use a wheeled trolley to overcome this problem
Patients often try to pull up on their frame to rise from a chair, which can cause them to fall
Frames may trip up patients and be difficult to manoeuvre with lots of furniture and thick carpets
Cannot be used on stairs, therefore patients may require two frames, one on each level
Beware bent frames, protruding screws, loose hand grips and worn ferrules
Other uses, drying underclothes

Ankle–foot orthosis or brace (see Fig. 15.14)
Usually made of thermoplastic construction and tailored to the individual
Occasionally useful in spastic foot drop where physiotherapy unsuccessful, but may exacerbate the problem
Beware in patients with oedema and tendency to leg ulcers

Knee brace
Occasionally required to prevent hyperextension of knee

Functional electrical stimulation
An experimental treatment which has been used to correct foot drop after stroke

Hand rails
Short grab rails can be useful to provide support, especially at thresholds and doorways
Full-length rails on staircases are invaluable to those with poor balance, confidence or vision
Advice on siting hand rails should be obtained from an occupational therapist. Poorly placed hand rails can cause accidents or may not be used

home. Two randomised trials which compared the effectiveness of home versus hospital-based physiotherapy showed that improvement in ADL function was slightly greater in those treated at home, but other outcomes were no different (Gladman *et al.*, 1995). Although the therapist may be able to reduce the patient's degree of impairment, even when intervention starts very late after a stroke, the therapist's main tool at this point is the provision of mobility aids (Tables 15.45 & 15.46). Where one prescribes an aid for patients it is important to provide them and any carers with training in its use, and to ensure that it is maintained in good order (Figs 15.13–15.19).

> *If one prescribes an aid one should teach the patient or carer how to use it, ensure that it solves the problem, ensure that it is maintained in good working order and provide follow-up to ensure its continued use or appropriate removal.*

Many patients do not use the aids provided which is both a waste of resources and an indication of the lack of value of that aid. It is important to follow-up patients who have been given aids to ensure they fit the patient's needs and are actually being used.

Patients who are unable to walk outside, have limited range or difficulty using their own or public transport may be helped by putting them in contact with any schemes which may be available locally to give assistance. For example, in the UK special financial allowances are available to help with the added cost of being immobile. In the last few years there has been a major campaign to improve access to public places for patients with disabilities.

15.32.2 Driving

Many people who have had a stroke do not return to driving (Legh-Smith *et al.*, 1986). The reasons are varied; severe residual motor, sensory, visual or cognitive impairments being the most common. In many countries the authorities place restrictions on driving after stroke, and particularly if the stroke is complicated by seizures (see Section 15.8). The variation in regulations probably reflects the dearth of relevant research in this area. Special, and usually more stringent regulations, sometimes apply to those who drive commercial vehicles and taxis.

In our experience, patients are often not asked whether they drive by their doctors so that many continue to drive and put lives at risk in contravention of their local regulations (Davenport *et al.*, 1995). It is the doctor's responsibility to ask patients whether or not they drive so they can be given the relevant information. Failure to do so might have serious consequences.

There appears to be little agreement about the optimal method of assessing a disabled patient's fitness to drive. Informal judgements are often made by patients or their family doctors. Bedside testing of patient's neurological impairments including cognitive function, assessments in

Table 15.46 Other aids to mobility.

Chairs (see Fig. 15.15)
Higher seats (but not so high as to cause the feet to dangle) without too much backward angle and firm armrests (of the correct height, shape and length) facilitate transfers
It is easier to stand from a chair if the patient can pull his/her heels under it
Chairs should be tailored to the individual's requirements but existing chairs may be raised or lowered
Chairs on castors can be dangerous

Ejector chairs (see Fig. 15.16)
The seat or chair may be sprung to provide an initial lift to allow the patient to rise
These must be tailored to the individual to avoid the patient being catapulted across the room
Electric chairs which slowly bring the patient to a semi-erect position are occasionally useful but are expensive, bulky and require training to use properly

Beds
A firm mattress at the correct height will facilitate transfers from a bed
Blocks or leg extensions can be used to modify an existing bed
A grab rail attached to the bed's frame or floor can facilitate independent transfers (see Fig. 15.17)
It may be impossible to attach aids to a divan-style bed
Mechanical devices which help the patient to sit in bed can occasionally be helpful (see Fig. 15.17)

Wheelchairs
An invaluable means to improve mobility
Many hundreds of designs including self-propelled, carer-propelled and electric chairs
Need to be tailored to individual's requirements
Must be kept in good working order (see Fig. 15.18)

Ramps
Useful to those in wheelchairs and their carers
Many designs available for different situations

Lifts
Many types, including
    Domestic stair-lifts (see Fig. 15.19) for those who can not manage stairs
    Through-the-floor lifts for accessing upper floors in wheelchairs
    Short rise lifts for accessing vehicles in wheelchairs or where there is insufficient space for a ramp
Lifts are expensive and may require structural alterations to accommodate them

---

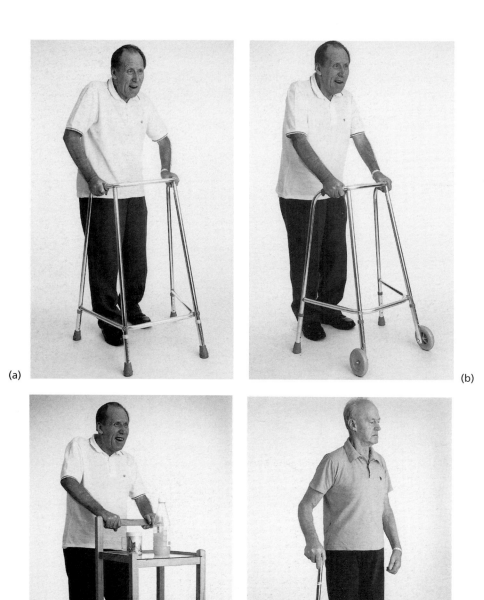

(a)

(b)

(c)

(d)

Figure 15.13 Walking aids. (a) A typical light-weight walking frame of adjustable height which may be useful if a patient has poor balance but reasonable arm and hand function. (b) A walking frame with wheels which may be better than (a) in patients who tend to fall backwards or who have Parkinson's disease. (c) A tea trolley which will provide the patient with support but also allow them to take things from place to place. (d) A long walking stick can be used to encourage the patient to put more of their weight through their affected leg.

driving simulators and road tests have all been advocated. Since none is perfect it is likely that a combination will prove the most effective. For instance, one might start with a bed-side assessment to demonstrate any physical, and probably more importantly cognitive impairments, which would make safe driving very unlikely (Nouri *et al.*, 1987). Patients who pass on the bedside testing could then be assessed on a driving simulator or an 'off-road' test which would be used to identify those who are clearly unsafe to drive (Nouri & Tinson, 1988). The remainder could then be given a road test

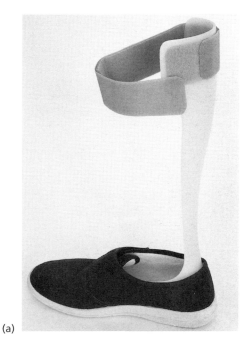

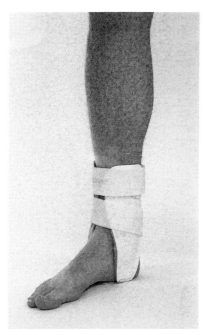

Figure 15.14 Ankle supports. (a) A thermoplastic ankle–foot orthosis: the famous AFO splint. Although this is very useful in patients with foot drop secondary to lower motor neurone lesions, in stroke patients it can sometimes increase the tendency to plantar flexion by stimulating the sole of the foot. (b) A lateral ankle support may be useful in patients who have a tendency to invert their foot when walking. (a)

(b)

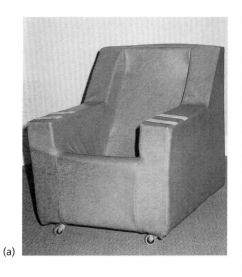

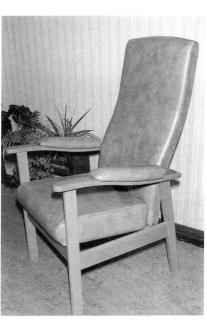

(a)

(b)

Figure 15.15 Choosing an appropriate chair for a stroke patient who has difficulties getting from sitting to standing. (a) A bad chair to ensure the user never escapes! The seat is low and slopes backwards, the arms are soft and offer little resistance to allow the person to push up on them, the base is solid so they cannot pull their legs under them and this chair is on castors so that if they eventually manage to stand the chair slides away and causes them to fall backwards. Note the Velcro pads on the arms to allow a tray to be fixed across the user's escape route. (b) A good chair to facilitate easy transfers. This chair is of reasonable height, is upright, has firm but padded arms and allows the user to pull their legs underneath them which makes it easier to get their weight over their feet. This chair does not have wings which may provide support for the user's head when sleeping but can stop interaction with other people sitting to either side.

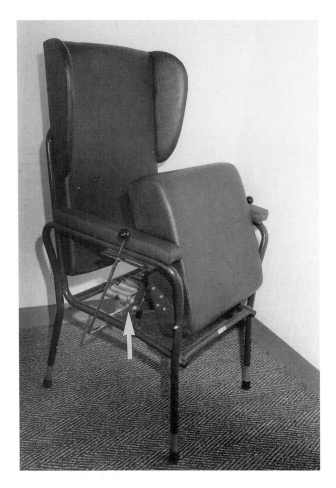

Figure 15.16 An ejector chair. The number of springs (arrow) can be altered depending on the weight of the user. Some patients find that this type of chair pushes them off balance.

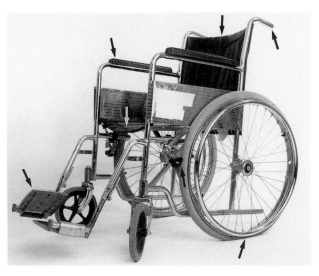

Figure 15.18 Things to look for when examining a wheelchair. This wheelchair has many hazardous and uncomfortable features. Note the white sticky tape covering the name of the hospital on the side of this wheelchair, which wished, very reasonably, to remain anonymous. 1, check that the tyres are properly inflated (arrow). Flat tyres make the wheelchair hard work to propel and the brakes inoperative. 2, check the brakes work (arrow). 3, check that the sides and arms (arrow) are removable to facilitate transfers onto toilets, into cars, etc. 4, check that the foot plates are not fixed (arrow) or flapping about. Both may cause injury. The foot plates should fold neatly and securely out of the way when not in use. 5, check that the arms (arrow) are properly padded to avoid discomfort and compression neuropathy of the ulnar nerve. 6, check that the back (arrow) and seat (arrow) are not sagging and that the appropriate cushion is being used to reduce the risk of pressure sores. 7, check that the grips on the handles are in good order (arrow).

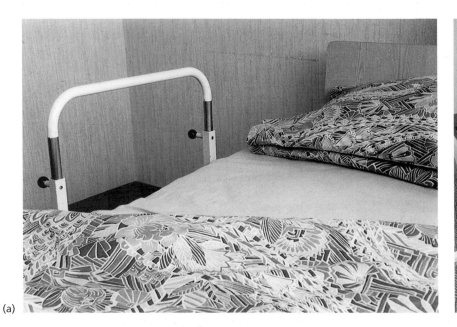
(a)

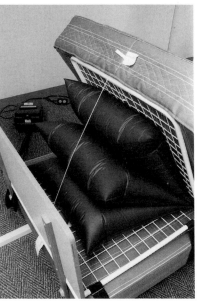
(b)

Figure 15.17 Aids to getting out of bed. Although many people can get out of a bed independently during a therapy session when they are 'warmed up' they may need aids to get out in the middle of the night or first thing in the morning. (a) A grab rail attached to the bed can facilitate transfers from lying to standing and may therefore prevent incontinence at night. The height of this model can be adjusted to suit the individual. (b) A pneumatic mattress elevator can be helpful in getting patients from lying to sitting.

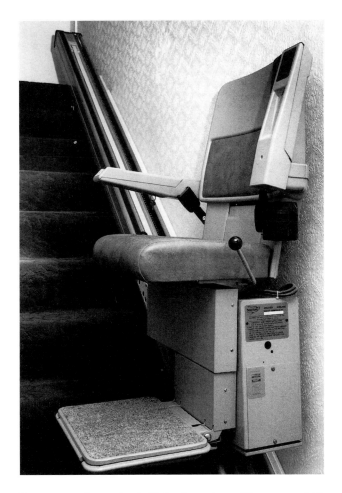

Figure 15.19 A typical stair-lift for domestic use. The armrests fold out of the way to facilitate transfers. The foot rest and seat fold up when not in use. The controls are on the armrests.

in a dual-control car with an appropriately trained instructor. This stepwise approach should minimise the risk of injury to the patient, instructor and other road users. Many countries provide specialist centres for the assessment of disabled drivers. These centres not only assess driving skills but also provide advice on the available vehicle adaptations which can allow patients with severe physical disability to drive.

15.32.3 Toileting

The problems of urinary and faecal incontinence have been discussed in Sections 15.14 and 15.15, respectively. In the Oxfordshire Community Stroke Project, 12% of patients were still dependent in toileting 1 year after their first stroke (see Table 15.43). Dependency may be due to an inability to transfer independently, walk or dress and undress. For the cognitively intact patient this may be an embarrassing disability which severely damages their self-esteem.

An assessment by an occupational therapist should define the severity and cause of the problem. The patient's ability to toilet themselves is very dependent on the environment so that a home assessment may be particularly useful. Simple factors such as the width of the door to the toilet or bathroom, the position and height of the toilet, and the position of the toilet roll holder can make a crucial difference to whether or not the patient can use the toilet independently.

Therapy aimed at improving performance in mobility, transfers and dressing will all facilitate independence in toileting. Table 15.47 lists some common problems and some simple solutions, and Fig. 15.20 shows some simple toilet aids.

15.32.4 Washing and bathing

About 11% and 36% of patients 1 year after a first-ever stroke are dependent in washing and bathing, respectively (see Table 15.43). Motor, sensory, visuospatial and cognitive impairments contribute most to these disabilities. Although poor arm function makes washing and grooming more difficult, most patients can perform these tasks with their unaffected arm, but patients with visuospatial and cognitive deficits, even when arm function seems quite good, may be unable to wash and groom themselves independently. Independence in bathing obviously requires some independence in mobility and transfers. Other disabling

Table 15.47 Toileting problems and solutions.

Can not get to toilet because of mobility or access problems
Solutions
    Urinal (see Fig. 15.5)
    Commode, many designs to suit individual needs (see Fig. 15.20)
    Chemical toilet, useful where regular emptying is not possible

Can not transfer on and off the toilet, or poor balance making manipulation of clothes difficult
Solutions
    Grab rails
    Toilet frame (see Fig. 15.20)
    Raised or adjustable toilet seat (see Fig. 15.20)

Can not clean myself
Solutions
    Toilet paper holder on the unaffected side which can be used with one hand
    Large aperture toilet seat
    Self-cleaning toilet, like a bidet and toilet in one

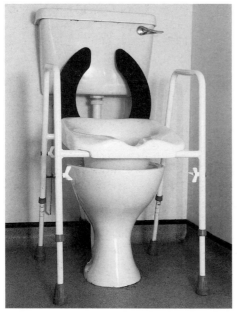
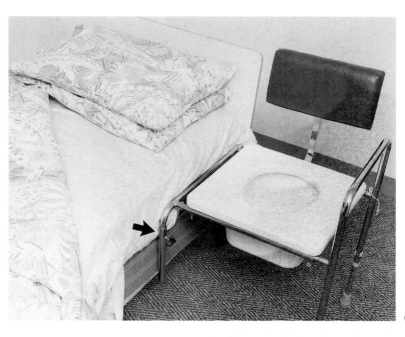

(a)
(b)

Figure 15.20 Simple toilet aids. (a) A raised toilet seat with a frame. (b) A commode. This one attaches securely to the bed (arrow) for use at night.

conditions in the elderly (e.g. painful arthritis) often contribute to the problems.

A skilled assessment by an occupational therapist, preferably in the patient's own home, will delineate the problem. This assessment can ensure that there is adequate access to the bathroom (e.g. for a wheelchair) and the size and layout of the bathroom will determine which aids can be used.

Therapy aimed at improving those impairments, especially motor impairments, which are contributing to the disability in bathing and washing may be of some help but, again, the provision of aids to allow the patient to compensate for their impairment is more effective. There are a wide range of aids and adaptations to overcome most problems with bathing (Table 15.48 & Fig. 15.21). Of course, in many countries patients prefer to take showers rather than a bath which generally reduces the difficulty. One general point is that patients who have trouble bathing should ensure that somebody else is in the house and that the bathroom door is left unlocked.

> *Patients who have difficulties bathing independently should not be left in their house alone whilst bathing. Some form of alarm or even a cordless telephone will increase safety.*

Some bathroom adaptations are expensive and cause considerable disruption to the patient's home. It is important that a proper assessment is done to avoid unnecessary building work and to ensure that any modifications really are likely to help the patient and/or carer. For some patients who live alone, or where aids and adaptations are not appropriate, it may be necessary to recommend either a simple strip wash or to introduce a nurse, care assistant or family member to help with bathing and so allow the patient to remain in their own home.

Table 15.48 Problems with grooming or bathing/showering and possible solutions.

Can not brush my dentures with one hand
Solutions
    Half fill sink with water
    Attach brush with a suction pad to the sink
    Brush dentures with functioning hand

Can not get into, and even more important, out of the bath
Solutions
    Grab rails appropriately mounted around bath
    Non-slip bath mat
    Bath stool
    Bath board
    Inflatable or hydraulic bath seats which can lower patients into or raise them out of the bath (see Fig. 15.21)
    Hoists
    Replace bath with shower

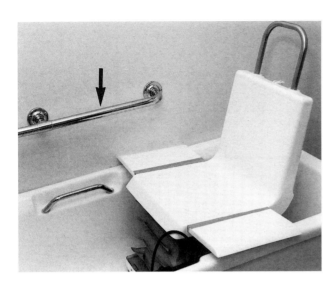

Figure 15.21 A pneumatic bath aid to lower patients into and to lift them out of a bath. However, the humble bath rail (arrow) with some other simple aids is very commonly all that is needed to allow the person to use a bath independently.

15.32.5 Dressing

About 22% of patients needed help from another person to dress 1 year after their first-ever stroke in the Oxfordshire Community Stroke Project (see Table 15.43). Dependency in dressing is usually due to a combination of arm weakness or incoordination, inability to stand independently to pull up lower garments, cognitive and visuospatial problems (Walker & Lincoln, 1991). A painful shoulder makes dressing even more difficult (see Section 15.24). A detailed assessment by an occupational therapist should elucidate the cause and define the degree of disability.

Occupational therapists spend a considerable proportion of their time training patients to dress themselves. If the disability is due simply to a motor deficit, then 'dressing practice' where the patient is taught to compensate for their impairments, is often successful (Walker *et al.*, 1994). If the patient has cognitive or visuospatial problems, or other non-stroke problems (e.g. arthritis), the benefit of this type of therapy is less obvious. There has been little formal evaluation of dressing therapy.

Advice on the best type of clothes can allow patients to become independent, i.e. avoidance of tight clothes with small buttons or zips, and shoes with laces. Some of the common problems and possible solutions are shown in Table 15.49 and Fig. 15.22. If the patient still cannot dress themself, then a care assistant or member of the family will be needed to help.

15.32.6 Feeding

One year after a first-ever stroke about 18% of patients in the Oxfordshire Community Stroke Project needed some help from another person to feed (see Table 15.43). Dependency in feeding is one of the most demeaning problems because of its associations with infancy. Impaired function of the arm and hand are the most common causes, although problems with sitting balance, facial weakness,

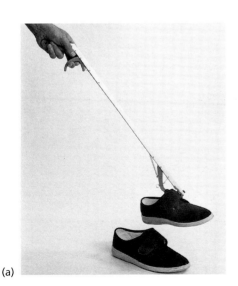

(a)

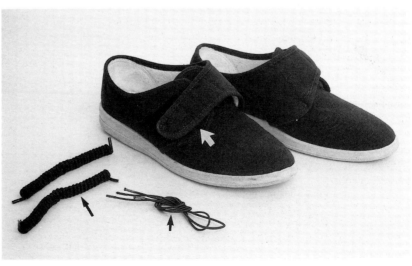

(b)

Figure 15.22 Simple dressing aids. (a) A reaching aid. (b) Elastic laces (short black arrow), spiral laces which one simply pulls tight (long black arrow) and Velcro fasteners (white arrow) are invaluable dressing aids for those with only one functioning hand or poor manual dexterity.

Table 15.49 Problems with dressing and possible solutions (see Fig. 15.22).

Can not manage zips or buttons
Solutions
    Button hook or toggle button hook allows patient to fasten
      buttons with one hand
    Hook to pull up zip
    Replace zips and buttons with Velcro

Can not get shoes on or tie shoe laces
Solutions
    Long-handled shoe horn
    Replace shoe laces with elastic ones or Velcro straps
    Shoe ties

Can not reach or pull up clothes
Solutions
    Dressing hook or even a walking stick
    Reaching aid

---

visuospatial and sensory function may be important as well. A small number of patients may have residual problems swallowing (see Section 15.17). Most problems can be identified simply by talking to the patient and/or carer, but often it is useful for a trained observer, usually an occupational therapist, to assess the patient.

Intensive therapy may improve arm function (see Section 15.21), but the provision and training in the use of feeding aids probably has more to offer late after the stroke. However, sometimes very simple problems, which require very simple solutions, are overlooked. For instance, it is important that any dentures are in good working order, that the patient is sitting at a table on a chair of appropriate height and that the knife is sharp. The type of food can be a crucial determinant of feeding dependency. A hemiplegic patient may be independent eating sandwiches but dependent for eating a steak. Some of the more common feeding problems and the aids which can help are shown in Table 15.50 and Fig. 15.23.

15.32.7 Preparing food

Many patients are unable to prepare food for themselves or their family because of a wide variety of post-stroke impairments. Cognitive and visuospatial problems may put patients, and others living in the same building, in danger from fires and explosions. Again, problems are easily identified by talking to, or observing the patient in the kitchen. An occupational therapist may be able to teach patients alternative methods of performing certain tasks and for many with physical rather than cognitive problems there is a large variety of kitchen aids available to help with specific difficulties (Table 15.51). Patients with cognitive problems may be helped by things such as electric kettles which turn themselves off and gas stoves which automatically ignite, but for those with severe cognitive problems it may

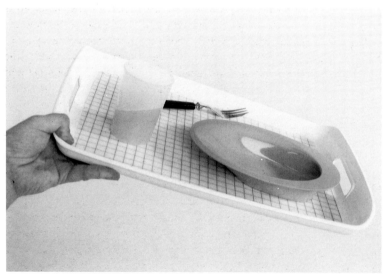

(a)

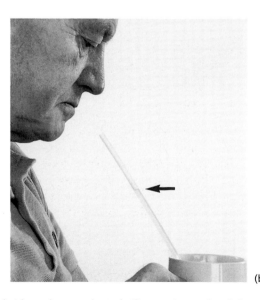

(b)

Figure 15.23 Simple feeding aids. (a) A combined fork and knife and a plate with a high side or plate guard may facilitate eating one handed. The non-slip tray also helps by fixing the plate and also reduces the risk of spills. (b) This drinking straw has a one-way valve so that when the user stops sucking the fluid does not fall back into the beaker (arrow). This may be useful in patients with facial weakness and poor lip closure but who have a normal swallow.

Table 15.50 Feeding problems and solutions (see Fig. 15.23).

Can not cut up food because of poor arm function
Solutions
   If moderate hand weakness a large-handled sharp knife may be
      enough
   Alternatively, a combined knife and spoon or fork may help, but
      warn the patient to be careful not to cut their mouth

Can not hold bowl or plate still when cutting or spooning
Solution
   A non-slip mat or tray, or containers with suction pads on

Can not push peas onto fork or spoon
Solution
   Provide a dish with a raised side or rim

Dribbling due to facial weakness
Solutions
   A mug with a spout or a straw may help. Straws are available
      with a non-return valve if the patient cannot suck using a
      conventional one because of facial weakness, but has an intact
      swallow

Table 15.51 Problems with food preparation and possible
solutions.

Can not open cans with one functional hand
Solution
   Wall-mounted (electric) tin opener

Can not open bottles with one functional hand
Solution
   A bottle or jar stabiliser to fix the bottles to work surface

Can not cut up or peel ingredients with one functional hand
Solution
   A plate or board with spikes on which to impale the item to
      be cut

be necessary to ban them from the kitchen or to remove
cookers, etc.

Where patients cannot prepare food for themselves it is
obviously important to ensure delivery of prepared meals to
their homes, or to provide a care assistant who can prepare
meals. Often, relatives and social services provide these
services.

15.33   Social difficulties

We have seen how stroke-related impairments result in disability or dependency in ADL. However, there is more to life
than just these basic activities. Environmental factors

become extremely important in determining the effect of the
stroke on a person's role in society and their handicap. This
section will address some of the social factors which are
often of greatest concern to patients and their carers.

15.33.1   Accommodation

About 50% of the patients who survive a stroke are dependent in ADL (see Table 15.43). Some patients with complex
or worsening disability may not, if admitted to hospital, be
able to return to their own home. In the Oxfordshire
Community Stroke Project, 643 (95%) of 675 people were
living at home before their first-ever in a lifetime stroke and
at 1 year 418 (89%) of the 467 survivors were able to live at
home. Thus, the proportion of patients in institutions had
not increased greatly, but many of the 32 patients who had
lived in an institution before their stroke had died. Patients'
ability to return home will depend on the answers to the following questions, amongst others.
1 Is the disability likely to improve or worsen with time?
2 Will aids and adaptations reduce dependency?
3 What does the patient's accommodation comprise?
4 What level of informal support is available, e.g. family?
5 What level of community support is available?

Any assessment has to identify the needs of the patient
and try to determine whether those needs can be practically
provided in the patient's current accommodation, or
whether alternative or modified accommodation will be
needed. This may involve one or more visits home with the
patient and carer to establish exactly what the practical
problems are. If a short visit is not enough, then home visits
for a few days and nights can be useful to predict how the
patient and carer will cope in the longer term. The layout of
the home is obviously important. Are there steps up to the
front door which make access difficult? Are the toilet and
bathroom upstairs? Is the house cluttered with furniture?
Are the carpets deep pile which may cause difficulty for a
patient with a foot drop? Some stroke units have pre-
discharge apartments in the hospital which allow the team
and the patient to assess under supervision how well they
cope. This may not be the same as discharge into the community, however.

The timing of accomodation assessment is difficult
because it often takes a considerable time to find alternative
accommodation or to make major structural changes to
the patient's current home. Thus, if one is going to avoid
unnecessary delays in hospital, one has to make a decision
before the patient has achieved their optimal functional
status. Considerable judgement is required to 'best guess' the
patient's final functional level and to identify their accommodation needs well in advance of hospital discharge.

After a thorough assessment the patient and their family, with help from the team, need to decide where they wish to live, taking into account all the practical issues including any financial constraints. After all, given unlimited funds, it is almost always possible to maintain even the most severely disabled patient at home. The final decision is often a result of negotiation between the patient, carer and team members. For instance, patients with visuospatial problems may not appreciate the likely problems which will face their carers after discharge. For these sorts of reasons it is not always possible to fulfil the wishes of both patient and carer.

Options for alternative accommodation and the availability of support in the community vary from place to place, and from country to country. It is therefore not relevant to go into detail about accommodation in any one country. However, in general, one needs a range of accommodation offering a variety of levels of support and supervision to meet the needs of individual patients.

15.33.2 Employment

About one-third of patients who have a stroke are of employment age. In Oxfordshire, 76 (24%) of 318 men and 39 (11%) of 357 women were in paid employment before their stroke. Of these, 68 (59%) returned to work at some stage, the majority within 6 months of the stroke. Obviously, the nature of previous employment, residual impairments and disabilities, and the patient's own wishes will determine whether return to employment is feasible. It is also likely that the local arrangements for paying sickness benefit will influence whether patients return to work, and the timing of their return (Saeki *et al.*, 1995). Of course, many patients who are approaching retirement age may not want to return to work anyway.

Assessment of the patient's ability to return to work is often left to the patient and family, but involvement of members of the team (i.e. occupational therapist, speech and language therapist, physiotherapist and social worker) can be very useful to help explore the possible work options. Some employers have occupational health departments which can provide further specialist advice on specific regulations covering return to work and on any alterations to the working environment or job itself which would facilitate this.

It is important that patients and their families are counselled about the patient's limitations. Many patients and families are under the misconception that patients should rest after a stroke and that physical activity will bring on another stroke (Wellwood *et al.*, 1994). This misconception may have made them rule out the possibility of return to work.

> *Many patients and their carers are under the misconception that exercise, hard work or stress will bring on another stroke. They should be counselled to dispel these myths.*

Patients may require specific occupational therapy to improve physical skills required for particular posts, and/or retraining to change employment. A return to part-time work, at least initially, is often more successful than the patient struggling to cope with full-time work. Patients often find that although they can perform the physical aspects of their work, their concentration may be impaired. In many countries, special schemes are available to provide employment for disabled people.

15.33.3 Leisure

Two-thirds of stroke patients are retired from employment. For them, resumption of a leisure activity is more important than work. Restriction in leisure activities may be the result of physical or cognitive impairments but may also be caused by psychological factors and even fear that an activity may bring on a further stroke. Many disabled stroke patients are unable to continue with their normal leisure activities and do not take up new ones which are within their abilities (Sjogren, 1982; Drummond, 1990). Reduction in leisure activities will exacerbate social isolation, lower mood and adversely affect relationships with carers (Sjogren, 1982; Feibel & Springer, 1982).

The level of social activities, including leisure, can be measured using the Frenchay Activities Index but a more specific measure of leisure function has recently been developed (Holbrook & Skilbeck, 1983; Schuling *et al.*, 1993; Drummond & Walker, 1994a).

Counselling the patient and their carers about the importance of maintaining leisure activities and social contacts may be useful, and can have dramatic consequences (Fig. 15.24), along with practical help in achieving them. The efficacy of therapy specifically directed at improving participation in leisure activities or using leisure goals to improve ADL function is uncertain, having only been tested in small randomised trials (Jongbloed & Morgan, 1991; Drummond & Walker, 1994b).

15.33.4 Sex

Although many stroke patients are elderly, they were often sexually active before their stroke. Limited information from formal research suggests that sexual activity is reduced after stroke along with the patient's and their partner's feelings of sexual satisfaction (Angeleri *et al.*, 1993). Obviously, severe

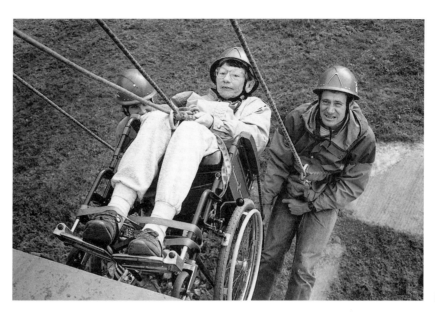

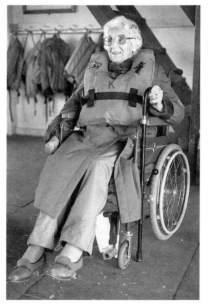

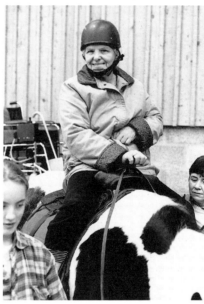

Figure 15.24 Leisure activities for patients with mobility problems after stroke. (a) Abseiling in a wheelchair; (b) canoeing; (c) horse riding. (Photographs taken by Renzo Mazzolini for the Chest Heart and Stroke Association, Scotland.)

physical disability can make sexual intercourse difficult but other factors may be even more important (Table 15.52). Reduced sexual activity may contribute to a worsening emotional relationship with a partner.

A patient and their partner may believe that reduced satisfaction with their sexual relationship is an inevitable consequence of the stroke. Although we often feel embarrassed about talking to people about these aspects of their lives it is important that sexual problems are addressed. Physical difficulties related to the patient's impairments can often be overcome with a little commonsense and some of the common causes of sexual dysfunction after stroke are easily dealt with (Table 15.52). It is the psychological factors which are often the most difficult to sort out. Sometimes patients and their partners simply need to be reassured that sexual activity, like any other physical activity, will not precipitate another stroke. Verbal information may usefully be supplemented by leaflets, supplied by charities and patients' organisations, which include advice for patients and carers (Duddle, 1993). We encourage patients to resume sexual activity as soon as they wish to after a stroke. One exception might be a patient with a recent rupture of a saccular aneurysm which has not

533

Table 15.52 Causes of dissatisfaction with sexual relationships after a stroke.

Emotional changes may adversely affect the relationship
Physical disability may make sexual intercourse difficult or
    impossible, e.g. indwelling catheter, contractures
Fear of bringing on another stroke
Impotence and reduced libido due to drugs, diabetes, etc.

---

for some reason been surgically or radiologically treated. One might imagine that the increase in blood pressure associated with orgasm could cause a rebleed. Unfortunately, strokes can put tremendous strains on a relationship which are more difficult to manage. Referral to a sexual dysfunction clinic, or for marital guidance, may be useful if problems persist after attending to the simple and obvious.

15.33.5 Finance

Stroke places a considerable financial burden on patients and their families, although these costs are difficult to quantify. Employment, and therefore income, may be affected (Holbrook, 1982). Disability, and the aids and adaptations needed to overcome it, may also be costly. Even when the patient is still in hospital, carers may have difficulty meeting the costs of transport to visit the patient. This is important because the patient's morale may suffer if regular visiting is not possible and this may adversely affect outcome. Of course, in some unenlightened health systems, the patient or family may have to pay directly for their health care and financial constraints may even prevent patients from receiving the necessary treatment.

The professionals involved must be alert to the financial problems which affect patients and be ready to offer help as required. In the UK, and other countries, where the level of government support for home care is dependent on the patient's personal finances, a financial assessment may be necessary for planning care. In the UK, social workers are responsible for these assessments although other agencies may become involved.

Depending on assessment of the patient's and carer's needs, and sometimes a financial assessment, patients or carers may be eligible for financial benefits from government, charitable and other sources (e.g. superannuation schemes, insurance policies, etc.).

15.34 Carers

Looking after a patient with disability places considerable physical and emotional strains on the carer (Anderson et al.,

1995). It may limit the carer's employment and leisure activities and lead to social isolation. Carers of disabled stroke patients are more often depressed, have more physical symptoms and are more dissatisfied with their jobs and social life than controls of similar age and sex (Carnwath & Johnson, 1987). The extent of these difficulties appears to be related to the patient's level of dependency and psychological problems (Wade et al., 1986; Carnwath & Johnson, 1987). The impact that a stroke has on the family changes over time. Periods which are likely to cause carers particular stress and when extra support may be needed are listed below.

1 Immediately after the stroke when the carer has to come to terms with what is potentially a life-threatening event and one which may have a major effect on the patient's and potential carer's future life together.

2 During a prolonged period of in-patient care. Visiting may be difficult because of travelling and also because the patient's behaviour may put emotional pressure on the carer.

3 Around the period of hospital discharge. Suddenly the patient who has been looked after by a team of highly skilled professionals appears, at least to the carer, to be the carer's sole responsibility.

4 During the weeks and months following hospital discharge when professional support dwindles (sometimes inappropriately and abruptly), friends stop calling and the carer becomes physically and emotionally exhausted.

Holbrook (1982) made some useful observations of the stages which families typically go through in adjusting to the change in their lives (Table 15.53). Although these do not apply to all carers, it is useful to be aware of them in managing patients and their families.

Although the physical aspects of caring for a person with a disabling stroke are hard it is often the patient's psychological and resulting behavioural problems which cause most distress to carers (Brocklehurst et al., 1981). Carers note a change in personality; the patient may become short tempered and irritable, depressed or apathetic (Angeleri et al., 1993). Such changes may lead to a deterioration in their relationship which may be compounded by a cessation or disturbance of their sexual relationship (see Section 15.33.4).

Carers often have feelings of guilt which add to their distress. They worry that they contributed to the stroke, perhaps by giving the patient the wrong diet or because of some petty incident which the carer feels they should have avoided. They feel guilty about not visiting enough or for not having the patient home soon enough. After hospital discharge they feel guilty about wanting to carry on with their own lives. They often worry that the patient will fall,

Table 15.53 Stages of adjustment amongst families of patients with a stroke. (From Holbrook, 1982.)

Stage 1
Crisis
  Shock
  Confusion
  High anxiety

Stage 2
Treatment stage
  High expectation of recovery
  Denial that disability is permanent
  Periods of grieving
  Fears for the future
    Job
    Mobility
    Lifestyle
    About coping

Stage 3
Realisation of disability
  Anger
  Feelings of rejection
  Despair
  Frustration
  Depression

Stage 4
Adjustment

---

have another stroke or even die unless they are in constant attendance. These fears, apart from adding to the distress of carers, may also cause the carers to become overprotective towards the patient, which may prejudice the patient's outcome.

It is important that all those involved in managing a stroke patient are aware of the burden that caring for a disabled patient places on the family or other carers. The carer should be invited to discuss *their* problems. This is usually best done when the patient is absent since carers often feel uncomfortable or guilty when talking about *their* own problems if the patient is present. Indeed, carers often need a lot of encouragement to discuss *their* problems. However, they should be encouraged to do so not only for their own sake, but also for the patient's. If they are not coping this will adversely affect the patient.

It is important to assess the carer's physical and mental ability to go on providing the necessary care. If the patient is in hospital it is often useful to get the carer to help with the patient's nursing care and attend their therapy sessions. This gives the carer an indication of what caring may involve, it can help the carer and team members to identify and hopefully resolve problems before discharge, and it provides a

valuable opportunity to 'train' the carer. Pre-discharge visits home for 1 day or a weekend fulfil similar functions.

Carers may need physical or simply psychological support.

Physical support

Physical support is usually limited whilst the patient is in hospital, although some carers may need help with finances (see Section 15.33.5) and visiting. However, physical support is likely to become more important after the patient is discharged home. Examples include:
1 providing help with housework to give the carer more time for providing personal care;
2 providing a care assistant or district nurse to help with the patient's personal care;
3 providing a laundry service if the patient has persisting urinary or faecal incontinence;
4 arranging for the patient to attend a day hospital or day centre or arranging 'patient sitting' services to allow the carer to go shopping, have their hair done or attend some social function;
5 arranging regular respite admissions to a hospital or nursing home to allow the carer to go on holiday, or simply to give them a well-earned rest.

Such services may be expensive but they probably prevent or delay the need for long-term institutional care which may be even more expensive.

Psychological support

Carers often need help coming to terms with the changes in the person who has had a stroke. They have many questions and sources of concern (Table 15.54). Support is needed whilst the patient is in hospital and thereafter. It may take a variety of forms.
1 An informal talk with the consultant, nurse, therapist or social worker. These are valuable opportunities for carers to ask questions.
2 A carers' group where they can ask team members questions, share experiences and provide mutual support (Mykyta *et al.*, 1976; Holbrook, 1982).
3 Formal sessions with a counsellor which may help them come to terms with their problems.

The setting in which support is given needs to be tailored to the individual since, for example, not everybody wants to attend a group.

The need for these sorts of services may not be apparent whilst patients are in hospital or when they attend an outpatient department. Also, for patients who are not admitted after their stroke, or who remain in hospital for just a few

Table 15.54 Common questions asked by carers.

Acutely
What is a stroke?
Will they die?
Will they be disabled?
Why did this happen?
Was it my fault?
Will it happen again?

After hospital discharge
How long will they keep improving for?
Will their speech get better?
Why is he/she not the person I knew before?
Can I leave them alone to go out?
Can they exercise, will it bring on another stroke?
Will I always feel so tired?
Where can I get help with money?
Where can I get help with bathing?
Can I have a rest or holiday, i.e. respite?

---

days, the opportunities for the patient and their carer to ask questions and obtain advice are often limited. One approach, which is currently being evaluated, is to provide a dedicated stroke family support worker who can identify the physical and emotional needs of patients and their families and try to meet them using all available resources. In many places this role is already, at least partially, carried out by social workers and other members of the team, but there are often difficulties in bridging the gap between hospital and community care.

Giving information

Carers may know little about stroke, its causes and consequences and have often received misleading information from families and friends (Wellwood *et al.*, 1994). Carers, like patients, vary in the amount, type and format of information they want about stroke. Information giving therefore needs to be tailored to the individual. Leaflets, audio or video tapes may usefully reinforce verbal transfer of information but more formal evaluation of their relative effectiveness is required (Lomer & McLennan, 1987). It is important that patients and carers are given consistent information and advice to avoid confusion. Good communication between potential providers of information is therefore vital.

References

Agrell B, Dehlin O (1989). Comparison of six depression rating scales in geriatric stroke patients. *Stroke* 20: 1190–4.

Albiin N, Asplund K, Bjermer L (1982). Nutritional status of medical patients on emergency admission to hospital. *Acta Med Scand* 212: 151–6.

Allen CMC (1983). Clinical diagnosis of the acute stroke syndrome. *Quart J Med* 208: 515–23.

Allman RM, Walker JM, Hart MK, Lapsade CA, Noel LB, Smith CR (1987). Air fluidised beds or conventional therapy for pressure sores. *Ann Intern Med* 107: 641–8.

Anderson G, Vestergaard K, Ingeman-Nielsen M (1995). Post-stroke pathological crying: frequency and correlation to depression. *Eur J Neurol* 2: 45–50.

Andersen G, Vestergaard K, Lauritzen L (1994). Effective treatment of post stroke depression with the selective serotonin reuptake inhibitor citalopram. *Stroke* 25: 1099–104.

Andersen G, Vestergaard K, Riis JO (1993). Citalopram for post-stroke pathological crying. *Lancet* 342: 837–9.

Anderson CS, Linto J, Stewart-Wynne EG (1995). A population-based assessment of the impact and burden of caregiving for long-term stroke survivors. *Stroke* 26: 843–9.

Angeleri F, Angeleri VA, Foschi N, Giaquinto S, Nolfe G (1993). The influence of depression, social activity and family stress on functional outcome after stroke. *Stroke* 24(10): 1478–83.

Arden M, Mayou R, Feldman E, Hawton K (1993). Cognitive impairment in the elderly medically ill: how often is it missed? *Intern J Geriatr Psychiatr* 8: 929–37.

Ashburn A, Lynch M (1988). Disadvantages of the early use of wheelchairs in the treatment of hemiplegia. *Clin Rehabil* 2: 327–31.

Ashworth B (1964). Preliminary trial of carisoprodol in multiple sclerosis. *Practitioner* 192: 540–2.

Askenasy JJ, Goldhammer I (1988). Sleep apnea as a feature of bulbar stroke. *Stroke* 19: 637–9.

Asplund K (1992). Any progress on progressing stroke? *Cerebrovasc Dis* 2: 317–19.

Astrom M, Adolfsson R, Asplund K (1993). Major depression in stroke patients. A 3 year longitudinal study. *Stroke* 24: 976–82.

Axelsson K, Asplund K, Norberg A, Alafuzoff I (1988). Nutritional status in patients with acute stroke. *Acta Med Scand* 224: 217–24.

Azzimondi G, Bassein L, Nonino F *et al.* (1995). Fever in acute stroke worsens prognosis. A prospective study. *Stroke* 26: 2040–3.

Bainbridge W, Reding M (1994). Full-field prisms for hemi-field visual impairments following stroke: a controlled trial. *Neurology* 44 (Suppl. 2): A312 (abstract).

Bainton T, Fox M, Bowsher D, Wells C (1992). A double blind trial of naxolone in central post-stroke pain. *Pain* 48: 159–62.

Barer DH (1989a). Continence after stroke: useful predictor or goal of therapy? *Age Ageing* 18: 183–91.

Barer DH (1989b). The natural history and functional consequences of dysphagia after hemispheric stroke. *J Neurol Neurosurg Psychiatr* 52: 236–41.

Barratt E (1988). A review of risk assessment methods. *Care Sci Pract* 6: 49–52.

Bastow MD, Rawlings J, Allison SP (1983). Benefits of

supplementary tube feeding after fractured neck of femur: a randomised controlled trial. *Br Med J* 287: 1589–92.

Belfield PW (1989). Urinary catheters. In: Mulley GP, ed. *Everyday Aids and Appliances*. London: BMJ, 55–9.

Ben-Menachem T, Fogel R, Patel RV *et al.* (1994). Prophylaxis for stress-related gastric hemorrhage in the medical intensive care unit. A randomized, controlled, single-blind study. *Ann Intern Med* 121: 568–75.

Benbow S, Sangster G, Barer D (1991). Incontinence after stroke. *Lancet* 338: 1602–3.

Berkovic SF, Bladin P, Darby DG (1984). Metabolic disorders presenting as stroke. *Med J Aust* 140(7): 421–4.

Bhakta B, Cozens JA, Bamford JM, Chamberlain MA (1996). Use of botulinum toxin in stroke patients with severe upper limb spasticity. *J Neurol Neurosurg Psychiatr* (in press).

Bliss MR (1995). Preventing pressure sores in elderly patients: a comparison of seven mattress overlays. *Age Ageing* 24: 297–302.

Bliss MR, McLaren R, Exton-Smith AN (1967). Preventing pressure sores in hospital: controlled trial of a large-celled rippled mattress. *Br Med J* 1: 394–7.

Bobath B (1978). *Adult Hemiplegia Evaluation and Treatment*, 2nd edn. London: Heinemann.

Boeer A, Voth E, Prange HW (1991). Early heparin therapy in patients with spontaneous intracerebral haemorrhage. *J Neurol Neurosurg Psychiatr* 54: 466–7.

Bohannon RW, Smith MB (1987). Interrater reliability of a modified Ashworth spastic scale of muscle spasticity. *Phys Therapy* 67: 206–7.

Borrie MJ, Campbell A, Caradoc-Davies TH, Spears GFS (1986). Urinary incontinence after stroke: a prospective study. *Age Ageing* 15: 177–81.

Bounds JV, Wiebers DO, Whisnant JP, Okazaki H (1981). Mechanisms and timing of deaths from cerebral infarction. *Stroke* 12(4): 474–7.

Braus DF, Krauss JK, Strobel J (1994). The shoulder hand syndrome after stroke: a prospective clinical trial. *Ann Neurol* 36: 728–33.

Britton M, Carlsson A, De Faire U (1986). Blood pressure course in patients with acute stroke and matched controls. *Stroke* 17: 861–4.

Britton M, De Faire U, Helmers C, Miah K, Ryding C, Wester PO (1979). Arrhythmias in patients with acute cerebrovascular disease. *Acta Med Scand* 205: 425–8.

Brocklehurst JC, Andrews K, Richards B, Laycock PJ (1985). Incidence and correlates of incontinence in stroke patients. *J Am Geriatr Soc* 33: 540–2.

Brocklehurst JC, Morris P, Andrews K, Richards B, Laycock P (1981). Social effects of stroke. *Soc Sci Med* 15A: 35–9.

Brooke MM, de Lateur BJ, Diana-Rigby GC, Questad KA (1991). Shoulder subluxation in hemiplegia: effects of three different supports. *Arch Phys Med Rehabil* 72: 583–6.

Brown HW, Plum F (1961). The neurologic basis of Cheyne–Stokes respiration. *Am J Med* 30: 849–60.

Brunnstrom S (1970) *Movement Therapy in Hemiplegia*. New York: Harper and Row.

Burcar PJ, Notenberg MD, Yarnell PR (1977). Hyponatraemia and central pontine myelinolysis. *Neurology* 27: 223–6.

Burt AA, Currie S (1978). A double blind controlled trial of baclofen and diazepam in spasticity due to cerebrovascular lesions. In: Jukes AM, ed. *Spasticity and Cerebral Pathology*. Cambridge: Cambridge Medical Publications, 77–9.

Burvill P, Johnson G, Anderson C, Chakera T, Jamrozik K, Stewart-Wynne E (1994). Post stroke depression and lesion location. *Cerebrovasc Dis* 4: 234 (abstract).

Burvill PW, Johnson GA, Jamrozik KD, Anderson CS, Stewart-Wynne EG, Chakera TMH (1995a). Prevalence of depression after stroke: the Perth Community Stroke Study. *Br J Psychiatr* 166: 320–7.

Burvill PW, Johnson GA, Jamrozik KD, Anderson CS, Stewart-Wynne EG, Chakera TMH (1995b). Anxiety disorders after stroke: results from the Perth Community Stroke Study. *Br J Psychiatr* 166: 328–32.

Busto R, Dietrich D, Globus MYT, Ginsberg MD (1989). The importance of brain temperature in cerebral ischaemic injury. *Stroke* 20(8): 1113–14.

Busto R, Dietrich WD, Globus MYT, Valdes I, Scheinberg P, Ginsberg MD (1987). Small differences in intra-ischemic brain temperature critically determine the extent of ischemic neuronal injury. *J Cereb Blood Flow Metab* 7: 729–38.

Candelise L, Landi G, Orazio EN, Boccardi E (1985). Prognostic significance of hyperglycaemia in acute stroke. *Arch Neurol* 42: 661–3.

Carlberg B, Asplund K, Hagg E (1991). Course of blood pressure in different subsets of patients after acute stroke. *Cerebrovasc Dis* 1: 281–7.

Carlsson A, Britton M (1993). Blood pressure after stroke. A one-year follow-up study. *Stroke* 24: 195–9.

Carnwath TCM, Johnson DAW (1987). Psychiatric morbidity among spouses of patients with stroke. *Br Med J* 294: 409–11.

Carr EK, Kenney FD (1992). Positioning of the stroke patient: a review of the literature. *Int J Nurs Stud* 29(4): 355–69.

Castillo J, Martinez F, Leira R, Prieto JM, Lema M, Noya M (1994). Mortality and morbidity of acute cerebral infarction related to temperature and basal analytic parameters. *Cerebrovasc Dis* 4: 66–71.

Cederholm T, Hellstrom K (1992). Nutritional status in recently hospitalized and free-living elderly subjects. *Gerontology* 38: 105–10.

Challiner Y, Hayward M, Al-Jubouri M, Julious S (1992). Is subcutaneous rehydration as effective as intravenous in elderly stroke patients? *Age Ageing* 21: 1–17 (abstract).

Chen H, Chopp M, Welch KMA (1991). Effect of mild hyperthermia on the ischaemic infarct volume after middle cerebral artery occlusion in the rat. *Neurology* 41: 1133–5.

Cheyne J (1818). A case of apoplexy in which the fleshy part of the heart was converted to fat. *Dublin Hosp Rep* 2: 216.

Chiu KY, Pun WK, Luk KDK, Chow SP (1992). A prospective study on hip fractures in patients with previous cerebrovascular accidents. *Injury* 23(5): 297–9.

Clough NP (1994). The cost of pressure area management in an intensive care unit. *J Wound Care* 3(1): 33–5.

Collen FM, Wade DT (1991). Residual mobility problems after stroke. *Int Disabil Studies* 13: 12–15.

Collen FM, Wade DT, Robb GF, Bradshaw CM (1991). The Rivermead Mobility Index: a further development of the Rivermead Motor Assessment. *Int Disabil Studies* 13: 50–4.

Cook DJ, Fuller HD, Guyatt GH *et al.* (1994). Risk factors for gastrointestinal bleeding in critically ill patients. *N Engl J Med* 330(6): 377–81.

Cope C, Tyrone MR, Skversky NJ (1973). Phlebographic analysis of the incidence of thrombosis in hemiplegia. *Radiology* 109: 581–4.

Cornall C (1991). Self propelling wheelchairs: the effect on spasticity in hemiplegic patients. *Physiother Theory Pract* 7: 13–21.

Counsell C, Sandercock P (1995). The efficacy and safety of anticoagulant therapy in patients with acute presumed ischaemic stroke: a systematic review of the randomized trials comparing anticoagulants with control. In: Warlow C, van Gijn J, Sandercock P, eds. *Stroke Module of the Cochrane Database of Systematic Reviews*. London: BMJ Publishing Group.

Cullum N, Deeks J, Fletcher A *et al.* (1995). The prevention and treatment of pressure sores. *Effect Health Care* 2: 1–16.

Davalos A, Ricart W, Gonzalez-Huix F, Molins A, Genis D (1994). Nutritional status and clinical outcome in acute cerebral infarct. *Cerebrovasc Dis* 4: 239 (abstract).

Davenport RJ, Dennis MS, Warlow CP (1995). Improving the recording of the clinical assessment of stroke patients using a clerking proforma. *Age Ageing* 24: 43–8.

Davenport RJ, Dennis MS, Warlow CP (1996a). Gastrointestinal haemorrhage following acute stroke. *Stroke* 27: 421–4.

Davenport RJ, Dennis MS, Wellwood I, Warlow CP (1996b). Complications following acute stroke. *Stroke* 27: 415–20.

David R, Enderby P, Bainton D (1982). Treatment of acquired aphasia: speech therapists and volunteers compared. *J Neurol Neurosurg Psychiatr* 45: 957–61.

Demeurisse G, Demol O, Robaye E (1980). Motor evaluation in vascular hemiplegia. *Eur Neurol* 19: 382–9.

Denes G, Semenza C, Stoppa E, Lis A (1982). Unilateral spatial neglect and recovery from hemiplegia: a follow up study. *Brain* 105: 543–52.

DePippo KL, Holas MA, Reding MJ (1992). Validation of the 3-oz water swallow test for aspiration following stroke. *Arch Neurol* 49: 1259–61.

DePippo KL, Holas MA, Reding MJ, Mandel FS, Lesser ML (1994). Dysphagia therapy following stroke: a controlled trial. *Neurology* 44: 1655–60.

Desmond DW, Tetemichi TK, Figueroa M, Gropen TI, Stern Y (1994). Disorientation following stroke: frequency, course, and clinical correlates. *J Neurol* 241: 585–91.

Desmukh M, Bisignani M, Landau P, Orchard TJ (1991). Deep vein thrombosis in rehabilitating stroke patients. Incidence, risk factors and prophylaxis. *Am J Phys Med Rehabil* 70: 313–16.

Dickmann U, Voth E, Schicha H, Henze T, Prange H, Emrich D (1988). Heparin therapy, deep vein thrombosis and pulmonary embolism after intracerebral haemorrhage. *Klin Wochenschr* 66: 1182–3.

Dickstein R, Hocherman S, Pillar T, Shaham R (1986). Stroke rehabilitation. Three exercise therapy approaches. *Phys Therapy* 66(8): 1233–8.

Dimant J, Grob D (1977). Electrocardiographic changes and myocardial damage in patients with acute cerebrovascular accidents. *Stroke* 8(4): 448–55.

Downes B, Rooney V, Roper-Hall A, Oyebode J, Main A, Mayer P (1993). The effectiveness of counselling stroke survivors and their carers in the community. *Br Geriatr Soc Conf Papers* April (abstract).

Dromerick A, Reding M (1994). Medical and neurological complications during in-patient stroke rehabilitation. *Stroke* 25: 358–61.

Drummond A (1990). Leisure activity after stroke. *Int Disabil Studies* 12(4): 157–60.

Drummond A, Walker MF (1994b). Leisure therapy after stroke. *Clin Rehabil* 8: 86 (abstract).

Drummond AER, Walker MF (1994a). The Nottingham Leisure Questionnaire for stroke patients. *Br J Occup Therapy* 57: 414–18.

Duddle M (1993). Sex after stroke illness. *Stroke Assoc Leaflet* S16.

Duncan PW, Goldstein LB, Horner RD, Landsman PB, Samsa GP, Matchar DB (1994). Similar motor recovery of upper and lower extremities after stroke. *Stroke* 25: 1181–8.

Elizabeth J, Singarayar J, Ellul J, Barer D, Lye M (1993). Arterial oxygen saturation and posture in acute stroke. *Age Ageing* 22: 269–72.

Ellul J, Barer D (1993). Detection and management of dysphagia in patients with acute stroke. *Age Ageing* 22 (Suppl. No. 2): 17 (abstract).

Enderby PM, Wood VA, Wade DT, Langton Hewer R (1986). The Frenchay Aphasia Screening Test: a short, simple test for aphasia appropriate for non-specialists. *Intern Rehabil Med* 8: 166–70.

Exton-Smith AN, Overstall PW, Wedgewood J, Wallace G (1982). Use of 'air wave system' to prevent pressure sores in hospital. *Lancet* June: 1288–90.

Faghri PD, Rodgers MM, Glaser RM, Bors JG, Ho C, Akuthota P (1994). The effects of functional electrical stimulation on shoulder subluxation, arm function recovery, and shoulder pain in hemiplegic patients. *Arch Phys Med Rehabil* 75: 73–9.

Feibel JH, Springer CJ (1982). Depression and failure to resume social activities after stroke. *Arch Phys Med Rehabil* 63: 276–8.

Feldman Z, Kanter MJ, Robertson CS *et al.* (1992). Effect of head elevation on intracranial pressure, cerebral perfusion pressure, and cerebral blood flow in head-injured patients. *J Neurosurg* 76: 207–11.

Ferrell BA, Osterweil D, Christensen P (1993). A randomised trial of low air loss beds for treatment of pressure ulcers. *J Am Med*

Assoc 269: 494–7.

Finucane P, Aslan SM, Duncan D (1991). Percutaneous endoscopic gastrostomy in elderly patients. *Postgrad Med J* 67: 371–3.

Flanagan EM (1967). Methods for facilitation and inhibition of motor activity. *Am J Phys Med* 46: 1006–11.

Folstein MF, Folstein SE, McHugh PR (1975). 'Mini-Mental State': a practical method for grading cognitive state of patients for clinicians. *J Psychiatr Res* 12: 189–98.

Forster A, Young J (1995). Incidence and consequences of falls due to stroke: a systematic inquiry. *Br Med J* 311: 83–6.

Fotherby MD, Potter JF, Panayiotou B, Harper G (1993). Blood pressure changes after stroke: abolishing the white-coat effect. *Stroke* 24: 1422 (letter) .

Friedland J, McColl M-A (1987). Social support and psychological dysfunction after stroke: buffering effects in a community sample. *Arch Phys Med Rehabil* 68: 475–80.

Gautier JC (1985). Stroke in progression. *Stroke* 16: 729–33.

Gelber DA, Good DC, Herrmann D (1993). Comparisons of two physical therapy approaches in the treatment of the pure motor hemiparetic patient. *Neurology* 43: A234 (abstract).

Gelber DA, Good DC, Laven LJ, Verhulst SJ (1993). Causes of urinary incontinence after acute hemispheric stroke. *Stroke* 24(3): 378–82.

Gladman J, Forster A, Young J (1995). Hospital- and home-based rehabilitation after discharge from hospital for stroke patients: analysis of two trials. *Age Ageing* 24: 49–53.

Glanz M, Klawansky S, Stason W et al. (1995). Biofeedback therapy in poststroke rehabilitation: a meta-analysis of the randomized controlled trials. *Arch Phys Med Rehabil* 76: 508–15.

Gordon C, Langton Hewer R, Wade DT (1987). Dysphagia in acute stroke. *Br Med J* 295: 411–14.

Gordon WA, Hibbard MR, Egelko S et al. (1985). Perceptual remediation in patients with right brain damage: a comprehensive program. *Arch Phys Med Rehabil* 66: 353–9.

Gottlieb JE, Menashe PI, Cruz E (1986). Gastrointestinal complications in critically ill patients: the intensivists overview. *Am J Gastroenterol* 81: 227–38.

Grace J, Nadler JD, White DA et al. (1995). Folstein vs modified mini-mental state examination in geriatric stroke. Stability, validity and screening utility. *Arch Neurol* 52: 477–84.

Gray CS, French JM, Bates D, Cartlidge NEF, James OFW, Venables G (1990). Motor recovery following acute stroke. *Age Ageing* 19: 179–84.

Gray CS, French JM, Bates D, Cartlidge NEF, Venables GS, James OFW (1989) Recovery of visual fields in acute stroke: homonymous hemianopia associated with adverse prognosis. *Age Ageing* 18: 419–21.

Gray JM, Robertson IH, Pentland B, Anderson SI (1992). Microcomputer based cognitive rehabilitation for brain damage; a randomised group controlled trial. *Neuropsychol Rehabil* 2: 97–116.

Gross CR, Lindquist RD, Wooley AC, Granier R, Allard K, Webster B (1992). Clinical indicators of dehydration severity in elderly patients. *J Emerg Med* 10: 267–74.

Hagen C (1973). Communication abilities in hemiplegia: effect of speech therapy. *Arch Phys Med Rehabil* 54: 454–63.

Hajek VE, Kates MH, Donnelly R, McGree S (1993). The effect of visuo-spatial training in patients with right hemisphere stroke. *Can J Rehabil* 6: 175–86.

Hamdy RC, Krishnaswamy G, Canellaro V, Whalen K, Harvill L (1993). Changes in bone mineral content and density after stroke. *Am J Phys Med Rehabil* 72: 188–91.

Han-Hwa H, Chung C, Tcho JL et al. (1993). A randomized controlled trial on the treatment for acute partial ischemic stroke with acupuncture. *Neuroepidemiology* 12: 106–13.

Harris CP, Townsend JJ, Baringer SR (1993). Symptomatic hyponatraemia: can myelinolysis be prevented by treatment? *J Neurol Neurosurg Psychiatr* 56(6): 626–32.

Hartman J, Landau WM (1987). Comparison of formal language therapy with supportive counseling for aphasia due to acute vascular accident. *Arch Neurol* 44: 646–9.

Herrmann M, Bartels C, Schumacher M, Wallesch C-W (1995). Poststroke depression. Is their a pathoanatomic correlate for depression in the postacute stage of stroke? *Stroke* 26: 850–6.

Hesse S, Lucke D, Malezic M et al. (1994). Botulinum toxin treatment for lower limb extensor spasticity in chronic hemiparetic patients. *J Neurol Neurosurg Psychiatr* 57: 1321–4.

Hibbard MR, Grober SE, Gordon WA, Aletta EG, Freeman A (1990). Cognitive therapy and the treatment of post-stroke depression. *Topics Geriatr Rehabil* 5(3): 43–55.

Hindfelt B (1976). The prognostic significance of subfebrility and fever in ischaemic cerebral infarction. *Acta Neurol Scand* 53: 72–9.

Hodkinson HM (1972). Evaluation of a mental test score for assessment of mental impairment in the elderly. *Age Ageing* 1: 233–8.

Hofman A, Geelkerkern RH, Willie J, Hamming JJ, Herman J, Breslau PJ (1994). Pressure sores and pressure decreasing mattresses: controlled clinical trial. *Lancet* 343: 568–71.

Holas MA, DePippo KL, Reding MJ (1994). Aspiration and relative risk of medical complications following stroke. *Arch Neurol* 51: 1051–3.

Holbrook M (1982). Stroke: social and emotional outcome. *J Roy Coll Phys Lond* 116(2): 100–4.

Holbrook M, Skilbeck CE (1983). An activities index for use with stroke patients. *Age Ageing* 12: 166–70.

Horner J, Brazer SR, Massey EW (1993). Aspiration in bilateral stroke patients: a validation study. *Neurology* 43: 430–3.

House A (1987a). Mood disorders after stroke: a review of the evidence. *Intern J Geriatr Psychiatry* 2: 211–21.

House A (1987b). Depression after stroke. *Br Med J* 294: 76–8.

House A, Dennis, M, Hawton K, Warlow C (1989a). Methods of identifying mood disorders in stroke patients: experience in the Oxfordshire Community Stroke Project. *Age Ageing* 18: 371–9.

House A, Dennis M, Molyneux A, Warlow C, Hawton K (1989b). Emotionalism after stroke. *Br Med J* 298: 991–4.

House A, Dennis M, Warlow C, Hawton K, Molyneux A (1990). Mood disorders after stroke and their relation to lesion location.

Brain 113: 1113–29.

House A, Dennis M, Mogridge L, Warlow C, Hawton K, Jones L (1991). Mood disorders in the year after first stroke. *Br J Psychiatry* 158: 83–92.

Inaba M, Piorkowski M (1972). Ultrasound in treatment of painful shoulders in patients with hemiplegia. *Phys Ther* 52(7): 737–41.

Inaba M, Edberg E, Montgomery J, Gillis MK (1973). Effectiveness of functional training, active exercise and resistive exercise for patients with hemiplegia. *Phys Therapy* 53(1): 28–35.

Johnstone AJ, Lohlun JC, Miller JD *et al.* (1993). A comparison of the Glasgow Coma Scale and the Swedish Reaction Level Scale. *Brain Injury* 7(6): 501–6.

Jongbloed L, Morgan D (1991). An investigation of involvement in leisure activities after a stroke. *Am J Occup Ther* 45(5): 420–7.

Jongbloed L, Stacey S, Brighton C (1989). Stroke rehabilitation: sensorimotor integrative treatment versus functional treatment. *Am J Occup Ther* 43: 391–7.

Joynt RJ, Feibel JH, Sladek CM (1981). Antidiuretic hormone levels in stroke patients. *Ann Neurol* 9: 182–4.

Kaldor A, Berlin I (1981). Pneumonia, stroke, and laterality. *Lancet* 1: 843.

Kalra L, Yu G, Wilson K, Roots P (1995). Medical complications during stroke rehabilitation. *Stroke* 26: 990–4.

Karp HR, Sieker HO, Heyman A (1961). Cerebral circulation and function in Cheyne–Stokes respiration. *Am J Med* 30: 861–70.

Kaste M, Fogelholm R, Erila T *et al.* (1994). A randomised, double-blind, placebo-controlled trial of nimodipine in acute ischemic hemispheric stroke. *Stroke* 25: 1348–53.

Katrak PH, Cole AMD, Poulos CJ, McCauley JCK (1992). Objective assessment of spasticity, strength and function with early exhibition of Dantrolene sodium after cerebrovascular accident: a randomized double-blind study. *Arch Phys Med Rehabil* 73: 4–9.

Kemp MG, Kopanke D, Tordecilla L *et al.* (1993). The role of surfaces and patients attributes in preventing pressure ulcers in elderly patients. *Res Nurs Health* 16: 89–96.

Ketel WB, Kolb ME (1984). Long-term treatment with dantrolene sodium of stroke patients with spasticity limiting the return of function. *Curr Med Res Opin* 8: 161–9.

Kidd D, Lawson J, Nesbitt R, MacMahon J (1993). Aspiration in acute stroke: a clinical study with videofluroscopy. *Quart J Med* 86: 825–9.

Kilpatrick CJ, Davis SM, Hopper JL, Rossiter SC (1992). Early seizures after acute stroke. Risk of late seizures. *Arch Neurol* 49: 509–11.

Kilpatrick DJ, Davis SM, Tress BM, Rossiter SC, Hopper JL, Vandendriesen ML (1990). Epileptic seizures in acute stroke. *Arch Neurol* 47: 157–60.

Kinsella G, Ford B (1985). Hemi-inattention and the recovery patterns of stroke patients. *Intern Rehabil Med* 7: 102–6.

Kolodzik PW, Eilers MA (1991). Hiccups (Singultus): review and approach to management. *Ann Emerg Med* 20: 565–73.

Kusuda K, Saku Y, Sadoshima S, Kozo I, Fujishima M (1989). Disturbances of fluid and electrolyte balance in patients with acute stroke. *Nippon Ronen Igakkai Zasshi* 26: 223–7.

Launois S, Bizec JL, Whitelaw WA, Cabane J, Derenne JPh (1993). Hiccups in adults: an overview. *Eur Respir J* 6: 563–75.

Lauritzen L, Bjerg Bendsen B, Vilmar T, Bjerg Bendsen E, Lunde M, Bech P (1994). Post-stroke depression: combined treatment with imipramine or desipramine and mianserin. A controlled clinical study. *Psychopharmacology* 114: 119–22.

Lavy S, Yaar I, Melamed E (1974). The effect of acute stroke on cardiac functions in an intensive care stroke unit. *Stroke* 5: 775–80.

Leandri M, Parodi CI, Corrieri N, Rigardo S (1990). Comparison of TENS treatments in hemiplegic shoulder pain. *Scand J Rehabil Med* 22(2): 69–71.

Legh-Smith J, Wade DT, Langton Hewer R (1986). Driving after a stroke. *J Roy Soc Med* 79: 200–3.

Leijon G, Bovie J (1989). Central post-stroke pain—a controlled trial of amitriptyline and carbamazepine. *Pain* 36: 27–36.

Leijon G, Boivie J, Johansson I (1989). Central post-stroke pain—neurological symptoms and pain characteristics. *Pain* 36: 13–25.

Lincoln NB, Gamlen R, Thomason H (1989). Behavioural mapping of patients on a stroke unit. *Int Disabil Studies* 11(4): 149–54.

Lincoln NB, Whiting SE, Cockburn J, Bhavnani G (1985). An evaluation of perceptual training. *Int Rehabil Med* 7(3): 99–109.

Lincoln NB, Mulley GP, Jones AC, McGuirk E, Lendrem W, Mitchell RA (1984). Effectiveness of speech therapy for aphasic stroke patients. A randomised controlled trial. *Lancet* June: 1197–1200.

Lipsey JR, Robinson RG, Pearlson GD, Rao K, Price TR (1984). Nortriptyline treatment of post-stroke depression: a double-blind study. *Lancet* Feb: 297–300.

Lisk DR, Grotta JC, Lamki L *et al.* (1993). Should hypertension be treated after acute stroke. A randomized controlled trial using single photon emission computed tomography. *Arch Neurol* 50: 855–62.

Lomer M, McLellan DL (1987). Informing hospital patients and their relatives about stroke. *Clin Rehabil* 1: 33–7.

Loverro J, Reding M (1988). Bed orientation and rehabilitation outcome for patients with stroke and hemianopsia or visual neglect. *J Neurol Rehab* 147: 150.

McCarthy ST, Turner J (1986). Low-dose subcutaneous heparin in the prevention of deep vein thrombosis and pulmonary emboli following acute stroke. *Age Ageing* 15: 85–8.

Machfoed MH, Herainy, Eko T (1993). Cimetidine paraenteral for prevention of acute upper gastrointestinal bleeding in acute stroke patients. *Can J Neurol Sci* 20 (Suppl. 4): S247.

Magnusson M, Johansson K, Johansson BB (1994). Sensory stimulation promotes normalization of postural control after stroke. *Stroke* 25: 1176–80.

Marshall RC, Wertz RT, Weiss DG *et al.* (1989). Home treatment for aphasic patients by trained non-professionals. *J Speech Hearing Disord* 54: 462–70.

Martin J, Meltzer H, Elliot D (1988). *The Prevalence of Disability Among Adults*. London: Office of Population Censuses and Surveys, HMSO.

Matsumoto N, Whisnant JP, Kurland LT, Okazaki H (1973).

Natural history of stroke in Rochester, Minnesota, 1995 through 1969: an extension of a previous study, 1945 through 1954. *Stroke* 4: 20–9.

Medical Research Council (1982). *Aids to the Examination of the Peripheral Nervous System*. Grimsby: Albert Gait Ltd, Castle Press, 1–60.

Meikle M, Wechsler E, Tupper A-M *et al.* (1979). Comparative trial of volunteer and professional treatments of dysphasia after stroke. *Br Med J* 2: 87–9.

Melo TP, de Mendonca A, Crespo M, Carvalho M, Ferro JM (1992). An emergency room-based study of stroke coma. *Cerebrovasc Dis* 2: 93–101.

Messer J, Reitman D, Sacks HS, Smith H, Chalmers TC (1983). Association of adrenocorticosteroid therapy and peptic-ulcer disease. *N Engl J Med* 309: 21–4.

Metz CA, Livinston DH, Smith JS, Larson GM, Wilson TH (1993). Impact of multiple risk factors and ranitidine prophylaxis on the development of stress-related upper gastrointestinal bleeding: a prospective, multicentre, double-blind, randomized trial. The Ranitidine Head Injury Study Group. *Crit Care Med* 21: 1844–9.

Mikolich JR, Jacobs WC, Fletcher GF (1981). Cardiac arrhythmias in patients with acute cerebrovascular accidents. *J Am Med Assoc* 246: 1314–17.

Moyer DJ, Welsh FA, Zager EL (1992). Spontaneous cerebral hypothermia diminishes focal infarction in rat brain. *Stroke* 23: 1812–16.

Mulley G (1982). Associated reactions in the hemiplegic arm. *Scand J Rehabil Med* 14: 117–20.

Mulley G (1991) Walking frames. In: Mulley G, ed. *More Everyday Aids and Appliances*. London: BMJ, 174–81.

Mulley GP (1981). Pneumonia, stroke and laterality. *Lancet* May: 1051 (letter).

Murray GB, Shea V, Conn DK (1986). Electroconvulsive therapy for post stroke depression. *J Clin Psychiatr* 47: 258–60.

Myers MG, Norris JW, Hachinski VC, Sole MS (1981). Plasma norepinephrine in stroke. *Stroke* 12(2): 200–4.

Mykyta LJ, Bowling JH, Nelson DA, Lloyd EJ (1976). Caring for relatives of stroke patients. *Age Ageing* 5: 87–90.

Nachtmann A, Siebler M, Rose G, Sitzer M, Steinmetz H (1995). Cheyne–Stokes respiration in ischemic stroke. *Neurology* 45: 820–1.

Norris JW, Groggatt GM, Hachinski VC (1978). Cardiac arrhythmias in acute stroke. *Stroke* 9(4): 392–6.

Norris JW, Hachinski VC, Myers MG, Callow J, Wong T, Moore RW (1979). Serum cardiac enzymes in stroke. *Stroke* 10(5): 548–53.

North JB, Jennett S (1974). Abnormal breathing patterns associated with acute brain damage. *Arch Neurol* 31: 338–44.

Norton B, Homer-Ward M, Donnelly MT, Long RG, Holmes GKT (1996). A randomised prospective comparison of percutaneous endoscopic gastrostomy and nasogastric tube feeding after acute dysphagic stroke. *Br Med J* 312: 13–16.

Nouri FM, Tinson DJ (1988). A comparison of a driving simulator and a road test in the assessment of driving ability after a stroke. *Clin Rehabil* 2: 99–104.

Nouri FM, Tinson DJ, Lincoln NB (1987). Cognitive ability and driving after stroke. *Intern Disabil Studies* 9: 110–115.

Nyberg L, Gustafson Y (1995). Patient falls in stroke rehabilitation. A challenge to rehabilitation strategies. *Stroke* 26: 838–42.

Nyswonger GD, Helmchen RH (1992). Early enteral nutrition and length of stay in stroke patients. *J Neurosci Nurs* 24: 220–3.

O'Neill PA, McLean KA (1992). Water homeostasis and ageing. *Med Lab Sci* 49: 291–8.

O'Neill PA, Davies I, Fullerton KJ, Bennett D (1991). Stress hormone and blood glucose response following acute stroke in the elderly. *Stroke* 22: 842–7.

O'Neill PA, Cheadle B, Wyatt R, McGuffog J, Fullerton KJ (1990). The value of the Frenchay Aphasia Screening Test for dysphasia: better than the clinician? *Clin Rehabil* 4: 123–8.

O'Rourke S, McHale S, Slattery J, Dennis M (1995). Detecting depression after stroke: a comparison of the General Health Questionnaire and the Hospital Anxiety and Depression Scale. *Proc Br Psychol Soc* 3(2): 138.

O'Rourke SJ, Dennis MS, Slattery J, Warlow CP (1995). Preliminary results from a randomised trial of a stroke family support worker; patients' outcome at six months post stroke. *Age Ageing* 25 (Suppl. 1): 32 (abstract).

O'Sullivan CE, Issa FG, Berthon-Jones M, Saunders NA (1984). Pathophysiology of sleep apnea. In: Saunders NA, Sullivan CE, eds. *Sleep and Breathing*. New York/Basel: Marcek Dekker Inc, 299–363.

Oczkowski WJ, Ginsberg JS, Shin A, Panju A (1992). Venous thromboembolism in patients undergoing rehabilitation for stroke. *Arch Phys Med Rehabil* 73: 712–16.

Olsen TS, Hogenhaven H, Thage O (1987). Epilepsy after stroke. *Neurology* 37: 1209–11.

Oppenheimer SM, Hoffbrand BI, Oswald GA, Yudkin JS (1985). Diabetes mellitus and early mortality from stroke. *Br Med J* 291: 1014–15.

Panayiotou BN, Harper GD, Fotherby MD, Potter JF, Castleden CM (1993). Interarm blood pressure difference in acute hemiplegia. *J Am Geriatr Soc* 41: 422–3.

Partridge CJ, Edwards SM, Mee R, Van Langenberghe HVK (1990). Hemiplegic shoulder pain: a study of two methods of physiotherapy treatment. *Clin Rehabil* 4: 43–9.

Pender SM, Courtney MG, Rajan E, McAdam B, Fielding JF (1993). Percutaneous endoscopic gastrostomy—results of an Irish single unit series. *Ir J Med Sci* 162: 452–5.

Phillips SJ (1994). Pathophysiology and management of hypertension in acute ischemic stroke. *Hypertension* 23(1): 131–6.

Plum F, Posner JB (1980). Supratentorial lesions causing coma. In: Plum F, McDowell FH, eds. *The Diagnosis of Stupor and Coma*. Philadelphia: FA Davis Company, 134–6.

Powers WJ (1993). Acute hypertension after stroke: the scientific basis for treatment decisions. *Neurology* 43: 461–7.

Prasad BK, Banarjee AK, Howard H (1982). Incidence of deep vein thrombosis and the effect of pneumatic compression of the calf in elderly hemiplegics. *Age Ageing* 11: 42–4.

Przelomski MM, Roth RM, Gleckman RA, Marcus EM (1986). Fever in the wake of a stroke. *Neurology* 36: 427–9.

Raha SK, Woodhouse K (1994). The use of percutaneous endoscopic gastrotomy (PEG) in 161 consecutive elderly patients. *Age Ageing* 23: 162–3.

Reinstein L, Gracey JG, Kline JA, Van Buskirk C (1972). Cardiac monitoring in the acute stroke patient. *Arch Phys Med Rehabil* 53: 311–14.

Reith J, Jorgensen HS, Pedersen PM *et al.* (1996). Body temperature in acute stroke, relation to stroke: severity, infarct size, mortality, and outcome. *Lancet* 347: 422–5.

Rem JA, Hachinski VC, Boughner DR, Barnett HJM (1985). Value of cardiac monitoring and echocardiography in TIA and stroke patients. *Stroke* 16(6): 950–6.

Robertson IH (1993). Cognitive rehabilitation in neurologic disease. *Curr Opin Neurol* 6: 756–60.

Robertson IH, Gray JM, Pentland B, Waite LJ (1990). Microcomputer-based rehabilitation for unilateral left visual neglect; a randomised controlled trial. *Arch Phys Med Rehabil* 71: 663–8.

Robinson RG, Price TR (1982). Poststroke depressive disorders: a follow-up study of 103 patients. *Stroke* 13: 635–41.

Robinson RG, Szetela B (1981). Mood change following left hemisphere brain injury. *Ann Neurol* 40: 195–202.

Robinson RG, Kubos KL, Starr LB, Rao K, Price TR (1984). Mood disorders in stroke patients: importance of location of lesion. *Brain* 107: 81–93.

Robinson RG, Parikh RM, Lipsey JR, Starkstein SE, Price TR (1993). Pathological laughing and crying following stroke: validation of a measurement scale and a double-blind treatment study. *Am J Psychiatr* 150: 286–93.

Roderick P, Wilkes HC, Meade TW (1993). The gastrointestinal toxicity of aspirin: an overview of randomised controlled trials. *Br J Clin Pharmacol* 35: 219–26.

Rossi PW, Kheyets S, Reding MJ (1990). Fresnels prisms improve visual perception in stroke patients with homonymous hemianopia or unilateral visual neglect. *Neurology* 40(10): 1597–9.

Roth EJ, Mueller K, Green D (1988). Stroke rehabilitation outcome: impact of coronary artery disease. *Stroke* 19: 42–7.

Rout MW, Lane DJ, Wollner L (1971). Prognosis in acute cerebrovascular accidents in relation to respiratory pattern and blood gas tensions. *Br Med J* 3: 7–9.

Roy CW (1988). Shoulder pain in hemiplegia: a literature review. *Clin Rehabil* 2: 35–44.

Saeki S, Ogata H, Okubo T, Takahashi K, Hoshuyama T (1995). Return to work after stroke. A follow-up study. *Stroke* 26: 399–401.

Sandercock P, Van den Velt AGM, Lindley RI, Slattery J (1993). Antithrombotic therapy in acute ischaemic stroke: an overview of the completed randomised trials. *J Neurol Neurosurg Psychiatr* 56: 17–25.

Sandercock P, Bamford J, Dennis M *et al.* (1992). Atrial fibrillation and stroke: prevalence in different types of stroke and influence on early and long term prognosis (Oxfordshire Community Stroke Project). *Br Med J* 305: 1460–5.

Sandercock PAG, Warlow CP, Jones LN, Starkey IR (1989). Predisposing factors for cerebral infarction: the Oxfordshire Community Stroke Project. *Br Med J* 298: 75–80.

Sandstrom B, Alhaug J, Einarsdottir K, Simpura E-M, Isaksson B (1985). Nutritional status, energy and protein intake in general medical patients in three Nordic hospitals. *Hum Nutr: Appl Nutr* 39A: 87–94.

Scales JT, Lowthian PT, Poole AG, Ludman WR (1982). 'Vaperm' patient support system: a new general purpose hospital mattress. *Lancet* II: 1150–2.

Schiffer RB, Herndon RM, Rudick RA (1985). Treatment of pathologic laughing and weeping with amitriptyline. *N Engl J Med* 312: 1480–2.

Schleenbaker RE, Mainous AGI (1993). Electromyographic biofeedback for the neuromuscular re-education in the hemiplegic stroke patient: a meta analysis. *Arch Phys Med Rehabil* 74: 1301–4.

Schuling J, de Haan R, Limburg M, Groenier KH (1993). The Frenchay Activities Index. Assessment of functional status in stroke patients. *Stroke* 24: 1173–7.

Schuster DP, Rowley H, Feinstein S, McGue MK, Zuckerman GR (1984). A prospective evaluation of the risk of upper gastrointestinal bleeding after admission to a medical intensive care unit. *Am J Med* 76: 623–30.

Sharpe M, Hawton K, House A *et al.* (1990). Mood disorders in long-term survivors of stroke: associations with brain lesion location and volume. *Psychol Med* 20: 815–28.

Shea JD (1975). Pressure sores: classification and management. *Clin Orthopaed* 112: 89–100.

Shieff C, Nashold BSJ (1987). Stereotactic mesencephalic tractotomy for thalamic pain. *Neurol Res* 9: 101–4.

Shinar D, Gross CR, Price TR, Banko M, Bolduc PL, Robinson RG (1986). Screening for depression in stroke patients: the reliability and validity of the center for epidemiologic studies depression scale. *Stroke* 17(2): 241–5.

Sinyor D, Jacques P, Kalouper DG, Becker R, Goldenberg M, Coopersmith H (1986). Poststroke depression and lesion location. *Brain* 109: 537–46.

Sjogren K (1982). Leisure after stroke. *Intern Rehabil Med* 4(2): 80–7.

Sloan RL, Brown KW, Pentland B (1992). Fluoxetine as a treatment for emotional lability after brain injury. *Brain Inj* 6: 315–19.

Small SL (1994). Pharmacotherapy of aphasia. A critical review. *Stroke* 25: 1282–9.

Smith DS, Goldenberg E, Ashburn A *et al.* (1981). Remedial therapy after stroke: a randomised controlled trial. *Br Med J* 282: 517–20.

Smith N (1989). Aids for urinary incontinence. In: Mulley GP, ed. *Everyday Aids and Appliances*. London: BMJ, 50–4.

Smithard DG, Renwick D, O'Neill PA (1993). Change in nutritional status following acute stroke. *Age Ageing* 22 (Suppl. No. 3): 11 (abstract).

Somerville K, Faulkner G, Langman MJS (1986). Non-steroidal

anti-inflammatory drugs and bleeding peptic ulcer. *Lancet* i: 462–4.

Song F, Freemantle N, Sheldon TA *et al.* (1993). Selective serotonin reuptake inhibitors: meta-analysis of efficacy and acceptability. *Br Med J* 306: 683–7.

Splaingard ML, Hutchins B, Sulton LD, Chaudhuri G (1988). Aspiration in rehabilitation patients: videofluoroscopy vs bedside clinical assessment. *Arch Phys Med Rehabil* 69: 637–40.

Sprecht H, Fruhmann G (1972). Incidence of periodic breathing in 2000 subjects without pulmonary or neurological disease. *Bull Physiopath Respir* 8: 1075–83.

St Clair M (1992). Survey of the uses of the Pegasus Airwave System in the United Kingdom. *J Tissue Viability* 2: 9–16.

Starmark JE, Stalhammar S, Holmgren E (1988). The reaction level scale (RLS85): manual and guidelines. *Acta Neurochir* 91: 12–20.

Stanners AJ, Chapman AN, Bamford JM (1993). Clinical predictors of aspiration soon after stroke. *Age Ageing* 22 (Suppl. No. 2): 17 (abstract).

Stern PH, McDowell F, Miller JM, Robinson M (1970). Effects of facilitation exercise techniques in stroke rehabilitation. *Arch Phys Med Rehabil* 50(6): 526–31.

Stone SP, Halligan PW, Greenwood RJ (1993). The incidence of neglect phenomena and related disorders in patients with an acute right or left hemisphere stroke. *Age Ageing* 22: 46–52.

Stone SP, Patel P, Greenwood RJ, Halligan PW (1992). Measuring visual neglect in acute stroke and predicting its recovery: the visual neglect recovery index. *J Neurol Neurosurg Psychiatr* 55: 431–6.

Sunderland A, Tinson D, Bradley L, Langton Hewer R (1989). Arm function after stroke. An evaluation of grip strength as a measure of recovery and a prognostic indicator. *J Neurol Neurosurg Psychiatr* 52: 1267–72.

Sunderland A, Fletcher D, Bradley L, Tinson D, Langton Hewer R, Wade DT (1994). Enhanced physical therapy for arm function after stroke: a one year follow up study. *J Neurol Neurosurg Psychiatr* 57: 856–8.

Sunderland A, Tinson DJ, Bradley EL, Fletcher D, Langton Hewer R, Wade DT (1992). Enhanced physical therapy improves recovery of arm function after stroke. A randomised controlled trial. *J Neurol Neurosurg Psychiatr* 55: 530–5.

Tatemichi TK, Paik M, Bagiella E, Desmond DW, Pirro M, Hanzawa LK (1994). Dementia after stroke is a predictor of long term survival. *Stroke* 25: 1915–19.

Taylor TV, Rimmer S, Day B, Butcher J, Dymock IW (1974). Ascorbic acid supplementation in the treatment of pressure sores. *Lancet* ii: 544–6.

ter Reit G, Kessels GH, Knipschild P (1995). Randomised clinical trial of ultrasound treatment for pressure ulcers. *Br Med J* 310: 1040–1.

ter Reit G, Van Houten H, Knipschild P (1992). Health care professionals' view of the effectiveness of pressure ulcer treatments: a survey among nursing home physicians,

dermatologists and nursing staff in the Netherlands. *Clin Exp Dermatol* 17: 328–31.

Towle D, Lincoln NB, Mayfield LM (1989). Evaluation of social work on depression after stroke. *Clin Rehabil* 3: 89–96.

Turney TM, Garraway WM, Whisnant JP (1984). The natural history of hemispheric and brainstem infarction in Rochester, Minnesota. *Stroke* 15(5): 790–4.

Unosson M, Ek AC, Bjurulf P, von Schenck H, Larsson J (1994). Feeding dependence and nutritional status after acute stroke. *Stroke* 25: 366–71.

van Kooten F, Hoogerbrugge N, Naarding P, Koudstaal PJ (1993). Hyperglycaemia in the acute phase of stroke is not caused by stress. *Stroke* 24: 1129–32.

Van Langenberghe HVK, Partridge CJ, Edwards MS, Mee R (1988). Shoulder pain in hemiplegia—a literature review. *Physiother Pract* 4: 155–62.

Veis SL, Logemann JA (1985). Swallowing disorders in persons with cerebrovascular accident. *Arch Phys Med Rehabil* 66: 372–5.

Wade DT (1992). Measures of motor impairment. In: *Measurement in Neurological Rehabilitation*. Oxford: Oxford Medical Publications, 147–74.

Wade DT, Langton Hewer R (1985). Outlook after an acute stroke: urinary incontinence and loss of consciousness compared in 532 patients. *Quart J Med* 56: 601–8.

Wade DT, Legh-Smith J, Langton Hewer R (1985). Social activities after stroke: measurement and natural history using the Frenchay Activities Index. *Int Rehabil Med* 7: 176–81.

Wade DT, Legh-Smith J, Langton Hewer R (1986). Effects of living with and looking after survivors of a stroke. *Br Med J* 293: 418–20.

Wade DT, Collen FM, Robb GF, Warlow CP (1992). Physiotherapy intervention late after stroke and mobility. *Br Med J* 304: 609–13.

Wagenaar RC, Meijer OG, van Wieringen PCW *et al.* (1990). The functional recovery of stroke: a comparison between neuro-developmental treatment and the Brunnstrom method. *Scand J Rehabil Med* 22: 1–8.

Wahlgren NG, MacMahon DG, De Keyser J, Indredavik B, Ryman T (1994). Intravenous Nimodipine West European Stroke Trial (INWEST) of Nimodipine in the treatment of acute ischaemic stroke. *Cerebrovasc Dis* 4: 204–10.

Walker MF, Lincoln NB (1991). Factors influencing dressing performance after stroke. *J Neurol Neurosurg Psychiatr* 54: 699–701.

Walker MF, Drummond A, Lincoln NB (1994). Dressing after stroke. *Clin Rehabil* 8: 86 (abstract).

Wallace JD, Levy LL (1981). Blood presure after stroke. *J Am Med Assoc* 246: 2177–80.

Wanklyn P, Ilsley DW, Greenstein D *et al.* (1994). The cold hemiplegic arm. *Stroke* 25: 1765–70.

Wardlaw JM (1993). Cheyne–Stokes respiration in patients with acute ischaemic stroke: observations on middle cerebral artery blood velocity changes using transcranial doppler ultrasound. *Cerebrovasc Dis* 3: 377–80.

Warlow C, Ogston D, Douglas AS (1976). Deep venous thrombosis of the legs after strokes. Part 1. Incidence and predisposing factors. *Br Med J* 1: 1178–81.

Webb P (1974). Periodic breathing during sleep. *J Appl Physiol* 37: 899–903.

Weinberg J, Diller L, Gordon WA *et al.* (1979). Training sensory awareness and spatial organization in people with right brain damage. *Arch Phys Med Rehabil* 60: 491–6.

Weinmann EE, Salzman EW (1994). Deep vein thrombosis (review). *N Engl J Med* 331: 1630–41.

Wells PS, Lensing AWA, Hirsh J (1994). Graduated compression stockings in the prevention of postoperative venous thromboembolism: a meta analysis. *Arch Intern Med* 154: 67–72.

Wellwood I, Dennis MS, Warlow CP (1994). Perceptions and knowledge of stroke among surviving patients with stroke and their carers. *Age Ageing* 23: 293–8.

Wertz RT, Weiss DG, Aten JL *et al.* (1986). Comparison of clinic, home and deferred language treatment for aphasia. A veterans administration cooperative study. *Arch Neurol* 43: 653–7.

Whurr R, Perlman Lorch M, Nye C (1992). A meta-analysis of studies carried out between 1946 and 1988 concerned with the efficacy of speech and language therapy treatment for aphasic patients. *Eur J Disord Commun* 27: 1–17.

Wijdicks EFM, Fulgham JR, Batts KP (1994). Gastrointestinal bleeding in stroke. *Stroke* 25: 2146–8.

Wills EE, Anderson TW, Beattie BL, Scott A (1983). A randomised placebo-controlled trial of ultraviolet light in the treatment of superficial pressure sores. *J Am Geriatr Soc* 31: 131–3.

Wilson B, Cockburn J, Halligan P (1987). Behavioural inattention test. *Thames Valley Test Company*. Titchfield, Hants.

Yekutiel M, Guttman E (1993). A controlled trial of the retraining of the sensory function of the hand in stroke patients. *J Neurol Neurosurg Psychiatr* 56: 241–4.

Preventing recurrent stroke and other serious vascular events

16

16.1 Prognosis and prediction of future vascular events

The prognosis for early death and disability after stroke has been discussed in Section 10.2. This section describes the long-term prognosis of patients with transient ischaemic attacks (TIAs) and stroke for important future vascular events, particularly those, such as recurrent stroke, that might be prevented by appropriate treatment strategies. As highlighted in Section 10.2, much of the information we have about the prognosis of these patients comes from following large cohorts of patients over time. But, because the prognosis of each individual patient may vary considerably from the prognosis of all patients 'en masse' (because of the different underlying causes of the TIA/stroke and different co-morbidities, etc.; see below), it is important that the prognostic data from cohort studies are interpreted in their proper context. This section is therefore structured to help apply the results of cohort studies to individual patients to answer the question 'what is the risk of another important vascular event for *this* patient?' and thereby to be able to identify the appropriate goals and treatments for *this* patient.

16.1.1 Prognosis after TIA and mild ischaemic stroke

Patients with TIA and mild ischaemic stroke are not only *qualitatively* similar in terms of age, sex and prevalence of co-existent vascular diseases and risk factors, but they also share a similar prognosis for future stroke and death and will therefore be considered together (see Section 3.1.3) (Wiebers *et al.*, 1982; Dennis *et al.*, 1989; Koudstaal *et al.*, 1992b).

Cohorts of patients with TIA and mild ischaemic stroke

The prognosis of patients with TIA and mild ischaemic stroke, as a group, varies considerably amongst different studies due to differences in study methodology and case mix (Table 16.1) (Hankey *et al.*, 1993a). Before the results of the different studies can be accepted and validly compared, they should ideally meet most, if not all, of the criteria listed in Table 16.1. The few prognostic studies which are comparable indicate that the prognosis of hospital-referred TIA patients is better than of community-based patients (Dennis *et al.*, 1990; Hankey *et al.*, 1991; Hankey & Warlow, 1994). This is mainly because hospital series tend not to include patients in whom a very early stroke occurred (at home) before they had time to reach the hospital, and because older patients (who have a worse prognosis because of a greater prevalence of adverse prognostic factors) are less likely to be

Table 16.1 Methodological explanations which might account for the different prognosis of patients with TIA and mild ischaemic stroke in different studies (see Sackett *et al.*, 1991).

Study nature (e.g. prospective or retrospective)
Referral patterns
Sample size
Case selection
Diagnostic criteria
Time delay between the last TIA and entry into the study
Pathogenesis of TIA
Prevalence and level of important prognostic factors
Treatments
Adequacy of follow-up
Outcome criteria
Methods of survival analysis

referred to hospital (Hankey *et al.*, 1993a). Even so, TIA patients as a group, whether hospital or community based, have an increased absolute risk of stroke and other serious vascular events compared with age- and sex-matched controls (Howard *et al.*, 1994) (Table 16.2). This is because patients with symptomatic cerebrovascular disease almost always have co-existent symptomatic or asymptomatic vascular disease elsewhere, such as in the coronary, peripheral and renal arteries (see Section 6.2.1).

The risk of stroke is highest soon after the TIA; in the *first* year, the absolute risk of stroke is about 12% in community

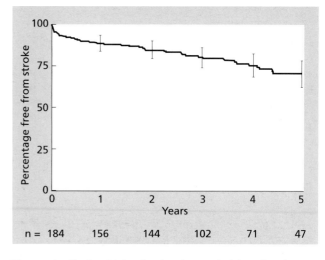

Figure 16.1 Kaplan–Meier plot showing survival free of stroke in 184 TIA patients in the Oxfordshire Community Stroke Project. The vertical bars indicate 95% confidence intervals of the Kaplan–Meier estimate. The numbers along the *x*-axis indicate the number of people at risk of stroke at the beginning of each year of follow-up. (From Dennis *et al.*, 1990; reprinted with permission from *Stroke*.)

Table 16.2 Absolute average annual risk and relative risk of important outcome events after TIA and stroke. (From Dennis *et al.*, 1993*; Hankey & Warlow, 1994†; Burn *et al.*, 1994‡.)

	Absolute annual risk (%)		
	Hospital referred	Community	Relative risk
After TIA†			
Death	5	8	1.4
Stroke			
0–1 year	7	12	12
0–5 years	4	7	7
Myocardial infarction	3	3	Unknown
Stroke, myocardial infarction or vascular death	6	9	Unknown
Stroke, myocardial infarction or death	8	10	Unknown
After stroke			
Death			
0–30 days		20 (PICH 50%, CI 10%)	Unknown
30 days–1 year		10	3
0–1 year		30	8
30 days–5 years		9	2
Recurrent stroke‡			
0–1 year		10–16	15
1–5 years		4	Unknown
0–5 years		4–8	9

CI, cerebral infarction; PICH, primary intracerebral haemorrhage.

studies and 7% in hospital series (Table 16.2; Fig. 16.1). The relative risk is about 12 times that of people of the same age and sex who have not had a TIA (Dennis *et al.*, 1990). This higher early risk of stroke reflects not just iatrogenic post-angiographic and post-carotid endarterectomy strokes in some patients, but presumably the presence of unstable and 'active' arterial embolic sources, such as a fissured atherosclerotic plaque which has released a small embolus which is soon to be followed by a larger one, before the endothelium heals (Whisnant & Wiebers, 1987; Dennis *et al.*, 1990; Hankey *et al.*, 1991).

> *After transient ischaemic attacks and ischaemic stroke the risk of recurrent stroke is highest within the first few weeks and months: about 10% in the first year, and then about 5%/year.*

Table 16.2 lists the approximate average annual risk and relative risk (compared with people of the same age and sex who have not had a TIA) of each of the important outcome events over the first 5 years after a TIA (Hankey & Warlow,

1994). Heart disease is the most common cause of death amongst TIA patients; about 40% of deaths after TIA are due to heart disease, 25% to stroke, 5% to other vascular diseases such as ruptured aortic aneurysm and 30% to non-vascular disorders (Hankey & Warlow, 1994). Data on the site, nature and severity of stroke after TIA are limited but it seems that most strokes are ischaemic, about two-thirds are major disabling strokes, about one-half to two-thirds occur in the same vascular territory as the presenting TIA (particularly carotid territory events), and about 20% of the latter (i.e. strokes in the same vascular territory) are lacunar infarcts (Dennis *et al.*, 1990; Hankey *et al.*, 1991; Cillessen *et al.*, 1993).

> *After transient ischaemic attacks and ischaemic stroke it is important to recognise the importance of non-stroke vascular events such as myocardial infarction; indeed, coronary heart disease is a more likely cause of death than stroke.*

Individual TIA patients

Although TIA patients as a *group* have an increased risk of stroke and other serious vascular events, the prognosis of TIA patients as *individuals* is extremely variable; some have a benign prognosis and others a poor prognosis. This is because of differences in 'case mix', i.e. differences in the causes and treatment of TIAs amongst different patients and also differences in the presence and level of important prognostic factors (Hankey *et al.*, 1993a; Landi *et al.*, 1993). An example of different prognoses for TIA patients with presumed different causes comes from the Dutch TIA trial: although TIA patients with 'atypical' symptoms (episodes of cerebral or visual dysfunction that were not fully compatible with the internationally accepted criteria for a TIA) were found to have a similar overall risk of major vascular events as patients with 'typical' symptoms, they had a lower risk of stroke and a higher risk of major cardiac events than patients with 'typical' symptoms, suggesting that 'atypical' TIAs may have been due to heart disease, perhaps a cardiac arrhythmia (Koudstaal *et al.*, 1992a). On the other hand, the nature of the symptomatic vascular disease did not seem to be relevant to the prognosis: patients with TIA and mild ischaemic stroke who were thought to have intracranial small vessel disease on the basis of their clinical features and cranial computerised tomography (CT) scan at baseline had an identical annual stroke rate of 3.6% as those with presumed large vessel disease (Kappelle *et al.*, 1995).

Table 16.3 lists the important independent adverse prognostic factors for stroke, coronary events and the composite outcome event of non-fatal stroke, non-fatal myocardial

Table 16.3 Important independent predictors of major vascular events in TIA patients. (From Hankey *et al.*, 1992; Dutch TIA Trial Study Group, 1993; Pop *et al.*, 1994.) These studies aimed to investigate the relationship between each of several potential prognostic variables and the occurrence of stroke in TIA patients. Multiple regression analysis was used to examine the independent effect of each of the variables on the subsequent risk of stroke by taking into account and adjusting for the effect of the other variables.

Stroke
Increasing number of TIAs in the 3 months before presentation (multiple attacks)
Increasing age
Peripheral vascular disease
TIAs of the brain (compared with the eye)

Coronary event
Increasing age
Male sex
Ischaemic heart disease (angina pectoris, anterior myocardial infarction or T-wave inversion on electrocardiogram)

Stroke, myocardial infarction or vascular death
Increasing age
Peripheral vascular disease
Increasing number of TIAs in the 3 months before presentation (multiple attacks)
Male sex
TIAs of the brain (compared with the eye)
Left ventricular hypertrophy on the electrocardiogram

---

infarction and vascular death (whichever occured first) that have been identified in each of two large studies (Hankey *et al.*, 1992, 1993b; Dutch TIA Trial Study Group, 1993; Pop *et al.*, 1994; van Latum *et al.*, 1995). The combined outcome event of non-fatal stroke, non-fatal myocardial infarction or vascular death is used because the underlying arterial pathology is usually the same (atherothromboembolism), this underlying pathology is likely to respond to the same treatment (e.g. antithrombotic drugs); combining the outcome events generates the biggest number and with that comes greater statistical power and therefore certainty about what the exact risks are, and what the treatment effect really is. Based on the presence and power of the significant prognostic factors in one of these studies (Hankey *et al.*, 1993b), prediction models (equations) of both the relative risk and absolute risk of stroke (Table 16.4) and of all serious vascular events (Table 16.5) have been developed. These models have been applied to two independent cohorts of TIA patients to test their external validity and are fairly reliable predictors of outcome, particularly for patients predicted to be at low risk. Similar prediction models have been developed for survival after TIA (Hankey *et al.*, 1992; Evans *et al.*,

1994). Hopefully, these prediction models can be applied in clinical practice as an aid to identifying which TIA patients are at high (and low) risk of serious vascular events, so that only high-risk patients are exposed to costly and risky (but effective) investigations and treatments (such as carotid angiography and endarterectomy), and low-risk patients are not exposed to treatments that are potentially dangerous and which consume medical resources unnecessarily. Prediction models should be used with caution, however; they should not lead to overemphasis on the need to identify and treat *only* high-risk patients because most strokes, and other vascular outcome events, occur in patients who are predicted to be at lower risk (in the same way that most strokes occur in people with 'normal' blood pressure and plasma cholesterol, who are considered to be at low risk) (see Section 18.4).

16.1.2 Prognosis after stroke (ischaemic and haemorrhagic stroke combined)

Most of the data about the prognosis after stroke come from studies that have examined 'all stroke', not particular stroke types such as ischaemic stroke or even mild ischaemic stroke compared with primary intracerebral haemorrhage (PICH). These data are useful for clinicians who, for whatever reason, are not able to classify strokes into pathological types.

Cohorts of stroke patients (see Table 16.2)

Community studies indicate that about 20% of all patients with a first-ever in a lifetime stroke die within 1 month (see Section 10.2.3). After the first month, the average annual risk of death falls appreciably to about 9%/year over the next few years (see Fig. 10.2). Although some studies have shown a greater risk of dying over the first 5 years after stroke (i.e. >9%/year), the poorer survival may have been, in part, because these studies included patients with recurrent strokes (and not just first-ever in a lifetime strokes) in their inception cohort (Schmidt *et al.*, 1988; Kojima *et al.*, 1990). However, there is in fact remarkably little information about case fatality rates amongst patients with first-ever in a lifetime and recurrent stroke (see Section 10.2.3).

Amongst the 80% or so of stroke patients who survive the first 30 days after stroke, the relative risk of dying is about twice the risk of people in the general population (see Fig. 10.2) (Dennis *et al.*, 1993). This excess risk of death persists for several years, probably because stroke patients have co-existent vascular risk factors and diseases such as hypertension and coronary heart disease (Sacco *et al.*, 1982).

It is not always easy to distinguish a recurrent stroke from other causes of worsening in the first week or so after a

Table 16.4 Prediction equation for survival free of stroke.

Age in years −60	Multiplied by	4.5
Female	Subtract	36
TIA of the eye (amaurosis fugax) only	Subtract	72
Carotid and vertebrobasilar TIAs	Add	53
Number of TIAs in the last 3 months (n)	Add	$1.6 \times (n-1)$
Peripheral vascular disease	Add	76
Left ventricular hypertrophy (ECG)	Add	68
Residual neurological signs	Add	74

Total score = y

Divide y by 100 and exponentiate ($e^{y/100}$) = x

Probability of survival free of stroke
At 1 year = 0.96^x
At 5 years = 0.88^x

Example: 65-year-old woman with five episodes of amaurosis fugax only in last 3 months and ECG shows left ventricular hypertrophy

			Cumulative score
65 − 60 years = 5	Multiplied by	4.5	22.5
Female	Subtract	36	−13.5
TIA of the eye (amaurosis fugax) only	Subtract	72	−85.5
Five TIAs in the last 3 months	Add	$1.6 \times (5-1)$	−79.1
Left ventricular hypertrophy (ECG)	Add	68	−11.1

Total score = −11.1

Divide −11.1 by 100 and exponentiate ($e^{-0.111}$)
$e^{-0.111} = 1/(e^{0.111})$
$\qquad\quad = 1/1.117$
$\qquad\quad = 0.895$

Probability of survival free of stroke
At 1 year = $0.96^{0.895}$ = 0.96 or 96%
At 5 years = $0.88^{0.895}$ = 0.89 or 89%

ECG, electrocardiography.

stroke (see Section 15.5). Bearing this in mind, it seems that the risk of recurrent stroke is greatest early after the first stroke: about 2–3% of survivors of first-ever in a lifetime stroke have a recurrent stroke within the first 30 days, about 9% in the first 6 months and 10–16% within 1 year, which is about 15 times greater than the risk in the general population of the same age and sex (see Table 16.2; Fig. 16.2) (Matsumoto *et al.*, 1973; Viitanen *et al.*, 1988; Terent, 1989; Broderick *et al.*, 1992; Burn *et al.*, 1994). After the first year, the average annual risk of recurrent stroke for the next 4 years falls to about 5% (and about 40% of these recurrences are not of functional significance to the patient) (Marquardsen, 1969; Matsumoto *et al.*, 1973; Sacco *et al.*, 1982; Sage & van Uitert, 1983; Dombovy *et al.*, 1987; Meissner *et al.*, 1988; Schmidt *et al.*, 1988; Viitanen *et al.*, 1988; Terent, 1989; Broderick *et al.*, 1992; Burn *et al.*, 1994). This risk is very similar to that of TIA patients and is about nine times the risk of stroke in the general population of the same age and sex (see Table 16.2) (Burn *et al.*, 1994).

Although the decision to treat with secondary prevention measures, and for how long, is based on the absolute risk of recurrent stroke for a patient rather than the relative risk (see Section 16.2), these data emphasise that these measures should be started as soon as possible and continued for at least 4 years, if not longer.

Individual stroke patients

As with TIA patients, the prognosis of individual stroke patients is extremely variable: some patients die immediately, some die later, some survive and are left with a permanent disability and some recover completely. Factors that increase the risk of a first-ever in a lifetime stroke may not necessarily be so important in predicting a recurrent stroke. Unfortunately, the data we have on the long-term follow-up of community-based stroke patients are limited and so the results of statistical analyses of prognostic variables are not robust and are hence inconsistent. An increased risk of recur-

549

Table 16.5 Prediction equation for survival free of stroke, myocardial infarction or vascular death.

Age in years −60	Multiplied by	6
Female	Subtract	68
TIA of the eye (amaurosis fugax) only	Subtract	56
Number of TIAs in the last 3 months (n)	Add	$1.5 \times (n − 1)$
Carotid and vertebrobasilar TIAs	Add	71
Peripheral vascular disease	Add	84
Residual neurological signs	Add	66
Left ventricular hypertrophy (ECG)	Add	54

Total score = y

Divide y by 100 and exponentiate $(e^{y/100}) = x$

Probability of survival free of stroke, myocardial infarction or vascular death
At 1 year $= 0.95^x$
At 5 years $= 0.79^x$

Example: 65-year-old woman with five episodes of amaurosis fugax only in last 3 months and ECG shows left ventricular hypertrophy

			Cumulative score
65 − 60 years = 5	Multiplied by	6	30
Female	Subtract	68	−38
TIA of the eye (amaurosis fugax) only	Subtract	56	−94
Five TIAs in the last 3 months	Add	$1.5 \times (5 − 1)$	−88
Left ventricular hypertrophy (ECG)	Add	54	−34

Total score = −34

Divide −34 by 100 and exponentiate $(e^{-0.34})$
$$e^{-0.34} = 1/(e^{0.34})$$
$$= 1/1.4$$
$$= 0.7$$

Probability of survival free of stroke, myocardial infarction or vascular death
At 1 year $= 0.95^{0.7} = 0.96$ or 96%
At 5 years $= 0.79^{0.7} = 0.85$ or 85%

ECG, electrocardiography.

rent stroke has been associated with high blood pressure (Hier *et al.*, 1991; Alter *et al.*, 1994; Lai *et al.*, 1994), low blood pressure (Irie *et al.*, 1993), valvular heart disease and congestive heart failure (Broderick *et al.*, 1992), atrial fibrillation (Lai *et al.*, 1994), an abnormal initial brain CT scan and a history of diabetes mellitus (Hier *et al.*, 1991). A lower risk of recurrent stroke has been associated with a low diastolic blood pressure, no history of stroke, no history of diabetes and an infarct of unknown cause (Hier *et al.*, 1991). In the Oxfordshire Community Stroke Project, the risk of recurrent stroke did not appear to be related to age, sex or the pathological type of stroke (Burn *et al.*, 1994), and a previous history of ischaemic heart disease or atrial fibrillation was not associated with a definite excess risk of recurrent stroke, whether within 30 days or within the first few years (Sandercock *et al.*, 1992; Burn *et al.*, 1994).

16.1.3 Prognosis after ischaemic stroke

Cohorts of ischaemic stroke patients

The overall case fatality of patients with first-ever ischaemic stroke is about 10% at 30 days, 20% at 6 months and 25% at 1 year (see Fig. 10.3). Young adults (<45 years of age) have a better prognosis with a lower overall case fatality of about 2% at 30 days and a low risk of subsequent fatal events (Abraham *et al.*, 1971; Marshall, 1982; Lanzino *et al.*, 1991; Ferro & Crespo, 1994); a recent long-term follow-up study of 296 young adults with ischaemic stroke over a mean of 6 years reported an annual mortality rate from vascular death of 1.7% (Kappelle *et al.*, 1994). The overall risk of recurrent stroke in the first 2 years after a first-ever ischaemic stroke varies in different studies from about 4 to 14% (Bamford *et al.*, 1987, 1990, 1991; Hier *et al.*, 1991).

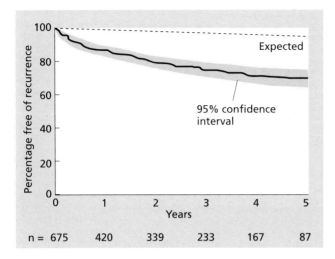

Figure 16.2 Kaplan–Meier plot showing the probability that, given survival, first-ever in a lifetime stroke patients will remain free from recurrent stroke, compared with the expected probability of people in the same general population remaining free from a first-ever in a lifetime stroke (derived from Oxfordshire Community Stroke Project incidence data 1981–86). The shading indicates 95% confidence intervals. The numbers along the *x*–axis indicate the number of people at risk of recurrent stroke at the beginning of each year of follow-up. (From Burn *et al.*, 1994; reprinted with permission from *Stroke*.)

Individual ischaemic stroke patients

Amongst patients with ischaemic stroke, the location and size of the infarct is a major prognostic factor; about 90% of patients with infarction of the whole middle cerebral artery territory are dead or dependent at 1 year post-stroke compared with 50% of those with restricted cortical, lacunar or brainstem infarcts (Wade & Langton Hewer, 1987; Dombovy *et al.*, 1987; Bamford *et al.*, 1991). In the Oxfordshire Community Stroke Project, the 1-year rates of recurrent stroke varied amongst the four clinical subtypes of cerebral infarction: total anterior circulation infarction (TACI) 6%, lacunar infarction (LACI) 9%, partial anterior circulation infarction (PACI) 17% and posterior circulation infarction (POCI) 20% (Bamford *et al.*, 1991). Furthermore, there were three different patterns of recurrence (Fig. 16.3); patients with PACI had a high early recurrence rate (suggesting an active source of recurrent embolism), patients with POCI had a moderately high early recurrence rate with further episodes throughout the first year, and those with LACI had a low and fairly constant recurrence rate, supporting the notion that LACIs occur as a result of occlusion of a single perforating artery and are not usually due to an active source of recurrent embolism (Bamford *et al.*, 1987, 1991; Sacco *et*

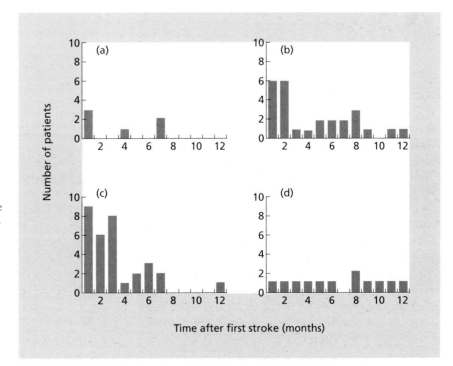

Figure 16.3 The timing of recurrent stroke in different subtypes of cerebral infarction. (a) TACI; (b) POCI; (c) PACI; (d) LACI. These histograms show the number of patients who experienced a first recurrent stroke at different time intervals (months) after an initial first-ever in a lifetime ischaemic stroke of each clinical subtype. These data come from the Oxfordshire Community Stroke Project. (From Bamford *et al.*, 1991; reproduced with permission from the *Lancet*.)

al., 1989). There is some evidence that recurrent infarcts in patients with LACI are lacunar again, also supporting the hypothesis that LACIs are usually caused by a general disorder of intracranial small vessels (Boiten & Lodder, 1993), but other studies have found that recurrent LACIs account for no more than about 25% of recurrences (which is similar to the proportion of patients with first-ever in a lifetime ischaemic stroke who are found to have a LACI) (Gandolfo *et al.*, 1986; Sacco *et al.*, 1991; Clavier *et al.*, 1994; Kappelle *et al.*, 1995).

16.1.4 Prognosis after primary intracerebral haemorrhage (PICH)

Cohorts of primary intracerebral haemorrhage patients

There have been many studies on the prognosis of PICH, but most were retrospective hospital-based studies of selected patients, some before the era of CT scanning, or prospective hospital-based studies with short follow-up. Such hospital-based studies may be biased by omitting patients with milder strokes who do not require admission, severely ill patients who die before they can be admitted and elderly patients who remain in nursing homes. A few community-based studies have provided information on PICH, but most were undertaken before the era of freely available CT scans, or only reported relatively short follow-up. Therefore, although much is now known about the long-term risk of death, disability and subsequent vascular events in patients with ischaemic stroke, there have been very few community-based studies of the long-term follow-up of patients with brain CT scan evidence of PICH. A population study in the Jyvaskyla region, Central Finland, of 158 patients with CT or autopsy-confirmed PICH, all of whom were followed up for a median of 32 months, found that the 30-day case fatality rate was 50%, but that after the first month the probability of survival did not differ from an age- and sex-matched normal population (Fogelholm *et al.*, 1992). In the Oxfordshire Community Stroke Project, which registered 66 patients with PICH, the 30-day case fatality rate was also about half (52%) (Counsell *et al.*, 1995a), but the long-term case fatality was worse than in Finland; all surviving patients were followed for up to 6 years and the average death rate for those surviving 30 days was 8%/year for the first 5 years, which is similar to that for patients with ischaemic stroke (Dennis *et al.*, 1993; Counsell *et al.*, 1995a). The main causes of 'late' deaths (>30 days) were extracranial vascular disease such as myocardial infarction (55%) and the complications of immobility due to the initial or recurrent stroke (45%).

The long-term risk of death or of recurrent stroke after primary intracerebral haemorrhage is not precisely known because there have been no large and community-based studies.

The risk of recurrent stroke following PICH is poorly documented in many studies due to varying duration and intensity of follow-up. In the Oxfordshire Community Stroke Project, each patient was carefully assessed for recurrent stroke, but the numbers were quite small. Amongst those surviving 30 days, the annual risk of recurrent stroke was about 7% and, of death and/or recurrent stroke about 11% (Fig. 16.4) (Counsell *et al.*, 1995a). These rates are similar to those following ischaemic stroke (Hier *et al.*, 1991; Burn *et al.*, 1994). At least 25% of the recurrences were definite haemorrhages, and in those patients there was a high chance of underlying amyloid angiopathy (see Section 8.2.3). The population study in the Jyvaskyla region, Central Finland, found that amongst patients who had survived 10 days or more, six (4%) had a recurrent PICH (diagnosed by CT or autopsy) and another five had a recurrent ischaemic or non-defined acute stroke at some time between 36 and 1210 days after the initial bleed (Fogelholm *et al.*, 1992).

Of course, recurrence depends on aetiology. Haemorrhages due to arteriovenous malformations and amyloid angiopathy (which are commonly lobar haemorrhages) more commonly recur, whereas it is said that patients with hypertensive haemorrhages tend not to rebleed if their blood pressure is well controlled (Lee *et al.*, 1990; Passero *et al.*, 1995).

Individual primary intracerebral haemorrhage patients

There have not been any prospective community-based follow-up studies of patients with PICH which have recorded sufficient numbers of recurrent strokes to have the statistical power to identify reliably any predictive factors. If it were possible to predict those at low risk of recurrent haemorrhage, it may then be possible to identify subgroups of patients who would benefit from aspirin to prevent fatal *cardio*vascular disease or recurrent *ischaemic* stroke. However, at the moment aspirin should not be given to PICH patients for fear of causing recurrent intracerebral bleeding (see Section 16.4).

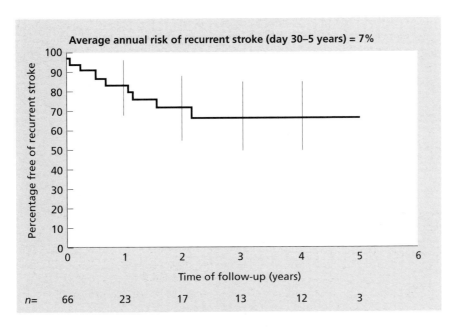

Figure 16.4 Kaplan–Meier plot showing the percentage of patients free of recurrent stroke after PICH, censored for deaths not due to recurrent stroke. The vertical error bars indicate the 95% confidence interval. The numbers along the x-axis indicate the number of people at risk of recurrent stroke at the beginning of each year of follow-up. These data come from the Oxfordshire Community Stroke Project. (From Counsell *et al.*, 1995a; reproduced with permission of *Cerebrovascular Diseases*.)

16.2 The general approach to preventing recurrent stroke and other serious vascular events

There are two approaches to stroke prevention: the *mass* and the *high-risk* strategy. The mass strategy involves making small changes to every member of the general stroke-free population (such as a reduction by a few millimetres of mercury of diastolic blood pressure), which has the effect of reducing the mean blood pressure of the entire population (see Section 18.6). Such changes are achieved by alterations in lifestyle or in the environment. The high-risk strategy is to seek out individuals with high levels of risk, such as those labelled as having hypertension, and then to give them medical or surgical treatments to reduce that risk (see Section 18.4). It seems at first counter-intuitive, but it is nonetheless true, that the mass strategy is likely to have as great an impact on stroke incidence as all the medical activity entailed in the high-risk strategy (Rose, 1992). This is not to belittle the efforts of doctors but merely to point out that their efforts must be supported by wider, population-based efforts.

Primary prevention is in the hands of primary health care doctors, governmental public health departments and politicians. Politicians have a much greater influence than doctors over the measures which are central to the success of primary stroke prevention (i.e. the measures which could improve the health of the entire population: a ban on tobacco advertising, a reduction in the salt content of processed foods, reduced social deprivation and poverty, to name but a few). Since we are primarily physicians and not politicians, this chapter deals only with the *secondary* prevention of stroke; in other words, preventing stroke after TIA or a first-ever in a lifetime stroke. Throughout the chapter we will emphasise that the decision whether or not to apply a preventive measure should be based mostly on the likely *absolute* benefit (e.g. avoid 50 events per 1000 patients treated, or treat 20 patients to avoid one event) rather than on the *relative* reduction; even an impressive 50% relative reduction will only yield an absolute benefit of 10 per 1000 patients treated (treat 100 patients to avoid one event) if the patient is, anyway, at low risk of the event (e.g. 2% in controls reduced to 1% in the treated group). Strategies for secondary stroke prevention are divided into: (i) risk factor modification, which applies to all stoke and TIA patients (see Section 16.3); (ii) antiplatelet therapy (see Section 16.4); (iii) anticoagulants (see Section 16.5); and (iv) vascular surgical procedures which apply only to patients with confirmed ischaemic events (i.e. intracranial haemorrhage has been ruled out by appropriately timed brain CT or magnetic resonance imaging (MRI)) (see Section 16.7).

> *The decision to treat a patient depends more on the absolute benefit of treatment than the relative reduction of risk provided by the treatment. Patients at very low absolute risk of recurrent stroke (e.g. 1%) are still at low absolute risk, even if the treatment reduces their risk by 50% (i.e. to 0.5%); the 0.5% absolute reduction in risk of recurrent stroke (or absolute benefit) means 200 patients have to be treated to prevent one having a stroke (i.e. 100/0.5).*

Treat any underlying cause

It goes without saying that if a specific treatable cause for the cerebral ischaemia has been identified, such as arteritis or infective endocarditis, then specific treatment should be given (see Section 16.6). However, this is likely to apply to less than 5% of unselected patients with cerebral ischaemia (see Chapter 7). Of course, patients with stroke often have other vascular disorders which require specific treatment or preventative action in their own right; the assessment and treatment of angina, heart failure, cardiac arrhythmias, valvular heart disease, abdominal aortic aneurysm and peripheral vascular disease may not directly reduce the risk of further stroke, but should at least improve quality of life and reduce the risk of other serious vascular events.

16.3 Risk-factor control (for patients with TIA, ischaemic stroke and primary intracerebral haemorrhage (PICH))

This section deals with the interventions which are applica-ble to all patients with acute cerebrovascular disease irre-spective of pathological type; for example, long-term blood pressure reduction applies to patients with hypertension whether the event was ischaemic or haemorrhagic. Smoking cessation is important for any patient with symptomatic vas-cular disease (even if cessation may not definitely reduce the risk of recurrent stroke).

16.3.1 Blood pressure reduction

Raised blood pressure is the most important treatable and causal risk factor for stroke (see Section 6.2.3). This relation-ship is much stronger than had previously been realised. Two things have clarified the relationship: (i) systematic reviews of the observational epidemiological studies; and (ii) the realisation that random error in the measurement of the baseline blood pressure should be corrected for (MacMahon *et al.*, 1990; Collins & MacMahon, 1994). The technical term for this error is the 'regression–dilution bias' and its importance (and how to correct for it) are explained in detail elsewhere (MacMahon *et al.*, 1990; MacMahon & Rodgers, 1994a). A systematic review, correcting for this error, showed that for each 7.5-mmHg rise in usual diastolic blood pressure there is a *doubling* in the risk of stroke (Collins & MacMahon, 1994; MacMahon & Rodgers, 1994a) (see Fig. 6.7). There is rather more limited evidence about the rela-tionship between usual diastolic blood pressure and the risk of subsequent stroke amongst survivors of stroke (MacMahon & Rodgers, 1994a). However, the UK-TIA Aspirin trial data strongly suggest that, after correction for the regression–dilution bias, there is a strong linear relation-ship between usual diastolic blood pressure and risk of stroke amongst survivors of minor ischaemic stroke and TIA

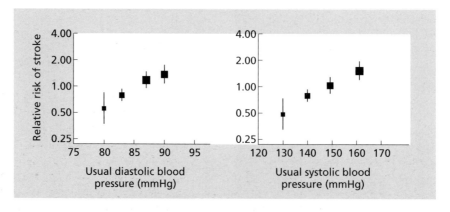

Figure 16.5 Relative risk of stroke by approximate mean usual systolic and diastolic blood pressure amongst 2201 patients with a history of TIA or minor stroke. Solid squares represent stroke risk in each category relative to the risk in the whole study population. The sizes of the squares are proportional to the number of events in each category of usual diastolic blood pressure. The vertical lines indicate the 95% confidence intervals. (From S. MacMahon, personal communication, 1996; reproduced by permission of Dr S. MacMahon.)

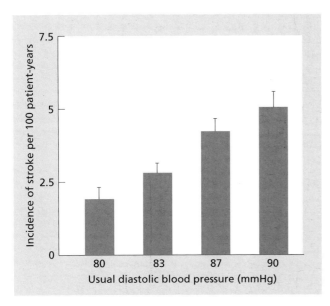

Figure 16.6 Absolute risk of stroke by approximate mean usual diastolic blood pressure amongst 2201 patients with a history of TIA or minor stroke. The vertical error bars indicate one standard deviation. (From S. MacMahon, personal communication, 1996; reproduced by permission of Dr S. MacMahon.)

(Rodgers *et al.*, 1996) (Fig. 16.5). These observational data highlight the high absolute risk (see Section 16.1.1) of stroke in such patients and that blood pressure reduction *might* lead to worthwhile absolute reduction in the risk of recurrent stroke even amongst individuals whose blood pressure is apparently 'normal', or only modestly elevated (Fig. 16.6) (MacMahon & Rodgers, 1994a).

Evidence from randomised trials

Antihypertensive drug therapy in primary stroke prevention amongst patients with moderate to severe hypertension has been evaluated in trials which recruited almost 50 000 individuals (MacMahon & Rodgers, 1994a). Conventional antihypertensive drugs reduced the risk of stroke by about 38%, and most of the benefit becomes apparent within 1–2 years of starting treatment (Collins & MacMahon, 1994; MacMahon & Rodgers, 1994a,b) (Figs 16.7 & 16.8). There have been only two small trials, with a total of 549 patients, evaluating the effect of antihypertensive drugs amongst stroke survivors (i.e. of secondary stroke prevention). A systematic review of these two trials showed that treatment was similarly associated with a 38% reduction in the risk of (recurrent) stroke, but the confidence interval was wide and included both the possibility that blood pressure reduction more than halved the risk of stroke or gave almost no benefit

at all (see Fig. 16.7). The addition of data from two other trials evaluating beta-blockers (not primarily designed to reduce blood pressure), the Treatment of Easy Stroke Trial (TEST) study and the beta-blocker component of the Dutch TIA trial, increased the amount of data available. Putting these four studies together, with a total of 2742 patients, the relative reduction in the risk of stroke was 19%, which was not statistically significant (Fig. 16.9) (MacMahon & Rodgers, 1994a,b).

The absolute benefits of blood pressure reduction might be substantial amongst individuals with a history of stroke or TIA, in whom the annual incidence of the stroke is about 10% in the first year after the event and about 5%/year thereafter. If blood pressure treatment reduced this risk by 40%, only about 50 patients would have to be treated to avoid one stroke in 1 year. But, whilst blood pressure reduction in hypertensive patients may confer a similar proportional reduction in primary and secondary stroke incidence, the true size of the benefit for secondary prevention is somewhat uncertain and the benefits could be much smaller (MacMahon & Rodgers, 1994b).

Individuals with recent stroke or transient ischaemic attack have a much higher absolute risk of stroke than most individuals in the general population. Because of this, even patients with relatively 'normal' blood pressure may benefit substantially from blood pressure reduction after stroke. It seems likely that benefits from blood pressure reduction will be determined more by the patient's general characteristics and mix of risk factors for vascular disease than by their absolute level of blood pressure. Which individuals with 'normal blood pressure' and 'mild elevations' of blood pressure benefit most from blood pressure reduction after stroke will be determined by trials currently in progress.

Who to treat: implications for practice

The evidence is not strong and does not support long-term routine use of antihypertensive drugs therapy in every stroke and TIA patient. The decision on whether or not to use antihypertensive drugs in a given individual should be based, not on their level of blood pressure, but rather on that individual's absolute risk of a serious vascular event, cardiac as well as cerebral. In general, patients with a blood pressure of 150–170 mmHg systolic, or 90–100 mmHg diastolic, or both, should be given treatment to lower blood pressure if the risk of a major vascular event in the next 10 years is more than 20% (Jackson *et al.*, 1993) (see Section 16.1.1 on how to identify such individuals). The results of clinical trials indicate that, at this level of absolute risk, about 150 people

Trials or subsets of trials	n	Events Treatment (%)	Control (%)	Odds ratio and CI	Reduction (%) ±SD
HDFP	10 940	1.9	2.9		
MRC younger adults	17 354	0.7	1.3		
EWPHE	840	7.7	11.3		
SHEP	4736	4.4	6.8		
STOP-H	1627	3.7	6.7		
MRC older adults	4396	4.6	6.1		
11 smaller trials	7760	2.4	4.4		
Total	47 653	2.2	3.5		38±4
All entry DBP < 110	35 139	1.3	2.2		39±6
Some ≥ 110, all ≤ 115	7669	4.6	6.5		32±8
Some or all > 115	4845	4.7	8.2		45±9
Fatal stroke	47 653	0.6	1.0		40±8
Non-fatal stroke	47 653	1.6	2.5		37±5
Primary prevention	47 104	2.0	3.2		38±5
Secondary prevention	549	18.8	27.3		38±16

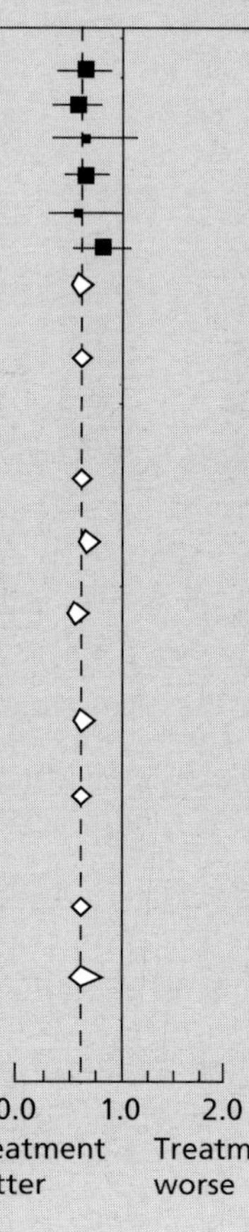

Overall treatment effect 2P < 0.0001
χ^2 test for heterogeneity; 15.8, P = 0.5

0.0   1.0   2.0
Treatment better   Treatment worse

Figure 16.7 Overview of the results from 17 randomised trials of the effects of antihypertensive therapy on stroke risk. The ratio of odds of stroke in the treatment group compared with the control group is plotted for each trial (black square: area proportional to number of strokes), along with the 99% confidence interval (horizontal line). The presence of a black square to the left of the solid vertical line suggests benefit but this benefit is significant at the level of 2P < 0.01, only if the entire confidence interval is to the left of the solid vertical line. An overview of all of the trial results (and 95% confidence interval) is represented by a diamond, beside which is given the overall relative reduction in stroke risk. (From MacMahon & Rodgers, 1994a; reproduced with permission of the authors and *Hypertension Research*.)

would require treatment for 2 or 3 years to reduce the annual number of vascular events by one (Table 16.6). Since the absolute risk of stroke rises with age, and since antihypertensive therapy is effective in older people, elderly hypertensive stroke patients stand to gain as much (or even more) from blood pressure reduction as younger patients (MacMahon & Rodgers, 1994a,b). Until the results of current trials in stroke and TIA survivors are available (see below), we use antihypertensive durgs only in patients at highest risk, and remain uncertain about how to treat lower risk individuals (and how best to define 'high' and 'low' risk). In particular,

we will need to have a clearer idea whether the *relative* benefits of treatment vary with the level of *absolute* risk defined at baseline. For example, carotid endarterectomy is certainly ineffective or even harmful amongst individuals at low absolute risk, whilst aspirin may possibly be beneficial only amongst low-risk individuals (Rothwell, 1995). This explains our caution in extrapolating too far from the available blood pressure lowering trial data in primary prevention, to help us to decide how to manage stroke and TIA survivors.

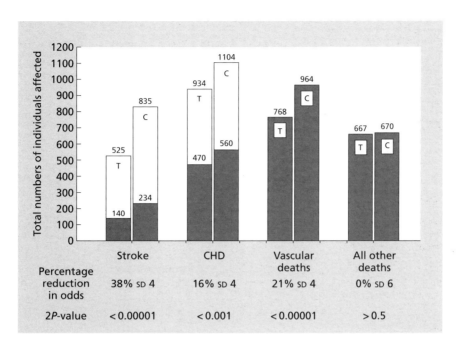

Figure 16.8 Absolute benefit of antihypertensive drug treatment over 5 years. Overview of the results of 17 randomised trials of blood pressure lowering including a total of 47 667 individuals in whom there was a mean diastolic blood pressure difference between treated patients and controls, during follow-up, of 5–6 mmHg. Fatal events are represented by shaded columns. C, control; CHD, coronary heart disease; T, treatment. (From Collins & MacMahon, 1994; reproduced with permission of the authors and of the *British Medical Bulletin*.)

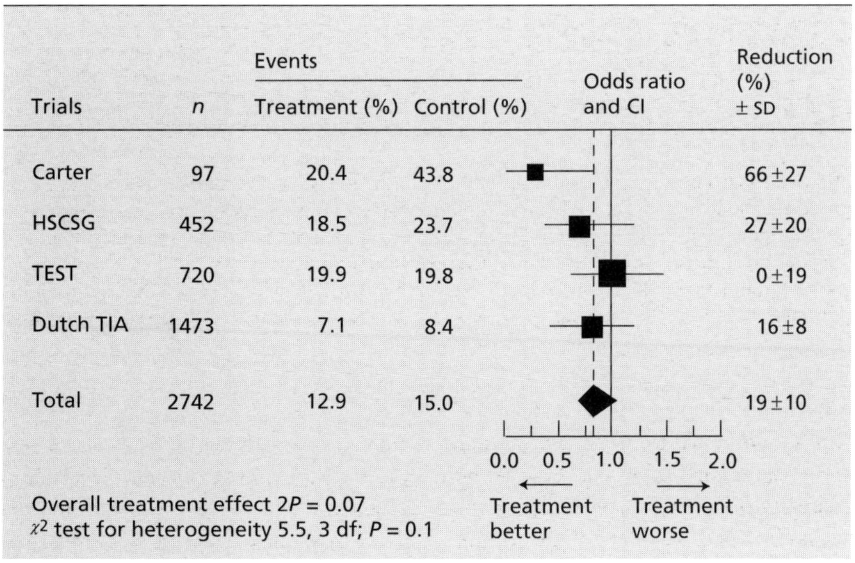

Trials	n	Events Treatment (%)	Control (%)	Odds ratio and CI	Reduction (%) ± SD
Carter	97	20.4	43.8		66 ± 27
HSCSG	452	18.5	23.7		27 ± 20
TEST	720	19.9	19.8		0 ± 19
Dutch TIA	1473	7.1	8.4		16 ± 8
Total	2742	12.9	15.0		19 ± 10

0.0 0.5 1.0 1.5 2.0

Treatment better Treatment worse

Overall treatment effect $2P = 0.07$
χ^2 test for heterogeneity 5.5, 3 df; $P = 0.1$

Figure 16.9 The results of a systematic review of four randomised trials to estimate the reduction in stroke risk with blood pressure reduction in stroke and TIA patients with (and without) hypertension. The ratio of odds of stroke in the treatment group compared with the control group is plotted for each trial (black square: area proportional to number of strokes), along with the 99% confidence interval (horizontal line). The presence of a black square to the left of the solid vertical line suggests benefit, but this benefit is significant at the level of $2P < 0.01$ only if the entire confidence interval is to the left of the solid vertical line. An overview of all of the trial results (and 95% confidence interval) is represented by a diamond, beside which is given the overall relative reduction in stroke risk. (From S. MacMahon, personal communication, 1996; reproduced with permission of S. MacMahon.)

Table 16.6 Relative and absolute reduction in risk achievable if diastolic blood pressure is reduced by 5–6 mmHg.

	60-year-old woman with initial diastolic blood pressure of 100 mmHg and no other risk factors for vascular disease	70-year-old man with initial diastolic blood pressure of 95 mmHg and multiple risk factors for vascular disease
Absolute risk of serious vascular event in next 10 years (%) (i.e. of stroke, myocardial infarction or vascular death)		
Without treatment	10	50
With treatment	7	33
Absolute reduction in risk (per 1000 patients)	30 (i.e. 10–7%)	170 (i.e. 50–33%)
Relative reduction in risk	One-third	One-third
Need to treat this number of similar individuals to avoid one serious vascular event within the next 10 years*	33	6

* This is the 'number needed to treat'. (Modified from Jackson *et al.*, 1993.)

Who to treat: implications for research

There are substantial uncertainties about the wisdom of blood pressure reduction in patients after stroke, mainly because of concerns that this may precipitate a further stroke. Whether this risk applies to the generality of stroke and TIA survivors or just to a particular subset (e.g. those with severe carotid or vertebral artery stenosis) is not known. In the light of these uncertainties, a large trial evaluating the balance of risk and benefits of blood pressure reduction in a wide variety of TIA and stroke survivors is now under way (the Protection against Recurrent Stroke Study (PROGRESS) trial; A. Rodgers, personal communication, 1995). The principal eligibility criterion is that the responsible physician is substantially uncertain about whether or not to give antihypertensive drugs. Therefore, patients with blood pressure which would conventionally be considered 'normal', and patients with only moderate elevations of blood pressure, are likely to be included. There may even be some individuals with quite high levels of blood pressure in whom the clinicians are uncertain about the value of treatment for some reason. About 6000 patients will be ran-

domised between a regimen consisting of an angiotensin-converting enzyme inhibitor combined with diuretic, and a placebo control. The results should be available within 4 or 5 years. A similar study is being conducted in China (PATS Collaborating Group, 1995).

When to start after an acute stroke

There are enormous variations in clinical practice. Some clinicians prefer to start treatment for hypertension almost immediately, within hours of stroke onset, whereas others prefer to delay treatment by at least 1 or 2 weeks (Lindley *et al.*, 1995a,b). Our own practice is equally variable since there is no good evidence to guide us. As a practical point, blood pressure tends to fall spontaneously without treatment over the first 2 weeks after stroke onset, and so provided there is no evidence that the patient has accelerated hypertension it may be best to defer any treatment decision for 1–2 weeks (see Sections 11.12 and 15.7). Sometimes, however, patients whose blood pressure has fallen to apparently normal levels by the time of hospital discharge are found to have raised blood pressures at their post-discharge clinic visit. This may be a spurious elevation of blood pressure due to the 'white coat effect' (i.e. the stress of seeing a doctor), but the rise does highlight the need to check the blood pressure amongst stroke survivors on more than one occasion after discharge from hospital.

> *It is unclear when raised blood pressure should be lowered after acute stroke. Unless the patient has accelerated hypertension, we tend to wait for 1–2 weeks.*

Dietary salt reduction

Analysis of the observational data relating salt intake to blood pressure, and of the randomised trials of different interventions to reduce salt intake, has quite clearly shown that a reduction in dietary salt has substantial promise as an effective means of blood pressure control (Frost *et al.*, 1991; Law *et al.*, 1991a,b). This holds true both for whole populations and for individuals. A relatively simple modification of the diet (not adding salt at the table, avoiding salty foods) can lead to a reduction in salt intake of up to 100 mmol/day. This degree of salt reduction in a 20–29 year old on the fifth centile of the blood pressure distribution is likely to lead to a 1-mmHg fall in diastolic blood pressure. By contrast, the same reduction in dietary salt intake in a patient aged 60–69 years on the 95th centile is likely to lead to a 7-mmHg fall in diastolic blood pressure, comparable to the reduction which can be achieved with diuretics or beta-blockers. It therefore seems reasonable to advise older hypertensive stroke survivors to reduce their dietary salt intake. This can be achieved without major discomfort and, in the patients most likely to benefit from it (i.e. elderly hypertensive stroke survivors), is likely to lead both to a worthwhile reduction in diastolic blood pressure and to minimise the need for drug therapy with all the attendant adverse effects.

> *Reducing dietary salt intake reduces blood pressure, particularly in older people with high blood pressure.*

Reduce alcohol intake

Very high levels of alcohol intake are associated with sustained rises in blood pressure (see Section 6.2.3). Therefore, avoidance of such high levels is likely to lead to blood pressure reduction. Whether this reduces the risk of stroke is not known, but we suspect it does.

Which antihypertensive drug?

In the absence of specific contraindications, low-dose diuretics or low-dose beta-blockers should be considered for first-line treatment, although their use is supported only by indirect evidence from the randomised trials in primary stroke prevention (Jackson *et al.*, 1993). Evidence from the randomised comparisons of newer agents such as angiotensin-converting enzyme inhibitors, suggests that they cause less in the way of adverse effects, but they are a great deal more expensive. There is, as yet, no clear evidence that these more expensive agents are any more effective in reducing the risk of stroke and coronary disease than the older, cheaper agents. Ferner and Neil (1995) calculated, using data from the Medical Research Council (MRC) trial of treatment of mild hypertension, that to treat 800 patients with bendrofluazide for 1 year in order to prevent one vascular event would cost £1400 per event prevented. If the efficacy is similar, treating the same number of the patients with angiotensin-converting enzyme inhibitors would cost approximately £100 000 per vascular event prevented (Ferner & Neil, 1995).

Exercise, weight reduction and *lifestyle changes* are discussed later (see Section 16.3.5).

16.3.2 Cholesterol reduction

The relationship between plasma cholesterol and ischaemic stroke is unclear (see Section 6.2.3), and it is therefore difficult to predict what lowering plasma cholesterol might do

to stroke risk. On the other hand, a systematic review of the relationship between baseline cholesterol and the risk of subsequent coronary heart disease, corrected for regression–dilution bias, has shown that the association is strong (and much stronger than that directly inferred from individual prospective studies) (Law *et al.*, 1994a,b). From these observational cohort studies (which included about 500 000 men and 18 000 coronary heart disease events) it is estimated that a long-term reduction in plasma cholesterol of 0.6 mmol/L (about 10%), which can be achieved by modest dietary change, lowers the relative risk of ischaemic heart disease by 50% at age 40 years, falling to 20% at age 70 years. The randomised controlled trials (RCTs) (based on 45 000 men and 4000 ischaemic heart disease events) showed that the full effect of reduction in risk is achieved by 5 years (Law *et al.*, 1994a,b; Wald & Thomson, 1994). Because TIA patients and survivors of ischaemic stroke are at high risk of coronary events (see Section 16.1.1), it seems reasonable to reduce their plamsa cholesterol, if not to reduce the risk of stroke, at least to reduce the risk of coronary events.

Evidence from randomised trials

There has been considerable debate whether or not cholesterol reduction reduces death from all causes, and whether the reduction in death from coronary heart disease is offset by an increase in death from cancer, suicide and other non-vascular causes. However, a careful and systematic review of all the observational data and the relevant RCTs did not support this concern (Iso *et al.*, 1989; Law *et al.*, 1994a,b). The only cause of death attributable to low serum cholesterol concentration was haemorrhagic stroke, and the excess risk only appeared amongst individuals with baseline cholesterol concentrations below about 5 mmol/L (relative risk 1.9, 95% confidence interval (CI): 1.4–2.5). However, only about 6% of people in Western populations have a cholesterol level in this range and so, overall, any excess risk of haemorrhagic stroke will be outweighed by the benefits from the lower risk of coronary events. Cholesterol reduction may of course have other benefits too. There is accumulating evidence that substantial reductions in cholesterol, maintained for a few years, may reduce the risk of progression of coronary atheroma, thereby reducing the need for vascular surgical procedures (Scandinavian Simvastatin Survival Study Group, 1994). It is not yet known whether plasma cholesterol reduction, by preventing progression (or possibly even by causing regression) of atheroma in the carotid and verte-bral arteries, could reduce the need for vascular surgical procedures on these arteries (Mack *et al.*, 1993; Adams *et al.*, 1995; Crouse *et al.*, 1995). As might be anticipated from the confused observational data, a systematic review of the RCTs of cholesterol reduction in the primary prevention of coronary heart disease showed that cholesterol reduction did not clearly reduce the risk of fatal or non-fatal stroke (Herbert *et al.*, 1995). However, the confidence interval was wide and it is still possible that cholesterol reduction might give a moderate reduction or a moderate increase in the risk of stroke. The Scandinavian Simvastatin Survival (4S) Study Group did show a trend towards a reduction in non-fatal plus fatal stroke which was marginally statistically significant, but the analysis included the rather less relevant TIAs as a major outcome event (Scandinavian Simvastatin Survival Study Group, 1994). When the results of this study were added to the overview already undertaken (Table 16.7) there are two conclusions:

1 there is no clear evidence of any reduction in fatal stroke (and there was a possibility of a small increase);
2 the estimate of a 10% relative reduction in the risk of fatal plus non-fatal stroke is not precise and the upper confidence interval includes the possibility of no effect.

The British Heart Foundation (BHF)/MRC Heart Protection Study should help to resolve at least some of these uncertainties (Keech *et al.*, 1994). About 18 000 patients at high risk of serious vascular events (because of a history of past myocardial infarction, stroke, TIA or other vascular disease) will be randomised between cholesterol reduction with simvastatin and control and then followed for at least 5 years. About 6000 patients with a past history of stroke or TIA will be included. This study will have sufficient power to detect worthwhile reductions in death from all causes, and should determine whether or not there is a clear reduction in total stroke risk (i.e. whether any increase in haemorrhagic stroke is offset by a greater reduction in ischaemic stroke). The value of antioxidant vitamins seperately and in combination with cholesterol reduction will also be evaluated at the same time by means of a factorial design (Keech *et al.*, 1994).

Who to treat

As with blood pressure, there is no threshold level of cholesterol below which the risk of coronary heart disease does not fall so, in general, 'the lower the cholesterol the better'. It therefore seems prudent to advise all survivors of ischaemic stroke (almost all of whom have a cholesterol higher than 3 mmol/L) to reduce their dietary intake of saturated fat. Moderate dietary change, which can reduce plasma cholesterol by 0.6 mmol/L, can lead to a worthwhile reduction in the risk of coronary heart disease (Law *et al.*, 1994a,b). Patients are more likely to achieve cholesterol reduction by diet if they have been told their cholesterol level, or at least been informed that it is high (Elton *et al.*, 1994). The rationale for suggesting dietary cholesterol reduction in survivors of ischaemic stroke and TIA is simply that their *cerebrovascular* event immediately identifies them as being at higher risk of all vascular events, including coronary events, than normal people (Figs 16.10 & 16.11). The presence of symptomatic vascular disease (i.e. the stroke) shifts the relationship between cholesterol and coronary heart disease to the left. So that, for a given level of cholesterol, the risk of a coronary heart disease event is substantially higher. This is confirmed by the lipid research clinic programme data (Fig. 16.11) showing the difference in risk of future coronary heart disease events in individuals with and without symptomatic coronary heart disease at the baseline in relation to their plasma cholesterol levels (Pekkanen *et al.*, 1990). Thus, the emphasis is not so much on the level of cholesterol, but

Study	Treated (*n/N*)	Control (*n/N*)	O − E	V	OR (95% CI)
Fatal stroke					
Overview*	70/17 971	67/18 451	+3.3	33.7	1.1 (0.8–1.6)
4S Study†	14/2221	12/2223	+1.0	6.5	1.2 (0.5–2.5)
Total	84/20 192	79/20 674	+4.3	40.2	1.1 (0.8–1.5)
Non-fatal plus fatal stroke					
Overview*	209/17 971	226/18 451	−0.7	99.3	1.0 (0.8–1.2)
4S Study†	70/2221	98/2223	−14.0	40.4	0.7 (0.5–1.0)
Total	279/20 192	324/20 674	−14.7	139.7	0.9 (0.8–1.0)

Table 16.7 Effects of cholesterol reduction on fatal and non-fatal stroke; evidence from all available randomised trials.

* Herbert *et al.*, 1995.
† Scandinavian Simvastatin Survival Study Group, 1994. Non-fatal events included TIAs in the analysis.
CI, 95% confidence interval; *n/N*, number of events/number allocated to that treatment group; O − E, observed minus expected number of events; OR, odds ratio; V, variance.

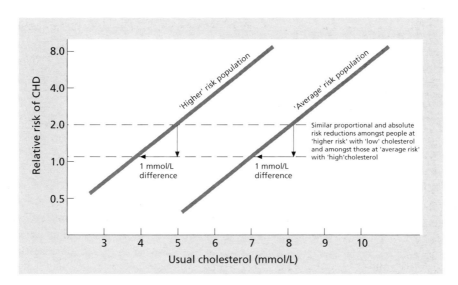

Figure 16.10 Relative risk of coronary heart disease (CHD) at various levels of plasma cholesterol (millimoles per litre). The right-hand regression line indicates the relationship between usual cholesterol and CHD in an 'average risk population' (generally individuals who are free of vascular disease at baseline). The left-hand regression line (higher risk population) represents the relationship between CHD and cholesterol amongst individuals at higher risk, usually because of the presence of symptomatic vascular disease at baseline. In both categories of patients a similar reduction in cholesterol (1.0 mmol) leads to an approximate halving of the risk of CHD. However, in high-risk populations, a cholesterol of 5.0 mmol/L is associated with a fourfold higher risk of CHD than a similar cholesterol in the average risk population. (J. Armitage, personal communication, 1996.)

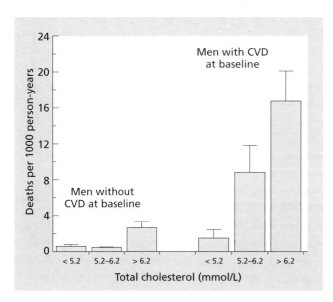

Figure 16.11 Lipid research clinics programme prevention study. This figure further illustrates the difference between high- and low-risk populations. Amongst a high-risk population (men with symptomatic cardiovascular disease (CVD) at baseline) a given level of cholesterol is associated with a substantially higher risk of future death from coronary heart disease than in a low-risk population (men without symptomatic CVD at baseline). (From Pekkanen *et al.*, 1990; reproduced with permission of the authors and the *New England Journal of Medicine*.)

on the presence of other clinical predictors of outcome such as symptomatic vascular disease (e.g. claudication) and other risk factors (e.g. increasing age, increasing blood pressure, etc.).

Agent/dose/adverse effects

Given that all patients should consider reducing their cholesterol by diet, it seems reasonable to tell people their cholesterol level and give simple dietary advice. Dieticians in different hospitals have different criteria (i.e. different levels of cholesterol) for accepting referrals for dietary intervention. Many different organisations produce appropriate leaflets on suitable dietary change. The results of the 4S study suggest that any patient with a history of ischaemic stroke or TIA *and* a previous myocardial infarction *and* a cholesterol level greater than 5.2 mmol/L is likely to benefit from cholesterol reduction with a statin (Scandanavian Simvastatin Survival Study Group, 1994). We would not recommend *routine* use of cholesterol-lowering drugs in all TIA and stroke patients until the results from the MRC/BHF Heart Protection Study are available; in the interim, useful guidelines on assessment and management of hyperlipidaemia are published in the National Heart Foundation of New Zealand guidelines (Mann *et al.*, 1993).

Cholesterol reduction by dietary means is advisable in all patients with recent stroke or transient ischaemic attack. This should reduce the risk of myocardial infarction. Which patients benefit the most from cholesterol reduction with drugs will be determined by current trials.

16.3.3 Smoking cessation

In 1995, smoking caused three million deaths and it is forecast that by the year 2025 smoking could cause perhaps 10 million deaths per year worldwide (Peto, 1994). Long-term follow-up studies, started in the 1950s, have shown that the association between smoking and deaths from cancer and vascular diseases is far stronger than had previously been thought. The old statement, based partly on the first 20 years of the Study of British Doctors, that 'at least a quarter' of all regular cigarette smokers would be killed by the habit now needs revision. In fact, the proportion is about 50% (Peto, 1994). Smoking is clearly a risk factor for ischaemic stroke (see Section 6.2.3) and for subarachnoid haemorrhage (see Section 9.1.1); its effect on the risk of PICH is less clear (Shinton & Beevers, 1989; Donnan *et al.*, 1993).

There have been no satisfactory controlled trials randomising people between 'continue smoking' and 'stop smoking', but the adverse health effects of smoking are so clearly established that all who use tobacco in any form (cigarettes, pipe, cigars or chewing tobacco) should be advised to stop (Peto, 1994). There is now clear evidence that nicotine replacement therapy is a useful aid to smoking cessation (Table 16.8) (Silagy *et al.*, 1994; Tang *et al.*, 1994). A formal review of the RCTs evaluating different forms of nicotine replacement therapy showed that it is effective, achieving abstinence rates of 19%, compared with about 10% in control subjects. Smoking clinics seem to achieve higher abstinence rates than smoking cessation managed in primary care, but the intervention is worthwhile in both settings (Silagy *et al.*, 1994). For patients who are particularly nicotine dependent, nico-

Table 16.8 Effectiveness of nicotine replacement therapy (NRT) in achieving smoking cessation (quitting). (Modified from Silagy *et al.*, 1994.)

NRT preparation	Proportion quitting		
	NRT (%)	Control (%)	OR (95% CI)
Gum	18	11	1.6 (1.5–1.8)
Patches	20	11	2.1 (1.6–2.6)
Nasal spray	26	10	2.9 (1.5–5.7)
Inhaler	15	5	3.0 (1.4–6.6)
All NRT trials	19	11	1.7 (1.6–1.9)

OR, odds ratio.

tine chewing gum seems to be the most effective replacement therapy (Tang *et al.*, 1994). In less highly dependent smokers, the different preparations are comparable in their efficacy, but nicotine patches offer greater convenience and minimal need for instruction. Inhalers and nasal sprays have not been adequately assessed but may be useful in patients with a particularly severe nicotine craving.

Smoking cessation, aided by nicotine replacement therapy if necessary, is advisable for all smokers whether they have had a stroke or not.

16.3.4 Reduction in alcohol intake

Particularly high levels of alcohol consumption have been associated with stroke in a number of observational studies (see Section 6.2.3). However, some studies have suggested that people who abstain completely from alcohol have a somewhat higher risk of cardiovascular events (possibly including stroke) than individuals who drink a modest to a moderate amount of alcohol regularly (see Section 6.2.3). A systematic review of these observational studies is clearly required before firm conclusions about the relationship between alcohol and the risk of stroke can be drawn. Regular moderate to heavy intake of alcohol can increase blood pressure, so moderation of alcohol intake may help to lower blood pressure, particularly amongst individuals whose blood pressure is sufficiently high to warrant drug therapy (Rose, 1992). There have been no RCTs on the effect of alcohol reduction and the risk of subsequent stroke.

16.3.5 Lifestyle changes

Diet

Reduction in the total fat content of the diet to no more than 30% of calorie intake, and a switch from saturated animal fat to unsaturated vegetable fats, along with an attempt to increase the intake of vegetables and fresh fruit and dietary fibre, and to reduce the consumption of low-residue processed foods are part of current national UK dietary guidelines. The role of increased vitamin C and fish consumption in the prevention of stroke and vascular disease remains unclear, but a diet rich in these nutrients has the potential to be protective; as ever, further evidence is required (Khaw & Woodhouse, 1995; Morris *et al.*, 1995).

Exercise

Observational studies have confirmed that individuals who are more active have a lower risk of subsequent coronary disease (see Section 6.2.3). It is not known whether adopting a policy of increased physical activity after a stroke or TIA provides significant protection, although a recent meta-analysis of physical rehabilitation programmes following myocardial infarction suggested a reduction in mortality with exercise (Antman *et al.*, 1992). Patients should be encouraged to return to normal physical activities and take regular moderate exercise, if only to help their self-confidence and indepedence (see Section 15.33.3). The combination of brisk walking and dietary salt reduction is more effective than brisk walking alone in blood pressure reduction (Arroll & Beaglehole, 1995).

16.4 Antiplatelet therapy (for patients with TIA and ischaemic stroke only)

Patients with a history of symptomatic vascular disease (i.e. myocardial infarction, stroke, TIA, angina intermittent claudication, etc.) are at particular risk of vascular death or of further cardiac or cerebrovascular events. Platelets are involved in the pathophysiology, not just of acute thrombosis occurring in arteries and veins, but possibly also in the process of atherogenesis in arterial walls (see Section 6.2.2). Antiplatelet therapy should therefore reduce the risk of recurrent vascular events.

16.4.1 Evidence

A systematic review of the RCTs available in 1994 (Antiplatelet Trialists' Collaboration, 1994a) has provided clear evidence of the benefits of antiplatelet therapy. Two hundred and fifty-seven eligible trials included approximately 150 000 patients. One hundred and fifty-nine RCTs of prolonged antiplatelet therapy (for 1 month or more) versus control amongst approximately 100 000 patients formed the bulk of the data. More detailed analyses were possible on individual patient data from 32 of these trials amongst 74 000 patients. Since antiplatelet therapy may prevent not just ischaemic stroke, but also myocardial infarction and other vascular deaths, the most appropriate analysis of efficacy is based on the composite outcome of stroke, myocardial infarction or vascular death (whichever occurs first); this composite outcome will be referred to as 'serious vascular events'. Amongst a wide variety of individuals at high risk for different reasons, antiplatelet therapy reduced the risk of serious vascular events by about 25% and this proportional risk reduction was remarkably consistent across different categories of high-risk patients (Fig. 16.12). The studies evaluating antiplatelet therapy in patients with a history of past stroke or TIA suggested that antiplatelet therapy reduced the 3-year risk of serious vascular events from about 22% to

about 18%, equivalent to the avoidance of 40 serious vascular events per 1000 patients treated, i.e. about 25 of these high vascular risk individuals need to receive antiplatelet therapy for 3 years to avoid one serious vascular event (Fig. 16.13). The similar absolute benefits for antiplatelet therapy amongst patients who were at risk for other reasons are also shown in Fig. 16.13. It is clear that individuals who are free of vascular risk factors and of symptomatic vascular disease (low-risk primary prevention) are at extremely low risk without treatment, with a 5-year risk of a serious vascular event of approximately 5%; such individuals have very little to gain from antiplatelet therapy even if this does reduce vascular risk, which is uncertain.

It should not be forgotten that antiplatelet therapy is anti-haemostatic and so, not surprisingly, it is associated with a small but definite excess of haemorrhagic strokes. In the overview, haemorrhagic strokes occurred in 0.4% of controls and 0.6% of treated patients, i.e. an excess of about two per 1000 patients treated. However, this small but definite hazard is enormously outweighed by the reduction of recurrent ischaemic stroke (12.2% in controls reduced to 9.7% in treated patients). The balance of risk and benefit is therefore favourable for most individuals at high vascular risk as a result of a TIA or an ischaemic stroke (see also adverse effects, Section 16.4.4).

16.4.2 Who to treat

Selection of high-risk individuals

The relative (proportional) reductions in the risk of serious vascular events were identical in patients presenting with TIAs and with completed ischaemic stroke (Antiplatelet Trialists' Collaboration, 1994a). These proportional reductions in serious vascular events were approximately similar in males and females, diabetics and non-diabetics, older patients and younger patients, and in patients with and without hypertension (Fig. 16.14). The relative reduction observed with atrial fibrillation was not significantly different from that observed in other high-risk groups, but because the numbers of events in the trials evaluating antiplatelet therapy in atrial fibrillation were small, the confidence interval was wide (Antiplatelet Trialists' Collaboration, 1994a; Atrial Fibrillation Investigators, 1994). A suggestion from the Stroke Prevention in Atrial Fibrillation Investigators Group (Stroke Prevention in Atrial Fibrillation Investigators, 1994) that aspirin was ineffective amongst the subgroup of older patients may have been due to the play of chance since, in general, antiplatelet therapy appeared equally effective in older and younger patients (Antiplatelet Trialists' Collaboration, 1994a) (Fig. 16.14).

Category of trial	Number of trials with data	MI, stroke or vascular death		Stratified statistics		Odds ratio and CI (antiplatelet : control)	Odds reduction (%) (SD)
		Anti-platelet	Adjusted controls*	O–E	Variance		
Prior MI	11	1331/9877	1693/9914	−158.5	561.6	■	25% (4)
Acute MI	9	992/9388	1348/9385	−177.9	510.3	■	29% (4)
Prior stroke/TIA	18	1076/5837	1301/5870	−98.5	386.5	■	22% (4)
Acute stroke	1	2/15	3/14	−0.6	1.1		
Other cardiac disease							
Unstable angina	7	182/1991	285/2027	−49.1	89.7	■	
Post–CABG	19	124/2529	127/2546	−4.1	38.0	■	
Post–PTCA	4	32/663	61/669	−13.0	18.2	■	
Stable angina/CAD	5	27/278	42/273	−7.5	14.6	■	
Atrial fibrillation	2	82/888	113/904	−14.6	43.5	■	
Rheumatic valve disease	1	9/78	17/76	−4.2	5.4	■	
Valve surgery	6	46/602	79/642	−13.8	27.3	■	
Peripheral vascular disease							
Intermittent claudication	22	160/1646	195/1649	−15.7	63.6	■	
Peripheral grafts	9	65/771	69/768	−4.6	27.3	■	
Peripheral angioplasty	2	5/194	8/195	−1.0	1.9		
Other high risk							
Renal dialysis	10	2/256	6/269	−1.8	1.9		
Diabetes	7	34/687	30/678	0.9	12.1	■	
Other	9	14/836	23/832	−5.0	7.9	■	
■ All trials*	142	4183/36 536 (11.4%)	5400/36 711 (14.7%)	−568.8	1810.9	◇	27% (2)

Treatment effect 2P < 0.00001
Test for heterogeneity: χ^2_{16} = 18.9; P > 0.1; NS
*Crude, unadjusted control total = 4706/32 278

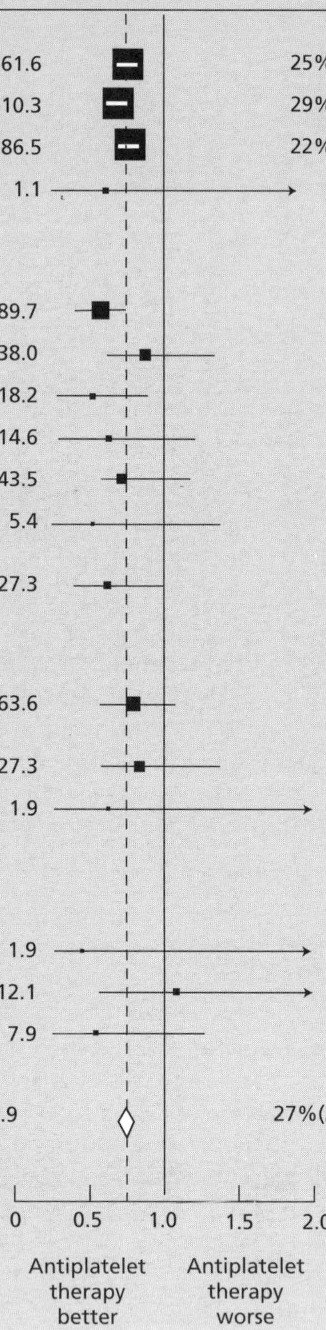

Odds ratio scale: 0 0.5 1.0 1.5 2.0

Antiplatelet therapy better — Antiplatelet therapy worse

Figure 16.12 Proportional effects of antiplatelet therapy on serious vascular events in 142 trials of antiplatelet therapy versus control in patients subdivided by type of trial. CABG, coronary artery bypass grafting; CAD, coronary artery disease; MI, myocardial infarction; PTCA, percutaneous transluminal coronary angioplasty. In most trials, patients were allocated roughly evenly between treatment groups, but in some more were deliberately allocated to active treatment; to allow direct comparisons between percentages having an event in each treatment group, in this figure and elsewhere, adjusted totals have been calculated after converting any unevenly randomised trials to even ones by counting control patients more than once. Statistical calculations are, however, based on actual numbers from individual trials. The ratio of the odds of an event in the treatment group compared with that in the control group is plotted for each trial (black square: area proportional to amount of statistical information contributed by trial) along with its 99% confidence interval (horizontal line). Stratified overview of results of all trials (and 95% confidence interval) is represented by open diamond, indicating odds ratio of 0.73 (SD 0.02) or, equivalently, an odds reduction of 27% (SD 2). (Reproduced by permission of the Antiplatelet Trialists' Collaboration, 1994a and *British Medical Journal*.)

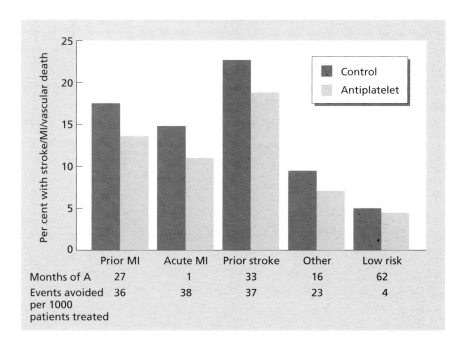

Figure 16.13 Absolute effects of antiplatelet therapy (145 trials) on serious vascular events (myocardial infarction (MI), stroke or vascular death) in four high-risk categories of patient (secondary prevention) and in low-risk people (primary prevention). Adjusted totals calculated after converting any unevenly randomised trials to even ones by counting control patients more than once. Statistical significance (2P) based on stratified analyses of original, unadjusted numbers in each trial. Months of A, means of scheduled antiplatelet therapy duration. No trial lasted under 1 month. (Reproduced by permission of the Antiplatelet Trialists' Collaboration, 1994a and *British Medical Journal*.)

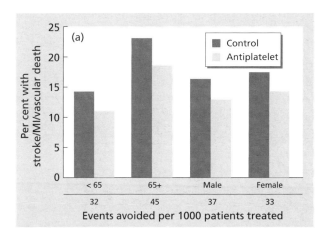
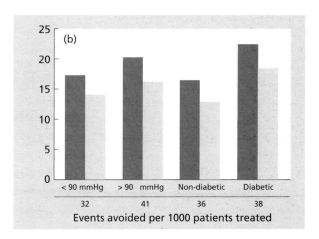

Figure 16.14 Absolute effects of antiplatelet therapy on serious vascular events in the 29 trials in high-risk patients with information available on each individual patient. Adjusted totals calculated after converting any unevenly randomised trials to even ones by counting control patients more than once. Statistical significance (2P) based on stratified analyses of original, unadjusted numbers in each trial. (a) Subdivided by age and sex; (b) subdivided by diastolic blood pressure and diabetes. MI, myocardial infarction. (Reproduced by permission of the Antiplatelet Trialists' Collaboration, 1994a and *British Medical Journal*.)

> *In general, most patients with symptomatic vascular disease—including ischaemic stroke and transient ischaemic attack—should be treated with antiplatelet drugs because all these patients are at high risk of serious vascular events.*

There is some debate about whether patients with asymptomatic carotid stenosis have a sufficiently high risk of stroke to justify antiplatelet therapy and a trial is under way. A recent small trial did not provide clear evidence of benefit (Cote *et al.*, 1995). Since many individuals with asymptomatic bruits have coronary heart disease or peripheral vascular disease (and such patients clearly benefit from antiplatelet therapy) the decision about whether or not to use antiplatelet therapy should be governed not so much by the presence or absence of the bruits, but by any *symptomatic* vascular disease the patient reports.

What to do with cardiac lesions other than atrial fibrillation?

Some patients with potential cardiac sources of embolism other than atrial fibrillation, first identified after an initial stroke or TIA, may benefit from antiplatelet therapy. The list is extensive and includes patent foramen ovale, mitral annulus calcification, left-ventricular aneurysm, etc. However, there have been no RCTs and probably never will be if for no other reason than the number of available patients is so small. The risk of recurrent vascular events in most individuals with mitral valve prolapse and TIA or stroke is low, so antiplatelet therapy is probably adequate (Orencia *et al.*, 1995). We would seldom use antiplatelet therapy in a patient under the age of 40 years with an asymptomatic cardiac abnormality other than atrial fibrillation, and no evidence of symptomatic vascular disease in the heart, legs or brain. In older patients, aged over 40 years with such cardiac lesions, we would be more likely to use antiplatelet therapy, particularly if there were also evidence of symptomatic atherosclerotic vascular disease.

Antiphospholipid antibody syndrome and the lupus anticoagulant (see also Section 7.6)

Another vexed question and one where there are no RCTs. It is probably reasonable to use antiplatelet therapy in the first instance and then only use oral anticoagulants if the patient continues to have vascular events. A recent non-randomised retrospective study suggested that warfarin was superior to aspirin, but the difference in vascular event rates between warfarin-treated patients and controls may have been related more to patient selection than to the treatment itself; anticoagulant therapy needs to be evaluated by a randomised trial (Khamashta *et al.*, 1995).

16.4.3 Who not to treat

It seems illogical to treat somebody with a primary haemorrhagic stroke (PICH or subarachnoid haemorrhage before the aneurysm is clipped) with an antihaemostatic drug like aspirin. Patients with a history of recent gastrointestinal bleeding (haematemesis or malaena) or with symptoms suggestive of active peptic ulceration should probably not receive antiplatelet therapy. Those with a definite allergy to aspirin should obviously avoid this drug.

16.4.4 Agent/dose/duration/adverse effects

Although there is a lot of information about the benefits of antiplatelet therapy compared with control there is far less comparing one form of antiplatelet therapy with another. In the Antiplatelet Trialists' Collaboration (1994a) there were only 32 trials (with approximately 14 000 patients) of direct randomised comparisons of one antiplatelet regimen with another (Fig. 16.15). From these direct comparisons, no agent was clearly superior to medium-dose aspirin (75–325 mg daily). However, the confidence intervals were wide and one can not exclude the possibility that a low dose of aspirin, 30–50 mg daily, is better (or worse) than medium-dose aspirin. The addition of dipyridamole to aspirin confers no definite extra benefit (but does seem to cause an excess of adverse effects such as headache). Ticlopidine is not clearly superior to aspirin. Indirect comparisons are a less reliable means of comparing one antiplatelet regimen with another since patient characteristics differ from one study to another (Antiplatelet Trialists' Collaboration, 1994a). Figure 16.16 illustrates the available data in which each different regimen has been compared with control; again, there was no significant heterogeneity of treatment effect, suggesting that the effects of these agents were not importantly different. The selection of agent must therefore be based on safety, cost and side effects. Aspirin appears to have the best safety and adverse effect profile. Since the adverse effects of aspirin (principally nausea, dyspepsia and probably constipation) are dose related (UK-TIA Study Group, 1991), we think it is preferable to opt for a dose which is known to be effective (75–300 mg) and less likely to be associated with adverse effects. Others feel differently and strongly support the idea that only high-dose aspirin (>1 g/day) has been proven to be effective (Dyken *et al.*, 1992). For patients who develop adverse effects on 300 mg daily the dose may be progressively reduced to 30 mg daily (Dutch TIA Trial Study Group, 1991; SALT Collaborative Group, 1991). For patients who experience adverse effects even on low doses, enteric-coated preparations of aspirin are now available. For the few patients who are genuinely completely intolerant of aspirin, ticlopidine is an effective alternative. Its use is associated

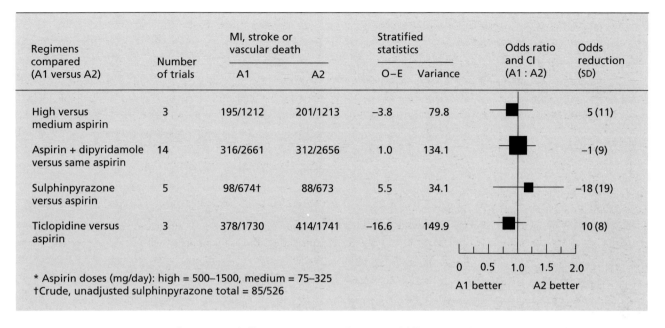

Regimens compared (A1 versus A2)	Number of trials	MI, stroke or vascular death		Stratified statistics		Odds ratio and CI (A1 : A2)	Odds reduction (SD)
		A1	A2	O–E	Variance		
High versus medium aspirin	3	195/1212	201/1213	–3.8	79.8		5 (11)
Aspirin + dipyridamole versus same aspirin	14	316/2661	312/2656	1.0	134.1		–1 (9)
Sulphinpyrazone versus aspirin	5	98/674†	88/673	5.5	34.1		–18 (19)
Ticlopidine versus aspirin	3	378/1730	414/1741	–16.6	149.9		10 (8)

* Aspirin doses (mg/day): high = 500–1500, medium = 75–325
†Crude, unadjusted sulphinpyrazone total = 85/526

0   0.5   1.0   1.5   2.0
A1 better   A2 better

Figure 16.15 Direct comparisons of proportional effects on serious vascular events of different antiplatelet regimens in trials in over 1000 high-risk patients. The ratio of the odds of an event in the treatment group compared with that in control group is plotted for each group of trials (black square: area proportional to amount of statistical information available) along with its 95% confidence interval (horizontal line). (Reproduced by permission of the Antiplatelet Trialists' Collaboration, 1994a and *British Medical Journal*.)

with neutropenia which is usually reversible, but reports of irreversible agranulocytosis and aplastic anaemia have appeared recently (Shear & Apple, 1995). A number of other antiplatelet agents are currently in clinical development; the largest study (Clopidogrel versus Aspirin in the Prevention of Recurrent Ischaemic Events (CAPRIE)) is comparing aspirin with clopidogrel and will report results in 1996/97 (M. Gent, personal communications).

Patients (and their doctors) often become quite worried if they have had a stroke or TIA and are completely aspirin intolerant. It is worth remembering that, for such patients, the benefits of aspirin are only moderate and that blood pressure reduction, smoking cessation and modification of cholesterol levels may produce benefits which are at least as big as, if not bigger than, the effects of antiplatelet therapy. These other aspects of secondary prevention should always be dealt with whether or not the patient is being given aspirin. Whether or not anticoagulants are superior to aspirin is discussed below (see Section 16.5.4).

16.4.5 How long should treatment continue?

Most of the trials evaluating aspirin in high-risk patients lasted just 2–3 years (Antiplatelet Trialists' Collaboration, 1994a). The benefits of continuing aspirin beyond this

period have therefore not been evaluated formally. There was clear evidence of benefit for up to 2 years treatment with probable additive benefit between years 2 and 3. Although there is no firm evidence from RCTs to support this, it seems highly likely that individuals who are at continuing high risk because of past stroke or TIA should probably continue aspirin lifelong, provided there are no adverse effects.

> *Medium-dose aspirin (75–300 mg daily) is advisable for most patients with a history of recent transient ischaemic attack or ischaemic stroke and should be continued for life.*

16.5 Anticoagulants (for patients with TIA and ischaemic stroke only)

Emboli arising in the heart, extracranial arteries or elsewhere often contain fibrin and because inhibitors of the coagulation cascade prevent conversion of fibrinogen to fibrin, anticoagulant drugs should reduce the thromboembolic complications of occlusive arterial disease. Anticoagulants were first available for clinical use in the 1950s and have been extensively used (but not extensively tested in large reliable RCTs) in patients with stroke and TIA ever since.

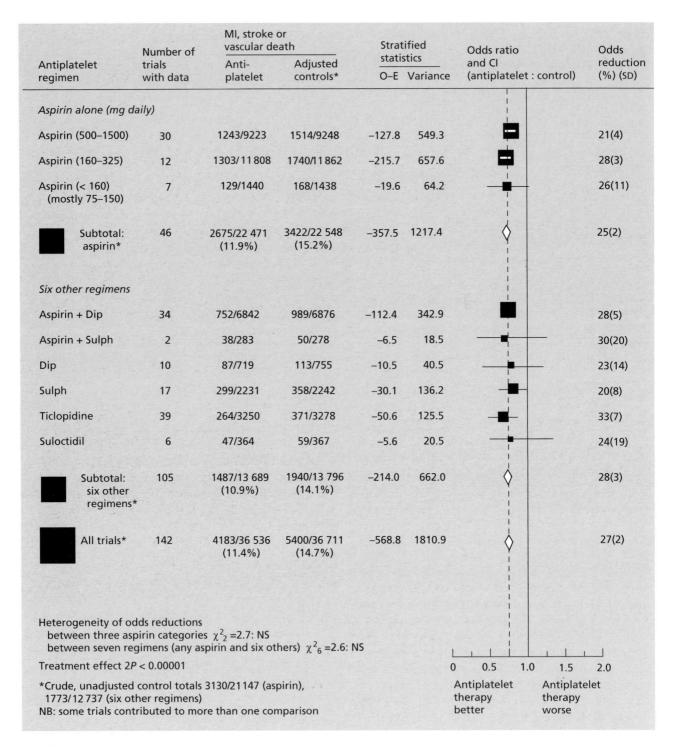

Antiplatelet regimen	Number of trials with data	MI, stroke or vascular death		Stratified statistics		Odds ratio and CI (antiplatelet : control)	Odds reduction (%) (SD)
		Anti-platelet	Adjusted controls*	O–E	Variance		
Aspirin alone (mg daily)							
Aspirin (500–1500)	30	1243/9223	1514/9248	−127.8	549.3		21(4)
Aspirin (160–325)	12	1303/11808	1740/11862	−215.7	657.6		28(3)
Aspirin (< 160) (mostly 75–150)	7	129/1440	168/1438	−19.6	64.2		26(11)
Subtotal: aspirin*	46	2675/22 471 (11.9%)	3422/22 548 (15.2%)	−357.5	1217.4		25(2)
Six other regimens							
Aspirin + Dip	34	752/6842	989/6876	−112.4	342.9		28(5)
Aspirin + Sulph	2	38/283	50/278	−6.5	18.5		30(20)
Dip	10	87/719	113/755	−10.5	40.5		23(14)
Sulph	17	299/2231	358/2242	−30.1	136.2		20(8)
Ticlopidine	39	264/3250	371/3278	−50.6	125.5		33(7)
Suloctidil	6	47/364	59/367	−5.6	20.5		24(19)
Subtotal: six other regimens*	105	1487/13 689 (10.9%)	1940/13 796 (14.1%)	−214.0	662.0		28(3)
All trials*	142	4183/36 536 (11.4%)	5400/36 711 (14.7%)	−568.8	1810.9		27(2)

Heterogeneity of odds reductions
between three aspirin categories χ^2_2 =2.7: NS
between seven regimens (any aspirin and six others) χ^2_6 =2.6: NS

Treatment effect $2P < 0.00001$

*Crude, unadjusted control totals 3130/21147 (aspirin), 1773/12 737 (six other regimens)
NB: some trials contributed to more than one comparison

Figure 16.16 Indirect comparisons of proportional effects on serious vascular events of different antiplatelet regimens in 142 trials in high-risk patients. The ratio of odds of myocardial infarction (MI), stroke or vascular death in the treatment group compared with the control group is plotted for each trial (black square: area proportional to number of strokes), along with the 99% confidence interval (horizontal line). The presence of a black square to the left of the solid vertical line suggests benefit, but this benefit is significant at the level of $2P < 0.01$ only if the entire confidence interval is to the left of the solid vertical line. An overview of all of the trial results (and 95% confidence interval) is represented by a diamond, beside which is given the overall relative reduction in risk of MI, stroke or vascular death. Dip, dipyridamole; Sulph, sulphinpyrazone. (Reproduced by permission of the Antiplatelet Trialists' Collaboration, 1994a and *British Medical Journal*.)

16.5.1 Evidence

Patients without atrial fibrillation

A systematic review of the trials of anticoagulants in survivors of myocardial infarction suggested that long-term use reduced the risk of stroke and vascular death (Antman *et al.*, 1992; Vaitkus *et al.*, 1992; ASPECT Research Group, 1994). Further studies in survivors of myocardial infarction comparing anticoagulants with antiplatelet therapy are underway; at present, there is no clearcut evidence to suggest that anticoagulants are better than aspirin (Cairns, 1994). A systematic review of anticoagulants in the prevention of stroke amongst patients who have had a TIA or ischaemic stroke likewise suggested that the balance of risk and benefit from anticoagulants was unclear, that anticoagulants could not be recommended for routine practice and that further studies were required (Jonas, 1988). Two large RCTs are now under way: the Warfarin Aspirin Recurrent Stroke Study (WARSS) in the US which is comparing warfarin with aspirin in a double-blind placebo-controlled trial, and the Stroke Prevention in Recurrent Ischaemia Trial (SPIRIT) in Europe is also comparing, in a single-blind trial, warfarin with aspirin. The results will not be available for several years.

> *In ischaemic stroke and transient ischaemic attack patients who are in sinus rhythm it is not clear whether antithrombotic therapy with anticoagulants is as effective and safe as aspirin, but trials (WARSS and SPIRIT) comparing the two should provide useful information about which is the better regimen; for now, aspirin is the antithrombotic agent of choice.*

Patients with atrial fibrillation

A systematic review of the five studies on the value of anticoagulants in the primary prevention of stroke in patients with atrial fibrillation showed a reduction in the annual risk of stroke of 68% (Fig. 16.17), from 4.5% in control to 1.4% in the treated group (Atrial Fibrillation Investigators, 1994). However, the balance of risk and benefit from long-term anticoagulant therapy in primary stroke prevention can not be directly extrapolated to atrial fibrillation patients who have survived a TIA or ischaemic stroke, not least because their absolute risk of stroke is much higher. The average annual risk of stroke per year amongst control patients in the five primary prevention trials was just over 4%, compared with 12% amongst controls in the European Atrial Fibrillation Trial (EAFT) (European Atrial Fibrillation Trial Study Group, 1993; Atrial Fibrillation Investigators, 1994) (Figs 16.18 & 16.19). In the EAFT, anticoagulants reduced

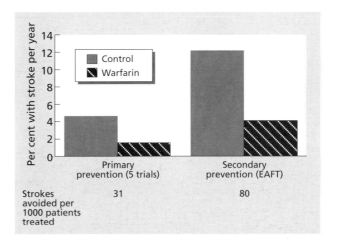

Figure 16.17 The absolute effect, in terms of stroke prevention, of anticoagulants in primary prevention of stroke in patients with atrial fibrillation, based on a systematic review of five trials compared with the effect in one secondary prevention trial. (Data from European Atrial Fibrillation Trial Study Group, 1993; Atrial Fibrillation Investigators, 1994.)

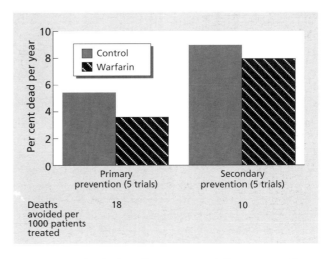

Figure 16.18 The absolute effects, in terms of all causes mortality, of anticoagulants in patients with atrial fibrillation based on a systematic review of five trials compared with the effect in one secondary prevention trial. (Data from European Atrial Fibrillation Trial Study Group, 1993; Atrial Fibrillation Trial Investigators, 1994.)

the risk of stroke by two-thirds, from 12 to 4%/year and of the primary outcome event (stroke, myocardial infarction, systemic embolism or vascular death) by about 50%, reducing the annual rate of events from 17% in control to 8% in anticoagulant-allocated patients. Anticoagulants appeared to be more effective than aspirin (Koudstaal, 1995d). The incidence of major bleeding complications was low, both on

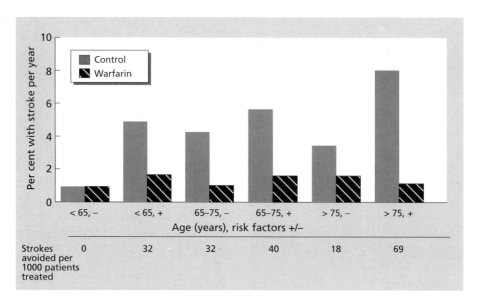

Figure 16.19 The absolute effect, in terms of stroke prevention, of anticoagulants in primary prevention of stroke in patients with atrial fibrillation based on a systematic review of five trials: absolute risk of stroke in relation to baseline risk and presence (+) or absence (−) of risk factors. (Data from Atrial Fibrillation Investigators, 1994.)

anticoagulation (2.8%/year) and on aspirin (0.9%/year) and, as it happened, no intracranial bleeds were identified. Forty-six patients in the Veterans Administration Stroke Prevention in atrial fibrillation (AV–SPINAF) study had a history of prior stroke or TIA at the time of randomisation. These two trials have been systematically reviewed (Koudstaal, 1995a). Thus, if 1000 patients are treated with anticoagulants for 1 year, about 90 serious vascular events (mostly strokes) are avoided; about 11 ischaemic stroke or TIA survivors need to be treated with anticoagulants to prevent one vascular event (stroke, myocardial infarction, systemic embolism or vascular death). However, translating these research findings into clinical practice has major implications for health care providers. A systematic review of the evidence from a public health perspective reached rather less optimistic conclusions (Green *et al.*, 1995). People with atrial fibrillation in the general population are likely to be less compliant with, and less carefully monitored than, patients within the trials; this may reduce the benefits and increase the risks (Green *et al.*, 1995). Green *et al.* (1995) calculated that it would require 112 patients to be treated to prevent one major stroke. One major bleed might occur for every 50 treated patients. Treatment of 1000 patients with warfarin would, therefore, prevent nine major strokes at a cost of about 20 major bleeds (Green *et al.*, 1995). It is also likely that, when applied to the generality of patients with ischaemic stroke and TIA, the benefits of anticoagulants may be less extreme than suggested by the trials. There will therefore need to be major changes in health service provision to match the increased need for anticoagulant therapy and to

ensure that it is delivered both effectively and safely (Sudlow *et al.*, 1995).

16.5.2 Who to treat

In general, we routinely use anticoagulants rather than antiplatelet agents for long-term secondary prevention after TIA or ischaemic stroke in patients in atrial fibrillation. However, ischaemic stroke survivors and TIA patients are a fairly heterogeneous group, and certain factors may make clinicans reluctant to prescribe long-term anticoagulants; for example, a history of uncontrolled hypertension, recent gastrointestinal bleeding, alcoholic liver disease, confusion or dementia, tendency to falls and difficulties with access to an anticoagulant clinic. These factors increase the likelihood of over-anticoagulation and the risk of intracranial bleeding (Hart *et al.*, 1995). On the other hand, some of the same factors that increase the risk of haemorrhage *with* treatment also increase the risk of stroke *without* treatment, particularly hypertension (Atrial Fibrillation Investigators, 1994; van Latum *et al.*, 1995). Many other factors have been identified which alone, or in combination with other factors, identify those patients with stroke (or TIA) and atrial fibrillation who are at highest risk of stroke without treatment (and therefore have the most to gain) (Atrial Fibrillation Investigators, 1994; Di Pasquale *et al.*, 1995; van Latum *et al.*, 1995) (Table 16.9; Fig. 16.19). For low-risk individuals aspirin is a reasonable alternative to anticoagulants (see Section 16.4.2).

Table 16.9 Annual rate of serious vascular events* in the 375 patients in the EAFT allocated placebo (all had had prior TIA or ischaemic stroke). (From van Latum *et al.*, 1995.)

| Number of risk factors† | Event rate (95% CI) | |
	Age <75 years	Age >75 years
0	6.3 (0.8–23.0)	0 (0–15.0)
1–2	15 (11–20)	16 (11–23)
>3	30 (21–42)	37 (26–53)

* Events were: vascular death, non-fatal stroke, non-fatal myocardial infarction and systemic embolism (whichever occured first).
† Risk factors were: ischaemic heart disease, previous thromboembolism, systemic blood pressure >160 mmHg, duration of atrial fibrillation >1 year, infarction visible on CT scan, cardiothoracic ratio >50% on chest X-ray.

> *Anticoagulants are indicated for many patients with recent transient ischaemic attack or ischaemic stroke who are in atrial fibrillation, provided there are no contraindications. It is important to assess the risk of anticoagulation for each individual patient.*

Cardioversion of patients in atrial fibrillation

There is no consensus amongst cardiologists on the comparative merits of cardioversion by electrical shock, cardioversion by drugs and long-term oral anticoagulants (Moreyra *et al.*, 1995). A decision analysis suggested that long-term anti-arrhythmic drugs such as amiodarone may be preferable to anticoagulants in primary prevention; no calculations were provided for secondary prevention (Middlekauff *et al.*, 1995). The selection of patients for cardioversion may be guided by the results of transoephageal echocardiography (Kinch & Davidoff, 1995; Di Pasquale *et al.*, 1995). We now quite often discuss whether or not to try and convert patients with atrial fibrillation and a recent TIA or ischaemic stroke to sinus rhythm with our local cardiological colleagues. Further trials to evaluate the best policy in this area are clearly needed.

Frequent TIAs or ischaemic strokes despite antiplatelet therapy and surgery

In our experience, this situation is relatively uncommon. The first step should be to verify again that the attacks are truly ischaemic in nature and do not represent structural brain disease, epilepsy, migraine, psychogenic disorder, etc. (see Chapter 3). If the diagnosis is correct, these admittedly rare patients are often very worried, as are their doctors. Of course, those with carotid ischaemic events and severe symp-tomatic carotid stenosis should be considered for endarterectomy but sometimes this is not possible or practical (see Section 16.7), and very occasionally the attacks continue after what appears to be a technically adequate operation. On the whole, 2–3 months of oral anticoagulants seems to reduce the frequency and severity of the attacks, which is comforting to the patient and reduces anxiety all round. We generally do this in the full knowledge that this treatment may not reduce the risk of stroke or vascular death (Jonas, 1988). It is purely given for symptom control. It is often possible to withdraw the anticoagulants gradually and replace them with aspirin therapy. In such cases, the fractured atheromatous plaque that was causing the frequent attacks has perhaps 'healed' and become covered with endothelium (see Section 6.2.2).

Other cardiac embolic sources

For patients who have cardiac disorders, other than atrial fibrillation and mechanical prosthetic valves, which have the *potential* to be a source of embolism, the place of anticoagulants has been less clearly established in stroke prevention. The management of stroke in patients with prosthetic mechanical valves already on anticoagulants was discussed in Sections 6.4 and 11.3. The criteria to select patients with lesions such as patent foramen ovale, atrial septal aneurysm, mitral valve prolapse and left ventricular aneurysms for long-term anticoagulants have not been defined by reliable large trials. Since the balance of risk and benefit of antiplatelet therapy is clearly established for a wide variety of cardiac conditions, aspirin is probably preferable to anticoagulants in most circumstances. The management of ischaemic stroke and other thromboembolic events amongst pregnant patients with prosthetic heart valves is highly controversial and has recently been discussed in detail (Greaves, 1993; Sbarouni & Oakley, 1994).

Dissection of the carotid and vertebral arteries

Thrombus may form at sites of intimal damage, and embolise to the brain, causing further infarction and a progressive stroke syndrome (see Section 7.1). If the dissection can be imaged by ultrasound, MR angiography or conventional angiography, the difficult decision about whether or not to give anticoagulants to prevent recurrent stroke often arises and has been discussed earlier (see Section 11.3.3).

Antiphospholipid antibody syndrome and the lupus anticoagulant (see also Section 7.6)

This acquired disorder of the clotting system which predisposes to thrombosis may be treated with antiplatelet or anticoagulant drugs. A recent non-randomised study suggested warfarin was the treatment of choice (Khamashta *et al.*, 1995), but this needs to be confirmed by randomised trials.

16.5.3 Who not to treat

CT scan not available

None of us starts anticoagulants without first doing a brain CT scan (or perhaps MRI) to exclude intracranial haemorrhage, because anticoagulation of a patient with a PICH is presumably unwise, at least in the short term, if not in the long term. It is not clear whether or not the presence of haemorrhagic transformation of a cerebral infarct is an absolute contraindication to the use of anticoagulants.

Infective endocarditis

Patients with active endocarditis should not be treated with oral anticoagulants because of their high risk of intracerebral haemorrhage (Hart *et al.*, 1995).

Other contraindications

These have all been mentioned previously but bear repeating (see Section 11.3.4 and Tables 11.5 and 11.7). The risk of complications from long-term anticoagulant therapy is likely to be higher in patients with uncontrolled hypertension, in elderly confused patients, patients with alcoholic liver disease, and in patients unable to attend for regular blood tests to monitor anticoagulant therapy. It is often difficult to judge whether or not a patient will be compliant with treatment, but clearly a history of poor compliance with some previous medication is at least an indicator.

16.5.4 Agent/dose/adverse effects

If anticoagulant therapy is to be used for long-term secondary prevention, a baseline full blood count, platelet count, international normalised ratio (INR) and liver function tests should be done—and the results known—before treatment is started. If there is urgency to anticoagulate, heparin can be given immediately, since oral anticoagulant therapy takes several days to become effective. Convenient heparin and warfarin dosing schedules are given in Tables 16.10 and 16.11. Patients should be followed up regularly. The frequency of follow-up will be determined by local facilities and by how far the patient lives from the hospital. Follow-up by the local general practitioner may be feasible.

Table 16.10 A schedule for dosage and monitoring of full-dose standard heparin therapy. (From Hirsh, 1991; Scottish Intercollegiate Guidelines Network, 1996.)

1 *Initial loading dose* 5000 IU (or 75 IU/kg body weight) intravenous bolus over 5 minutes

2 *Initial maintenance dose*

Intravenous infusion	Subcutaneous injection (12-hourly)
Add 25 000 IU heparin to 50 ml 0.9% saline (= 500 IU/ml)	Use 25 000 IU/ml
1000 IU/hour (= 2 ml/hour)	12 500 IU (or 80 IU/kg body weight)

3 *Measure APTT ratio* (at 4–6 hours, then at least daily)—adjust dose as follows

APTT ratio	Intravenous infusion	Subcutaneous injection (12-hourly)
over 7.0	Stop for 60 minutes and reduce by 500 IU/hour	Reduce to 7500 IU (or by 120 IU/kg)
5.1–7.0	Stop for 60 minutes and reduce by 500 IU/hour	
4.1–5.0	Stop for 60 minutes and reduce by 300 IU/hour	Reduce by 5000 IU (or by 80 IU/kg)
3.1–4.0	Stop for 60 minutes and reduce by 100 IU/hour	Reduce by 2500 IU (or by 40 IU/kg)
2.6–3.0	Stop for 60 minutes and reduce by 50 IU/hour	
1.5–2.5	No change	No change
1.2–1.4	If high-risk PE, give 3000 IU (or 75 IU/kg body weight) intravenous bolus over 5 minutes and: Increase by 200 IU/hour	Increase by 2500 IU (or by 40 IU/kg)
Under 1.2	If high-risk PE, give 5000 IU (or 75 IU/kg body weight) intravenous bolus over 5 minutes and: Increase by 400 IU/hour	Increase by 5000 IU (or by 40 IU/kg)

After each change in dose, repeat activated prothromboplastin time (APTT) between 6 and 10-hours later. When target therapeutic range achieved, monitor APTT daily whilst in range. Also monitor: INR if also on oral anticoagulants; blood count, anaemia due to bleeding; thrombocytopenia (if platelet count falls below 150 × 10^9/L or by more than 100 × 10^9/L from previous reading, stop heparin and consult haematologist). PE, pulmonary embolism.

The trials of anticoagulation in patients with atrial fibrillation evaluated oral anticoagulants aiming for an INR between 2.0 and 4.0 (European Atrial Fibrillation Trial Study Group, 1993; Atrial Fibrillation Trialists, 1994). Non-randomised evidence from the EAFT suggested than an INR

Table 16.11 A schedule for dosage and monitoring of full-dose warfarin therapy.(From Scottish Intercollegiate Guidelines Network, 1996.)

Day	INR (9–11 AM)	Warfarin dose (mg) given at 5–7 PM
1st	<1.4	10
2nd	<1.8	10
	1.8	1
	>1.8	0.5
3rd	<2.0	10
	2.0–2.1	5
	2.2–2.3	4.5
	2.4–2.5	4
	2.6–2.7	3.5
	2.8–2.9	3
	3.0–3.1	2.5
	3.2–3.3	2
	3.4	1.5
	3.5	1
	3.6–4.0	0.5
	>4.0	0
		Predicted maintenance dose
4th	<1.4	>8
	1.4	8
	1.5	7.5
	1.6–1.7	7
	1.8	6.5
	1.9	6
	2.0–2.1	5.5
	2.2–2.3	5
	2.4–2.6	4.5
	2.7–3.0	4
	3.1–3.5	3.5
	3.6–4.0	3
	4.1–4.5	Miss out next day dose then give 2 mg
	4.5	Miss out 2 days' doses then give 1 mg

Activated prothromboplastin time (APTT) should be within or below the therapeutic range (1.5–2.5 times control). If APTT is above this range the heparin effect on INR should be neutralised by adding protamine (0.4 µg/ml plasma) to the sample.

above 5.0 was associated with an unacceptably high risk of haemorrhage, and an INR below 2.0 carried a high risk of recurrent stroke because of inadequate treatment (European Atrial Fibrillation Trial Study Group, 1995). Therefore, aiming for an INR of about 3–4 is probably best. The EAFT also suggested that anticoagulants were superior to aspirin in patients with atrial fibrillation and recent TIA or ischaemic stroke (European Atrial Fibrillation Trial Study Group, 1993).

Long-term subcutaneous heparin therapy

A small trial in Italy is comparing antiplatelet therapy with once daily subcutaneous heparin in patients with TIA and minor stroke (D. Inzitari, personal communication, 1996). The results of this trial will be of some interest since heparin may be useful in patients who are truly aspirin intolerant, but also may be indirectly relevant to stroke prevention in pregnant women (who can not take oral anticoagulants because of fears of fetal damage). The hazards of heparin therapy are discussed in Section 11.3.6.

Mesoglycan

Mesoglycan is a novel antithrombotic drug consisting of dermatan sulphate and heparin sulphate. It has been compared with aspirin in 1398 patients with recent ischaemic stroke. There were no clear differences in major outcome events between the two groups (Forconi et al., 1995). The agent is worthy of further study, but can not be recommended for routine use at present.

The combination of aspirin with anticoagulants

One small trial compared the safety and efficacy of warfarin alone with 75 mg aspirin daily plus warfarin (Turpie et al., 1993). The combination therapy in patients with high-risk (mechanical heart valves) and low-risk (bioprosthetic valves) cardiac lesions was associated with fewer strokes and other thromboembolic events, without an apparent increase in haemorrhagic adverse effects. However, the number of cerebral haemorrhages was small, and the trial could not exclude a moderate excess of bleeds with the combination. Nonetheless, the trial was useful, since it suggested that combination therapy was at least reasonably safe for patients who continue to have attacks whilst on aspirin or warfarin alone. However, much more randomised evidence is required before this conclusion can be made definitely.

How long should treatment be continued?

Most of the trials have tested only a few years of anticoagulant therapy, and it is not yet known whether the balance of risk and benefit alters with prolonged therapy, particularly as the patient passes the age of 70 years. Further research is clearly required to determine the optimum duration of treatment.

16.6 Treatment of specific underlying causes

Homocystinuria

Observational epidemiological studies and case–control studies have suggested that a moderate increase in plasma homocystine is an independent risk factor for premature vascular disease and stroke (see Section 6.2.3). Treatment of young patients who have high levels of homocystine with high-dose oral folate, has been reported to yield some benefit in terms of neurological function, but whether this leads to a reduction in the risk of serious vascular events is not known.

Migraine

Migraine may be a modest independent risk factor for stroke, but the proportion of all strokes attributable to migraine is extremely small. The risk of stroke in an individual migraineur is so low that prophylactic treatment purely to prevent migrainous stroke is probably not justified (see Section 7.5). Patients who have frequent severe migraine *and* other vascular risk factors should of course have their vascular risk factors dealt with conventionally; those who have *symptomatic* vascular disease should be on aspirin anyway.

Arteritis

Arteritis is dealt with under the treatment of acute stroke (see Section 11.9).

Hyperviscosity

Stroke is a rare complication of hyperviscosity syndromes (see Section 7.6). Treatment should be guided by the treatment of the disorder causing the hyperviscosity (e.g. by the type and severity of the underlying pathology, e.g. myeloma), and not by the stroke.

Oral contraceptives and hormone replacement therapy (HRT)

Young women who have a stroke of any pathological type whilst on the oral contraceptive should probably stop (see Section 7.10). A substantial proportion of these women have other vascular risk factors (usually smoking but other factors may be present as well, such as hypertension) and these require attention in their own right. Alternative forms of contraception should be offered. A small proportion of post-menopausal women on HRT suffer a stroke. For them, the question that then arises is 'should the treatment be stopped or continued?'. Observational epidemiological data suggest that, amongst women free of vascular disease when they start treatment, HRT is more likely to prevent coronary heart disease events than cause cancer of the breast or uterine cavity and there may also be a small reduction in the risk of limb bone fractures. There are several ongoing randomised trials of HRT in primary and secondary prevention of vascular disease. The most relevant of these is the Womens Estrogen Stroke Trial (WEST) study, which is comparing, in post-menopausal women with recent stroke or TIA, HRT with control, to see whether there is a net reduction in the risk of stroke and other serious vascular events in such high-risk individuals (Horwitz & Brass, 1994). Pending the results of these trials in primary and secondary prevention, guidance for an individual woman having a stroke whilst on HRT must be based on guesswork rather than facts. In our experience, most women choose to stop treatment.

> *The role of hormone replacement therapy in post-menopausal women for primary and secondary stroke prevention is the subject of current research; firm guidelines can not be given at present.*

Infections

Less than 1% of all strokes are due to unusual infections, but if rare treatable conditions such as Lyme disease, human immunodeficiency virus (HIV) or syphilis are diagnosed clinically and confirmed serologically, then specific treatment is required (see Section 7.8).

16.7 Endarterectomy for symptomatic carotid stenosis

16.7.1 Introduction

Soon after the introduction of cerebral angiography and the appreciation that atherothrombotic stenosis at or near the origin of the internal carotid artery (ICA) might be responsible for ischaemic stroke, surgeons began to devise methods to remove or bypass the stenotic lesion. The first successful carotid endarterectomy was done in 1953, but lay unreported until 1975 (DeBakey, 1975), although there had been earlier surgical attempts in China (Chao *et al.*, 1938) and Argentina (Carrea *et al.*, 1955). However, it was the report of a successful carotid *reconstruction* in a patient with frequent low-flow TIAs (Eastcott *et al.*, 1954) that gave the impetus to what was to become, in North America at least, an epidemic of carotid endarterectomies for asymptomatic as well as symptomatic stenosis (Dyken & Pokras 1984). ICA occlusion generally came to be regarded as inoperable, and still is.

Innumerable surgical series have been published, and although they provide some idea of the risk of surgery and how it might be minimised, they can not demonstrate any certain benefit because most had no control group and the rest had only non-randomised controls. Two early randomised trials were inconclusive (Fields *et al.*, 1970; Shaw *et al.*, 1984). Not surprisingly, there were soon huge variations in surgery rates between countries and even within the same country (UK-TIA Study Group, 1983; Warlow, 1984). Under these highly unsatisfactory circumstances, neurologists began to question publicly the utility of carotid endarterectomy, inappropriate use of surgery was documented, and the number of operations—perhaps as a consequence—began to fall (Warlow, 1984; Barnett *et al.*, 1984; Pokras & Dyken, 1988; Winslow *et al.*, 1988). In the 1980s all these pressures persuaded surgeons and neurologists to mount randomised trials large enough to be conclusive, and in the early 1990s the first results in patients with *symptomatic* stenosis began to appear (European Carotid Surgery Trialists' Collaborative Group, 1991; North American Symptomatic Carotid Endarterectomy Trial Collaborators, 1991; Mayberg *et al.*, 1991). Surgery clearly does prevent stroke in patients with recently symptomatic severe ICA stenosis, but at a price: the risk of stroke as a consequence of surgery, the risk of the other complications of surgery, the cost of the surgery, and the risk and cost of the investigations to select suitable patients. However, the stage is now set for clinical guidelines supported by something other than whim (Brown & Humphrey, 1992; Moore *et al.*, 1995), the beginning of cost-effectiveness analyses (see Section 16.7.6) and an estimate of the public health impact of surgery (see Section 18.5).

16.7.2 The operation of carotid endarterectomy (Fig. 16.20)

Usually under general rather than local anaesthesia, the carotid bifurcation in the neck is exposed, gently mobilised, and slings are placed around the internal, external and common carotid arteries. During this exposure embolic material may be inadvertently dislodged from within the arterial lumen, and nerves which lie close to the artery can be damaged (see Section 16.7.4). After applying clamps to the three arteries, if possible away from any atheromatous plaque, the bifurcation is opened through a longitudinal incision, the entire stenotic lesion cored out, the distal intimal margin secured, the arteriotomy closed and the clamps released to restore blood flow to the brain. Clearly, there is a risk that the temporary reduction in the ICA blood flow will cause ipsilateral ischaemic stroke if the collateral supply from the contralateral ICA and the vertebrobasilar system, through the circle of Willis, is inadequate, particularly if there is already maximal vasodilatation in the area of brain supplied by the operated ICA (i.e. cerebrovascular reserve is exhausted). Also, emboli may be released by clamping the ICA, or from the endarterectomy site when the clamps are removed

at the end of the procedure (Gaunt *et al.*, 1994). Not just during the operation but even in the hours and days after surgery, the patient is still at risk of embolic stroke from thrombus forming at the operation site, particularly if the distal intimal flap left after the endarterectomy has not been controlled. Most patients should already be on antiplatelet drugs before surgery (see Section 16.4) and these should be continued afterwards (Lindblad *et al.*, 1993). In addition, most surgeons heparinise patients during the procedure itself. This then is the operation at its simplest and it should take only about 1.5 hours. For 40 years, surgeons have been attempting to make the operation safer by using various modifications on the basic technique, which itself has remained essentially unchanged (Loftus & Quest, 1987).

Cerebral protection (shunting)

In theory it should be possible to prevent cerebral ischaemia due to low flow during the operation by inserting a temporary intraluminal shunt from the common carotid artery (CCA) to the ICA whilst the endarterectomy is carried out at leisure. Some surgeons always use a shunt for this reason but there are potential problems: insertion of the shunt may be difficult and it can dissect the arterial wall or dislodge atherothrombotic material which embolises to the brain; clot may form in the shunt and embolise, or even occlude the shunt completely; the shunt may be obstructed by kinking, or if the end abuts against the arterial wall; the shunt can transmit emboli from thrombus in the CCA forming as a result of damage during shunt insertion; the shunt itself may get in the way making the operation longer and technically more difficult; and the more extensive surgical exposure required may increase the chance of nerve damage, postoperative haematoma and infection. A compromise is to shunt only patients likely to develop cerebral ischaemia as a result of low flow but this reduces the surgeon's experience of shunting, and so perhaps the required skills.

Enormous but inconclusive efforts have been made to identify those patients who should be selectively shunted to prevent cerebral ischaemia (Ferguson, 1986; Ojemann & Heros, 1986; Naylor *et al.*, 1992). Some believe that shunts should be used if a patient has contralateral ICA occlusion or has had a recent ischaemic stroke. Others shunt patients who have a low ICA 'stump' pressure (measured distal to the ICA clamp), which should indicate a poor collateral blood flow to the ipsilateral cerebral hemisphere. Collateralisation itself can possibly be predicted preoperatively with transcranial Doppler (Schneider *et al.*, 1988). Intraoperative monitoring of the electroencephalogram (EEG), sensory evoked potentials, regional cerebral blood flow or middle cerebral artery (MCA) blood flow, emboli detected with transcranial

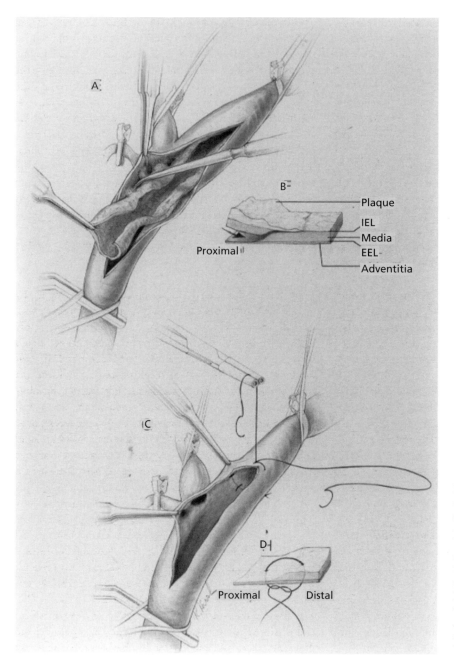

Figure 16.20 Illustration of a standard carotid endarterectomy. At A the atherothrombotic plaque is being cored out, the plane of the dissection usually being between the media and external elastic lamina (EEL) at B. In C the artery is being closed with particular attention to tacking down the distal intimal flap at D. IEL, internal elastic lamina. (Reproduced with permission from *Atlas of Vascular Surgery* edited by C.K. Zarins and B.L. Gewertz, Churchill Livingstone, New York, 1987.)

Doppler of the MCA, and the neurological state of the patient if operated under local anaesthesia, may all provide early warning of cerebral ischaemia. However, this may be too late for a quickly inserted shunt, or abandoned operation, to ameliorate the consequences of cerebral ischaemia which may not even be reversible at all if it is acutally due to embolism rather than low flow.

There is no standard method to predict which patients will have an ischaemic stroke as a result of carotid clamping and so due to low cerebral blood flow. It is, therefore, difficult to select patients who should be protected by a shunt during carotid endarterectomy which is why so many different techniques and criteria are in common use.

It is almost impossible to demonstrate reliably that any particular policy reduces perioperative stroke risk, because this risk is already so small that very large numbers are required to avoid random error (Schroeder, 1990; Halsey, 1992; Rothwell *et al.*, 1996b). Only two randomised trials have been done, both too small to be conclusive (Gumerlock & Neuwelt, 1988; Sandmann *et al.*, 1993). Furthermore, it is difficult to distinguish the rather small number of preventable (by shunting) strokes due to low flow from the larger number of unpreventable (by shunting) strokes due to embolism (see Section 16.7.3). As a result there is no standard policy for operative monitoring or the use of shunts, and surgeons have to rely on their own experience, commonsense and whatever technique of monitoring they have available and are comfortable with. All do agree, however, that controlling systemic blood pressure before, during and after surgery is crucial to avoid hypotension, which will make any cerebral ischaemia worse, and hypertension which may cause cerebral oedema or even intracerebral haemorrhage (see Section 16.7.3). Operative damage to the nerve to the carotid sinus, or changes in the carotid sinus itself, may make control of the postoperative blood pressure more of a problem, and may be the explanation for the small but definite long-term rise in blood pressure (Slattery & Warlow, 1996).

Re-stenosis and patch angioplasty

After successful carotid endarterectomy the risk of ischaemic stroke ipsilateral to be operated artery over the next few years is very low (see Section 16.7.5). So, in a sense, whether and how often carotid stenosis recurs is of little clinical concern because even if it does it seems not to matter. However, if recurrent stenosis does become symptomatic then a second carotid endarterectomy is more difficult and risky (Piepgras *et al.*, 1986). The rate of re-stenosis has been much studied using various non-invasive methods and the figures vary enormously depending on whether the study is prospective or retrospective, the completeness of follow-up, the sensitivity and specificity of the method used, the definition of re-stenosis and the length of follow-up. Certainly, recurrent atherothrombotic stenosis can occur, but usually not for some years after endarterectomy, whilst early re-stenosis (within 1 year or so) is more likely to be due to neointimal fibromuscular hyperplasia (Hunter *et al.*, 1987). Sometimes, however, a re-stenosis is not a re-stenosis at all but a residual stenosis from a technically inadequate carotid endarterectomy.

Some surgeons now routinely insert a patch of vein or synthetic material when closing the artery to enlarge the lumen and—as a result—perhaps to reduce the risk of re-stenosis and, more importantly, of stroke (Awad & Little, 1989). A meta-analysis of the few randomised trials has shown a pos-

sible reduction in re-stenosis and fewer perioperative arterial occlusions in the patched group but, not surprisingly, there were so few strokes that any effect on their risk was quite uncertain (Counsell *et al.*, 1995b). Patching does increase the surgery time and there are complications, albeit rarely: (i) the centre of a vein patch can become necrotic and rupture to cause a life-threatening neck haematoma; (ii) the patch may cause aneurysmal bulging and dilatation at the carotid bifurcation; and (iii) synthetic grafts can become infected. Also, it may be impossible to find enough saphenous vein left over by the coronary artery surgeons, and removing what vein there is can be complicated by local haematoma, infection, ulceration and discomfort. Further randomised trials are clearly required.

Early technical failure

Just occasionally the ICA occludes immediately, or a few days after surgery, as a result of thrombosis or dissection. This does not necessarily cause stroke if the collateral supply to the brain is sufficient. Both thrombosis and dissection are thought to be due to poor operative technique, particularly if the distal intimal flap has been left unsecured or there is a ridge of tissue due to faulty suturing. Therefore, before closing the skin some surgeons make considerable efforts to check the endarterectomy site with conventional ultrasonography, angiography, angioscopy or intravascular ultrasound imaging and, if necessary, they re-open the artery to improve the anatomical result. Whether this has much effect on the surgical or later stroke risk is unknown.

16.7.3 Perioperative stroke (Table 16.12)

The most feared complication of carotid endarterectomy is stroke, the very event the operation is designed to prevent. The reported risk of stroke ranges from an implausibly low 1% or less, to an unacceptably high of 20% or more. This variation may be explained by differences in: (i) the definition of stroke; (ii) the accuracy of stroke diagnosis; (iii) the completeness of the clinical details; (iv) whether the study was retrospective or prospective, and whether the diagnosis of stroke was based on patient observation or just medical record review; (v) variation in case selection, surgical and anaesthetic skills; and (vi), perhaps, publication bias (Campbell, 1993; Rothwell *et al.*, 1996b). Death is most unlikely after more than 20% of perioperative strokes (which are almost always TACIs or PACIs with a case fatality at 30 days of about 40% and 5%, respectively; see Table 10.2); therefore, studies which report less than four times as many non-fatal as fatal strokes are almost certainly undercounting mild strokes, a tendency which may well be due to

Table 16.12 Complications of carotid endarterectomy.

Ischaemic stroke (almost always ipsilateral to the operated artery)
   due to:
Embolism from the operation site during surgery
Embolism from the operation site after surgery
Carotid dissection
Perioperative carotid occlusion
Low cerebral blood flow during surgery
Perioperative systemic hypotension

Haemorrhagic stroke (almost always ipsilateral to the operated
   artery) due to:
Perioperative hypertension
Post-endarterectomy cerebral hyperperfusion

Death due to:
Stroke
Myocardial infarction
Pulmonary embolism
Rupture of arterial operation site

Myocardial infarction

Local complications
Nerve injury (vagal, hypoglossal, marginal mandibular branch
   of facial, spinal accessory, greater auricular, transverse
   cervical nerves)
Wound infection
Neck haematoma
Aneurysmal dilatation at operation site
Patch disruption and haemorrhage

Others
Deep venous thrombosis and pulmonary embolism
Transhemispheric cerebral oedema
Headache, focal motor seizures
Facial (parotid) pain
Pain at vein donor site after vein patch angioplasty

surgeons reporting their own results without the 'help' of any neurologists (Rothwell *et al.*, 1996b). Even though the size of the stroke risk depends on the study quoted, and this risk varies between different institutions, there is no doubt that there is a risk, which is realistically somewhere between 3 and 10%, depending on various factors (see Section 16.7.7).

There are several causes for perioperative stroke but these can be difficult to identify when the stroke occurs during general anaesthesia, and even afterwards when in an emergency situation in a surgical ward it may be impossible to get one or more of a neurologist, brain CT scan, carotid ultrasound and angiogram quickly enough to allow any useful corrective action (see below). Clinical details are often so poorly recorded that, in retrospect, it can be impossible to

establish a cause. Also, despite attempts to do so, it is difficult anyway to be sure whether *any* stroke, let alone a perioperative stroke, is due to embolism or low flow (see Section 6.5.5) (Steed *et al.*, 1982; Krul *et al.*, 1989; Riles *et al.*, 1994).

Embolism from the operation site

This is probably the most common cause of stroke *during* surgery. Atherothrombotic debris may be released whilst the carotid bifurcation is being mobilised, as the carotid clamps are applied, when any shunt is inserted and when the clamps are removed. Indeed, air bubbles or particulate emboli during surgery are very commonly detected by transcranial Doppler, although most seem to be of little clinical consequence (Spencer *et al.*, 1990; Gaunt *et al.*, 1994; Jansen *et al.*, 1994a). *Postoperative* stroke is usually due to: (i) embolism from residual but disrupted atheromatous plaque; (ii) thrombus forming on the endarterectomised surface or on suture lines, or more likely on a loose distal intimal flap where the lesion has been snapped off in the ICA and sometimes even in the external carotid artery; (iii) thrombus complicating damaged arterial wall as a result of the clamps; and (iv) thrombus complicating arterial dissection starting at a loose intimal flap of the ICA or as a result of shunt damage to the arterial wall.

> *Stroke complicating carotid endarterectomy is most commonly due to embolism from the operation site during or soon after surgery. Ischaemic stroke due to the interruption of carotid blood flow during surgery is less common and intracerebral haemorrhage is extremely rare.*

Acute internal carotid artery occlusion

This is caused by occlusive thrombosis or dissection as a result of the same mechanisms as those above. This may not cause stroke if the collateral blood supply is adequate.

Low-flow ischaemic stroke

This most commonly occurs if the ICA is clamped in the absence of adequate collateral blood flow and a shunt (see Section 16.7.2) and, occasionally, if there is severe systemic hypotension. Low-flow infarction contralateral to surgery can occur if the contralateral ICA is occluded.

Haemorrhagic stroke

This type of stroke is unusual. It occurs during surgery or up to about 1-week later. It may be due to the increase in perfusion pressure and cerebral blood flow that occurs after the removal of a severe ICA stenosis, particularly if cerebral autoregulation is defective as a consequence of a recent cerebral infarct. Antithrombotic drugs and uncontrolled hypertension may also play a part (Solomon *et al.*, 1986; Hafner *et al.*, 1987; Piepgras *et al.*, 1988; Jansen *et al.*, 1994b). Interestingly, transient cerebral hyperperfusion, even bilaterally, lasting some days is very common after carotid endarterectomy, particularly if the lesion was severely stenosing and cerebrovascular reserve was poor; this may be the cause of the occasional case of transhemispheric cerebral oedema as well as of intracerebral haemorrhage (Andrews *et al.*, 1987; Schroeder, 1988; Naylor *et al.*, 1993b; Chambers *et al.*, 1994).

Management

If cerebral ischaemia has not already been suspected by intraoperative monitoring, the first clue that a patient has had an intraoperative stroke is delay or failure to awaken from anaesthesia. It is vital to determine, within minutes if possible, whether the cause is thrombosis at the operation site, because this is amenable to correction. If transcranial Doppler monitoring has been used during the operation, a change in the MCA velocity signal may have suggested a problem at the endarterectomy site (any confusion with intracerebral haemorrhage distorting the MCA Doppler signal is most unlikely). Ideally, a rapid bedside duplex scan should be carried out and the neck immediately re-opened if ICA occlusion is confirmed or suspected. Passage of a Fogarty catheter, restoration of flow and correction of any technical fault which caused the thrombosis can, in some circumstances, be followed by complete neurological recovery. The later after operation a stroke occurs the less likely that return to theatre is either practical or effective, but how late is too late is a guess.

If the investigations show that the operated ICA is still patent then the next question to answer is whether the stroke is due to intracerebral haemorrhage. A brain CT scan is therefore needed and further management is the same as for spontaneous stroke (see Chapter 10).

16.7.4 Other complications (Table 16.12)

Death as a result of carotid surgery is very rare (perhaps about 1%) and is due to stroke, myocardial infarction or some other complication of the frequently associated coronary heart disease or, rarely, to pulmonary embolism.

Myocardial infarction during or in the days after surgery occurs in about 3% of patients, more often if there is symptomatic coronary heart disease, and particularly if myocardial infarction has occurred in the previous few months or the patient has unstable angina. Perioperative myocardial infarction can be painless so clues to the diagnosis are unexplained hypotension, tachycardia and arrhythmias. Congestive cardiac failure and cardiac arrhythmias are also occasional problems (Riles *et al.*, 1979; North American Symptomatic Carotid Endarterectomy Trial Collaborators, 1991; Urbinati *et al.*, 1994).

Nerve injuries, as a result of traction or pressure more often than transection, are common but not necessarily symptomatic, and usually of no long-term consequence. Depending on how hard one looks, a frequency of up to about 20% can be expected. Damage to the recurrent and superior laryngeal branches of the vagus, or more likely the vagus itself, causes change of voice quality, hoarseness, difficulty coughing and sometimes dyspnoea on exertion due to vocal cord paralysis. If a simultaneous or staged bilateral carotid endarterectomy is done and causes bilateral vocal cord paralysis then airway obstruction can occur. Hypoglossal nerve injury causes ipsilateral weakness of the tongue which can lead to temporary or even permanent dysarthria, difficulty with mastication or dysphagia. Again, bilateral damage causes much more serious speech and swallowing problems, and sometimes even upper airway obstruction. Damage to the marginal mandibular branch of the facial nerve causes rather trivial weakness at the corner of the mouth. Spinal accessory nerve injury is rare and causes pain and a feeling of stiffness in the shoulder and neck, along with weakness of the sternomastoid and trapezius muscles. A high incision can cut the greater auricular nerve to cause numbness over the ear lobe and angle of the jaw, which may persist. Damage to the transverse cervical nerves is almost inevitable and causes numbness around the scar area but this is seldom a problem. Clearly, permanent disability from a nerve injury is as bad as mild stroke and needs to be taken into account when considering the risks and benefits of surgery (Gutrecht & Jones, 1988; Maniglia & Han, 1991; Sweeney & Wilbourn, 1992).

> *Permanent disability from surgical injury to a nerve in the neck can be as bad or worse than many operative strokes, and must be taken into account when assessing the risk of surgery.*

Local wound complications include infection, haematoma or, rarely, major haemorrhage, due to leakage or rupture of the arteriotomy or patch, which can be life threatening if it causes tracheal compression, and aneurysm formation weeks or years later; all are rare (Graver & Mulcare, 1986). Although surgeons often notice the haemostatic defect caused by preoperative aspirin this probably does not increase the rate of re-operation for bleeding (Lindblad *et al.*, 1993).

Headache ipsilateral to the operation may occur and is perhaps related to transient cerebral hyperperfusion (see Section 16.7.3), uncontrolled hypertension or something akin to cluster headache due to subtle damage to the sympathetic plexus around the carotid artery (De Marinis *et al.*, 1991; Ille *et al.*, 1995). Very rarely, *focal motor seizures* occur as well as headache (Youkey *et al.*, 1984). Of course, seizures may occasionally complicate perioperative stroke, just like any other stroke (see Section 6.5.6).

Facial pain ipsilateral to surgery and related to eating is most unusual and may in some way be due to disturbance of the innervation of the parotid gland (Truax, 1989).

16.7.5 Evidence of benefit

As a result of the first reports of the large randomised trials in recently symptomatic patients with carotid distribution TIAs or mild ischaemic stroke with enough recovery to make the prevention of further stroke in the same vascular territory worthwhile, it is now quite clear that endarterectomy of *severe* ICA stenosis almost completely abolishes the risk of ischaemic stroke ipsilateral to the operated artery over the subsequent few years (European Carotid Surgery Trialists' Collaborative Group, 1991; North American Symptomatic Carotid Endarterectomy Trial Collaborators, 1991; Mayberg *et al.*, 1991). Indeed, the ipsilateral stroke risk becomes so low that presumably both embolic and low-flow strokes are being prevented (Fig. 16.21). Moreover, because most strokes in patients with recently symptomatic and severe carotid stenosis *are* ipsilateral and ischaemic, and taking account of the early risk of surgical death or stroke, the balance of surgical risk and long-term benefit is clearly in favour of surgery combined with best medical treatment compared with best medical treatment alone (i.e. treatment of hypertension, stopping smoking, antithrombotic drugs, etc.) (Fig. 16.22).

The higher ipsilateral ischaemic stroke risk in the no-surgery group in the North American Symptomatic Carotid Endarterectomy Trial (NASCET) compared with the European Carotid Surgery Trial (ECST) is mostly explained by the fact that a stenosis measured as 70% using the NASCET method is equivalent to a stenosis of about 82% using the ECST method (see Section 6.6.4); the 'severe stenosis' NASCET patients had, therefore, more severe stenosis than the 'severe stenosis' ECST patients. If one compares the ECST patients with 82–99% stenosis (by the ECST method) the results become much more like the NASCET results (Table 16.13), not surprisingly as the risk of ipsilateral ischaemic stroke increases with the amount of stenosis, particularly above about 80% (ECST method) (Fig. 16.23). In the NASCET, patients were randomised and operated sooner after the last ischaemic event than in the ECST, and stroke outcome was defined as symptoms lasting more than 24 hours rather than more than 7 days; adjustment for these differences would somewhat inflate the stroke risk in the no-surgery and surgery patients in the ECST.

From inspection of Fig. 16.21 it seems as though the risk of ipsilateral ischaemic stroke in the no-surgery patients flat-

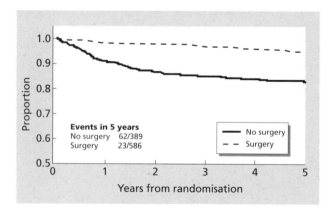

Figure 16.21 European Carotid Surgery Trial results in patients with 70–99% stenosis of a recently symptomatic ICA. The solid line indicates the survival free of ipsilateral ischaemic stroke lasting more than 7 days (censoring non-stroke death) in patients randomised to no-surgery and the dotted line in those surviving surgery without a stroke. (Unpublished information from the European Carotid Surgery Trialists' Collaborative Group, 1996, with permission.)

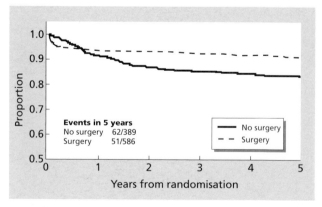

Figure 16.22 The overall results of the European Carotid Surgery Trial in patients with severe (70–99%) stenosis of a recently symptomatic ICA. The solid line indicates the survival free of stroke lasting more than 7 days, or any surgical death (censoring non-stroke deaths) in patients randomised to no-surgery and the dotted line in those randomised to surgery. (Unpublished information from the European Carotid Surgery Trialists' Collaborative Group, 1996, with permission.)

Table 16.13 Comparison of the ECST patients with recently symptomatic severe carotid artery stenosis (70–99% and 82–99% by ECST method) with patients in the NASCET with severe symptomatic stenosis (70–99% by NASCET method). (From unpublished ECST information; Barnett & Warlow, 1993.)

	ECST (70–99%) (%)	ECST (82–99%) (%)	NASCET (70–99%) (%)
Stroke or death within 30 days of surgery	6	4	6
Ipsilateral ischaemic stroke in 2 years in no-surgery patients	13	19	26

tens out after 2 or 3 years, so that the benefit of surgery will be felt mostly in that period, once the patient has survived the early risk of surgery. Where the curves cross (see Fig. 16.22) the risk of stroke is equal in surgical and non-surgical patients but, because the surgical strokes have occurred earlier and may have caused persisting disability, the surgery group is not really advantaged until about 6–12 months after this point, when the two groups have about the same total number of 'stroke–disability' years.

After succesful surgery for severe and recently symptomatic carotid stenosis the high risk of ischaemic stroke ipsilateral to the operated artery is almost completely removed. For patients with mild and moderate recently symptomatic stenosis the unoperated risk of stroke is not high enough to make the immediate risk of surgery worthwhile.

For patients with mild (0–29% ECST) stenosis of the symptomatic ICA, the unoperated ipsilateral ischaemic stroke rate is so low that the risk of surgery is not worthwhile because any potential benefit is cancelled out by the risk of surgery (European Carotid Surgery Trialists' Collaborative Group, 1991) (Fig. 16.24). Presumably, most of these patients have had TIAs due to intracranial small vessel disease and not embolism from the mildly diseased carotid bifurcation. Even in the moderate (30–69% ECST) stenosis patients the unoperated risk of stroke is still not, on average, high enough to make the risk of surgery worthwhile (European Carotid Surgery Trialists' Collaborative Group, 1996b) (Fig. 16.25). Whether moderate stenosis patients should be followed up with duplex in case the stenosis becomes greater than 70% is unclear; if the patient has no symptoms at that stage, the stenosis although severe is essentially asymptomatic when the advantage of surgery is much less than it is for severe symptomatic stenosis (see Section 16.12). It is probably preferable to ask the patient to return if there are any further cerebrovascular symptoms and if, *then*, the carotid stenosis is severe it would be reasonable to recommend carotid endarterectomy.

Attempts to show that carotid endarterectomy does not merely reduce stroke risk but improves cognitive performance, perhaps by increasing blood flow to the brain, or by

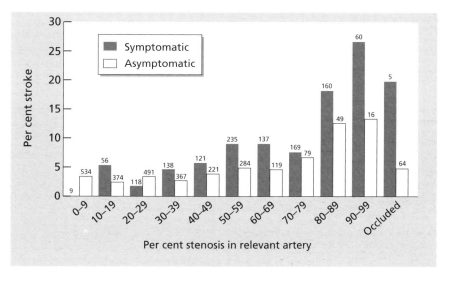

Figure 16.23 The actuarial 3-year risk of an ischaemic stroke in the distribution of a recently symptomatic carotid stenosis (solid bars), and of an asymptomatic carotid stenosis contralateral to a symptomatic ICA (open bars). The numbers on the bars refer to the number of patients in each stenosis group. The stenosis is measured using the ECST method. (Unpublished information from the European Carotid Surgery Trialists' Collaborative Group, 1996, with permission.)

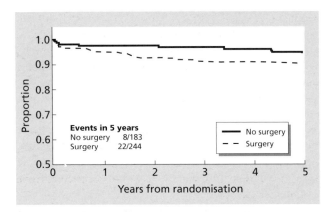

Figure 16.24 The overall results of the ECST in patients with mild (0–29%) stenosis of a recently symptomatic ICA. The solid line indicates survival free of stroke lasting more than 7 days, or any surgical death (censoring non-stroke deaths) in patients randomised to no-surgery and the dotted line to those randomised to surgery. (Unpublished information from the European Carotid Surgery Trialists' Collaborative Group, 1996, with permission.)

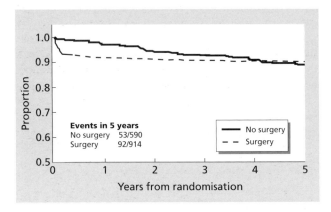

Figure 16.25 The overall results of the ECST in patients with moderate (30–69%) stenosis of a recently symptomatic ICA. The solid line indicates the survival free of stroke lasting more than 7 days, or any surgical death (censoring non-stroke deaths) in patients randomised to no-surgery and the dotted line to those randomised to surgery. (Unpublished information from the European Carotid Surgery Trialists' Collaborative Group, 1996, with permission.)

reducing the frequency of subclinical emboli which can often be demonstrated before but seldom after surgery (Markus *et al.*, 1995; van Zuilen *et al.*, 1995), have been beset with methodological difficulties and no conclusions can be drawn (Hemmingsen *et al.*, 1982; Parker *et al.*, 1983).

Attempts to correct surgically what are thought to be symptomatic carotid coils, kinks and fibromuscular dysplasia are not supported by any good evidence.

16.7.6 The selection of patients for carotid endarterectomy

Carotid endarterectomy is not only inconvenient and frightening for patients, but there are a number of usually trivial and temporary problems such as nerve palsies, and there is always some risk of stroke and even death. To these must be added the risk of, at present, the preceding angiography since most but not all surgeons feel it is unsafe to operate on the basis of ultrasonography alone (Strandness, 1995). However, the combination of MR angiography with good quality ultrasound or spiral CT may soon get rid of the need for angiography in most, if not all, cases (see Section 6.6.4). Clearly, several essential conditions must be fulfilled before even recommending cerebral angiography, let alone surgery (Table 16.14).

We are not dealing with a simple, cheap, safe and widely available treatment such as aspirin and it is therefore essential that safe surgery is offered to patients who have the most to gain (i.e. those at highest risk of ipsilateral ischaemic stroke) and who are most likely to survive to enjoy that gain for a number of years. For example, if the combined angiographic and surgical risk of stroke is 10%, if the unoperated risk of stroke is 20% after 2 years, and if successful surgery reduces this risk of stroke to zero, then doing 10 operations would cause one stroke, avoid two and the net gain would be one stroke avoided. This kind of very approximate calcula-

Table 16.14 Conditions to be fulfilled before cerebral angiography with a view to selecting patients for carotid endarterectomy.

---

1 A patient with one or more carotid distribution* TIAs or non-disabling ischaemic strokes in the previous few months and who has, therefore, everything or almost everything to lose from a major hemisphere stroke. Vascular risk factors should be under control (see Section 16.3) and most patients should be taking antiplatelet therapy (see Section 16.4)

2 Duplex sonography shows severe carotid bifurcation disease in the symptomatic artery (likely to be at least 70% stenosis by ECST measurement on a subsequent angiogram)

3 The patient is prepared to consider and accept the early risk and inconvenience of angiography and surgery for long-term benefit

4 The patient is fit for surgery: no recent myocardial infarction; angina controlled; no cardiac failure; hypertension controlled; reasonable lung function; and biologically not too aged

5 The institution has an experienced cerebral angiography team with a low complication rate, preferably kept under prospective and independent audit

6 The institution has an experienced surgical and anaesthetic team with a low surgical complication rate, preferably kept under prospective and independent audit

---

* For distinction between carotid and vertebrobasilar distribution attacks, see Table 4.12.

tion can be done for various surgical and angiographic risks, for various survival periods and for various stroke risks without surgery (Table 16.15). Clearly, to reduce the number of patients that have to be operated on to prevent one having a stroke, and therefore to maximise cost-effectiveness, we need to know who is at highest risk of surgical stroke, and who will survive to be at high risk of ipsilateral ischaemic stroke if surgery is not done; after all, surgery is not cheap, the charges in 1985 being US$4000 and $6000 in a private and University Hospital, respectively (Green & McNamara, 1987) and the cost in Sweden in 1991 was estimated at US$11 602 (Asplund et al., 1993).

16.7.7 Who is at high (or low) risk of surgery?

Perioperative stroke risk (and the risk of the few non-stroke deaths which are usually cardiac in origin) is presumably related to: (i) the skill of the surgeon; (ii) the skill of the anaesthetist; (iii) aspects of the surgical technique; (iv) patient demographic factors; (v) co-existing pathology, such as coronary heart disease; (vi) the state of the brain and any ischaemic damage; and (vii) the state of the arterial supply to the brain. Although surgical and anaesthetic skill must be important, the risk of surgery is not necessarily related to the

number of operations done. In any event, the risk is difficult to quantify accurately, particularly when the risk of surgical stroke is so low and when most surgeons operate on a relatively small number of patients every year. A surgeon doing as many as one operation per week might not expect to have more than five stroke complications in 2 years, i.e. 5%, but with a 95% confidence interval of about 2–11% so that in the next 2 years his or her complication rate might, just by chance alone, be as good as 2% or as bad as 11%. Variation in surgical technique—the use of shunts, patches, etc.—are all of uncertain benefit with respect to perioperative stroke risk (see Section 16.7.2).

Very few serious attempts have been made to sort out which patient-related factors affect perioperative stroke risk and so help guide selection of patients for surgery (Sundt et al., 1975; McCrory et al., 1993; Riles et al., 1994). In general, the highest surgical risk is predicted by female sex, hypertension, infarct on CT, ischaemia of the brain rather than the eye and contralateral ICA occlusion (Fig. 16.26). Unfortunately, as is so often the case in preventive medicine (see Section 18.4), most events occur in patients at medium rather than high risk (of perioperative stroke), so that by avoiding operating on the highest surgical risk patients one would not have a large impact on overall surgical risk (McCrory et al., 1993). In clinical practice it is, therefore, not really possible to know exactly whether an individual patient is at particularly high or at particularly low risk of perioperative stroke or death.

> *Perioperative stroke risk depends not just on the skill of the surgeon and anaesthetist, but also on various patient-related factors such as age, female sex, contralateral internal carotid occlusion and hypertension.*

Recent myocardial infarction, or current unstable angina, are both thought to increase the risk of perioperative cardiac complications (see Section 16.7.4). But, if coronary artery bypass surgery is deemed necessary for *symptomatic* coronary heart disease it is profoundly unclear whether this should be done before carotid endarterectomy (and risk a stroke during the procedure), after carotid endarterectomy (and risk cardiac complications during carotid endarterectomy) or simultaneously under the same general anaesthetic (Graor & Hertzer, 1988; Akins, 1995; Davenport et al., 1995). The risk of the last option may be unacceptable, although a small quasi-randomised trial suggests otherwise (Hertzer et al., 1989). Which of the first two options to choose depends on the individual patient and close collaboration between neurologist, cardiologist and surgeon; there is no clear guidance from randomised trials.

Table 16.15 The approximate number of patients with severe and recently symptomatic carotid stenosis who must have a carotid endarterectomy to avoid one having a stroke depends on the angiographic (see Section 6.6.4) and surgical risk, the duration of survival and the stroke rate without surgery (assuming all strokes are abolished after the patient survives surgery without a stroke).

Surgical and angiographic stroke risk (%)	Survival (years)				
	1	2	3	4	
5	10	4	2	2	If unoperated,
10	20	5	3	2	stroke risk 15%/year
15		7	3	2	
20		10	4	2	
5	20	7	4	3	If unoperated,
10		10	5	3	stroke risk 10%/year
15		20	7	4	
20			10	5	
5		20	10	7	If unoperated,
10			20	10	stroke risk 5%/year
15				20	

Note: the assumption that unoperated stroke risk remains constant with time may not be correct. At present, the flattening of the survival free of ipsilateral ischaemic stroke curve in Fig. 16.21 suggests that annual stroke risk declines so that the 'cost-effectiveness' of surgery may not increase as much as the table indicates in the third and fourth postoperative years.

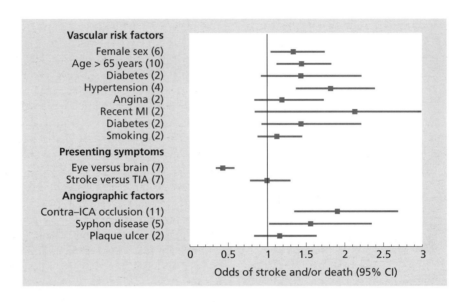

Figure 16.26 Risk factors for operative stroke derived from a systematic review of the literature. The numbers in brackets refer to the number of relevant studies identified. The solid black square indicates the odds ratio and the horizontal line the 95% confidence interval. An odds ratio greater than 1 indicates an increased risk of operative stroke in the presence of that risk factor. The increased risk is statistically significant ($P < 0.05$) if the confidence interval does not cross the vertical line. MI, myocardial infarction. (From P. Rothwell, unpublished observations.)

It is uncertain whether carotid endarterectomy should precede, follow or be combined with coronary artery bypass surgery in patients who have both cerebrovascular and cardiac symptoms severe enough to require surgery.

It is completely impossible to compare surgical morbidity between surgeons or institutions, or in the same place at different times, or before and after the introduction of a particular technique, without adjusting for case mix: in other words, for the patient's inherent surgical risk. In addition, large enough numbers have to be collected to avoid random error (Rothwell *et al.*, 1996b). This level of sophistication has never been achieved (Michaels, 1988; Brook *et al.*, 1990). It is clearly important, however, to know the risk of surgery in one's own hospital (*and* of any preceding angiography; see Section 6.6.4) in the sort of patients that are usually operated on; risks reported in the literature are not generalisable to one's own institution and anyway tend to be lower than the real risk in the community at large (Hsia *et al.*, 1992).

Valid comparison of surgical stroke risk between different surgeons or institutions, or in the same place at different times, is impossible without both adjustment for case mix and several hundred patients in each comparison period. Such an ideal has never been, and may never be, achieved.

If a patient has symptoms referable to *both* severely stenosed ICAs, requiring, therefore, a bilateral carotid endarterectomy, it is probably safer to do the operations a few weeks apart rather than under the same anaesthetic. This is partly because of the dangers of bilateral hypoglossal or vagal nerve damage (see Section 16.7.4).

Even before a staged second carotid endarterectomy it is always wise to inspect the tongue and vocal cords to ensure there has been no subclinical unilateral nerve damage from the first operation because, if so, the second operation should be postponed.

16.7.8 Who will survive to be at high (or low) risk of ipsilateral ischaemic stroke without surgery?

Both the ECST and NASCET have shown very clearly how important the severity of carotid stenosis ipsilateral to the cerebral or ocular symptoms is in the prediction of ischaemic stroke in the same arterial distribution (see Fig. 16.23). Furthermore, even within the category of 'severe' stenosis there is increasing risk with worsening stenosis, and angiographically demonstrated 'ulceration' or 'irregularity' increases the risk even more; other angiographic features of the symptomatic and asymptomatic ICA do not improve prediction further, and there is uncertainty about the influence of various plaque characteristics seen on ultrasound (Barnett & Meldrum, 1994; Rothwell *et al.*, 1995). However, not *all* patients with even extremely severe symptomatic stenosis go on to have an ipsilateral ischaemic stroke and it is unclear what additional factors place some patients at particularly high risk; these factors will not necessarily be the same as those derived from a general TIA population (see Section 16.1.1), although we would not be surprised if they were similar (i.e. increasing risk with age, frequency of TIAs, claudication and brain rather than eye attacks) (North American Symptomatic Carotid Endarterectomy Trial Collaborators, 1991; Streifler et al., 1995).

The risk of ischaemic stroke ipsilateral to symptomatic carotid stenosis increases as the stenosis becomes more severe, particularly when it is more than about 80% of the vessel diameter, whereas the risk of perioperative stroke is largely independent of the amount of stenosis. Therefore, the more severe the stenosis, the more a patient has to gain from successful carotid endarterectomy. In practice, the risk of surgery is unacceptable if the stenosis is less than about 70–80%, but the exact breakeven point must depend on other factors which predict stroke without surgery, such as ischaemia in the brain rather than in the eye and being male rather than female.

Some argue that almost everyone with severe (>70% ECST) stenosis is at a high enough risk to warrant surgery because as a group they have, on average, a 20% ipsilateral ischaemic stroke risk at about 2 years, and if the risk of surgery could be reduced to 5% then one would have to operate on only seven patients to avoid one having a stroke (Table 16.15). But, within this 'on-average' high-risk group there must be some patients whose estimated risk (on the basis of prognostic models) of ipsilateral ischaemic stroke is so low that surgery is not worthwhile, even though the stenosis is severe, and the challenge is to identify them reliably so they can be spared what for them would turn out to be unecessary surgery (Rothwell, 1995).

It is conceivable that patients with poor cerebral reactivity are at particularly high risk of low-flow strokes and it seems that this impairment can be corrected by carotid endarterectomy (Bishop et al., 1987; Schroeder, 1988; Naylor et al., 1993a; Hartl et al., 1994). However, we do not know what proportion of strokes in severe carotid stenosis patients are actually due to low flow and what proportion to embolism, and whether correcting impaired cerebral reactivity will indeed reduce ipsilateral ischaemic stroke risk anymore than in those without such an impairment.

A considerable difficulty is that many of the predictive factors for ipsilateral ischaemic stroke in an unoperated patient are likely to be similar to those that predict a high risk of stroke as a consequence of surgery. It may be, of course, that

one might be prepared to accept an apparently rather high risk of surgery (say because of an occluded contralateral ICA) if the patient's risk without surgery was even higher than usual. To confuse matters further one also has to avoid offering surgery to patients unlikely to survive long enough to enjoy any benefit of stroke prevention and therefore to make the surgical risks worthwhile; clearly, that would include patients with advanced cancer, but most non-stroke deaths in the first year after TIA are due to coronary heart disease which are probably predicted by factors which are very similar to those factors that predict stroke (i.e. age, claudication, etc.) (Hankey et al., 1992).

An occasional patient with a lacunar ischaemic stroke or TIA may have severe carotid stenosis (see Section 6.3) and the question then arises whether the stenosis is 'symptomatic' (i.e. small vessel occlusion has, unusually, been caused by embolism or low flow) or 'asymptomatic' (i.e. the stenosis is a coincidental bystander and the cerebral ischaemia was really due to intracranial small vessel disease). Unfortunately, but not surprisingly, the number of such patients in the randomised trials is so small that it is not certain what effect surgery has (Boiten et al., 1996). Under the circumstances we suspect that most people would recommend surgery, particularly if the stenosis is *very* severe (>90%), because even if the artery was asymptomatic at least with this degree of stenosis there is some evidence that the risk of ipsilateral ischaemic stroke is high enough to justify the risk of surgery (see Section 16.12.2). The same arguments probably apply if there is a major co-existing source of embolism from the heart (such as non-rheumatic atrial fibrillation), in which case the patient may be reasonably anticoagulated as well as being offered surgery (see also Section 6.7.3).

16.7.9 Balancing competing risks

Ideally, one would like to know, for an individual patient, their risk of ipsilateral ischaemic stroke over the next few years, their risk of carotid endarterectomy and their chance of surviving long enough to make the risk of surgery worthwhile in the sense of enjoying a stroke-free life. At present, we certainly do not know these risks for individuals and only have an approximate idea what they may be in groups of individuals. Another difficulty is that the risk of stroke declines with time after a TIA (see Section 16.1.1) so if diagnosis is delayed by several months, then the risk of surgery may no longer be justifiable; exactly how many months delay is allowable in this situation is uncertain and one can but recommend that patients be investigated quickly and efficiently to minimise the problem. Resolving all these uncertainties will be difficult and perhaps impossible because we are dealing with events which may be unpredictable and also with prognostic factors which may be the same for two or even all three of the events of interest (e.g. age and severity of symptomatic carotid stenosis are certainly risk factors for stroke in unoperated patients and perhaps also for coronary events). Also, even if we can direct safe surgery to patients at highest unoperated stroke risk, we may have to face the prevention paradox that most strokes occur in those at moderate rather than in those at highest risk (see Table 18.4d).

> *In severe symptomatic carotid stenosis patients the risk of stroke is highest within weeks or months of the most recent cerebrovascular event. It follows, therefore, that the benefit of surgery is maximised if it is done quickly after patients present to medical attention.*

Deciding who should have surgery is difficult enough, but explaining the various competing risks to a worried patient and how taking an early risk might prevent later stroke is much more difficult. The way in which this is done will make a great difference as to how a patient reacts. A risk reduction of 50% (i.e. from 20 to 10% stroke risk) is more likely to lead to operative consent than the equivalent absolute risk reduction of 10% or the statement that 'operating on 10 patients like you will prevent one having a stroke'. One cannot assume that an apparently rational clinical decision will reflect what a patient wants done.

16.8 Carotid angioplasty

If endarterectomy of a severe symptomatic carotid stenosis more or less abolishes the risk of ipsilateral ischaemic stroke, then other methods to remove the lesion might, in theory, have the same effect. Clearly, percutaneous transluminal balloon angioplasty is one such potential method (Brown, 1992) (Fig. 16.27). At present, however, it is not clear how risky the procedure is because not very many patients have been reported (Brown *et al.*, 1990; Porta *et al.*, 1991). The major concerns are: (i) the angioplasty balloon dislodges atherothrombotic debris to embolise to the brain or eye; (ii) the procedure causes arterial wall dissection at the time or afterwards; (iii) thrombus forms on the stretched and so damaged plaque, and then embolises; (iv) the angioplasty balloon obstructs carotid blood flow for long enough to cause low-flow ischaemic stroke; (v) dilatation of the balloon causes bradycardia or hypotension due to carotid sinus stimulation; (vi) overdistention of the arterial wall causes aneurysm formation and even arterial rupture; and (vii) that angioplasty precipitates vasospasm. Even if the immediate risk of angioplasty turns out to be acceptable there is no reliable information on the long-term outcome, particularly with respect to the risk of ischaemic stroke in the distribution of the relevant ICA, because no randomised trials are yet complete. Of course, angioplasty should be less unpleasant and is less invasive than carotid endarterectomy, and it is most unlikely to cause nerve injuries, wound infection, venous thromboembolism or myocardial infarction. So, if the benefits do turn out to be greater than the risks, it may be applicable not just to patients presently eligible for carotid endarterectomy but also to those who are unfit for surgery because of coronary heart disease or other problems, and also for stenoses too distal for direct surgery. At present, angioplasty should only be undertaken in the context of RCTs.

> *At present, there is no evidence to support the use of carotid angioplasty outside well-conducted randomised trials.*

16.9 Extra-to-intracranial bypass surgery

About 10% of patients with carotid TIA or mild ischaemic stroke have occlusion of the ICA, or stenosis of the ICA well distal to the bifurcation, or MCA occlusion or stenosis, all of which are inoperable, or out of reach of the vascular surgeon, if not of the angioplasty enthusiast's balloon. These lesions can all be bypassed by anastomosing a branch of the external carotid artery (usually the superficial temporal) via a burr hole to a cortical branch of the MCA. This 'surgical collateral' was reckoned to improve the cerebral blood supply to the MCA bed distal to the inoperable or inaccessible stenosis or occlusion and so reduce the risk of stroke, as well as to reduce the severity of any stroke that did occur. However, there are several reasons why the procedure might not work:

1 the artery feeding the anastomosis can take months to dilate into an effective collateral channel;

2 many patients have good collateral flow already from orbital collaterals or the circle of Willis;

3 not all strokes distal to ICA/MCA occlusion or inaccessible stenosis are due to low flow (see Section 6.2.3);

4 the risk of stroke in patients with ICA occlusion is not that high (about 7%/year) and, anyway, not all of these strokes are ipsilateral to the occlusion;

5 neither resting cerebral blood flow nor cerebral reactivity are necessarily depressed in these patients;

6 the risk of surgery may outweigh the benefit, if any (Latchaw *et al.*, 1979; Hankey & Warlow, 1991; Karnik *et al.*, 1992).

The risk–benefit relationship has been evaluated in only one randomised trial but this was large enough to demonstrate

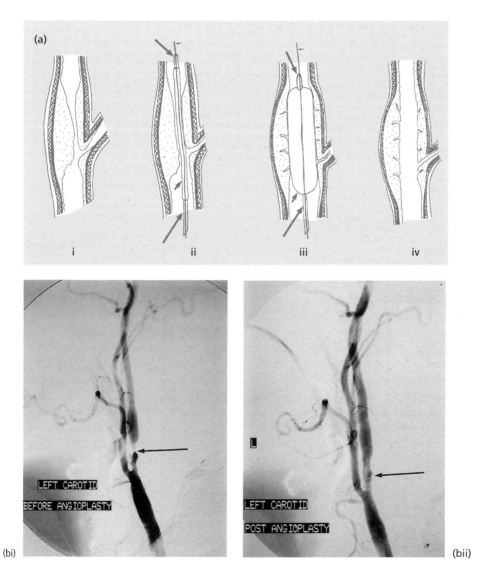

Figure 16.27 Percutaneous transluminal balloon angioplasty of the carotid artery. (a) Diagram to show the principle of angioplasty: (i) the carotid bifurcation with a large atherothrombotic stenosis; (ii) the guidewire (short arrow) with the (deflated—thick arrow) balloon catheter (long arrows) is passed across the stenosis; (iii) the balloon is inflated (in some systems the guidewire may be withdrawn prior to inflation, in others left in) and the plaque is pushed outwards so stretching the arterial wall and cracking the plaque; (iv) after the balloon is deflated and removed the lumen has been widened, the arterial wall remains stretched and the plaque remains. (b) Carotid angiogram to show stenosis (i) before (arrow) and (ii) after (arrow) angioplasty; the tight stenosis (arrow) has been converted to a more normal (looking) lumen.

reasonably conclusively that, in general, there was no benefit from extra-to-intracranial bypass (EC–IC Bypass Study Group, 1985; Haynes *et al.*, 1987). However, it has been argued that patients with impaired cerebrovascular reactivity were not identifiable in the whole extra-to-intracranial study population and perhaps it is *these* patients who *might* be benefited by surgery (Warlow, 1986). But, even though surgery may reverse such impaired reactivity, to show whether stroke is prevented would require another randomised trial in this specific subgroup (Karnik *et al.*, 1992).

At present, therefore, extra-to-intracranial bypass surgery can not be recommended as a routine method of stroke prevention.

16.10 Surgery and angioplasty for vertebrobasilar ischaemia

There is no good evidence (i.e. there are no randomised trials) that surgery improves the prognosis for patients with vertebrobasilar TIAs or ischaemic strokes. There is, however, no shortage of ingenious, if technically demanding, techniques which are far from risk free: (i) endarterectomy of severe carotid stenosis to improve collateral blood flow, via the circle of Willis, to the basilar artery distal to severe vertebral or basilar artery stenosis or occlusion; (ii) resection and anastomosis, resection and reimplantation, bypass or endarterectomy of proximal vertebral artery stenosis; (iii) release of the vertebral artery from compressive fibrous bands or osteophytes; and (iv) various extra-to-intracranial procedures to bypass vertebral artery stenosis or occlusion (Thevenet & Ruotolo, 1984; Diaz *et al.*, 1984; Harward *et al.*, 1984; Hopkins *et al.*, 1987; Spetzler *et al.*, 1987). Angioplasty of vertebral and even basilar artery stenosis has also been tried but there is no good evidence that the risks outweigh the benefits, if any.

Subclavian (and *innominate*) *steal*, although commonly detected with ultrasonography, very rarely causes neurological symptoms and does not seem to lead on to ischaemic stroke. However, incapacitatingly frequent vertebrobasilar TIAs in the presence of demonstrated unilateral or bilateral retrograde vertebral artery flow distal to severe subclavian or innominate disease may sometimes be relieved by: (i) endarterectomy or angioplasty of the subclavian artery; (ii) carotid to subclavian or femoral to subclavian bypass; (iii) transposition of the subclavian artery to the CCA; (iv) transposition of the vertebral artery to the CCA; and (v) axillary-to-axillary artery bypass grafting. All these procedures carry a risk and it is not clear which is the most sensible. Irrespective of the neurological situation, some kind of vascular surgical procedure may be needed if the hand and arm become ischaemic distal to subclavian or innominate artery disease (see Section 6.6.4) (Fields & Lemak, 1972; Bohmfalk *et al.*, 1979; Grosveld *et al.*, 1988; Hennerici *et al.*, 1988).

16.11 Other surgical procedures

Aortic arch atheroma is now increasingly diagnosed by transoesophageal echocardiography in patients with TIAs or ischaemic stroke but there seem to be no surgical, or indeed medical, treatment options over and above controlling vascular risk factors (see Section 16.3) and using antiplatelet drugs (see Section 16.4), or anticoagulants perhaps (see Section 16.5).

Innominate or *proximal CCA stenosis* or *occlusion* is quite often seen on angiograms in symptomatic patients but, unless very severe, does not influence the decision about endarterectomy for any ICA stenosis. Although it is possible to bypass such lesions it is highly doubtful whether this reduces the risk of stroke unless, perhaps, several major neck vessels are involved and the patient has low-flow cerebral or ocular symptoms (see Section 6.5.5); this very rare situation can be due to atheroma, Takayasu's disease or aortic dissection. Clearly, close consultation between neurologists and vascular surgeons is needed to sort out, on an individual patient basis, what to do for the best.

16.12 Endarterectomy for asymptomatic carotid stenosis

As far as one can tell, less than 20% of ischaemic stroke patients have had any preceding TIAs even when the stroke is likely to have been due to the embolic or low-flow consequences of severe carotid stenosis, i.e. TACIs or PACIs (see Table 6.2). Therefore, a large proportion of such strokes are unheralded by TIAs and, until the moment of stroke, any stenosis was 'asymptomatic'. If these asymptomatic stenoses could be detected before the stroke, then might not unheralded (by TIA) stroke be preventable by carotid endarterectomy, particularly as surgery is beneficial in patients whose stenoses have revealed themselves by becoming 'symptomatic' with TIAs (see Section 16.7)?

It is not difficult to identify asymptomatic carotid stenosis, and to quantify its extent by duplex sonography, in several categories of patient: (i) during screening programmes of normal people when a carotid bruit is heard and/or duplex is being used routinely; (ii) as a result of hearing a carotid bruit or doing a duplex examination during the course of working up patients with non-cerebral symptoms, particularly if they are presenting with vascular disease below the neck (angina, claudication, etc.); (iii) when bilateral carotid imaging is done in patients with unilateral carotid symptoms; and (iv) when patients are being worked up for major surgery below the neck and a carotid bruit is heard or a duplex ultrasound reveals carotid stenosis. One might also argue that a carotid stenosis is, or might well be, 'asymptomatic' in a patient with a lacunar TIA or ischaemic stroke (see Section 6.7.2), or in a fibrillating ischaemic stroke or TIA patient (see Section 6.7.3), even if the cerebral ischaemia was in the distribution of the stenosed artery. However, having identified asymptomatic carotid stenosis, several questions arise.

1 What is the risk of operating on it?
2 What is the risk (of stroke) if the stenosis is left unoperated?
3 Does surgery reduce any risk of stroke?
4 What is the balance of surgical risk versus long-term benefit from surgery, if any?

16.12.1 The risk of carotid endarterectomy for asymptomatic carotid stenosis

As in symptomatic carotid stenosis, there are a large number of case series with very different surgical risks of stroke and death depending on: (i) whether all strokes or only some strokes are included; (ii) the definition of stroke; (iii) the accuracy of stroke diagnosis; (iv) whether the study is prospective or retrospective; and (v), importantly, the type of patient (rather than type of lesion) that is being considered. Although surgical risk is about 50% of that for symptomatic carotid stenosis (Rothwell *et al.*, 1996a), there is still *some* risk and it may not necessarily be very low in, e.g. patients with angina whose carotid stenosis was discovered in preparation for coronary artery surgery, or in patients who have already had an endarterectomy on one side and are at risk of bilateral vagal or hypoglossal nerve palsies if both sides are operated on (see Section 16.7.4). As for symptomatic stenosis, the risk of surgery can not be generalised from the literature to a particular institution, and this risk must be known locally. In competent institutions, the risk of stroke and/or death within 30 days of surgery is probably about 5%, but it might well be lower in patients with no cardiac or respiratory symptoms, or higher in patients with, e.g. angina and contralateral carotid occlusion (Towne *et al.*, 1990).

16.12.2 The prognosis of asymptomatic carotid stenosis

There have not been many prospective studies of large numbers of patients in which all or most of them did not have a carotid endarterectomy at some stage during follow-up, and which used actuarial analysis stratified by degree of stenosis at study entry. In particular, one needs to know the risk of ischaemic stroke ipsilateral to the asymptomatic stenosis since, by analogy with symptomatic stenosis, endarterectomy is unlikely to reduce the risk of any other type or distribution of stroke. In fact, it seems that the absolute risk of stroke is quite low, considerably lower than in symptomatic stenosis: for *severe* asymptomatic stenosis, i.e. a stenosis of at least 70% of the arterial lumen, the annual risk of any stroke is perhaps 3%/year, and of ipsilateral ischaemic stroke about 2%/year (Bogousslavsky *et al.*, 1986; Meissner *et al.*, 1987; Norris *et al.*, 1991; Hobson *et al.*, 1993; European Carotid Surgery Trialists' Collaborative Group, 1995) (see Table 18.7b). With extreme (>90%) stenosis there is some evidence that the risk of ipsilateral ischaemic stroke becomes rather more significant, but this information is based on small numbers (see Fig. 16.23). There is no useful information whether other factors such as sex, age, etc., influence

these risks. It is in fact surprising how low the reported risk of ipsilateral ischaemic stroke seems to be, but perhaps even severely stenosed arteries are relatively benign unless either the atherothrombotic lesion breaks down and symptomatic embolisation occurs, or a fall in systemic blood pressure causes focal cerebral ischaemia; interestingly, asymptomatic stenosis is less likely than symptomatic stenosis to be associated with Doppler-detected 'embolic' signals in the MCA (Markus *et al.*, 1995).

The available studies also emphasise that the risk of coronary as well as cerebrovascular events increases with the severity of asymptomatic carotid stenosis. Therefore, a patient at risk of stroke is quite likely to die a cardiac death, possibly before the benefit (if any) of carotid endarterectomy has had time to occur (Chimowitz *et al.*, 1994). In patients having major surgery below the neck, asymptomatic carotid stenosis has little impact, if any, on the stroke risk (see Section 7.14) (Ivey *et al.*, 1984; Yatsu & Fields, 1985).

16.12.3 Surgical benefit

By extrapolating from the trials in symptomatic carotid stenosis (see Section 16.7.5) one would expect endarterectomy of severe asymptomatic stenosis to reduce the risk of ischaemic stroke ipsilateral to the operation. Until recently there was no evidence from randomised trials that this expectation was correct, perhaps because the trials were too small and because the unoperated stroke risk was so low (Clagett *et al.*, 1984; CASANOVA Study Group, 1991; Mayo Asymptomatic Carotid Endarterectomy Study Group, 1992; Hobson *et al.*, 1993). Including TIAs in any analysis is unhelpful because these events are, by definition, trivial in comparison with the risk of surgical stroke and, in any event, immediately move the patient into the symptomatic stenosis category where surgery becomes worthwhile. Surgery for severe asymptomatic carotid stenosis must be shown to reduce the risk of *stroke*, accepting that many severe stenoses that *become* symptomatic should be operated on. To some extent the Asymptomatic Carotid Artherosclerosis Study has now achieved this, but the overall risk of stroke in those randomised to no-surgery was so low (11.0% at 5 years) that even the considerable relative reduction in risk in those randomised to surgery preceded by angiography (to 5.1% at 5 years) conferred a mere 5.9% absolute benefit; in other words, about 85 patients must be operated on to prevent one having a stroke in the next year (Asymptomatic Carotid Artherosclerosis Group, 1995). This is hardly cost-effective medicine, particularly because the risk of a serious cardiac event is considerably higher than the risk of stroke (see above) and many of the strokes prevented are relatively mild. To prevent one *disabling* stroke in 1 year, about 170 patients must be submitted to the anxiety, discomfort, risk and costs of angiography and surgery.

16.12.4 The balance of surgical risk and benefit

Given the uncertain surgical risk (which to some extent must depend on the type of patient under consideration), and what appears to be a remarkably good prognosis for stroke in unoperated patients (even when they have major surgery below the neck), there is clearly no reason to recommend routine carotid endarterectomy for asymptomatic stenosis. Possible exceptions are patients with extreme stenosis who may have a higher unoperated ipsilateral ischaemic stroke risk then the average 2%/year of severe stenosis patients in general, and the very rare patient with an unbearable self-audible bruit due to the stenosis. Under these circumstances, it is highly unlikely that screening for asymptomatic stenosis is worthwhile, either for the individual or in the context of public health programmes to reduce stroke incidence (see Section 18.4).

Although carotid endarterectomy about halves the risk of stroke in patients with severe asymptomatic stenosis, the absolute risk of stroke is usually so low in these patients that surgery is hardly ever worthwhile. Rare exceptions might be patients with extremely severe stenosis and those with an unbearable self-audible bruit as a result of the stenosis.

References

Abraham J, Shetty G, Jose CJ (1971). Strokes in the young. *Stroke* 2: 258–67.

Adams HP, Byington RP, Hoen H, Dempsey R, Furberg CD (1995). Effect of cholesterol lowering medications on progression of mild atherosclerotic lesions of the carotid arteries and on the risk of stroke. *Cerebrovasc Dis* 5: 171–7.

Akins CW (1995). The case for concomitant carotid and coronary artery surgery. *Br Heart J* 74: 97–8.

Alter M, Friday G, Lai SM, O'Connell J, Sobel E (1994). Hypertension and risk of stroke recurrence. *Stroke* 25: 1605–10.

Andrews BT, Levy ML, Dillon W, Weinstein PR (1987). Unilateral normal perfusion pressure breakthrough after carotid endarterectomy: case report. *Neurosurgery* 21: 568–71.

Antiplatelet Trialists' Collaboration (1994). Collaborative overview of randomised trials of antiplatelet therapy. I. Prevention of death, myocardial infarction, and stroke by prolonged antiplatelet therapy in various categories of patients.

Br Med J 308: 81–106.

Antman EM, Lau J, Kupelnick B, Mosteller F, Chalmers TC (1992). A comparison of results of meta-analyses of randomised control trials and recommendations of clinical experts. Treatments for myocardial infarction. *J Am Med Assoc* 268(2): 240–8.

Arroll B, Beaglehole R (1995). Salt restriction and physical activity in treated hypertensives. *N Z Med J* 108: 266–8.

ASPECT Research Group (1994). Effect of long term oral anticoagulant treatment on mortality and cardiovascular morbidity after myocardial infarction. *Lancet* 343: 499–503.

Asplund K, Marke L-A, Terent A, Gustafsson C, Wester PO (1993). Costs and gains in stroke prevention: European perspective. *Cerebrovasc Dis* 3: 34–42.

Asymptomatic Carotid Atherosclerosis Group (1995). Carotid endarterectomy for patients with asymptomatic internal carotid artery stenosis. *J Am Med Assoc* 273: 1421–8.

Atrial Fibrillation Investigators (1994). Risk factors for stroke and efficacy of antithrombotic therapy in atrial fibrillation. Analysis of pooled data from five randomised controlled trials. *Arch Intern Med* 154: 1449–57.

Awad IA, Little JR (1989). Patch angioplasty in carotid endarterectomy: advantages, concerns and controversies. *Stroke* 20: 417–22.

Bamford J, Sandercock P, Jones L, Warlow C (1987). The natural history of lacunar infarction: the Oxfordshire Community Stroke Project. *Stroke* 18: 545–51.

Bamford J, Sandercock P, Dennis M, Burn J, Warlow C (1990). A prospective study of acute cerebrovascular disease in the community: the Oxfordshire Community Stroke Project— 1981–1986. Incidence, case fatality rates and overall outcome at one year of cerebral infarction, primary intracerebral haemorrhage and subarachnoid haemorrhage. *J Neurol Neurosurg Psychiatr* 53: 16–22.

Bamford J, Sandercock P, Dennis M, Burn J, Warlow C (1991). Classification and natural history of clinically identifiable subtypes of cerebral infarction. *Lancet* 337: 1521–6.

Barnett HJM, Meldrum H (1994). Status of carotid endarterectomy. *Curr Opin Neurol* 7: 54–9.

Barnett HJM, Warlow CP (1993). Carotid endarterectomy and the measurement of stenosis. *Stroke* 24: 1281–4.

Barnett HJM, Plum F, Walton JN (1984). Carotid endarterectomy —an expression of concern. *Stroke* 15: 941–3.

Bishop CCR, Butler L, Hunt T, Burnand KG, Browse NL (1987). Effect of carotid endarterectomy on cerebral blood flow and its response to hypercapnia. *Br J Surg* 74: 994–6.

Bogousslavsky J, Despland P-A, Regli F (1986). Asymptomatic tight stenosis of the internal carotid artery: long-term prognosis. *Neurology* 36: 861–3.

Bohmfalk GL, Story JL, Brown WE, Marlin AE (1979). Subclavian steal syndrome. Part I: proximal vertebral to common carotid artery transposition in three patients, and historical review. *J Neurosurg* 51: 628–40.

Boiten J, Lodder J (1993). Prognosis for survival, handicap and recurrence of stroke in lacunar and superficial infarction. *Cerebrovasc Dis* 3: 221–6.

Boiten J, Rothwell PM, Slattery J, Warlow CP, for the European Carotid Surgery Trialists' Collaborative Group (1996). Lacunar stroke in the European Carotid Surgery Trial: risk factors, distribution of carotid stenosis, effect of surgery and type of recurrent stroke. *Cerebrovasc Dis* (in press).

Broderick JP, Phillips SJ, O'Fallon WM, Frey RL, Whisnant JP (1992). Relationship of cardiac disease to stroke occurrence, recurrence, and mortality. *Stroke* 23: 1250–6.

Brook RH, Park RE, Chassin MR, Kosecoff J, Keesey J, Solomon DH (1990). Carotid endarterectomy for elderly patients: predicting complications. *Ann Intern Med* 113: 747–53.

Brown MM (1992). Balloon angioplasty for cerebrovascular disease. *Neurol Res* 14: 159–63.

Brown MM, Humphrey PRD, on behalf of the Association of British Neurologists (1992). Carotid endarterectomy: recommendations for management of transient ischaemic attack and ischaemic stroke. *Br Med J* 305: 1071–4.

Brown MM, Butler P, Gibbs J, Swash M, Waterston J (1990). Feasibility of percutaneous transluminal angioplasty for carotid artery stenosis. *J Neurol Neurosurg Psychiatr* 53: 238–43.

Burn J, Dennis M, Bamford J, Sandercock P, Wade D, Warlow C (1994). Long-term risk of recurrent stroke after a first-ever stroke. The Oxfordshire Community Stroke Project. *Stroke* 25: 333–7.

Cairns JA (1994). Oral anticoagulants or aspirin after myocardial infarction? *Lancet* 343: 497–8.

Campbell WB (1993). Can reported carotid surgical results be misleading? In: Greenhalgh RM, Hollier LH, eds. *Surgery for Stroke*. London: Saunders, 331–7.

Carrea R, Molins M, Murphy G (1955). Surgical treatment of spontaenous thrombosis of the internal carotid artery in the neck. Carotid-carotideal anastomosis. Report of a case. *Acta Neurol Latin Am* 1: 71–8.

CASANOVA Study Group (1991). Carotid surgery versus medical therapy in asymptomatic carotid stenosis. *Stroke* 22: 1229–35.

Chambers BR, Smidt V, Koh P (1994). Hyperfusion post-endarterectomy. *Cerebrovasc Dis* 4: 32–7.

Chao WH, Kwan ST, Lyman RS, Loucks HH (1938). Thrombosis of the left internal carotid artery. *Arch Surg* 37: 100–11.

Chimowitz MI, Weiss DG, Cohen SL, Starling MR, Hobson RW, Veterans Affairs Cooperative Study Group 167 (1994). Cardiac prognosis of patients with carotid stenosis and no history of coronary artery disease. *Stroke* 25: 759–65.

Cillessen JPM, Kappelle LJ, van Swieten JC, Algra A, van Gijn J (1993). Dose cerebral infarction after a previous warning occur in the same vascular territory? *Stroke* 24: 351–4.

Clagett GP, Youkey JR, Brigham RA *et al.* (1984). Asymptomatic cervical bruit and abnormal ocular pneumoplethysmography: a prospective study comparing two approaches to management. *Surgery* 96: 823–30.

Clavier I, Hommel M, Besson G, Noelle B, Perret JEF (1994). Long-term prognosis of symptomatic lacunar infarcts. *Stroke* 25: 2005–9.

Collins R, MacMahon S (1994) Blood pressure, antihypertensive drug treatment and the risks of stroke and of coronary heart disease. *Br Med Bull* 50(2): 272–98.

Cote R, Bathsta M, Abramowicz M, Langlois Y, Bourque F, Mackey A (1995). Lack of effect of aspirin in patients with carotid bruits and substantial carotid narrowing. The asymptomatic cervical study group. *Ann Int Med* 123: 720–2.

Counsell C, Salinas R, Warlow CP, Naylor AR (1995b). The role of routine patch angioplasty in carotid endarterectomy: a systematic review of the randomised controlled trials. Electronic publication in: *Cochrane Database of Systematic Reviews, Disk Issue 1.*

Counsell C, Boonyakarnkul S, Dennis M *et al.* (1995a). Primary intracerebral haemorrhage in the Oxfordshire Community Stroke Project 2. Prognosis. *Cerebrovasc Dis* 5: 26–34.

Crouse JR, Byington RP, Bond MG *et al.* (1995). Pravastatin, lipids and atherosclerosis in the carotid arteries (PLAC-II). *Am J Cardiol* 75: 455–9.

Davenport RJ, Starkey IR, Ruckley CV, Dennis M, Sandercock PAG, Warlow CP (1995). A difficult case: how should a patient presenting with unstable angina and a recent stroke be managed? *Br Med J* 310: 1449–52.

De Marinis M, Zaccaria A, Faraglia V, Fiorani P, Maira G, Agnoli A (1991). Post-endarterectomy headache and the role of the oculosympathetic system. *J Neurol Neurosurg Psychiatr* 54: 314–7.

DeBakey ME (1975). Successful carotid endarterectomy for cerebrovascular insufficiency. Nineteen-year follow-up. *J Am Med Assoc* 233: 1083–5.

Dennis M, Bamford J, Sandercock P, Warlow C (1990). Prognosis of transient ischaemic attacks in the Oxfordshire Community Stroke Project. *Stroke* 21: 848–53.

Dennis MS, Bamford JM, Sandercock PAG, Warlow CP (1989). A comparison of risk factors and prognosis for transient ischaemic attacks and minor ischaemic strokes. The Oxfordshire Community Stroke Project. *Stroke* 20: 1494–9.

Dennis MS, Burn JPS, Sandercock PAG, Bamford JM, Wade DT, Warlow CP (1993). Long-term survival after first-ever stroke: the Oxfordshire Community Stroke Project. *Stroke* 24: 796–800.

Di Pasquale G, Urbinatti S, Pinelli G (1995). New echocardiographic markers of embolic risk in atrial fibrillation. *Cerebrovasc Dis* 5: 315–22.

Diaz FG, Ausman JI, de los Reyes RA *et al.* (1984). Surgical reconstruction of the proximal vertebral artery. *J Neurosurg* 61: 874–81.

Dombovy M, Basford J, Whisnant J, Bergstrahl E (1987). Disability and use of rehabilitation services following stroke in Rochester, Minnesota, 1975–1979. *Stroke* 18: 830–6.

Donnan GA, You R, Thrift A, McNeil JJ (1993). Smoking as a risk factor for stroke. *Cerebrovasc Dis* 3: 129–38.

Dutch TIA Trial Study Group (1991). A comparison of two doses of aspirin (30 mg versus 283 mg a day) in patients after a transient ischaemic attack or minor ischaemic stroke. *N Engl J Med* 325(18): 1261–6.

Dutch TIA Trial Study Group (1993). Predictors of major vascular events in patients with a transient ischaemic attack of non-disabling stroke. *Stroke* 24: 527–31.

Dyken ML, Pokras R (1984). The performance of endarterectomy for disease of the extracranial arteries of the head. *Stroke* 15: 948–50.

Dyken ML, Barnett HJM, Easton JD *et al.* (1992). Low dose aspirin and stroke. 'It ain't necessarily so'. *Stroke* 23(10): 1395–9.

Eastcott HHG, Pickering GW, Rob CG (1954). Reconstruction of internal carotid artery in a patient with intermittent attacks of hemiplegia. *Lancet* 2: 994–6.

EC–IC Bypass Study Group (1985). Failure of extracranial–intracranial arterial bypass to reduce the risk of ischaemic stroke: results of an international randomised trial. *N Engl J Med* 313: 1191–200.

Elton PJ, Ryman A, Hammer M, Page F (1994). Randomised controlled trial in northern England of the effect of a person knowing their own serum cholesterol concentration. *J Epidemiol Commun Health* 48: 22–5.

European Atrial Fibrillation Trial Study Group (1993). Secondary prevention in nonrheumatic trial fibrillation after transient ischaemic attack or minor stroke. *Lancet* 342: 1255–62.

European Atrial Fibrillation Trial Study Group (1995). Optimal oral anticoagulant therapy in patients with nonrheumatic atrial fibrillation and recent cerebral ischaemia. *N Engl J Med* 333(1): 5–10.

European Carotid Surgery Trialists' Collaborative Group (1991). MRC European Carotid Surgery Trial: interim results for symptomatic patients with severe (70–99%) or with mild (0–29%) carotid stenosis. *Lancet* 337: 1235–43.

European Carotid Surgery Trialists' Collaborative Group (1995). Risk of stroke in the distribution of an asymptomatic carotid artery. *Lancet* 345: 209–12.

European Carotid Surgery Trialists' Collaborative Group (1996). Endarterectomy of moderate symptomatic carotid stenosis: interim results from the MRC European Carotid Surgery Trial. *Lancet* (in press).

Evans BA, Sicks JD, Whisnant JP (1994). Factors affecting survival and occurrence of stroke in patients with transient ischaemic attacks. *Mayo Clin Proc* 69: 416–21.

Ferguson GG (1986). Carotid endarterectomy. To shunt or not to shunt? *Arch Neurol* 43: 615–18.

Ferner RE, Neil HAW (1995). A suitable case for treatment. *Lancet* 345: 1051.

Ferro JM, Crespo M (1994). Prognosis after transient ischaemic attack and ischaemic stroke in young adults. *Stroke* 25: 1611–16.

Fields WS, Lemak NA (1972). Joint study of extracranial arterial occlusion. VII. Subclavian steal—a review of 168 cases. *J Am Med Assoc* 222: 1139–43.

Fields WS, Maslenikov V, Meyer JS, Hass WK, Remington RD, Macdonald M (1970). Joint study of extracranial arterial occlusion. V. Progress report of prognosis following surgery or nonsurgical treatment for transient cerebral ischaemic attacks and cervical carotid artery lesions. *J Am Med Assoc* 211: 1993–2003.

Fogelholm R, Nuutila M, Vuorela AL (1992). Primary intracerebral haemorrhage in the Jyvaskyla region, Central Finland, 1985–1989: incidence, case fatality rate, and functional outcome. *J Neurol Neurosurg Psychiatr* 55: 546–52.

Forconi S, Battistini N, Guerrini M, Passero SG (1995). A randomised, ASA-controlled trial of mesoglycan in secondary prevention after cerebral ischaemic events. *Cerebrovasc Dis* 5: 334–41.

Frost CD, Law MR, Wald NJ (1991). II Analysis of observational data within populations. *Br Med J* 302: 815–19.

Gandolfo C, Moretti C, Dall Agata D *et al.* (1986). Long-term prognosis of patients with lacunar syndromes. *Acta Neurol Scand* 74: 224–9.

Gaunt ME, Martin PJ, Smith JL *et al.* (1994). Clinical relevance of intraoperative embolization detected by transcranial Doppler ultrasonography during carotid endarterectomy: a prospective study of 100 patients. *Br J Surg* 81: 1435–9.

Graor RA, Hertzer NR (1988). Management of coexistent carotid artery and coronary artery disease. *Stroke* 19: 1441–3.

Graver LM, Mulcare RJ (1986). Pseudoaneurysm after carotid endarterectomy. *J Cardiovasc Surg* 27: 294–7.

Greaves M. (1993). Anticoagulants in pregnancy. *Pharmacol Ther* 59: 311–27.

Green CJ, Hadorn D, Kazanjian A (1995). Anticoagulation for stroke prevention in chronic non-valvular atrial fibrillation. Vancouver, BC: BC Office of Health Technology Assessment. Discussion Paper Series BCOHTA95: 2D. Centre for Health Services and Policy Research, University of British Columbia.

Green RM, McNamara J (1987). Optimal resources for carotid endarterectomy. *Surgery* 102: 743–8.

Grosveld WJHM, Lawson JA, Eikelboom BC, Windt JMvd, Ackerstaff RGA (1988). Clinical and hemodynamic significance of innominate artery lesions evaluated by ultrasonography and digital angiography. *Stroke* 19: 958–62.

Gumerlock MK, Neuwelt EA (1988). Carotid endarterectomy: to shunt or not to shunt. *Stroke* 19: 1485–90.

Gutrecht JA, Jones HR (1988). Bilateral hypoglossal nerve injury after bilateral carotid endarterectomy. *Stroke* 19: 261–2.

Hafner DH, Smith RB, King OW *et al.* (1987). Massive intracerebral haemorrhage following carotid endarterectomy. *Arch Surg* 122: 305–7.

Halsey JH for the International Transcranial Doppler Collaborators (1992). Risk and benefits of shunting in carotid endarterectomy. *Stroke* 23: 1583–7.

Hankey GJ, Warlow CP (1991). Prognosis of symptomatic carotid artery occlusion. An overview. *Cerebrovasc Dis* 1: 245–56.

Hankey GJ, Warlow CP (1994). *Transient Ischaemic Attacks of the Brain and Eye.* London: WB Saunders Co Ltd.

Hankey GJ, Slattery JM, Warlow CP (1991). The prognosis of hospital-referred transient ischaemic attacks. *J Neurol Neurosurg Psychiatr* 54: 793–802.

Hankey GJ, Slattery JM, Warlow CP (1992). Transient ischaemic attacks: which patients are at high (and low) risk of serious vascular events? *J Neurol Neurosurg Psychiatr* 55: 640–52.

Hankey GJ, Slattery JM, Warlow CP (1993b). Can the long term outcome of individual patients with transient ischaemic attacks be predicted accurately? *J Neurol Neurosurg Psychiatr* 56:

752–9.

Hankey GJ, Dennis MS, Slattery JM, Warlow CP (1993a). Why is the outcome of transient ischaemic attacks different in different groups of patients? *Br Med J* 306: 1107–11.

Hart RG, Boop BS, Anderson DC (1995). Oral anticoagulants and intracranial haemorrhage. Facts and hypotheses. *Stroke* 26: 1471–7.

Hartl WH, Janssen I, Furst H (1994). Effect of carotid endarterectomy on patterns of cerebrovascular reactivity in patients with unilateral carotid artery stenosis. *Stroke* 25: 1952–7.

Harward TRS, Wickbom IG, Otis SM, Bernstein EF, Dilley RB (1984). Posterior communicating artery visualization in predicting results of carotid endarterectomy for vertebrobasilar insufficiency. *Am J Surg* 148: 43–8.

Haynes RB, Mukherjee J, Sackett DL, Taylor DW, Barnett HJM, Peerless SJ for the EC/IC Bypass Study Group (1987). Functional status changes following medical or surgical treatment for cerebral ischaemia. Results of the extracranial–intracranial bypass study. *J Am Med Assoc* 257: 2043–6.

Hemmingsen R, Mejsholm B, Boysen G, Engell HC (1982). Intellectual function in patients with transient ischaemic attacks (TIA) or minor stroke. Long-term improvement after carotid endarterectomy. *Acta Neurol Scand* 66: 145–59.

Hennerici M, Klemm C, Rautenberg W (1988). The subclavian steal phenomenon: a common vascular disorder with rare neurologic deficits. *Neurology* 38: 669–73.

Herbert PR, Gazinao JM, Hennekens CH (1995). An overview of trials in cholesterol lowering and risk of stroke. *Arch Intern Med* 155: 50–5.

Hertzer NR, Loop FD, Beven EG, O'Hara PJ, Krajewski LP (1989). Surgical staging for simultaneous coronary and carotid disease: a study including prospective randomisation. *J Vasc Surg* 9: 455–63.

Hier DB, Edelstein G (1991). Deriving clinical prediction rules from stroke outcome research. *Stroke* 22: 1431–6.

Hier DB, Foulkes MA, Swiontoniowski M *et al.* (1991). Stroke recurrence within 2 years after ischaemic infarction. *Stroke* 22: 155–61.

Hirsh J (1991). Heparin. *N Engl J Med* 324: 1565–74.

Hobson RW, Weiss DG, Fields WS *et al.* (1993). Efficacy of carotid endarterectomy for asymptomatic carotid stenosis. *N Engl J Med* 328: 221–7.

Hopkins LN, Martin NA, Hadley MN, Spetzler RF, Budny J, Carter LP (1987). Vertebrobasilar insufficiency. Part 2: microsurgical treatment of intracranial vertebrobasilar disease. *J Neurosurg* 66: 662–74.

Horwitz RI, Brass LM (1994). Women's Estrogen for Stroke Trial (WEST). *Stroke* 25: 545 (abstract).

Howard G, Evans GW, Crouse JR *et al.* (1994). A prospective reevaluation of transient ischaemic attacks as a risk factor for death and fatal or nonfatal cardiovascular events. *Stroke* 25: 342–5.

Hsia DC, Krushat WM, Moscoe LM (1992). Epidemiology of carotid endarterectomies among Medicare beneficiaries. *J Vasc*

Surg 16: 201–8.

Hunter GC, Palmaz JC, Hayashi HH, Raviola CA, Vogt PJ, Guernsey JM (1987). The etiology of symptoms in patients with recurrent carotid stenosis. *Arch Surg* 122: 311–15.

Ille O, Woimant F, Pruna A, Corabianu O, Idatte JM, Haguenau M (1995). Hypertensive encephalopathy after bilateral carotid endarterectomy. *Stroke* 26: 488–91.

Irie K, Yamaguchi T, Minematsu K, Omae T (1993). The J-curve phenomenon in stroke recurrence. *Stroke* 24: 1844–9.

Iso H, Jacobs DR, Wentworth D, Neaton JD, Cohen JD (1989). Serum cholesterol levels and six year mortality from stroke in 350 977 men screened for the multiple risk factor intervention trial. *N Engl J Med* 320: 904–10.

Ivey TD, Strandness DE, Williams DB, Langlois Y, Misbach GA, Kruse AP (1984). Management of patients with carotid bruit undergoing cardiopulmonary bypass. *J Thorac Cardiovasc Surg* 87: 183–9.

Jackson R, Barham P, Bills J *et al.* (1993). Management of raised blood pressure in New Zealand: a discussion document. *Br Med J* 307: 107–10.

Jansen C, Ramos LMP, van Heesewijk JPM, Moll FL, van Gijn J, Ackerstaff RGA (1994a). Impact of microembolism and hemodynamic changes in the brain during carotid endarterectomy. *Stroke* 25: 992–7.

Jansen C, Sprengers AM, Moll FL *et al.* (1994b). Prediction of intracerebral haemorrhage after carotid endarterectomy by clinical criteria and intraoperative transcranial Doppler monitoring. *Eur J Vasc Surg* 8: 303–8.

Jonas S (1988). Anticoagulant therapy in cerebrovascular disease: review and meta-analysis (published erratum appears in *Stroke* 20(4): 562). *Stroke* 19: 1043–8.

Kappelle LJ, Adams HP Jr, Heffner ML, Torner JC, Gomez F, Biller J (1994). Prognosis of young adults with ischaemic stroke. *Stroke* 25: 1360–5.

Kappelle LJ, van Latum JC, van Swieten JC, Algra A, Koudstaal PJ, van Gijn J for the Dutch TIA Trial Study Group (1995). Recurrent stroke after transient ischaemic attack or minor ischaemic stroke: does the distinction between small and large vessel disease remain true to type? *J Neurol Neurosurg Psychiatr* 59: 127–31.

Karnik R, Valentin A, Ammerer H-P, Donath P, Slany J (1992). Evaluation of vasomotor reactivity by Transcranial Doppler and Acetazolamide test before and after extracranial–intracranial bypass in patients with internal carotid artery occlusion. *Stroke* 23: 812–17.

Keech A, Collins R, MacMahon S *et al.* (1994). Three year follow up of the Oxford Cholesterol Study: assessment of the efficacy and safety in simvastatin in preparation for a large mortality study. *Eur Heart J* 15: 255–69.

Khamashta MA, Cuadrado MJ, Mujic F, Taub NA, Hunt BJ, Hughes GRV (1995). The management of thrombosis in the antiphospholipid-antibody syndrome. *N Engl J Med* 332(15): 993–7.

Khaw KT, Woodhouse P (1995). Interrelation of vitamin C, infection, haemostatic factors and cardiovascular disease.

Br Med J 310: 1559–63.

Kinch JW, Davidoff R (1995). Prevention of embolic events after cardioversion of atrial fibrillation. Current and evolving strategies. *Arch Intern Med* 155: 1353–60.

Kojima S, Omura T, Wakamatsu W *et al.* (1990). Prognosis and disability of stroke patients after 5 years in Akita, Japan. *Stroke* 21: 72–7.

Koudstaal PJ (1995a). Secondary prevention following stroke or transient ischaemic attack in patients with nonrheumatic atrial fibrillation: anticoagulant therapy versus control. In: Warlow C, van Gijn J, Sandercock P, eds. *The Cochrane Database of Systematic Reviews 1995 (Issue 1)*. London: British Medical Journal Publishing.

Koudstaal PJ (1995b). Secondary prevention following stroke or transient ischaemic attack in patients with nonrheumatic atrial fibrillation: antiplatelet therapy versus control. In: Warlow C, van Gijn J, Sandercock P, eds. *The Cochrane Database of Systematic Reviews 1995 Issue 1*. London: British Medical Journal Publishing.

Koudstaal PJ (1995c). Effect of atrial fibrillation on early deaths and recurrent strokes in the International Stroke Trial. *Cerebrovasc Dis* 5(4): 232 (abstract).

Koudstaal PJ (1995d). Secondary prevention following stroke or transient ischaemic attack in patients with nonrheumatic atrial fibrillation: anticoagulant versus antiplatelet therapy. In: Warlow C, van Gijn J, Sandercock P, eds. *The Cochrane Database of Systematic Reviews 1995 Issue 1*. London: British Medical Journal Publishing.

Koudstaal PJ, Algra A, Pop GAM, Kappelle LJ, van Latum JC, van Gijn J for the Dutch TIA Study Group (1992b). Risk of cardiac events in atypical transient ischaemic attack or minor stroke. *Lancet* 340: 630–3.

Koudstaal PJ, van Gijn J, Frenken CWGM *et al.* for the Dutch Transient Ischaemic Attack Group (1992a). TIA, RIND, minor stroke: a continuum, or different subgroups? *J Neurol Neurosurg Psychiatr* 55: 95–7.

Krul JMJ, van Gijn J, Ackerstaff RGA, Eikelboom BC, Theodorides T, Vermeulen FEE (1989). Site and pathogenesis of infarcts associated with carotid endarterectomy. *Stroke* 20: 324–8.

Lai SM, Alter M, Friday G, Sobel E (1994). A multifactorial analysis of risk factors for recurrence of ischaemic stroke. *Stroke* 25: 958–62.

Landi G, Motto C, Cella E *et al.* (1993). Pathogenetic and prognostic features of lacunar transient ischaemic attack syndromes. *J Neurol Neurosurg Psychiatr* 56: 1265–70.

Lanzino G, Andreoli A, di Pasquale G *et al.* (1991). Aetiopathogenesis and prognosis fo cerebral ischaemia in young adults. A survey of 155 treated patients. *Acta Neurol Scand* 84: 321–5.

Latchaw RE, Ausman JI, Lee MC (1979). Superficial temporal-middle cerebral artery bypass. A detailed analysis of multiple pre- and postoperative angiograms in 40 consecutive patients. *J Neurosurg* 51: 455–65.

Law MR, Frost CD, Wald NJ (1991a). III Analysis of data from trials of salt reduction. *Br Med J* 302: 819–24.

Law MR, Frost CD, Wald NJ (1991b). I Analysis of observational data among populations. By how much does dietary salt reduction lower blood pressure? *Br Med J* 302: 811–15.

Law MR, Thomson SG, Wald NJ (1994). Assessing possible hazards of reducing serum cholesterol. *Br Med J* 308: 373–9.

Law MR, Wald NJ, Wu T, Hackshaw A, Bailey A (1994). Systematic underestimation of association between serum cholesterol concentration and ischaemic heart disease in observational studies: data from the BUPA study. *Br Med J* 308: 363–79.

Lee KS, Bae HG, Yun IG (1990). Recurrent intracerebral haemorrhage due to hypertension. *Neurosurgery* 26: 586–90.

Lindblad B, Persson NH, Takolander R, Bergqvist D (1993). Does low-dose acetylsalicylic acid prevent stroke after carotid surgery? A double-blind, placebo-controlled randomised trial. *Stroke* 24: 1125–8.

Lindley RI, Amayo EO, Marshall J, Sandercock P, Warlow C (1995b). Acute stroke treatment in UK hospitals: the Stroke Association Survey of Consultant Opinion. *J Roy Coll Phys* (in press).

Lindley RI, Amayo EO, Marshall J, Sandercock P, Dennis M, Warlow C (1995a). Hospital services for patients with acute stroke in the United Kingdom. The Stroke Association Survey of Consultant Opinion. *Age Ageing* 24: 525–32.

Loftus CM, Quest DO (1987). Technical controversies in carotid artery surgery. *Neurosurgery* 20: 490–5.

McCrory DC, Goldstein LB, Samsa GP *et al.* (1993). Predicting complications of carotid endarterectomy. *Stroke* 24: 1285–91.

Mack WJ, Selzer RH, Hodis HN *et al.* (1993). One year reduction and longitudinal analysis of carotid intima-media thickness associated with colestipol/niacin therapy. *Stroke* 24: 1779–83.

MacMahon S, Rodgers A (1994a). The epidemiological association between blood pressure and stroke: implications for primary and secondary prevention. *Hypertens Res* 17 (Suppl. I): S23–32.

MacMahon S, Rodgers A (1994b). Blood pressure, antihypertensive treatment and stroke risk. *J Hypertens* 12 (Suppl. 10): S5–14.

MacMahon S, Peto R, Cutler J *et al.* (1990). Blood pressure, stroke, and coronary heart disease Part 1—prolonged differences in blood pressure: prospective observational studies corrected for the regression dilution bias. *Lancet* 335: 765–74.

Maniglia AJ, Han DP (1991). Cranial nerve injuries following carotid endarterectomy: an analysis of 336 procedures. *Head Neck* 13: 121–4.

Mann GI, Crooke M, Fear H *et al.* (1993). Guidelines for detection and management of dyslipidaemia. *N Z Med J* 106: 133–42.

Markus HS, Thomson ND, Brown MM (1995). Asymptomatic cerebral embolic signals in symptomatic and asymptomatic carotid artery disease. *Brain* 118: 1005–11.

Marquardsen J (1969). The natural history of acute cerebrovascular disease: a retrospective study of 769 patients. *Acta Neurol Scand Suppl* 45 (Suppl. 38): 11–155.

Marshall J (1982). The cause and prognosis of strokes in people under 50 years. *J Neurol Sci* 53: 473–88.

Matsumoto N, Whisnant JP, Kurland LT, Okazaki H (1973). Natural history of stroke in Rochester, Minnesota 1955–1969: an extension of a previous study 1945–1954. *Stroke* 4: 20–9.

Mayberg MR, Wilson E, Yatsu F *et al.* for the Veterans Affairs Cooperative Studies Programe 309 Trialist Group (1991). Carotid endarterectomy and prevention of cerebral ischaemia in symptomatic carotid stenosis. *J Am Med Assoc* 266: 3289–94.

Mayo Asymptomatic Carotid Endarterectomy Study Group (1992). Results of a randomised controlled trial of carotid endarterectomy for asymptomatic carotid stenosis. *Mayo Clin Proc* 67: 513–18.

Meissner I, Whisnant JP, Garraway WM (1988). Hypertension management and stroke recurrrence in a community (Rochester, Minnesota, 1950–1979). *Stroke* 19: 459–63.

Meissner I, Wiebers DO, Whisnant JP, O'Fallon WM (1987). The natural history of asymptomatic carotid artery occlusive lesions. *J Am Med Assoc* 258: 2704–7.

Michaels JA (1988). Surgical audit and carotid endarterectomy. *Lancet* 2: 110–11.

Middlekauff HR, Stevenson WG, Gornbein JA (1995). Antiarrhythmic prophylaxis versus warfarin anticoagulation to prevention thromboembolic events among patients with atrial fibrillation. *Arch Intern Med* 155: 913–20.

Moore WS, Barnett HJM, Beebe HG *et al.* (1995). Guidelines for carotid endaterectomy. A multidisciplinary consensus statement from the Ad hoc committee, American Heart Association. *Stroke* 26: 188–201.

Moreyra E, Omron EM, Jeffrey M, Katz R (1995). Treatment of atrial fibrillation: European versus US practice—are we oceans apart? *Br J Cardiol* 73–6.

Morris MC, Mandson JE, Rosner B, Buring JE, Willett WC, Hennekens CH (1995). Fish consumption and cardiovascular disease in the Physicians' Health Study. A prospective study. *Am J Epidemiol* 14(2): 166–75.

Naylor AR, Bell PRF, Ruckley CV (1992). Monitoring and cerebral protection during carotid endarterectomy. *Br J Surg* 79: 735–41.

Naylor AR, Merrick MV, Sandercock PAG *et al.* (1993b). Serial imaging of the carotid bifurcation and cerebrovascular reserve after carotid endarterectomy. *Br J Surg* 80: 1278–82.

Naylor AR, Whyman MR, Wildsmith JAW *et al.* (1993a). Factors influencing the hyperaemic response after carotid endarterectomy. *Br J Surg* 80: 1523–7.

Norris JW, Zhu CZ, Bornstein NM, Chambers BR (1991). Vascular risks of asymptomatic carotid stenosis. *Stroke* 22: 1485–90.

North American Symptomatic Carotid Endarterectomy Trial Collaborators (1991). Beneficial effect of carotid endarterectomy in symptomatic patients with high-grade carotid stenosis. *N Engl J Med* 325: 445–53.

Ojemann RG, Heros RC (1986). Carotid endarterectomy. To shunt or not to shunt? *Arch Neurol* 43: 617–18.

Orencia AJ, Petty GW, Khandheria BK *et al.* (1995). Risk of stroke with mitral valve prolapse in population-based cohort study. *Stroke* 26: 7–13.

Parker JC, Granberg BW, Nichols WK, Jones JG, Hewett JE

(1983). Mental status outcomes following carotid endarterectomy: a six-month analysis. *J Clin Neuropsychol* 5: 345–53.

Passero S, Burgalassi L, D'Andrea P, Battistini N (1995). Recurrence of bleeding in patients with primary intracerebral haemorrhage. *Stroke* 26: 1189–92.

Patrono C (1994). Aspirin as an antiplatelet drug. *N Engl J Med* 330: 1287–94.

PATS Collaborating Group (1995). Epidemiology Survey. Post-stroke antihypertensive treatment study. *Chinese Med J* 108(9): 710–17.

Pekkanen J, Linn S, Heiss G *et al.* (1990). Ten year mortality from cardiovascular disease in relation to cholesterol level among men with and without preexisting cardiovascular disease. *N Engl J Med* 322: 1700–7.

Peto R (1994). Smoking and death: the past 40 years and the next 40. *Br Med J* 309: 937–9.

Piepgras DG, Marsh WR, Mussman LA, Sundt TM, Fode NC (1986). Recurrent carotid stenosis. Results and complications of 57 operations. *Ann Surg* 203: 205–13.

Piepgras DG, Morgan MK, Sundt TM, Yanagihara T, Mussman LM (1988). Intracerebral haemorrhage after carotid endarterectomy. *J Neurosurg* 68: 532–6.

Pokras R, Dyken ML (1988). Dramatic changes in the performance of endarterectomy for diseases of the extracranial arteries of the head. *Stroke* 19: 1289–90.

Pop GAM, Koudstaal PJ, Meeder HJ, Algra A, van Latum JC, van Gijn for the Dutch TIA Trial Study Group (1994). Predictive value of clinical history and electrocardiogram in patients with transient ischaemic attack or minor ischaemic stroke for subsequent cardiac and cerebral ischaemic events. *Arch Neurol* 51: 333–41.

Porta M, Munari LM, Belloni G, Moschini L, Bonaldi G (1991). Percutaneous angioplasty of atherosclerotic carotid arteries. *Cerebrovasc Dis* 1: 265–72.

Riles TS, Kopelman I, Imparato AM (1979). Myocardial infarction following carotid endarterectomy. A review of 683 operations. *Surgery* 85: 249–52.

Riles TS, Imparato AM, Jacobowitz GR *et al.* (1994). The cause of perioperative stroke after carotid endarterectomy. *J Vasc Surg* 19: 206–16.

Rodgers A, MacMahon S, Gamble G, Slattery J, Sandercock P, Warlow C (1996). Blood pressure is an important predictor of future stroke risk in individuals with cerebrovascular disease. *Br Med J* (in press).

Rose G (1992). *The Strategy of Preventive Medicine*. Oxford: University Press.

Rothwell PM (1995). Can overall results of clinical trials be applied to all patients? *Lancet* 345: 1616–19.

Rothwell PM, Slattery J, Warlow CP (1996a). A systematic comparison of the risk of stroke and death due to carotid endarterectomy for symptomatic and asymptomatic stenosis. *Stroke* 27: 266–9.

Rothwell PM, Slattery J, Warlow CP (1996b). A systematic review of the risk of stroke and death due to carotid endarterectomy.

Stroke 27: 260–5.

Rothwell PM, Salinas R, Ferrando LA, Slattery J, Warlow CP (1995). Does the angiographic appearance of a carotid stenosis predict the risk of stroke independently of the degree of stenosis? *Clin Radiol* 50: 830–3.

Sacco RL, Wolf PA, Kannel WB, McNamara PM (1982). Survival and recurrence following stroke: the Framingham study. *Stroke* 13: 290–5.

Sacco RJ, Foulkes MA, Mohr JP, Wolf PA, Hier DB, Price TR (1989). Determinants of early recurrence of cerebral infarction: the Stroke Data Bank. *Stroke* 20: 983–9.

Sacco SE, Whisnant JP, Broderick JP, Phillips SJ, O'Fallon WM (1991). Epidemiological characteristics of lacunar infarcts in a population. *Stroke* 22: 1236–41.

Sackett DL, Haynes RB, Guyatt GH, Tugwell P (1991). *Clinical Epidemiology. A Basic Science for Clinical Medicine*, 2nd edn. Boston: Little, Brown and Company, 173–85.

Sage JI, van Uitert RL (1983). Risk of recurrent stroke with atrial fibrillation: differences between rheumatic and atherosclerotic heart disease. *Stroke* 14: 537–40.

SALT Collaborative Group (1991). Swedish Aspirin low-dose Trial (SALT) of 75 mg aspirin as secondary prophylaxis after cerebrovascular ischaemic events. *Lancet* 338(8779): 1345–9.

Sandercock P, Bamford J, Dennis M *et al.* (1992). Atrial fibrillation and stroke: prevalence in different types of stroke and influence on early and long term prognosis (Oxfordshire Community Stroke Project). *Br Med J* 305: 1460–5.

Sandmann W, Willeke F, Kolvenbach R, Benecke R, Godehardt E (1993). To shunt or not to shunt: the definite answer with a randomised study. In: Veith FJ, ed. *Current Critical Problems in Vascular Surgery*, 5. St Louis: Quality Medical Publishing Inc, 434–40.

Sbarouni E, Oakley CM (1994). Outcome of pregnancy in women with valve prostheses. *Br Heart J* 71: 196–201.

Scandinavian Simvastatin Survival Study Group (1994). Randomised trial of cholesterol lowering in 4444 patients with coronary heart disease: the Scandinavian Simvastatin Survival Study (4S). *Lancet* 344: 1383–9.

Schmidt EV, Smirnov VE, Ryabova VS (1988). Results of the seven year prospective study of stroke patients. *Stroke* 19: 942–9.

Schneider PA, Ringelstein B, Rossman ME *et al.* (1988). Importance of cerebral collateral pathways during carotid endarterectomy. *Stroke* 19: 1328–34.

Schroeder T (1988). Hemodynamic significance of internal carotid artery disease. *Acta Neurol Scand* 77: 353–72.

Schroeder T (1990). How to predict which patient with carotid atherosclerosis is 'high risk'. *Acta Chir Scand Suppl* 555: 209–22.

Scottish Intercollegiate Guidelines Network (1996). Antithrombotic therapy. A national clinical guideline recommended for use in Scotland by the Scottish Intercollegiate Guidelines Network. HMSO, Edinburgh (in press).

Shaw DA, Venables GS, Cartlidge NEF, Bates D, Dickinson PH (1984). Carotid endarterectomy in patients with transient cerebral ischaemia. *J Neurol Sci* 64: 45–53.

Shear NH, Appel C (1995). Prevention of ischemic stroke. *N Engl J Med* 333: 460.

Shinton R, Beevers G (1989). Meta-analysis of relation between cigarette smoking and stroke. *Br Med J* 298: 789–94.

Siebler M, Sitzer M, Rose G, Bendfeldt D, Steinmetz H (1993). Silent cerebral embolism caused by neurologically symptomatic high-grade carotid stenosis. Event rates before and after carotid endarterectomy. *Brain* 116: 1005–15.

Silagy C, Mant D, Fowler G, Lodge M (1994). Meta analysis on efficacy of nicotine replacement therapies in smoking cessation. *Lancet* 343: 139–42.

Slattery JM, Warlow CP (1996). Long term raised blood pressure following carotid endarterectomy. *Br Med J* (submitted).

Solomon RA, Loftus CM, Quest DO, Correll JW (1986). Incidence and etiology of intracerebral haemorrhage following carotid endarterectomy. *J Neurosurg* 64: 29–34.

Spencer MP, Thomas GI, Nicholls SC, Sauvage LR (1990). Detection of middle cerebral artery emboli during carotid endarterectomy using transcranial Doppler ultrasonography. *Stroke* 21: 415–23.

Spetzler RF, Hadley MN, Martin NA, Hopkins LN, Carter LP, Budny J (1987). Vertebrobasilar insufficiency. Part 1: microsurgical treatment of extracranial vertebrobsilar disease. *J Neurosurg* 66: 648–61.

Steed DL, Peitzman AB, Grundy BL, Webster MW (1982). Causes of stroke in carotid endarterectomy. *Surgery* 92: 634–9.

Strandness DE (1995). Angiography before carotid endarterectomy —no. *Arch Neurol* 52: 832–3.

Streifler JY, Eliasziw M, Benavente OR *et al.* for the North American Symptomatic Carotid Endarterectomy Trial (1995). The risk of stroke in patients with first-ever retinal vs hemispheric transient ischaemic attacks and high-grade carotid stenosis. *Arch Neurol* 52: 246–9.

Stroke Prevention in Atrial Fibrillation Investigators (1994). Warfarin versus aspirin for prevention of thrombo embolism in atrial fibrillation: Stroke Prevention in Atrial Fibrillation II Study. *Lancet* 343: 687–91.

Sudlow CM, Rodgers H, Kenny RA, Thomson RG (1995). Service provision and use of anticoagulants in atrial fibrillation. *Br Med J* 311: 558–61.

Sundt TM, Sandok BA, Whisnant JP (1975). Carotid endarterectomy. Complications and preoperative assessment of risk. *Mayo Clin Proc* 50: 301–6.

Sweeney PJ, Wilbourn AJ (1992). Spinal accessory (11th) nerve palsy following carotid endarterectomy. *Neurology* 42: 674–5.

Tang JL, Law M, Wald N (1994). How effective is nicotine replacement therapy in helping people to stop smoking? *Br Med J* 308: 21–6.

Terent A (1989). Survival after stroke and TIA during the 1970s and 1980s. *Stroke* 20: 1320–6.

Thevenet A, Ruotolo C (1984). Surgical repair of vertebral artery stenoses. *J Cardiovasc Surg* 25: 101–10.

Towne JB, Weiss DG, Hobson RW (1990). First phase report of cooperative Veterans Administration asymptomatic carotid stenosis study—operative morbidity and mortality. *J Vasc Surg*

11: 252–9.

Truax BT (1989). Gustatory pain: a complication of carotid endarterectomy. *Neurology* 39: 1258–60.

Turpie AGG, Gent M, Laupacis A, Latour Y, Gunnstensen J, Basile F (1993). A comparison of aspirin with placebo in patients treated with warfarin after heart valve replacement. *N Engl J Med* 329: 524–9.

UK-TIA Study Group (1983). Variation in the use of angiography and carotid endarterectomy by neurologists in the UK-TIA aspirin trial. *Br Med J* 286: 514–17.

UK-TIA Study Group (1991). The United Kingdom transient ischaemic attack (UK-TIA) aspirin trial: final results. *J Neurol Neurosurg Psychiatr* 54: 1044–54.

Urbinati S, di Pasquale G, Andreoli A *et al.* (1994). Preoperative noninvasive coronary risk stratification in candidates for carotid endarterectomy. *Stroke* 25: 2022–7.

Vaitkus PT, Berlin JA, Schwartz JS, Barnathan ES (1992). Stroke complicating acute myocardial infarction. A meta-analysis of risk modification by anticoagulation and thrombolytic therapy. *Arch Int Med* 152: 2020–4.

van Latum JC, Koudstaal PJ, Venables GS, van Gijn J, Kappelle LJ, Algra A for the European Atrial Fibrillation Trial (EAFT) Study Group (1995). Predictors of major vascular events in patients with a transient ischaemic attack or minor ischaemic stroke and with nonrheumatic atrial fibrillation. *Stroke* 16: 801–6.

van Zuilen EV, Moll FL, Vermeulen FEE, Mauser HW, van Gijn J, Ackerstaff RGA (1995). Detection of cerebral microemboli by means of transcranial Doppler monitoring before and after carotid endarterectomy. *Stroke* 26: 210–13.

Viitanen M, Eriksson S, Asplund K (1988). Risk of recurrent stroke, myocardial infarction and epilepsy during long term follow up after stroke. *Eur Neurol* 28: 227–31.

Wade DT, Langton Hewer R (1987). Functional abilities after stroke: measurement, natural history and prognosis. *J Neurol Neurosurg Psychiatr* 50: 177–82.

Warlow CP (1984). Carotid endarterectomy: does it work? *Stroke* 15: 1068–76.

Warlow CP (1986). Extracranial to intracranial bypass and the prevention of stroke. *J Neurol* 233: 129–30.

Whisnant JP, Wiebers DO (1987). Clinical epidemiology of transient cerebral ischaemic attacks (TIA) in the anterior and posterior cerebral circulation. In: Sundt TM Jr, ed. *Occlusive Cerebrovascular Disease, Diagnosis and Surgical Management.* Philadelphia: Saunders, 60–5.

Wiebers DO, Whisnant JP, O'Fallon WM (1982). Reversible ischaemic neurological deficit (RIND) in a community: Rochester, Minnesota, 1955–1974. *Neurology* 32: 459–65.

Winslow CM, Solomon DH, Chassin MR, Kosecoff J, Merrick NJ, Brook RH (1988). The appropriateness of carotid endarterectomy. *N Engl J Med* 318: 721–7.

Yatsu FM, Fields WS (1985). Asymptomatic carotid bruit. Stenosis or ulceration, a conservative approach. *Arch Neurol* 42: 383–5.

Youkey JR, Clagett GP, Jaffin JH, Parisi JE, Rich NM (1984). Focal motor seizures complicating carotid endarterectomy. *Arch Surg* 119: 1080–4.

Zarins CK, Gewertz BL (eds) (1987). *Atlas of Vascular Surgery.* New York: Churchill Livingstone.

The organisation of stroke services

17

17.1 Introduction

Stroke is the third most common cause of death in most Western countries, after coronary heart disease and cancer. It accounts for 12% of all deaths in England and Wales (Secretary of State for Health, 1992) and is one of the most important causes of severe disability (Martin *et al.*, 1988). In Scotland, about 7% of all hospital-bed days are accounted for by stroke patients, who represent 2% of all hospital discharges. Stroke accounts for 6% of hospital costs and 4.6% of all National Health Service costs in Scotland (Isard & Forbes, 1992). Although the direct hospital costs are important early after a stroke, it is the costs related to long-term care of disabled survivors which dominate the lifetime costs (Bergman *et al.*, 1995). The financial burden on our society as a whole is likely to be huge but is extremely difficult to estimate because it is borne by patients' families (e.g. lost

income) and, in many countries, by social services. Approximately 25% of people who have a stroke are of working age so that we also have to consider its indirect costs such as the impact on national productivity. Studies from some countries (e.g. Sweden, US and Canada) suggest that the financial burden may be greater than in the UK, possibly because of greater expenditure on health services (Mills & Thompson, 1978; Hartunian *et al.*, 1980; Adelman, 1981; Terent, 1983; Persson *et al.*, 1990; Smurawska *et al.*, 1994). Even if the incidence is falling (see Section 18.2.2), the burden of stroke is likely to remain very substantial for the foreseeable future because of the increasing numbers of elderly people.

Governments, and in particular those responsible for providing health care, have become increasingly aware of the impact that stroke has on the health of the population and the cost to the community. In the UK, relatively little attention was paid to stroke until the publication of the King's Fund Consensus Conference (1988) on the treatment of stroke. This highlighted the many deficiencies in the services provided for stroke patients, concluding that 'services were often haphazard and poorly tailored to the patient's needs.' In England, stroke has moved up the political agenda and has been identified as one of the five key areas for improving the health of the nation over the next decade (Secretary of State for Health, 1992). These changes have lead to a tremendous surge of interest in stroke in general, and in stroke services in particular. Over the last few years there has been an increasing amount of research carried out to determine the best and most cost-effective ways of providing care for stroke patients. This chapter will cover the organisation of services for people who have had a stroke. Inevitably, the discussion will reflect the UK and to some extent the Australian and Dutch models of care, but we hope it will have some relevance for services elsewhere.

Aims of stroke services

The overall aim of stroke services is to deliver the care required by patients, and their families, in the most efficient and humane manner as possible. Services may not be stroke specific but comprise those for internal medicine, care of the elderly, neurology, rehabilitation and continuing care. It is the fact that they ought to be organised which is probably the most important factor in determining their effectiveness. When considering exactly how stroke services should best be organised it is useful to consider the main components of caring for patients with stroke and transient ischaemic attack (TIA) (Table 17.1). Stroke services should also provide information, support and sympathy to the patients and their families. In addition, given the lack of evidence for many of our interventions, services should facilitate research and education.

We have not included primary prevention amongst the components of care, despite this being potentially the most

Table 17.1 The components of the management of patients with TIA and stroke.

Prompt and accurate diagnosis
Assessment of patients' problems
Specific acute medical and surgical treatment
General care including interventions to resolve problems (includes
    many aspects of rehabilitation)
Terminal care of patients who are unlikely to survive
Hospital discharge and placement
Continuing or long-term care for severely disabled patients
Follow-up to detect and manage late-onset problems
Secondary prevention of further vascular events

effective method of reducing stroke-related death, disability and handicap (see Chapter 18). Primary stroke prevention has so much in common with the prevention of other vascular diseases that it would seem to make more sense to link these preventative services together, especially as their success depends more on political and social change than on health services.

A comprehensive stroke service has to provide the facilities and expertise to fulfil all of these functions. The manner in which the service is best provided will depend on local history, geography, needs, resources, people and politics. Therefore, any stroke service must be tailored to the local conditions to achieve maximum effectiveness. For this reason, it is difficult to be dogmatic about exactly how services should be organised. However, in this chapter we will attempt to provide general guidance and elucidate the principles which should be of use to the clinician, public health physician or health service manager (administrator) in planning a service. In planning or reviewing stroke services it is useful to start by trying to answer several questions.

1 What are the needs of the population to be served by the stroke service?
2 Assuming that resources are limited, to what extent can the needs of the population realistically be met?
3 What are the *current* resources, people and facilities, committed to the management of patients with TIAs and stroke?
4 What is the evidence for the cost-effectiveness of the various components of the stroke service?
5 What are the major gaps in the present provision of services (i.e. unmet needs and failure to provide cost-effective interventions)?
6 What resources, people and facilities are needed to meet the needs of the population?
7 How should these resources best be organised?
8 How can performance of the stroke services be monitored?

> Local stroke services must be tailored to local conditions; there is no perfect blueprint that can be applied everywhere.

17.2 Determining the needs of the population

If the aim of the service is to provide care for all those in the population who require care, not just those who can afford to pay for it, then the first factor to consider is the incidence of stroke and TIA in that population. This information should be the basis of a 'needs assessment' which those responsible for ensuring adequate health care provision must develop. This is fundamental to determining *how much* stroke service should be provided.

17.2.1 Incidence of acute cerebrovascular disease

Despite the huge burden that cerebrovascular disease places on communities throughout the world, there is less reliable data on its incidence than one might expect. Although a large number of 'incidence' studies have appeared in the literature over the past 30 years, the majority have had methodological weaknesses which make their results, at least in part, unreliable. The criteria for an 'ideal' stroke and TIA incidence study are listed in Table 17.2. The age-specific incidence rates provided by the 'ideal' studies are given in Table 17.3, all of which are in Caucasian populations because no reasonably up-to-date and more or less 'ideal' studies are available in other populations.

> *There are quite good data on the incidence of stroke in many Caucasian populations except in the Americas, some data in Orientals, and no reliable data at all in other parts of Asia and in the whole of Africa.*

Possible approaches to assessing need

Because of the dearth of reliable incidence data (i.e. the number of first-ever in a lifetime cases of stroke occurring in the population over a defined time period), those planning stroke services may decide to base their estimates of need on routinely collected mortality data (i.e. the number of deaths attributed to stroke in the population over a defined time period). They should, however, be aware of the potential problems of adopting this policy.

Mortality statistics depend on the collation of data from death certificates. They are thus dependent on the accuracy of death certification, which in countries with quite low autopsy rates, such as the UK and US, is known to be poor (see Section 18.2.1). The accuracy of mortality statistics also depends on the accuracy of the population denominators used and thus on the reliability and timing of the most recent census. Also, mortality statistics only include the deaths attributed to stroke (and not the number of stroke episodes) and are not in themselves of much value in estimating the need for health services. Although they are bound to reflect, at least indirectly, the incidence of stroke in the population, the case fatality rate may differ from place to place and so there will not be a uniform relationship between stroke mortality and incidence. There is some evidence that the case fatality rate is falling whilst the incidence is not (see Section 18.2).

Table 17.2 Criteria for an 'ideal' stroke and TIA incidence study. (From Malmgren *et al.*, 1987.)

Well-defined study population; the number and sex of the people in the population should be available in at least 10-year age intervals during the study

Complete ascertainment of all cases of both stroke and TIA occurring in that population, whether referred to hospital or not. This requires multiple overlapping methods to detect cases including contacting primary health teams, review of hospital admissions and death certificates

First-ever in a lifetime strokes and TIAs should be distinguished from first during the study period and recurrent strokes and TIAs

Accurate assessment of the cross-boundary flows in both directions

Prospective assessment of all suspected cases so that standard diagnostic criteria can be applied rigorously soon after the patient presents to medical attention (i.e. 'hot pursuit')

Studies should register patients with 'TIAs' as well as strokes to ensure that mild strokes, which may be misclassified as TIAs by referring doctors in routine clinical practice, are not under-represented

Use of diagnostic techniques, and especially brain computerised tomography scanning to determine the pathological type of stroke

Case ascertainment over whole years to avoid bias due to any seasonal fluctuations in incidence

Hospital activity is an alternative source of information which may reflect the incidence of stroke in hospital admission or discharge statistics. Out-patient attendances are seldom recorded. Again, inaccuracies in diagnostic codes may limit their usefulness but the major problem is that these data only include those patients who are admitted to the hospital with a stroke (Panayiotou *et al.*, 1993; Leibson *et al.*, 1994). This is therefore a better measure of the hospital service that is currently provided than the population's needs. The relationship between stroke incidence and hospitalisation can only be known with certainty where a reliable stroke incidence study has been performed to determine the proportion of stroke patients which attend hospital. Where hospital admission rates have been determined they have been shown to vary considerably between places, 55% to over 95% in developed countries, whilst there is no information from Asia and Africa (Bamford *et al.*, 1986; Asplund *et al.*, 1995). There is also no information about changes in admission rates with time. The hospital admission rate depends on several factors which are independent of population need:

1 the quality and availability of primary health care facilities;

2 the quality and availability of hospital facilities;

Table 17.3 Annual age specific incidence per 100 000 population in the 1980s and 1990s.

Place (mid-year) of study	Age (years)						45–84 (age adjusted)	45–74 (age adjusted) excluding subarachnoid haemorrhage
	0–44	45–54	55–64	65–74	75–84	85+		
1 Oxfordshire, England (1984) Bamford *et al.*, 1988	9	57	291	690	1428	2009	375	260
2 Soderhamn, Sweden (1990) Terent, 1988	12	67	313	976	2056	2995	481	324
3 Frederiksberg, Denmark (1989) Jorgensen *et al.*, 1992	4	104	306	712	1298	1599	386	295
4 Dijon, France (1987) Giroud *et al.*, 1989a,b	10	62	119	410	979	1641	223	151
5 Umbria, Italy (1988) Ricci *et al.*, 1991	5	115	280	541	1458	2180	367	249
6 Aosta, Italy (1989) D'Alessandro *et al.*, 1992	13	82	255	707	1607	3237	389	267
7 Warsaw, Poland* (1991) Czlonkowska *et al.*, 1994	14	76	268	408	901†	1355‡		215
8 Novosibirsk, Russia (1992) Feigin *et al.*, 1995	28	246	496	1060	1554	1513	596	486
9 Rochester, US (1988) Broderick *et al.*, 1989	9	62	269	642	1272	2111	352	246
10 Perth, Australia (1989) Anderson *et al.*, 1993a,b	17	98	207	511	1679	2369	349	209
11 Auckland, New Zealand (1991) Bonita *et al.*, 1993	18§	82	253	647	1267	1967	348	240

* Subarachnoid haemorrhage excluded; † age group 75–79 years; ‡ age group 80+ years; § age group 15–44 years.
Based on published data along with some unpublished data kindly made available to us from the authors and collated by Dr Cathie Sudlow.

3 the population's expectations—do people expect to be hospitalised after a stroke or does the culture allow for care in the community?
4 the availability of support services which may be informal (i.e. the extended family) or formal (i.e. community services);
5 the relative cost to the patient and their family of home versus hospital care;
6 the perceived value of hospital admission by doctors.

17.2.2 Stroke prevalence

Another measure of the frequency of stroke which some suggest is useful in planning services is stroke prevalence, i.e. the number of people who have ever had a stroke living in the population at one point in time. They argue that the prevalence of stroke is more important than the incidence in determining the needs for long-term support services in the community. However, we would argue that the greater the time which elapses following an acute stroke or TIA the less important disease-specific services become. If one is interested in determining the need for long-term support services it is

more useful to estimate the prevalence of disability due to all causes, rather than that related just to stroke. Patients with stroke are often elderly and suffer from other disabling conditions (e.g. arthritis, dementia), so that it is almost impossible to tease out what disability is attributable to stroke rather than these other causes. In addition, stroke prevalence can never reflect the true burden of stroke because the patients who die soon after stroke are not represented. There are also a number of important methodological difficulties associated with measuring the prevalence of stroke and TIA, not least the need to make accurate diagnoses sometimes years after the actual event and to survey thousands of people.

Stroke prevalence is difficult to measure and uninteresting.

17.2.3 A practical approach to needs assessment

The vast majority of health service planners are not fortunate enough to have had a recent, methodologically sound, stroke incidence study performed in the population they serve. Rather than carrying out their own incidence study, which is time consuming and expensive (but technically not that difficult), we recommend the following approach to determining local needs which uses both local data and information from incidence studies from other areas. If one looks at the results of the most reliable (i.e. those fulfilling most of the criteria of an 'ideal' study) stroke incidence studies (Table 17.3) it is surprising how little they vary (given the limits of their precision). However, it is important to point out that these are based mainly on Caucasian populations. One should start with the age- and sex-specific stroke incidence in the population which is closest to that locally in terms of geography, race and culture. These rates can then be applied to the local population numbers to obtain an age- and sex-standardised incidence rate (Table 17.4). A comparison of routinely collected data from the area in which the stroke incidence study was performed with similar data from one's own vicinity may give further evidence of the relevance of the incidence data. The cause-specific mortality rates are likely to be the most reliable and easily obtained. A large dif-

Table 17.4 A step-by-step guide to estimating approximately the number of strokes in a local population of interest.

Step 1	Obtain the most accurate census data for the population of interest for each sex and age category
Step 2	Identify the 'ideal' incidence study which is likely to have been done in a similar population to the one of interest (e.g. geography, race)
Step 3	Multiply each age- and sex-specific incidence rate by the number of people of that age and sex in the population of interest, e.g. if incidence in men of 65–74 years old is 690/100 000 and there are 11 000 men in this age band in the population of interest one would expect about 76 men (i.e. (690 × 11 000)/100 000) between 65 and 74 years old to suffer a stroke each year in the population of interest
Step 4	Sum the numbers of patients of each sex in each age band expected to have stroke to obtain the total number expected in the population
Step 5	Consider making an adjustment for any marked differences in, for example, the cause-specific mortality between the population of interest and the population where the incidence study was done
Step 6	If one is interested in TIA then their incidence is usually about 20% that of stroke (Dennis *et al.*, 1989a)
Step 7	The number of recurrent strokes is of the order of 30% of first-ever in a lifetime strokes, so that to estimate the total number of strokes likely to occur in the population of interest, the number of incident strokes should be inflated by 30%

ference compared with one's own area should alert one to potential differences in stroke incidence, although this may be related to the accuracy of death certification or different case fatality rates. One can then judge whether the incidence locally is likely to be greater or less than that from the available incidence study.

An alternative approach might be to use local hospital admission or discharge data and to adjust them to take account of the likely proportion of stroke patients admitted. This will be more reliable for stroke than for TIAs. One could estimate this proportion by surveying the local primary health teams and asking them to report the proportion of patients with acute stroke they refer to hospital. This may be reliable enough if they report that they refer virtually all cases (as in Sweden), but if the proportion is smaller their estimate may be misleading (Asplund *et al.*, 1995). Also, hospital discharge data may be very inaccurate for a number of reasons (Panayiotou *et al.*, 1993; Leibson *et al.*, 1994):

1 inaccuracy of routine clinical diagnosis, especially of TIAs;
2 lack of brain computerised tomography (CT) scans to confirm the stroke diagnosis, exclude other diagnoses or distinguish pathological types reliably;
3 coding errors;
4 failure to distinguish acute stroke admissions from those due to complications of an earlier stroke;
5 failure to code strokes occurring in hospital or in the context of another diagnosis.

The crude incidence of stroke tells one how common the problem is, but in itself is not sufficient to determine the health service needs of the population. Before one can plan a service one needs to have estimates of the following.

Age- and sex-specific incidence

Younger patients require different facilities from older ones, e.g. retraining for employment. Older women more often live alone and may require more formal support in the community. Table 17.3 shows the age-specific incidence rates from those studies which have used satisfactory or 'ideal' methodology. There does not appear to be a consistent difference in incidence between the sexes in these studies, females having a slightly higher incidence at young ages (where numbers are small) and at very old ages (see Section 6.2.3).

Type-specific incidence

(That is TIA, ischaemic stroke, primary intracerebral haemorrhage and subarachnoid haemorrhage.) These data may be

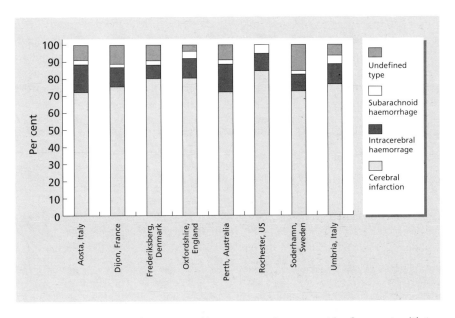

Figure 17.1 Histogram showing the proportions of patients aged between 45 and 84 years with a first-ever in a lifetime stroke due to cerebral infarction, primary intracerebral haemorrhage, subarachnoid haemorrhage and uncertain in 'ideal' incidence studies. Only studies with a CT scan rate of more than 70% which included subarachnoid haemorrhage are included. The study from Rochester did not have an uncertain category because the small proportion of patients who did not have a CT scan or autopsy were counted as cerebral infarctions. (Published data supplemented by unpublished data provided by Dr Cathie Sudlow.)

useful in more detailed planning of the population's needs. Patients with TIA and minor ischaemic stroke require prompt diagnosis, investigation and initiation of secondary prevention but do not require prolonged in-patient care, rehabilitation or community support services. Patients with subarachnoid haemorrhage usually require emergency hospitalisation and neurosurgical facilities (see Chapter 13). Haemorrhagic strokes have a higher early case fatality rate, so although they may require more care in the very early stages the longer term burden of severe disability may be less than patients with ischaemic stroke (see Table 10.2).

The estimates of the relative frequency of the pathological type of stroke are remarkably similar in most of the published incidence studies which come from predominantly Caucasian populations (Fig. 17.1). Although the proportion which are haemorrhagic is probably larger in Orientals, it is difficult to be certain because there are no recent more or less 'ideal' studies from non-Caucasian populations.

The prognosis of stroke and its subtypes

From the type-specific incidence and prognosis one can estimate the likely requirements for acute, diagnostic and assessment services, rehabilitation and terminal care services, long-term care, community support and secondary prevention. The prognosis of stroke and its subtypes has been dis-

cussed earlier (see Sections 10.2 and 16.1). Incidentally, one can also estimate the approximate prevalence of stroke in the population using the 'bath principle' (Fig. 17.2).

Changes over time

If one is planning a stroke service one has to take account of changes which may occur in the future, because one's service will need to alter to take these into account. Trends in stroke mortality and incidence are discussed later (see Section 18.2) and there is some evidence that the incidence, and maybe even the severity, of stroke is falling in many Western populations. Apart from the changing incidence one also has to take into account changing demographics. In most developed countries older people account for an increasing proportion of the population. Therefore, in a disease such as stroke where the incidence is much higher in older people (see Table 17.3), the total number of strokes will increase unless offset by a falling incidence rate. However, one has to remember that case fatality is higher in older patients (see Fig. 10.8) and in those with prior disability and, therefore, fewer of these older stroke patients will survive to require long-term care. Malmgren *et al.* (1989) calculated that over the next 30 years the number of new strokes occurring each year in the UK may well increase but there may be fewer *newly* disabled survivors. These sorts of forecasts are obvi-

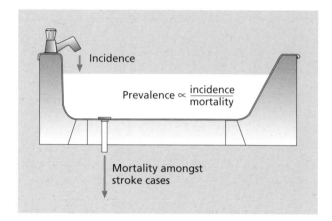

Figure 17.2 A bath with water running in (representing incident cases), the water level (representing prevalence) and water going down the plug hole (representing deaths in prevalent cases). The prevalence is directly proportional to the incidence and inversely proportional to the mortality amongst prevalent cases, although the mathematical relationship is quite complex.

ously important in determining the services one plans for the future. If there are going to be more acute strokes one will need to plan for more acute services, but if fewer survive the acute stage, rehabilitation and long-term care facilities may not need to increase to the same degree.

Changes in clinical practice may force rapid alterations in the shape of clinical services for stroke. For example, if a highly cost-effective acute treatment for ischaemic stroke was identified, but could only be given in hospital, this would markedly increase the hospitalisation rate in those countries where a sizeable proportion of strokes are currently managed at home. Conversely, if rehabilitation at home was demonstrated to be more cost-effective than that in hospital, this would require a transfer of hospital-based resources into the community. The changes in management of stroke have, until now, been small and gradual but with recent increases in research efforts major changes are more likely and the needs of the population could alter rapidly and unpredicatably.

17.2.4 Assuming that resources are limited, to what extent will the needs of the population be met?

Having obtained an estimate of one's local age-, sex- and type-specific incidence and outcome of stroke and TIA one is still a long way from determining the actual needs of the population. After all, this estimate does not indicate the actual resources these people will require and, of course, at some stage somebody has to make a political decision about how completely the population's needs are to be met.

Inevitably, where there are limited resources for health services, choices have to be made about allocating resources between areas (e.g. should one build a new hospital or a new school?). Having been given limited resources, however, it is important that those planning stroke services use them in as an efficient manner as possible and prioritise (i.e. ration) to make sure that sufficient funds are available for whatever are perceived to be the most important aspects of the service. These decisions are usually taken by politicians but, because they depend on information about the effectiveness of components of the stroke services, it is vital that the politicians receive sound medical advice.

17.3 Planning a service

Having established the aims of the service, the needs of the population and to what degree one expects to fulfil these, one can then plan the development of services. Usually one starts with the existing services even if these are inadequate and chaotic. It is then useful to consider the following questions prior to making any changes: (i) what are the current resources committed to the management of patients with TIAs and stroke?; and (ii) what are the major gaps (i.e. unmet needs and failure to provide cost-effective interventions) in the present provision of services? One needs to establish the strengths and weaknesses of the current services to identify the most important areas for improvement. Priority should be given to providing patients with basic care (e.g. nursing to provide for basic needs) and to delivering those interventions which are of proven effectiveness.

Although information regarding current services may already be available it is likely that in addition to routinely collected data it will be useful to carry out a survey to determine the following.

1 How many and what sort of patients are currently being managed (i.e. demographic and clinical data)?
2 Where are they being managed (i.e. hospital or community, neurology, internal medicine or geriatric medicine)?
3 By whom are they being managed (i.e. general practitioner, neurologst, general physician)?
4 How are they being managed (i.e. the process of care)?
5 What resources are currently being used?

A community-based register which identified all patients in the population who had a stroke or TIA would be an ideal but expensive and impractical way of answering these questions. A hospital-based stroke register is a practical alternative which can help answer most of the questions, although clearly it can not provide detailed information about patients who are not referred to hospital. A register is an invaluable tool for monitoring the performance of services as well as planning them (see Section 17.6). Such a survey will identify areas of strength and weakness and may determine which area to concentrate on first. This decision will also depend on how easily or cheaply a particular problem can be solved. For instance, poor standards of medical assessment may be improved by the introduction of a protocol and education for junior medical staff with little implication for resources, whilst the provision of an occupational therapy department where this is lacking will have major resource implications.

> *Set up a hospital-based stroke register to get some idea of the current state of the local stroke service, however fragmented and chaotic it is.*

What is the evidence for the cost-effectiveness of the various components of the stroke service?

Stroke services should first concentrate on providing basic care for the patients and their families and then aim to give priority to those aspects of care which are generally accepted as being, or have been proven to be, effective. Evidence from randomised trials and formal statistical overviews of groups of trials provide the most reliable unbiased evidence. The Stroke Review Group of the Cochrane Collaboration will become an excellent source of this type of information (see Section 11.2.1) even though at present not many reviews are available (Counsell *et al.*, 1995). It is important that those who are responsible for planning services are aware of all the available evidence concerning the effectiveness of interventions and the methods of delivering those interventions to the appropriate patients. If there are data concerning the cost of interventions and various other aspects of the service this may allow health care planners to make more informed choices about which services should be provided.

> *The best and quickest way to access information on the effectiveness of interventions in stroke will soon be the regularly updated electronic database provided by the Cochrane Collaboration.*

17.4   Where should stroke patients be managed?

17.4.1   Caring for stroke patients in the community

Why admit stroke patients to hospital?

The vast majority of patients who have a stroke have it in the community and not in hospital. Many of them require help from medical and social services. However, in some societies, most notably the UK, as many as 45% of patients with acute stroke are managed without ever being admitted to hospital, whilst in others, e.g. Sweden, almost everyone who has a stroke and many who have a TIA are immediately admitted to hospital for diagnosis, assessment and treatment (Bamford *et al.*, 1986; Asplund *et al.*, 1995).

The main reason for referral to hospital in the UK is for nursing care rather than diagnosis and treatment (Brocklehurst *et al.*, 1978; Wade & Langton Hewer, 1983; Bamford *et al.*, 1986). Social factors, in particular, the support available in the community, the housing and the wishes of the patients and their family have some influence on the general practitioner in the decision whether to refer or not. The low hospital referral rate in Oxfordshire may therefore reflect: the relatively good support which was available in that semirural community; the general practitioners' confidence in diagnosing, assessing and treating patients; and the wishes or expectations of the patients and their families. It may be that in societies where a much higher proportion of patients are hospitalised, the primary care services are less well developed and the primary care physicians (as well as their patients) less confident in their ability to manage stroke patients. It may also reflect the patient's expectations or wishes. After all stroke is a serious and potentially life-threatening illness.

Is care in the community safe, effective and less costly than hospital-based care?

It is interesting that in the UK, which already has a lower hospital admission rate for stroke than most other developed countries, there is a move to admit even fewer patients to hospital (Wade, 1992c). This is probably based on two assumptions: (i) that care in the community is at least as effective as care in hospital and may be cheaper; and (ii) that patients and families would prefer to be cared for at home. The adoption of a policy of non-admission for stroke patients carries the considerable risk that 'community care' may become synonymous with 'inadequate care'. It is far easier, and cheaper, to overlook the needs of patients when they are at home rather than in hospital, and it is far harder to monitor what is going on.

> *Do not move the care of stroke patients into the community until there is reliable evidence that this is at least as cost-effective as hospital-based care, or that it is preferred by patients and their families.*

There have been no randomised studies comparing the effectiveness or cost of care at home with that in hospital, and little evidence concerning patients' and families' preferences. Therefore, it would be unwise to introduce a major shift in the pattern of where patients are managed before more evidence about cost-effectiveness is available.

How feasible is community-based care?

Certainly, many of the components of care shown in Table 17.1 can very reasonably be provided without admission to hospital. We will discuss how each of these can be provided in the community.

Diagnosis and assessment. The clinical diagnosis and initial assessment of stroke, including simple blood tests and an electrocardiogram (ECG), do not in themselves require referral to hospital. Assuming a reasonable level of knowledge and competence, all this could be done by a primary care physician. CT brain scanning is an out-patient procedure and although a relatively small proportion of patients will need a CT scan to confirm the diagnosis, the majority will need one to plan further treatment, in particular secondary prevention (see Section 5.3.3). However, one will probably need to restructure the service to ensure that CT scans are performed within days of stroke onset to ensure reliable differentiation of haemorrhage from infarction (see Section 5.3.4). Other investigations (e.g. duplex sonography, echocardiography) can also be performed as out-patient procedures. But, all this does rely on an efficient means of transporting patients, some of whom may be disabled, to and from hospital and once they get there on having an efficient and streamlined system to look after them.

Transient events, TIAs and episodes which may be confused with them, are less reliably diagnosed and more often require the input from a specialist, especially where the diagnosis is crucial to future decision making, i.e. the distinction between carotid and posterior circulation TIAs in a patient with severe carotid stenosis. The large range of final diagnoses in patients referred to the Oxfordshire Community Stroke Project with 'probable TIAs' by general practitioners is shown in Table 17.5 (see Section 3.3.1).

Although the clinical diagnosis of stroke may be quite straightforward, the assessment which then guides further management needs to be both thorough and accurate (see Section 10.3.2). There is evidence from audits of case notes that even hospital-admitted patients often have incomplete and inaccurate assessments (Davenport *et al.*, 1995a). Evidence from our own studies of the assessments in primary care indicate that these are often superficial and even less complete. Of course, there is as yet little evidence that improving the completeness of assessment significantly alters outcome but, equally, no evidence exists that sloppy assessment is as effective as a good assessment. Also, one must not

Table 17.5 Final diagnoses of 512 patients referred as probable TIAs to the Oxfordshire Community Stroke Project by their general practitioner. (From Dennis *et al.*, 1989a.)

	Per cent
TIAs	38
Migraine	10
Syncope/pre-syncope	9
Possible TIA	9
'Funny turn' (no focal symptoms)	9
Isolated vertigo	6
Epileptic seizures	6
Transient global amnesia	3
Lone bilateral blindness*	3
Isolated diplopia	<1
Drop attacks	<1
Meningiomas	<1
Miscellaneous	5

* We later demonstrated that these patients had a risk of subsequent stroke which was at least that of the average patient with a TIA; we would now classify these as definite TIAs, probably due to ischaemia in the posterior circulation (see Section 3.2.2).

overlook the possibility that a thorough assessment of the patient's and carer's problems and needs has advantages beyond those measured by crude clinical outcome (e.g. patient's perception of self-value, etc.).

Acute specific treatment. In some societies the high hospital admission rates may, in part, reflect the belief, amongst both physicians and the public, that specific acute therapy is effective. Certainly in Italy, where the admission rate is probably about 85%, acute treatments such as glycerol are much more in vogue than in the UK (Ricci *et al.*, 1991; D'Alessandro *et al.*, 1992; Ricci, 1995) (see Table 11.3). However, since no routine acute medical treatment has yet been shown to be effective in improving the outcome after stroke, it is not necessary to admit patients for this reason. But, if effective acute treatments are found then this will have a profound effect on where stroke patients are managed. For example, if a treatment has to be preceded by brain CT or another hospital-based procedure, or if it is given by intravenous infusion, more stroke patients will have to be admitted to hospital. Also, it seems likely that hospital admission will normally be required to enter the randomised trials which are needed to test the effectiveness of novel therapies. Of course, if the treatment could be administered in the community, and haemorrhage did not have to be excluded by brain CT prior to administration, the hospital admission rate might actually fall since a proportion of patients might improve to such an extent that they did not require admission.

General care may be provided either in hospital or in the community, although most patients who have had a severe stroke will need admission to hospital unless considerably more support services are available in the community than currently. Wade *et al.* (1985) tested whether hospital admission could be prevented by providing a rapid response service in the community to support patients in their own home. Although this was not a randomised trial, the results did not suggest that this was possible, although this may have been because the service was unable to overcome the delays in providing enough community support. However, the potential bias in this non-random comparison could easily have obscured a real benefit, or harm, from the team.

Rehabilitation. It is possible to rehabilitate as patients outpatients either in their own homes or in hospital-based facilities such as day hospitals. Recent randomised trials have compared the effectiveness of domiciliary physiotherapy with that provided in a day hospital (Young & Forster, 1992, 1993; Gladman *et al.*, 1993; Gladman & Lincoln, 1994). A combined analysis demonstrated only small differences in outcome in patients randomised between the two methods of delivering physiotherapy (Gladman *et al.*, 1995). Certainly in patients with complex disability after a stroke, apart from the practical problems of providing enough care in the community, one also has the difficulty of coordinating a multidisciplinary team which is working over a wide geographical area.

Continuing care and maintenance, almost by definition, is provided in the community, although certain aspects may be hospital based, i.e. day hospital, respite care, etc. The emphasis on long-term institutional care varies from country to country.

Secondary prevention. There is little doubt that most of this aspect of stroke care can be very effectively managed in the community. However, there are now several effective options for the secondary prevention of stroke (see Chapter 16) and some (e.g. anticoagulation and carotid surgery) need detailed assessment prior to implementation. Those with TIAs and mild stroke can usually be managed mainly as outpatients or day patients. By providing rapid and easy access to a specialist opinion in out-patients it may be possible to avoid unnecessary hospital admission which will save resources. Some centres are able to offer a one visit assessment when patients can be assessed clinically and all the non-invasive investigations (e.g. blood tests, ECG, carotid duplex, brain CT) performed to allow the clinician to plan secondary prevention. It makes no sense to admit patients as the only way to obtain rapid access to investigatory facilities.

After all, the common investigations, except for conventional catheter angiography, can all be routinely performed on an out-patient basis. Hopefully in the next few years non-invasive arterial imaging with ultrasound and magnetic resonance will completely replace the more invasive and hazardous techniques (see Section 6.6.4). Those responsible for organising stroke services should ensure that patients have rapid access to investigations on an out-patient or day case basis and so avoid unnecessary admissions to hospital, and that there is an efficient system to process the patients, get the results back to the physician, and then translate them into advice for the patient.

The risk of stroke after a TIA, or recurrent stroke after a first stroke, is much higher in the early period and tails off later. The risk is approximately 4% in the first month, 9% in 6 months and 13% in the first year (see Section 16.1.1) (Dennis *et al.*, 1989b, 1990; Burn *et al.*, 1994). Thus, one has most to gain from starting secondary prevention as early as possible. Also, since the accurate diagnosis of TIAs depends on a good history it makes sense to assess the patients as soon after the event as possible.

In many centres so-called neurovascular, TIA or stroke clinics have been set up which are characterised by:
1 providing rapid access to a specialist opinion regarding TIAs, strokes and those episodes which may mimic them;
2 streamlined access to the necessary investigations;
3 close links with vascular surgeons or neurosurgeons who can offer carotid endarterectomy.
These clinics should avoid many of the shortcomings of traditional models of TIA and stroke care. In our experience, however, such clinics attract patients with a wide range of neurological conditions (Table 17.6), so the clinician must have neurological training or at least easy access to sound neurological advice.

Neurovascular clinics should provide rapid clinical assessment of patients who may have had a transient ischaemic attack or minor stroke, streamlined and cost-effective investigations, and early intervention to reduce the risk of a serious vascular event.

Coordination of care by a multidisciplinary team. There is now evidence that care in a dedicated stroke unit which is coordinated by a specialist with an interested multidisciplinary team is more effective than care provided in general wards (Langhorne *et al.*, 1993; Dennis & Langhorne, 1994; Stroke Unit Trialists' Collaboration, 1996). It therefore seems likely that specialist care would be superior to non-specialist care delivered in the community. It is even conceivable that care in the community could be coordinated by a specialist multidisciplinary team, but this would need to be

Table 17.11 Common problems which arise late after a stroke, often when the patient is no longer in hospital.

Patient
Deteriorating function due to
  Overprotective carer
  Progressing co-morbidities
  Lack of continuing therapy?
Depression or anxiety, even agoraphobia (see Section 15.31)
Social isolation
Financial difficulties
Sexual dysfunction (see Section 15.33.4)
Undetected rise in blood pressure
Central post-stroke pain (see Section 15.23)

Carer
Physical ill health due to the strain of caring
Depression or anxiety
Poor relationship with patient because of personality change
Social isolation because unable to get out to meet people
Financial difficulties

Table 17.12 A stroke follow-up checklist.

Review	
Impairments	Weakness, balance, speech, etc.
Disabilities	What can you do for yourself?
	Do you need help with any everyday activities?
	Ask specifically about 'activities of daily living' functions
Aids and adaptation	Have they been delivered yet?
	Is the patient or carer using them?
	Are they in good working order?
Support services	Are they happening?
	Are they appropriate and adequate?

Have any new problems arisen since last seen (see Table 17.11)?

How is any carer coping?

Is everything being done to prevent a recurrent vascular event?	Check the blood pressure
	Enquire about smoking, diet and exercise
	Check compliance with medication

---

method of delivering continuing therapy, i.e. domiciliary or day hospital (see Section 17.4.1).

Although secondary prevention should be started as soon after the stroke as possible, for the reasons outlined in Chapter 16, the interventions (e.g. modification of blood pressure, cholesterol, control of diabetes and antiplatelet therapy) need to be continued and monitored. This can be done in a hospital-based clinic but would be better and more conveniently (for the patient) managed in the primary health care sector since many of these interventions will be lifelong. A follow-up checklist should ensure that late problems are not overlooked (Table 17.12).

17.5.5 Information for patients and carers

Studies of the attitudes of patients and their carers to medical services in general, and stroke services in particular, have demonstrated that one of the greatest sources of dissatisfaction is with communication (Pound *et al.*, 1994; Wellwood *et al.*, 1995a). Patients and carers may receive very little information about the nature of stroke, its cause, management and likely prognosis (Wellwood *et al.*, 1994). Even where information is provided it may be in a form which is difficult to understand or retain.

The patient's, and their carer's, perception of the stroke service is likely to depend not just on the degree of recovery but also on the quality of communication. Although it is easy to show that many patients receive little information one must also remember that for some it may be enough. We have shown that some patients do not want a lot of information, preferring to trust in the professionals' judgement (Wellwood *et al.*, 1994). This will undoubtedly vary from place to place and may change over time. It is therefore important to tailor one's information giving to the individual's needs and wishes. This information should probably be provided using a number of different media including:
1 a noticeboard on the unit (Fig. 17.5);
2 an information pack containing appropriate leaflets;
3 audio and video tapes;
4 individual interviews with patients and carers;
5 patient and carer groups.
However, there is probably no substitute for one of the team sitting down with the patient and their family on one or more occasions to explain the situation and answer any specific questions. This can then be backed up with written

Table 17.13 Tips on improving communication with carers of hospitalised stroke patients.

Provide a noticeboard at the entrance to the unit introducing staff and informing relatives about how to contact members of the team
Hold ward rounds during visiting times
Invite carers to participate in patient care
Invite carers to therapy sessions
Set up a carers' group
Document the content of any discussions with relatives in the notes and report these at team meetings to ensure consistency
Arrange pre-discharge case conferences or family meetings
Back up verbal communication with written or audio material

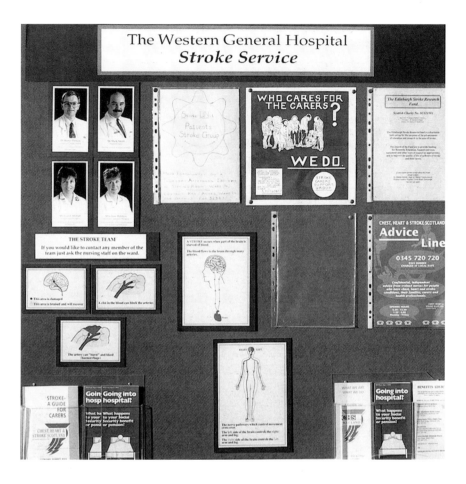

Figure 17.5 A noticeboard at the entrance to a stroke unit. Typically it introduces the members of the stroke team, indicating how they might be contacted. It presents, in simple terms, what a stroke is and how it might affect the patient. We also include useful pamphlets and information relating to patient and carer groups.

material. One novel approach, which has been used in other areas (e.g. oncology), is to record the interview and give the recording to the patient or family so that they can review what has been said as they wish. This might overcome the problem of patients and families only taking in a small proportion of the information given to them.

Like all other areas of stroke care a service needs to establish a system for ensuring that input, in this case information giving, is tailored to the individual needs of patients and carers (Table 17.13).

17.6 Monitoring and evaluating stroke services

We believe that the most reliable way of determining the relative effectiveness of interventions is an appropriately designed randomised trial, or a meta-analysis if more than one trial is available. Unfortunately, this is not a very practical option in the evaluation of a local stroke service rather than stroke services in general (Table 17.14), so we have to rely on less robust methodology.

Non-randomised comparisons of the process of care, or of patient and carer outcomes achieved by services, in different places at the same time or in the same place over time, are the only practical methods of evaluation. If one was to set up a new service in a hospital one could compare the process or outcomes with those in a nearby hospital without a new service. Alternatively, one could measure the process and outcomes achieved by the existing service and then measure whether these are improved after the new service has been established (i.e. a before-and-after study). However, such evaluations can be misleading. They may be able to demonstrate improvements (or worsening) or differences in the process or outcome of care but they can not provide reliable data to indicate that any changes are due to the new service (see Section 17.6.3). There may be systematic differences in the patients treated by services in different hospitals or in the same hospital over time. For example, in one of our own hospitals the development of a new stroke service was accompanied by closure of the accident and emergency department which may have accounted for fewer severe strokes being admitted. We observed a marked fall in case fatality and length of stay, but was this due to our new stroke

Table 17.14 Reasons why it is not practical to perform a randomised controlled trial to evaluate a new stroke unit.

In a single institution it may be impossible to isolate the treatment and control groups. Thus, there may be contamination of the control group which will reduce the power of the study to demonstrate significant differences in outcomes. Where one is comparing services in several institutions it may become difficult to distinguish the effects of the services from the effects of the individuals involved in the services

In a single institution it is often impractical to randomise sufficient patients to provide a statistically robust result

Although the benefits of a service may be measured in terms of crude outcomes, e.g. death, more subtle, but valuable benefits, such as patient satisfaction are less easily measured

Randomised trials need resources, e.g. randomisation services, maintenance of at least two parallel services, blinded assessments, data collection, storage and analysis which make them relatively unattractive to purchasers of health care. For example, in a recently completed trial of a stroke family support worker the trial cost as much as the intervention itself (O'Rourke *et al.*, 1995)

Some would argue that given the strong evidence for the effectiveness of organised stroke care it is ethically unacceptable to randomise patients to disorganised care

---

service (Davenport *et al.*, 1995b). Other changes might influence the results of any evaluation. For example, new legislation concerning care in the community accompanied the setting up of our unit. Could this account for our reduced length of stay?

Clearly, one can not rely on such non-randomised evaluations to influence practice elsewhere but they may fulfil important local functions. One could reasonably argue that, as long as the new service is not much more expensive to run, it does not matter whether any improvements observed can be attributed directly to that service. Obviously, if the new service was very costly one would want reassurance that the improvements would not have occurred spontaneously. Also, if a non-randomised evaluation demonstrates either no improvement or even a worse outcome, it is difficult to know how to respond. Were the changes due to the new service, in which case it ought to be modified, or were they due to some unforeseen confounding factor?

There are several other methodological problems, which can affect randomised as well as non-randomised comparisons, and which need to be considered.
1 Small numbers of patients so that any change observed may be accounted for by the play of chance.
2 Missing a moderate but real change because too few patients were studied.
3 Observer bias in assessing process or outcome. Often, the

observers have an interest in the result of the evaluation which may influence their judgements.

What aspects of a service can we measure? A stroke service may include some components for which there is little doubt of their effectiveness, but many others of uncertain benefit. When assessing performance it is therefore most important to monitor how well the service delivers those components whose effectiveness is established (e.g. aspirin for secondary prevention; see Section 16.4).

The simplest way to monitor the service is to measure the amount of work being carried out. Unfortunately, politicians and those who fund health care, place too much emphasis on the volume rather than quality of service. The number of cases managed by a service tells one very little about the quality of care given to those patients. In assessing the quality of care (or clinical audit as it tends to be called) one should consider three aspects of the service (Donabedian, 1988): (i) the structure, or facilities available; (ii) the process of care; and (iii) the outcomes of those treated.

17.6.1 Structure

From all that has gone previously it should be fairly obvious that a stroke service needs certain facilities to provide all the components necessary to care for patients with strokes and TIAs. This makes the setting of standards and the measurement of performance for structure relatively straightforward. Some basic standards for structure might include:
1 an identified individual who is responsible for the organisation of services;
2 a multidisciplinary team (see Section 10.3.5);
3 immediate access to acute hospital beds;
4 prompt out-patient assessment by a specialist for patients not needing admission to hospital (i.e. a neurovascular clinic; see Section 17.4.1);
5 prompt access to CT scanning for in-patients and out-patients (see Section 17.4.1);
6 prompt access to non-invasive vascular imaging, carotid angiography and surgery if necessary (see Section 16.7);
7 a stroke unit (see Section 17.4.2);
8 continuing care facilities, both community based and institutional.

However, care has to be taken in defining these standards. For example, what does 'prompt access' mean? There is also an inevitable overlap with measures of process and outcome when defining the quality of these elements. For example, the multidisciplinary team will only be effective if it meets regularly, the non-invasive vascular imaging must be accurate (see Section 6.6.4) and the carotid angiography and surgery must be delivered at low risk (see Section 16.7).

17.6.2 Process

Although some aspects of the process of care are easily monitored, e.g. waiting times for appointments, those relating to clinical care are more difficult. It may be relatively easy to define a standard (e.g. patients with TIAs and ischaemic strokes should be given aspirin to reduce the risk of further vascular events unless there are contraindications) but for others, for which there is less scientific justification, it is more difficult. The lack of scientific justification can, and frequently is, overcome by using the combined views of recognised experts, i.e. consensus. Thus, it is possible, by one means or another, to produce standards to which we may aspire even when there is limited evidence on which to base clinical practice. But, as we have already stressed, the care an individual receives should be based on a thorough assessment and tailored to their particular condition and needs (see Section 10.3.2). So, for example, one might set the standard that all patients should have a thorough assessment of their visuospatial function on admission because this may have important effect on their function and prognosis. However, the detailed testing of visuospatial function can not be done in unconscious patients nor in those who can not communicate or use their dominant hand. Thus, what appears to be a fairly straightforward standard can not be applied sensibly to every patient. To overcome this difficulty one has to develop standards with criteria attached where lower standards may be acceptable. The Royal College of Physicians *Stroke Audit Package* (1994) has addressed this problem by having a 'no but' clause attached to each standard (Fig. 17.6). This is essential for the process of care to be compared in different groups of patients so that, for example, if there is a higher proportion of unconscious patients in one group (i.e. a difference in case mix), the process with regard to assessing visuospatial function will not necessarily be worse.

> *Monitoring the process of care by case note review raises a number of important methodological problems which must be addressed if one's assessment is to be useful and valid.*

Another difficulty with measuring the process of care is that, by directly observing the care, one is likely to alter its delivery (the so-called Hawthorne effect). For example, if one was to watch junior doctors performing an assessment they are likely to take extra care in doing so. Also, such an approach is likely to be very costly if performed on all stroke admissions. The alternative is to audit the records of care but this immediately raises the question of the validity of the medical record, i.e. whether the records reflect the actual care provided. However, most people would agree that good

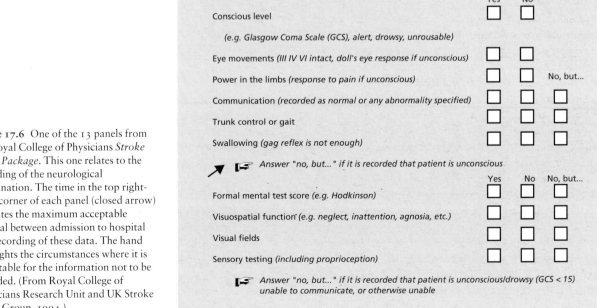

Figure 17.6 One of the 13 panels from the Royal College of Physicians *Stroke Audit Package*. This one relates to the recording of the neurological examination. The time in the top right-hand corner of each panel (closed arrow) indicates the maximum acceptable interval between admission to hospital and recording of these data. The hand highlights the circumstances where it is acceptable for the information not to be recorded. (From Royal College of Physicians Research Unit and UK Stroke Audit Group, 1994.)

Table 17.15 Important methodological issues in the audit of case notes.

Patient selection bias
The case notes audited should be a representative sample of all those treated. Thus, it might be a consecutive series or a random sample

Case note retrieval bias
Poor quality case notes or those of dead patients may be more difficult to retrieve which might bias the audit in a favourable direction. A high rate of retrieval is an important step in reducing bias (Vickers & Pollock, 1993)

Lack of precision
A sufficiently large number of case notes should be audited to provide a precise estimate of performance and to allow valid comparisons to be made with other centres or with audits performed at different times in the same centre

Observer bias
An auditor may have an interest in the result of the audit which may influence their assessment of performance. Blinded, or at least impartial, observers should be employed if possible

Poor inter-rater reliability of measure
If the measure of performance is not reliable then it will be more difficult to demonstrate real differences between centres. Also, if there is a consistent difference in the way an audit measure is applied by different auditors this may produce invalid comparisons

Differences in case mix
A standard which is applicable to one patient may not apply to another. It is important that standards are adjusted for difference in case mix

---

records probably do reflect good care given and that this is a reasonable method to measure the process of care. The other methodological problems involved in audits of case notes are summarised in Table 17.15.

Although one may be measuring the performance against some 'ideal' standard one is likely to want to compare the performance in the same service over time, or that between services. To do this meaningfully one has to have a valid and reliable measure of performance, to audit enough cases to produce statistically robust results and to be able to take into account differences in case mix between services or changes over time. The Royal College of Physicians *Stroke Audit Package* (1994) has been developed to overcome these methodological problems and enable valid comparisons to be made (Gompertz *et al.*, 1994). Unfortunately, this package only addresses a limited number of the more medical aspects of care so there still remains a need to develop audit tools which address other important aspects of care delivered by the different members of the multidisciplinary team.

17.6.3 Outcome

The term outcome causes confusion because of variation in usage. Clinicians use the term to refer to the clinical outcome of the patient or carer. Therefore, outcomes include survival, functional status, complications or less easily defined concepts such as quality of life. Other people, in particular those with a management background, use the term outcome to refer to any result of an intervention, e.g. reduced waiting times, readmission rates. Certain aspects, such as patient satisfaction with care, are referred to as indicators of process or outcome. In this section we use outcomes to refer to the clinical outcome of patients (i.e. physical, functional, cognitive, emotional, etc.).

Since the main aim of stroke services is to optimise the outcome of patients and carers the measurement of outcome is obviously the most relevant criterion by which to judge the performance of a service. Unfortunately, the use of outcomes to reflect the quality of care is the most challenging area of stroke audit (Gompertz *et al.*, 1995). The difficulties in using outcome data to reflect the quality of care have been extensively studied in the US (Daley *et al.*, 1988; Jencks *et al.*, 1988; Kahn *et al.*, 1988). Until these can be overcome, those involved in providing and monitoring health services must be wary of misinterpreting outcome data. The observed outcome in a group of patients treated by a particular service will be determined by four factors.

1 The quality and effectiveness of the care provided

This is the aspect which we hope outcomes will reflect.

2 The method of measurement of outcome

There are a large number of available measures of relevant aspects of outcome which may reflect the quality of care (Table 17.16). However, it is important that they have acceptable validity (i.e. they measure what they are intended to measure) and reliability (i.e. they are reproducible in different settings and when used by different people). A number of different types of scale have been developed and used to measure outcome after stroke. The choice of scale will depend on the question being asked but there are a number of features which one should look for in choosing an outcome measure (Table 17.17) (van Gijn & Warlow, 1992). One can loosely categorise the measures of outcome after stroke under the following headings.

Stroke scales. So-called 'stroke scales' (e.g. Mathews Scale, Scandinavian Stroke Scale, Canadian Stroke Scale, National

Table 17.16 Aspects of outcome which might be relevant in assessing stroke services, and some tools to measure these outcomes.

Outcome	Promising measurement tools
Survival	Case fatality during a defined time period, e.g. 30 days or 6 months post-stroke onset
Complications	Proportion of patients developing pressure sores or fractures
	There are difficulties in defining these and reliably recording them. Better services may identify more and record them more often (Davenport et al., 1996)
Residual impairments	Probably not very useful and not easily collected after hospital discharge
Mobility	10-m walking speed
Arm function	Nine-hole peg test
Psychological outcome	Hospital anxiety and depression scale General health questionnaire (see Table 15.42)
	Many of the most disabled patients will not be capable of responding to measures of psychological outcome
Disability	Barthel Index (see Table 17.18) Functional Independence Measure (FIM) Simple questions (see Fig. 17.7) Office of Population Censuses and Surveys disability scale Oxford Handicap Scale (see Table 17.20)
	Should be measured at defined point after the stroke, e.g. 6 months. Easily collected after hospital discharge
Handicap	London Handicap Scale
	A difficult area with no well-tested measures. The Oxford Handicap Scale does not really address handicap in isolation
Patient or carer satisfaction with care	Hospsat and Homesat (Pound et al., 1994)
	Is this an outcome or process measure? There are no well-tested measures available
General health	Nottingham Health Profile Short Form 36 EuroQol
	Potentially interesting because could allow comparisons with other disease states. However, many stroke patients can not complete the questionnaires because of cognitive problems

Institute of Health Stroke Scale) were largely developed to describe the severity of acute stroke and to monitor changes in the patient's condition (Mathew et al., 1972; Scandinavian Stroke Study Group, 1985; Cote et al., 1986, 1989; Brott et al., 1989). Most concentrate on the type and severity of the neurological impairments, although some (e.g. Mathews Scale) also includes a disability element (Mathew et al., 1972). They have been criticised for lacking relevance for patients, being complex and therefore impractical, and for summing 'apples and pears' (van Gijn & Warlow, 1992). They rely on a clinical examination and therefore can not be used other than in a 'face-to-face'

Table 17.17 Important features of scales for the measurement of outcome after stoke.

Validity
The scale should measure that aspect of outcome which it purports to measure. Different types of validity include: criterion validity when the measure is related to an accepted gold standard; construct validity where the measure is related to existing measures of similar aspects of outcome; content (or face) validity which relies on expert agreement that the measure is reasonable. There are considerable difficulties in demonstrating the validity of a particular measure (Lyden & Lau, 1991)

Reliability
This refers to the reproducibility of a measurement, most commonly between observers (interobserver reliability) and over time (intraobserver or test–retest reliability)

Relevance
The scale should measure some aspect of outcome which is relevant to the patient or carer as well as to the doctor. Thus, the size of a cerebral infarct on a CT scan is of little relevance whilst the patient's ability to look after themselves is very important to the patient and carer

Practicality
Scales vary in their complexity and the time taken to complete an assessment. Studies of long-term outcome involving hundreds of patients need very simple measures which can be completed by postal or telephone questionnaire, whilst smaller studies in hospital can afford to use more complex measures

Sensitivity
It is important that a scale can distinguish patients who have different outcomes or can detect important changes in a particular patient. Usually, more sensitive scales are more complex and unfortunately less reliable

Communicability
It is useful if the measure means something to other health professions or even patients. It is more useful to know that a patient feels 'fine' than to be told that their score on a particular stroke scale was, for example, 23

Table 17.18 Barthel Index showing two alternative scoring systems. (From Mahoney & Barthel, 1965.)

Item	Score	Score	Categories
Bowels	0	0	Incontinent or needs enemas
	5	1	Occasional incontinence (< once per week)
	10	2	Continent
Bladder	0	0	Incontinent/unable to manage catheter
	5	1	Occasional accident (< once per day)
	10	2	Continent
Grooming	0	0	Needs help with shaving, washing, hair or teeth
	5	1	Independent
Toilet use	0	0	Dependent
	5	1	Needs some help
	10	2	Independent on, off, dressing and cleaning
Feeding	0	0	Dependent
	5	1	Needs some help (e.g. with cutting, spreading)
	10	2	Independent if food provided within reach
Transfer	0	0	Unable and no sitting balance
(e.g. bed	5	1	Needs major help
to chair)	10	2	Needs minor help
	15	3	Independent
Mobility	0	0	Unable
	5	1	Wheelchair independent indoors
	10	2	Walks with help or supervision
	15	3	Independent (but may use aid)
Dressing	0	0	Dependent
	5	1	Needs some help
	10	2	Independent including fasteners
Stairs	0	0	Unable
	5	1	Needs some help or supervision
	10	2	Independent up and down
Bathing	0	0	Dependent
	5	1	Independent in bath or shower
Total	**100**	**20**	

situation. We do not think they are useful in evaluating stroke services. They might be used as a measure of case mix and they may be useful in describing short-term changes early after acute stroke where measuring disability, handicap or quality of life is both difficult and inappropriate.

> *It is better to have an imprecise answer to the right question than a precise answer to the wrong question.*

Functional scales include measures of disability or dependence in activities of daily living (ADL) such as the Barthel Index (Table 17.18), Nottingham ADL Scale and the Functional Independence Measure (FIM) (Mahoney & Barthel, 1965; Ebrahim *et al.*, 1985; State University of New York at Buffalo, 1993). One could also include the so-called extended ADL scales which identify whether patients are participating in more complex activities, e.g. shopping, leisure or work. These last include scales such as the Frenchay Activities Index and the Nottingham Extended ADL Scale (Holbrook & Skilbeck, 1983; Nouri & Lincoln, 1987; Schuling *et al.*, 1993). They appear to measure relevant aspects of outcome although some demonstrate ceiling effects (e.g. the Barthel Index) and may not pick up prolems in particular areas, e.g. communication (Wellwood *et al.*, 1995b). They are in general 'ordinal scales' so that care must be taken in choosing the appropriate statistical methods to describe or compare groups of patients (Table 17.19). One disability scale, the Office of Population Censuses and Surveys (OPCS) disability instrument, could be considered an 'interval' scale (Table 17.19) and appears to cover most aspects of disability (Martin *et al.*, 1988). However, it is probably too complex for routine use in large studies (McPherson *et al.*, 1993; Wellwood *et al.*, 1995b). Some of these scales are simple enough to incorporate into a postal or telephone questionnaire and therefore may be used in large studies of long-term outcome (Shinar *et al.*, 1987).

Handicap, and the closely allied concept of *quality of life*, are difficult to define and therefore difficult to measure, but are undoubtedly of relevance to stroke patients and their carers. The Oxford Handicap Scale (Table 17.20), which is a modification of the Rankin Scale, sounds as if it measures handicap but probably does not (Rankin, 1957; Bamford *et al.*, 1989). It includes reference to symptoms, dependency and lifestyle. However, it has been widely used, is relevant and simple enough to be used reliably over the telephone and is therefore useful in large studies (Candelise *et al.*, 1994). The London Handicap Scale has recently been developed and appears to be a promising measure of handicap after stroke but requires further evaluation (Harwood *et al.*, 1994).

> *Like motherhood, quality of life is much admired, difficult to define and even more difficult to measure.*

Generic measures (otherwise known as multidimensional measures) attempt to measure outcomes with respect to various aspects including physical function, psychological function, pain and social function. They include the Short

Table 17.19 Levels of measurement scales and their properties. (Adapted from Wade, 1992a.)

Level	Nominal	Ordinal	Interval	Ratio
Features	Categories for classification with no order	Rank order but non-uniform intervals	Uniform intervals but no zero	Uniform intervals with zero
General example	Rainy, snowy and windy	Hot, warm, cool and cold	Degrees centigrade	Degrees Kelvin
Stroke example	Total anterior circulation infarct, lacunar infarct	Oxford Handicap Scale	OPCS disability measure	Timed 10-m walk
Use of numbers	Descriptive only	Put in order	Indicate order or difference	Indicate order, difference or absolute value
Group description	Frequencies Proportions Mode	Median Range	Mean (Variance)	Mean (Variance) Coefficient of variation
Group comparison	Chi-square Odds ratio	Mann–Whitney Wilcoxon	t-test Analysis of variance	t-test Analysis of variance

OPCS, Office of Population Censuses and Surveys.

Table 17.20 Oxford Handicap Scale.

Grade	Description
0	No symptoms
1	Minor symptoms which do not interfere with lifestyle
2	Minor handicap. Symptoms which lead to some restriction in lifestyle but do not interfere with the patients' ability to look after themselves
3	Moderate handicap. Symptoms which significantly restrict lifestyle and prevent totally independent existence
4	Moderately severe handicap. Symptoms which clearly prevent independent existence although not needing constant care and attention
5	Severe handicap. Totally dependent, requiring constant attention day and night

Form 36, Nottingham Health Profile and EuroQol and Sickness Impact Profile (Bergner et al., 1981; Hunt et al., 1985; Ebrahim et al., 1986; EuroQol Group, 1990; Ware & Sherbourne, 1992; Brazier et al., 1992; De Haan et al., 1993). They provide information about relevant aspects of patients' lives but most provide a profile of outcome rather than an overall measure. This makes group comparisons complex. Because they are generic, i.e. can be used across many different health states, they do offer health economists and others the opportunity to compare the utility of different health outcomes in different diseases. Unfortunately, they tend to be complex and rely on patient's views of their health status which limits their use in patients with severe communication and cognitive difficulties, and they may not be practical in very large studies.

Simple questions. We have recently used two simple questions to categorise patients into those with poor, fair and good outcomes after stroke (Fig. 17.7) (Lindley et al., 1994). This approach to the measurement of outcome after stroke appears to be reasonably valid, reliable and is certainly practical where the outcome of very large numbers of patients needs to be measured. Further work is required to establish the optimal wording of the simple questions and to test them in different languages and settings.

Patient satisfaction. Many health care systems are being influenced by market forces and the idea that patients are consumers. This has placed increasing importance on the satisfaction of our 'clients' with their health care. Many health service managers regard patient satisfaction as being an important outcome, although some would consider satisfaction to be a measure of process. Pound et al. (1994) have developed measures of patient and carer satisfaction with hospital and home care. However, these measures need to be evaluated further in different settings before they can be recommended for general use. Unfortunately, patient and carer satisfaction may not reflect their outcome very well and patients are often satisfied with what professionals would regard as poor treatment (Wellwood et al., 1995a).

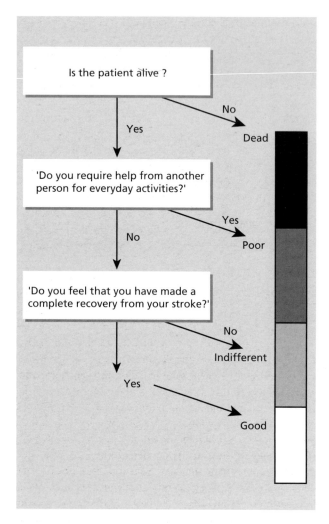

Figure 17.7 Simple questions which can be used to place stroke patients into four different outcome categories. The wording of these simple questions has since been modified to reduce ambiguity, i.e. 'Do you require help from anybody for everyday activities?' and 'Has the stroke left you with any problems?'. (From Lindley *et al.*, 1994.)

When should we measure outcome? Outcomes some months after the stroke are probably most relevant to patients but are more difficult and expensive to measure than at an earlier stage. Many services monitor the patient's functional status at the time of discharge and this information is easily and cheaply collected. However, because patients usually improve for several months after a stroke, the longer they stay in hospital the better their outcome at discharge. Thus, such measures are easily manipulated and impossible to interpret. It is more relevant to measure the outcome at a fixed interval from the stroke, but if this is after discharge this will inevitably be more time consuming and expensive.

However, some of the simpler measures can be made by telephone or postal questionnaire (Shinar *et al.*, 1987; Candelise *et al.*, 1994; Lindley *et al.*, 1994).

How to score dead patients? Because many patients die after stroke, outcome measurements can only be applied to the survivors. If these measures are averaged, and groups of patients compared, then there may be a serious problem of interpretation if there are more survivors in one group than in the other. Some workers attempt to get round this by giving the worst score to the dead patients and then including them in the analysis but, depending on the scale used, this is not necessarily valid. One solution is to measure the proportion of patients who are 'dead or disabled/handicapped', but this may sacrifice sensitivity.

3 Luck

With small numbers the imprecision of the estimate of performance may prevent useful comparisons being made. Thus, it is important to measure outcomes in a large, representative sample of patients or carers. This has implications for the type of measure of outcome used since it must be simple and practical to administer to large numbers. In Scotland the government has published the 30-day case fatality for patients admitted to 32 major hospitals over a 3-year period (The Scottish Office, 1994). The case fatality varied between 20.7% (95% confidence interval (CI): 17.8–23.9) and 37.6% (95% CI: 33.2–42.4) with a mean for Scotland of 28.4%. However, much of this observed variation in case fatality could be explained by chance alone. After all, with 32 hospitals one would expect at least one and perhaps two to have an average case fatality where the 95% confidence interval did not include the national mean. For example, we calculated that if one studied 50 hospitals, each treating 200 patients per year and the mean 30-day case fatality overall was 25%, then by chance alone one would expect the observed individual hospital case fatality to vary between 18 and 32%. A consequence of the need to have adequate numbers of patients to give precise estimates of outcomes is that it may take several years for a hospital to accumulate enough data to provide such a precise estimate of its case fatality rate.

> *If the outcomes are measured in a relatively small number of patients or carers, bad outcomes may reflect bad luck rather than bad care and, conversely, good outcomes may reflect good luck rather than good care.*
>
> *When planning an audit, estimate the likely number of cases which will need to be included to reliably identify a difference (i.e. do a power calculation).*

Thus, patient outcomes may not be seen to improve significantly for a considerable time after the development of a more effective stroke service. We suggest that power calculations should be performed (as for randomised trials) before instigating any audit to demonstrate changes in the outcomes following changes in a service.

4 Case mix

The most important determinant of outcome is probably not the *quality* or *effectiveness* of care, but rather the type of patient. The patient's pre-stroke status and the severity of the stroke are bound to have an overwhelming effect on outcome and may obscure any real effect that our treatments may have. The case mix can vary considerably in different services and in the same service over time, which means that raw outcome data can not be used to reflect the quality or effectiveness of care; they have to be adjusted for differences in case mix. Rockall *et al.* (1995) illustrated this point when they studied the variation in outcome from acute upper gastrointestinal haemorrhage in 74 hospitals in the UK. Marked differences in outcome were observed but many of these differences disappeared after adjusting for case mix differences, and the position of individual hospitals in the 'league tables' changed considerably depending on whether crude or adjusted outcomes were used to rank them. Unfortunately, this assumes that we know how to adjust for case mix in stroke which is not the case. Good case mix descriptors include those factors which are highly predictive of outcome. But, as we have already seen, our ability to predict outcome after stroke, even in terms of survival, is relatively poor (see Section 10.2.7). Also, we can only correct for those prognostic factors which we can identify and measure reliably. After all, this is the main reason why we rely on randomised controlled trials to provide evidence of effectiveness of interventions. The process of randomisation ensures that the different treatment groups are balanced for recognised, unrecognised and unmeasurable prognostic factors. In the report comparing outcomes after stroke in Scottish hospitals the only prognostic factors which were routinely collected, and could therefore be adjusted for, were age and sex (The Scottish Office, 1994). We are still struggling to identify factors that predict death and which could be used to adjust mortality data. The problems are even greater if one considers other relevant outcomes such as quality of life where we know almost nothing about the factors which predict this. We demonstrated some of the problems when we identified significant differences in the prognosis of different cohorts of TIA patients, which could not be fully explained on the basis of different treatments or case mix described using a wide range of prognostic variables (Hankey *et al.*, 1993). This,

despite using sophisticated mathematical techniques to, unsuccessfully, adjust for baseline differences in the cohorts. Because treatment effects (such as those observed with aspirin) are moderate compared with the effects of case mix, they are very difficult and even impossible to identify in the non-randomised studies that may be carried out to measure the effectiveness of a new stroke service. Before we use outcomes to reflect the effectiveness and quality of care, and to alter services as a consequence of these, we have to develop reliable methods to interpret them. It will be interesting to see whether this will ever be possible.

> *Crude measures of patient outcome do not necessarily reflect the quality or effectiveness of the care provided. Even adjusting for case mix may not solve this problem.*

Measuring the 'efficiency' of a service. Rather than attempting to interpret measures of outcome at a particular interval after the stroke, the change in the patient's condition can be used as an 'outcome'. Thus, people have measured the FIM on admission to and discharge from a treatment programme. Other measures such as the Barthel Index could be used in the same way. Any change in the FIM might be considered, at least in part, to be a measure of the effectiveness of the treatment programme, although most of the improvement may actually be spontaneous. The change in FIM can be divided by some measure of the amount of treatment provided, e.g. length of stay, to give an idea of 'efficiency'. In some ways this approach is similar to that described above since one could consider the FIM on admission to be a case mix descriptor. Unfortunately, differences in case mix, such as age, severity and location of the brain lesion and other medical problems, are likely to influence the rate of change in the FIM. Thus, to interpret the change in the FIM as a reflection of effectiveness or efficiency would still require a measure of case mix (Alexander, 1994). Another problem is that measures such as the FIM are not 'interval' scales (see Table 17.19). Thus, a change of 10 points at one end of the scale is not equivalent to a 10-point change at the other. This makes changes in score difficult to interpret.

17.6.4 A practical approach

Given our limited knowledge about how best to monitor the quality and effectiveness of stroke services we suggest the following approach, although this will inevitably change as our understanding improves.

1 Ensure that services include access to the facilities shown in Table 17.21.

2 Perform a regular audit of a representative sample of case notes using a well-tested and reliable audit instrument which

Table 17.21 Facilities needed for a comprehensive stroke service.

Primary care physicians
Access to acute hospital beds
Rapid access to neurovascular clinic
Rapid access to diagnostic imaging, e.g. brain CT, duplex
  sonography
Access to vascular surgery and other specialties which have
  occasional input (see Table 10.9)
Stroke rehabilitation unit with multidisciplinary team
Ability to perform pre-discharge home assessments
Facilities to continue therapy after hospital discharge which might
  include out-patients, day hospital and domiciliary
Facilities to follow patients up medically
Outreach multidisciplinary team or a community team which can
  link with hospital-based team
Resources to provide personal care to dependent patients living in
  the community
Long-term institutional care for patients with severe disability who
  can not be managed in the community

will allow comparisons to be made with other units or in the same unit over time, e.g. Royal College of Physicians *Stroke Audit Package* (1994).

3 Do not waste valuable resources on measuring outcome after stroke until we have the methods to interpret the data. If those funding health care demand that outcome data are collected these should be kept simple, to minimise the cost and because they are likely to be the easiest to interpret. However, any interpretation will require more complex data about the patients which the service treats. The case mix and outcome data together could form the basis for a minimum data set. Our suggestions as to what this might include are outlined in Table 17.22 and are based on some preliminary work in trying to interpret stroke outcomes. These items include some demographic data which are usually collected routinely (e.g. age, marital status) and which are likely to relate to outcome, the latter probably having an influence on place of residence since having a potential carer may increase the likelihood of returning home. Pre-stroke function, which will also reflect co-morbidity, is bound to relate closely to functional outcome, and pre-stroke dependence is known to increase the risk of death. One could suggest a wide range of different indicators of stroke severity such as conscious level, urinary incontinence, severity of motor weakness or the proportion of patients with total anterior circulation syndromes (see Section 4.4.8).

The frequency of complications after stroke is unlikely to provide any quantitative information about the quality of care but might be used to identify problems. For example, a high or rising proportion of patients with pressure sores may indicate inadequate numbers of nurses or poor-quality nursing care. Unfortunately, there are considerable problems in defining complications and in providing reliable diagnostic criteria to allow monitoring (Kalra *et al.*, 1995; Davenport *et al.*, 1996). Pressure sores and fractures are probably the most reliably monitored, but both are uncommon.

> *It is essential that health service managers understand the difficulties in interpreting measures of process or outcome and their limitations. They must not make important decisions about the distribution of resources on the basis of simplistic analyses of these crude types of data. However, large discrepancies in the apparent performance of different stroke services should trigger a detailed enquiry to look into the possible explanation. Also, it is important not to use the results of a non-randomised evaluation of a local stroke service to guide service development elsewhere.*

Table 17.22 Minimum data set for stroke. This reflects known factors which influence outcome after stroke and also what data are routinely available to health service workers.

Case mix data
Age
Sex
Marital status or living alone before the stroke
Pre-stroke function, i.e. was the patient independent in ADL?
Stroke severity
  Conscious level (normal or reduced?)
  Severity of weakness (can they lift an affected limb against
    gravity?)
  Urinary incontinence during first 7 days after the stroke

Process
Number of physicians responsible for stroke care. A lower number
  suggests more specialisation
Proportion of patients discussed by multidisciplinary teams
Proportion of patients CT scanned
Proportion of patients with ischaemic stroke on aspirin at discharge

Outcomes
Survival to 30 days
Independence/dependence in ADL at 6 months
Complications, e.g. pressure sores
Place of residence at 6 months

Note: there is little point routinely collecting other outcomes, even if they are as relevant to patients and their carers, since we know even less about the factors which predict them and can not, therefore, make any adjustments for case mix.

17.7   Cost-effectiveness of stroke services

Because of its frequency in most populations, the resulting severe disability and the need for prolonged institutional care, stroke represents a very considerable financial burden on most societies (see Section 17.1). Therefore, when planning stroke services it is important to not only aim for maximum effectiveness in terms of achieving the best possible outcomes for the patients and their families, but also to do this as efficiently as possible. As we have seen, there is little reliable information about the effectiveness of many interventions but there is even less about the cost-effectiveness of treatment. However, using data from a variety of sources one might make some informed guesses about the most cost-effective means of providing stroke services, at least from the health service perspective.

The major health service costs relating to acute stroke are those from hospital care (Terent *et al.*, 1994). Figure 17.8 shows the relative size of the components of the cost of hospital care for acute stroke patients in one of our institutions. It appears that at least in the British, and probably in other models of care as well, most of the direct hospital costs are attributed to nursing salaries and hospital overheads with relatively little being spent on investigation or specific treatment (Bowen & Yaste, 1994; Smurawska *et al.*, 1994; Dennis *et al.*, 1995). Thus, the cost to the health service of managing a patient with stroke is highly dependent on the length of hospital stay, assuming that the intensity of nursing input remains constant.

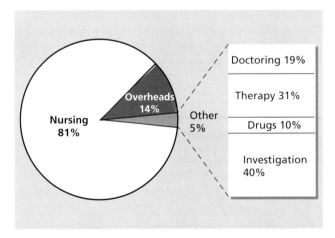

Figure 17.8 The proportion of direct hospital costs attributable to different aspects of care provided in Edinburgh, Scotland. These data relate to a period before stroke services were organised. The development of a stroke team and unit may have altered the proportions, although probably not by very much. (From Dennis *et al.*, 1995.)

Where most of the cost of stroke care in hospital is accounted for by nursing services and overheads, it does not make sense to argue about even quite large changes in the cost of investigations and treatment.

Attempts to restrict or rationalise the use of investigations or drug therapies can only have a marginal effect on the overall hospital costs. On the other hand, a policy of accelerated discharge (see Section 17.5.3) is likely to reduce the per capita costs considerably, although, depending on funding arrangements, this is likely to be transferred onto another budget, e.g. community care. However, interventions which promote more rapid or complete recovery may be very cost-effective as long as they are not themselves very expensive. The evidence from the systematic review of stroke unit trials suggests that patients not only more often survive but also have a better functional outcome (Dennis & Langhorne, 1994; Stroke Unit Trialists' Collaboration, 1996). In those trials which compared length of stay in an institution this was usually shorter in patients cared for in a stroke unit. Also, the total amount of therapy, where this was measured, was not significantly greater. Thus, it seems likely that by providing better coordinated stroke care in units that the cost of managing a case of stroke in hospital can be reduced. Of course, what we do not know is whether, for example, by doubling the amount of therapy patients receive we might increase the rate of recovery and thus shorten the length of hospital admission so that the increased therapy pays for itself.

A practical approach to monitoring the cost-effectiveness of a stroke service might include collecting data about the total length of stay in hospital (i.e. in both the acute and rehabilitation units) since this appears to be, at least in the UK, a reasonable reflection of direct hospital costs (Dennis *et al.*, 1995). However, note would have to be taken of any major changes in nursing costs or those related to investigations and treatment. The length of stay needs to be interpreted in the light of data about the destination on discharge and the patient's functional status. It is easy to reduce length of stay by discharging patients into nursing homes instead of to their own homes, and by discharging more severely dependent patients into the community, which will add to the cost (financial, physical and emotional) to the family and social services. Setting up systems to collect detailed data about exactly what investigations, drugs and therapy patients receive will be time consuming and expensive and probably provide very little more information about the cost of care. Reducing the length of stay by just 1 day would probably pay for all the investigations and drugs the average patient would consume.

> *An organised stroke service may be cheaper than a disorganised one and may release resources for other areas.*

References

Adelman SM (1981). The economic impact: national survey of stroke. *Stroke* 12 (Suppl. 1): 69–78.

Alberts MJ, Perry A, Dawson DV, Bertels C (1992). Effects of public and professional education on reducing the delay in presentation and referral of stroke patients. *Stroke* 23: 352–6.

Alexander MP (1994). Stroke rehabilitation outcome: a potential use of predictive variables to establish levels of care. *Stroke* 25: 128–34.

Anderson CS, Jamrozik KD, Burvill PW, Chakera TM, Johnson GA, Stewart-Wynne EG (1993a). Ascertaining the true incidence of stroke: experience from the Perth Community Stroke Study, 1989–1990. *Med J Aust* 158: 80–4.

Anderson CS, Jamrozik KD, Burvill PW, Chakera TM, Johnson GA, Stewart-Wynne EG (1993b). Determining the incidence of different subtypes of stroke: results from the Perth Community Stroke Study, 1989–1990. *Med J Aust* 158: 85–9.

Asplund K, Bonita R, Kuulasmaa K *et al.* (1995). Multinational comparisons of stroke epidemiology. Evaluation of case ascertainment in the WHO MONICA Stroke Study. *Stroke* 26: 355–60.

Bamford J, Sandercock P, Warlow C, Gray M (1986). Why are patients with acute stroke admitted to hospital? *Br Med J* 292: 1369–72.

Bamford J, Sandercock P, Dennis M *et al.* (1988). A prospective study of acute cerebrovascular disease in the community: the Oxfordshire Community Stroke Project 1981–86. 1. Methodology, demography and incident cases of first-ever stroke. *J Neurol Neurosurg Psychiatr* 51: 1373–80.

Bamford JL, Sandercock PAG, Warlow CP, Slattery J (1989). Interobserver agreement for the assessment of handicap in stroke patients (letter). *Stroke* 20: 828.

Bergman L, van de Meulen JHP, Limburg M, Habbema DF (1995). Costs of medical care after first-ever stroke in the Netherlands. *Stroke* 26: 1830–6.

Bergner M, Bobbitt RA, Carter WB, Gilson BS (1981). The Sickness Impact Profile: development and final revision of a health status measure. *Med Care* 19: 787–805.

Bonita R, Broad JB, Beaglehole R (1993). Changes in stroke incidence and case-fatality in Auckland, New Zealand, 1981–91. *Lancet* 342: 1470–3.

Bowen J, Yaste C (1994). Effect of a stroke protocol on hospital costs of stroke patients. *Neurology* 44: 1961–4.

Brazier JE, Harper R, Jones NMB *et al.* (1992). Validating the SF-36 health survey questionnaire: new outcome measure for primary care. *Br Med J* 305: 160–4.

Brocklehurst JC, Andrews K, Morris P, Richards BR, Laycock PL (1978). Why admit stroke patients to hospital. *Age Ageing* 7: 100–8.

Broderick JP, Phillips SJ, Whisnant JP, O'Fallon WM, Bergstrahl EJ (1989). Incidence rates of stroke in the eighties: the end of the decline in stroke? *Stroke* 20: 577–82.

Brott T, Adams HP, Olinger CP *et al.* (1989). Measurements of acute cerebral infarction: a clinical examination scale. *Stroke* 20: 864–70.

Burn J, Dennis M, Bamford J, Sandercock PAG, Wade D, Warlow CP (1994). Long-term risk of recurrent stroke after a first-ever stroke. The Oxfordshire Community Stroke Project. *Stroke* 25: 333–7.

Candelise L, Pinardi G, Aritzu E, Musicco M (1994). Telephone interview for stroke outcome assessment. *Cerebrovasc Dis* 4: 341–3.

Cote R, Hachinski VC, Shurvell BL, Norris JW, Wolfson C (1986). The Canadian Neurological Scale: a preliminary study in acute stroke. *Stroke* 17(4): 731–7.

Cote R, Battista RNN, Wolfson C, Boucher J, Adam J, Hachinski V (1989). The Canadian Neurological Scale: validation and reliability assessment. *Neurology* 39: 638–43.

Counsell C, Warlow C, Sandercock P, Fraser H, van Gijn J (1995). The Cochrane Collaboration Stroke Review Group. Meeting the need for systematic reviews in stroke care. *Stroke* 26: 498–502.

Czlonkowska A, Ryglewicz D, Weissbein T, Baranska-Gieruszczak M, Hier DB (1994). A prospective community-based study of stroke in Warsaw, Poland. *Stroke* 25: 547–51.

D'Alessandro G, Di Giovanni G, Roveyaz L *et al.* (1992). Incidence and prognosis of stroke in the Valle d'Aosta, Italy. First-year results of a community-based study. *Stroke* 23: 1712–15.

Daley J, Jencks S, Draper D, Lenhart G, Thomas N, Walker J (1988). Predicting hospital-associated mortality for medicare patients. A method for patients with stroke, pneumonia, acute myocardial infarction and congestive heart failure. *J Am Med Assoc* 260: 3617–24.

Davenport RJ, Dennis MS, Warlow CP (1995a). Improving the recording of the clinical assessment of stroke patients using a clerking proforma. *Age Ageing* 24: 43–8.

Davenport RJ, Dennis MS, Warlow CP (1995b). Assessing the effect of an inpatient stroke service. British Geriatric Society 1995, London Abstract in *Age Ageing* 1996; 25 (Suppl. 1): 32.

Davenport RJ, Dennis MS, Wellwood I, Warlow CP (1996). Complications following acute stroke. *Stroke* 27: 415–20.

De Haan R, Horn J, Limburg M, Van Der Meulen J, Bossuyt P (1993). A comparison of five stroke scales with measures of disability, handicap, and quality of life. *Stroke* 24: 1178–81.

Dennis M, Bamford J, Sandercock P, Warlow C (1990). Prognosis of transient ischemic attacks in the Oxfordshire Community Stroke Project. *Stroke* 21: 848–53.

Dennis M, Wellwood I, McGregor K, Dent J, Forbes J (1995). What are the major components of the cost of caring for stroke patients in hospital in the UK? In Proceedings of 4th European Stroke Conference, Bordeaux, France. *Cerebrovasc Dis* 5: 243 (abstract).

Dennis MS, Langhorne P (1994). So stroke units save lives: where do we go from here? *Br Med J* 309: 1273–7.

Dennis MS, Bamford JM, Sandercock PAG, Warlow CP (1989a). Incidence of transient ischemic attacks in Oxfordshire, England. *Stroke* 20: 333–9.

Dennis MS, Bamford JM, Sandercock PAG, Warlow CP (1989b). A comparison of risk factors and prognosis for transient ischemic attacks and minor ischemic strokes. The Oxfordshire Community Stroke Project. *Stroke* 20: 1494–9.

Donabedian A (1988). The quality of care: how can it be assessed? *J Am Med Assoc* 260: 19–26.

Donald IP, Baldwin N, Bannerjee M (1995). Gloucester Hospital-at-Home: a randomised controlled trial. *Age Ageing* 24: 434–9.

Drake WE, Hamilton MJ, Carlsson M, Kand F, Blumenkrantz J (1973). Acute stroke management and patient outcome: the value of neurovascular care units (NCU). *Stroke* 4: 933–45.

Ebrahim S, Barer D, Nouri F (1986). Use of the Nottingham Health Profile with patients after a stroke. *J Epidemiol Commun Health* 40: 166–9.

Ebrahim SB, Nouri F, Barer D (1985). Measuring disability after a stroke. *J Epidemiol Commun Health* 39: 86–9.

EuroQol Group (1990). EuroQol—a new facility for the measurement of health-related quality of life. *Health Policy* 16: 199–208.

Feigin VL, Wiebers DO, Nikitin YP, O'Fallon WM, Whisnant JP (1995). Stroke epidemiology in Novosibirsk, Russia: a population-based study. *Mayo Clin Proc* 70: 847–52.

Feldmann E, Gordon N, Brooks JM *et al.* (1993). Factors associated with early presentation of acute stroke. *Stroke* 24: 1805–10.

Garraway WM, Akhtar AJ, Prescott RJ, Hockey L (1980). Management of acute stroke in the elderly: preliminary results of a controlled trial. *Br Med J* April: 1040–3.

Giroud M, Gras P, Chadan N *et al.* (1991a). Cerebral haemorrhage in a French prospective population study. *J Neurol Neurosurg Psychiatr* 54: 595–8.

Giroud M, Milan C, Beuriat P *et al.* (1991b). Incidence and survival rates during a two-year period of intracerebral and subarachnoid haemorrhages, cortical infarcts, lacunes and transient ischaemic attacks. The stroke registry of Dijon: 1985–1989. *Int J Epidemiol* 20: 892–9.

Gladman J, Forster A, Young J (1995). Hospital- and home-based rehabilitation after discharge from hospital for stroke patients: analysis of two trials. *Age Ageing* 24: 49–53.

Gladman JRF, Lincoln NB (1994). Follow-up of a controlled trial of domiciliary stroke rehabilitation (DOMINO Study). *Age Ageing* 23: 9–13.

Gladman JRF, Lincoln NB, Barer DH (1993). A randomised controlled trial of domiciliary and hospital-based rehabilitation for stroke patients after discharge from hospital. *J Neurol Neurosurg Psychiatr* 56: 960–6.

Gompertz P, Dennis M, Hopkins A, Ebrahim S (1994). Development and reliability of the Royal College of Physicians Stroke Audit Form. *Age Ageing* 22: 378–83.

Gompertz P, Pound P, Briffa J, Ebrahim S (1995). How useful are non-random comparisons of outcomes and quality of care in purchasing hospital stroke services. *Age Ageing* 24: 137–41.

Hacke W, Schwab S, De Georgia M (1994). Intensive care of acute ischemic stroke. *Cerebrovasc Dis* 4: 385–92.

Hankey GJ, Dennis MS, Slattery JM, Warlow CP (1993). Why is the outcome of transient ischaemic attacks different in different groups of patients. *Br Med J* 306: 1107–11.

Harper GD, Haigh RA, Potter JF, Castleden CM (1992). Factors delaying hospital admission after stroke in Leicestershire. *Stroke* 23: 835–8.

Hartunian NS, Smart CN, Thompson MS (1980). The incidence and economic costs of cancer, motor vehicle injuries, coronary heart disease and stroke: a comparative analysis. *Am J Public Health* 70: 1249–60.

Harwood RH, Gompertz P, Ebrahim S (1994). Handicap one year after a stroke: validity of a new scale. *J Neurol Neurosurg Psychiatr* 57: 825–9.

Holbrook M, Skilbeck CE (1983). An activities index for use with stroke patients. *Age Ageing* 12: 166–70.

Hunt S, McEwan J, McKenna S (1985). Measuring health status: a new tool for clinicians and epidemiologists. *J Roy Coll Gen Pract* 35: 185–8.

Indredavik B, Bakke F, Solberg R, Rokseth R, Haaheim LL, Holme I (1991). Benefit of a stroke unit: a randomized controlled trial. *Stroke* 22: 1026–31.

Isard PA, Forbes JF (1992). The cost of stroke to the National Health Service in Scotland. *Cerebrovasc Dis* 2: 47–50.

Jencks SF, Daley J, Draper D, Thomas N, Lenhart G, Walker J (1988). Interpreting hospital mortality data. The role of clinical risk adjustment. *J Am Med Assoc* 260: 3611–16.

Jorgensen HS, Plesner AM, Hubbe P, Larsen K (1992). Marked increase of stroke incidence in men between 1972 and 1990 in Frederiksberg, Denmark. *Stroke* 23: 1701–4.

Kahn KL, Brook RH, Draper D *et al.* (1988). Interpreting hospital mortality data. How can we proceed? *J Am Med Assoc* 260: 3625–8.

Kalra L, Dale P, Crome P (1993). Improving stroke rehabilitation. A controlled study. *Stroke* 24: 1462–7.

Kalra L, Yu G, Wilson K, Roots P (1995). Medical complications during stroke rehabilitation. *Stroke* 26: 990–4.

Kaste M, Palomaki H, Sarna S (1995). Where and how should elderly stroke patients be treated? A randomised trial. *Stroke* 26: 249–53.

Kelly-Hayes M, Wolf PA, Kase CS, Brand FN, McGuirk JM, D'Agostino RB (1995). Temporal patterns of stroke onset. The Framingham study. *Stroke* 26: 1343–7.

Kennedy FB, Pozen TJ, Gabelman EH, Tuthill JE, Zaentz SD (1970). Stroke intensive care—an appraisal. *Am Health J* 80(2): 188–96.

King's Fund Consensus Conference (1988). Treatment of stroke. *Br Med J* 297: 126–8.

Langhorne P (1995). What is a stroke unit? A survey of the randomised trials. In proceedings of 4th European Stroke Conference, Bordeaux, France. *Cerebrovasc Dis* 5: 288 (abstract).

Langhorne P, Williams BO, Gilchrist W, Howie K (1993). Do stroke units save lives? *Lancet* 342: 395–8.

Leibson CL, Naessens JM, Brown RD, Whisnant JP (1994). Accuracy of hospital discharge abstracts for identifying stroke. *Stroke* 25: 2348–55.

Lindley RI, Waddell F, Livingstone M *et al.* (1994). Can simple questions assess outcome after stroke? *Cerebrovasc Dis* 4: 314–24.

Lyden PD, Lau GT (1991). A critical appraisal for stroke evaluation and rating scales. *Stroke* 22: 1345–52.

McPherson K, Sloan R, Hunter J, Dowell C (1993). Validation studies of the OPCS scale—more useful than the Barthel Index? *Clin Rehabil* 7: 105–12.

Mahoney F, Barthel D (1965). Functional evaluation: the Barthel Index. *Md State Med J* 14: 61–5.

Malmgren R, Warlow C, Bamford J, Sandercock P (1987). Geographical and secular trends in stroke incidence. *Lancet* Nov: 1196–1200.

Malmgren R, Bamford J, Warlow C, Sandercock P, Slattery J (1989). Projecting the number of patients with first-ever strokes and patients newly handicapped by stroke in England and Wales. *Br Med J* 298: 656–60.

Martin F, Oyewole A, Moloney A (1994). A randomized controlled trial of a high support hospital discharge team for elderly people. *Age Ageing* 23: 228–34.

Martin J, Meltzer H, Elliot D (1988). *The Prevalence of Disability Among Adults.* London: Office of Population Censuses and Surveys: HMSO.

Mathew NT, Meyer JS, Rivera VM, Charney JZ, Hartmann A (1972). Double-blind evaluation of glycerol therapy in acute cerebral infarction. *Lancet* December: 1327–9.

Melin AL, Bygren LO (1992). Efficacy of the rehabilitation of elderly primary health care patients after short-stay hospital treatment. *Med Care* 30(11): 1004–15.

Mills E, Thompson M (1978). The economic costs of stroke in Massachusetts. *N Engl J Med* 299(8): 415–18.

Nouri FM, Lincoln NB (1987). An extended activities of daily living scale for stroke patients. *Clin Rehabil* 1: 301–5.

O'Mahony PG, Dobson R, Thompson R, Rodgers H, James OFW (1995). Satisfaction with information and advice received by stroke patients. In Proceedings of 4th European Stroke Conference, Bordeaux, France. *Cerebrovasc Dis* Jul–Aug: 229 (abstract).

O'Rourke SJ, Dennis MS, Slattery J, Warlow CP (1996). Preliminary results from a randomised trial of a stroke family support worker: patients' outcome at six months post stroke. *Age Ageing* 25 (Suppl. 1): 32.

Panayiotou BN, Fotherby MD, Potter JF, Castleden CM (1993). The accuracy of diagnostic coding of cerebrovascular disease. *Med Audit News* 3(10): 153–5.

Persson U, Silverberg R, Lindgren B *et al.* (1990). Direct costs of stroke for a Swedish population. *Intern J Technol Assess Health Care* 6: 125–37.

Pitner SE, Mance CJ (1973). An evaluation of stroke intensive care: results of a municipal hospital. *Stroke* 4: 737–41.

Pound P, Gompertz P, Ebrahim S (1994). Patients' satisfaction with stroke services. *Clin Rehabil* 8: 7–17.

Rankin J (1957). Cerebral vascular accidents in people over the age of 60. II Prognosis. *Scot Med J* 2: 200–15.

Ricci S (1995). Between-country variations in the use of medical treatments for acute stroke. In Procedings of 4th European Stroke Conference, Bordeaux, France. *Cerebrovasc Dis* Jul-Aug: 272 (abstract).

Ricci S, Celani MG, La Rosa F *et al.* (1991). SEPIVAC: a community-based study of stroke incidence in Umbria, Italy. *J Neurol Neurosurg Psychiatr* 54: 695–8.

Rockall TA, Logan RFA, Devlin HB, Northfield TC (1995). Variation in outcome after acute upper gastrointestinal haemorrhage. *Lancet* 346: 346–50.

Rothwell PM, Wroe SJ, Slattery J, Warlow CP (1996). Is stroke incidence related to season or temperature? *Lancet* 347: 934–6.

Royal College of Physicians Research Unit, and UK Stroke Audit Group (1994). *Stroke Audit Package.* London: Royal College of Physicians.

Scandinavian Stroke Study Group (1985). Multicenter trial of hemodilution in ischemic stroke: background and study protocol. *Stroke* 16: 885–90.

Schuling J, De Haan R, Limburg M, Groenier KH (1993). The Frenchay Activities Index. Assessment of functional status in stroke patients. *Stroke* 24: 1173–7.

Secretary of State for Health (1992). *The Health of the Nation.* London: HMSO.

Shinar D, Gross CR, Bronstein KS *et al.* (1987). Reliability of the activities of daily living scale and its use in telephone interview. *Arch Phys Med Rehabil* 68: 723–8.

Smurawska LT, Alexandrov AV, Bladin CF, Norris JW (1994). Cost of acute stroke care in Toronto, Canada. *Stroke* 25: 1628–31.

State University of New York at Buffalo (1993). *Guide for Use of the Uniform Data Set for Medical Rehabilitation (Adult FIM), Version 4.0.* Buffalo, NY.

Stevens RS, Ambler NR, Darren MD (1984). A randomized controlled trial of a stroke rehabilitation ward. *Age Ageing* 13: 65 75.

Stroke Units Trialists' Collaboration (1996). A systematic review of specialist multidisciplinary team (stroke unit) care for stroke in patients. In: Warlow C, van Gijn J, Sandercock P, eds. *Stroke Module of the Cochrane Database of Systematic Reviews, 1996* (updated 23 February 1996). Available in the Cochrane Library. London: BMJ Publishing Group.

Terent A (1983). Medico-social consequences and direct costs of stroke in a Swedish community. *Scand J Rehab Med* 15: 165–71.

Terent A (1988). Increasing incidence of stroke amongst Swedish women. *Stroke* 19: 598–603.

Terent A, Marke L-A, Asplund K, Norrving B, Jonsson E, Wester P-O (1994). Costs of stroke in Sweden. A National perspective. *Stroke* 25: 2363–9.

The Scottish Office (1994). Clinical Outcome Indicators I. Mortality after admission of stroke. II. Discharge home after admission of stroke. Edinburgh: HMSO.

Townsend J, Piper M, Frank AO, Dyer S, North WRS, Meade TW (1988). Reduction in hospital admission stay of elderly patients by a community based hospital discharge scheme: a randomised controlled trial. *Br Med J* 297: 544–7.

van Gijn J, Warlow CP (1992). Down with Stroke Scales. *Cerebrovasc Dis* 2: 239–47.

Vickers N, Pollock A (1993). Incompleteness and retrieval of case note in a case note audit of colorectal cancer. *Qual Health Care* 2: 170–4.

Wade DT (1992a). Measures of motor impairment. In: *Measurement in Neurological Rehabilitation*. Oxford: Oxford Medical Publications, 147–65.

Wade DT (1992b). Stroke: rehabilitation and long-term care. *Lancet* 339: 791–3.

Wade DT (1992c). *Epidemiologically based needs assessment, Report 3: Stroke*. London: NHS Management Executive.

Wade DT, Langton-Hewer R (1983). Why admit stroke patients to hospital. *Lancet* i: 807–9.

Wade DT, Langton-Hewer R, Skilbeck CE, Bainton D, Burns-Cox C (1985). Controlled trial of a home-care service for acute stroke patients. *Lancet* i: 323–6.

Ware JE, Sherbourne CD (1992). The MOS 36-item short form health survey (SF-36) I. Conceptual framework and item selection. *Med Care* 30: 473–83.

Wellwood I, Dennis M, Warlow C (1995a). Patients' and carers' satisfaction with acute stroke management. *Age Ageing* 24: 519–24.

Wellwood I, Dennis MS, Warlow CP (1994). Perceptions and knowledge of stroke among surviving patients with stroke and their carers. *Age Ageing* 23: 293–8.

Wellwood I, Dennis MS, Warlow CP (1995b). A comparison of the Barthel Index and the OPCS disability instrument used to measure outcome after acute stroke. *Age Ageing* 24: 54–7.

Wood-Dauphinee S, Shapiro S, Bass E *et al.* (1984). A randomized trial of team care following stroke. *Stroke* 15(5): 864–72.

Wroe SJ, Sandercock P, Bamford J, Dennis M, Slattery J, Warlow C (1992). Diurnal variation in incidence of stroke: Oxfordshire Community Stroke Project. *Br Med J* 304: 155–7.

Young J, Forster A (1993). Day hospital and home physiotherapy for stroke patients: a comparative cost-effectiveness study. *J Roy Coll Phys Lond* 27(3): 252–7.

Young JB, Forster A (1992). The Bradford community stroke trial: results at six months. *Br Med J* 304: 1085–9.

Reducing the burden of stroke and improving the public health

18

18.1   Introduction

The burden of stroke on patients, their families and society in general is constantly and correctly being re-emphasised: in most Western populations it is the third most common cause of death after coronary heart disease and cancer, and the most common life-threatening neurological condition; in the UK, stroke disability is both common and the most important single cause of severe disability in people living in their own homes (Harris, 1971; Martin *et al.*, 1988); and, in Scotland, stroke consumes almost 5% of the entire National Health Service budget (Isard & Forbes, 1992). In descending order of interest to most clinicians, but, as we shall see, in roughly ascending order of likely impact on the public health, there are four strategies which will reduce stroke burden: (i) treating first-ever in a lifetime and recurrent strokes to reduce case fatality and increase the independence and quality of life of the survivors; (ii) reducing the risk of stroke after transient ischaemic attack (TIA), and of recurrent stroke after a first-ever in a lifetime stroke; (iii) seeking out and treating people at particularly high risk of stroke to reduce their risk of stroke; and (iv) reducing the average level of causative risk factors in the whole population to reduce

the incidence of stroke (Fig. 18.1). The effectiveness, practicability and cost of these four strategies must be compared. First, however, one must consider how the burden of stroke can be monitored routinely over time so that goals to reduce this burden can be set, and then worked towards by implementing one or more of the strategies to reduce that burden.

> *Stroke is the third most common cause of death in most Western populations, the most common life-threatening neurological condition and the most important single cause of severe disability in people living in their own homes.*

18.2   Changes in the burden of stroke with time

Mortality statistics are at present the only *routinely* available method for monitoring the burden of stroke with time. No country in the world has a routine method of monitoring stroke *incidence* (hospital discharge rates are no substitute because the proportion of strokes admitted is mostly

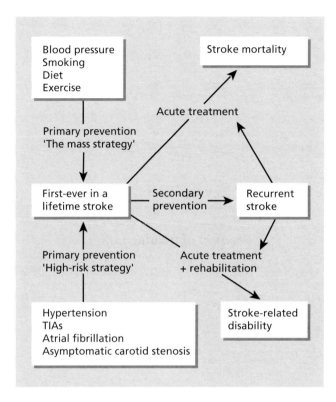

| Blood pressure
Smoking
Diet
Exercise | | Stroke mortality |

Figure 18.1 Strategies for reducing the burden of stroke. (From Dennis & Warlow, 1991.)

unknown and could change unpredictably and unmeasurably with time; see Section 17.2.1); nor for monitoring stroke case fatality and outcome in the survivors; and certainly not for monitoring the cost of stroke which is so difficult to measure at one point in time, let alone at several (see Section 17.7). At present, therefore, the only way in which the success of strategies for reducing stroke burden can be assessed is by monitoring stroke mortality, e.g. as in the UK Governmental target set out in *The Health of the Nation* (Secretary of State for Health, 1992). So, how reliable are stroke mortality statistics, what do they mean and is stroke mortality changing?

18.2.1 Time trends in stroke mortality

There is no doubt that there have been substantial changes in stroke mortality in both men and women and at all ages over the past few decades (Fratiglioni *et al.*, 1983; Bonita & Beaglehole, 1993). In most Western countries and Japan, rates have fallen by up to 7%/year in parallel with falling (but not so fast) mortality for coronary heart disease (Fig. 18.2). However, in some countries, particularly in Eastern

Europe, stroke and coronary heart disease mortality have both been rising from an already high level (Fig. 18.2). What explains these changing rates? Is stroke incidence changing, the most common assumption, or are there other plausible explanations such as the following.

Changes in diagnostic accuracy

The clinical diagnosis of stroke versus not stroke should be reasonably secure in countries with good health care for the majority of its population, even though autopsy to confirm the diagnosis has declined precipitously (Lanska, 1993). It is thus unlikely that inaccurate diagnosis wholly explains changing mortality, particularly in patients under 75 years old where the diagnosis is rather easier and, rightly or wrongly, more likely to be attempted carefully than in the very elderly. Of course, the World Health Organization (WHO) clinical definition of stroke (Hatano, 1976) must be adhered to rigidly and at present we can see no compelling reason for any modification based on brain imaging, or on any other criteria. A stroke definition based on imaging would be doomed to change with time because imaging technology improves with time, as does its availability (see Section 3.1).

Arithmetic error

Clearly, older populations have a higher stroke mortality than younger populations, but the decline observed in stroke mortality is seen *within* age strata, and also when the age of the population is standardised to some standard population such as that of the UK or Europe. However, if the age band strata are too wide then any change in the number of people within various substrata of a single stratum could lead to apparent rather than real changes in stroke mortality: after all, even across a mere 10-year age difference there can be a more than doubling of stroke mortality and incidence (see Section 17.2.1) (Bonita & Beaglehole, 1993). This problem is particularly pertinent, and may be obscured, in the oldest age stratum with an open upper end, because this stratum might contain people of very different ages and the proportion of people at these different ages may change with time.

Changes in death certification practice

The decline in stroke mortality has been so consistent in so many countries that it is unlikely to be due to a *systematic* drift in how death certificates are completed and then coded. However, the documented inaccuracy of death certification of stroke, particularly in the elderly, does lead to some con-

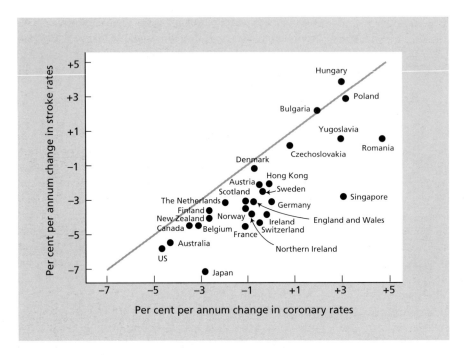

Figure 18.2 A comparison of the annual percentage decline of age-standardised mortality due to stroke and coronary heart disease in men aged 40–69 years between 1970 and 1985 in 27 countries with reasonably reliable data. (From Bonita *et al.*, 1990; reproduced with permission from the authors and *Stroke.*)

cern, even though accuracy may be improving at least when stroke patients are admitted to hospitals with computerised tomography (CT) scanning facilities (Corwin *et al.*, 1982; Hasuo *et al.*, 1989; Iso *et al.*, 1990). In times past, sudden death may have been certified as due to stroke even though it is now known that stroke is very seldom the cause of death within minutes of the onset of symptoms (except in the case of subarachnoid haemorrhage, which causes only about 5% of first-ever in a lifetime strokes; see Fig. 17.1) and that the much more common explanation is some complication of coronary heart disease, particularly an arrhythmia (Phillips *et al.*, 1977; Thomas *et al.*, 1988). Recognising and then avoiding this artefact may explain some of the decline in stroke mortality, particularly in Japan in the early post-war years (Netsky & Miyaji, 1976), but is unlikely to be the explanation for the continuing fall in stroke mortality in Japan as well as in Western European and North American countries.

Competing causes of death

It has been argued that declining stroke mortality is because those likely to die of stroke are now dying earlier of coronary heart disease or some other non-stroke cause. This is unlikely because in countries where stroke mortality is falling, coronary heart disease mortality and overall mortality are also falling (Fig. 18.2).

Changes in the mixture of stroke types

Certain types of stroke are far more likely to cause early death than others; for example, the 30-day case fatality after lacunar infarction is less than 5%, whereas after total anterior circulation infarction it is about 40% (see Table 10.2). If, therefore, the proportion of strokes due to lacunar infarction is increasing and the proportion due to total anterior circulation infarction is decreasing, then stroke mortality would fall even if stroke incidence remained constant. This kind of detail of stroke pathological type, and ischaemic stroke subtype, is simply not available or accurate in routine mortality statistics and even in incidence studies it is very difficult to achieve (see Section 17.2.3).

Changes in case fatality

There is some evidence that stroke patients are surviving longer (Garraway *et al.*, 1983; Bonita *et al.*, 1993). If so, this would have the effect of reducing stroke mortality (but not incidence) because patients would then be alive longer and so more likely to die of an intercedent event, such as myocardial infarction, than of the stroke itself. Improved survival could be due to: (i) a change in the proportion of various stroke types (see above) for which there is no evidence one way or the other; (ii) improvements in stroke treatment which is unlikely because there is still no routine treatment that is definitely effective (see Chapter 11); (iii) improvements in nursing care which is plausible but unproven; and (iv) the introduction of stroke units (see Section 17.4.2), but this is only a very recent and as yet far from widespread development. Of course, another explanation is that more milder strokes are now being *identified* and then included in studies of survival, and perhaps what were called TIAs are now called strokes.

In summary, therefore, there are several more or less plausible reasons for changes in stroke mortality which are nothing to do with changes in overall stroke incidence. A fall (or a rise) in stroke mortality does not necessarily mean that there has been a fall (or a rise) in stroke incidence. Unfortunately, stroke incidence is tedious and expensive to measure at one point in time (see Section 17.2.1) and even more so at several points in time (see Section 18.2.2), and nowhere does this approach routine practice, even in public health departments. It might be more cost-effective to improve on all the possible biases and inaccuracies of routinely collected mortality statistics and then to use them as a surrogate for stroke incidence. At present, however, we are very uncertain whether stroke mortality can be safely extrapolated to stroke incidence, particularly when it seems as though changes in stroke mortality have been more dramatic than changes in stroke incidence (see Section 18.2.2).

Stroke mortality is declining in many Western countries and in Japan, but it is unclear whether this is due to a decline in incidence, lower case fatality or an artefact of mortality statistics.

18.2.2 Time trends in stroke incidence

Measuring stroke incidence accurately is not technically difficult but does require more resources than are available in routine clinical and public health practice, and it is time consuming (Bonita *et al.*, 1983). As a consequence there are rather few stroke incidence studies which can be said to be ideal, or more or less ideal, when set against standard methodological criteria (see Section 17.2.1) (Sudlow & Warlow, 1996). Not surprisingly, these studies have only been done in developed countries. Very few 'ideal' stroke incidence studies have been repeated, or continued for long enough, to provide reliable time trend information.

The most widely quoted time trend information comes from Rochester, Minnesota where stroke incidence did decline remarkably in the 1950s and 1960s, but since then it has stabilised and even increased (Broderick *et al.*, 1989). One can not, however, assume that similar changes in incidence have occurred elsewhere, indeed they may not have done: although incidence rates have fallen in Hisayama,

Japan (Ueda *et al.*, 1981) and in Novosibirsk, Russia (Feigin *et al.*, 1995), they have not in Auckland, New Zealand (Bonita *et al.*, 1993), and they have actually risen in Soderhamn, Sweden (Terent, 1988) and in Denmark (Jorgensen *et al.*, 1992). For other parts of the world there is simply no information available. None of the studies can provide reliable information for different pathological types of stroke because brain CT to differentiate primary intracerebral haemorrhage from ischaemic stroke has either not been practicable in community-based incidence studies (and no other method is reliable for measuring stroke incidence), or it has become available so recently that time trend studies have simply not yet been possible. It does seem, however, that the incidence of subarachnoid haemorrhage, which does not require CT for accurate diagnosis, has not changed, at least not in Rochester, Minnesota (Ingall *et al.*, 1989).

In the few places where it has been measured, stroke incidence has declined, stayed the same or increased.

It is distinctly odd that stroke mortality has fallen so much in places such as Sweden and New Zealand, whereas stroke *incidence* has not, even though in Auckland it seems as though stroke severity has declined which could provide one explanation for the difference between mortality and incidence time trends (Bonita *et al.*, 1993). Another explanation is not the inaccuracy of mortality statistics discussed earlier, but the possible inaccuracy of incidence studies which have to be sustained over time without any change in their methodology, and which may be based on a rather small number of strokes, and so lack precision (Asplund *et al.*, 1995).

18.2.3 Is stroke burden changing?

Although stroke mortality is almost certainly declining in most developed countries it is not at all clear that this is a reflection of declining stroke incidence. It could be that the burden of stroke is not changing at all, at least in terms of incidence; of course, because most populations are ageing the *number* of stroke patients will certainly increase. However, the number of *newly* dependent stroke survivors will not necessarily increase in parallel because elderly dependent people who have strokes are more likely to die as a consequence than young independent people (Malmgren *et al.*, 1989). It is also conceivable that strokes are becoming milder, perhaps because there has been a decline in the incidence of the more severe stroke types (see Section 18.2.1). Finally, it may be that stroke patients are surviving longer, either because of better nursing care or because strokes are becoming milder. We have no idea if the cost of stroke is changing, or indeed what it really is (see Section 17.7). There are, therefore, far more questions than answers in this area and it is hardly surprising that, at present, no goals are being set by the UK, or any other Government, which are based on stroke incidence, severity, outcome or cost. Only mortality goals are being set, despite their well-appreciated imperfections.

18.2.4 Why is stroke burden changing, if it really is?

If we do not really know whether or not stroke burden is changing, then it is perhaps premature to ask *why* it is changing. However, many people have assumed, perhaps wrongly, that because stroke mortality is declining, then stroke incidence *must* be declining and have then attempted to provide an explanation. A further assumption is often made that the explanation is to do with the medical treatment of causative risk factors, particularly hypertension (Whisnant, 1984). However, calculations have shown that the drug treatment of hypertension can not possibly explain all of the decline in stroke mortality, even if this really reflects declining incidence: at most, only 25% of the decline can be explained this way (Bonita & Beaglehole, 1989). Nor can the identification and treatment of TIAs have had much impact on stroke incidence, largely because only a small proportion of strokes are preceded by TIAs (Whisnant, 1983) (see Section 18.5). A general population decline in the prevalence and level of causative risk factors, such as high blood pressure, has been suggested and there is some evidence for an effect on stroke mortality but not—curiously—on stroke incidence, and there is some evidence for coronary heart disease mortality (Tuomilehto *et al.*, 1991; Vartiainen *et al.*, 1994, 1995); it is conceivable that the reduction of the salt content of preserved food as a consequence of refrigeration *might* have lowered the average population blood pressure, but we can not be sure.

Rather than attempt to look backwards to explain, with difficulty, any change in stroke burden which may or may not have occurred, it could be more productive to look forwards and consider what strategies *might* reduce stroke burden in the future, whether such strategies could be implemented and how the effects—if any—could be monitored.

18.3   Likely effect of acute stroke treatment on morbidity and mortality

Enormous efforts are now being devoted to developing and testing promising new treatments for acute stroke, particularly for ischaemic stroke (see Chapter 11). In addition, it is highly likely that reorganising haphazard stroke care into stroke units is an effective strategy to reduce case fatality and dependency (see Section 17.4.2).

What impact might treatment of acute stroke have on the overall burden of stroke? Clearly, it will have no effect on stroke incidence and, unfortunately, any impact on stroke mortality will be small; even with an optimistic scenario, in which all stroke patients get a treatment which reduces case fatality by 25%, stroke mortality would still only be reduced by about 9% (Table 18.1) and with a more realistic scenario, in which only about 50% of ischaemic strokes get a treatment which reduces case fatality by 15%, any reduction would be nearer 1% (Table 18.1). This rather gloomy mes-

Table 18.1 The estimated effect of the treatment of acute stroke on stroke mortality in England and Wales.

Optimistic (unrealistic?) scenario

About 130 000 patients per annum have a first-ever in a lifetime or recurrent stroke in the UK*†, of whom about 24 700 (i.e. 19%) die in the first month‡. If treatment reduced case fatality by about 25%, from 19 to 14%, and could be applied to all patients, then only 18 500 would die in the first month

Therefore, 6200 deaths avoided

However, stroke mortality in England and Wales is recorded as about 68 000 deaths per annum§

Therefore, the proportion of stroke mortality avoided by the treatment of acute stroke would be $\frac{6200}{68\,000} \times 100 =$ about 9%

Pessimistic (realistic?) scenario

About 130 000 patients per annum have a first-ever in a lifetime or recurrent stroke in the UK*†, of whom about 105 300 (i.e. 81%) are due to cerebral infarction‡. Of these ischaemic stroke patients, about 10% (10 530) die in the first month‡

If treatment could be delivered to 50%, i.e. about 52 650 of these ischaemic stroke patients, and if it reduced case fatality by 15%, from 10 to 8.5%, then not 5265 but about 4475 would die in the first month

Therefore, 790 deaths avoided

However, stroke mortality in the UK is recorded as about 68 000 deaths per annum§

Therefore, the proportion of stroke mortality avoided by the treatment of acute ischaemic stroke would be

$\frac{790}{68\,000} \times 100 = 1.2\%$

---

* From Bamford *et al.*, 1988.
† From Malmgren *et al.*, 1987.
‡ From Bamford *et al.*, 1990.
§ From Secretary of State for Health, 1992.

sage for the public health (notwithstanding the useful impact treatment would have on treated *individuals*) is because: (i) patients may die before treatment can be started; (ii) treatment is likely to be far from completely effective; (iii) treatment may be contraindicated in various types of patients and may have risks; (iv) treatment may only work if given within a few hours of stroke onset; and (v) much of overall stroke mortality is due not to the immediate causes of brain damage but to later complications such as pneumonia. Of course, if the treatment reduced dependency, it is likely that later complications, including some of those causing death, might be reduced but what impact this would have on stroke burden is impossible to say. Even if treatment were to reduce dependency in stroke survivors, we can not predict by what proportion total stroke dependency would be reduced, because we have no methodology to measure the prevalence of this specific type of dependency in the community.

> *The treatment of acute stroke will have surprisingly little impact on stroke mortality, optimistically reducing it by about 10%.*

It is conceivable that the mortality statistics are wrong and that many people coded as dying of stroke are in fact dying of something else, a problem that has been discussed earlier (see Section 18.2.1); if so, the proportionate reduction in stroke mortality attributable to acute stroke treatment would be higher than that calculated here.

18.4 Likely effect of the 'high-risk' strategy for primary stroke prevention

For some years it has been axiomatic that it is sensible to identify people who are at the highest risk of a disorder and then to attempt to reduce, often successfully, their individual risks. So, attempts are made to identify and treat people with severe hypertension to reduce their risk of stroke, people with familial hypercholesterolaemia to reduce their risk of coronary events, and people who drink alcohol heavily, people who are obese, people who smoke, and so on. This strategy requires major efforts, particularly in general practice, to identify the 'cases' by either systematic screening of all potentially at-risk people on the practice register, or by opportunistic 'case' finding (for example, by measuring the blood pressure of all adults attending the practice for whatever reason) (Holmen *et al.*, 1991). This activity in itself requires considerable resources but these pale into insignificance when set against the resources required to treat those at high risk of stroke (i.e. the 'cases'), so often for years, if not for ever, with non-pharmacological advice, or with drugs, to reduce their individual risk (in the stroke context

we are almost entirely concerned with the treatment of hypertension and of atrial fibrillation) (Family Heart Study Group, 1994). Moreover, there is increasing evidence that, for many reasons, compliance with treatment in 'real life' is considerably less than it is in randomised controlled trials, so the overall effectiveness of any treatment is attenuated (Andrade *et al.*, 1995). After all, it is unethical to go to the effort of screening and identifying an individual as high risk and then be unable to reduce that risk through lack of resources; the individual has gained nothing and may even have lost something by being labelled as 'sick' (Rose, 1991).

Naturally, the 'high-risk' strategy becomes harder to sustain as one attempts to identify not just those at highest risk of stroke (e.g. people with a diastolic blood pressure >120 mmHg), but also the many more at somewhat lower risk but still clearly *at risk* (e.g. people with a diastolic blood pressure of 110–120 mmHg) (Fig. 18.3). Also, to make matters worse, the lower the risk of stroke in a group of people (e.g. with moderate rather than severe hypertension), the greater the number who have to be detected and treated to prevent one of them having a stroke; in other words, the less cost-effective treatment becomes (see Table 16.6). Indeed, it becomes extraordinarily expensive to prevent one stroke if, for example, middle-aged patients with moderate hypertension are treated with even quite inexpensive drugs (Table 18.2). Treating atrial fibrillation with long-term anticoagulation is reasonably cost-effective, particularly if the coagulation control is good enough to keep the risk of intracranial haemorrhage low (see Section 16.5; Table 18.2); aspirin may be almost as effective for some patients, it is certainly less costly and less risky (see Section 16.4.2).

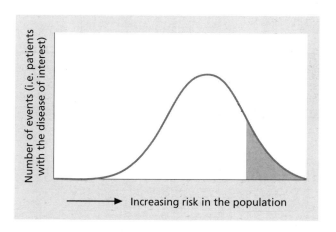

Figure 18.3 Most cases of a disease occur in people at moderate risk, rather few (shaded) in people at highest risk.

Table 18.2 Estimated costs of various preventative strategies for stroke. (From Asplund *et al.*, 1993.)

	Number of strokes avoided per million population per annum	Net cost per stroke avoided (US$) 1991
Drug treatment of hypertension (diuretics or beta-blockers)		
70–80 years old	420	Net gain
45–55 years old	10	500 000
Anticoagulation for atrial fibrillation		
0.3% risk of intracranial haemorrhage	79	Net gain
1.3% risk of intracranial haemorrhage	53	Net gain
2.0% risk of intracranial haemorrhage	27	2630
Aspirin for minor stroke/TIA	21	Net gain
Carotid endarterectomy for minor stroke/TIA	10	145 000

> The 'high-risk' strategy for stroke prevention requires the identification and treatment of people at particularly high risk of stroke; in other words, those with hypertension or in atrial fibrillation.

Despite considerable effort, the effect of the 'high-risk' strategy on modifiable vascular risk has been disappointingly small, at least in Europe if not in the US, even when this strategy has been attempted in the context of well-funded and organised randomised trials run by enthusiasts (Rose *et al.*, 1983; Fries *et al.*, 1993; Family Heart Study Group, 1994; Imperial Cancer Research Fund OXCHECK Study Group, 1995; Lindholm *et al.*, 1995). Indeed, it has proved exceptionally difficult to demonstrate that the 'high-risk' strategy reduces all cause mortality at all, perhaps because the required sample size is all but impossible to achieve rather than because the 'high-risk' strategy is flawed (McCormick & Skrabanek, 1988).

The higher an individual's risk of the disease to be prevented, and assuming the same proportional reduction in risk achievable from treatment at all levels of baseline risk, then the more such individuals have to gain from prevention, and the more cost-effective the intervention becomes (Field *et al.*,

1995). In other words, given a constant proportional risk reduction, those individuals at highest absolute risk gain the most from treatment and the fewer need to be treated to prevent one having a preventable event (Jackson *et al.*, 1993; Table 18.3). The assumption that the *proportional* risk reduction conferred by a treatment remains similar at all levels of baseline risk has not, it must be admitted, been tested in detail. It seems to be true for the prevention of serious vascular events by antiplatelet drugs where at least prior disease category and patient demographics do not influence the proportional risk reduction (Antiplatelet Trialists' Collaboration, 1994), but estimated baseline risk might (Rothwell, 1995), and for blood pressure lowering whose effect is the same at different levels of baseline blood pressure (Collins & MacMahon, 1994). But, the assumption may not be true for cholesterol lowering (Davey Smith *et al.*, 1993). The assumption is clearly *not* true if there is a similar high risk of treatment at all levels of baseline risk of the disease to be prevented; for example, the risk of carotid endarterecto-

Table 18.3 The number needed to treat to prevent one patient having an event depends on the baseline absolute risk of the disorder to be prevented as well as the relative reduction in risk due to the treatment.

(a) The effect of increasing baseline risk of stroke (as age and blood pressure increase) on the number of men who need to be treated each year (over the ensuing decade) to prevent one of them having a stroke (assuming a 39% relative, i.e. proportional, risk reduction due to treatment at all levels of baseline risk) (Kawachi & Purdie, 1989)

Age (years)	Diastolic blood pressure (mmHg)		
	90	100	110
30	4292	3217	2423
40	1746	1315	997
50	1059	654	398
60	540	403	281

(b) The effect of increasing baseline risk of coronary death (as age increases, and given the higher risk in men than women) on the number of people who need to be screened and then, if plasma cholesterol ≥ 6.5 mmol/L, treated to prevent one of them dying a coronary death in the next 5 years (assuming a 20% relative, i.e. proportional, risk reduction due to treatment at all levels of baseline risk) (Khaw & Rose, 1989)

Age (years)	Men	Women
25–34	21 067	137 320
35–44	2 463	23 244
45–54	586	2 224
55–64	231	450

Table 18.4 Examples to show that only a small proportion of events occur in people at the highest risk of those events, and that most events occur in people at moderate risk.

(a) Systolic blood pressure and the risk of stroke in men aged 40–49 years. The prevalence of various levels of blood pressure and the incidence and expected number of cases of stroke arising in each blood pressure stratum over 24 years, using Framingham Study data (Ebrahim, 1990)

Systolic blood pressure (mmHg)	Prevalence (%)	Stroke incidence per 100/24 years	Expected number of strokes (%)
<120	16	1.7	27 (5)
120–139	43	3.6	155 (27)
140–159	29	5.6	162 (28)
160–179	8	12.8	102 (18)
180+	4	31.8	127 (22)
Total	100		573 (100)

i.e. 78% of strokes occur in people with systolic blood pressure less than 180 mmHg, and over half of all strokes (60%) in people with levels of less than 160 mmHg

(b) Maternal age and Down's syndrome, in England and Wales, 1979–85. The birth prevalence of Down's syndrome, percentage of all births with Down's syndrome, and percentage of all Down's syndrome births arising in each maternal age stratum (Rose, 1992)

Maternal age (years)	Prevalence of Down's syndrome per 1000 pregnancies	Percentage of all births occurring in each age stratum	Percentage of Down's syndrome births in each age stratum
<20	0.4	9	5
20–24	0.4	30	17
25–29	0.5	34	25
30–34	1.0	19	27
35–39	2.2	6	18
40–44	5.1	1	7
45+	8.1	0.1	1
All ages	0.7	100	100

i.e. about half (47%) of Down's syndrome births occur in mothers under the age of 30 years

(c) The estimated number and proportion of serious vascular events (stroke, myocardial infarction and vascular death) that arise in the 5 years after a TIA or mild ischaemic stroke stratified by the baseline level of risk. (From Hankey et al., 1993, using UK-TIA Aspirin Trial patients)

Predicted risk of serious vascular events within 5 years (%)	Number of patients in each predicted risk stratum	Number (and %) of serious vascular events arising in stratum
0–10	236	17 (5)
11–20	509	86 (23)
21–30	389	92 (25)
31–40	220	61 (16)
41–50	117	49 (13)
51–60	73	24 (6)
61–70	42	16 (4)
71–80	30	14 (4)
81–90	24	10 (3)
91–100	13	4 (1)
Total	1653	373 (100)

i.e. only 68 out of 373 (18%) events are likely to arise in patients at greater than 50% risk of a serious vascular event

(d) The number and proportion of ipsilateral ischaemic strokes estimated to arise over 5 years in carotid TIA patients without carotid surgery, stratified by extent of symptomatic carotid stenosis (measured by the European Carotid Surgery Trial method; see Section 6.6.4)

Symptomatic carotid stenosis (%)	Number of patients in each stenosis stratum*	Per cent risk of stroke in 5 years ipsilateral to the symptomatic carotid artery†	Number (and cumulative %) of all strokes calculated from 2nd and 3rd columns
0–9	47	0	0 (0)
10–19	37	7.9	3 (9)
20–29	27	6.6	2 (15)
30–39	22	8.2	2 (21)
40–49	4	20.9	1 (24)
50–59	18	13.5	2 (30)
60–69	17	22.6	4 (42)
70–79	18	18.9	3 (52)
80–89	15	27.1	4 (64)
90–99	9	40	4 (76)
Occluded	15	50	8 (100)
Total	229	14.4	33 (100)

i.e. about 40% of strokes occurred in patients with less than 70% stenosis, and only about one-third of the strokes (33%) arose in patients with severe carotid stenosis (70–99%), which is in the range in which carotid endarterectomy is beneficial (see Section 16.7.5)

* Unpublished data from Hankey et al., 1991: a hospital-referred cohort of 229 TIA patients fit enough to be considered for carotid angiography with a view to carotid endarterectomy and studied before the availability of non-invasive carotid tests to screen out from angiography those patients without severe carotid stenosis.
† From the European Carotid Surgery Trial, no-surgery patients, unpublished interim results in 1995.

my is not worthwhile in patients at low risk of stroke so that the proportional risk reduction conferred by surgery is low or even negative in such patients, whilst it is clearly large in patients at high baseline risk of stroke, i.e. those with severe recently symptomatic carotid stenosis and with other poor prognostic factors (Rothwell, 1995).

The paradox is that, unfortunately, the more one refines the 'high-risk' strategy to make it cost-effective (i.e. by focusing preventive efforts on those individuals at highest risk and so reducing the number of patients who need to be treated to prevent one having a stroke), the smaller becomes the proportion of *all* events that is prevented. This is because most events occur *not* in those at highest risk (because their numbers are small) but in those at moderate risk (because their numbers are very much greater, even though their absolute risk is less than that in individuals at highest risk) (Fig. 18.3; Table 18.4) (Whelton, 1994). After all, even if as many as one-third of all strokes arise from about 20% of the population at highest risk (identified on the basis of a combination of various risk factors), it would be enormously expensive to find and treat them all successfully and we would still be failing to prevent the other two-thirds of the strokes (D'Agostino *et al.*, 1994). Recently, however, it has been claimed that 80% of all strokes can be expected to arise in the 20% predicted to be at highest risk in a population (Coppola *et al.*, 1995). Inevitably, the 'high-risk' strategy which concentrates on the right-hand end of the normal distribution (i.e. the deviants) misses out the large middle portion (i.e. the normals), a paradox which has been repeatedly emphasised by Rose (1992) (Fig. 18.3). Moreover, those proclaimed to be at less than highest risk may think it is safe to smoke and indulge in other 'unhealthy' activities, as may their general practitioners (Kinlay & Heller, 1990).

> *Because most strokes arise in people at moderate risk of stroke, concentrating preventive measures only on those at highest risk will have rather little effect on stroke incidence.*

In the context of treating hypertension, if drug treatment reduces an individual's stroke risk by about 38% (which is a reasonable expectation; Collins & MacMahon, 1994), and somehow is given to *all* those people with a systolic blood pressure of 160 mmHg or more (which would be impossible to achieve in practice, probably undesirable in the very elderly, as well as costly), then stroke incidence would be reduced by only 15% (Table 18.5).

Applying the same principles to atrial fibrillation, one can see that because only about 20% of patients are in atrial fibrillation at or before presentation with first-ever in a lifetime stroke (Sandercock *et al.*, 1992), the treatment of fibrillating people could not possibly prevent more than 20% of all

Table 18.5 The estimated effect of treating hypertension (defined as systolic blood pressure ≥160 mmHg) and so reducing the risk of stroke by 38%, using population data from Framingham (see Table 18.4a). (From Ebrahim, 1990.)

Systolic blood pressure (mmHg)	Prevalence (%)	Expected number of strokes before treatment	Expected number of strokes after treatment
Not treated			
<120	16	27	27
120–139	43	155	155
140–159	29	162	162
Treated			
160–179	8	102	63
180+	4	127	79
Total		573	486

i.e. a proportional (relative) reduction of $\frac{(573 - 486)}{573} \times 100 =$ 15% in stroke numbers (and in stroke incidence)

Note: Ebrahim provided data on treatment producing 25% and 50% relative risk reductions of stroke, whilst we have used 38% in line with the recent meta-analysis of the available randomised controlled trials (Collins & MacMahon, 1994).

strokes. In fact, the likely proportion prevented would be more like 5% if anticoagulation could be given to about 50% of the fibrillating people under the age of 80 years (Table 18.6). Because aspirin can be given to more people than warfarin, where the difficulties and risks are higher, it might also reduce stroke incidence by 5% even though it is relatively less effecive than warfarin, or even by about 8% if it were given to all age groups and not just to those under the age of 80 years (Table 18.6).

Although carotid endarterectomy does seem to about halve the risk of stroke ipsilateral to 'severe' asymptomatic carotid stenosis, the cost-effectiveness is highly questionable (see Section 16.12.3); about 85 patients must be operated to prevent one having a stroke in 1 year. Some would advocate screening the population for carotid stenosis and then offering surgery to those fit for surgery (perhaps under the age of 80 years). Not only would this be hugely expensive (about 60 000 carotid endarterectomies would be needed in Scotland to clear the prevalent backlog of 'cases', a country with only about 5 million people and 30 vascular surgeons), but even if surgery was done on *all* those aged 50–79 years, stroke incidence would only be reduced by about 6%, less as the years go by (Table 18.7).

Because smoking and cholesterol are uncertain risk factors for stroke (see Section 6.2.3), and it is unclear whether quitting smoking and lowering cholesterol has any influence on

Table 18.6 The estimated effect that the treatment of atrial fibrillation should have on stroke incidence.

(a) The prevalence (per 100 population) of patients with atrial fibrillation (AF) by age in various community-based studies, both sexes combined

	Age (years)*			
Reference	50–59	60–69	70–79	80+
Ostrander *et al.* (1965) Michigan	0.5	1.3	4.1	2.9
Rose *et al.* (1978) Male London civil servants	0.4	N/A	N/A	N/A
Evans (1985) South Tyneside, England	N/A	N/A	3.2	8.0
Hill *et al.* (1987) British General Practice	N/A	N/A	3.0	5.6
Wolf *et al.* (1991) Framingham, US	0.5	1.8	4.8	8.8
Langenberg *et al.* (1994) Dutch General Practice	N/A	2.8	6.6	10.0
Furberg *et al.* (1994) US	N/A	N/A	5.8	7.3
Overall approximation†	0.5	2.0	5.0	8.0

(b) The estimated number of strokes in Scotland with and without anticoagulation or aspirin for patients in AF

				Expected number of strokes in 1 year in people in AF		
Age (years)	Number of people in Scotland‡	Prevalence of AF/ 100 population§	Number of people with AF (from column 2 and 3)	No treatment¶	Anticoagulation** (and number of strokes prevented)	Aspirin†† (and number of strokes prevented)
50–59	556 956	0.5	2785	139	45 (93)	89 (50)
60–69	515 593	2.0	10 312	516	165 (351)	330 (186)
70–79	345 859	5.0	17 293	865	277 (588)	554 (311)
80+	168 247	8.0	13 460	673	215 (458)	431 (242)
Total 50+	1 586 655	2.8	43 850	2193	702 (1491)	1404 (789)

(c) Calculation of the proportional impact of treatment on stroke incidence

About 30 000 people in Scotland under the age of 80 years are in AF (over that age, anticoagulation would seldom be used because of the risks) (see Table 18.6b)
Perhaps 50%, i.e. 15 000 might have no contraindications and be suitable and willing for anticoagulation with warfarin
Of these, about 5% will have a stroke per annum, i.e. 750 (see Section 16.5.1)
This could be reduced by 68% with warfarin, i.e. to about 250 (see Section 16.5.1)
∴ 750 − 250 = 500 strokes avoided

In Scotland, there are about 10 000 first-ever in a lifetime strokes per annum (National Medical Advisory Committee, 1993)

∴ Warfarin might reduce stroke incidence by about $\frac{500}{10\,000} \times 100 = 5\%$

Or, if aspirin were given to all 30 000 fibrillating people under the age of 80 years, strokes could be reduced by 36%, i.e. from about 1500 to 960 (see Section 16.4.2)

∴ Aspirin might reduce stroke incidence by about $\frac{540}{10\,000} \times 100 = $ about 5%

If aspirin were to be given to the 44 000 patients at *all* ages, then the percentage reduction in stroke incidence would be about 8%

---

* Prevalence below the age of 50 years so low that any data are unreliable.
† Formal analysis not possible because not all the studies provided numerators and denominators.
‡ Official Scottish Population Statistics for 1990, General Registrar for Scotland.
§ From Table 18.6a.
¶ Assuming risk of first-ever in a lifetime stroke of about 5%/year at all ages, and that most fibrillation is 'non-rheumatic' (see Section 16.5.1).
** Relative risk reduction of 68% (see Section 16.5.1).
†† Relative risk reduction of 36% (see Section 16.4.2).
N/A, not available.

Table 18.7 The estimated public health impact of carotid endarterectomy for asymptomatic carotid stenosis.

(a) Prevalence of carotid stenosis (about 50–99%) in various studies* by age, males and females combined

| Reference | Age (years) | | | |
	50–59	60–69	70–79	80+
Ricci et al. (1991) Italy	1/138 (0.7%)	1/101 (1%)	9/60 (15%)	4/21 (19%)
O'Leary et al. (1992) US	N/A	N/A	73/1458 (5%)	28/322 (7%)
Prati et al. (1992) Italy	1/236 (0.4%)	8/194 (4%)	13/139 (9%)	5/47 (11%)
Willeit & Kiechl (1993) Austria	6/228 (3%)	22/232 (10%)	25/206 (12%)	N/A
Total	8/602 (1.3%)	31/527 (5.9%)	120/1863 (6.4%)	37/390 (9.5%)

(b) Some studies† reporting the risk of stroke in the distribution of an asymptomatic carotid stenosis

Reference	Number	Mean age (years)	Per cent stenosis‡	Approximate risk of stroke (%)
Meissner et al. (1987)	292	67	≈80+	2.1/year
Norris et al. (1991)	177	64	75–99	2.5/year
Hobson et al. (1993)	233	65	50–99	9.4 in 4 years
European Carotid Surgery Trialists' Collaborative Group (1995)	127	64	70–99	5.7 in 3 years
Asymptomatic Carotid Atherosclerosis Study Group (1995)	834	67	60–99	11.0 in 5 years

(c) Estimate of the number of strokes avoided if all patients in Scotland with asymptomatic and 'severe' carotid stenosis were operated on

| Age (years) | Population in Scotland§ | Per cent with asymptomatic 50–99% carotid stenosis¶ | Number with asymptomatic 50–99% carotid stenosis from column 1 and 2 | Number with strokes related to asymptomatic carotid stenosis per annum | | Strokes avoided |
				No-surgery**	Surgery††	
50–59	556 956	1.3	7240	145	72	73
60–69	515 593	5.9	30 420	608	304	304
70–79	345 859	6.4	22 135	443	222	221
80+	168 247	9.5	15 983	320	160	160
Total	1 586 655	—	75 778	1516	758	758

(d) Proportion of first-ever in a lifetime strokes which might be prevented by a policy of screening for asymptomatic carotid stenosis and offering surgery to all those under the age of 80 years

Number of people in Scotland between the ages of 50 and 80 years (above this age surgery not usually recommended) (from Table 18.7c) 1 418 408

Number of people with approximately 50–99% asymptomatic carotid stenosis (from Table 18.7c) 59 795

Assuming a 2% per annum risk of stroke in the asymptomatic carotid stenosis distribution (see Table 18.7b, c), then the number of people with such a stroke each year would be 1196

Assuming about a 50% reduction in stroke risk with carotid endarterectomy preceded by angiography (from Table 18.7c), then the number of strokes avoided per annum would be $\frac{1196}{100} \times 50 = 598$

In Scotland about 10 000 first-ever in a lifetime strokes per annum‡‡

∴ Surgery would avoid about $\frac{598}{10\,000} \times 100$ of all first strokes in the next year = 6%§§

* Studies selected were reasonably large, gave age bands in decades, recorded carotid stenosis at about 50–99% by age, and were population based but usually without exclusion of any symptomatic patients.
† The selected studies were reasonably large ($n > 100$), mostly prospective, the carotid stenosis was 'severe' and usually unoperated unless it became symptomatic.
‡ Stenosis measured in various different ways.
§ Official Scottish Population Statistics for 1990, General Registrar for Scotland.
¶ From Table 18.7a.
** About 2% per annum, from Table 18.7b.
†† Approximate 50% relative risk reduction derived from the Asymptomatic Carotid Atherosclerosis (ACAS) and Veterans Administration trials (see Section 16.12.3).
‡‡ National Medical Advisory Committee (1993).
§§ It is not possible to calculate the annual figure because the incidence of the development of severe asymptomatic carotid stenosis is unknown.
N/A, not available.

the risk of stroke rather than coronary events (see Sections 16.3.2 and 16.3.3), and at present there are no definitely effective and routine treatments for a raised plasma fibrinogen level (Cook & Ubben, 1990), no calculations have been done to examine the impact of the treatment of these risk factors on stroke incidence.

In summary, therefore, treating patients at particularly high risk of stroke is a reasonably cost-effective method to prevent strokes and will benefit those individuals. However, because most strokes do not occur in those at highest risk, and in many of those at highest risk treatment itself is impracticable or too risky, the 'high-risk' strategy will not have a major impact on stroke incidence.

18.5 Likely effect of treating transient ischaemic attacks (TIAs) (and minor ischaemic strokes) on stroke incidence

TIA patients are certainly at high risk of stroke; about 25% will have a stroke in 5 years and as many or more a serious cardiac event (see Section 16.1.1). For these individual patients, a treatment such as aspirin, which reduces stroke risk by about 25% (see Section 16.4), or carotid endarterectomy which reduces stroke risk in suitable TIA patients by about 70% (see Section 16.7), is clearly reasonable. Aspirin is cost-effective, largely because it is cheap and non-toxic, whereas it does cost several thousand pounds to prevent a stroke with carotid endarterectomy (see Table 18.2).

But, what impact will these effective treatments for individuals have at the population level? Neither aspirin nor carotid endarterectomy are likely to prevent more than about 4% of all strokes (Tables 18.8 & 18.9), and nor will lowering the blood pressure of hypertensive TIA patients (Table 18.10). The reasons are that only about 15% of strokes are preceded by TIAs (see Table 6.2); of these only about 50% come to medical attention (see Dennis et al., 1989a). Strokes can occur so quickly after TIA presentation that treatment can not be started in time (see Section 16.1.1), treatment is less than 100% effective (see above), there are risks of treatment (see Chapter 16) and not all patients will comply with treatment. Also, although most TIA patients are eligible for aspirin (see Section 16.4.2), and most hypertensive TIA patients for blood pressure control (see Section 16.3.1), the same can not be said for carotid endarterectomy which is only indicated in recently symptomatic patients who are fit enough for surgery and who have severe carotid stenosis; perhaps about 10% of all hospital-referred TIA cases (Hankey et al., 1991).

So, once again we are confronted by the paradox. Treatment for a relatively small number of high-risk (TIA)

Table 18.8 The estimated public health impact, in terms of first-ever in a lifetime strokes prevented, of treating all prevalent TIA patients in England and Wales with aspirin.

Number of incident TIA patients per annum* is about 21 000
Mortality about 50% at 10 years†

∴ Prevalence of TIA patients is about 21 000 × 10 = 210 000

Of whom about 6% have a stroke each year† 12 600

This can be reduced with aspirin by about 25%‡ to 9450

∴ Aspirin prevents about 3150 strokes per annum

But, in England and Wales there are about 100 000 first-ever in a lifetime strokes per annum§

∴ Aspirin for TIA patients would reduce the incidence of stroke by about 3% at best

* From Dennis et al., 1989a.
† From Hankey et al., 1991.
‡ From Antiplatelet Trialists' Collaboration, 1994.
§ From Bamford et al., 1988.
Note: this calculation for stroke *incidence* omits the added effect that aspirin would have in preventing some recurrent strokes after a first ischaemic stroke. It also ignores the impact that aspirin would have on reducing the risk of coronary events in TIA patients.

Table 18.9 The estimated public health impact, in terms of all strokes prevented, of treating recently symptomatic patients with severe carotid stenosis in England and Wales with carotid endarterectomy.

Number of incident TIA patients per annum* is about 21 000
Number of incident minor ischaemic stroke patients per annum† is about 30 000
Total 51 000

About 65% under the age of 75 years 33 150
About 80% have 'carotid' attacks* 26 520
About 20% have 70–99% carotid stenosis‡ 5304

If treating 10 patients avoids one stroke in 2 years (see Section 16.7.6), then treating 5304 patients will avoid about 530 strokes

i.e. <1% of all the 130 000 first-ever in a lifetime and recurrent strokes in England and Wales per annum (see Table 18.1).

* From Dennis et al., 1989a.
† From Dennis et al., 1989b.
‡ From Hankey et al., 1991.

patients will be reasonably effective for those individuals, but will have surprisingly little impact on overall stroke incidence in the population. Of course, aspirin and carotid endarterectomy are also appropriate after mild first-ever in a lifetime ischaemic stroke and will therefore reduce the risk of recurrent stroke, but this will have no effect on stroke incidence (i.e. the frequency of first-ever in a lifetime stroke).

Table 18.10 The estimated public health impact, in terms of first-ever in a lifetime strokes prevented, of treating all prevalent hypertensive TIA patients in England and Wales with blood-pressure-lowering drugs.

Number of incident TIA patients per annum* is about 21 000
Mortality about 50% at 10 years†

∴ Prevalence of TIA patients is about 21 000 × 10 = 210 000

About 50% of TIA patients are hypertensive = 105 000
  (systolic blood pressure ⩾160/90 mmHg twice)‡
of whom about 6%§ have a stroke each year† = 6300

Treatment reduces stroke risk by about 38%¶

∴ $\frac{6300 \times 38}{100}$ strokes avoided = 2394

But, in England and Wales there about 100 000 first-ever in a lifetime strokes per annum (see Table 18.1)

∴ Treatment of hypertension in TIA patients reduces stroke incidence by about 2%

---

* Dennis *et al.*, 1989a.
† Hankey *et al.*, 1991.
‡ Dennis *et al.*, 1989b.
§ Hypertensive TIA patients probably have a higher risk of stroke than the average, so this 6% could be an underestimate.
¶ Collins & MacMahon, 1994.

Prevention of stroke after transient ischaemic attacks is an example of the 'high-risk' strategy and will have little effect on stroke incidence, even though the individual transient ischaemic attack patient will have much to gain from treatment.

18.6 Likely effect of the 'mass' strategy for primary stroke prevention

In recent years epidemiologists have begun to calculate what the effect might be of not just truncating the right-hand end of the tail of a risk distribution (see Fig. 18.3) by treating high-risk individuals, but of shifting the entire distribution slightly to the left (Fig. 18.4). This would not just reduce the mean of a continuously varying risk factor (such as blood pressure or cholesterol level) but also of reducing the number of patients at particularly high risk and who are therefore declared as diseased and so requiring treatment (Table 18.11). Of great consequence would also be the likely number of events prevented not just by reducing the small number of high-risk individuals but of the much larger number of people at moderate risk. As an example of what might happen, Ebrahim (1990) has calculated that reducing the population mean systolic blood pressure by a mere 2–3 mmHg

should reduce the incidence of stroke by about 10% (Table 18.12). This sort of reduction in blood pressure, or more, should be achievable by a public health strategy aimed at the *whole* population, so that everyone reduces their risk by just a little bit: a slightly lower blood pressure in everyone, less cigarettes smoked by all smokers, somewhat more exercise all round, a little less alcohol for all drinkers, a touch of weight reduction for all, and so on. Indeed, there have been remarkable falls in mean cholesterol, blood pressure and smoking in countries such as Iceland, US and Finland (Sytkowski *et al.*, 1990; Sigfusson *et al.*, 1991; Vartiainen *et al.*, 1994). Clearly, and luckily for us, an individual's blood pressure is not *entirely* a matter of genetics, if only because the mean population blood pressure is lower in the summer than in the winter (Khaw, 1994).

The 'mass' strategy for stroke prevention requires a small downward shift in the mean population blood pressure by a few millimetres of mercury. This should have a surprisingly large impact on stroke incidence.

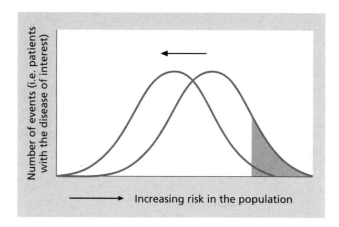

Figure 18.4 The 'mass' strategy of disease prevention involves a small left shift in the risk distribution.

Table 18.11 The estimated effect of reducing the mean level of a risk factor in the population on the prevalence of abnormally high values (i.e. of 'disease'). (From Rose & Day, 1990.)

Risk factor	Reduction in mean value	Predicted fall in prevalence of high values (%)	
		From	To
Systolic blood pressure	5 mmHg	15	11
Body weight	1 kg	6	4
Alcohol intake	15 ml/week	17	15

Table 18.12 The estimated effect of a downward shift in the population mean systolic blood pressure by 2–3 mmHg, using population data from Framingham (see Table 18.4a). (From Ebrahim, 1990.)

Systolic blood pressure (mmHg)	Prevalence before intervention (%)	Prevalence after intervention (%)	Expected number of strokes before intervention	Expected number of strokes after intervention
<120	16	17	27	29
120–139	43	44	155	158
140–159	29	26	162	146
160–179	8	7	102	90
180+	4	3	127	95
Total			573	518

i.e. a proportional reduction of $\frac{(573 - 518)}{573} \times 100 = 10\%$ in stroke numbers (and incidence)

It *may* be possible to lower the mean population blood pressure by several millimetres of mercury by any one of several non-pharmacological interventions: (i) a reduction in salt intake by a tolerable 3 g/day by means of a public health campaign and insistence on labelling the salt content of processed and other foods with a gradual reduction in the permitted concentration; (ii) facilitation of regular exercise by children and adults by discouraging car use, and provision of sports grounds and safe cycling facilities; (iii) reduced alcohol consumption by safe drinking campaigns; and (iv) a general emphasis on weight control by promoting exercise and calorie labelling of foods (Cutler, 1991; Law *et al.*, 1991; Arroll & Beaglehole, 1992; Alderman, 1994) (see also Sections 6.2.3 and 16.3.5). All these interventions depend on education and political action to improve the national health and very little, if at all, on action at the individual doctor level (Council on Scientific Affairs, 1990). Moreover, the political will must come not just from the Department of Health but also from the Treasury, the Departments of Education, Agriculture, Transport and the Environment; in other words, from across the whole of Government, a point so often missed by commentators who claim that any improvement in 'health' is inevitably something to do with the Department of Health. Naturally, one has to accept the so-called prevention paradox: a measure that brings large benefits to the community offers little to each participating individual (Rose, 1981). But, as such, these recommendations are no more invasive or prescriptive than providing a clean water supply or mass immunisation, both of which are clearly in the domain of public health services.

This 'mass' strategy is not amenable to evaluation by a randomised controlled trial, not because the outcome is not measurable or because the sample size would have to be too big or it would take too long to demonstrate an effect, but because this strategy requires everybody to be 'treated' and it would simply be impracticable to apply the 'treatment' to a random 50% of the population. The effectiveness has to be taken on trust. But, because it is simple, probably inexpensive and, in theory, makes sense, it would surely be worth pursuing. Of course, moving an entire distribution of a risk factor to the left would increase the number of individuals at very low risk of the disease in question and one would need to be reasonably confident that these individuals would not be systematically disadvantaged in some way.

1 If mean population blood pressure were lowered, would the larger number of patients with 'low' blood pressure be put at risk of some unexpected disorder, perhaps depression and fatigue, for example (Barrett-Connor & Palinkas, 1994)?
2 If the mean weight of the population was reduced, would the larger number of 'thin' people be put at risk in some way?
3 If the mean cigarette consumption was reduced what possible danger could there be for the larger number of ex-smokers and non-smokers?
4 Would the increased number of non-drinkers really have a higher mortality, particularly from coronary heart disease, than light drinkers (Marmot & Brunner, 1991; Doll *et al.*, 1994)?
5 Does very low cholesterol concentration really cause haemorrhagic stroke, or even suicide, if not cancer (Law & Thompson, 1991; Law *et al.*, 1994; Gallerani *et al.*, 1995)?
Because being simple goes against the grain of societies which believe in a quick technological fix for illness, and which may crave short-term results in the market place, and in societies which may exalt the individual over the community, the 'mass' strategy may be very difficult to implement. However, the argument in favour of this strategy of not just stroke prevention, but prevention of disease, in general, is persuasive, if not compelling (Rose, 1992).

18.7 Goals, strategies and measuring success (or failure)

Setting targets or goals in any human endeavour is surely reasonable provided they are not so easily achieved that no effort is required, or so difficult to achieve that demoralisation sets in. This certainly applies to stroke rehabilitation (see Section 10.3.3) and could be applied to reducing the burden of stroke in the whole community. The difficulty is in knowing what target to measure: (i) it has to be at the level of the whole community or a random sample of it to avoid selection bias; (ii) it has to be simple so that it is measurable in very large numbers of people at reasonable cost; (iii) it has to be robust so that it can be measured reliably at various points in time; (iv) it must be valid and so measure something meaningful; and (v) it almost certainly has to be measurable in routine practice to ensure complete coverage for the forseeable future. At present, the *only* measure which comes anywhere near fulfilling these criteria is stroke mortality, despite its imperfections. Anything else is impracticable at present (see Section 18.2.1) (Dennis & Warlow, 1991). However, one can reasonably hope, and even expect, that an intervention which reduces stroke incidence and disability would have *some* impact on stroke mortality, although this impact could well be attenuated by the fact that not all types of stroke are fatal, mortality statistics are inaccurate, and so on. One fear is that in our efforts to improve the accuracy of stroke mortality statistics we might cause an artefactual decline in stroke mortality simply by moving, appropriately, some patients to another more plausible category of cause of death. After all, there must be something wrong with the data if 1 year after stroke about 30% of the patients are dead (i.e. 39 000 out of 130 000 first and recurrent strokes in England and Wales; see Section 10.2.3), and yet stroke is noted on the death certificate in about 68 000 patients a year (Secretary of State for Health, 1992).

> At present, mortality statistics are, despite their imperfections, the only routinely available method to measure the success or failure of stroke prevention programmes.

In the meantime it is surely important to develop some *routine* method of measuring stroke incidence as well as of outcome and survival, which is both practicable and inexpensive, but this will take time to achieve. At the very least, routine measurement of stroke outcome is required to inform health care decisions, for how else can one system of care be compared with another (see Section 17.6.3)?

As to which stroke prevention strategy to choose, it seems sensible to pursue all of them whilst accepting that each one on its own would not have a dramatic effect (Table 18.13) (Dennis & Warlow, 1991). It would be impossible to deny an effective treatment to an individual if the benefits outweighed the risks and the cost was acceptable, either to the individual or to a third-party payer. It would be inconceivable not to continue to search for and evaluate treatments for acute stroke, and it would be unpardonable to ignore the theoretical attractions of the 'mass strategy' for stroke prevention.

Table 18.13 The estimated maximum effect of various interventions on stroke incidence, and the number of people who need to be treated to prevent one having a stroke in 1 year.

Intervention	Reduction in stroke incidence (%)	Number needed to be treated to prevent one stroke in 1 year
Treat systolic blood pressure ≥160 mmHg	15 (see Table 18.5)	Hundreds, depending on age
Reduce population mean systolic blood pressure by 2–3 mmHg	10 (see Table 18.12)	Thousands
Aspirin for atrial fibrillation, all ages	8 (see Table 18.6c)	30
Endarterectomy for asymptomatic severe carotid stenosis	6* (see Table 18.7d)	85
Aspirin for atrial fibrillation, age <80 years	5 (see Table 18.6c)	56
Anticoagulation for atrial fibrillation, age <80 years	5 (see Table 18.6c)	30
Aspirin for TIAs	3 (see Table 18.8)	67
Treatment of hypertension in TIA patients	2 (see Table 18.10)	44
Endarterectomy for recently symptomatic severe carotid stenosis	<1 (see Table 18.9)	20

* This figure would decline with time because it can be calculated only for the first year after surgery for all prevalent cases of asymptomatic carotid stenosis; the *incidence* of severe carotid stenosis is unknown and probably always will be.

Finally, *any* strategy for stroke prevention must be intimately linked with *any* strategy for the prevention of coronary heart disease and peripheral vascular disease, because they are all caused by the same underlying degenerative vascular disorders. So, stroke prevention should not be considered in isolation, but within a general strategy for the prevention of *all* forms of vascular disease, including stroke.

> Stroke prevention must not be seen in isolation but as part of a programme to prevent all forms of degenerative vascular disease.

References

Alderman MH (1994). Non-pharmacological treatment of hypertension. *Lancet* 344: 307–11.

Andrade SE, Walker AM, Gottlieb LK *et al.* (1995).

Discontinuation of antihyperlipidemic drugs—do rates reported in clinical trials reflect rates in primary care settings? *N Engl J Med* 332: 1125–31.

Antiplatelet Trialists' Collaboration (1994). Collaborative overview of randomised trials of antiplatelet therapy—I: prevention of death, myocardial infarction, and stroke by prolonged antiplatelet therapy in different categories of patients. *Br Med J* 308: 81–106.

Arroll B, Beaglehole R (1992). Does physical activity lower blood pressure: a critical review of the clinical trials. *J Clin Epidemiol* 45: 439–47.

Asplund K, Marke L-A, Terent A, Gustafsson C, Wester PO (1993). Costs and gains in stroke prevention: European perspective. *Cerebrovasc Dis* 3 (Suppl. 1): 34–42.

Asplund K, Bonita R, Kuulasmaa K *et al.* for the WHO MONICA Project (1995). Multinational comparisons of stroke epidemiology. Evaluation of case ascertainment in the WHO MONICA Stroke Study. *Stroke* 26: 355–60.

Asymptomatic Carotid Atherosclerosis Study Group (1995). Carotid endarterectomy for patients with asymptomatic internal carotid artery stenosis. *J Am Med Assoc* 273: 1421–8.

Bamford J, Dennis M, Sandercock P, Burn J, Warlow C (1990). The frequency, causes and timing of death within 30 days of a first stroke: the Oxfordshire Community Stroke Project. *J Neurol Neurosurg Psychiatr* 53: 824–9.

Bamford J, Sandercock P, Dennis M *et al.* (1988). A prospective study of acute cerebrovascular disease in the community: the Oxfordshire Community Stroke Project 1981–6. 1. Methodology, demography & incident cases of first-ever stroke. *J Neurol Neurosurg Psychiatr* 51: 1373–80.

Barrett-Connor E, Palinkas LA (1994). Low blood pressure and depression in older men: a population based study. *Br Med J* 308: 446–9.

Bonita R, Beaglehole R (1989). Increased treatment of hypertension does not explain the decline in stroke mortality in the United States, 1970–1980. *Hypertension* 13 (Suppl. I): I69–I73.

Bonita R, Beaglehole R (1993). Stroke mortality. In: Whisnant JP, ed. *Stroke: Populations, Cohorts and Clinical Trials.* Oxford: Heinemann, 59–79.

Bonita R, Beaglehole R, North JDK (1983). The long-term monitoring of cardiovascular disease: is it feasible? *Commun Health Studies* 7: 111–17.

Bonita R, Broad JB, Beaglehole R (1993). Changes in stroke incidence and case-fatality in Auckland, New Zealand, 1981–1991. *Lancet* 342: 1470–3.

Bonita R, Stewart A, Beaglehole R (1990). International trends in stroke mortality 1970–1985. *Stroke* 21: 989–92.

Broderick JP, Phillips SJ, Whisnant JP, O'Fallon WM, Bergstralh EJ (1989). Incidence rates of stroke in the eighties: the end of the decline of stroke? *Stroke* 20: 577–82.

Collins R, MacMahon S (1994). Blood pressure, antihypertensive drug treatment and the risks of stroke and of coronary heart disease. *Br Med Bull* 50: 272–98.

Cook NS, Ubben D (1990). Fibrinogen as a major risk factor in cardiovascular disease. *Trends Pharamacol Sci* 11: 444–51.

Coppola WGT, Whincup PH, Papacosta O, Walker M, Ebrahim S (1995). Scoring system to identify men at high risk of stroke: a strategy for general practice. *Br J Gen Pract* 45: 185–9.

Corwin LI, Wolf PA, Kannel WB, McNamara PM (1982). Accuracy of death certification of stroke: the Framingham Study. *Stroke* 13: 818–21.

Council on Scientific Affairs (1990). The Worldwide Smoking Epidemic. Tobacco trade, use, and control. *J Am Med Assoc* 263: 3312–18.

Cutler JA (1991). Randomised clinical trials of weight reduction in nonhypertensive persons. *Ann Epidemiol* 1: 363–70.

D'Agostino RB, Wolf PA, Belanger AJ, Kannel WB (1994). Stroke risk profile: adjustment for antihypertensive medication. The Framingham Study. *Stroke* 25: 40–3.

Davey Smith G, Song F, Sheldon TA (1993). Cholesterol lowering and mortality: the importance of considering initial level of risk. *Br Med J* 306: 1367–73.

Dennis M, Warlow C (1991). Strategy for Stroke. *Br Med J* 303: 636–8.

Dennis M, Bamford J, Sandercock P, Warlow C (1989a). Incidence of transient ischaemic attacks in Oxfordshire, England. *Stroke* 20: 333–9.

Dennis M, Bamford J, Sandercock P, Warlow C (1989b). A comparison of risk factors and prognosis for transient ischaemic attacks and minor ischaemic strokes. The Oxfordshire Community Stroke Project. *Stroke* 20: 1494–9.

Doll R, Peto R, Hall E, Wheatley K, Gray R (1994). Mortality in relation to consumption of alcohol: 13 years' observations on male British doctors. *Br Med J* 309: 911–18.

Ebrahim S (1990). *Clinical Epidemiology of Stroke.* Oxford: Oxford University Press.

European Carotid Surgery Trialists' Collaborative Group (1995). Risk of stroke in the distribution of an asymptomatic carotid artery. *Lancet* 345: 209–12.

Evans GJ (1985). Risk factors for stroke in the elderly. MD Thesis, University of Cambridge.

Family Heart Study Group (1994). Randomised controlled trial evaluating cardiovascular screening and intervention in general practice: principal results of British family heart study. *Br Med J* 308: 313–20.

Feigin VL, Wiebers DO, Whisnant JP, O'Fallon WM (1995). Stroke incidence and 30-day case fatality rates in Novosibirsk, Russia, 1982 through 1992. *Stroke* 26: 924–9.

Field K, Thorogood M, Silagy C, Normand C, O'Neill C, Muir J (1995). Strategies for reducing coronary risk factors in primary care: which is most cost effective? *Br Med J* 310: 1109–12.

Fratiglioni L, Massey EW, Schoenberg DG, Schoenberg BS (1983). Mortality from cerebrovascular disease; international comparisons and temporal trends. *Neuroepidemiology* 2: 101–16.

Fries JF, Bloch DA, Harrington H, Richardson N, Beck R (1993). Two year results of a randomised controlled trial of a health promotion programme in a retiree population: the Bank of America Study. *Am J Med* 94: 455–62.

Furberg CD, Psaty BM, Manolio TA, Gardin JM, Smith VE,

647

Rautaharju PM, for the CHS Collaborative Research Group (1994). Prevalence of Atrial Fibrillation in Elderly Subjects (the Cardiovascular Heath Study). *Am J Cardiol* 74: 236–41.

Gallerani M, Manfredini R, Caracciolo S, Scapoli C, Molinari S, Fersini C (1995). Serum cholesterol concentrations in parasuicide. *Br Med J* 310: 1632–6.

Garraway WM, Whisnant JP, Drury I (1983). The changing pattern of survival following stroke. *Stroke* 14: 699–703.

Hankey GJ, Slattery JM, Warlow CP (1991). The prognosis of hospital-referred transient ischaemic attacks. *J Neurol Neurosurg Psychiatr* 54: 793–802.

Hankey GJ, Slattery JM, Warlow CP (1993). Can the long term outcome of an individual patient with transient ischaemic attacks be predicted accurately. *J Neurol Neurosurg Psychiatr* 56: 752–9.

Harris AI (1971). *Handicapped and Impaired in Great Britain*. London: Her Majesty's Stationery Office.

Hasuo Y, Ueda K, Kiyohara Y *et al.* (1989). Accuracy of diagnosis on death certificates for underlying causes of death in a long-term autopsy-based population study in Hisayama, Japan; with special reference to cardiovascular diseases. *J Clin Epidemiol* 42: 577–84.

Hatano S (1976). Experience from a multicentre stroke register: a preliminary report. *Bull WHO* 54: 541–53.

Hill JD, Mottram EM, Killeen PD (1987). Study of the prevalence of atrial fibrillation in general practice patients over 65 years of age. *J Roy Coll Gen Practit* 37: 172–3.

Hobson RW, Weiss DG, Fields WS *et al.* and the Veterans Affairs Cooperative Study Group (1993). Efficacy of carotid endarterectomy for asymptomatic carotid stenosis. *N Engl J Med* 328: 221–7.

Holmen J, Forsen L, Hjort PF, Midthjell K, Waaler HT, Bjorndal A (1991). Detecting hypertension: screening versus case finding in Norway. *Br Med J* 302: 219–22.

Imperial Cancer Research Fund OXCHECK Study Group (1995). Effectiveness of health checks conducted by nurses in primary care: final results of the OXCHECK study. *Br Med J* 310: 1099–104.

Ingall TJ, Whisnant JP, Wiebers DO, O'Fallon, WM (1989). Has there been a decline in subarachnoid haemorrhage mortality? *Stroke* 20: 718–24.

Isard PA, Forbes JF (1992). The cost of stroke to the National Health Service in Scotland. *Cerebrovasc Dis* 2: 47–50.

Iso H, Jacobs DR, Goldman L (1990). Accuracy of death certificate diagnosis of intracranial haemorrhage and nonhaemorrhagic stroke. *Am J Epidemiol* 132: 993–8.

Jackson R, Barham P, Bills J *et al.* (1993). Management of raised blood pressure in New Zealand: a discussion document. *Br Med J* 307: 107–10.

Jorgensen HS, Plesner A-M, Hubbe P, Larsen K (1992). Marked increase of stroke incidence in men between 1972 and 1990 in Frederiksberg, Denmark. *Stroke* 23: 1701–4.

Kawachi I, Purdie G (1989). The benefits and risks of treating mild to moderate hypertension. *N Z Med J* 102: 377–9.

Khaw K-T (1994). Genetics and environment: Geoffrey Rose revisited. *Lancet* 343: 838–9.

Khaw K-T, Rose G (1989). Cholesterol screening programmes: how much potential benefit? *Br Med J* 299: 606–7.

Kinlay S, Heller RF (1990). Effectiveness and hazards of case finding for a high cholesterol concentration. *Br Med J* 300: 1545–7.

Langenberg M, Hellemons BSP, van Ree JW *et al.* (1994). Atrial fibrillation in elderly patients: prevalence and comorbidity in general practice. *Cerebrovasc Dis* 4: 229.

Lanska DJ (1993). Decline in autopsies for deaths attributed to cerebrovascular disease. *Stroke* 24: 71–5.

Law MR, Thompson SG (1991). Low serum cholesterol and the risk of cancer: an analysis of the published prospective studies. *Cancer Causes Control* 2: 253–9.

Law MR, Frost CD, Wald NJ (1991). By how much does dietary salt reduction lower blood pressure? III—analysis of data from trials of salt reduction. *Br Med J* 302: 819–24.

Law MR, Thompson SG, Wald NJ (1994). Assessing possible hazards of reducing serum cholesterol. *Br Med J* 308: 373–9.

Lindholm LH, Ekbom T, Dash C, Eriksson M, Tibblin G, Scherstein B on behalf of the CELL Study Group (1995). The impact of health care advice given in primary care on cardiovascular risk. *Br Med J* 310: 1105–9.

McCormick J, Skrabanek P (1988). Coronary heart disease is not preventable by population interventions. *Lancet* 2: 839–41.

Malmgren R, Warlow C, Bamford J, Sandercock P (1987). Geographical and secular trends in stroke incidence. *Lancet* 2: 1196–1200.

Malmgren R, Bamford J, Warlow C, Sandercock P, Slattery J (1989). Projecting the number of patients with first-ever strokes and patients newly handicapped by stroke in England and Wales. *Br Med J* 298: 656–60.

Marmot M, Brunner E (1991). Alcohol and cardiovascular disease: the status of the U shaped curve. *Br Med J* 303: 565–8.

Martin J, Meltzer H, Elliot D (1988). OPCS surveys of disability in Great Britain Report 1. The prevalence of disability among adults. Office of Population Censuses and Surveys. London: Her Majesty's Stationery Office.

Meissner I, Wiebers DO, Whisnant JP, O'Fallon M (1987). The natural history of asymptomatic carotid artery occlusive lesions. *J Am Med Assoc* 258: 2704–7.

National Medical Advisory Committee (1993). *The Management of Patients with Stroke*. Edinburgh: Her Majesty's Stationery Office.

Netsky MG, Miyaji T (1976). Prevalence of cerebral haemorrhage and thrombosis in Japan: study of the major causes of death. *J Chronic Disord* 29: 711–21.

Norris JW, Zhu CZ, Bornstein NM, Chambers BR (1991). Vascular risks of asymptomatic carotid stenosis. *Stroke* 22: 1485–90.

O'Leary DH, Polak JF, Kronmal RA *et al.* on behalf of the CHS Collaborative Research Group (1992). Distribution and correlates of sonographically detected carotid artery disease in the cardiovascular health study. *Stroke* 23: 1752–60.

Ostrander LD, Brandt RL, Kjelsberg MO, Epstein FH (1965). Electrocardiographic findings among the adult population of a total natural community, Tecumseh, Michigan. *Circulation* 31: 888–98.

Phillips LH, Whisnant JP, Reagan TJ (1977). Sudden death from stroke. *Stroke* 8: 392–5.

Prati P, Vanuzzo D, Casaroli M *et al.* (1992). Prevalence and determinants of carotid atherosclerosis in a general population. *Stroke* 23: 1705–11.

Ricci S, Flamini FO, Celani MG *et al.* (1991). Prevalence of internal carotid-artery stenosis in subjects older than 49 years: a population study. *Cerebrovasc Dis* 1: 16–19.

Rose G (1981). Strategy of prevention: lessons from cardiovascular disease. *Br Med J* 282: 1847–51.

Rose G (1991). Ancel Keys lecture. *Circulation* 84: 1405–9.

Rose G (1992). *The Strategy of Preventive Medicine.* Oxford: Oxford University Press.

Rose G, Day S (1990). The population mean predicts the number of deviant individuals. *Br Med J* 301: 1031–4.

Rose G, Tunstall-Pedoe HD, Heller RF (1983). UK heart disease prevention project: incidence and mortality results. *Lancet* 1: 1062–70.

Rose G, Baxter RJ, Reid DD, McCartney P (1978). Prevalence and prognosis of electrocardiographic findings in middle-aged men. *Br Heart J* 40: 636–43.

Rothwell P (1995). Can overall results of clinical trials be applied to all patients? *Lancet* 345: 1616–19.

Sandercock PAG, Bamford J, Dennis M *et al.* (1992). Atrial fibrillation and stroke: prevalence in different stroke types and influence on early and long term prognosis (Oxfordshire Community Stroke Project). *Br Med J* 305: 1460–5.

Secretary of State for Health (1992). *The Health of the Nation.* London: Her Majesty's Stationery Office.

Sigfusson N, Sigvaldason H, Steingrimsdottir L *et al.* (1991). Decline in ischaemic heart disease in Iceland and change in risk factor levels. *Br Med J* 302: 1371–5.

Sudlow C, Warlow C (1996). Comparing stroke incidence worldwide. What makes studies comparable? *Stroke* 27: 550–8.

Sytkowski PA, Kannel WB, D'Agostino RB (1990). Changes in risk factors and the decline in mortality from cardiovascular disease. The Framingham Heart Study. *N Engl J Med* 322: 1635–41.

Terent A (1988). Increasing incidence of stroke among Swedish women. *Stroke* 19: 598–603.

Thomas AC, Knapman PA, Krikler DM, Davies MJ (1988). Community study of the causes of 'natural' sudden death. *Br Med J* 297: 1453–6.

Tuomilehto J, Bonita R, Stewart A, Nissinen A, Salonen JT (1991). Hypertension, cigarette smoking, and the decline in stroke incidence in Eastern Finland. *Stroke* 22: 7–11.

Ueda K, Omae T, Hirota Y *et al.* (1981). Decreasing trend in incidence and mortality from stroke in Hisayama residents, Japan. *Stroke* 12: 154–60.

Vartiainen E, Sarti C, Tuomilehto J, Kuulasmaa K (1995). Do changes in cardiovascular risk factors explain changes in mortality from stroke in Finland? *Br Med J* 310: 901–4.

Vartiainen E, Puska P, Pekkanen J, Tuomilehto J, Jousilahti P (1994). Changes in risk factors explain changes in mortality from ischaemic heart disease in Finland. *Br Med J* 309: 23–7.

Whelton PK (1994). Epidemiology of hypertension. *Lancet* 344: 101–6.

Whisnant JP (1983). The role of the neurologist in the decline of stroke. *Ann Neurol* 14: 1–7.

Whisnant JP (1984). The decline of stroke. *Stroke* 15: 160–8.

Willeit J, Kiechl S (1993). Prevalence and risk factors of asymptomatic extracranial carotid artery atherosclerosis. A population-based study. *Arteriosclerosis Thrombosis* 13: 661–8.

Wolf PA, Abbott RD, Kannel WB (1991). Atrial fibrillation as an independent risk factor for stroke: the Framingham Study. *Stroke* 22: 983–8.

Index